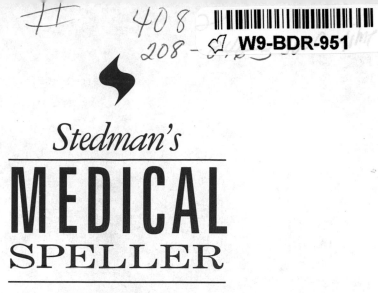

Stedman's
MEDICAL
SPELLER

SECOND EDITION

Stedman's

MEDICAL
SPELLER

SECOND EDITION

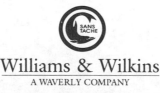

Williams & Wilkins
A WAVERLY COMPANY

BALTIMORE • PHILADELPHIA • LONDON • PARIS • BANGKOK
BUENOS AIRES • HONG KONG • MUNICH • SYDNEY • TOKYO • WROCLAW

Series Editor: Elizabeth B. Randolph
Associate Managing Editor: Maureen Barlow Pugh
Production Coordinator: Marette Magargle-Smith
Cover Design: Reuter & Associates

Copyright © 1996
Williams & Wilkins
351 West Camden Street
Baltimore, Maryland 21201-2436 USA

Printed in the United States of America

First Edition 1992

Library of Congress Cataloging-in-Publication Data

Stedman's medical speller. — 2nd ed.
    p.   cm.
    Developed from the database of Stedman's medical dictionary, 26th ed.
    ISBN 0-683-40023-1
    1. Medicine — Terminology.   2. English language — Orthography and spelling.
I. Stedman, Thomas Lathrop, 1853–1938.   Medical dictionary.   II. Williams & Wilkins.
    [DNLM: 1. Nomenclature.   W 15 S812 1996]
R123.S7 1996
610′.14 — dc20
DNLM/DLC
for Library of Congress
                                   96-7785
                                       CIP

97 98 99
2 3 4 5 6 7 8 9 10

Contents

Preface to the Second Edition

Users of the first edition of *Stedman's Medical Speller* know that sometimes it is helpful to refer to a word book that covers general medical language as opposed to one that contains only specialty-specific terms. The many requests we received for a new edition of this, our only word book that covers general medical terminology, played a large part in our decision to revise this text.

Unlike our other word books, *Stedman's Medical Speller, Second Edition,* comprises only terms from the 26th edition of *Stedman's Medical Dictionary.* We extracted the terms from the "big green" and then fully cross-indexed them for easy look-up. This compilation of more than 113,000 entries was built from a base vocabulary of more than 72,000 medical words, phrases, and acronyms.

For this second edition of *Stedman's Medical Speller,* we have eliminated the hyphenation that appeared in the first edition, because we felt that the hyphenation made the words difficult to read. In addition, we have included a more comprehensive listing of gross anatomy terms (including both Latin and English Nomina Anatomica names). For quick reference, hyphenation information and a list of medical prefixes, suffixes, and combining forms appear in the appendices in the back of the book.

Our goal has been to provide a comprehensive yet streamlined reference tool. Although this reference covers all major medical specialties, we have omitted terminology that we felt either would not be helpful to users of this word book or that were well represented in our other *Stedman's* word books. Specifically, we excluded biochemistry terms, pharmacology terms, veterinary terms, pathology terms, and combining forms. Abbreviations were also excluded from *Stedman's Medical Speller.* Note that pathology terms can be found in *Stedman's Pathology & Lab Medicine Words,* and a comprehensive listing of medical abbreviations can be found in *Stedman's Abbreviations, Acronyms & Symbols.*

We at Williams & Wilkins strive to provide you with the most up-to-date and accurate word references available. Your use of this word book will prompt new editions, which will be published as often as justified by updates and revisions. We welcome your suggestions for improvements, changes, corrections, and additions—whatever will make this *Stedman's* product more useful to you. Please use the postpaid card at the back of this book and send your recommendations in care of *"Stedman's"* at Williams & Wilkins.

Acknowledgments

Stedman's Medical Speller, Second Edition, benefits directly from the hard work and effort that went into the *Stedman's Medical Dictionary, 26th Edition.* We therefore would like to thank Marjory Spraycar, Editor of *Stedman's Medical Dictionary,* and the consultants, editors, database experts, and publishing experts who are responsible for the quality content contained in this word book.

Special thanks also go to Bonnie Montgomery, who copy edited the manuscript and ensured that the format was consistent with our other published word books.

As with all of our Stedman's word references, we have benefited from the suggestions and expertise of our many contacts in the medical transcriptionist community. Thanks to all of our advisory board participants, reviewers and editors, American Association of Medical Transcriptionists meeting attendees, and others who have written in with requests and comments—keep talking, and we will keep listening.

Explanatory Notes

Stedman's Medical Speller, Second Edition, is an up-to-date, authoritative assurance of quality and exactness of *general* medical language to the wordsmiths of the health care professions—medical transcriptionists, medical editors and copy editors, health information management personnel, court reporters, and the many other users and producers of medical documentation.

Medical transcription is an art as well as a science. Both are needed to correctly interpret a physician's dictation, whose language is a product of education, training, and experience. This variety in medical language means that there are several acceptable ways to express certain terms, including jargon. This second edition of *Stedman's Medical Speller* provides variant spellings and phrasings for many terms. This, in addition to complete cross-indexing, makes *Stedman's Medical Speller, Second Edition,* a valuable resource for determining the validity of terms as you encounter them.

Alphabetical Organization

Alphabetization of entries is letter by letter as spelled, ignoring punctuation, spaces, prefixed numbers, Greek letters, or other characters. For example:

acid-fast staining methods

acid formaldehyde hematin

α-acid glycoprotein

acid hematin

In subentries, the abbreviated singular form or the spelled-out plural form of the noun main entry word is ignored in alphabetization.

Format and Style

All main entries are in **boldface** to speed up location of a sought-after entry, to enhance distinction between main entries and subentries, and to relieve the textual density of the pages.

Irregular plurals and variant spellings are shown on the same line as the singular or preferred form of the word. For example:

scolex, pl. **scoleces**

curette, curet

Hyphenation

In this second edition, we did not retain the hyphenation that characterized every entry in the first edition, because we determined that the hyphenation made the words difficult to read. Ease of use is, of course, one of our primary goals, and we hope that this change will make this edition of *Stedman's Medical Speller* more user friendly. For information about the hyphenation of medical words, see the "Rules for Hyphenation" appendix in the back of this book or, for specific terms, see your *Stedman's Medical Dictionary, 26th edition.*

Possessives

This book is unique in our line of word books in that all of the terms have been taken directly from *Stedman's Medical Dictionary.* Use of possessives in this word book reflects the usage of its source (i.e., *Stedman's Medical Dictionary*). Note, however, that retaining the possessive is a question of style, not of accuracy, and thus is a matter of choice.

Cross-indexing

The word list is in an index-like main entry-subentry format that contains two combined alphabetical listings:

(1) A *noun* main entry-subentry organization typical of the A to Z section of medical dictionaries like **Stedman's:**

bubo
> bullet b.
> chancroidal b.
> malignant b.
> virulent b.

hand
> accoucheur's h.
> drop h.
> ghoul h.
> opera-glass h.

(2) An *adjective* main entry-subentry organization, which lists words and phrases as you hear them. The main entries are the adjectives or modifiers in a multiword term. The subentries are the nouns around which the terms are constructed and to which the adjectives or modifiers pertain:

bipolar
> b. cautery
> b. cell
> b. disorder
> b. taxis

Hamman's
> H. disease
> H. murmur
> H. sign
> H. syndrome

This format gives the user more than one way to locate and identify a multiword term. For example:

acne
> halogen a.

halogen
> h. acne

clamp
> Fogarty c.
> gingival c.

Fogarty
> F. balloon
> F. clamp

The format also allows the user to see together all terms that contain a particular descriptor as well as all types, kinds, or variations of a noun entity. For example:

birth
- b. amputation
- b. canal
- cross b.
- b. palsy
- premature b.

clasp
- c. arm
- bar c.
- circumferential c.
- extended c.
- c. guideline

A tortuous 2-words

α
α-1 antitrypsin deficiency panniculitis
α-1-proteinase deficiency
α chain disease
α fetoprotein
α granules
α hemolysin
α′ hemolysis
α thalassemia
α thalassemia intermedia

A
A bands
A bile
A cells
A disks
A fibers
A wave

Aaron's sign

Aarskog-Scott syndrome

abacterial thrombotic endocarditis

Abadie's sign of tabes dorsalis

abapical
a. pole

abarognosis

abarticular gout

abasia
atactic a., ataxic a.
choreic a.
spastic a.
a. trepidans

abasia-astasia

abasic

abaxial, abaxile

Abbe
A. flap
A. operation

Abbé's condenser

Abbott's
A. artery
A. method
A. stain for spores
A. tube

ABC leads

abdomen
acute a.
boat-shaped a.
carinate a.
navicular a.
a. obstipum
pendulous a.
protuberant a.
scaphoid a.
surgical a.

abdominal
a. angina
a. aorta
a. aortic plexus
a. apoplexy
a. ballottement
a. canal
a. cavity
a. dropsy
a. external oblique muscle
a. fibromatosis
a. fissure
a. fistula
a. guarding
a. hernia
a. hysterectomy
a. hysteropexy
a. hysterotomy
a. internal oblique muscle
a. migraine
a. muscle deficiency syndrome
a. myomectomy
a. nephrectomy
a. ostium of uterine tube
a. pad
a. part of aorta
a. part of esophagus
a. part of thoracic duct
a. part of ureter
a. pool
a. pregnancy
a. pressure
a. pulse
a. reflexes
a. regions
a. respiration
a. ring
a. sac
a. salpingectomy
a. salpingo-oophorectomy
a. salpingotomy
a. section
a. typhoid
a. zones

abdominocardiac reflex

abdominocentesis

abdominocyesis

abdominocystic

abdominogenital

abdominohysterectomy

abdominohysterotomy

abdominojugular reflux

abdominopelvic
a. cavity
a. splanchnic nerves

abdominoperineal
abdominoplasty
abdominoscopy
abdominoscrotal
abdominothoracic arch
abdominovaginal hysterectomy
abdominovesical
abduce
abducens
    a. eminence
    a. nucleus
    a. oculi
abducent nerve
abduct
abduction
abductor
    a. digiti minimi muscle of foot
    a. digiti minimi muscle of hand
    a. hallucis muscle
    a. muscle of great toe
    a. muscle of little finger
    a. muscle of little toe
    a. pollicis brevis muscle
    a. pollicis longus muscle
Abell-Kendall method
Abel's bacillus
Abelson murine leukemia virus
abembryonic
abenteric
Abernethy's fascia
aberrant
    a. artery
    a. bile ducts
    a. bundles
    a. complex
    a. ducts
    a. ductules
    a. ganglion
    a. goiter
    a. hemoglobin
    a. obturator artery
    a. regeneration
    a. ventricular conduction
aberration
    chromatic a.
    chromosome a.
    color a.
    coma a.
    curvature a.
    dioptric a.
    distortion a.
    lateral a.
    longitudinal a.
    mental a.
    meridional a.
    monochromatic a.
    newtonian a.
    optical a.

    spherical a.
    ventricular a.
aberrometer
abetalipoproteinemia
abeyance
abient
ability
abiotic
abiotrophy
abirritation
abl
ablastemic
ablastin
ablate
ablation
    electrode catheter a.
ablatio placentae
ABLB test
ablepharia
ablution
ablutomania
abnerval
abneural
abnormal
    a. cleavage of cardiac valve
    a. correspondence
    a. occlusion
abnormality
    figure-of-8 a.
    snowman a.
ABO
    ABO antigens
    ABO blood group
    ABO factors
    ABO hemolytic disease of the
      newborn
aboiement
aborad, aboral
abort
aborted
    a. ectopic pregnancy
    a. systole
aborticide
abortion
    accidental a.
    ampullar a.
    complete a.
    criminal a.
    elective a.
    habitual a.
    illegal a.
    imminent a.
    incipient a.
    incomplete a.
    induced a.
    inevitable a.
    infected a.
    menstrual extraction a.

missed a.
a. rate
septic a.
spontaneous a.
therapeutic a.
threatened a.
tubal a.
abortionist
abortive
a. neurofibromatosis
a. transduction
abortus bacillus
aboulia
abrachia
abrachiocephaly, abrachiocephalia
abrade
abraded wound
Abrahams' sign
Abrams' heart reflex
abrasion
brush burn a.
gingival a.
mechanical a.
tooth a.
abrasiveness
abrasive strip
ABR audiometry
abreact
abreaction
motor a.
abruption
abruptio placentae
abscess
acute a.
alveolar a.
amebic a.
apical a.
apical periodontal a.
appendiceal a.
Bartholin's a.
Bezold's a.
bicameral a.
bone a.
Brodie's a.
bursal a.
caseous a.
cheesy a.
cholangitic a.
chronic a.
cold a.
collar-button a.
crypt a.'s
dental a., dentoalveolar a.
diffuse a.
Douglas a.
dry a.
Dubois' a.'s
embolic a.

fecal a.
follicular a.
gas a.
gingival a.
gravitation a.
gummatous a.
hematogenous a.
hot a.
hypostatic a.
ischiorectal a.
lacunar a.
lateral alveolar a.
lateral periodontal a.
mastoid a.
metastatic a.
migrating a.
miliary a.
Munro's a.
orbital a.
otic a.
otogenous a.
palatal a.
pancreatic a.
parafrenal a.
parametric a., parametritic a.
paranephric a.
parotid a.
Pautrier's a.
pelvic a.
perforating a.
periapical a.
periappendiceal a.
periarticular a.
pericemental a.
pericoronal a.
perinephric a.
periodontal a.
perirectal a.
peritonsillar a.
periureteral a.
periurethral a.
phlegmonous a.
Pott's a.
premammary a.
psoas a.
pulp a.
pyemic a.
radicular a.
residual a.
retrobulbar a.
retrocecal a.
retropharyngeal a.
ring a.
root a.
satellite a.
septicemic a.
shirt-stud a.
stellate a.

abscess (*continued*)
    stercoral a.
    sterile a.
    stitch a.
    subdiaphragmatic a.
    subepidermal a.
    subhepatic a.
    subperiosteal a.
    subphrenic a.
    subungual a.
    sudoriparous a.
    syphilitic a.
    thecal a.
    thymic a.'s
    Tornwaldt's a.
    tropical a.
    tuberculous a.
    tubo-ovarian a.
    verminous a.
    wandering a.
    worm a.
abscissa
abscission
absconsio
abscopal effect
absence
    pure a.
    a. seizure
    simple a.
absent state
Absidia
absolute
    a. agraphia
    a. cell increase
    a. glaucoma
    a. hemianopia
    a. humidity
    a. hyperopia
    a. intensity threshold acuity
    a. leukocytosis
    a. refractory period
    a. scotoma
    a. terminal innervation ratio
    a. threshold
    a. viscosity
absorbable gelatin film
absorbed dose
absorbent
    a. points
    a. system
    a. vessels
absorber head
absorption
    a. collapse
    cutaneous a.
    disjunctive a.
    external a.
    a. fever

    interstitial a.
    a. lines
    parenteral a.
    pathologic a.
    percutaneous a.
    photoelectric a.
absorptive cells of intestine
abstinence symptoms
abstract
    a. intelligence
    a. thinking
abstriction
abterminal
abtropfung
abulia
abulic
abuse
    child a.
    elder a.
    sexual a.
    spouse a.
abutment
    auxiliary a.
    intermediate a.
    isolated a.
    splinted a.
acalculia
acampsia
acantha
acanthamebiasis
Acanthamoeba
acanthella
acanthesthesia
Acanthia lectularia
acanthion
Acanthocheilonema
acanthocyte
acanthocytosis with chorea
acanthoid
acantholysis
acanthoma
    a. adenoides cysticum
    clear cell a.
    Degos' a.
    a. fissuratum
acanthopodia
acanthor
acanthorrhexis
acanthosis
    glycogenic a.
    a. nigricans
acanthotic
acanthrocyte
acanthrocytosis
acapnia
acapnial alkalosis
acarbia
acardia

ACE inhibitors

acardiac
acardiotrophia
acardius
    a. acephalus
    a. amorphus
    a. anceps
acariasis
    demodectic a.
    psoroptic a.
    sarcoptic a.
acarid
Acaridae
acaridan
acaridiasis
Acarina
acarine
    a. dermatosis
acarinosis
acarodermatitis
    a. urticarioides
acaroid
acarology
acarophobia
Acarus
    A. balatus
    A. gallinae
    A. hordei
    A. rhizoglypticus hyacinthi
    A. scabiei
acaryote
acatamathesia
acataphasia
acathectic
acathexia
acathexis
acathisia
accelerans
accelerated
    a. conduction
    a. eruption
    a. hypertension
    a. reaction
    a. rejection
acceleration
    angular a.
    linear a.
    radial a.
accelerator
    a. factor
    a. fibers
    a. globulin
    linear a.
    a. nerves
    proserum prothrombin conversion a.
    prothrombin a.
    serum a.
    serum prothrombin conversion a.
accelerin

accelerometer
accentuator
accès pernicieux
access
    a. opening
accessorius
    a. willisii
accessory
    a. adrenal
    a. atrium
    a. auricles
    a. breast
    a. canal
    a. cartilage
    a. cephalic vein
    a. chromosome
    a. cramp
    a. cuneate nucleus
    a. flexor muscle of foot
    a. flocculus
    a. gland
    a. hemiazygos vein
    a. lacrimal glands
    a. ligaments
    a. meningeal branch of middle meningeal artery
    a. molecules
    a. nasal cartilages
    a. nerve
    a. nerve lymph nodes
    a. nerve trunk
    a. obturator artery
    a. olivary nuclei
    a. organs
    a. organs of the eye
    a. pancreas
    a. pancreatic duct
    a. parotid gland
    a. phrenic nerves
    a. placenta
    a. plantar ligaments
    a. portion of spinal accessory nerve
    a. process
    a. quadrate cartilage
    a. saphenous vein
    a. sign
    a. spleen
    a. suprarenal glands
    a. symptom
    a. thyroid
    a. thyroid gland
    a. tragus
    a. tubercle
    a. vertebral vein
    a. visual apparatus
    a. volar ligaments

accident
    cardiac a.
    cerebrovascular a.
    a. neurosis
    serum a.
accidental
    a. abortion
    a. host
    a. hypothermia
    a. image
    a. murmur
    a. symptom
accident-prone
acclimating fever
acclimation
acclimatization
accolé forms
accommodation
    amplitude of a.
    a. of eye
    histologic a.
    negative a.
    a. of nerve
    a. phosphene
    positive a.
    range of a.
    a. reflex
    relative a.
accommodative
    a. asthenopia
    a. convergence
    a. convergence-accommodation ratio
    a. strabismus
accompanying
    a. vein
    a. vein of hypoglossal nerve
accomplice
accordion graft
accouchement
    a. forcé
accoucheur
accoucheur's hand
accretio cordis
accretionary growth
accretion lines
accrochage
accumulation disease
accuracy
acedia
acellular
acelom
acelomate, acelomatous
acenesthesia
acentric
    a. chromosome
acephalia, acephalism
acephalic migraine
acephaline

acephalism (*var. of* acephalia)
acephalobrachia
acephalocardia
acephalocheiria, acephalochiria
acephalocyst
acephalogasteria
acephalopodia
acephalorrhachia
acephalostomia
acephalothoracia
acephalous
acephalus
    a. acormus
    a. dibrachius
    a. dipus
    a. monobrachius
    a. monopus
    a. paracephalus
    a. sympus
acephaly
acervuline
acervulus
acestoma
acetabula (*pl. of* acetabulum)
acetabular
    a. artery
    a. branch
    a. fossa
    a. labrum
    a. lip
    a. notch
acetabulectomy
acetabuloplasty
acetabulum, pl. acetabula
acetate
    cresyl violet a.
acetone
    a. fixative
    a. test
acetone-insoluble antigen
acetonemia
acetonemic
acetonuria
aceto-orcein stain
acetrizoate sodium
achalasia
    esophageal a.
Achard syndrome
Achard-Thiers syndrome
ache
    bone a.
    stomach a.
acheilia
acheilous, achilous
acheiria, achiria
acheiropody, achiropody
acheirous, achirous
Achenbach syndrome

achievement
    a. age
    a. motive
    a. quotient
    a. test
Achilles
    A. bursa
    A. reflex
    A. tendon
    A. tendon reflex
achillobursitis
achillodynia
achillorrhaphy
achillotenotomy
achillotomy
achilous (*var. of* acheilous)
achiria (*var. of* acheiria)
achiropody (*var. of* acheiropody)
achirous (*var. of* acheirous)
achlorhydria
achlorhydric anemia
achlorophyllous
Acholeplasma, pl. *Acholeplasmata*
    A. axanthum
    A. granularum
    A. laidlawii
acholia
acholic
acholuria
acholuric
    a. jaundice
achondrogenesis
achondroplasia
    homozygous a.
achondroplastic
    a. dwarfism
achoresis
Achorion
achrestic anemia
achroacyte
achroacytosis
achromacyte
achromasia
achromat
achromatic
    a. apparatus
    a. lens
    a. objective
    a. threshold
    a. vision
achromatin
achromatinic
achromatism
achromatocyte
achromatolysis
achromatophil
achromatophilia

achromatopsia, achromatopsy
    atypical a.
    complete a.
    incomplete a.
    typical a.
achromatosis
achromatous
achromaturia
achromia
    a. parasitica
    a. unguium
achromic
achromocyte
achromoderma
achromophil
achromophilic, achromophilous
achromotrichia
achylia
    a. gastrica
    a. pancreatica
achylous
acid
    a. agglutination
    a. cell
    a. dyspepsia
    a. etch cemented splint
    a. fuchsin
    a. gland
    a. indigestion
    a. intoxication
    a. perfusion test
    a. phosphatase test for semen
    a. red 87
    a. red 91
    a. reflux test
    a. stain
    a. tide
    a. wave
acidaminuria
acid-ash diet
acid-citrate-dextrose
acidemia
    lactic a.
acid-etched restoration
acid-fast
acidic dyes
acidified serum test
acidity
    total a.
acidocyte
acidophil, acidophile
    a. adenoma
    a. cell
    a. granule
acidophilic
    a. leukocyte
acidophilus milk

acidosis
  carbon dioxide a.
  compensated a.
  compensated respiratory a.
  diabetic a.
  hyperchloremic a.
  lactic a.
  metabolic a.
  primary renal tubular a.
  renal tubular a.
  respiratory a.
  secondary renal tubular a.
  starvation a.
  uncompensated a.
acidotic
aciduria
aciduric
acinar
  a. carcinoma
  a. cell
  a. cell tumor
Acinetobacter
  A. calcoaceticus
acini (*gen. and pl. of* acinus)
acinic
  a. cell adenocarcinoma
  a. cell carcinoma
aciniform
acinitis
acinose
  a. carcinoma
acinotubular gland
acinous
  a. carcinoma
  a. cell
  a. gland
a-c interval
acinus, gen. and pl. **acini**
  liver a.
  pulmonary a.
  Rappaport's a.
acknemia (*var. of* acnemia)
aclasia
aclasis
  diaphysial a.
  tarsoepiphyseal a.
acleistocardia
acme
acmesthesia
acne
  a. albida
  a. artificialis
  a. bacillus
  bromide a.
  a. cachecticorum
  chlorine a.
  a. ciliaris
  colloid a.

  a. conglobata
  a. cosmetica
  cystic a.
  a. decalvans
  a. erythematosa
  a. frontalis
  a. fulminans
  a. generalis
  halogen a.
  a. hypertrophica
  a. indurata
  iodide a.
  a. keloid
  a. keratosa
  a. medicamentosa
  a. necrotica
  a. neonatorum
  a. papulosa
  pomade a.
  a. punctata
  a. pustulosa
  a. rosacea
  a. scrofulosorum
  a. simplex, simple a.
  steroid a.
  a. syphilitica
  tar a.
  tropical a.
  a. urticata
  a. varioliformis
  a. venenata
  a. vulgaris
acneform
  a. syphilid
acnegenic
acneiform
acnemia, acknemia, aknemia
acolasia
acolous
acomia
aconative
acorea
acorn-tipped catheter
Acosta's disease
acouasm
acousma
acousmatamnesia
acoustic
  a. agraphia
  a. aphasia
  a. area
  a. cell
  a. crest
  a. enhancement
  a. impedance
  a. lemniscus
  a. lens
  a. meatus

a. nerve
a. neurilemoma
a. neurinoma
a. neuroma
a. papilla
a. pressure
a. radiation
a. reference level
a. schwannoma
a. shadow
a. spots
a. striae
a. tetanus
a. tolerance
a. trauma deafness
a. tubercle
a. vesicle
acousticofacial
a. crest
a. ganglion
acousticopalpebral reflex
acousticophobia
acoustics
acquired
a. agammaglobulinemia
a. centric relation
a. character
a. cuticle
a. drives
a. eccentric relation
a. enamel cuticle
a. epileptic aphasia
a. hemolytic anemia
a. hemolytic icterus
a. hyperlipoproteinemia
a. hypogammaglobulinemia
a. ichthyosis
a. immunity
a. immunodeficiency syndrome
(AIDS)
a. leukoderma
a. leukopathia
a. megacolon
a. methemoglobinemia
a. nevus
a. pellicle
a. reflex
a. sensitivity
a. toxoplasmosis in adults
a. trichoepithelioma
a. tufted angioma
acquisition
acquisitus
acral
a. lentiginous melanoma
acrania
acranial
acranius

Acrel's ganglion
Acremonium
acribometer
acridine
a. dyes
tetramethyl a.
acridine orange
acritical
acroagnosis
acroanesthesia
acroarthritis
acroasphyxia
acroataxia
acroblast
acrobrachycephaly
acrocentric
a. chromosome
acrocephalia
acrocephalic
acrocephalopolysyndactyly
acrocephalosyndactyly
type I a.
type II a.
type III a.
type IV a.
type V a.
acrocephalous
acrocephaly
acrochordon
acrocinesia, acrocinesis
acrocontracture
acrocyanosis
acrocyanotic
acrodermatitis
a. chronica atrophicans
a. continua
a. enteropathica
a. hiemalis
papular a. of childhood
a. perstans
a. vesiculosa tropica
acrodermatosis
acrodynic erythema
acrodysesthesia
acrodysostosis
acrodysplasia
acroedema
acroesthesia
acrofacial
a. dysostosis
a. syndrome
acrogenous
acrogeria
acrognosis
acrohyperhidrosis
acrokeratoelastoidosis
acrokeratosis
paraneoplastic a.

acrokeratosis verruciformis
acrokinesia
acroleukopathy
acromegalia
acromegalic
    a. gigantism
acromegalogigantism
acromegaloidism
acromegaly
acromelalgia
acromelic
    a. dwarfism
acromesomelia
acrometagenesis
acromial
    a. angle
    a. arterial network
    a. artery
    a. articular facies of clavicle
    a. articular surface of clavicle
    a. branch of suprascapular artery
    a. branch of thoracoacromial artery
    a. end of clavicle
    a. extremity of clavicle
    a. plexus
    a. process
    a. reflex
acromicria
acromioclavicular
    a. disk
    a. joint
    a. ligament
acromiocoracoid
acromiohumeral
acromion
    a. presentation
acromioscapular
acromiothoracic
    a. artery
acromphalus
acromyotonia
acromyotonus
acro-osteolysis
acropachy
acropachyderma
acroparesthesia
    a. syndrome
acropathy
acropetal
acrophobia
acropigmentation
acropleurogenous
acropustulosis
    infantile a.
acroscleroderma
acrosclerosis
acrosomal
    a. cap

a. granule
a. vesicle
acrosome
acrospiroma
    eccrine a.
acrostealgia
acroteric
Acrotheca
acrotheca
acrotic
acrotism
acrotrophodynia
acrotrophoneurosis
acrylic
    a. resin
    a. resin base
    a. resin tooth
    a. resin tray
ACTH-producing adenoma
ACTH stimulation test
actin filament
acting out
actinic
    a. cheilitis
    a. conjunctivitis
    a. dermatitis
    a. granuloma
    a. keratitis
    a. keratosis
    a. porokeratosis
    a. prurigo
    a. ray
    a. reticuloid
actinism
actinium emanation
actinodermatitis
actinogram
actinohematin
Actinomadura
    A. africana
    A. madurae
actinomycelial
Actinomyces
    A. bovis
    A. israelii
    A. naeslundii
    A. odontolyticus
    A. pyogenes
    A. viscosus
Actinomycetaceae
Actinomycetales
actinomycetes
actinomycoma
actinomycotic appendicitis
Actinomyxidia
actinoneuritis
actinophage
Actinopoda

actinotherapy
action
    ball valve a.
    a. current
    a. potential
    a. tremor
activated
    a. clotting time
    a. macrophage
    a. partial thromboplastin time
activation
    a. analysis
    EEG a.
activator
    polyclonal a.
active
    a. anaphylaxis
    a. caries
    a. chronic hepatitis
    a. congestion
    a. elcctrode
    a. hyperemia
    a. immunity
    a. immunization
    a. inflammation
    a. labor
    a. length-tension curve
    a. movement
    a. mutant
    a. placebo
    a. prophylaxis
    a. psychoanalysis
    a. splint
    a. treatmcnt
    a. vasoconstriction
    a. vasodilation
activities of daily living scale
activity
    blocking a.
    nonsuppressible insulin-like a.
    plasma renin a.
    triggered a.
actomyosin
    platelet a.
actual cautery
Acuaria spiralis
acuity
    absolute intensity threshold a.
    resolution a.
    spatial a.
    stereoscopic a.
    Vernier a.
    visibility a.
    visual a.
aculeate
acuminate
    a. papular syphilid
acuology

acupressure
acupuncture
    a. anesthesia
acus
acusection
acusector
acusis
acute
    a. abdomen
    a. abscess
    a. adrenocortical insufficiency
    a. African sleeping sickness
    a. alcoholism
    a. angle
    a. anterior poliomyelitis
    a. appendicitis
    a. ascending paralysis
    a. ataxia
    a. atrophic paralysis
    a. bacterial endocarditis
    a. brachial radiculitis
    a. bulbar poliomyelitis
    a. catarrhal conjunctivitis
    a. cellular rejection
    a. chalazion
    a. cholecystitis
    a. chorea
    a. compression triad
    a. contagious conjunctivitis
    a. crescentic glomerulonephritis
    a. cutaneous leishmaniasis
    a. decubitus ulcer
    a. delirium
    a. disseminated encephalomyelitis
    a. disseminated myositis
    a. epidemic conjunctivitis
    a. epidemic leukoencephalitis
    a. febrile neutrophilic dermatosis
    a. fibrinous pericarditis
    a. follicular conjunctivitis
    a. fulminating meningococcal
      septicemia
    a. fulminating meningococcemia
    a. glaucoma
    a. glomerulonephritis
    a. goiter
    a. hallucinatory paranoia
    a. hemorrhagic conjunctivitis
    a. hemorrhagic encephalitis
    a. hemorrhagic glomerulonephritis
    a. hemorrhagic leukoencephalitis
    a. hemorrhagic pancreatitis
    a. idiopathic polyneuritis
    a. inclusion body encephalitis
    a. infectious nonbacterial
      gastroenteritis
    a. inflammation
    a. inflammatory polyneuropathy

acute (*continued*)
 a. intermittent porphyria
 a. interstitial nephritis
 a. interstitial pneumonia
 a. interstitial pneumonitis
 a. isolated myocarditis
 a. lobar nephrosis
 a. lymphocytic leukemia
 a. malaria
 a. mania
 a. miliary tuberculosis
 a. necrotizing encephalitis
 a. necrotizing hemorrhagic
  encephalomyelitis
 a. necrotizing hemorrhagic
  leukoencephalitis
 a. necrotizing myelitis
 a. necrotizing ulcerative gingivitis
 a. nephritis
 a. nephrosis
 a. organic brain syndrome
 a. parenchymatous hepatitis
 a. phase protein
 a. phase reactants
 a. phase reaction
 a. porphyria
 a. post-streptococcal
  glomerulonephritis
 a. primary hemorrhagic
  meningoencephalitis
 a. promyelocytic leukemia
 a. pulmonary alveolitis
 a. pyelonephritis
 a. radiation syndrome
 a. recurrent rhabdomyolysis
 a. reflex bone atrophy
 a. rejection
 a. respiratory failure
 a. rheumatic arthritis
 a. rhinitis
 a. rickets
 a. scalp cellulitis
 a. schizophrenia
 a. schizophrenic episode
 a. situational reaction
 a. splenic tumor
 a. stress reaction
 a. transverse myelitis
 a. trypanosomiasis
 a. tuberculosis
 a. urticaria
 a. vascular purpura
 a. viral conjunctivitis
 a. yellow atrophy of the liver
acyanotic
acystia
adacrya
adactylous

adamantine
 a. membrane
adamantinoma
 a. of long bones
 pituitary a.
Adam's apple
Adams-Stokes
 A.-S. disease
 A.-S. syncope
 A.-S. syndrome
adansonian classification
adaptation
 dark a.
 a. diseases
 light a.
 photopic a.
 reality a.
 retinal a.
 scotopic a.
 social a.
 a. syndrome of Selye
adaptive
 a. behavior
 a. behavior scales
 a. hypertrophy
adaptometer
adaxial
addict
addiction
 alcohol a.
Addis
 A. count
 A. test
Addison-Biermer disease
addisonian
 a. anemia
 a. crisis
 a. syndrome
Addison's
 A. anemia
 A. clinical planes
 A. disease
additive model
additivity
 causal a.
 interlocal a.
 intralocal a.
addressing ligands
adducent
adduction
adductor
 a. brevis muscle
 a. canal
 a. hallucis muscle
 a. hiatus
 a. longus muscle
 a. magnus muscle
 a. minimus muscle

a. muscle of great toe
a. muscle of thumb
a. pollicis muscle
a. reflex
a. tubercle
adelomorphous
Aden
A. fever
A. ulcer
adenalgia
adendric
adendritic
adenectomy
adenectopia
adenemphraxis
adeniform
adenitis
adenization
adenoacanthoma
adenoameloblastoma
adeno-associated virus
adenoblast
adenocarcinoma
acinic cell a.
alveolar a.
a. in Barrett's esophagus
bronchiolar a.
bronchioloalveolar a.
clear cell a.
mesonephric a.
mucoid a.
papillary a.
renal a.
a. in situ
adenocellulitis
adenochondroma
adenocystoma
adenocyte
adenodiastasis
adenodynia
adenoepithelioma
adenofibroma
adenofibromyoma
adenofibrosis
adenogenous
adenohypophysial
adenohypophysis
adenohypophysitis
lymphocytic a.
adenoid
a. cystic carcinoma
a. facies
a. squamous cell carcinoma
a. tissue
a. tumor
adenoidal-pharyngeal-conjunctival virus
adenoidectomy
adenoiditis

adenoids
adenoleiomyofibroma
adenolipoma
adenolipomatosis
symmetric a.
adenolymphocele
adenolymphoma
adenoma
acidophil a.
ACTH-producing a.
adnexal a.
adrenocortical a.
apocrine a.
basal cell a.
basophil a.
bronchial a.
canalicular a.
carcinoma ex pleomorphic a.
chromophil a.
chromophobe a., chromophobic a.
colloid a.
embryonal a.
eosinophil a.
fibroid a., a. fibrosum
follicular a.
Fuchs' a.
gonadotropin-producing a.
growth hormone-producing a.
hepatic a.
hepatocellular a.
Hürthle cell a.
islet cell a.
lactating a.
Leydig cell a.
macrofollicular a.
microfollicular a.
monomorphic a.
nephrogenic a.
a. of nipple
null-cell a.
ovarian tubular a.
oxyphil a.
papillary cystic a.
papillary a. of large intestine
Pick's tubular a.
pituitary a.
pleomorphic a.
polypoid a.
prolactin-producing a.
prostatic a.
renal cortical a.
sebaceous a.
a. sebaceum
testicular tubular a.
thyrotropin-producing a.
tubular a.
undifferentiated cell a.
villous a.

adenomatoid
    a. odontogenic tumor
    a. tumor
adenomatosis
    erosive a. of nipple
    familial multiple endocrine a.
    fibrosing a.
    multiple endocrine a.
    pulmonary a.
adenomatous
    a. goiter
    a. polyp
adenomegaly
adenomere
adenomyoma
adenomyosarcoma
adenomyosis
    a. uteri
adenoneural
adenopathy
adenophlegmon
Adenophorasida
Adenophorea
adenophyma
adenosalpingitis
adenosarcoma
    müllerian a.
adenosatellite virus
adenose
adenosis
    blunt duct a.
    fibrosing a.
    microglandular a.
    sclerosing a.
adenosquamous carcinoma
adenotomy
adenotonsillectomy
adenous
Adenoviridae
adenovirus
    canine a. 1
    porcine a.'s
adeps, gen. **adipis, adipes**
    a. renis
adequal cleavage
adequate stimulus
adermia
adermogenesis
adherence
    immune a.
    a. syndrome
adherent
    a. leukoma
    a. pericardium
    a. placenta
adhesins
adhesio, pl. **adhesiones**
    a. interthalamica

adhesion
    amniotic a.'s
    a. dyspepsia
    fibrinous a.
    fibrous a.
    interthalamic a.
    a. molecules
    a. phenomenon
    primary a.
    secondary a.
    a. test
adhesiotomy
adhesive
    a. absorbent dressing
    a. arachnoiditis
    a. atelectasis
    a. bandage
    a. capsulitis
    a. inflammation
    a. otitis
    a. pericarditis
    a. peritonitis
    a. phlebitis
    a. pleurisy
    a. vaginitis
adiadochocinesia, adiadochocinesis
adiadochokinesis
adiaphoresis
adiaphoria
adiaspore
adiastole
adiathermancy
Adie
    A. pupil
    A. syndrome
adiemorrhysis
adient
    a. behavior
Adinida
adipectomy
adipes (*gen. of* adeps)
Adipiodone
adipis (*gen. of* adeps)
adipocellular
adipoceratous
adipocere
adipocyte
adipodermal graft
adipometer
adiponecrosis
adiposalgia
adipose
    a. capsule
    a. cell
    a. degeneration
    a. folds of the pleura
    a. fossae
    a. infiltration

a. tissue
a. tumor
adiposis
a. cerebralis
a. dolorosa
a. orchica
a. tuberosa simplex
a. universalis
adiposity
adiposogenital
a. degeneration
a. dystrophy
a. syndrome
adiposuria
adipsia, adipsy
aditus, pl. **aditus**
a. ad antrum
a. ad aqueductum cerebri
a. ad infundibulum
a. ad saccum peritonei minorem
a. glottidis inferior
a. glottidis superior
a. laryngis
a. orbitae
a. pelvis
adjacent angle
adjustable
a. articulator
a. axis face-bow
a. occlusal pivot
adjustment
a. disorders
occlusal a.
adjuvant
Freund's a.
Freund's incomplete a.
ADL
adlerian
a. psychoanalysis
a. psychology
Adler's test
admaxillary gland
admedial, admedian
adminiculum, pl. **adminicula**
a. lineae albae
adnerval
adneural
adnexa, sing. **adnexum**
a. oculi
a. uteri
adnexal
a. adenoma
a. carcinoma
adnexectomy
adnexitis
adnexopexy
adnexum (*sing. of* adnexa)
adnexum

adolescence
adolescent
a. albuminuria
a. crisis
a. medicine
a. round back
adoptive
a. immunity
a. immunotherapy
adoral
adrenal
accessory a.
a. androgen-stimulating hormone
a. apoplexy
a. body
a. capsule
a. cortex
a. cortex injection
a. cortical carcinomas
a. cortical syndrome
a. crisis
a. gland
a. hermaphroditism
a. hypertension
a. leukodystrophy
Marchand's a.'s
a. rest
a. virilism
a. virilizing syndrome
a. weight factor
adrenalectomy
adrenalism
adrenalitis
adrenalopathy
adrenarche
adrenergic fibers
adrenic
adrenoceptor
adrenocortical
a. adenoma
a. insufficiency
adrenocorticomimetic
adrenocorticotropic releasing factor
adrenogenic, adrenogenous
adrenogenital syndrome
adrenoleukodystrophy
adrenomedullary hormones
adrenomegaly
adrenomyeloneuropathy
adrenopathy
adrenoprival
adromia
Adson
A. forceps
A. maneuver
A. test
adsorption
immune a.

adsternal
adterminal
adult
    a. hypophosphatasia
    a. lactase deficiency
    a. medulloepithelioma
    a. pseudohypertrophic muscular
      dystrophy
    a. respiratory distress syndrome
    a. rickets
    a. T-cell leukemia
    a. T-cell lymphoma
    a. tuberculosis
    a. type
adultomorphism
adult-onset diabetes
advance
advanced life support
advanced multiple-beam equalization
  radiography
advancement
    capsular a.
    a. flap
    tendon a.
adventitia
adventitial
    a. cell
    a. neuritis
adventitious
    a. albuminuria
    a. bursa
    a. cyst
adversive movement
adynamia
    a. episodica hereditaria
adynamic
    a. ileus
Aeby's
    A. muscle
    A. plane
Aedes
    A. *aegypti*
    A. *albopictus*
    A. *leucocelaenus*
    A. *polynesiensis*
    A. *variegatus*
aelurophobia
Aelurostrongylus
aequorin
aerendocardia
aerial
    a. mycelium
    a. sickness
aeroatelectasis
Aerobacter
aerobe
    obligate a.
aerobic

aerobiology
aerobioscope
aerobiosis
aerobiotic
aerocele
Aerococcus
aerocolpos
aerodermectasia
aerodontalgia
    primary a.
    secondary a.
aerodontia
aeroemphysema
aerogastria
    blocked a.
aerogen
aerogenesis
aerogenic, aerogenous
    a. tuberculosis
aerohydrotherapy
aeromedicine
aeromonad
Aeromonas
aero-odontalgia
aero-odontodynia
aeropathy
aeropause
aerophil, aerophile
aerophilic, aerophilous
aerophobia
aeropiesotherapy
aeroplankton
aeroplethysmograph
aerosialophagy
aerosinusitis
aerosis
aerosolization
aerospace medicine
aerotherapeutics, aerotherapy
aerotitis media
aestival
aestivoautumnal fever
afebrile
afetal
affect
    blunted a.
    a. displacement
    flat a.
    a. hunger
    inappropriate a.
    labile a.
    a. memory
    a. spasms
affect display
affection
affective
    a. disorders
    a. personality disorder

A

a. psychosis
a. tone
affectivity
affectomotor
afferent
a. fibers
a. glomerular arteriole
a. loop syndrome
a. lymphatic
a. nerve
a. vessel
affinity antibody
affinous
affirmation
afflux, affluxion
affusion
afibrillar
a. cementum
afibrinogenemia
congenital a.
AFORMED phenomenon
African
A. endomyocardial fibrosis
A. hemorrhagic fever
A. histoplasmosis
A. horse sickness virus
A. sleeping sickness
A. tick fever
A. trypanosomiasis
afterbirth
aftercare
aftercataract
afterchroming
aftercontraction
aftercurrent
afterdischarge
aftereffect
aftergilding
afterimage
negative a.
positive a.
afterimpression
afterload
ventricular a.
afterloading screw
aftermovement
afterpains
afterperception
afterpotential
diastolic a.
positive a.
aftersensation
aftersound
aftertaste
aftertouch
afunctional occlusion
agalactia
agalactorrhea

agalactosis
agalactous
agamete
agamic
agammaglobulinemia
acquired a.
secondary a.
Swiss type a.
transient a.
agamocytogeny
Agamofilaria
agamogenesis
agamogenetic
agamogony
Agamomermis culicis
agamont
agamous
aganglionic
aganglionosis
agapism
agar
ascitic a.
bile salt a.
birdseed a.
blood a.
Bordet-Gengou potato blood a.
brain-heart infusion a.
brilliant green salt a.
chocolate a.
cholera a.
Conradi-Drigalski a.
cornmeal a.
Czapek's solution a.
Drigalski-Conradi a.
EMB a.
Endo a.
Endo's fuchsin a.
eosin-methylene blue a.
French proof a.
fuchsin a.
Guarnieri's gelatin a.
lactose-litmus a.
MacConkey a.
Mueller-Hinton a.
Novy and MacNeal's blood a.
nutrient a.
oatmeal-tomato paste a.
Pfeiffer's blood a.
potato dextrose a.
rice-Tween a.
Sabouraud's a.
Sabouraud's dextrose a.
serum a.
Thayer-Martin a.
yeast extract a.
Ag-AS stain
agastric
agastroneuria

age
  achievement a.
  anatomical a.
  basal a.
  Binet a.
  bone a.
  childbearing a.
  chronologic a.
  developmental a.
  emotional a.
  fetal a.
  gestational a.
  menstrual a.
  mental a.
  physical a.
  physiologic a.
agenesis
  gonadal a.
  renal a.
  thymic a.
agenitalism
agenosomia
agent
  Bittner a.
  chimpanzee coryza a.
  contrast a.
  delta a.
  Eaton a.
  embedding a.'s
  F a.
  fertility a.
  foamy a.'s
  high osmolar contrast a.
  initiating a.
  LDH a.
  luting a.
  MS-1 a.
  MS-2 a.
  Norwalk a.
  Pittsburgh pneumonia a.
  promoting a.
  reovirus-like a.
  transforming a.
  TRIC a.'s
agerasia
age-related macular degeneration
age-specific rate
ageusia
ageustia
agger, pl. **aggeres**
  a. nasi
  a. perpendicularis
  a. valvae venae
agglomerate, agglomerated
agglomeration
agglutinating antibody
agglutination
  acid a.

  bacteriogenic a.
  cold a.
  cross a.
  false a.
  group a.
  immune a.
  indirect a.
  mixed a.
  nonimmune a.
  passive a.
  spontaneous a.
  a. test
agglutinative thrombus
agglutinin
  blood group a.'s
  chief a.
  cold a.
  cross-reacting a.
  flagellar a.
  group a.
  H a.
  immune a.
  incomplete a.
  major a.
  minor a.
  O a.
  partial a.
  plant a.
  saline a.
  serum a.
  somatic a.
  warm a.'s
agglutinogen
  blood group a.'s
  T a.
agglutinogenic
agglutinophilic
agglutinoscope
agglutogen
agglutogenic
aggregate
  a. anaphylaxis
  a. glands
aggregated
  a. lymphatic follicles
  a. lymphatic follicles of vermiform
    appendix
  a. lymphatic nodules
aggregation
  familial a.
aggregometer
aggressin
aggression
aggressive
  a. infantile fibromatosis
  a. instinct
aging
  clonal a.

agitated depression
agitographia
agitolalia
agitophasia
aglobulia
aglobuliosis
aglobulism
aglossia
aglossia-adactylia syndrome
aglossostomia
aglutition
aglycosuria
aglycosuric
agmen, pl. agmina
    a. peyerianum
agminate, agminated
    a. glands
agnathia
agnathous
agnea
agnogenic
    a. myeloid metaplasia
agnosia
    auditory a.
    color a.
    finger a.
    localization a.
    optic a.
    position a.
    tactile a.
    visual a.
    visual-spatial a.
agomphious
agomphosis, agomphiasis
agonadal
agonal
    a. clot
    a. infection
    a. leukocytosis
    a. rhythm
    a. thrombus
agony
agoraphobia
agoraphobic
agraffe
agrammatica
agrammatism
agrammatologia
agranular
    a. cortex
    a. endoplasmic reticulum
    a. leukocyte
agranulocyte
agranulocytic angina
agranulocytosis
agranuloplastic
agraphia
    absolute a.

    acoustic a.
    amnemonic a.
    atactic a.
    cerebral a.
    constructional a.
    literal a.
    mental a.
    motor a.
    musical a.
    verbal a.
agraphic
agretope
agriothymia
agromania
agrypnia
agrypnocoma
ague
    brass founder's a.
agyiophobia
agyria
A-H
    A.-H. conduction time
    A.-H. interval
ahaustral
Ahumada-Del Castillo syndrome
ahylognosia
Aicardi's syndrome
aichmophobia
aid
    first a.
    hearing a.
AIDS
    acquired immunodeficiency syndrome
    AIDS dementia
    AIDS dementia complex
AIDS-related
    A.-r. complex
    A.-r. virus
ailurophobia
ainhum
air
    alveolar a.
    a. bronchogram
    a. cells
    a. cells of auditory tube
    complemental a.
    complementary a.
    a. conduction
    a. contrast barium enema
    a. contrast enema
    a. dose
    a. embolism
    functional residual a.
    a. hunger
    minimal a.
    reserve a.
    residual a.
    a. sickness

air *(continued)*
    a. splint
    supplemental a.
    a. syringe
    tidal a.
    a. tube
    a. vesicles
air-bone gap
airborne infection
airbrasive technique
air-conditioner lung
air-gap
    a.-g. radiography
    a.-g. technique
airplane splint
airsickness
airspace
airspace-filling pattern
airtrapping
airway
    anatomical a.
    conducting a.
    lower a.
    a. pattern
    a. resistance
    respiratory a.
    upper a.
Ajellomyces capsulatum
Ajellomyces dermatitidis
Akabane virus
akamushi disease
akanthion
akaryocyte
akaryote
akathisia
akembe
akeratosis
Akerlund deformity
akinesia
    a. algera
    a. amnestica
akinesic
akinesis
akinesthesia
akinetic
    a. mutism
    a. seizure
akiyami
aknemia *(var. of* acnemia)
aknemia
Akureyri disease
ala, gen. and pl. **alae**
    a. auris
    a. central lobule
    a. cerebelli
    a. cinerea
    a. cristae galli
    alae lingulae cerebelli

    a. lobuli centralis
    a. major ossis sphenoidalis
    a. minor ossis sphenoidalis
    a. nasi
    a. orbitalis
    a. ossis ilii
    a. sacralis
    a. temporalis
    a. vespertilionis
    a. vomeris
alactic oxygen debt
alalia
alalic
Alanson's amputation
alar
    a. artery of nose
    a. chest
    a. folds
    a. lamina of neural tube
    a. ligaments
    a. part of nasalis muscle
    a. plate of neural tube
    a. process
    a. spine
ALARA
alarm reaction
alaryngeal speech
alastrim
alba
Albarran's
    A. glands
    A. test
Albarran y Dominguez' tubules
albedo
    a. retinae
Albers-Schönberg disease
Albert's
    A. disease
    A. stain
    A. suture
albicans, pl. **albicantia**
albiduria
albidus
albinism
    cutaneous a.
    ocular a.
    oculocutaneous a., tyrosinase
      negative type, tyrosinase positive
      type
    rufous a.
Albini's nodules
albino
albinotic
albinuria
Albinus' muscle
albocinereous
Albrecht's bone

Albright's
   A. disease
   A. hereditary osteodystrophy
   A. syndrome
albuginea
albugineotomy
albugineous
albumin
   bovine serum a.
   a. Ghent
   a. Mexico
   a. Naskapi
   a. Reading
albuminaturia
albumin-globulin ratio
albuminocholia
albuminocytologic dissociation
albuminoid degeneration
albuminoptysis
albuminorrhea
albuminous
   a. cell
   a. degeneration
   a. gland
   a. swelling
albuminuria
   adolescent a.
   adventitious a.
   a. of athletes
   Bamberger's a.
   benign a.
   cardiac a.
   colliquative a.
   cyclic a.
   dietetic a., digestive a.
   essential a.
   false a.
   febrile a.
   functional a.
   intermittent a.
   lordotic a.
   neuropathic a.
   orthostatic a.
   physiologic a.
   postrenal a.
   postural a.
   prerenal a.
   recurrent a.
   regulatory a.
   transient a.
albuminuric
   a. retinitis
Alcaligenes
alcaptonuria, alkaptonuria
Alcian blue
Alcock's canal
alcohol
   a. addiction

   a. amnestic syndrome
   a. diuresis
   a. withdrawal delirium
alcoholic
   a. cardiomyopathy
   a. cirrhosis
   a. deterioration
   a. hyalin
   a. hyaline bodies
   a. myocardiopathy
   a. pneumonia
   a. polyneuropathy
   a. psychoses
   a. withdrawal tremor
alcoholism
   acute a.
   alpha a.
   beta a.
   chronic a.
   delta a.
   epsilon a.
   gamma a.
alcoholophobia
alcohol-soluble eosin
aldehyde fuchsin
Alder
   A. anomaly
   A. bodies
aldosterone antagonist
aldosteronism
   idiopathic a.
   primary a.
   secondary a.
aldosteronogenesis
Aldrich syndrome
alecithal
   a. ovum
Alectorobius talaje
alemmal
Aleppo boil
alethia
aleukemia
aleukemic
   a. leukemia
   a. myelosis
aleukemoid
aleukia
aleukocytic
aleukocytosis
aleurioconidium
aleuriospore
Aleutian mink disease virus
Alexander's
   A. deafness
   A. disease
alexia
   incomplete a.
   motor a.

alexia *(continued)*
    musical a.
    optical a.
    sensory a.
    visual a.
alexic
alexin
alexithymia
aleydigism
Alezzandrini's syndrome
algae
    blue-green a.
algal
algedonic
algesia
algesic
algesichronometer
algesidystrophy
algesimeter
algesiogenic
algesiometer
algesthesia
algesthesis
algetic
algid
    a. malaria
    a. pernicious fever
    a. stage
algiomotor
algiomuscular
algiovascular
algodystrophy
algogenesis, algogenesia
algogenic
algoid cell
algolagnia
algology
algometer
algometry
algophilia
algophobia
algopsychalia
algorithm
algospasm
algovascular
alible
Alice in Wonderland syndrome
alienation
alienia
alienist
aliform
alignment
    a. curve
    a. mark
aliment
alimentary
    a. apparatus
    a. canal

    a. diabetes
    a. glycosuria
    a. hyperinsulinism
    a. lipemia
    a. osteopathy
    a. pentosuria
    a. system
    a. tract
    a. tract smear
alimentation
    forced a.
    parenteral a.
    rectal a.
alinasal
alinement
alinjection
alisphenoid
    a. cartilage
alizarin
    a. cyanin
    a. indicator
    a. purpurin
    a. red S
alkalemia
alkali
    a. denaturation test
    a. therapy
alkaline
    a. reflux gastritis
    a. tide
    a. toluidine blue O
    a. wave
alkaline-ash diet
alkalinuria
alkalitherapy
alkalosis
    acapnial a.
    compensated a.
    compensated metabolic a.
    compensated respiratory a.
    metabolic a.
    respiratory a.
    uncompensated a.
alkalotic
alkaluria
alkannan
alkaptonuria *(var. of* alcaptonuria)
allachesthesia
allantochorion
allantoenteric diverticulum
allantogenesis
allantoic
    a. cyst
    a. diverticulum
    a. fluid
    a. sac
    a. stalk
    a. vesicle

A

allantoidoangiopagous twins
allantoidoangiopagus
allantoinuria
allaxis
allele
    codominant a.
    silent a.
allelic
    a. exclusion
    a. gene
allelism
allelocatalysis
allelomorph
allelomorphic
allelomorphism
allelotaxis, allelotaxy
Allen-Doisy test
Allen-Masters syndrome
Allen's test
allergen
allergenic
    a. extract
allergic
    a. angiitis
    a. conjunctivitis
    a. contact dermatitis
    a. coryza
    a. eczema
    a. extract
    a. granulomatosis
    a. granulomatous angiitis
    a. inflammation
    a. purpura
    a. reaction
    a. rhinitis
allergic salute
allergin
allergist
allergization
allergized
allergosis
allergy
    atopic a.
    bacterial a.
    cold a.
    contact a.
    delayed a.
    immediate a.
    latent a.
    physical a.
    polyvalent a.
Allescheria boydii
allesthesia
allied health professional
allied reflexes
alligator
    a. forceps
    a. skin

Allis forceps
Allis' sign
alliteration
all or none
all or none law
alloalbuminemia
alloantibody
alloantigen
allocentric
allochezia, allochetia
allochiria, allocheiria
allochroic
allochroism
allochromasia
allocortex
allodiploid
allodynia
alloerotic
alloeroticism
alloerotism
alloesthesia
allogamy
allogenic, allogeneic
allogotrophia
allograft
    a. rejection
allogroup
allohexaploid
allokeratoplasty
allokinesis
allolalia
allomeric function
allometron
allongement
allonomous
allopath
allopathic
    a. keratoplasty
allopathist
allopathy
allopentaploid
allophasis
allophenic
allophore
allophthalmia
alloplasia
alloplast
alloplasty
alloploid
alloploidy
allopolyploid
allopolyploidy
allopsychic
allorhythmia
allorhythmic
allosensitization

allosome
>paired a.
>unpaired a.

allotetraploid
allotope
allotopia
allotransplantation
allotrichia circumscripta
allotriodontia
allotriogeustia
allotriophagy
allotriosmia
allotriploid
allotropic personality
allotype
>Gm a.'s
>InV a.'s
>Km a.'s

allotypic
>a. determinants
>a. marker

alloxuremia
alloxuria
alloy
>chrome-cobalt a.'s
>eutectic a.
>gold a.
>silver-tin a.

Almeida's disease
Almén's test for blood
almond nucleus
alogia
alopecia
>a. adnata
>androgenic a.
>a. areata
>a. capitis totalis
>a. celsi
>Celsus' a.
>cicatricial a.
>a. cicatrisata
>a. circumscripta
>a. congenitalis
>congenital sutural a.
>a. disseminata
>female pattern a.
>a. follicularis
>a. hereditaria
>Jonston's a.
>a. leprotica
>a. liminaris frontalis
>lipedematous a.
>male pattern a.
>a. marginalis
>a. medicamentosa
>moth-eaten a.
>a. mucinosa
>a. neurotica

>patterned a.
>a. pityrodes
>postoperative pressure a.
>postpartum a.
>premature a., a. prematura
>a. presenilis
>pressure a.
>scarring a.
>a. senilis
>a. symptomatica
>a. syphilitica
>a. totalis
>a. toxica
>traction a.
>traumatic a.
>a. triangularis
>a. triangularis congenitalis
>a. universalis

alopecic
Alpers disease
alpha
>a. alcoholism
>a. angle
>a. blocking
>a. cells of anterior lobe of hypophysis
>a. cells of pancreas
>a. error
>a. fibers
>a. granule
>a. radiation
>a. rhythm
>a. substance
>A. test
>a. units
>a. wave

Alphavirus
alphos
Alpine scurvy
Alport's syndrome
Alström's syndrome
ALT:AST ratio
alteration
>modal a.
>qualitative a.
>quantitative a.

alterative inflammation
altercursive intubation
alteregoism
alternans
>auditory a.
>auscultatory a.
>concordant a.
>discordant a.
>electrical a.

Alternaria
alternate
>a. binaural loudness balance test

24

a. cover test
a. day strabismus
a. hemianesthesia
alternating
a. hemiplegia
a. light test
a. mydriasis
a. pulse
a. strabismus
a. tremor
alternation
cardiac a.
concordant a.
discordant a.
electrical a. of heart
a. of generations
mechanical a. of the heart
alternative
a. hypothesis
a. inheritance
a. medicine
a. tremor
alternator
alternocular
alteromonas
A. putrefaciens
altitude
a. chamber
a. disease
a. erythremia
altitudinal
a. hemianopia
Altmann-Gersh method
Altmann's
A. anilin-acid fuchsin stain
A. fixative
A. granule
A. theory
altrigendrism
alum
chrome a.
alum-hematoxylin
aluminosis
Alu sequences
alvei (*pl. of* alveus)
alveoalgia
alveolalgia
alveolar
a. abscess
a. adenocarcinoma
a. air
a. angle
a. arch of mandible
a. arch of maxilla
a. atrophy
a. body
a. bone
a. border

a. canals
a. cell
a. cell carcinoma
a. crest
a. dead space
a. duct
a. duct emphysema
a. foramina
a. gas
a. gas equation
a. gingiva
a. gland
a. hydatid cyst
a. index
a. macrophage
a. mucosa
a. osteitis
a. part of mandible
a. pattern
a. periosteum
a. point
a. process
a. ridge
a. sac
a. septum
a. soft part sarcoma
a. supporting bone
a. ventilation
a. yoke
alveolar-arterial oxygen difference
alveolate
alveolectomy
alveoli (*gen. and pl. of* alveolus)
alveolingual
alveolitis
acute pulmonary a.
chronic fibrosing a.
extrinsic allergic a.
fibrosing a.
alveolobuccal
a. groove
a. sulcus
alveolocapillary
a. block
a. membrane
alveoloclasia
alveolodental
a. canals
a. ligament
a. membrane
alveololabial
a. groove
a. sulcus
alveololabialis
alveololingual
a. groove
a. sulcus
alveolonasal line

alveolopalatal
alveoloplasty
    interradicular a., intraseptal a.
alveoloschisis
alveolotomy
alveolus, gen. and pl. **alveoli**
    a. dentalis, pl. alveoli dentales
    pulmonary a.
    alveoli pulmonis
alveoplasty
alveus, pl. **alvei**
    a. hippocampi
    a. of hippocampus
    a. urogenitalis
alvinolith
alymphia
alymphocytosis
alymphoplasia
    Nezelof type of thymic a.
    thymic a.
Alzheimer
    A. dementia
    A. disease
    A. sclerosis
    A. type I astrocyte
    A. type II astrocyte
AMA
amacrine
    a. cell
amalgam
    a. carrier
    a. matrix
    pin a.
    spherical a.
    a. strip
    a. tattoo
amalgamate
amalgamation
amalgamator
Am antigens
amastia
amastigote
amathophobia
amativeness
amaurosis
    a. congenita of Leber
    a. fugax
    pressure a.
    toxic a.
amaurotic
    a. cat's eye
    a. mydriasis
    a. nystagmus
    a. pupil
amaxophobia
amazia
ambageusia

Ambard's
    A. constant
    A. laws
Amberg's lateral sinus line
ambidexterity
ambidextrism
ambidextrous
ambient
    a. behavior
    a. cistern
ambiguous
    a. atrioventricular connections
    a. external genitalia
    a. nucleus
ambilateral
ambilevous
ambisexual
ambisinister
ambisinistrous
ambivalence
ambivalent
ambivert
amblyaphia
amblygeustia
Amblyomma
    A. americanum
    A. cajennense
    A. hebraeum
    A. maculatum
    A. variegatum
amblyopia
    anisometropic a.
    deprivation a.
    a. ex anopsia
    hysterical a.
    nocturnal a.
    nutritional a.
    refractive a.
    sensory a.
    strabismic a.
    suppression a.
    toxic a.
amblyopic
amblyoscope
    major a.
    Worth's a.
amboceptor
ambomalleal
ambos
Amboyna button
Ambu bag
ambulance
ambulatory, ambulant
    a. anesthesia
    a. automatism
    a. plague
    a. schizophrenia

a. surgery
a. typhoid
ambustion
ameba, pl. **amebae, amebas**
amebaism
amebiasis
    a. cutis
    hepatic a.
    pulmonary a.
amebic
    a. abscess
    a. colitis
    a. dysentery
    a. granuloma
    a. vaginitis
amebiform
amebiosis
amebism
amebocyte
ameboid
    a. cell
    a. movement
ameboididity
ameboidism
ameboma
amebula, pl. **amebulae**
amebule
ameburia
amelanotic
    a. melanoma
amelia
amelioration
ameloblast
ameloblastic
    a. adenomatoid tumor
    a. fibroma
    a. fibrosarcoma
    a. layer
    a. odontoma
    a. sarcoma
ameloblastoma
    pigmented a.
    pituitary a.
ameloblastomatous craniopharyngioma
amelodental junction
amelodentinal
    a. junction
amelogenesis
    a. imperfecta
amenia
amenorrhea
    dietary a.
    emotional a.
    exercise-induced a.
    hyperprolactinemic a.
    hypophysial a.
    hypothalamic a.
    lactation a.

    ovarian a.
    pathologic a.
    physiologic a.
    postpartum a.
    primary a.
    secondary a.
    traumatic a.
amenorrhea-galactorrhea syndrome
amenorrheal, amenorrheic
amentia
    nevoid a.
    phenylpyruvic a.
    Stearns alcoholic a.
amential
American
    A. Law Institute formulation
    A. Law Institute rule
    A. leishmaniasis
    A. tarantula
    A. trypanosomiasis
amerism
ameristic
Ames
    A. assay
    A. test
ametria
ametropia
    axial a.
    index a.
ametropic
amiantaceous
amianthoid
amicrobic
amicroscopic
amido black 10B
amidonaphthol red
Amidostomum anseris
amimia
aminoacidemia
aminoaciduria
aminobenzene
p-**aminohippurate clearance**
aminuria
amitosis
amitotic
ammonemia, ammoniemia
ammoniacal urine
ammonia rash
ammoniemia (*var. of* ammonemia)
ammoniuria
Ammon's
    A. fissure
    A. horn
    A. prominence
amnemonic agraphia
amnesia
    anterograde a.
    emotional a.

amnesia *(continued)*
    lacunar a., localized a.
    posthypnotic a.
    retrograde a.
    transient global a.
    traumatic a.
amnesiac
amnesic
    a. aphasia
amnestic
    a. aphasia
    a. psychosis
    a. syndrome
amniocardiac vesicle
amniocele
amniocentesis
amniochorial, amniochorionic
amnioembryonic junction
amniogenesis
amniogenic cells
amniography
amnioma
amnion
    a. nodosum
    a. ring
amnionic
amnionitis
amniorrhea
amniorrhexis
amnioscope
amnioscopy
amniotic
    a. adhesions
    a. amputation
    a. bands
    a. cavity
    a. corpuscle
    a. duct
    a. ectoderm
    a. fluid
    a. fluid embolism
    a. fluid syndrome
    a. sac
amniotome
amniotomy
A-mode
Amoeba
    A. buccalis
    A. coli
    A. dentalis
    A. dysenteriae
    A. histolytica
    A. meleagridis
    A. proteus
Amoebotaenia
amok
amorph
amorphagnosia

amorphia, amorphism
amorphosynthesis
amorphus
Amoss' sign
amotio placentae
amperometry
amphiarthrodial
amphiarthrosis
amphiaster
amphibolic fistula
amphibolous fistula
amphicelous
amphicentric
amphichroic
amphichromatic
amphicyte
amphikaryon
amphileukemic
Amphimerus
amphimicrobe
amphimixis
amphinucleolus
amphistome
amphithymia
amphitrichate, amphitrichous
amphitypy
amphochromatophil, amphochromatophile
amphochromophil, amphochromophile
amphocyte
amphodiplopia
amphophil, amphophile
    a. granule
amphophilic, amphophilous
amphoric
    a. rale
    a. resonance
    a. respiration
    a. voice
    a. voice sound
amphoriloquy
amphorophony
amphoteric reaction
amphotonia, amphotony
amphotropic virus
amplification
    genetic a.
amplifier
    a. host
    image a.
amplitude
    a. of accommodation
    a. of convergence
    a. of pulse
ampulla, gen. and pl. ampullae
    a. canaliculi lacrimalis
    a. chyli
    a. of ductus deferens
    a. ductus deferentis

A

a. ductus lacrimalis
duodenal a.
a. duodeni
a. of gallbladder
Henle's a.
hepatopancreatic a.
a. hepatopancreatica
a. of lacrimal canaliculus
a. lactifera
lactiferous a.
a. membranacea, pl. ampullae
  membranaceae
membranous a.
a. of milk duct
a. ossea, pl. ampullae osseae
osseous a.
phrenic a.
rectal a.
a. recti
a. of rectum
a. of the semicircular canals
a. of the semicircular ducts
Thoma's a.
a. tubae uterinae
a. of uterine tube
Vater's a.

ampullar
a. abortion
a. pregnancy

ampullary
a. aneurysm
a. crest
a. crura of semicircular ducts
a. folds of uterine tube
a. limbs of semicircular ducts
a. sulcus

ampullitis
ampullula
amputating ulcer
amputation
Alanson's a.
amniotic a.
aperiosteal a.
Bier's a.
birth a.
bloodless a.
Callander's a.
Carden's a.
central a.
cervical a.
Chopart's a.
cinematic a.
cineplastic a.
circular a.
congenital a.
consecutive a.
a. in continuity
double flap a.

dry a.
Dupuytren's a.
eccentric a.
elliptical a.
excentric a.
Farabeuf's a.
flap a.
flapless a.
forequarter a.
Gritti-Stokes a.
guillotine a.
Guyon's a.
Hancock's a.
Hey's a.
hindquarter a.
immediate a.
interilioabdominal a.
intermediate a.
interpelviabdominal a.
interscapulothoracic a.
intrapyretic a.
intrauterine a.
Jaboulay's a.
kineplastic a.
Kirk's a.
a. knife
Krukenberg's a.
Larrey's a.
Le Fort's a.
linear a.
Lisfranc's a.
Mackenzie's a.
major a.
Malgaigne's a.
mediotarsal a.
Mikulicz-Vladimiroff a.
minor a.
multiple a.
musculocutaneous a.
a. neuroma
oblique a.
osteoplastic a.
oval a.
pathologic a.
periosteoplastic a.
Pirogoff's a.
primary a.
pulp a.
quadruple a.
racket a.
rectangular a.
root a.
secondary a.
spontaneous a.
Stokes a.
subastragalar a.
subperiosteal a.
Syme's a.

amputation (*continued*)
    tarsotibial a.
    Teale's a.
    tertiary a.
    a. by transfixion
    transverse a.
    traumatic a.
    Tripier's a.
    Vladimiroff-Mikulicz a.
amputee
Amsler
    A. chart
    A. test
Amsterdam syndrome
amuck
amusia
    instrumental a.
    motor a.
    sensory a.
    vocal a.
Amussat's
    A. valve
    A. valvula
amychophobia
Amycolatopsis
    A. *orientalis* subsp. *lurida*
amyctic
amyelencephalia
amyelencephalic, amyelencephalous
amyelia
amyelic
amyelinated
amyelination
amyelinic
amyeloic, amyelonic
amyelous
amygdala, gen. and pl. **amygdalae**
    a. cerebelli
amygdaloid
    a. body
    a. complex
    a. fossa
    a. nucleus
    a. tubercle
amylaceous corpuscle
amylase-creatinine clearance ratio
amylasuria
amylemia
amyloid
    a. angiopathy
    a. bodies of the prostate
    a. corpuscle
    a. degeneration
    a. kidney
    a. nephrosis
    a. tumor
amyloidosis
    a. of aging

    a. cutis
    familial a.
    focal a.
    lichen a.
    lichenoid a.
    light chain-related a.
    macular a.
    a. of multiple myeloma
    nodular a.
    primary a.
    renal a.
    secondary a.
    senile a.
amylopectinosis
amylophagia
amylorrhea
amylosuria
amyluria
amyocardia
amyoesthesia, amyoesthesis
amyoplasia
    a. congenita
amyostasia
amyostatic
amyosthenia
amyosthenic
amyotaxy, amyotaxia
amyotonia
    a. congenita
amyotrophia
amyotrophic
amyotrophy
    diabetic a.
    hemiplegic a.
    neuralgic a.
    progressive spinal a.
amyous
amyxorrhea
Anabaena
anabiosis
anabiotic cells
anabrosis
anabrotic
anacamptometer
anacatadidymus (*var. of* anakatadidymus)
anacatesthesia
anacidity
anaclasis
anaclitic
    a. depression
    a. psychotherapy
anacmesis
anacrotic
    a. limb
    a. pulse
anacrotism
anacusis

A

anadenia
 a. ventriculi
anadicrotic
 a. pulse
anadicrotism
anadidymus
anadipsia
anadrenalism
anaerobe
 facultative a.
 obligate a.
anaerobic
 a. cellulitis
anaerobiosis
anaerogenic
anaerophyte
anaeroplasty
anagen
 a. effluvium
anagenesis
anagenetic
anagogy
anakatadidymus, anacatadidymus
anákhré
anakmesis
anakusis
anal
 a. atresia
 a. canal
 a. cleft
 a. columns
 a. crypts
 a. ducts
 a. erotism
 a. fascia
 a. fissure
 a. fistula
 a. membrane
 a. orifice
 a. pecten
 a. phase
 a. pit
 a. plate
 a. reflex
 a. region
 a. skin tag
 a. sphincter
 a. triangle
 a. valves
 a. verge
analbuminemia
analeptic enema
analgesia
 a. algera
 conduction a.
 a. dolorosa
 inhalation a.

 patient controlled a.
 spinal a.
analgesic
 a. cuirass
 a. nephritis
 a. nephropathy
analgesimeter
anality
anallergic
analphalipoproteinemia
analysand
analysis, pl. **analyses**
 activation a.
 bite a.
 blood gas a.
 bradykinetic a.
 cephalometric a.
 character a.
 cluster a.
 content a.
 decision a.
 didactic a.
 discriminant a.
 displacement a.
 distributive a.
 Downs' a.
 ego a.
 Fourier a.
 gastric a.
 interaction process a.
 linkage a.
 Northern blot a.
 occlusal a.
 path a.
 pedigree a.
 percept a.
 regression a.
 saturation a.
 segregation a.
 sequential a.
 Southern blot a.
 survival a.
 training a.
 transactional a.
 a. of variance
 Western blot a.
analytic
 a. psychiatry
 a. study
 a. therapy
analytical
 a. psychology
 a. sensitivity
 a. specificity
analyzer, analyzor
 pulse height a.
analyzing rod
anamnesis

anamnestic
   a. reaction
   a. response
anamnionic, anamniotic
anamorph
anamorphosis
ananaphylaxis
ananastasia
anancasm
anancastia
anancastic
   a. personality
anandria
anangioplasia
anangioplastic
anapeiratic
anaphase
   a. lag
anaphia
anaphrodisia
anaphylactic
   a. antibody
   a. intoxication
   a. reaction
   a. shock
anaphylactogen
anaphylactogenesis
anaphylactogenic
anaphylactoid
   a. crisis
   a. purpura
   a. shock
anaphylatoxin
anaphylatoxin inactivator
anaphylaxis
   active a.
   aggregate a.
   antiserum a.
   chronic a.
   generalized a.
   inverse a.
   local a.
   passive a.
   passive cutaneous a.
   reversed a.
   reversed passive a.
   systemic a.
anaphylotoxin
anaplasia
Anaplasma
anaplastic
   a. astrocytoma
   a. carcinoma
   a. cell
   a. large cell lymphoma
   a. oligodendroglioma
anaplasty
anapophysis

anaptic
anarithmia
anarthria
anarthritic rheumatoid disease
anasarca
   fetoplacental a.
anasarcous
anastigmatic
anastole
anastomose
anastomosed graft
anastomosing
   a. fibers
   a. vessel
anastomosis, pl. anastomoses
   arteriolovenular a.
   a. arteriovenosa
   arteriovenous a.
   Béclard's a.
   bevelled a.
   Billroth I a.
   Billroth II a.
   Braun's a.
   cavopulmonary a.
   circular a.
   Clado's a.
   conjoined a.
   cruciate a., crucial a.
   Damus-Stancel-Kaye a.
   elliptical a.
   Galen's a.
   Hofmeister-Pólya a.
   Hoyer's anastomoses
   Hyrtl's a.
   intermesenteric arterial a.
   intestinal a.
   isoperistaltic a.
   Jacobson's a.
   Martin-Gruber a.
   microvascular a.
   portacaval anastomoses
   portal-systemic anastomoses
   postcostal a.
   Potts' a.
   precapillary a.
   precostal a.
   Riolan's a.
   Roux-en-Y a.
   Schmidel's anastomoses
   Sucquet-Hoyer anastomoses
   Sucquet's anastomoses
   termino-terminal a.
   transureteroureteral a.
   uretero-ileal a.
   ureterosigmoid a.
   ureterotubal a.
   ureteroureteral a.

anastomotic
 a. branch
 a. branch of middle meningeal
  artery to lacrimal artery
 a. fibers
 a. stricture
 a. ulcer
 a. veins
anastral
anatomic
 a. rigidity
 a. teeth
anatomical
 a. age
 a. airway
 a. crown
 a. dead space
 a. element
 a. neck of humerus
 a. pathology
 a. position
 a. root
 a. snuffbox
 a. sphincter
 a. tubercle
 a. wart
anatomicomedical
anatomicopathological
anatomicosurgical
anatomist
anatomy
 applied a.
 artificial a.
 artistic a.
 clastic a.
 clinical a.
 dental a.
 descriptive a.
 functional a.
 general a.
 gross a.
 living a.
 macroscopic a.
 medical a.
 microscopic a.
 pathological a.
 physiological a.
 plastic a.
 practical a.
 radiological a.
 regional a.
 special a.
 surface a.
 surgical a.
 systematic a.
 systemic a.
 topographic a.

 transcendental a.
 ultrastructural a.
anatopism
anatricrotic
anatricrotism
anatripsis
anatrophic nephrotomy
anaxon, anaxone
anazoturia
ancestor
 leading a.
anchorage
 cervical a.
 extraoral a.
 intermaxillary a.
 intramaxillary a.
 intraoral a.
 multiple a.
 occipital a.
 reciprocal a.
 reinforced a.
 simple a.
 stationary a.
anchoring villus
anchor splint
ancillary
ancipital, ancipitate, ancipitous
ancon
anconad
anconal, anconeal
 a. fossa
anconeus
 a. muscle
anconitis
anconoid
Ancylostoma
 A. *braziliense*
 A. *caninum*
 A. *ceylanicum*
 A. *duodenale*
ancylostoma dermatitis
ancylostomatic
ancylostomiasis
 cutaneous a.
 a. cutis
ancyroid
Andernach's ossicles
Andersch's
 A. ganglion
 A. nerve
Anders' disease
Andersen's disease
Anderson
 A. and Goldberger test
 A. splint
Anderson-Collip test
Anderson-Hynes pyeloplasty
Andral's decubitus

andriatrics, andriatry
androblastoma
androgen binding protein
androgenesis
androgenic
    a. alopecia
    a. zone
androgenous
androgynism
androgynoid
androgynous
androgyny
android
    a. pelvis
andrology
andromania
andromorphous
andropathy
androphobia
anecdotal
anechoic
    a. chamber
anectasis
anelectrotonic
anelectrotonus
Anel's method
anemia
    achlorhydric a.
    achrestic a.
    acquired hemolytic a.
    addisonian a.
    Addison's a.
    angiopathic hemolytic a.
    aplastic a.
    asiderotic a.
    autoimmune hemolytic a.
    Bartonella a.
    Belgian Congo a.
    Biermer's a.
    brickmaker's a.
    cameloid a.
    chlorotic a.
    congenital a.
    congenital aplastic a.
    congenital dyserythropoietic a., type
      I, type II, type III
    congenital hemolytic a.
    congenital hypoplastic a.
    congenital nonregenerative a.
    Cooley's a.
    cow milk a.
    crescent cell a.
    deficiency a.
    Diamond-Blackfan a.
    dilution a.
    dimorphic a.
    diphyllobothrium a.
    drepanocytic a.

dyshemopoietic a.
Ehrlich's a.
elliptocytary a.
elliptocytic a.
elliptocytotic a.
erythroblastic a.
erythronormoblastic a.
essential a.
Faber's a.
false a.
familial erythroblastic a.
familial hypoplastic a.
familial microcytic a.
familial pyridoxine-responsive a.
familial splenic a.
Fanconi's a.
fish tapeworm a.
folic acid deficiency a.
globe cell a.
goat's milk a.
a. gravis
ground itch a.
Heinz body a.
hemolytic a.
hemorrhagic a.
hookworm a.
hyperchromic a., hyperchromatic a.
hypochromic a.
hypochromic microcytic a.
hypoferric a.
hypoplastic a.
icterohemolytic a.
infectious a.
intertropical a.
iron deficiency a.
isochromic a.
lead a.
Lederer's a.
leukoerythroblastic a.
local a.
macrocytic a.
macrocytic achylic a.
macrocytic a. of pregnancy
macrocytic a. tropical
malignant a.
Marchiafava-Micheli a.
megaloblastic a.
megalocytic a.
metaplastic a.
microangiopathic hemolytic a.
microcytic a.
microdrepanocytic a.
milk a.
mountain a.
myelophthisic a., myelopathic a.
normochromic a.
normocytic a.
nutritional a.

A

nutritional macrocytic a.
osteosclerotic a.
ovalocytic a.
pernicious a.
physiologic a.
polar a.
posthemorrhagic a.
primary erythroblastic a.
primary refractory a.
pure red cell a.
radiation a.
refractory a.
scorbutic a.
secondary refractory a.
sickle cell a.
sideroblastic a., sideroachrestic a.
slaty a.
spastic a.
spherocytic a.
splenic a.
target cell a.
toxic a.
traumatic a.
tropical a.
type I (*var. of* congenital
    dyserythropoietic a.)
type II (*var. of* congenital
    dyserythropoietic a.)
type III (*var. of* congenital
    dyserythropoietic a.)
unstable hemoglobin hemolytic a.

anemic
a. anoxia
a. halo
a. hypoxia
a. infarct
a. murmur

anemometer
anemophobia
anemotrophy
anencephalia
anencephalic
anencephalous
anencephaly
partial a.

anenterous
anenzymia
anephric
anepia
anergasia
anergastic
anergia
anergic
a. leishmaniasis

anergy
negative a.
nonspecific a.

positive a.
specific a.

aneroid
a. manometer

anerythroplasia
anerythroplastic
anerythroregenerative
anesthecinesia
anesthekinesia
anesthesia
acupuncture a.
ambulatory a.
axillary a.
balanced a.
basal a.
block a.
brachial a.
caudal a.
cervical a.
circle absorption a.
closed a.
compression a.
conduction a.
continuous epidural a.
continuous spinal a.
crossed a.
dental a.
diagnostic a.
differential spinal a.
dissociated a.
dissociative a.
a. dolorosa
electric a.
endotracheal a.
epidural a.
extradural a.
field block a.
fractional epidural a.
fractional spinal a.
general a.
girdle a.
glove a.
gustatory a.
high spinal a.
hyperbaric a.
hyperbaric spinal a.
hypobaric spinal a.
hypotensive a.
hypothermic a.
hysterical a.
infiltration a.
inhalation a.
insufflation a.
intercostal a.
intramedullary a.
intranasal a.
intraoral a.
intraosseous a.

anesthesia *(continued)*
    intraspinal a.
    intratracheal a.
    intravenous a.
    intravenous regional a.
    isobaric spinal a.
    local a.
    low spinal a.
    a. machine
    nerve block a.
    nonrebreathing a.
    open drop a.
    outpatient a.
    painful a.
    paracervical block a.
    paravertebral a.
    patient controlled a.
    peridural a.
    perineural a.
    periodontal a.
    presacral a.
    pressure a.
    pudendal a.
    rebreathing a.
    a. record
    rectal a.
    refrigeration a.
    regional a.
    retrobulbar a.
    sacral a.
    saddle a.
    saddle block a.
    segmental a.
    semi-closed a.
    semi-open a.
    spinal a.
    splanchnic a.
    stocking a.
    subarachnoid a.
    surgical a.
    tactile a.
    therapeutic a.
    thermal a., thermic a.
    to-and-fro a.
    topical a.
    total spinal a.
    traumatic a.
    unilateral a.
    visceral a.
anesthesiologist
anesthesiology
anesthetic
    a. circuit
    a. depth
    flammable a.
    a. gas
    general a.
    a. index

    inhalation a.
    intravenous a.
    a. leprosy
    primary a.
    secondary a.
    a. shock
    spinal a.
    a. vapor
    volatile a.
anesthetist
anesthetization
anesthetize
anestrum
anethopath
anetoderma
    Jadassohn-Pellizzari a.
    Schweninger-Buzzi a.
aneuploid
aneuploidy
    partial a.
aneurolemmic
aneurysm
    ampullary a.
    a. by anastomosis
    aortic a.
    aortic sinus a.
    arteriosclerotic a.
    arteriovenous a.
    atherosclerotic a.
    axial a.
    benign bone a.
    Bérard's a.
    berry a.
    cardiac a.
    Charcot-Bouchard a.
    cirsoid a.
    compound a.
    congenital cerebral a.
    consecutive a.
    coronary artery a.
    cylindroid a.
    diffuse a.
    ductal a.
    ectatic a.
    embolomycotic a.
    false a.
    fusiform a.
    hernial a.
    infraclinoid a.
    intracavernous a.
    intracranial a.
    miliary a.
    mural a.
    mycotic a.
    a. needle
    Park's a.
    peripheral a.
    phantom a.

Pott's a.
pulmonary artery a.
racemose a.
Rasmussen's a.
a. of the right ventricle or right
  ventricular outflow patch
ruptured a.
saccular a., sacculated a.
serpentine a.
a. of sinus of Valsalva
supraclinoid a.
syphilitic a.
traumatic a.
true a.
tubular a.
varicose a.
ventricular a.
a. of the ventricular portion of the
  membranous septum
aneurysmal, aneurysmatic
  a. bone cyst
  a. bruit
  a. cough
  a. murmur
  a. phthisis
  a. sac
  a. varix
aneurysmectomy
aneurysmogram
aneurysmograph
aneurysmoplasty
aneurysmorrhaphy
aneurysmotomy
Angelman syndrome
angel's wing
Angelucci's syndrome
Anger camera
Anghelescu's sign
angiectasia, angiectasis
  congenital dysplastic a.
angiectatic
angiectopia
angiitis, angitis
  allergic a.
  allergic granulomatous a.
  consecutive a.
  hypersensitivity a.
  a. livedo reticularis
  necrotizing a.
angina
  abdominal a., a. abdominis
  agranulocytic a.
  crescendo a.
  a. cruris
  a. decubitus
  a. diphtheritica
  a. of effort
  false a.

Heberden's a.
hypercyanotic a.
intestinal a.
a. inversa
Ludwig's a.
lymphatic a.
a. lymphomatosa
monocytic a.
necrotic a.
neutropenic a.
a. notha
a. pectoris
a. pectoris decubitus
a. pectoris sine dolore
a. pectoris vasomotoria
preinfarction a.
Prinzmetal's a.
reflex a.
a. scarlatinosa
a. sine dolore
a. spuria
unstable a.
variant a. pectoris
vasomotor a.
a. vasomotoria
Vincent's a.
walk-through a.
anginal
anginiform
anginoid
anginophobia
anginose, anginous
  a. scarlatina
angioarchitecture
angioblast
angioblastic
  a. cells
  a. cyst
angioblastoma
angiocardiography
  exercise radionuclide a.
  gated radionuclide a.
  radionuclide a.
angiocardiokinetic, angiocardiocinetic
angiocardiopathy
angiocholecystitis
angiocholitis
angiocyst
angioderm
angiodiascopy
angiodysgenetic myelomalacia
angiodysplasia
angiodystrophy, angiodystrophia
angioedema
  hereditary a.
angioelephantiasis
angioendotheliomatosis
  proliferating systematized a.

angiofibrolipoma
angiofibroma
    juvenile a.
angiofibrosis
angiofollicular mediastinal lymph node
  hyperplasia
angiogenesis
    a. factor
angiogenic
angioglioma
angiogliomatosis
angiogliosis
angiogram
angiographic
angiography
    biplane a.
    a. catheter
    cerebral a.
    closed a.
    coronary a.
    digital subtraction a.
    fluorescein a.
    interventional a.
    magnetic resonance a.
    magnification a.
    MR a.
    open a.
    radionuclide a.
    scintigraphic a.
    selective a.
    therapeutic a.
angiohyalinosis
angiohypertonia
angiohypotonia
angioid
    a. streaks
angioimmunoblastic lymphadenopathy
  with dysproteinemia
angioinvasive
angiokeratoma
    diffuse a.
    Fordyce's a.
    Mibelli's a.'s
angiokeratosis
angiokinesis
angiokinetic
angioleiomyoma
angiolipofibroma
angiolipoma
angiolith
angiolithic
    a. degeneration
    a. sarcoma
angiologia
angiology
angiolupoid
angiolymphoid hyperplasia with
  eosinophilia

angiolysis
angioma
    acquired tufted a.
    capillary a.
    cavernous a.
    cherry a.
    a. lymphaticum
    petechial a.'s
    a. serpiginosum
    spider a.
    superficial a.
    telangiectatic a.
    a. venosum racemosum
    venous a.
angiomatoid
    a. tumor
angiomatosis
    bacillary a.
    cephalotrigeminal a.
    cerebroretinal a.
    congenital dysplastic a.
    cutaneomeningospinal a.
    encephalotrigeminal a.
    oculoencephalic a.
    telangiectatic a.
angiomatous
angiomegaly
angiomyocardiac
angiomyofibroma
angiomyolipoma
angiomyoma
angiomyoneuroma
angiomyopathy
angiomyosarcoma
angiomyxoma
angioneurectomy
angioneuredema
angioneuromyoma
angioneuropathy
angioneuroses
angioneurosis
angioneurotic
    a. edema
angioneurotomy
angio-osteohypertrophy syndrome
angioparalysis
angioparalytic neurasthenia
angioparesis
angiopathic
    a. hemolytic anemia
    a. neurasthenia
angiopathy
    amyloid a.
    cerebral amyloid a.
    congophilic a.
    giant cell hyaline a.
angiophacomatosis, angiophakomatosis
angioplany

A

angioplasty
    a. balloon
    percutaneous transluminal a.
    percutaneous transluminal
      coronary a.
angiopoiesis
angiopoietic
angiorrhaphy
angiorrhexis
angiosarcoma
angioscope
angioscopy
angioscotoma
angioscotometry
angiosis
angiospasm
    labyrinthine a.
angiospastic
angiostenosis
Angiostrongylus
    A. cantonensis
    A. costaricensis
    A. malaysiensis
angiotelectasis, angiotelectasia
angiotomy
angiotonia
angiotrophic
angitis (*var. of* angiitis)
angle
    acromial a.
    acute a.
    adjacent a.
    alpha a.
    alveolar a.
    a. of anomaly, a. of abnormality
    anorectal a.
    a. of antetorsion
    a. of anteversion
    a. of aperture
    apical a.
    axial a.
    basilar a.
    Bennett a.
    beta a.
    biorbital a.
    Broca's a.'s
    Broca's basilar a.
    Broca's facial a.
    buccal a.'s
    bucco-occlusal a.
    cardiodiaphragmatic a.
    cardiohepatic a.
    cardiophrenic a.
    carrying a.
    cavity line a.
    cavosurface a.
    cephalic a.
    cephalomedullary a.

Boehler's Angle

    cerebellopontile a.
    cerebellopontine a.
    a. of convergence
    costal a.
    costophrenic a.
    craniofacial a.
    critical a.
    cusp a.
    Daubenton's a.
    a. of declination
    a. of depression
    a. of deviation
    disparity a.
    duodenojejunal a.
    a. of eccentricity
    a. of emergence
    epigastric a.
    ethmoid a.
    facial a.
    a. of femoral torsion
    filtration a.
    flip a.
    Frankfort-mandibular incisor a.
    frontal a. of parietal bone
    a. of Fuchs
    gamma a.
    hypsiloid a.
    impedance a.
    a. of incidence
    incident a.
    incisal guide a.
    a. of inclination
    inferior a. of scapula
    infrasternal a.
    iridocorneal a.
    a. of iris
    Jacquart's facial a.
    a. of jaw
    kappa a.
    lateral a. of eye
    lateral a. of scapula
    lateral a. of uterus
    limiting a.
    line a.
    Louis' a.
    Lovibond's a.
    Ludwig's a.
    lumbosacral a.
    a. of mandible
    mastoid a. of parietal bone
    maxillary a.
    medial a. of eye
    mesial a.
    metafacial a.
    meter a.
    a. of mouth
    neck-shaft a.
    occipital a. of parietal bone

angle *(continued)*
    olfactory a.
    ophryospinal a.
    parietal a.
    pelvivertebral a.
    phrenopericardial a.
    Pirogoff's a.
    point a.
    a. of polarization
    pontine a.
    pubic a.
    Q a.
    Quatrefages' a.
    Ranke's a.
    a. of reflection
    refracting a. of a prism
    a. of refraction
    Rolando's a.
    Serres' a.
    S-N-A a.
    S-N-B a.
    sphenoid a., sphenoidal a.
    sphenoidal a. of parietal bone
    sternal a.
    sternoclavicular a.
    subpubic a.
    substernal a.
    superior a. of scapula
    sylvian a.
    tentorial a.
    Topinard's facial a.
    a. of torsion
    venous a.
    Virchow-Holder a.
    Virchow's a.
    visual a.
    Vogt's a.
    Weisbach's a.
    Welcker's a.
    y-a.
angle-closure glaucoma
Angle's classification of malocclusion
angor
    a. animi
    a. pectoris
Angström's law
Anguillula
angular
    a. acceleration
    a. aperture
    a. artery
    a. cheilitis
    a. conjunctivitis
    a. convolution
    a. curvature
    a. gyrus
    a. notch
    a. sphincter

    a. spine
    a. stomatitis
    a. vein
angulation
angulus, gen. and pl. **anguli**
    a. acromialis
    a. costae
    a. frontalis ossis parietalis
    a. inferior scapulae
    a. infrasternalis
    a. iridis
    a. iridocornealis
    a. lateralis scapulae
    a. mandibulae
    a. mastoideus ossis parietalis
    a. occipitalis ossis parietalis
    a. oculi lateralis
    a. oculi medialis
    a. oculi nasalis
    a. oculi temporalis
    a. oris
    a. sphenoidalis ossis parietalis
    a. sterni
    a. subpubicus
    a. superior scapulae
anhaphia
anhedonia
anhepatic jaundice
anhepatogenous jaundice
anhidrosis
anhidrotic ectodermal dysplasia
anhistic, anhistous
ani (*gen. of* anus)
aniacinamidosis
aniacinosis
anicteric
    a. hepatitis
    a. leptospirosis
    a. virus hepatitis
anidean
anideus
    embryonic a.
anidous
anidrosis
anidrotic
anile
anilinction, anilinctus
aniline
    a. fuchsin
aniline blue
anilingus
anilinophil, anilinophile
anilinophilous
anility
anima
animal
    control a.
    conventional a.

a. force
a. graft
Houssay a.
a. magnetism
a. model
normal a.
a. pole
a. psychology
sentinel a.
a. viruses
animalcule
animation
animatism
animism
animus
A-N interval
anion gap
aniridia
anisakiasis
anisakid
Anisakidae
Anisakis
aniseikonia
anisoaccommodation
anisochromasla
anisochromatic
anisocoria
essential a.
physiologic a.
simple a.
simple-central a.
anisocytosis
anisodactylous
anisodactyly
anisogamy
anisognathous
anisokaryosis
anisomastia
anisomelia
anisometropia
anisometropic
a. amblyopia
anisopiesis
anisorrhythmia
anisosphygmia
anisosthenic
anisotonic
anisotropic disks
Anitschkow
A. cell
A. myocyte
ankle
a. bone
a. clonus
a. jerk
a. joint
a. reflex
a. region

ankyloblepharon
congenital a.
ankylocolpos
ankylodactyly, ankylodactylia
ankyloglossia
a. superior syndrome
ankylomele
ankylopoietic
ankyloproctia
ankylosed
a. tooth
ankylosing
a. hyperostosis
a. spondylitis
ankylosis
artificial a.
bony a.
dental a.
extracapsular a.
false a.
fibrous a.
intracapsulai a.
spurious a.
true a.
Ankylostoma
ankylostomiasis
ankylotic
ankyroid
anlage, pl. **anlagen**
annealing
a. lamp
a. tray
annectent
a. gyrus
Annelida
annelids
annellide
annelloconidium
annexa
annexal
annexectomy
annexitis
annexopexy
annihilation radiation
annular
a. band
a. cartilage
a. cataract
a. ligament
a. ligament of the radius
a. ligament of the stapes
a. ligaments of the trachea
a. pancreas
a. part of fibrous digital sheath
a. placenta
a. plexus
a. pulley
a. scleritis

annular *(continued)*
  a. scotoma
  a. sphincter
  a. staphyloma
  a. stricture
  a. synechia
  a. syphilid
annulate lamellae
annuloaortic ectasia
annuloplasty
  a. ring
annulorrhaphy
annulospiral
  a. ending
  a. organ
annulus
  a. abdominalis
  a. ciliaris
  a. conjunctivae
  a. femoralis
  a. fibrocartilagineus membranae
  tympani
  a. fibrosus
  a. fibrosus cordis
  a. fibrosus disci intervertebralis
  a. fibrosus of intervertebral disc
  a. of fibrous sheath
  Haller's a.
  a. hemorrhoidalis
  a. inguinalis profundus
  a. inguinalis superficialis
  a. iridis
  a. iridis major
  a. iridis minor
  a. lymphaticus cardiae
  a. ovalis
  a. tendineus communis
  a. tympanicus
  a. umbilicalis
  a. urethralis
  Vieussens' a.
anochlesia
anochromasia
anociassociation
anococcygeal
  a. body
  a. ligament
  a. nerves
anocutaneous line
anodal
  a. closure contraction
  a. closure tetanus
  a. current
  a. duration tetanus
  a. opening contraction
  a. opening tetanus

anode
  a. rays
  rotating a.
anoderm
anodontia
  partial a.
anodontism
anoetic
anogenital
  a. band
  a. raphe
anomalad
anomaloscope
anomalous
  a. atrioventricular excitation
  a. complex
  a. conduction
  a. correspondence
  a. mitral arcade
  a. trichromatism
  a. uterus
  a. viscosity
anomaly
  Alder's a.
  Aristotle's a.
  Chédiak-Steinbrinck-Higashi a.
  developmental a.
  Ebstein's a.
  eugnathic a.
  Freund's a.
  Hegglin's a.
  May-Hegglin a.
  morning glory a.
  Pelger-Huët nuclear a.
  Peters' a.
  Rieger's a.
  Shone's a.
  Uhl a.
anomia
anomic aphasia
anomie
anonychia, anonychosis
anonyma
anonymous veins
Anopheles
  A. albimanus
  A. albitarsus
  A. balabacensis
  A. culicifacies
  A. darlingi
  A. fluviatilis
  A. freeborni
  A. funestus
  A. gambiae
  A. labranchiae
  A. maculatus
  A. maculipennis
  A. minimus

A. *pseudopunctipennis*
A. *quadrimaculatus*
A. *stephensi*
A. *sundaicus*
A. *superpictus*
Anophelinae
anopheline
Anophelini
anophelism
anophthalmia
anoplasty
Anoplocephala
    A. *perfoliata*
Anoplura
anorchia
anorchism
anorectal
    a. angle
    a. flexure
    a. junction
    a. lymph nodes
    a. spasm
    a. syndrome
anorexia
    a. nervosa
anorgasmy, anorgasmia
anorthography
anoscope
    Bacon's a.
anosigmoidoscopy
anosmia
anosmic
anosodiaphoria
anosognosia
anosognosic
    a. epilepsy
    a. seizures
anospinal
    a. center
anosteoplasia
anostosis
anotia
anovesical
anovular
    a. menstruation
    a. ovarian follicle
anovulation
anovulational menstruation
anovulatory
    a. cycle
anoxemia
    a. test
anoxia
    anemic a.
    anoxic a.
    diffusion a.
    histotoxic a.
    a. neonatorum

    oxygen affinity a.
    stagnant a.
anoxic
    a. anoxia
ANP
    ANP clearance receptors
    ANP receptors
Anrep
    A. effect
    A. phenomenon
ansa, gen. and pl. **ansae**
    a. cervicalis
    Haller's a.
    Henle's a.
    a. hypoglossi
    lenticular a.
    a. lenticularis
    ansae nervorum spinalium
    peduncular a.
    a. peduncularis
    Reil's a.
    a. sacralis
    a. subclavia
    Vieussens' a.
ansate
anserine
    a. bursa
    a. bursitis
ansiform
    a. lobule
ansotomy
ant
    harvester a.
    velvet a.
antagonism
    bacterial a.
antagonist
    aldosterone a.
    associated a.
antagonistic
    a. muscles
    a. reflexes
antalgesia
antalgic gait
antebrachial
    a. fascia
    a. flexor retinaculum
antebrachium
antecardium
antecedent
    plasma thromboplastin a.
    a. sign
antecubital
    a. space
antefebrile
anteflex
anteflexion
    a. of iris

antegonial notch
antegrade
- a. cardioplegia
- a. conduction
- a. cystography
- a. pyelography
- a. urography

antemortem
- a. clot
- a. thrombus

antenatal
- a. diagnosis

antepartum
anteposition
anteprostate
antepyretic
anterior
- a. ampullar nerve
- a. antebrachial nerve
- a. antebrachial region
- a. aphasia
- a. arch of atlas
- a. articular surface of dens
- a. asynclitism
- a. atlanto-occipital membrane
- a. auricular branches of superficial temporal artery
- a. auricular groove
- a. auricular muscle
- a. auricular nerves
- a. auricular vein
- a. axillary fold
- a. axillary line
- a. basal branch
- a. basal segment
- a. belly of digastric muscle
- a. border
- a. border of eyelids
- a. border of fibula
- a. border of lung
- a. border of pancreas
- a. border of radius
- a. border of testis
- a. border of tibia
- a. border of ulna
- a. brachial region
- a. branch
- a. canaliculus of chorda tympani
- a. cardiac veins
- a. cardinal veins
- a. carpal region
- a. cecal artery
- a. cells
- a. central convolution
- a. central gyrus
- a. centriole
- a. cerebellar notch
- a. cerebral artery

- a. cerebral vein
- a. cervical intertransversarii muscles
- a. cervical intertransverse muscles
- a. cervical lymph nodes
- a. chamber cleavage syndrome
- a. chamber of eye
- a. chamber trabecula
- a. choroidal artery
- a. choroiditis
- a. ciliary artery
- a. circumflex humeral artery
- a. clear space
- a. column
- a. column of medulla oblongata
- a. commissure
- a. communicating artery
- a. component of force
- a. condyloid canal of occipital bone
- a. condyloid foramen
- a. conjunctival artery
- a. coronary plexus
- a. corticospinal tract
- a. costotransverse ligament
- a. cranial base
- a. cranial fossa
- a. cruciate ligament
- a. crural nerve
- a. crural region
- a. crus of stapes
- a. cubital region
- a. curvature
- a. cusp of atrioventricular valve
- a. cutaneous branches of intercostal nerves
- a. cutaneous branch of iliohypogastric nerve
- a. cutaneous nerves of abdomen
- a. deep cervical lymph nodes
- a. descending artery
- a. elastic layer
- a. embryotoxon
- a. epithelium of cornea
- a. ethmoidal air cells
- a. ethmoidal artery
- a. ethmoidal nerve
- a. extremity
- a. extremity of caudate nucleus
- a. facial height
- a. facial vein
- a. femoral cutaneous nerves
- a. focal point
- a. fontanel
- a. fovea
- a. funiculus
- a. gray column
- a. ground bundle
- a. group of axillary lymph nodes

a. guide
a. horn
a. horn cell
a. humeral circumflex artery
a. hypothalamic region
a. inferior cerebellar artery
a. inferior iliac spine
a. inferior segment
a. inferior segmental artery of kidney
a. intercondylar area of tibia
a. intercostal arteries
a. intercostal branches of internal thoracic artery
a. intercostal veins
a. intermediate groove
a. intermediate sulcus
a. interosseous artery
a. interosseous nerve
a. interventricular artery
a. interventricular groove
a. intestinal portal
a. intraoccipital joint
a. intraoccipital synchondrosis
a. jugular lymph nodes
a. jugular vein
a. junction line
a. knee region
a. labial arteries
a. labial commissure
a. labial nerves
a. labial veins
a. lacrimal crest
a. lateral malleolar artery
a. layer of rectus abdominis sheath
a. ligament of head of fibula
a. ligament of Helmholtz
a. ligament of malleus
a. limb of internal capsule
a. limb of stapes
a. limiting layer of cornea
a. limiting ring
a. lingual gland
a. lip of uterine os
a. lobe of hypophysis
a. longitudinal ligament
a. lunate lobule
a. margin
a. medial malleolar artery
a. median fissure of medulla oblongata
a. median fissure of spinal cord
a. median line
a. mediastinal arteries
a. mediastinal lymph nodes
a. mediastinotomy
a. mediastinum
a. medullary velum

a. megalophthalmos
a. meningeal artery
a. meniscofemoral ligament
a. myocardial infarction
a. naris
a. nasal aperture
a. nasal spine
a. neuropore
a. notch of cerebellum
a. notch of ear
a. nuclei of thalamus
a. occlusion
a. ocular segment
a. palatine arch
a. palatine foramen
a. parietal artery
a. parolfactory sulcus
a. part
a. part of anterior commissure of brain
a. part of diaphragmatic surface of liver
a. part of fornix of vagina
a. part of pons
a. pelvic exenteration
a. perforated substance
a. peroneal artery
a. pillar of fauces
a. pillar of fornix
a. piriform gyrus
a. pole of eyeball
a. pole of lens
a. pontomesencephalic vein
a. primary division
a. process of malleus
a. pyramid
a. pyramidal fasciculus
a. pyramidal tract
a. quadrigeminal body
a. recess
a. recess of tympanic membrane
a. rectus muscle of head
a. region of arm
a. region of elbow
a. region of forearm
a. region of leg
a. region of neck
a. region of thigh
a. rhinoscopy
a. rhizotomy
a. root
a. sacrococcygeal ligament
a. sacroiliac ligaments
a. sacrosciatic ligament
a. scalene muscle
a. scleritis
a. sclerotomy

anterior *(continued)*
a. scrotal branch of external pudendal artery
a. scrotal nerves
a. scrotal veins
a. segment
a. semicircular canals
a. serratus muscle
a. sinuses
a. spinal artery
a. spinocerebellar tract
a. spinothalamic tract
a. staphyloma
a. sternoclavicular ligament
a. superficial cervical lymph nodes
a. superior alveolar arteries
a. superior alveolar branches of infraorbital nerve
a. superior dental arteries
a. superior iliac spine
a. superior segment
a. superior segmental artery of kidney
a. supraclavicular nerve
a. surface
a. surface of arm
a. surface of cornea
a. surface of elbow
a. surface of eyelids
a. surface of forearm
a. surface of iris
a. surface of kidney
a. surface of leg
a. surface of lens
a. surface of lower limb
a. surface of maxilla
a. surface of pancreas
a. surface of patella
a. surface of petrous part of temporal bone
a. surface of prostate
a. surface of radius
a. surface of suprarenal gland
a. surface of thigh
a. surface of ulna
a. symblepharon
a. synechia
a. talar articular surface of calcaneus
a. talofibular ligament
a. talotibial ligament
a. teeth
a. temporal artery
a. thalamic radiations
a. thalamic tubercle
a. tibial artery
a. tibial bursa
a. tibial compartment syndrome

a. tibial lymph node
a. tibial muscle
a. tibial nerve
a. tibial node
a. tibial recurrent artery
a. tibial veins
a. tibiofibular ligament
a. tibiotalar ligament
a. tibiotalar part of deltoid ligament
a. triangle of neck
a. tubercle of atlas
a. tubercle of cervical vertebrae
a. tubercle of thalamus
a. tympanic artery
a. urethra
a. urethral valve
a. urethritis
a. uveitis
a. vein of septum pellucidum
a. vertebral vein
a. vitrectomy
a. wall of middle ear
a. wall of stomach
a. wall of tympanic cavity
a. wall of vagina
a. white commissure

anterodorsal thalamic nucleus
anteroexternal
anterofacial dysplasia
anterograde
a. amnesia
a. block
a. conduction
a. memory
anteroinferior
a. myocardial infarction
anterointernal
anterolateral
a. central arteries
a. column of spinal cord
a. cordotomy
a. fontanel
a. groove
a. myocardial infarction
a. striate arteries
a. sulcus
a. surface of shaft of humerus
a. system
a. thalamostriate arteries
a. tractotomy
anteromedial
a. central arteries
a. central branches
a. surface of shaft of humerus
a. thalamic nucleus
a. thalamostriate arteries

A

anteromedian
    a. groove
anteroposterior
    a. diameter of the pelvic inlet
    a. dysplasia
    a. facial dysplasia
    a. projection
anteroseptal myocardial infarction
anterosuperior
anterotic
anteroventral thalamic nucleus
antesystole
anteversion
anteverted
anthelix
anthema
antheridium
anthocyanins
Anthomyia
    A. canicularis
anthracemia
anthracic
anthracoid
anthracosilicosis
anthracosis
anthracotic
    a. tuberculosis
anthramucin
anthrapurpurin
anthrax
    cerebral a.
    cutaneous a.
    intestinal a.
    a. pneumonia
    pulmonary a.
    a. septicemia
anthropobiology
anthropocentric
anthropogenesis
anthropogenic, anthropogenetic
anthropogeny
anthropogony
anthropography
anthropoid pelvis
anthropology
    applied a.
    criminal a.
    cultural a.
    physical a.
anthropometer
anthropometric
anthropometry
anthropomorphism
anthroponomy
anthroponotic cutaneous leishmaniasis
anthropopathy
anthropophilic
anthropophobia

anthroposcopy
anthroposomatology
antiagglutinin
antialexin
antiallergic
antianaphylaxis
antianemic
antiantibody
antiantitoxin
antiarrhythmic
antiautolysin
antibacterial
anti-basement
    a.-b. membrane antibody
    a.-b. membrane glomerulonephritis
    a.-b. membrane nephritis
antibiogram
antibiont
antibiosis
antibiotic
    a. enterocolitis
    a. sensitivity
    a. sensitivity test
antibiotic-resistant
antibody
    affinity a.
    agglutinating a.
    anaphylactic a.
    anti-basement membrane a.
    anticardiolipin a.'s
    anti-idiotype a.
    antinuclear a.
    antiphospholipid a.'s
    avidity a.
    bivalent a.
    blocking a.
    blood group a.'s
    cell-bound a.
    CF a.
    chimeric a.'s
    cold a.
    cold-reactive a.
    a. combining site
    complement-fixing a.
    complete a.
    cross-reacting a.
    cytophilic a.
    cytotropic a.
    a. deficiency disease
    a. deficiency syndrome
    a. excess
    fluorescent a.
    Forssman a.
    heterocytotropic a.
    heterogenetic a.
    heterophil a.
    heterophile a.
    homocytotropic a.

antibody *(continued)*
  idiotype a.
  immobilizing a.
  incomplete a.
  inhibiting a.
  lymphocytotoxic a.'s
  monoclonal a.
  natural a.
  neutralizing a.
  nonprecipitable a.
  nonprecipitating a.
  normal a.
  P-K a.'s
  polyclonal a.
  Prausnitz-Küstner a.
  precipitating a.
  reaginic a.
  treponema-immobilizing a.
  treponemal a.
  univalent a.
  Vi a.
  Wassermann a.
antibody-dependent cell-mediated cytotoxicity
antibrachial
antibrachium
anticardiolipin antibodies
anticarious
anticathexis
anticipate
anticipation
anticlinal
anticnemion
anticoagulant
  lupus a.
  a. therapy
anticomplement
anticomplementary
  a. serum
anticontagious
anticus
anticytotoxin
antidiuresis
antidromic
antidysrhythmic
antienergic
antiepithelial serum
antifibrillatory
antifibrinolysin
anti-G
  a.-G. suit
antigen
  ABO a.'s
  acetone-insoluble a.
  allogeneic a.
  Am a.'s
  Au a.
  Aus a.

Australia a.
Be^a a.'s
Becker a.
Bi a.
Bile's a.
blood group a.
By a.
capsular a.
carcinoembryonic a.
C carbohydrate a.
CDE a.'s
cholesterinized a.
Chr^a a.'s
class I a.'s
class II a.'s
class III a.'s
common a.
complete a.
conjugated a.
D a.
delta a.
Dharmendra a.
Di a.
Duffy a.'s
a. excess
flagellar a.
Forssman a.
Fy a.'s
G a.
Ge a.
Gm a.'s
Good a.
Gr a.
group a.'s
H a.
H-2 a.'s
He a.'s
heart a.
hepatitis-associated a.
hepatitis B core a.
hepatitis B e a.
hepatitis B surface a.
heterogeneic a.
heterogenetic a.
heterogenic enterobacterial a.
heterophil a.
heterophile a.
hexon a.
histocompatibility a.
HL-A a.'s
Ho a.
homologous a.
Hu a.'s
human leukemia-associated a.'s
human lymphocyte a.'s
H-Y a.
I a.'s
incomplete a.

a. interferon
InV group a.
Jk a.'s
Jobbins a.
Js a.
K a.'s
Km a.
Kveim a.
Kveim-Stilzbach a.
Lan a.
Le a.'s
leukocyte common a.
Levay a.
Lu a.'s
lymphocyte function associated a.
lymphogranuloma venereum a.
Lyt a.'s
M a.
M_1 a., M_2 a., M^g a., M^c a.
Mitsuda a.
MNSs a.'s
Mu a.
mumps skin test a.
O a.
oncofetal a.'s
organ-specific a.
Ot a.
P a.'s
partial a.
penton a.
pollen a.
private a.'s
prostate-specific a.
public a.'s
R a.
Rh a.'s
Rhus toxicodendron a.
Rhus venenata a.
S a.
sensitized a.
shock a.
Sm a.
soluble a.
somatic a.
species-specific a.
specific a.'s
Stobo a.
Streptococcus M a.
Sw^a a.
Swann a.'s
T a.'s
Tac a.
T-dependent a.
theta a.
thymus-independent a.
tissue-specific a.
Tj a.
Tr^a a.

transplantation a.
tumor a.'s
tumor-associated a.
tumor-specific transplantation a.'s
V a.
Vel a.
Ven a.
Vi a.
Vw a.
Webb a.
Wr^a a.
Wright a.'s
Xg a.
Yt^a a.
antigen-antibody complex
antigen-binding site
antigen-combining site
antigenemia
antigenic
a. competition
a. complex
a. determinant
a. drift
a. shift
antigenicity
antigen-presenting cells
antigen-responsive cell
antigen-sensitive cell
antiglobulin test
antigravity
a. muscles
anti-HB$_s$
anti-HB$_c$
anti-IIB$_e$
antihelix
antihemagglutinin
antihemolysin
antihemolytic
antihemophilic
a. factor A
a. factor B
a. globulin A
a. globulin B
antihormones
antihuman
a. globulin
a. globulin test
antihypotensive
anti-idiotype
a.-i. antibody
a.-i. autoantibody
anti-insulin
anti-kidney serum nephritis
antileukocidin
antileukotoxin
antilobium
antilymphocyte serum
antilysin

antimesenteric
antimetropia
antimicrobial spectrum
antimongoloid
anti-Monson curve
antimutagen
antimutagenic
antineurotoxin
antiniad
antinial
antinion
antinomy
antinuclear
    a. antibody
    a. factor
antioncogene
antiparastata
antiperistalsis
antiperistaltic
antiphospholipid antibodies
antiplasmin
antiplatelet
antipodal
    a. cone
anti-Pr cold autoagglutinin
antiprecipitin
antiprostate
antiprothrombin
antipyresis
antireflection coating
antireticular cytotoxic serum
antiricin
antiruminant
anti-S
antisense therapy
antisepsis
antiseptic dressing
antiserum
    a. anaphylaxis
    blood group a.s
    heterologous a.
    homologous a.
    monovalent a.
    nerve growth factor a.
    NGF a.
    polyvalent a.
    specific a.
antishock garment
antisocial
    a. personality
    a. personality disorder
antistaphylococcic
antistaphylolysin
antisteapsin
antistreptococcic
antistreptokinase
antistreptolysin
antisubstance

anti-tac
antithenar
antithrombin
    a. III
    normal a.
    a. test
antitonic
antitoxigen
antitoxinogen
antitoxin rash
antitragicus
    a. muscle
antitragohelicine
    a. fissure
antitragus
antitrismus
antitrope
antitropic
antitrypsin deficiency
antitryptic index
antitumorigenesis
antiviral
    a. immunity
    a. protein
Antoni
    A. type A neurilemoma
    A. type B neurilemoma
Anton's syndrome
antra
antra (*pl. of* antrum)
antral
    a. pouch
    a. sphincter
antrectomy
antri (*gen. of* antrum)
antroduodenectomy
antronasal
antrophose
antropyloric
antroscope
antroscopy
antrostomy
    intraoral a.
antrotomy
antrotonia
antrotympanic
antrum, gen. antri, pl. antra
    a. auris
    a. cardiacum
    antra ethmoidalia
    follicular a.
    a. of Highmore
    mastoid a.
    a. mastoideum
    maxillary a.
    pyloric a.
    a. pyloricum

tympanic a.
Valsalva's a.
Antyllus' method
anular
anulus, pl. **anuli**
anuresis
anuretic
anuria
anuric
anus, gen. **ani**, pl. **anus**
artificial a.
Bartholin's a.
a. cerebri
imperforate a.
a. vesicalis
vesicalis a.
vestibular a., vulvovaginal a.
anvil
a. sound
anxiety
a. attack
castration a.
a. disorders
a. dream
free-floating a.
a. hysteria
a. neurosis
noetic a.
a. reaction
separation a.
situation a.
a. syndrome
a. tension state
anxious delirium
aorta, gen. and pl. **aortae**
abdominal a.
a. abdominalis
a. angusta
a. ascendens
ascending a.
buckled a.
a. descendens
descending a.
dynamic a.
kinked a.
overriding a.
primitive a.
pseudocoarctation of the a.
shaggy a.
thoracic a.
a. thoracica
ventral aortas
aortal
aortalgia
aortarctia
aortartia
aortectasis, aortectasia
aortectomy

aortic
a. aneurysm
a. arch
a. arches
a. arch syndrome
a. area
a. atresia
a. bodies
a. body tumor
a. bulb
a. dissection
a. dwarfism
a. facies
a. foramen
a. hiatus
a. incompetence
a. insufficiency
a. knob
a. knuckle
a. lymphatic plexus
a. murmur
a. nerve
a. nipple
a. notch
a. opening
a. orifice
a. ostium
a. reflex
a. regurgitation
a. sac
a. septal defect
a. sinus
a. sinus aneurysm
a. spindle
a. stenosis
a. sulcus
a. valve
a. vestibule
a. window
aortica, gen. **corporis**, pl. **corpora**
glomera a., gen. corporis,
pl. corpora
aortic curtain
aortico-left ventricular tunnel
aorticopulmonary
a. septal defect
a. window
aorticorenal
a. ganglia
aortic-pulmonic window
aortitis
giant cell a.
syphilitic a.
aortoannular ectasia
aortocoronary
a. bypass
aortogram

aortography
    retrograde a.
    translumbar a.
aortoiliac
    a. bypass
    a. occlusive disease
aortopathy
aortopexy
aortoplasty
aortoptosia, aortoptosis
aortopulmonary
    a. septum
    a. window
aortorenal bypass
aortorrhaphy
aortosclerosis
aortostenosis
aortotomy
APACHE score
apallesthesia
apallic
    a. state
    a. syndrome
apancreatic
aparalytic
aparathyreosis
aparathyroidism
apareunia
apathetic
    a. thyrotoxicosis
apathism
apathy
apatite calculus
A-pattern strabismus
A-P-C
    A-P-C virus
ape hand
apeidosis
apellous
apenteric
apepsinia
aperiodic
aperiosteal amputation
aperistalsis
apertognathia
Apert's
    A. hirsutism
    A. syndrome
apertura, pl. aperturae
    a. externa aqueductus vestibuli
    a. externa canaliculi cochleae
    a. lateralis ventriculi quarti
    a. mediana ventriculi quarti
    a. pelvis inferior
    a. pelvis minoris
    a. pelvis superior
    a. piriformis
    a. sinus frontalis
    a. sinus sphenoidalis
    a. thoracis inferior
    a. thoracis superior
    a. tympanica canaliculi chordae tympani
aperture
    angular a.
    anterior nasal a.
    a. diaphragm
    external a. of cochlear canaliculus
    external a. of vestibular aqueduct
    frontal sinus a.
    inferior pelvic a.
    inferior thoracic a.
    laryngeal a.
    lateral a. of the fourth ventricle
    a. of mastoid antrum
    medial a. of the fourth ventricle
    median a. of the fourth ventricle
    numerical a.
    a. of orbit
    sphenoidal sinus a.
    superior pelvic a.
    superior thoracic a.
apex, gen. apicis, pl. apices
    a. of arytenoid cartilage
    a. auriculae
    a. beat
    a. capitis fibulae
    a. cartilaginis arytenoideae
    a. cordis
    a. cornus posterioris
    a. cuspidis dentis
    a. of cusp of tooth
    a. of dens
    a. dentis
    a. of head of fibula
    a. of heart
    a. impulse
    a. linguae
    a. of lung
    a. nasi
    a. of orbit
    a. ossis sacri
    a. partis petrosae ossis temporalis
    a. of patella
    a. patellae
    a. of petrous part of temporal bone
    a. pneumonia
    a. of the posterior horn
    a. prostatae
    a. of prostate
    a. pulmonis
    a. radicis dentis
    root a.
    a. of sacrum
    a. satyri

a. of urinary bladder
a. vesicae
apexcardiogram
apexcardiography
apexification
apexigraph
Apgar score
aphagia
aphakia
aphakic
a. eye
a. glaucoma
aphalangia
aphanisis
aphasia
acoustic a.
acquired epileptic a.
amnestic a., amnesic a.
anomic a.
anterior a.
associative a.
ataxic a.
auditory a.
Broca's a.
conduction a.
crossed a.
expressive a.
fluent a.
functional a.
global a.
graphic a.
graphomotor a.
impressive a.
jargon a.
Kussmaul's a.
mixed a.
motor a.
nominal a.
nonfluent a.
pathematic a.
posterior a.
psychosensory a.
pure a.'s
receptive a.
semantic a.
sensory a.
syntactical a.
total a.
transcortical a.
visual a.
Wernicke's a.
aphasiac, aphasic
aphasiologist
aphasiology
aphasmid
Aphasmidia
apheliotropism
aphemesthesia

aphemia
aphemic
aphephobia
apheresis
aphilopony
aphonia
hysterical a.
nonorganic a.
a. paralytica
spastic a.
aphonic pectoriloquy
aphonogelia
aphonous
aphotesthesia
aphrasia
aphrodisia
aphrodisiac
aphrodisiomania
aphtha, pl. **aphthae**
Bednar's aphthae
herpetiform aphthae
aphthae major
Mikulicz' aphthae
aphthae minor
recurrent scarring aphthae
aphthoid
aphthosis
aphthous stomatitis
aphylactic
aphylaxis
apical
a. abscess
a. angle
a. area
a. branch
a. branch of inferior lobar branch
of right pulmonary artery
a. cap
a. complex
a. dendrite
a. dental foramen
a. ectodermal ridge
a. foramen of tooth
a. gland
a. granuloma
a. group of axillary lymph nodes
a. infection
a. ligament of dens
a. lordotic projection
a. periodontal abscess
a. periodontal cyst
a. periodontitis
a. pneumonia
a. process
a. segment
a. space
apical-aortic conduit
apicalis

apicectomy
apiceotomy
apices (*pl. of* apex)
apicis (*gen. of* apex)
apicitis
apicoectomy
apicolocator
apicolysis
Apicomplexa
apicoposterior
    a. artery
    a. branch of left superior
      pulmonary vein
    a. segment
apicostome
apicostomy
apicotomy
apiculate
apiculus
apicurettage
apinealism
apiphobia
apituitarism
aplanatic
    a. lens
aplanatism
aplasia
    congenital a. of thymus
    a. cutis congenita
    germinal a.
    gonadal a.
    pure red cell a.
aplastic
    a. anemia
    a. lymph
apleuria
apnea
    central a.
    deglutition a.
    induced a.
    obstructive a., peripheral a.
    sleep a.
    sleep-induced a.
apneic
    a. oxygenation
    a. pause
apneumatosis
apneumia
apneusis
apneustic
    a. breathing
apobiosis
apocarteresis
apochromatic
    a. lens
    a. objective
apocleisis

apocrine
    a. adenoma
    a. carcinoma
    a. chromhidrosis
    a. gland
    a. metaplasia
    a. miliaria
    a. sweat glands
apodal
apodemialgia
apodia
apodous
apody
apogamia, apogamy
apogee
apolar
    a. cell
apomixia
aponeurectomy
aponeurorrhaphy
aponeurosis, pl. aponeuroses
    bicipital a., a. bicipitalis
    Denonvilliers' a.
    epicranial a.
    a. epicranialis
    extensor a.
    a. of external abdominal oblique
      muscle
    a. of insertion
    a. of internal abdominal oblique
      muscle
    a. of investment
    a. linguae
    lingual a.
    a. musculi bicipitis brachii
    a. of origin
    a. palatina
    palatine a.
    palmar a.
    a. palmaris
    Petit's a.
    a. pharyngea
    plantar a.
    a. plantaris
    Sibson's a.
    temporal a.
    thoracolumbar a.
    a. of vastus muscles
aponeurositis
aponeurotic
    a. fibroma
    a. reflex
aponeurotome
aponeurotomy
apopathetic
apophylaxis
apophysary
    a. point

apophysial, apophyseal
    a. fracture
    a. point
apophysis, pl. **apophyses**
    basilar a.
    a. conchae
    a. helicis
    Ingrassia's a.
    lenticular a.
    temporal a.
apophysitis
    a. tibialis adolescentium
apoplasmia
apoplectic
    a. cyst
    a. retinitis
apoplectiform
apoplexy
    abdominal a.
    adrenal a.
    bulbar a.
    cutaneous a.
    functional a.
    heat a.
    labyrinthine a.
    neonatal a.
    pituitary a.
    spinal a.
    uteroplacental a.
apoptosis
aporia
aporioneurosis
aposome
apostaxis
aposthia
apostilb
apothanasia
apoxesis
apparatus
    accessory visual a.
    achromatic a.
    alimentary a.
    attachment a.
    Barcroft-Warburg a.
    Beckmann's a.
    Benedict-Roth a.
    central a.
    chromatic a.
    chromidial a.
    dental a.
    digestive a.
    a. digestorius
    genitourinary a.
    Golgi a.
    Haldane's a.
    Heyns' abdominal decompression a.
    juxtaglomerular a.
    Kirschner's a.

    lacrimal a.
    a. lacrimalis
    a. ligamentosus colli
    a. ligamentosus weitbrechti
    masticatory a.
    mental a.
    pyriform a.
    a. respiratorius
    respiratory a.
    Roughton-Scholander a.
    Sayre's suspension a.
    Scholander a.
    subneural a.
    a. suspensorius lentis
    Taylor's a.
    urinary a.
    urogenital a.
    a. urogenitalis
    Van Slyke a.
    vestibular a.
    Warburg's a.
apparent
    a. leukonychia
    a. origin
    a. viscosity
appendage
    atrial a.
    auricular a.
    drumstick a.
    epiploic a.
    a.'s of eye
    a.'s of the fetus
    left auricular a.
    right auricular a.
    a.'s of skin
    testicular a.
    uterine a.'s
    vermiform a.
    vesicular a.
appendalgia
appendectomy
    auricular a.
appendical
appendiceal
    a. abscess
appendicectasis
appendicectomy
appendices (*pl. of* appendix)
appendicis (*gen. of* appendix)
appendicism
appendicitis
    actinomycotic a.
    acute a.
    bilharzial a.
    chronic a.
    focal a.
    foreign-body a.
    gangrenous a.

appendicitis (*continued*)
  left-sided a.
  lumbar a.
  obstructive a.
  perforating a.
  recurrent a.
  relapsing a.
  stercoral a.
  subperitoneal a.
  suppurative a.
  verminous a.
appendiclausis
appendicocele
appendicoenterostomy
appendicolith
appendicolithiasis
appendicolysis
appendicostomy
appendicovesicostomy
appendicular
  a. artery
  a. colic
  a. lymph nodes
  a. muscle
  a. skeleton
  a. vein
appendix, gen. **appendicis**, pl. **appendices**
  auricular a.
  a. ceci
  a. epididymidis
  a. of epididymidis
  epiploic a.
  a. epiploica, pl. appendices
    epiploicae
  a. fibrosa hepatis
  fibrous a. of liver
  Morgagni's a.
  a. testis
  a. of the testis
  a. ventriculi laryngis
  vermiform a.
  a. vermiformis
  vesicular appendices of uterine
    tube
  a. vesiculosa, pl. appendices
    vesiculosae
apperception
apperceptive
  a. mass
appersonation, appersonification
appestat
appetite
  a. juice
appetition
appetitive behavior
applanation
  a. tonometer
applanometry

apple jelly nodules
appliance
  craniofacial a.
  edgewise a.
  extraoral fracture a.
  Hawley a.
  intraoral fracture a.
  labiolingual a.
  light wire a.
  obturator a.
  orthodontic a.
  ribbon arch a.
  Roger-Anderson pin fixation a.
  surgical a.
  universal a.
applicator
applied
  a. anatomy
  a. anthropology
appliqué forms
appositional growth
apposition suture
appraisal
  health risk a.
approach
  idiographic a.
  nomothetic a.
  regressive-reconstructive a.
approach-approach conflict
approach-avoidance conflict
AP projection
approximate
approximation
  a. suture
apractagnosia
apractic
apragmatism
apraxia
  a. algera
  constructional a.
  cortical a.
  gait a.
  ideational a., ideatory a.
  ideokinetic a., ideomotor a.
  innervation a.
  limb-kinetic a.
  motor a.
  ocular motor a.
  transcortical a.
  verbal a.
apraxic
aproctia
aprophoria
aprosexia
aprosody
aprosopia
apthovirus
aptitude test

Apt test
apyknomorphous
apyretic
    a. tetanus
    a. typhoid
apyrexia
apyrexial
aquagenic pruritus
aquaphobia
aquapuncture
Aquaspirillum
aqueduct
    cerebral a.
    a. of cerebrum
    cochlear a.
    Cotunnius' a.
    fallopian a.
    sylvian a.
    a. veil
    a. of vestibule
aqueductal intubation
aqueductus, pl. aqueductus
    a. cerebri
    a. cochleae
    a. cotunnii
    a. fallopii
    a. sylvii
    a. vestibuli
aqueous
    a. chambers
    a. flare
    a. humor
    a. influx phenomenon
    a. vein
aquiparous
arabinosis
arabinosuria
arachnephobia
Arachnia
    A. *propionica*
Arachnida
arachnodactyly
arachnoid
    arachnoid a.
    a. of brain
    a. cyst
    a. foramen
    a. granulations
    a. mater cranialis
    a. mater encephali
    a. membrane
    a. of spinal cord
    a. trabecula
    a. villi
arachnoidal
    a. granulations
arachnoidea, arachnoides
    a. encephali

    a. mater spinalis
    a. spinalis
arachnoiditis
    adhesive a.
    neoplastic a.
    obliterative a.
arachnolysin
arachnophobia
Aran-Duchenne disease
Arantius'
    A. ligament
    A. nodule
    A. ventricle
araphia
arbor, pl. arbores
    a. vitae
    a. vitae uteri
arborescent
    a. cataract
arborization
    a. block
arborize
arboroid
arborvirus
arbovirus
arc
    auricular a., binauricular a.
    bregmatolambdoid a.
    crater a.
    flame a.
    interauricular a.
    longitudinal a. of skull
    mercury a.
    nasobregmatic a.
    naso-occipital a.
    a. perimeter
    pulmonary a.
    reflex a.
    Riolan's a.
arcade
    anomalous mitral a.
    arterial a.'s
    Flint's a.
    intestinal arterial a.'s
    pancreaticoduodenal arterial a.'s
    Riolan's a.'s
Arcanobacterium
    A. *haemolyticum*
arcate
arc-flash conjunctivitis
arch
    abdominothoracic a.
    alveolar a. of mandible
    alveolar a. of maxilla
    anterior a. of atlas
    anterior palatine a.
    a. of the aorta
    aortic a.

arch *(continued)*
    aortic a.'s
    arterial a.'s of colon
    arterial a.'s of ileum
    arterial a.'s of jejunum
    arterial a. of lower eyelid
    arterial a. of upper eyelid
    axillary a.
    a. bar
    branchial a.'s
    carpal a.'s
    coracoacromial a.
    cortical a.'s of kidney
    Corti's a.
    costal a.
    a. of cricoid cartilage
    crural a.
    deep crural a.
    deep palmar (arterial) a.
    deep palmar venous a.
    dental a.
    dorsal venous a. of foot
    double aortic a.
    expansion a.
    fallen a.'s
    fallopian a.
    femoral a.
    a.'s of the foot
    a. form
    glossopalatine a.
    Gothic a.
    Haller's a.'s
    hemal a.'s
    hyoid a.
    iliopectineal a.
    inferior dental a.
    jugular venous a.
    labial a.
    Langer's a.
    lateral longitudinal a. of foot
    lateral lumbocostal a.
    a. length
    a. length deficiency
    lingual a.
    longitudinal a. of foot
    malar a.
    mandibular a.
    medial longitudinal a. of foot
    medial lumbocostal a.
    nasal a.
    nasal venous a.
    neural a.
    a. of the palate
    palatoglossal a.
    palatopharyngeal a.
    pharyngeal a.'s
    pharyngopalatine a.
    plantar a.

    plantar arterial a.
    plantar venous a.
    popliteal a.
    posterior a. of atlas
    posterior palatine a.
    postoral a.'s
    primitive costal a.'s
    pubic a.
    ribbon a.
    superciliary a.
    superficial palmar (arterial) a.
    superficial palmar venous a.
    superior dental a.
    supraorbital a.
    tarsal a.
    tendinous a.
    tendinous a. of levator ani muscle
    tendinous a. of pelvic fascia
    tendinous a. of soleus muscle
    a. of thoracic duct
    transverse a. of foot
    Treitz's a.
    vertebral a.
    visceral a.'s
    W-a.
    a. wire
    wire a.
    zygomatic a.

archaeocerebellum
archaic
archaic-paralogical thinking
arched crest
archenteric canal
archenteron
archeocerebellum
archeokinetic
archetype
archicerebellum
archicortex
archil
archipallium
architectonics
architecture
    bone a.
arch-loop-whorl system
archwire
arciform
    a. arteries
    a. veins of kidney
arcon articulator
arctation
arcual
arcuate
    a. arteries of kidney
    a. artery
    a. crest
    a. crest of arytenoid cartilage
    a. eminence

a. fasciculus
a. fibers
a. fibers of cerebrum
a. line
a. line of ilium
a. line of rectus sheath
a. nuclei
a. nucleus
a. nucleus of thalamus
a. popliteal ligament
a. pubic ligament
a. scotoma
a. uterus
a. veins of kidney
a. zone
arcuation
arcus
a. adiposus
a. alveolaris mandibulae
a. alveolaris maxillae
a. anterior atlantis
a. aortae
a. cartilaginis cricoideae
a. cornealis
a. costalis
a. costarum
a. dentalis inferior
a. dentalis superior
a. ductus thoracici
a. glossopalatinus
a. iliopectineus
a. inguinalis
a. juvenilis
a. lipoides
a. lumbocostalis lateralis
a. lumbocostalis medialis
a. palatini
a. palatoglossus
a. palatopharyngeus
a. palmaris profundus
a. palmaris superficialis
a. palpebralis inferior
a. palpebralis superior
a. pedis longitudinalis
a. pedis longitudinalis pars lateralis
a. pedis longitudinalis pars medialis
a. pedis transversalis
a. plantaris
a. posterior atlantis
a. pubis
a. raninus
a. senilis
a. superciliaris
a. tarseus
a. tendineus
a. tendineus fasciae pelvis
a. tendineus musculi levatoris ani
a. tendineus musculi solei

a. tendineus of obturator fascia
a. unguium
a. venosus dorsalis pedis
a. venosus juguli
a. venosus palmaris profundus
a. venosus palmaris superficialis
a. venosus plantaris
a. vertebrae
a. volaris profundus
a. volaris superficialis
a. zygomaticus
ardanesthesia
ardent fever
ardor
area, pl. **areae**
acoustic a.
a. acustica
anterior intercondylar a. of tibia
aortic a.
apical a.
association areas
auditory a.
bare a. of liver
bare a. of stomach
basal seat a.
Broca's a.
Broca's parolfactory a.
Brodmann's areas
a. of cardiac dullness
catchment a.
Celsus' a.
a. centralis
a. cochleae
cochlear a.
Cohnheim's a.
contact a.
cribriform a. of the renal papilla
a. cribrosa papillae renalis
denture-bearing a.
denture foundation a.
denture-supporting a.
dermatomic a.
embryonal a., embryonic a.
entorhinal a.
excitable a.
a. of facial nerve
Flechsig's areas
frontal a.
fronto-orbital a.
fusion a.
gastric a.
a. gastrica
germinal a., a. germinativa
Head's areas
impression a.
inferior vestibular a.
insular a.
a. intercondylaris anterior tibiae

area *(continued)*
    a. intercondylaris posterior tibiae
    Jonston's a.
    Kiesselbach's a.
    lateral hypothalamic a.
    Little's a.
    macular a.
    Martegiani's a.
    mitral a.
    motor a.
    a. nervi facialis
    a. nuda hepatis
    olfactory a.
    oval a. of Flechsig
    Panum's a.
    parastriate a.
    a. parolfactoria, a. parolfactoria
      Brocae
    parolfactory a.
    pear-shaped a.
    peristriate a.
    piriform a.
    Pitres' a.
    postcentral a.
    post dam a.
    posterior hypothalamic a.
    posterior intercondylar a. of tibia
    posterior palatal seal a.
    postpalatal seal a.
    a. postrema
    precentral a.
    precommissural septal a.
    prefrontal a.
    premotor a.
    preoptic a.
    prestriate a.
    pretectal a.
    primary visual a.
    pulmonary a.
    relief a.
    rest a.
    retention a.
    Rolando's a.
    secondary aortic a.
    secondary visual a.
    sensorial areas, sensory areas
    sensorimotor a.
    septal a.
    silent a.
    skip areas
    somesthetic a.
    stress-bearing a.
    striate a.
    Stroud's pectinated a.
    a. subcallosa
    subcallosal a.
    superior vestibular a.
    supporting a.

    tissue-bearing a.
    tricuspid a.
    trigger a.
    vagus a.
    vestibular a.
    a. vestibularis inferior
    a. vestibularis superior
    visual a.
    Wernicke's a.
areatus, areata
areflexia
    detrusor a.
arenaceous
Arenaviridae
Arenavirus
areola, pl. **areolae**
    Chaussier's a.
    a. mammae
    a. of nipple
    a. papillaris
    a. umbilicus
areolar
    a. choroiditis
    a. choroidopathy
    a. glands
    a. tissue
    a. venous plexus
argasid
argentaffin, argentaffine
    a. cells
    a. granules
argentaffinoma
Argentinean hemorrhagic fever
Argentine hemorrhagic fever virus
argentophil, argentophile
argininosuccinicaciduria
Argonz-Del Castillo syndrome
Argyll Robertson pupil
argyrophil, argyrophile
argyrophilic
    a. cells
    a. fibers
arhigosis
arhinencephaly (*var. of* arrhinencephaly)
arhinia
Arias-Stella
    A.-S. effect
    A.-S. phenomenon
    A.-S. reaction
ariboflavinosis
Arie-Pitanguy
    A.-P. mammaplasty
    A.-P. operation
aristotelian method
Aristotle's anomaly
arithmetic mean
arithmomania

Arizona
>A. hinshawii

Arlt's
>A. operation
>A. sinus

arm
>bar clasp a.
>brawny a.
>circumferential clasp a.
>clasp a.
>dynein a.
>a. phenomenon
>reciprocal a.
>retentive a., retention a.
>retentive circumferential clasp a.
>stabilizing circumferential clasp a.

armamentarium
Armanni-Ebstein
>A.-E. change
>A.-E. kidney

armarium
armed
>a. macrophage
>a. rostellum

Armillifer
armor
>character a.
>a. heart

armored heart
armpit
Army
>A. Alpha tests
>A. Beta tests
>A. General Classification Test

Arndt-Gottron syndrome
Arndt's law
Arneth
>A. classification
>A. count
>A. formula
>A. index
>A. stages

Arnold-Chiari
>A.-C. deformity
>A.-C. malformation
>A.-C. syndrome

Arnold's
>A. bodies
>A. bundle
>A. canal
>A. ganglion
>A. nerve
>A. tract

arousal
>a. function
>a. reaction

arrector, pl. **arrectores**
>a. pili muscles
>arrectores pilorum

arrest
>cardiac a.
>cardioplegic a.
>cardiopulmonary a.
>circulatory a.
>deep hypothermic a.
>epiphysial a.
>heart a.
>maturation a.
>sinus a.

arrested
>a. dental caries
>a. tuberculosis

arrhaphia
Arrhenius-Madsen theory
arrhenoblastoma
arrhinencephaly, arhinencephaly, arrhinencephalia
arrhinia
arrhythmia
>cardiac a.
>continuous a.
>juvenile a.
>nonphasic sinus a.
>perpetual a.
>phasic sinus a.
>respiratory a.
>sinus a.

arrhythmic
arrhythmogenic
arrow point tracing
Arruga's forceps
arsenical
>a. keratosis
>a. polyneuropathy
>a. tremor

arsenic pigmentation
arsenotherapy
artefact
arteria, gen. and pl. **arteriae**
>a. acetabuli
>arteriae alveolares superiores
> anteriores
>a. alveolaris inferior
>arteriae alveolaris inferioris
>a. alveolaris superior posterior
>a. anastomotica auricularis magna
>a. anastomotica magna
>a. angularis
>a. aorta
>a. appendicularis
>a. arcuata
>arteriae arcuatae renis
>a. articularis azygos
>a. ascendens
>arteriae atriales

arteria *(continued)*
a. auditiva interna
a. auricularis posterior
a. auricularis profunda
a. axillaris
a. basilaris
a. brachialis
a. brachialis superficialis
a. buccalis
a. bulbi penis
a. bulbi urethrae
a. bulbi vaginae
a. bulbi vestibuli
a. calcarina
a. callosomarginalis
a. canalis pterygoidei
arteriae caroticotympanicae arteriae
  carotidis internae
a. carotis communis
a. carotis externa
a. carotis interna
a. caudae pancreatis
a. cecalis anterior
a. cecalis posterior
a. celiaca
arteriae centrales anterolaterales
arteriae centrales anteromediales
arteriae centrales posterolaterales
arteriae centrales posteromediales
a. centralis brevis
a. centralis longa
a. centralis retinae
a. cerebelli inferior anterior
a. cerebelli inferior posterior
a. cerebelli superior
a. cerebri anterior
a. cerebri media
a. cerebri posterior
a. cervicalis ascendens
a. cervicalis profunda
a. cervicalis superficialis
a. cervicovaginalis
a. choroidea anterior
a. choroidea posterior
a. ciliaris anterior
a. ciliaris posterior brevis
a. ciliaris posterior longa
a. circumflexa femoris lateralis
a. circumflexa femoris medialis
a. circumflexa humeri anterior
a. circumflexa humeri posterior
a. circumflexa iliaca profunda
a. circumflexa iliaca superficialis
a. circumflexa scapulae
a. colica dextra
a. colica media
a. colica sinistra
a. collateralis media

a. collateralis radialis
a. collateralis ulnaris inferior
a. collateralis ulnaris superior
a. comes nervi phrenici
a. comitans nervi ischiadici
a. comitans nervi mediani
a. communicans anterior
a. communicans posterior
a. conjunctivalis anterior
a. conjunctivalis posterior
a. coronaria dextra
a. coronaria sinistra
a. cremasterica
a. cystica
a. deferentialis
a. digitalis dorsalis
a. digitalis palmaris communis
a. digitalis palmaris propria
a. digitalis plantaris communis
a. digitalis plantaris propria
a. dorsalis clitoridis
a. dorsalis nasi
a. dorsalis pedis
a. dorsalis penis
a. dorsalis scapulae
a. ductus deferentis
a. epigastrica inferior
a. epigastrica superficialis
a. epigastrica superior
a. episcleralis
a. ethmoidalis anterior
a. ethmoidalis posterior
a. facialis
a. femoralis
a. fibularis
a. frontalis
a. frontobasalis lateralis
a. frontobasalis medialis
a. gastrica dextra
arteriae gastricae breves
a. gastrica sinistra
a. gastroduodenalis
a. gastroepiploica dextra
a. gastroepiploica sinistra
a. gastro-omentalis dextra
a. gastro-omentalis sinistra
a. genus descendens
a. genus inferior lateralis
a. genus inferior medialis
a. genus media
a. genus superior lateralis
a. genus superior medialis
a. glutea inferior
a. glutea superior
a. gyri angularis
arteriae helicinae penis
a. hepatica communis
a. hepatica propria

a. hyaloidea
a. hypogastrica
a. hypophysialis inferior
a. hypophysialis superior
arteriae ileales
a. ileocolica
a. iliaca communis
a. iliaca externa
a. iliaca interna
a. iliolumbalis
a. infraorbitalis
arteriae insulares
arteriae intercostales posteriores I
 et II
arteriae intercostales posteriores III-
 XI
a. intercostalis suprema
arteriae interlobares renis
arteriae interlobulares
a. interlobulares (hepatis)
a. interlobulares (renis)
a. intermesenterica
a. interossea anterior
a. interossea communis
a. interossea posterior
a. interossea recurrens
a. interossea volaris
arteriae intestinales
a. ischiadica, a. ischiatica
arteriae jejunales
arteriae labiales anteriores
a. labialis inferior
a. labialis superior
a. labyrinthi
a. lacrimalis
a. laryngea inferior
a. laryngea superior
a. lienalis
a. ligamenti teretis uteri
a. lingualis
a. lobi caudati
arteriae lumbales imae
a. lumbalis
a. lusoria
arteriae malleolares posteriores
 laterales
arteriae malleolares posteriores
 mediales
a. malleolaris anterior lateralis
a. malleolaris anterior medialis
a. mammaria interna
a. masseterica
a. maxillaris
a. maxillaris externa
a. mediana
arteriae mediastinales anteriores
a. meningea anterior
a. meningea media

a. meningea posterior
a. mentalis
a. mesenterica inferior
a. mesenterica superior
a. metacarpea dorsalis
a. metacarpea palmaris
a. metatarsae
a. metatarsea dorsalis
a. metatarsea plantaris
a. musculophrenica
arteriae nasales posteriores laterales
a. nasalis posterior septi
a. nasi externa
a. nervorum
a. nutricia
arteriae nutriciae humeri
a. nutriens fibulae
a. nutriens tibialis
a. obturatoria
a. obturatoria accessoria
a. occipitalis
arteriae occipitalis
a. occipitalis lateralis
a. occipitalis medialis
a. ophthalmica
a. ovarica
a. palatina ascendens
a. palatina descendens
a. palatina major
a. palatina minor
arteriae palpebrales
a. pancreatica dorsalis
a. pancreatica inferior
a. pancreatica magna
a. pancreaticoduodenalis inferior
a. pancreaticoduodenalis superior
a. paracentralis
arteriae parietales
a. parietales anterior
a. parietales posterior
a. parieto-occipitalis
arteriae perforantes
a. pericallosa
a. pericardiacophrenica
a. perinealis
a. peronea
a. pharyngea ascendens
a. phrenica inferior
a. phrenica superior
a. plantaris lateralis
a. plantaris medialis
arteriae pontis
a. poplitea
a. precunealis
a. princeps pollicis
a. profunda brachii
a. profunda clitoridis
a. profunda femoris

arteria *(continued)*
a. profunda linguae
a. profunda penis
arteriae pudendae externae
a. pudenda interna
a. pulmonalis
a. pulmonalis dextra
a. pulmonalis sinistra
a. radialis
a. radialis indicis
a. radicularis magna
a. ranina
a. rectalis inferior
a. rectalis media
a. rectalis superior
a. recurrens
a. recurrens radialis
a. recurrens tibialis anterior
a. recurrens tibialis posterior
a. recurrens ulnaris
a. renalis
arteriae renis
a. retinae centralis
a. retroduodenalis
a. sacralis lateralis
a. sacralis mediana
a. scapularis descendens
a. scapularis dorsalis
a. segmenti anterioris inferioris renis
a. segmenti anterioris superioris renis
a. segmenti inferioris renis
a. segmenti posterioris renis
a. segmenti superioris renis
arteriae sigmoideae
a. spermatica interna
a. sphenopalatina
a. spinalis anterior
a. spinalis posterior
a. splenica
a. stylomastoidea
a. subclavia
a. subcostalis
a. sublingualis
a. submentalis
a. subscapularis
a. sulci centralis
a. sulci postcentralis
a. sulci precentralis
a. supraduodenalis
a. supraorbitalis
arteriae suprarenales superiores
a. suprarenalis inferior
a. suprarenalis media
a. suprascapularis
a. supratrochlearis
a. suralis

a. tarsea lateralis
a. tarsea medialis
a. temporalis anterior
a. temporalis intermedia
a. temporalis media
a. temporalis posterior
a. temporalis profunda
a. temporalis superficialis
a. testicularis
arteriae thalamostriatae anterolaterales
arteriae thalamostriatae anteromediales
a. thoracica interna
a. thoracica lateralis
a. thoracica superior
a. thoracoacromialis
a. thoracodorsalis
arteriae thymicae
a. thyroidea ima
a. thyroidea inferior
a. thyroidea superior
a. tibialis anterior
a. tibialis posterior
a. transversa cervicis
a. transversa colli
a. transversa faciei
a. tympanica anterior
a. tympanica inferior
a. tympanica posterior
a. tympanica superior
a. ulnaris
a. umbilicalis
a. urethralis
a. uterina
a. vaginalis
arteriae ventriculares
a. vertebralis
a. vesicalis inferior
a. vesicalis superior
a. vitellina
a. volaris indicis radialis
a. zygomatico-orbitalis

arterial
a. arcades
a. arches of colon
a. arches of ileum
a. arches of jejunum
a. arch of lower eyelid
a. arch of upper eyelid
a. blood
a. bulb
a. canal
a. capillary
a. circle of cerebrum
a. cone
a. duct
a. flap

a. forceps
a. grooves
a. hyperemia
a. hypotension
a. ligament
a. line
a. murmur
a. nephrosclerosis
a. sclerosis
a. segments of kidney
a. spider
a. switch operation
a. tension
a. thoracic outlet syndrome
a. transfusion
a. vein
a. wave
arterialization
arteriarctia
arteriectasis, arteriectasia
arteriectomy
arterioatony
arteriocapillary
a. sclerosis
arteriococcygeal gland
arteriogram
arteriographic
arteriography
bronchial a.
cerebral a.
arteriola, pl. **arteriolae**
a. glomerularis afferens
a. glomerularis efferens
a. macularis inferior
a. macularis superior
a. medialis retinae
a. nasalis retinae inferior
a. nasalis retinae superior
arteriolae rectae
a. temporalis retinae inferior
a. temporalis retinae superior
arteriolar
a. nephrosclerosis
a. network
a. sclerosis
arteriole
afferent glomerular a.
capillary a.
efferent glomerular a.
inferior macular a.
inferior nasal a. of retina
inferior temporal a. of retina
medial a. of retina
superior macular a.
superior nasal a. of retina
superior temporal a. of retina
arteriolith

arteriolitis
necrotizing a.
arteriology
arteriolonecrosis
arteriolonephrosclerosis
arteriolosclerosis
arteriolosclerotic kidney
arteriolovenous
arteriolovenular
a. anastomosis
a. bridge
arteriomalacia
arteriometer
arteriomotor
arteriomyomatosis
arterionephrosclerosis
arteriopalmus
arteriopathy
hypertensive a.
plexogenic pulmonary a.
arterioplania
arterioplasty
arteriopressor
artcriorrhaphy
arteriorrhexis
arteriosclerosis
coronary a.
hyperplastic a.
hypertensive a.
medial a.
Mönckeberg's a.
nodular a.
a. obliterans
peripheral a.
senile a.
arteriosclerotic
a. aneurysm
a. gangrene
a. kidney
a. psychosis
a. retinopathy
arteriospasm
arteriostenosis
arteriotomy
arteriotony
arteriovenous
a. anastomosis
a. aneurysm
a. carbon dioxide difference
a. fistula
a. nicking
a. oxygen difference
a. shunt
arteritis
brachiocephalic a.
coronary a.
cranial a.
extracranial a.

arteritis *(continued)*
    giant cell a.
    granulomatous a.
    Heubner's a.
    Horton's a.
    intracranial granulomatous a.
    neurocranial granulomatous a.
    a. nodosa
    a. obliterans, obliterating a.
    rheumatic a.
    rheumatoid a.
    Takayasu's a.
    temporal a.

artery
    Abbott's a.
    aberrant a.
    aberrant obturator a.
    accessory obturator a.
    acetabular a.
    acromial a.
    acromiothoracic a.
    a. of Adamkiewicz
    alar a. of nose
    angular a.
    a. of angular gyrus
    anterior cecal a.
    anterior cerebral a.
    anterior choroidal a.
    anterior ciliary a.
    anterior circumflex humeral a.
    anterior communicating a.
    anterior conjunctival a.
    anterior descending a.
    anterior ethmoidal a.
    anterior humeral circumflex a.
    anterior inferior cerebellar a.
    anterior inferior segmental a. of kidney
    a. of anterior inferior segment of kidney
    anterior intercostal a.'s
    anterior intercostal branches of internal thoracic a.
    anterior interosseous a.
    anterior interventricular a.
    anterior labial a.'s
    anterior lateral malleolar a.
    anterior medial malleolar a.
    anterior mediastinal a.'s
    anterior meningeal a.
    anterior parietal a.
    anterior peroneal a.
    anterior spinal a.
    anterior superior alveolar a.'s
    anterior superior dental a.'s
    anterior superior segmental a. of kidney

a. of anterior superior segment of kidney
anterior temporal a.
anterior tibial a.
anterior tibial recurrent a.
anterior tympanic a.
anterolateral central a.'s
anterolateral striate a.'s
anterolateral thalamostriate a.'s
anteromedial central a.'s
anteromedial thalamostriate a.'s
apicoposterior a.
appendicular a.
arciform a.'s
arcuate a.
arcuate a.'s of kidney
ascending a.
ascending cervical a.
ascending palatine a.
ascending pharyngeal a.
atrial a.'s
a. to atrioventricular node
axillary a.
azygos a. of vagina
basilar a.
brachial a.
bronchial a.'s
buccal a., buccinator a.
a. of bulb of penis
a. of bulb of vestibule
calcaneal a.'s
calcarine a.
a. of calf
callosomarginal a.
caroticotympanic a.'s
carotid a.'s
carpal a.
caudal pancreatic a.
a. of caudate lobe
cavernous a.'s
cecal a.'s
celiac a.
central a.
central a. of retina
central sulcal a.
a. of central sulcus
cerebellar a.'s
cerebral a.'s
a.'s of cerebral hemorrhage
cervicovaginal a.
Charcot's a.
chief a. of thumb
circumflex femoral a.'s
circumflex fibular a.
circumflex humeral a.'s
circumflex iliac a.'s
circumflex scapular a.
coiled a. of the uterus

colic a.'s
collateral a.
collateral digital a.
common carotid a.
common hepatic a.
common iliac a.
common interosseous a.
common palmar digital a.
common plantar digital a.
communicating a.
companion a. to sciatic nerve
conjunctival a.'s
coronary a.
cortical a.'s
costocervical a.
cremasteric a.
cricothyroid a.
cystic a.
deep auricular a.
deep brachial a.
deep cervical a.
deep circumflex iliac a.
deep a. of clitoris
deep epigastric a.
deep lingual a.
deep a. of penis
deep temporal a.
deep a. of thigh
deep a. of tongue
deferential a.
descending genicular a.
descending a. of knee
descending palatine a.
descending scapular a.
digital collateral a.
distributing a.
dolichoectatic a.
dorsal a. of clitoris
dorsal digital a.
dorsal a. of foot
dorsal interosseous a.
dorsalis pedis a.
dorsal metacarpal a.
dorsal metatarsal a.
dorsal nasal a.
dorsal a. of nose
dorsal pancreatic a.
dorsal a. of penis
dorsal scapular a.
dorsal thoracic a.
a. of Drummond
a. of ductus deferens
elastic a.
end a.
episcleral a.
esophageal a.'s
external carotid a.
external iliac a.

external mammary a.
external maxillary a.
external a. of nose
external pudendal a.'s
external spermatic a.
facial a.
femoral a.
fibular a.
frontal a.
gastric a.'s
gastroduodenal a.
gastroepiploic a.'s
gastro-omental a.'s
genicular a.'s
glaserian a.
great anastomotic a.
greater palatine a.
great pancreatic a.
great radicular a.
great superior pancreatic a.
helicine a.'s of the penis
hepatic a.'s
a. of Heubner
highest intercostal a.
highest thoracic a.
humeral a.
hyaloid a.
hypogastric a.
ileal a.'s
ileocolic a.
iliac a.'s
iliolumbar a.
inferior alveolar a.
inferior dental a.
inferior epigastric a.
inferior gluteal a.
inferior hemorrhoidal a.
inferior hypophysial a.
inferior internal parietal a.
inferior labial a.
inferior laryngeal a.
inferior lateral genicular a.
inferior medial genicular a.
inferior mesenteric a.
inferior pancreatic a.
inferior pancreaticoduodenal a.
inferior phrenic a.
inferior rectal a.
inferior segmental a. of kidney
a. of inferior segment of kidney
inferior suprarenal a.
inferior thyroid a.
inferior tympanic a.
inferior ulnar collateral a.
inferior vesical a.
infraorbital a.
infrascapular a.
innominate a.

artery *(continued)*
   insular a.'s
   intercostal a.'s
   interlobar a.
   interlobar a.'s of kidney
   interlobular a.'s
   interlobular a.'s of kidney
   interlobular a.'s of liver
   intermediate temporal a.
   internal auditory a.
   internal carotid a.
   internal iliac a.
   internal mammary a.
   internal maxillary a.
   internal pudendal a.
   internal spermatic a.
   internal thoracic a.
   intestinal a.'s
   jejunal a.'s
   a.'s of kidney
   Kugel's anastomotic a.
   a. of labyrinth
   labyrinthine a.
   lacrimal a.
   lateral circumflex femoral a.
   lateral circumflex a. of thigh
   lateral femoral circumflex a.
   lateral frontobasal a.
   lateral inferior genicular a.
   lateral malleolar a.'s
   lateral nasal a.
   lateral occipital a.
   lateral plantar a.
   lateral sacral a.
   lateral splanchnic a.'s
   lateral striate a.'s
   lateral superior genicular a.
   lateral tarsal a.
   lateral thoracic a.
   left colic a.
   left coronary a.
   left gastric a.
   left gastroepiploic a.
   left gastro-omental a.
   left hepatic a.
   left pulmonary a.
   lenticulostriate a.'s
   lesser palatine a.
   lienal a.
   lingual a.
   long central a.
   long posterior ciliary a.
   long thoracic a.
   lowest lumbar a.'s
   lowest thyroid a.
   lumbar a.
   macular a.'s
   marginal a. of colon

   masseteric a.
   mastoid a.
   maxillary a.
   medial circumflex femoral a.
   medial circumflex a. of thigh
   medial femoral circumflex a.
   medial frontobasal a.
   medial inferior genicular a.
   medial malleolar a.'s
   medial occipital a.
   medial plantar a.
   medial striate a.
   medial superior genicular a.
   medial tarsal a.
   median a.
   median sacral a.
   mediastinal a.'s
   medium a.
   medullary a.'s of brain
   medullary spinal a.'s
   mental a.
   metatarsal a.
   middle cerebral a.
   middle colic a.
   middle collateral a.
   middle genicular a.
   middle hemorrhoidal a.
   middle meningeal a.
   middle rectal a.
   middle sacral a.
   middle suprarenal a.
   middle temporal a.
   muscular a.
   musculophrenic a.
   mylohyoid a.
   myometrial arcuate a.'s
   myometrial radial a.'s
   a. needle
   Neubauer's a.
   nutrient a.
   nutrient a. of femur
   nutrient a. of fibula
   nutrient a.'s of humerus
   nutrient a. of the tibia
   obturator a.
   occipital a.
   omphalomesenteric a.
   ophthalmic a.
   orbital a.
   orbitofrontal a.
   ovarian a.
   palmar interosseous a.
   palmar metacarpal a.
   palpebral a.'s
   a. of the pancreatic tail
   paracentral a.
   parent a.
   parietal a.'s

A

parieto-occipital a.
a.'s of penis
perforating a.'s
perforating a.'s of foot
perforating a.'s of hand
perforating a.'s of internal
  mammary
perforating peroneal a.
pericallosal a.
pericardiacophrenic a.
perineal a.
peroneal a.
pipestem a.'s
plantar metatarsal a.
pontine a.'s, a.'s of pons
popliteal a.
postcentral a.
postcentral sulcal a.
a. of postcentral sulcus
posterior alveolar a.
posterior auricular a.
posterior cecal a.
posterior cerebral a.
posterior choroidal a.
posterior circumflex humeral a.
posterior communicating a.
posterior conjunctival a.
posterior dental a.
posterior descending a.
posterior ethmoidal a.
posterior humeral circumflex a.
posterior inferior cerebellar a.
posterior intercostal a.'s 1–2
posterior intercostal a.'s 3-11
posterior interosseous a.
posterior interventricular a.
posterior labial a.'s
posterior lateral nasal a.'s
posterior mediastinal a.'s
posterior meningeal a.
posterior pancreaticoduodenal a.
posterior parietal a.
posterior peroneal a.'s
posterior segmental a. of kidney
a. of posterior segment of kidney
posterior septal a. of nose
posterior spinal a.
posterior superior alveolar a.
posterior temporal a.
posterior tibial a.
posterior tibial recurrent a.
posterior tympanic a.
posterolateral central a.'s
posteromedial central a.'s
precentral a.
precentral sulcal a.
a. of precentral sulcus
precuneal a.

pre-Rolandic a.
princeps cervicis a.
princeps pollicis a.
principal a. of thumb
profunda brachii a.
profunda femoris a.
proper hepatic a.
proper palmar digital a.
proper plantar digital a.
a. of pterygoid canal
pubic a.'s
pulmonary a.
a. of pulp
pyloric a.
radial a.
radial collateral a.
radial index a.
radialis indicis a.
radial recurrent a.
radicular a.'s
ranine a.
recurrent a.
recurrent a. of Heubner
recurrent interosseous a.
recurrent radial a.
recurrent ulnar a.
renal a.
retroduodenal a.
right colic a.
right coronary a.
right gastric a.
right gastroepiploic a.
right gastro-omental a.
right hepatic a.
right pulmonary a.
Rolandic a.
a. of round ligament of uterus
a. to sciatic nerve
screw a.'s
scrotal a.'s
segmental a.'s of kidney
septal a.
sheathed a.
short central a.
short gastric a.'s
short posterior ciliary a.
sigmoid a.'s
sinoatrial nodal a.
sinuatrial node a.
a. to the sinuatrial (S-A) node
sinus node a.
small a.'s
somatic a.'s
sphenopalatine a.
spinal a.'s
spiral a.
splenic a.
stapedial a.

artery *(continued)*
sternal a.'s
sternomastoid a.
stylomastoid a.
subclavian a.
subcostal a.
sublingual a.
submental a.
subscapular a.
sulcal a.
superficial brachial a.
superficial cervical a.
superficial circumflex iliac a.
superficial epigastric a.
superficial palmar a.
superficial temporal a.
superficial volar a.
superior cerebellar a.
superior epigastric a.
superior gluteal a.
superior hemorrhoidal a.
superior hypophysial a.
superior intercostal a.
superior internal parietal a.
superior labial a.
superior laryngeal a.
superior lateral genicular a.
superior medial genicular a.
superior mesenteric a.
superior pancreaticoduodenal a.
superior phrenic a.
superior rectal a.
superior segmental a. of kidney
a. of superior segment of kidney
superior suprarenal a.'s
superior thoracic a.
superior thyroid a.
superior tympanic a.
superior ulnar collateral a.
superior vesical a.
supraduodenal a.
supraorbital a.
suprascapular a.
supratrochlear a.
supreme intercostal a.
sural a.
terminal a.
testicular a.
thoracoacromial a.
thoracodorsal a.
thymic a.'s
thyroid ima a.
transverse cervical a.
transverse facial a.
transverse a. of neck
transverse pancreatic a.
transverse scapular a.
ulnar a.

umbilical a.
urethral a.
uterine a.
vaginal a.
venous a.
ventral splanchnic a.'s
ventricular a.'s
vertebral a.
vidian a.
vitelline a.
volar interosseous a.
Wilkie's a.
Zinn's a.
zygomatico-orbital a.
arthragra
arthral
arthralgia
intermittent a.
periodic a.
arthralgic
arthrectomy
arthresthesia
arthritic
a. atrophy
a. calculus
a. general pseudoparalysis
arthritide
arthritis, pl. **arthritides**
acute rheumatic a.
atrophic a.
chronic absorptive a.
chylous a.
a. deformans
degenerative a.
enteropathic a.
filarial a.
gonococcal a.
gonorrheal a.
gouty a.
hemophilic a.
hypertrophic a.
Jaccoud's a.
juvenile a., juvenile rheumatoid a.
juvenile chronic a.
Lyme a.
a. mutilans
neuropathic a.
a. nodosa
ochronotic a.
proliferative a.
psoriatic a.
pyogenic a.
rheumatoid a.
suppurative a.
Arthrobacter
arthrocele
arthrocentesis
arthrochondritis

A

arthroclasia
arthroconidium
Arthroderma
arthrodesis
   triple a.
arthrodia
arthrodial
   a. articulation
   a. cartilage
   a. joint
arthrodynia
arthrodynic
arthrodysplasia
arthroendoscopy
arthroereisis
arthrogenous
arthrogram
arthrography
arthrogryposis
   a. multiplex congenita
arthrokatadysis
arthrolith
arthrolithiasis
arthrologia
arthrology
arthrolysis
arthrometer
arthrometry
arthronosos
arthro-ophthalmopathy
   hereditary progressive a.-o.
arthropathia
   a. psoriatica
arthropathology
arthropathy
   diabetic a.
   Jaccoud's a.
   long-leg a.
   neuropathic a.
   static a.
   tabetic a.
arthrophyma
arthroplasty
   Charnley hip a.
   gap a.
   interposition a.
   intracapsular temporomandibular
     joint a.
   total joint a.
arthropneumoradiography
arthropod
Arthropoda
arthropodic, arthropodous
arthropyosis
arthrorisis
arthrosclerosis
arthroscope
arthroscopy

arthrosis
   temporomandibular a.
arthrospore
arthrosteitis
arthrostomy
arthrosynovitis
arthrotome
arthrotomy
arthrotropic
arthrotyphoid
arthroxesis
Arthus
   A. phenomenon
   A. reaction
articular
   a. branches
   a. capsule
   a. cartilage
   a. cavity
   a. chondrocalcinosis
   a. circumference of radius
   a. circumference of ulna
   a. corpuscles
   a. crepitus
   a. crescent
   a. crests
   a. disc
   a. disc of acromioclavicular joint
   a. disc of distal radioulnar joint
   a. disc of sternoclavicular joint
   a. disc of temporomandibular joint
   a. disk
   a. eminence of temporal bone
   a. facet
   a. fossa of temporal bone
   a. fracture
   a. gout
   a. labrum
   a. lamella
   a. leprosy
   a. lip
   a. margin
   a. meniscus
   a. muscle
   a. muscle of elbow
   a. muscle of knee
   a. nerve
   a. network
   a. pit of head of radius
   a. process
   a. rheumatism
   a. sensibility
   a. surface
   a. surface of acromion
   a. surface of arytenoid cartilage
   a. surface of head of fibula
   a. surface of head of rib
   a. surface of patella

articular *(continued*
  a. surface c temporal bone
  a. surface f tubercle of rib
  a. tubercle of temporal bone
  a. vascul circle
  a. vascur network
  a. vascar network of elbow
  a. vaslar network of knee
articulare
articularis
  a. iti muscle
  a. nu muscle
articula
articul skeleton
  ng **paper**
artic io, pl. **articulationes**
arti a. acromioclavicularis
  a. atlantoaxialis lateralis
  a. atlantoaxialis mediana
  a. atlanto-occipitalis
  a. bicondylaris
  a. calcaneocuboidea
  a. capitis costae
  articulationes carpometacarpeae
  a. carpometacarpea pollicis
  a. cartilaginis
  articulationes cinguli membri inferioris
  articulationes cinguli membri superioris
  a. complexa
  a. composita
  a. condylaris
  a. costotransversaria
  articulationes costovertebrales
  a. cotylica
  a. coxae
  a. cricoarytenoidea
  a. cricothyroidea
  a. cubiti
  a. cuneonavicularis
  a. dentoalveolaris
  a. ellipsoidea
  a. fibrosa
  a. genus
  a. humeri
  a. humeroradialis
  a. humeroulnaris
  a. incudomallearis
  a. incudostapedia
  articulationes intercarpeae
  articulationes interchondrales
  articulationes intermetacarpeae
  articulationes intermetatarseae
  articulationes interphalangeae manus
  articulationes interphalangeae pedis
  articulationes intertarseae

  a. lumbosacralis
  a. mandibularis
  articulationes manus
  a. mediocarpea
  articulationes membri inferioris liberi
  articulationes membri superioris liberi
  articulationes metacarpophalangeae
  articulationes metatarsophalangeae
  articulationes ossiculorum auditus
  a. ossis pisiformis
  a. ovoidalis
  articulationes pedis
  a. plana
  a. radiocarpea
  a. radioulnaris distalis
  a. radioulnaris proximalis
  a. sacrococcygea
  a. sacroiliaca
  a. sellaris
  a. simplex
  a. spheroidea
  a. sternoclavicularis
  articulationes sternocostales
  a. subtalaris
  a. synovialis
  a. talocalcaneonavicularis
  a. talocruralis
  a. tarsi transversa
  articulationes tarsometatarseae
  a. temporomandibularis
  a. tibiofibularis
  a. trochoidea
  articulationes zygapophyseales
articulation
  arthrodial a.
  atlanto-occipital a.
  balanced a.
  bicondylar a.
  carpal a.
  cartilaginous a.
  compound a.
  condylar a.
  confluent a.
  cricoarytenoid a.
  cricothyroid a.
  cuneonavicular a.
  dental a.
  distal radioulnar a.
  a.'s of foot
  glenohumeral a.
  a.'s of hand
  humeral a.
  humeroradial a.
  incudomalleolar a.
  incudostapedial a.
  interchondral a.'s

intermetatarsal a.'s
interphalangeal a.'s
intertarsal a.'s
metacarpophalangeal a.'s
metatarsophalangeal a.'s
peg-and-socket a.
a. of pisiform bone
proximal radioulnar a.
radiocarpal a.
sacroiliac a.
spheroid a.
sternocostal a.'s
superior tibial a.
talocrural a.
temporomandibular a.
transverse tarsal a.
trochoid a.
articulator
adjustable a.
arcon a.
non-arcon a.
articulatory
articulostat
articulus
artifact
chemical shift a.
artifactitious
artifactual
artificial
a. active immunity
a. anatomy
a. ankylosis
a. anus
a. crown
a. dentition
a. eye
a. fever
a. heart
a. insemination
a. intelligence
a. kidney
a. pacemaker
a. passive immunity
a. pneumothorax
a. pupil
a. radioactivity
a. respiration
a. sphincter
a. tears
a. ventilation
artistic anatomy
arycorniculate synchondrosis
aryepiglottic
a. fold
a. muscle
arytenoepiglottidean
a. fold

arytenoid
a. cartilage
a. glands
a. swelling
arytenoidal articular surface of cricoid
arytenoidectomy
arytenoideus
arytenoiditis
arytenoidopexy
asbestoid
asbestos
a. bodies
a. corn
a. liner
a. wart
asbestosis
ascariasis
ascarid
Ascaridae
Ascaridata
Ascaridida
Ascarididae
Ascarididea
Ascaridoidea
Ascaridorida
Ascaris
A. equorum
Ascaroidea
Ascarops strongylina
ascendens
ascending
a. anterior branch
a. aorta
a. artery
a. branch
a. branch of the inferior mesenteric artery
a. cervical artery
a. cholangitis
a. colon
a. current
a. degeneration
a. frontal convolution
a. frontal gyrus
a. lumbar vein
a. myelitis
a. neuritis
a. palatine artery
a. paralysis
a. parietal convolution
a. parietal gyrus
a. part of aorta
a. part of duodenum
a. pharyngeal artery
a. pharyngeal plexus
a. posterior branch
a. process
a. pyelonephritis

ascensus
ascertainment
        complete a.
        incomplete a.
        single a.
        total a.
        truncate a.
Aschelminth
Ascher's
        A. aqueous influx phenomenon
        A. syndrome
Aschheim-Zondek test
Aschner-Dagnini reflex
Aschner
        A. phenomenon
        A. reflex

Aschoff
        A. bodies
        A. cell
        A. nodules
        (pl. of ascus)
ascites
        a. adiposus
        chyliform a.
        chylous a., a. chylosus
        fatty a.
        gelatinous a.
        hemorrhagic a.
        milky a.
        pseudochylous a.
ascitic
        a. agar
ascitogenous
ascocarp
ascogenous
ascogonium
Ascoli reaction
Ascoli's test
Ascomycetes
ascomycetous
Ascomycota
ascorbate-cyanide test
ascospore
ascus, pl. asci
asecretory
Aselli's pancreas
asemasia, asemia
asepsis
aseptate
aseptic
        a. fever
        a. necrosis
        a. surgery
asepticism
asequence
asexual
        a. dwarfism

        a. generation
        a. reproduction
Ashby method
ashen
        a. tuber
        a. tubercle
        a. wing
Asherman's syndrome
Ashman's phenomenon
ashy dermatosis
Asian influenza
Asiatic
        A. cholera
        A. schistosomiasis
asiderotic anemia
asitia
Askanazy cell
Ask-Upmark kidney
asocial
asoma, pl. asomata
aspalasoma
aspartylglycosaminuria
aspect
aspergilloma
aspergillomycosis
aspergillosis
        bronchopneumonic a.
        bronchopulmonary a.
        disseminated a.
        invasive a.
        pulmonary a.
Aspergillus
        A. clavatus
        A. flavus
        A. fumigatus
        A. nidulans
        A. niger
        A. terreus
aspermatogenic
        a. sterility
aspermia
aspersion
aspheric
        a. lens
asphygmia
asphyxia
        blue a.
        cyanotic a.
        a. livida
        local a.
        a. neonatorum
        a. pallida
        symmetric a.
        traumatic a.
asphyxial
asphyxiant
asphyxiate

asphyxiating
    a. thoracic chondrodystrophy
    a. thoracic dysplasia
asphyxiation
Aspiculuris tetraptera
aspirate
aspirating needle
aspiration
    a. biopsy
    meconium a.
    a. pneumonia
aspirator
    vacuum a.
    water a.
asplenia
    functional a.
    a. syndrome
asplenic
asporogenous
asporous
asporulate
Assam fever
assay
    Ames a.
    clonogenic a.
    competitive binding a.
    complement binding a.
    double antibody sandwich a.
    EAC rosette a.
    enzyme-linked immunosorbent a.
    Grunstein-Hogness a.
    hemizona a.
    immunochemical a.
    immunoradiometric a.
    indirect a.
    radioreceptor a.
    Raji cell radioimmune a.
assertive
    a. conditioning
    a. training
Assézat's triangle
assident
    a. sign
    a. symptom
assimilable
assimilation
    a. pelvis
    reproductive a.
    a. sacrum
assist-control ventilation
assisted
    a. cephalic delivery
    a. circulation
    a. reproductive technology
    a. respiration
    a. ventilation
assistive movement
Assmann's tuberculous infiltrate

associate
    paired a.'s
associated
    a. antagonist
    a. macrophage
    a. movements
association
    a. areas
    clang a.
    a. constant
    a. cortex
    dream a.'s
    a. fibers
    free a.
    genetic a.
    loose a.'s
    a. mechanism
    a. neurosis
    a. system
    a. test
    a. time
    a. tract
associationism
associative
    a. aphasia
    a. strength
assortative mating
assortment
    independent a.
assumption
astacoid rash
astasia
astasia-abasia
astatic
asteatodes
asteatosis
    a. cutis
aster
    sperm a.
astereognosis
asterion
asterixis
asternal
asternia
asteroid
    a. body
    a. hyalosis
asthenia
    neurocirculatory a.
asthenic
    a. personality
    a. personality disorder
asthenopia
    accommodative a.
    muscular a.
    nervous a.
asthenopic
asthenospermia

asthma
  atopic a.
  bronchial a.
  bronchitic a.
  cardiac a.
  catarrhal a.
  cotton-dust a.
  a. crystals
  dust a.
  extrinsic a.
  food a.
  hay a.
  intrinsic a.
  miller's a.
  miner's a.
  nervous a.
  reflex a.
  spasmodic a.
  steam-fitter's a.
  stripper's a.
  summer a.
asthmatic
  a. bronchitis
asthmatoid wheeze
asthmogenic
astigmatic
  a. dial
  a. lens
astigmatism
  a. against the rule
  compound hyperopic a.
  compound myopic a.
  corneal a.
  hyperopic a.
  irregular a.
  lenticular a.
  mixed a.
  myopic a.
  a. of oblique pencils
  regular a.
  simple hyperopic a.
  simple myopic a.
  a. with the rule
astigmatometry, astigmometry
astigmia
astomatous
astomia
astomous
astragalar
astragalectomy
astragalocalcanean
astragalofibular
astragaloscaphoid
astragalotibial
astral
astrapophobia
astroblast
astroblastoma

astrocele
astrocyte
  Alzheimer type I a.
  Alzheimer type II a.
  fibrillary a., fibrous a.
  gemistocytic a.
  protoplasmic a.
  reactive a.
astrocytoma
  anaplastic a.
  cerebellar a.
  desmoplastic cerebral a.
  fibrillary a.
  gemistocytic a.
  grade I a.
  grade II a.
  grade III a.
  grade IV a.
  juvenile cerebellar a.
  low grade a.
  piloid a.
  plocytic a.
  protoplasmic a.
  subependymal giant cell a.
astrocytosis
  a. cerebri
astroependymoma
astroglia
  a. cell
astroid
astrokinetic
astrosphere
Astwood's test
asyllabia
asylum
asymbolia
asymmetric
  a. motor neuropathy
asymmetrical chondrodystrophy
asymmetry
asymptomatic
  a. coccidioidomycosis
  a. neurosyphilis
asymptotic
asynchronous pulse generator
asynclitism
  anterior a.
  posterior a.
asyndesis
asynechia
asynergia
asynergic
asynergy
asynesia, asynesis
asystematic
asystole
asystolia
asystolic

atactic
    a. abasia
    a. agraphia
atactilia
ataraxia
atavism
atavistic
    a. epiphysis
ataxia
    acute a.
    Briquet's a.
    Bruns a.
    cerebellar a.
    chronic a.
    a. cordis
    Friedreich's a.
    hereditary cerebellar a.
    hereditary spinal a.
    hysterical a.
    kinetic a.
    Leyden's a.
    locomotor a.
    Marie's a.
    moral a.
    motor a.
    optic a.
    respiratory a.
    sensory a.
    spinal a.
    spinocerebellar a.
    static a.
    a. telangiectasia, a.-telangiectasia
    a. telangiectasia syndrome
    vasomotor a.
    vestibulocerebellar a.
ataxiadynamia
ataxiagram
ataxiagraph
ataxiameter
ataxiaphasia
ataxic
    a. abasia
    a. aphasia
    a. breathing
    a. dysarthria
    a. gait
    a. paramyotonia
    a. paraplegia
    a. tremor
ataxiophemia
ataxiophobia
ataxy
atelectasis
    adhesive a.
    cicatrization a.
    parenchymal a.
    passive a.
    patchy a.

    platelike a.
    primary a.
    resorption a.
    round a.
    secondary a.
    segmental a.
    subsegmental a.
atelectatic
    a. rale
atelia
ateliosis
ateliotic
    a. dwarfism
A$_2$ thalassemia
athelia
atherectomy
    coronary a.
    directional a.
athermancy
athermanous
athermosystaltic
atheroembolism
atherogenesis
atherogenic
atheroma
    a. embolism
atheromatous
    a. degeneration
    a. plaque
atherosclerotic
    a. aneurysm
atherosis
atherothrombosis
atherothrombotic
athetoid
athetosic, athetotic
athetosis
    double a.
    double congenital a.
    posthemiplegic a.
athlete's
    a. foot
    a. heart
athletic heart
athrepsia, athrepsy
athrocytosis
athrombia
athymia
athymism
athyrea
athyroidism
athyrosis
athyrotic
atlantad
atlantal
atlantic part of vertebral artery
atlantoaxial
    a. joint

atlantodidymus
atlantoepistrophic
atlanto-occipital
    a.-o. articulation
    a.-o. joint
    a.-o. membrane
atlanto-odontoid
atlas
atloaxoid
atlodidymus
atloid
atlo-occipital
atmosphere
    ICAO standard a.
atmospherization
atomism
atomistic
    a. psychology
atonia
atonic
    a. bladder
    a. dyspepsia
    a. ectropion
    a. entropion
    a. epiphora
    a. seizure
    a. ulcer
atonicity
atony
atopen
atopic
    a. allergy
    a. asthma
    a. cataract
    a. dermatitis
    a. eczema
    a. keratoconjunctivitis
    a. reagin
atopognosia, atopognosis
atopy
atrabiliary
    a. capsule
atraumatic
    a. needle
    a. suture
atrepsy
atresia
    anal a., a. ani
    aortic a.
    biliary a.
    bronchial a.
    choanal a.
    esophageal a.
    a. folliculi
    intestinal a.
    a. iridis
    laryngeal a.
    pulmonary a.

A TORTUOUS 2 words

    tricuspid a.
    vaginal a.
atresic
    a. teratosis
atretic
    a. corpus luteum
    a. ovarian follicle
atretoblepharia
atretocystia
atretogastria
atretopsia
atria (*pl. of* atrium)
atrial
    a. appendage
    a. arteries
    a. auricle
    a. auricula
    a. bigeminy
    a. branches
    a. capture
    a. capture beat
    a. chaotic tachycardia
    a. complex
    a. diastole
    a. dissociation
    a. echo
    a. extrasystole
    a. fibrillation
    a. flutter
    a. fusion beat
    a. gallop
    a. kick
    a. myxoma
    a. natriuretic factor
    a. natriuretic peptide
    a. septal defect
    a. sound
    a. standstill
    a. synchronous pulse generator
    a. systole
    a. tachycardia
    a. transport function
    a. triggered pulse generator
    a. ventricular canal defect
atrial-well technique
atrichia
atrichosis
atrichous
atriocarotid interval
atriomegaly
atrionector
atriopeptin
atrioseptoplasty
atrioseptostomy
    balloon a.
atriosystolic murmur
atriotomy

atrioventricular
  a. band
  a. block
  a. bundle
  a. canal
  a. canal cushions
  a. conduction
  a. connections
  a. dissociation
  a. extrasystole
  a. gradient
  a. groove
  a. interval
  a. junctional bigeminy
  a. junctional rhythm
  a. junctional tachycardia
  a. nodal branch
  a. nodal extrasystole
  a. node
  a. septum
  a. sulcus
  a. valves
atrlplicism
atrium, pl. **atria**
  accessory a.
  auricle of a.
  a. cordis
  a. dextrum cordis
  a. glottidis
  a. of heart
  left a. of heart
  a. meatus medii
  nasal a.
  a. pulmonale
  right a. of heart
  a. sinistrum cordis
atrophedema
atrophia
  a. cutis
  a. maculosa varioliformis cutis
  a. pilorum propria
atrophic
  a. arthritis
  a. excavation
  a. gastritis
  a. glossitis
  a. heterochromia
  a. inflammation
  a. kidney
  a. pharyngitis
  a. rhinitis
  a. thrombosis
  a. vaginitis
atrophie blanche
atrophied
atrophoderma
  a. albidum
  a. biotripticum

  a. diffusum
  a. maculatum
  a. neuriticum
  a. of Pasini and Pierini
  a. reticulatum symmetricum faciei
  senile a., a. senilis
  a. striatum
  a. vermiculatum
atrophodermatosis
atrophy
  acute reflex bone a.
  acute yellow a. of the liver
  alveolar a.
  arthritic a.
  blue a.
  brown a.
  Buchwald's a.
  central areolar choroidal a.
  cerebellar a.
  choroidal vascular a.
  compensatory a.
  congenital cerebellar a.
  cyanotic a.
  cyanotic a. of the liver
  dentatorubral cerebellar a. with
    polymyoclonus
  disuse a.
  Erb a.
  essential progressive a. of iris
  exhaustion a.
  facioscapulohumeral a.
  familial spinal muscular a.
  fatty a.
  gingival a.
  Hoffmann's muscular a.
  horizontal a.
  Hunt's a.
  idiopathic muscular a.
  infantile muscular a.
  infantile progressive spinal
    muscular a.
  infantile spinal muscular a.
  ischemic muscular a.
  juvenile muscular a.
  juvenile spinal muscular a.
  Kienböck's a.
  Leber's hereditary optic a.
  linear a.
  macular a.
  marantic a.
  muscular a.
  myopathic a.
  neuritic a.
  neurogenic a.
  neurotrophic a.
  nutritional type cerebellar a.
  olivopontocerebellar a.
  periodontal a.

atrophy *(continued)*
  peroneal muscular a.
  Pick's a.
  postmenopausal a.
  pressure a.
  primary idiopathic macular a.
  primary macular a. of skin
  progressive choroidal a.
  progressive circumscribed
    cerebral a.
  progressive infantile spinal
    muscular a.
  progressive muscular a.
  progressive spinal muscular a.
  pulp a.
  red a.
  scapulohumeral a.
  senile a.
  serous a.
  striate a. of skin
  Sudeck's a.
  traction a.
  transneuronal a.
  trophoneurotic a.
  villous a.
  Vulpian's a.
  Werdnig-Hoffmann muscular a.
  yellow a. of the liver
  Zimmerlin's a.
atropine test
attached
  a. cranial section
  a. craniotomy
  a. gingiva
attachment
  a. apparatus
  bar clip a.'s
  bar-sleeve a.'s
  epithelial a.
  frictional a.
  internal a.
  key a.
  keyway a.
  muscle-tendon a.
  parallel a.
  pericemental a.
  precision a.
  slotted a.
attack
  drop a.
  panic a.
  salaam a.
  transient ischemic a.
  uncinate a.
  vagal a.
  vasovagal a.
attending
  a. physician

  a. staff
  a. surgeon
attention
  a. deficit disorder
  a. deficit hyperactivity disorder
attenuated
  a. tuberculosis
  a. vaccine
  a. virus
attenuation compensation
attic
  tympanic a.
atticomastoid
atticotomy
attitude
  emotional a.'s
  fetal a.
  passional a.'s
attitudinal
  a. reflexes
attollens
  a. aurem, a. auriculam
  a. oculi
attraction
  neurotropic a.
  a. sphere
attrahens
attributable risk
attrition
atypia
atypical
  a. absence seizure
  a. achromatopsia
  a. facial neuralgia
  a. fibroxanthoma
  a. gingivitis
  a. lipoma
  a. measles
  a. melanocytic hyperplasia
  a. mycobacteria
  a. pneumonia
  a. trigeminal neuralgia
  a. verrucous endocarditis
atypism
Au antigen
Aub-DuBois table
Auberger blood group, Au blood group
Aubert's phenomenon
Auchmeromyia
  A. luteola
audile
audioanalgesia
audiogenic
  a. seizure
audiogram
  pure tone a.
  speech a.
audiologist

audiology
audiometer
    automatic a.
    Békésy a.
    limited range a.
    pure-tone a.
    speech a.
audiometric
audiometrist
audiometry
    auditory brainstem response a.,
      ABR a.
    automatic a.
    Békésy a.
    brainstem evoked response a.,
      BSER a.
    cortical a.
    diagnostic a.
    electrodermal a.
    electrophysiologic a.
    evoked response a.
    pure-tone a.
    screening a.
    speech a.
audiovisual
audit
audition
    chromatic a.
auditive
auditory
    a. agnosia
    a. alternans
    a. aphasia
    a. area
    a. brainstem response audiometry
    a. canal
    a. capsule
    a. cortex
    a. fatigue
    a. field
    a. ganglion
    a. hairs
    a. hallucination
    a. hyperesthesia
    a. lemniscus
    a. localization
    a. nerve
    a. nucleus
    a. oculogyric reflex
    a. organ
    a. ossicles
    a. pathway
    a. pits
    a. placodes
    a. pore
    a. process
    a. receptor cells
    a. reflex

    a. striae
    a. strings
    a. teeth
    a. threshold
    a. tract
    a. tube
    a. vertigo
    a. vesicle
Auenbrugger's sign
Auer
    A. bodies
    A. rods
Auerbach's
    A. ganglia
    A. plexus
Aufrecht's sign
augmentation
    a. graft
    a. mammaplasty
augmented
    a. histamine test
    a. lead
augmentor
    a. fibers
    a. nerves
augnathus
Aujeszky's disease virus
aura, pl. **aurae**
    intellectual a.
    kinesthetic a.
    reminiscent a.
aural
    a. myiasis
    a. vertigo
auramine
    a. O
    a. O fluorescent stain
aurantiasis cutis
aures (*pl. of* auris)
auriasis
auricle
    accessory a.'s
    atrial a.
    a. of atrium
    cervical a.
    a. of left atrium
    a. of right atrium
auricula, pl. **auriculae**
    atrial a.
    a. atrialis
    a. dextra
    a. sinistra
auricular
    a. appendage
    a. appendectomy
    a. appendix
    a. arc
    a. branch of occipital artery

auricular *(continued)*
    a. branch of vagus nerve
    a. canaliculus
    a. cartilage
    a. complex
    a. extrasystole
    a. fibrillation
    a. fissure
    a. flutter
    a. ganglion
    a. index
    a. ligaments
    a. notch
    a. point
    a. reflex
    a. standstill
    a. surface of ilium
    a. surface of sacrum
    a. systole
    a. tachycardia
    a. triangle
    a. tubercle
    a. veins
auriculare, pl. **auricularia**
auriculocranial
auriculo-infraorbital plane
auriculopalpebral reflex
auriculopressor reflex
auriculotemporal
    a. nerve
    a. nerve syndrome
auriculoventricular
    a. groove
    a. interval
aurid, pl. **aurides**
auriform
auris, pl. **aures**
    a. externa
    a. interna
    a. media
aurochromoderma
auropalpebral reflex
aurotherapy
Aus antigen
auscultate, auscult
auscultation
    immediate a., direct a.
    mediate a.
auscultatory
    a. alternans
    a. gap
    a. percussion
    a. sound
aussage test
Austin
    A. Flint murmur
    A. Flint phenomenon
Australia antigen

Australian
    A. Q fever
    A. tick typhus
    A. X disease
    A. X disease virus
    A. X encephalitis
autacoid
    a. substance
autecic, autecious
autemesia
authenticity
authoritarian personality
authority figure
autism
    early infantile a.
    infantile a.
autistic
    a. disorder
    a. parasite
autoagglutination
autoagglutinin
    anti-Pr cold a.
    cold a.
autoallergic
autoallergization
autoallergy
autoanalysis
autoanaphylaxis
autoantibody
    anti-idiotype a.
    cold a.
    Donath-Landsteiner cold a.
    hemagglutinating cold a.
    idiotype a.
    warm a.
autoanticomplement
autoantigen
autoassay
autoaugmentation
autoblast
autocatheterization, autocatheterism
autochthonous
    a. ideas
    a. malaria
    a. parasite
autoclasis, autoclasia
autoclave
autocrine
    a. hypothesis
autocystoplasty
autocytolysin
autocytotoxin
autodermic
    a. graft
autodiploid
autodrainage
autoecholalia
autoerotic

autoeroticism
autoerotism
autoerythrocyte
    a. sensitization
    a. sensitization syndrome
autofluoroscope
autogamous
autogamy
autogeneic graft
autogenesis
autogenetic, autogenic
autogenous
    a. keratoplasty
    a. union
autognosis
autograft
autografting
autogram
autographism
autohemagglutination
autohemolysin
autohemolysis
    a. test
autohemotransfusion
autohexaploid
autohypnosis
autohypnotic
autohypnotism
autoimmune
    a. disease
    a. hemolytic anemia
    a. neonatal thrombocytopenia
    a. thyroiditis
autoimmunity
autoimmunization
autoimmunocytopenia
autoinfection
autoinfusion
autoinoculable
autoinoculation
autoisolysin
autokeratoplasty
autokinesia, autokinesis
autokinetic
    a. effect
autolesion
autologous
    a. graft
autolysin
automallet
automated differential leukocyte counter
automatic
    a. audiometer
    a. audiometry
    a. beat
    a. condenser
    a. contraction

    a. epilepsy
    a. plugger
automatism
    ambulatory a.
    immediate posttraumatic a.
automatograph
automixis
automnesia
automysophobia
autonomic
    a. disorder
    a. epilepsy
    a. ganglia
    a. imbalance
    a. motor neuron
    a. motor neurons
    a. nerve
    a. nervous system
    a. neurogenic bladder
    a. nuclei
    a. part
    a. plexuses
autonomotropic
autonomous
    a. psychotherapy
autonomy
    functional a.
autoparenchymatous metaplasia
autopathic
autopentaploid
autopepsia
autophagia
autophagic
    a. vacuole
autophagolysosome
autophagy
autophilia
autophobia
autophony
autoplast
autoplastic
    a. graft
autoplasty
autoploid
autoploidy
autoplugger
autopod
autopodium, pl. **autopodia**
autopoisonous
autopolyploid
autopolyploidy
autopsy
autoradiogram
autoradiograph
autoradiography
autoregulation
    heterometric a.
    homeometric a.

autoreinfection
autorrhaphy
autoscopic phenomenon
autosensitize
autosepticemia
autoserotherapy
autoserum
    a. therapy
autosexualism
autosite
autosmia
autosomal
    a. gene
autosomatognosis
autosomatognostic
autosome
autosuggestibility
autosuggestion
autosynnoia
autotelic
autotemnous
autotetraploid
autotherapy
autotomy
autotopagnosia
autotoxemia
autotoxic
autotoxicosis
autotransfusion
autotransplant
autotransplantation
autotriploid
autotroph
autotrophic
autovaccination
autozygous
autumn fever
auxanogram
auxanographic
    a. method
auxanography
auxanology
auxesis
auxetic growth
auxiliary
    a. abutment
auxiliomotor
auxilytic
auxocardia
auxodrome
auxotonic
auxotroph
auxotrophic
    a. strains
A-V
    A-V block
    A-V conduction
    A-V dissociation

A-V extrasystole
A-V interval
A-V junction
A-V junctional rhythm
A-V junctional tachycardia
A-V nodal extrasystole
A-V strabismus syndrome
available arch length
avalanche conduction
avalvular
avascular
    a. necrosis
avascularization
Avellis' syndrome
average
    a. flow rate
    a. pulse magnitude
aversion therapy
aversive
    a. behavior
    a. conditioning
    a. control
    a. stimulus
    a. training
Aviadenovirus
avian
    a. encephalomyelitis virus
    a. erythroblastosis virus
    a. influenza virus
    a. leukosis-sarcoma virus
    a. lymphomatosis virus
    a. myeloblastosis virus
    a. neurolymphomatosis virus
    a. pneumoencephalitis virus
    a. sarcoma
    a. sarcoma virus
    a. viral arthritis virus
aviation
    a. medicine
    a. otitis
aviator's
    a. disease
    a. ear
avidity
    a. antibody
Avipoxvirus
avirulent
avitaminosis
    conditioned a.
avivement
avoidance
    a. conditioning
    a. training
avoidance-avoidance conflict
avoidant
    a. disorder of adolescence
    a. disorder of childhood

a. personality
a. personality disorder
avulsed wound
avulsion
    a. fracture
    nerve a.
    root a.
    tooth a.
axes (*pl. of* axis)
axial
    a. ametropia
    a. aneurysm
    a. angle
    a. cataract
    a. current
    a. filament
    a. hyperopia
    a. illumination
    a. muscle
    a. myopia
    a. neuritis
    a. pattern flap
    a. plane
    a. plate
    a. point
    a. projection
    a. section
    a. skeleton
    a. surface
    a. view
    a. walls of the pulp chambers
axifugal
axil
axile
    a. corpuscle
axilla, gen. and pl. **axillae**
    a. thermometer
axillary
    a. anesthesia
    a. arch
    a. arch muscle
    a. artery
    a. cavity
    a. fascia
    a. fold
    a. fossa
    a. glands
    a. hair
    a. line
    a. lymph nodes
    a. nerve
    a. plexus
    a. region
    a. sheath
    a. space
    a. sweat glands
    a. thermometer

    a. triangle
    a. vein
axiobuccal
axiobuccogingival
axioincisal
axiolabial
axiolabiolingual
    a. plane
axiolingual
axiolinguocervical
axiolinguoclusal
axiolinguogingival
axiomesial
axiomesiocervical
axiomesiodistal
    a. plane
axiomesiogingival
axiomesioincisal
axion
axio-occlusal
axioplasm
axiopodium, pl. **axiopodia**
axiopulpal
axioversion
axipetal
axiramificate
axis, pl. **axes**
    basibregmatic a.
    basicranial a.
    basifacial a.
    biauricular a.
    a. bulbi externus
    a. bulbi internus
    celiac a.
    cephalocaudal a.
    cerebrospinal a.
    condylar a.
    conjugate a.
    a. corpuscle
    craniofacial a.
    a. cylinder
    a. deviation
    electrical a.
    embryonic a.
    encephalomyelonic a.
    external a. of eye
    facial a.
    hinge a.
    instantaneous electrical a.
    internal a. of eye
    a. of lens
    a. lentis
    a. ligament of malleus
    long a.
    long a. of body
    mandibular a.
    mean electrical a.
    neural a.

axis *(continued)*
  neutral a. of straight beam
  normal electrical a.
  opening a.
  optic a.
  a. opticus
  orbital a.
  pelvic a.
  a. pelvis
  principal optic a.
  pupillary a.
  rotational a.
  sagittal a.
  secondary a.
  a. shift
  a. of symmetry
  thoracic a.
  thyroid a.
  a. traction
  transporionic a.
  transverse horizontal a.
  vertical a.
  visual a.
  Y-a.
axis-traction forceps
axoaxonic
  a. synapse
axodendritic
  a. synapse
axofugal
axograph
axolemma
axolysis
axon
  a. degeneration
  a. hillock
  a. loss polyneuropathy
  a. reflex
  a. terminals
axonal
  a. degeneration
  a. polyneuropathy
  a. process
  a. terminal boutons
axoneme
axonography
axonopathy
axonotmesis
axopetal
axoplasm
axoplasmic transport
axopodium, pl. **axopodia**
axosomatic
  a. synapse

axostyle
axotomy
Ayala's
  A. index
  A. quotient
Ayerza's
  A. disease
  A. syndrome
Ayre brush
azin dyes
azobilirubin
azocarmine
  a. dyes
azocarmine B, azocarmine G
azoic
azo itch
azolitmin
azoospermia
azophloxin
Azorean disease
azotemia
  nonrenal a., prerenal a.
azotemic
  a. retinitis
azothermia
azovan blue
Aztec ear
A.-Z. test
azul
azure
  a. A
  a. B
  a. C
  a. I
  a. II
  a. lunula of nails
azuresin
azurophil, azurophile
  a. granule
azurophilia
azygoesophageal recess
azygogram
azygography
azygos
  a. artery of vagina
  a. continuation (of the inferior
    vena cava)
  a. fissure
  a. lobe of lung
  a. vein
  a. vein principle
azygous

β

β corynebacteriophage
β hemolysin
β hemolysis
β phage
β thalassemia

B

B bile
B cell
B cell antigen receptors
B cell differentiation/growth factors
B fibers
B lymphocyte
B virus
B wave

B6 bronchus sign
B19 virus
Babbitt metal
Babcock tube
Babès-Ernst bodies
Babesiidae
Babès' nodes
Babinski

B. phenomenon
B. reflex
B. sign
B. syndrome

baby

blue b.
blueberry muffin b.
b. bottle syndrome
collodion b.
test-tube b.
b. tooth

baccate
Baccelli's sign
bacciform
Bachmann's bundle
Bachman-Pettit test
Bachman test
Bacillaceae
bacillar, bacillary
Bacille bilié de Calmette-Guérin, Bacille Calmette-Guérin
bacillemia
bacilli (*pl. of* bacillus)
bacilliform
bacillin
bacillomyxin
bacillosis
bacilluria
Bacillus

B. amyloliquefaciens
B. anthracis
B. brevis

B. cereus
B. hemolyticus
B. histolyticus
B. megaterium
B. polymyxa
B. sphaericus
B. subtilis
B. thuringiensis

bacillus, pl. **bacilli**

Abel's b.
abortus b.
acne b.
Bang's b.
Battey b.
blue pus b.
Bordet-Gengou b.
Calmette-Guérin b.
cholera b.
coliform bacilli
colon b.
comma b.
Döderlein's b.
Ducrey's b.
dysentery b.
Eberth's b.
Flexner's b.
Friedländer's b.
Gärtner's b.
gas b.
Ghon-Sachs b.
glanders b.
grass b.
Hansen's b.
hay b.
Hofmann's b.
influenza b.
Johne's b.
Klebs-Loeffler b.
Koch's b.
Koch-Weeks b.
lactic acid b.
leprosy b.
Loeffler's b.
mist b.
Moeller's grass b.
Morgan's b.
Much's b.
necrosis b.
paracolon b.
paradysentery b.
paratyphoid b.
Park-Williams b.
Pfeiffer's b.
plague b.
Plaut's b.

B

bacillus *(continued)*
    Plotz b.
    Preisz-Nocard b.
    Sachs' b.
    Schmorl's b.
    Schottmueller's b.
    Shiga b.
    Shiga-Kruse b.
    Sonne b.
    timothy-hay b.
    tubercle b.
    typhoid b.
    Vincent's b.
    vole b.
    Weeks' b.
    Welch's b.
    Whitmore's b.
back
    adolescent round b.
    b. cross
    b. of foot reflex
    hollow b.
    b. mutation
    poker b.
    b. pressure
    saddle b.
    b. teeth
    b. vertex power
backache
back-action plugger
backboard splint
backbone
backflow
    pyelovenous b.
background
    b. level
    b. radiation
backing
back-knee
backprojection
backscatter
backward
    b. curvature
    b. heart failure
backwash ileitis
Bacon's anoscope
bacteremia
bacteria (*pl. of* bacterium)
bacteria
    coryneform b.
bacteria-free stage of bacterial endocarditis
bacterial
    b. allergy
    b. antagonism
    b. capsule
    b. cast
    b. cystitis

    b. encephalitis
    b. endarteritis
    b. endocarditis
    b. food poisoning
    b. hemolysin
    b. interference
    b. peliosis
    b. pericarditis
    b. plaque
    b. pneumonia
    b. vaginosis
    b. vegetations
    b. virus
bactericholia
bactericidal
bactericide
    specific b.
bacterid
bacteriemia
bacterioagglutinin
bacteriocidal
bacteriocidin
bacteriocin factors
bacteriocinogenic plasmids
bacteriocinogens
bacteriocins
bacterioclasis
bacteriofluorescin
bacteriogenic
    b. agglutination
bacteriogenous
bacteriologic, bacteriological
bacteriologist
bacteriology
    systematic b.
bacteriolysin
bacteriolysis
bacteriolytic
    b. serum
bacteriolyze
bacteriopexy
bacteriophage
    defective b.
    filamentous b.
    b. immunity
    mature b.
    b. plaque
    b. resistance
    temperate b.
    typhoid b.
    b. typing
    vegetative b.
    virulent b.
bacteriophagia
bacteriophagology
bacteriophytoma
bacterioprotein
bacteriopsonin

bacteriosis
bacteriospermia
bacteriostasis
bacteriostat
bacteriostatic
bacteriotoxic
bacteriotropic
    b. substance
bacteriotropin
bacteriotrypsin
Bacterium
bacterium, pl. **bacteria**
    Binn's b.
    blue-green b.
    Chauveau's b.
    endoteric b.
    exoteric b.
    lysogenic b.
    pyogenic b.
bacteriuria
bacteroid
Bacteroidaceae
Bacteroides
    B. *bivius*
    B. *capillosus*
    B. *corrodens*
    B. *disiens*
    B. *fragilis*
    B. *furcosus*
    B. *melaninogenicus*
    B. *nodosus*
    B. *oralis*
    B. *oris*
    B. *pneumosintes*
    B. *praeacutus*
    B. *putredinis*
    B. *thetaiotamicron*
    B. *ureolyticus*
baculiform
Baculoviridae
baculovirus
Baehr-Lohlein lesion
Baelz' disease
Baer's
    B. law
    B. vesicle
bag
    Ambu b.
    breathing b.
    colostomy b.
    Douglas b.
    nuclear b.
    Petersen's b.
    Politzer b.
    reservoir b.
    b. of waters
bagassosis
Bagdad boil

bag-gel implant
Baggenstoss change
Bagolini test
bahnung
Baillarger's
    B. bands
    B. lines
Bailliart's ophthalmodynamometer
Bainbridge reflex
baked tongue
Baker's
    B. acid hematein
    B. cyst
    B. pyridine extraction
baker's
    b. eczema
    h. itch
balance
    occlusal b.
    b. theory
    Wilhelmy b.
balanced
    b. anesthesia
    b. articulation
    b. bite
    b. diet
    b. occlusion
    b. polymorphism
    b. translocation
balancing
    b. contact
    b. occlusal surface
    b. side
    b. side condyle
balanic
    b. hypospadias
balanitic epispadias
balanitis
    b. circumscripta plasmacellularis
    b. diabetica
    plasma cell b.
    b. xerotica obliterans
    b. of Zoon
balanoplasty
balanoposthitis
balantidial dysentery
balantidiasis
Balantidium
    B. *coli*
    B. *suis*
balantidosis
balanus
BALB test
bald
    b. tongue
baldness
    common b.
    congenital b.

baldness *(continued)*
    male pattern b.
    pubic b.
Baldy's operation
Balint's syndrome
Balkan
    B. beam
    B. frame
    B. nephropathy
    B. splint
ball
    chondrin b.
    b. of the foot
    fungus b.
    b. thrombus
    b. valve
    b. valve action
    b. variance
Ballance's sign
ball-and-socket joint
ballerina-foot pattern
ballet
    cardiac b.
ballism
ballismus
ballistocardiogram
ballistocardiograph
ballistocardiography
ballistophobia
balloon
    angioplasty b.
    b. atrioseptostomy
    b. catheter
    b. cell
    b. cell nevus
    b. counter pulsation
    detachable b.
    intra-aortic b.
    b. sickness
ballooning degeneration
balloonseptostomy
balloon-tip catheter
ballottable
ballottement
    abdominal b.
    renal b.
Ball's operation
ball-valve thrombus
balneotherapeutics, balneotherapy
Baló's disease
Baltic myoclonus disease
Bamberger-Marie
    B.-M. disease
    B.-M. syndrome
Bamberger's
    B. albuminuria
    B. disease
    B. sign

bamboo
    b. hair
    b. spine
bancroftian filariasis
bancroftiasis, bancroftosis
band
    A b.'s
    amniotic b.'s
    annular b.
    anogenital b.
    atrioventricular b.
    Baillarger's b.'s
    b. bands
    Bechterew's b.
    Broca's diagonal b.
    b. cell
    chromosome b.
    Clado's b.
    b.'s of colon
    contraction b.
    Essick's cell b.'s
    Gennari's b.
    b. of Giacomini
    H b.
    His' b.
    Hunter-Schreger b.'s
    I b.
    iliotibial b.
    b. of Kaes-Bechterew
    Ladd's b.
    Lane's b.
    longitudinal b.'s of cruciform
      ligament
    M b.
    Mach's b.
    Maissiat's b.
    matrix b.
    Meckel's b.
    moderator b.
    b. neutrophil
    oligoclonal b.
    orthodontic b.
    pecten b.
    Reil's b.
    silastic b.
    Simonart's b.'s
    Soret b.
    Streeter's b.'s
    uncus b. of Giacomini
    ventricular b. of larynx
    Z b.
    zonular b.
bandage
    adhesive b.
    Barton's b.
    capeline b.
    circular b.
    cravat b.

crucial b.
demigauntlet b.
Desault's b.
elastic b.
Esmarch b.
figure-of-8 b.
four-tailed b.
gauntlet b.
gauze b.
Gibney's fixation b.
Gibson's b.
hammock b.
immovable b.
Martin's b.
oblique b.
plaster b.
roller b.
scarf b.
Scultetus' b.
b. sign
spica b.
spiral b.
suspensory b.
T-b.
triangular b.
Velpeau's b.
bandbox resonance
banding
BrDu-b.
high-resolution b.
NOR-b.
prometaphase b.
pulmonary artery b.
reverse b.
Bandl's ring
bandpass filter
band-shaped keratopathy
bandwidth
bandy-leg
Bang's bacillus
bank
blood b.
eye b.
Bannister's disease
Bannwarth's syndrome
Banti's
B. disease
B. syndrome
bar
arch b.
b. of bladder
clasp b.
b. clasp
b. clasp arm
b. clip attachments
b. joint denture
labial b.
lingual b.

median b. of Mercier
Mercier's b.
occlusal rest b.
palatal b.
Passavant's b.
prism b.
sternal b.
terminal b.
baragnosis
Bárány's
B. caloric test
B. sign
barba
Barbados leg
barbed broach
barber's
b. itch
b. pilonidal sinus
barbiero
barbotage
barbula hirci
Barclay-Baron disease
Barcoo
B. rot
B. vomit
Barcroft-Warburg
B.-W. apparatus
B.-W. technique
Bardet-Biedl syndrome
Bardinet's ligament
bare
b. area of liver
b. area of stomach
b. lymphocyte syndrome
baresthesia
baresthesiometer
bariatric
bariatrics
baritosis
barium
b. enema
b. meal
b. swallow
Barkan's operation
Barkman's reflex
Barkow's ligaments
Barlow
B. disease
B. syndrome
Barnes
Barnes'
B. curve
B. dystrophy
B. zone
baroceptor
barognosis
barograph
barometrograph

B

91

barophilic
baroreceptor
    b. nerve
baroreflex
baroscope
barosinusitis
barostat
barotaxis
barotitis media
barotrauma
    otic b.
    sinus b.
barotropism
Barraquer's
    B. disease
    B. method
Barr chromatin body
barrel chest
barrel-shaped thorax
barren
Barré's sign
Barrett's
    B. epithelium
    B. esophagus
    B. syndrome
barrier
    blood-air b.
    blood-aqueous b.
    blood-brain b.
    blood-cerebrospinal fluid b., blood-
      CSF b.
    b. contraceptive
    incest b.
    placental b.
bar-sleeve attachments
bartholinitis
Bartholin's
    B. abscess
    B. anus
    B. cyst
    B. cystectomy
    B. duct
    B. gland
Barth's hernia
Bartonella
    B. anemia
    B. bacilliformis
bartonellosis
Barton's
    B. bandage
    B. forceps
    B. fracture
Bart's syndrome
Bartter's syndrome
Baruch's law
baruria
basad

basal
    b. age
    b. anesthesia
    b. body
    b. body temperature
    b. bone
    b. cell
    b. cell adenoma
    b. cell carcinoma
    b. cell epithelioma
    b. cell hyperplasia
    b. cell layer
    b. cell nevus
    b. cell nevus syndrome
    b. cell papilloma
    b. cistern
    b. corpuscle
    b. diet
    b. ganglia
    b. gland
    b. granule
    b. joint reflex
    b. lamina
    b. lamina of choroid
    b. lamina of ciliary body
    b. lamina of cochlear
    b. lamina of neural tube
    b. lamina of semicircular duct
    b. layer
    b. layer of choroid
    b. layer of ciliary body
    b. membrane of semicircular duct
    b. nuclei
    b. nucleus of Ganser
    b. part of occipital bone
    b. part of pulmonary artery
    b. plate of neural tube
    b. ridge
    b. rod
    b. seat
    b. seat area
    b. skull fracture
    b. sphincter
    b. squamous cell carcinoma
    b. striations
    b. surface
    b. tentorial branch of internal
      carotid artery
    b. tuberculosis
    b. vein of Rosenthal
    b. veins
basalioma
basalis
    norma b.
basaloid
    b. carcinoma
    b. cell
basaloma

basal ration
Basan's syndrome
base
    acrylic resin b.
    anterior cranial b.
    b. of arytenoid cartilage
    b. of bladder
    b. of brain
    cavity preparation b.
    cement b.
    b. of cochlea
    cranial b.
    b. deficit
    denture b.
    b. excess
    external b. of skull
    b. of heart
    b. hospital
    b. of hyoid bone
    internal b. of skull
    b. line
    b. of lung
    b. of mandible
    b. material
    b. of metacarpal bone
    metal b.
    b. of metatarsal bone
    b. of modiolus
    b. of patella
    b. of phalanx
    b. plate
    b. projection
    b. of prostate
    record b.
    b. of renal pyramid
    b. of sacrum
    shellac b.
    b. of skull
    b. of stapes
    temporary b.
    tinted denture b.
    b. of tongue
    tooth-borne b.
    trial b.
    b. view
baseball finger
basedoid
basedowian
Basedow's
    B. disease
    B. goiter
    B. pseudoparaplegia
baseline
    b. fetal heart rate
    b. tonus
    b. variability of fetal heart rate

basement
    b. lamina
    b. membrane
baseplate
    stabilized b.
    b. wax
base-stacking
bas-fond
basialis
basialveolar
basibregmatic axis
basic
    b. diet
    b. dyes
    b. electrical rhythm
    b. esotropia
    b. exotropia
    b. fuchsin
    b. fuchsin-methylene blue stain
    b. life support
    b. personality
    b. personality type
    b. stain
basicranial
    b. axis
    b. flexure
basidia (*pl. of* basidium)
Basidiobolus
Basidiomycetes
Basidiomycota
basidiospore
basidium, pl. basidia
basifacial
    b. axis
basihyal
basihyoid
basilar, basilaris
    b. angle
    b. apophysis
    b. artery
    b. bone
    b. cartilage
    b. cell
    b. crest of cochlear duct
    b. fibrocartilage
    b. impression
    b. index
    b. invagination
    b. lamina
    b. leptomeningitis
    b. membrane
    b. meningitis
    b. migraine
    b. part of the occipital bone
    b. part of pons
    b. plexus
    b. pontine sulcus
    b. process

basilar *(continued)*
    b. process of occipital bone
    b. prognathism
    b. sinus
    b. sulcus
    b. vertebra
basilateral
basilemma
basilicus
basilic vein
basin
    emesis b., kidney b.
    pus b.
basinasal
    b. line
basioccipital
    b. bone
basiocciput
basioglossus
basion
basipetal
basipharyngeal canal
basiphobia
basis
    b. cartilaginis arytenoideae
    b. cerebri
    b. cochleae
    b. cordis
    b. cranii
    b. cranii externa
    b. cranii interna
    b. mandibulae
    b. modioli
    b. ossis metacarpalis
    b. ossis metatarsalis
    b. ossis sacri
    b. patellae
    b. pedunculi
    b. phalangis
    b. prostatae
    b. pulmonis
    b. pyramidis renis
    b. stapedis
basisphenoid
    b. bone
basisquamous carcinoma
basitemporal
basivertebral
    b. vein
basket
    b. cell
    fibrillar b.'s
    stone b.
Basle Nomina Anatomica
basocyte
basocytopenia
basocytosis
basoerythrocyte

basoerythrocytosis
basograph
basolateral
basometachromophil,
    basometachromophile
basopenia
basophil, basophile
    b. adenoma
    b. cell of anterior lobe of
      hypophysis
    b. granule
    b. substance
    tissue b.
basophilia
    Grawitz' b.
    punctate b.
basophilic
    b. degeneration
    b. leukemia
    b. leukocyte
    b. leukocytosis
    b. leukopenia
    b. substance
basophilism
    Cushing's b.
    Cushing's pituitary b.
basophilocyte
basophilocytic leukemia
basoplasm
basosquamous carcinoma
Bassen-Kornzweig syndrome
Bassini's operation
Bassler's sign
Bastedo's sign
bat ear
bath
    colloid b.
    contrast b.
    douche b.
    dousing b.
    electric b., electrotherapeutic b.
    Greville b.
    hafussi b.
    hydroelectric b.
    immersion b.
    b. itch
    light b.
    Nauheim b.
    needle b.
    b. pruritus
    sitz b.
bathing trunk nevus
bathmotropic
    negatively b.
    positively b.
bathophobia
bathyanesthesia
bathycardia

B

bathyesthesia
bathygastry
bathyhyperesthesia
bathyhypesthesia
Batson's plexus
Batten disease
Batten-Mayou disease
battered
    b. child syndrome
    b. spouse syndrome
battery
    Halstead-Reitan b.
Battey bacillus
battle
    b. fatigue
    b. neurosis
battledore placenta
Battle's sign
Baudelocque's
    B. diameter
    B. operation
    B. uterine circle
Bauer's
    B. chromic acid leucofuchsin stain
    B. syndrome
Bauhin's
    B. gland
    B. valve
Baumès symptom
Baumgarten's
    B. glands
    B. veins
bauxite pneumoconiosis
bay
    celomic b.
    lacrimal b.
    b. sore
Bayesian hypothesis
Bayes theorem
Bayle's disease
Bayley Scales of Infant Development
bayonet
    b. forceps
    b. hair
Bazett's formula
Bazex's syndrome
Bazin's disease
B-cell
    B.-c. differentiating factor
    B.-c. stimulatory factor 2
Be^a antigens
beaded
    b. hair
beading
    b. of the ribs
beak
    b. sign
beaked pelvis

beaker cell
Beale's cell
beam
    Balkan b.
    cantilever b.
    continuous b.
    electron b.
    restrained b.
    simple b.
bearing
    central b.
bearing down
bearing-down pain
beat
    apex b.
    atrial capture b.
    atrial fusion b.
    automatic b.
    combination b.
    coupled b.'s
    dependent b.
    Dressler b.
    dropped b.
    echo b.
    ectopic b.
    escape b., escaped b.
    forced b.
    fusion b.
    heart b.
    interference b.
    mixed b.
    paired b.'s
    parasystolic b.
    premature b.
    pseudofusion b.
    reciprocal b.
    retrograde b.
    summation b.
    ventricular fusion b.
beat-to-beat variability of fetal heart rate
Beau's lines
Beauvaria
Bechterew-Mendel reflex
Bechterew's
    B. band
    B. disease
    B. nucleus
    B. sign
Becker
    B. antigen
    B. disease
    B. nevus
    B. stain for spirochetes
    B. type muscular dystrophy
    B. type tardive muscular dystrophy
Becker's
Beckmann's apparatus

95

Beck's
 B. method
 B. triad
Beckwith-Wiedemann syndrome
Béclard's
 B. anastomosis
 B. hernia
 B. triangle
Becquerel rays
bed
 b. of breast
 capillary b.
 fracture b.
 Gatch b.
 mud b.
 nail b.
 parotid b.
 b. rest
 b. sore
 b. of stomach
 water b.
bedbug
bedlam
bedlamism
Bednar
 B. aphthae
 B. tumor
bedside radiography
bedsore
bed-wetting
beer heart
Beer's
 B. knife
 B. law
beeturia
Beevor's sign
Begbie's disease
**Begg light wire differential force
 technique**
Béguez César disease
behavior
 adaptive b.
 adient b.
 ambient b.
 appetitive b.
 aversive b.
 b. chain
 coronary-prone b.
 b. disorder
 health b.
 hookean b.
 b. modification
 molar b.
 molecular b.
 obsessive b.
 operant b.
 passive-aggressive b.
 b. reflex

 respondent b.
 ritualistic b.
 target b.
 b. therapy
 type A b.
 type B b.
behavioral
 b. epidemic
 b. genetics
 b. health
 b. immunogen
 b. manifestation
 b. medicine
 b. pathogen
 b. psychology
behavioral sciences
behaviorism
behaviorist
behavioristic psychology
Behçet's
 B. disease
 B. syndrome
Behring's law
Behr's
 B. disease
 B. syndrome
being
 b. beaten
 b. buried alive
 b. dirty
 b. locked in
 b. stared at
 b. touched
BEI test
bejel
Békésy
 B. audiometer
 B. audiometry
bel
belching
belemnoid
Belgian Congo anemia
bell
 b. clapper deformity
 b. sound
 b. stage
bell-crowned
belle indifference
Bellini's
 B. ducts
 B. ligament
Bell-Magendie law
bellmetal resonance
bellows murmur
Bell's
 B. law
 B. muscle
 B. palsy

B. phenomenon
B. respiratory nerve
B. spasm
bell-shaped crown
belly
anterior b. of digastric muscle
b. button
b.'s of digastric muscle
frontal b. of occipitofrontalis
  muscle
inferior b. of omohyoid b.
occipital b. of occipitofrontalis
  muscle
b.'s of omohyoid muscle
posterior b. of digastric muscle
prune b.
superior b. of omohyoid muscle
bellyache
belonephobia
Belsey
B. Mark IV operation
B. Mark IV procedure
B. Mark V procedure
belt test
Bence
B. Jones cylinders
B. Jones myeloma
B. Jones proteinuria
bench testing
Bender
B. gestalt test
B. Visual Motor Gestalt test
bending fracture
bends
beneceptor
Benedek's reflex
Benedict-Roth
B.-R. apparatus
B.-R. calorimeter
Benedict's
B. solution
B. test for glucose
Benedikt's syndrome
beneficence
benign
b. albuminuria
b. bone aneurysm
b. cementoblastoma
b. childhood epilepsy with
  centrotemporal spikes
b. dry pleurisy
b. dyskeratosis
b. essential tremor
b. familial chorea
b. familial chronic pemphigus
b. familial icterus
b. giant lymph node hyperplasia
b. glycosuria

b. hypertension
b. inoculation lymphoreticulosis
b. inoculation reticulosis
b. juvenile melanoma
b. lymphadenosis
b. lymphocytoma cutis
b. lymphoepithelial lesion
b. lymphoma of the rectum
b. mesenchymoma
b. mesothelioma
b. mesothelioma of genital tract
b. migratory glossitis
b. mucosal pemphigoid
b. myalgic encephalomyelitis
b. neonatal convulsions
b. nephrosclerosis
b. paroxysmal peritonitis
b. paroxysmal postural vertigo
b. positional vertigo
b. prostatic hypertrophy
b. stupor
b. tertian malaria
b. tetanus
b. tumor
Bennett
B. angle
B. fracture
B. movement
Bennhold's Congo red stain
Bensley's specific granules
bentiromide
b. test
bentonite flocculation test
benzeneamine
benzidine test
benzopurpurin 4B
Beradinelli's syndrome
Bérard's aneurysm
Béraud's valve
bereavement
Berger
B. cells
B. disease
B. focal glomerulonephritis
B. rhythm
B. space
Bergmann's
B. cords
B. fibers
Bergmeister's papilla
Berg's stain
beriberi, beri beri
dry b.
b. heart
infantile b.
ship b.
wet b.
Berkefeld filter

Berlin
    B. blue
    B. edema
berlock dermatitis
berloque dermatitis
Bernard-Horner syndrome
Bernard's
    B. canal
    B. duct
    B. puncture
Bernard-Sergent syndrome
Bernard-Soulier syndrome
Bernays' sponge
Bernhardt-Roth syndrome
Bernhardt's
    B. disease
    B. formula
Bernheim's syndrome
Bernoulli
    B. distribution
    B. trial
Bernstein test
berry
    b. aneurysm
    b. cell
Berry's ligaments
Berson test
Berthelot reaction
Bertin's
    B. bones
    B. columns
    B. ligament
    B. ossicles
beryllium granuloma
Besnier-Boeck-Schaumann
    B.-B.-S. disease
    B.-B.-S. syndrome
Besnier's prurigo
Besnoitia
Besnoitiidae
bestiality
Best's
    B. carmine stain
    B. disease
beta
    b. alcoholism
    b. angle
    b. cell of anterior lobe of
      hypophysis
    b. cell of pancreas
    b. error
    b. fibers
    b. granule
    b. radiation
    b. rhythm
    b. sheets
    B. tests
    b. wave

betacism
betacyaninuria
betatron
betel cancer
Bethesda
    B. system
    B. unit
Bethesda-Ballerup Group
Betke-Kleihauer test
Bettendorff's test
Betz cells
Beuren syndrome
Bevan-Lewis cells
bevel
    cavosurface b.
    reverse b.
bevelled anastomosis
Bezold-Jarisch reflex
Bezold's
    B. abscess
    B. ganglion
    B. mastoiditis
    B. sign
    B. symptom
    B. triad
BH interval
Bianchi's
    B. nodule
    B. valve
Bi antigen
biarticular
bias
biasterionic
biauricular
    b. axis
biaxial joint
bibliomania
bicameral
    b. abscess
bicanalicular sphincter
BICAP cautery
bicapsular
bicarbonate
    standard b.
bicardiogram
bicellular
bicephalus
biceps
    b. brachii muscle
    b. femoris muscle
    b. femoris reflex
    b. muscle of arm
    b. muscle of thigh
    b. reflex
Bichat's
    B. canal
    B. fat-pad
    B. fissure

B. foramen
B. fossa
B. ligament
B. membrane
B. protuberance
B. tunic
bicho
biciliate
bicipital
    b. aponeurosis
    b. fascia
    b. groove
    b. rib
    b. ridges
    b. tuberosity
bicipitoradial bursa
Bickel's ring
biclonal
    b. gammopathy
    b. peak
biclonality
biconcave
    b. lens
bicondylar
    b. articulation
    b. joint
biconvex
    b. lens
bicornous, bicornate, bicornuate
bicoudate catheter
bicuspid
    b. aortic valve
    b. tooth
    b. valve
bicuspidization
bidactyly
bidet
bidirectional ventricular tachycardia
bidiscoidal
    b. placenta
biduous
Biebl loop
Biederman's sign
Bielschowsky's
    B. disease
    B. sign
    B. stain
Biemond syndrome
Biermer's
    B. anemia
    B. disease
    B. sign
Biernacki's sign
Bier's
    B. amputation
    B. hyperemia
    B. method
Biesiadecki's fossa

bifascicular
bifid
    b. cranium
    b. penis
    b. rib
    b. thumb
    b. tongue
    b. uterus
    b. uvula
Bifidobacterium
    B. bifidum
bifidus factor
bifocal
    b. lens
    b. spectacles
biforate
    b. uterus
bifoveal fixation
bifurcate, bifurcated
    b. ligament
bifurcatio
    b. aortae
    b. tracheae
    b. trunci pulmonalis
bifurcation
    b. of aorta
    b. lymph nodes
    b. of pulmonary trunk
    b. of trachea
Bigelow's
    B. ligament
    B. septum
bigemina
bigeminal
    b. bodies
    b. pregnancy
    b. pulse
    b. rhythm
bigemini
bigeminum
bigeminy
    atrial b.
    atrioventricular junctional b.
    escape-capture b.
    nodal b.
    reciprocal b.
    ventricular b.
bigerminal
bilabe
bilaminar blastoderm
bilateral
    b. hermaphroditism
    b. left-sidedness
    b. lithotomy
    b. medial orbital ecchymoses
    b. pleurisy
    b. synchrony
bilateralism

bile
A b.
b. acid tolerance test
B b.
C b.
b. capillary
b. cyst
b. duct
b. esculin test
b. gastritis
b. papilla
b. peritonitis
b. salt agar
b. solubility test
b. thrombus
white b.
bi-leaflet valve
Bile's antigen
Bilharzia
bilharzial
b. appendicitis
b. dysentery
b. granuloma
bilharziasis
bilharzioma
bilharziosis
biliary
b. atresia
b. calculus
b. canaliculus
b. cirrhosis
b. colic
b. duct
b. ductules
b. dyskinesia
b. fistula
b. steatorrhea
b. xanthomatosis
bilifaction, bilification
biliferous
biligenesis
biligenic
bilious
b. headache
b. pneumonia
b. remittent fever
b. remittent malaria
b. typhoid of Griesinger
b. vomit
biliousness
biliptysis
bilirachia
bilirubin
conjugated b.
direct reacting b.
b. encephalopathy
indirect reacting b.
unconjugated b.

bilirubinemia
bilirubinuria
bilitherapy
biliuria
billowing mitral valve syndrome
Billroth
B. cords
B. I anastomosis
B. II anastomosis
B. operation I
B. operation II
B. venae cavernosae
Bill's maneuver
bilobate, bilobed
bilobectomy
bilobular
bilocular, biloculate
b. femoral hernia
b. joint
b. stomach
bimanual
b. palpation
b. percussion
b. version
bimastoid
bimaxillary
b. dentoalveolar protrusion
b. protrusion
b. protrusive occlusion
binangle
b. chisel
binary
b. combination
b. digit
b. fission
b. process
binasal hemianopia
binaural
b. alternate loudness balance test
b. stethoscope
binauricular arc
bind
double b.
binder
obstetrical b.
T-b.
binding constant
Binet
B. age
B. scale
B. test
Binet-Simon scale
Bingham
B. flow
B. model
B. plastic
Bing's reflex
Binn's bacterium

binocular
    b. fixation
    b. heterochromia
    b. loupe
    b. microscope
    b. ophthalmoscope
    b. parallax
    b. rivalry
    b. vision
binomial
    b. distribution
binotic
Binswanger's
    B. disease
    B. encephalopathy
binuclear, binucleate
binucleolate
Binz' test
bioacoustics
bioastronautics
biochemical
    b. metastasis
    b. profile
biochemical pathway (*var. of* pathway)
biocidal
bioelectric potential
bioengineering
biofeedback
    EMG b.
biogenetic
    b. law
biogravics
bioinstrument
biokinetics
biologic
    b. evolution
    b. hemolysis
    b. time
biological
    b. coefficient
    b. half-life
    b. immunotherapy
    b. psychiatry
    b. sampling
    b. vector
biology
    cellular b.
    oral b.
    radiation b.
biomechanics
    dental b.
biomedical
    b. engineering
    b. model
biometrical school
biometry
    b. fetal
biomicroscope

biomicroscopy
Biomphalaria
Biondi-Heidenhain stain
bionecrosis
biophage
biophagism
biophagous
biophagy
biophilia
biophotometer
biophylactic
biophylaxis
biophysical profile
biophysics
    dental b.
bioplasm
bioplasmic
biopsy
    aspiration b.
    brush b.
    chorionic villus b.
    endoscopic b.
    excision b.
    fine needle b.
    incision b.
    needle b.
    b. needle
    open b.
    punch b.
    shave b.
    sponge b.
    trephine b.
    wedge b.
biopsychology
biopsychosocial
    b. model
bioptome
biopyoculture
biorbital
    b. angle
biorheology
biorhythm
bioroentgenography
biosafety
biosocial
biostatics
biotelemetry
biotic
    b. factors
    b. potential
biotropism
Biot's
    B. breathing
    B. breathing sign
    B. respiration
    B. sign
biotype
biovar

biovular
biparasitism
biparietal
    b. diameter
bipartite
    b. uterus
    b. vagina
bipedicle flap
bipennate, bipenniform
    b. muscle
biperforate
biphasic response
biphenotypic
biphenotypy
biplane angiography
bipolar
    b. cautery
    b. cell
    b. disorder
    b. lead
    b. neuron
    b. psychosis
    b. taxis
    b. version
bipotentiality
biramous
Birbeck's granule
Birch-Hirschfeld stain
bird
    b. face
    b. nest filter
    b. shot retinochoroiditis
bird-breeder's
    b.-b. disease
    b.-b. lung
bird-fancier's lung
birdseed agar
Bird's sign
birefringence
birefringent
Birnaviridae
Birnavirus
birth
    b. amputation
    b. canal
    b. certificate
    b. control
    cross b.
    b. defect
    b. fracture
    b. of malformed fetus
    b. palsy
    premature b.
    b. rate
    b. trauma
    b. weight
birthmark
    strawberry b.

bisacromial
bisalbuminemia
bisaxillary
Bischof's myelotomy
biscuit
    b. bite
biscuit-bake
biscuit-firing
bisexual
bisferient
bisferious
    b. pulse
Bishop's sphygmoscope
bisiliac
Biskra
    B. boil
    B. button
Bismarck
    B. brown R
    B. brown Y
bismuth
    b. iodide
    b. line
    b. triiodide
bistephanic
bistoury
bistratal
bit
bite
    b. analysis
    balanced b.
    biscuit b.
    close b.
    closed b.
    deep b.
    edge-to-edge b.
    end-to-end b.
    b. fork
    b. gauge
    jumping the b.
    locked b.
    normal b.
    open b.
    b. plane
    rest b.
    b. rim
    working b.
bitemporal
    b. hemianopia
biteplate, biteplane
bites
bitewing
    b. film
    b. radiograph
biting
    b. louse
    b. pressure
    b. strength

Bitot's spots
bitrochanteric
bitropic
Bittner
    B. agent
    B. milk factor
    B. virus
Bittorf's reaction
biundulant meningoencephalitis
biuret test
bivalent
    b. antibody
    b. chromosome
bivalve speculum
biventer
    b. cervicis
    b. lobule
    b. mandibulae
biventral
    b. lobule
biventricular
Bixler type hypertelorism
bizygomatic
Bizzozero's
    B. corpuscle
    B. red cells
Bjerrum
    B. scotoma
    B. screen
    B. sign
Bjork-Shiley valve
Bjornstad's syndrome
BK virus
black
    b. box
    b. cataract
    b. currant rash
    b. death
    b. eye
    b. fever
    b. heel
    b. line
    b. lung
    b. measles
    b. piedra
    b. plague
    b. sickness
    b. spore
    b. tarantula
    b. tongue
    b. urine
    b. vomit
black-dot ringworm
blackout
    visual b.
Black's
    B. classification
    B. formula

blackwater fever
bladder
    atonic b.
    autonomic neurogenic b.
    b. calculi
    b. compliance
    gall b.
    hyperreflexic b.
    hypertonic b.
    ileal b.
    neurogenic b.
    neuropathic b.
    nonneurogenic neurogenic b.
    poorly compliant b.
    pseudoneurogenic b.
    b. reflex
    reflex neurogenic b.
    b. schistosomiasis
    b. stone
    trabeculated b.
    uninhibited neurogenic b.
    unstable b.
    urinary b.
bladderworm
blade bone
bladevent
blain
Blainville ears
Blair-Brown graft
Blalock-Hanlon operation
Blalock shunt
Blalock-Taussig
    B.-T. operation
    B.-T. shunt
bland
    b. diet
    b. embolism
    b. infarct
Blandin's gland
blank
blanket suture
Blasius' duct
blast
    b. cell
    b. crisis
    b. injury
blastema
    metanephric b.
    nephric b.
blastemic
blastic
blastocele
blastocelic
blastocoele
blastocoelic
Blastoconidium
blastocyst

B

Blastocystis
 B. hominis
blastocyte
blastocytoma
blastoderm, blastoderma
 bilaminar b.
 embryonic b.
 extraembryonic b.
 trilaminar b.
blastodermal, blastodermic
blastodisk
blastogenesis
blastogenetic, blastogenic
blastolysis
blastolytic
blastoma
blastomere
blastomerotomy
blastomogenic
Blastomyces dermatitidis
blastomycetic dermatitis
blastomycosis
 Brazilian b.
 cutaneous b.
 North American b.
 South American b.
 systemic b.
blastoneuropore
blastophore
blastopore
blastoporic canal
blastospore
blastotomy
blastula
blastular
blastulation
Blatin's syndrome
Blatta
Blattella
Blattidae
blear eye
bleary eye
bleb
bleed
bleeder
bleeding
 dysfunctional uterine b.
 occult b.
 b. polyp
 b. time
blemish
blending inheritance
blennadenitis
blennemesis
blennogenic
blennogenous
blennoid
blennophthalmia

blennorrhagia
blennorrhagic
blennorrhea
 b. conjunctivalis
 inclusion b.
 b. neonatorum
 Stoerk's b.
blennorrheal
 b. conjunctivitis
blennostasis
blennostatic
blennuria
blepharadenitis
blepharal
blepharectomy
blepharedema
blepharitis
 b. acarica
 b. angularis
 ciliary b.
 demodectic b.
 b. follicularis
 marginal b.
 b. marginalis
 meibomian b.
 b. oleosa
 b. parasitica
 pediculous b.
 b. phthiriatica
 pustular b.
 b. rosacea
 seborrheic b.
 b. sicca
 b. squamosa
 b. ulcerosa
blepharoadenitis
blepharoadenoma
blepharochalasis
blepharochromidrosis
blepharoclonus
blepharocoloboma
blepharoconjunctivitis
 seborrheic b.
blepharodiastasis
blepharokeratoconjunctivitis
blepharon
blepharophimosis
blepharoplast
blepharoplastic
blepharoplasty
blepharoplegia
blepharoptosis, blepharoptosia
 b. adiposa
 false b.
blepharospasm, blepharospasmus
blepharostat
blepharostenosis
blepharosynechia

blepharotomy
blighted ovum
blind
    b. boil
    b. enema
    b. fistula
    b. foramen of frontal bone
    b. foramen of the tongue
    b. gut
    b. headache
    b. loop syndrome
    b. nasotracheal intubation
    b. passage
    b. spot
    b. study
    b. test
blinding
    b. disease
    b. glare
blindness
    color b.
    cortical b.
    day b.
    eclipse b.
    flash b.
    flight b.
    functional b.
    hysterical b.
    legal b.
    letter b.
    mind b.
    music b.
    night b.
    note b.
    object b.
    psychic b.
    river b.
    sight b.
    sign b.
    snow b.
    solar b.
    taste b.
    text b., word b.
blister
    blood b.
    fever b.
    fly b.
    flying b.
blistering
    b. distal dactylitis
Bloch-Sulzberger
    B.-S. disease
    B.-S. syndrome
block
    alveolocapillary b.
    b. anesthesia
    anterograde b.
    arborization b.

    atrioventricular b., A-V b.
    bone b.
    bundle-branch b.
    complete A-V b.
    conduction b.
    congenital heart b.
    depolarizing b.
    b. design test
    entrance b.
    epidural b.
    exit b.
    fascicular b.
    field b.
    first degree A-V b.
    heart b.
    incomplete atrioventricular b.
    intra-atrial b.
    intraventricular b., I-V b.
    Mobitz b.
    Mobitz types of atrioventricular b.
    nerve b.
    nondepolarizing b.
    partial heart b.
    peri-infarction b.
    phase I b.
    phase II b.
    protective b.
    retrograde b.
    second degree A-V b.
    sinoatrial b., S-A b., sinus b.
    sinoauricular b.
    spinal b.
    stellate b.
    suprahisian b.
    unidirectional b.
    b. vertebrae
    Wenckebach b.
    Wilson b.
    Wolff-Chaikoff b.
blockade
    virus b.
blocked aerogastria
blocking
    b. activity
    alpha b.
    b. antibody
block-out
Blocq's disease
blood
    b. agar
    arterial b.
    b. bank
    b. blister
    b. calculus
    b. capillary
    b. cast
    b. cell
    b. circulation

blood *(continued)*
    b. clot
    cord b.
    b. corpuscle
    b. count
    b. crisis
    b. crystals
    b. cyst
    b. disk
    b. dust
    b. dyscrasia
    b. gas analysis
    b. gases
    b. group
    b. group agglutinins
    b. group agglutinogens
    b. group antibodies
    b. group antigen
    b. group antiserums
    b. grouping
    b. group substance
    b. group systems
    b. island
    b. islet
    laky b.
    b. lymph
    b. mole
    b. motes
    occult b.
    b. pH
    b. plasma fractions
    b. plastid
    b. plate
    b. pool imaging
    b. pressure
    b. puzzles
    b. relationship
    b. relative
    b. serum
    sludged b.
    b. spots
    b. substitute
    b. tumor
    b. type
    b. urea nitrogen
    venous b.
    b. vessel
    b. volume nomogram
blood-air barrier
blood-aqueous barrier
blood-brain barrier
blood-cerebrospinal fluid barrier
blood count
    complete b. c.
    differential white b. c.
    Schilling's b. c.
blood-CSF barrier

blood group
    ABO b. g.
    Auberger b. g., Au b. g.
    CDE b. g.
    Diego b. g.
    Dombrock b. g.
    Duffy b. g.
    Fy b. g.
    Jk b. g.
    K b. g., k b. g.
    Kell b. g.
    Kidd b. g.
    Lewis B. g., Le B. g.
    Lutheran B. g., Lu B. g.
    MNSs b. g.
    private b. g.
    Sutter b. g.
    Xg b. g.
bloodless
    b. amputation
    b. decerebration
    b. operation
    b. phlebotomy
bloodletting
    general b.
    local b.
bloodshot
bloodstream
blood-vascular system
blood vessel
    retinal b. v.'s
bloodworm
Bloom's syndrome
blot
blotch
blotting
Blount-Barber disease
Blount's disease
blowfly
blow-out fracture
blowout pipette
blubber finger
blue
    b. asphyxia
    b. atrophy
    b. baby
    bromphenol b.
    b. cataract
    b. cone monochromatism
    b. disease
    b. dome cyst
    b. dot sign
    b. edema
    b. fever
    b. line
    b. nevus
    b. pus
    b. pus bacillus

B

b. rubber-bleb nevi
b. sclera
b. spot
b. toe syndrome
b. vision
blueberry muffin baby
blue-green
b.-g. algae
b.-g. bacterium
bluetongue virus
Blumberg's sign
Blumenau's nucleus
Blumenbach's clivus
Blumer's shelf
blunt duct adenosis
blunted affect
blush
B-mode
B.-m. echocardiography
boat-shaped abdomen
bobbing
inverse ocular b.
ocular b.
Bochdalek's
B. foramen
B. ganglion
B. gap
B. hernia
B. muscle
B. valve
Bockhart's impetigo
Bock's
B. ganglion
B. nerve
Bödecker index
Bodian's copper-PROTARGOL stain
Bodo
B. caudatus
B. saltans
B. urinarius
body
adrenal b.
alcoholic hyaline b.'s
Alder b.'s
alveolar b.
amygdaloid b.
amyloid b.'s of the prostate
anococcygeal b.
anterior quadrigeminal b.
aortic b.'s
Arnold's b.'s
asbestos b.'s
Aschoff b.'s
asteroid b.
Auer b.'s
Babès-Ernst b.'s
Barr chromatin b.
basal b.

bigeminal b.'s
brassy b.
b. burden
Cabot's ring b.'s
Call-Exner b.'s
cancer b.'s
carotid b.
b. of caudate nucleus
cavernous b. of clitoris
cavernous b. of penis
b. cavity
cell b.
central b.
central fibrous b.
chromaffin b.
chromatin b.
ciliary b.
Civatte b.'s
b. of clavicle
b. of clitoris
coccygeal b.
colloid b.'s
compressible cavernous b.'s
conchoidal b.'s
Councilman b., Councilman hyaline b.
Cowdry's type A inclusion b.'s
Cowdry's type B inclusion b.'s
creola b.'s
cyanobacterium-like b.'s
cytoid b.'s
cytoplasmic inclusion b.'s
Deetjen's b.'s
demilune b.
Döhle b.'s
Donovan's b.'s
b. dysmorphic disorder
Ehrlich's inner b.
elementary b.'s
b. of epididymis
epithelial b.
fat b. of cheek
fat b. of ischiorectal fossa
fat b. of orbit
ferruginous b.'s
foreign b.
b. of fornix
fruiting b.
fuchsin b.'s
b. of gallbladder
Gamna-Favre b.'s
Gamna-Gandy b.'s
Gandy-Gamna b.'s
geniculate b.
glass b.
glomus b.
Guarnieri b.'s
Halberstaedter-Prowazek b.'s

body (*continued*)

Hassall-Henle b.'s
Hassall's b.'s
Heinz b.'s
Heinz-Ehrlich b.
hematoxylin b.'s, hematoxyphil b.'s
Herring b.'s
Highmore's b.
Howell-Jolly b.'s
hyaline b.'s
hyaline b.'s of pituitary
hyaloid b.
b. of hyoid bone
b. of ilium
b. image
inclusion b.'s
b. of incus
infrapatellar fat b.
intercarotid b.
intermediate b. of Flemming
b. of ischium
Jaworski's b.'s
Jolly b.'s
juxtaglomerular b.
juxtarestiform b.
Lafora b.
Lallemand's b.'s
b. language
lateral geniculate b.
L-D b.
LE b.
Leishman-Donovan b.
Lewy b.'s
Lieutaud's b.
Lindner's b.'s
loose b.
Luse b.'s
Luys' b.
Mallory b.'s
malpighian b.'s
mamillary b.
b. of mammary gland
b. of mandible
b. mass index
b. of maxilla
b. mechanics
medial geniculate b.
melon-seed b.
metachromatic b.'s
Michaelis-Gutmann b.
Miyagawa b.'s
molluscum b.
Mooser b.'s
multilamellar b.
multivesicular b.'s
myelin b.
b. of nail
Negri b.'s

nerve cell b.
neuroepithelial b.
Nissl b.'s
nodular b.
nuclear inclusion b.'s
Odland b.
olivary b.
onion b.'s
pacchionian b.'s
pampiniform b.
b. of pancreas
Pappenheimer b.'s
para-aortic b.'s
parabasal b.
paranephric b.
paranuclear b.
paraphysial b.
paraterminal b.
Paschen b.'s
b. of penis
perineal b.
b. of phalanx
Pick's b.'s
pineal b.
b. plethysmograph
Plimmer's b.'s
polar b.
polyhedral b.
pontobulbar b.
posterior quadrigeminal b.
Prowazek b.'s
Prowazek-Greeff b.'s
psammoma b.'s
psittacosis inclusion b.'s
pubic b., b. of pubic bone
b. of pubis
quadrigeminal b.'s
Renaut b.
residual b.
residual b. of Regaud
rest b.
restiform b.
b. of rib
rice b.
b. righting reflexes
Rushton b.
Russell b.'s
sand b.'s
Sandström's b.'s
Savage's perineal b.
Schaumann b.'s
b. schema
sclerotic b.'s
segmenting b.
b. of sphenoid bone
spongy b. of penis
b. stalk
b. of sternum

b. of stomach
striate b.
suprarenal b.
b. of sweat gland
Symington's anococcygeal b.
b. of talus
b. of thigh bone
threshold b.
thyroid b.
b. of tibia
tigroid b.'s
b. of tongue
trachoma b.'s
trapezoid b.
Trousseau-Lallemand b.'s
tuffstone b.
turbinated b.
tympanic b.
b. of ulna
ultimobranchial b.
b. of urinary bladder
b. of uterus
vaccine b.'s
Verocay b.'s
b. of vertebra
Virchow-Hassall b.'s
vitreous b.
Weibel-Palade b.'s
wolffian b.
Wolf-Orton b.'s
X b.
Y b.
yellow b.
zebra b.
Zuckerkandl's b.'s
body-weight ratio
Boeck's
B. disease
B. sarcoid
Boehmer's hematoxylin
Boerhaave's
B. glands
B. syndrome
Bogros'
B. serous membrane
B. space
Bohn's nodules
Bohr's equation
boil
Aleppo b.
Bagdad b.
Biskra b.
blind b.
date b.
Delhi b.
Jericho b.
Madura b.
Oriental b.

salt water b.'s
tropical b.
boilermaker's deafness
Boley gauge
Bolivian
B. hemorrhagic fever
B. hemorrhagic fever virus
Boll's cells
Bolognini's symptom
bolometer
bolster finger
Bolton-Broadbent plane
Bolton-nasion
B.-n. line
B.-n. plane
Bolton plane
bolus dressing
bombard
Bombay
B. phenomenon
B. trait
bone
b. abscess
b. ache
b. age
Albrecht's b.
alveolar b.
alveolar supporting b.
ankle b.
b. architecture
basal b.
basilar b.
basioccipital b.
basisphenoid b.
Bertin's b.'s
blade b.
b. block
breast b.
Breschet's b.'s
brittle b.'s
bundle b.
calcaneal b.
calf b.
b. canaliculus
cancellous b.
capitate b.
carpal b.'s
cartilage b.
cavalry b.
b. cell
central b.
central b. of ankle
cheek b.
b. chips
coccygeal b.
collar b.
compact b.
b. conduction

bone *(continued)*
    convoluted b.
    b. corpuscle
    cortical b.
    coxal b.
    cranial b.'s
    cubital b.
    cuboid b.
    cuneiform b.
    b. cyst
    dermal b.
    b.'s of digits
    dorsal talonavicular b.
    ear b.'s
    elbow b.
    endochondral b.
    epactal b.'s
    epihyal b.
    epipteric b.
    episternal b.
    ethmoid b.
    exercise b.
    exoccipital b.
    facial b.'s
    first cuneiform b.
    flank b.
    b. flap
    flat b.
    Flower's b.
    b. forceps
    fourth turbinated b.
    frontal b.
    Goethe's b.
    b. graft
    greater multangular b.
    hamate b.
    heel b.
    highest turbinated b.
    hip b.
    hollow b.
    hooked b.
    iliac b.
    incarial b.
    incisive b.
    b. infarct
    b.'s of inferior limb
    inferior turbinated b.
    innominate b.
    intermaxillary b.
    intermediate cuneiform b.
    interparietal b.
    irregular b.
    ischial b.
    b. island
    jaw b.
    jugal b.
    Krause's b.
    lacrimal b.

lamellar b.
lateral cuneiform b.
lenticular b.
lentiform b.
lesser multangular b.
lingual b.
long b.
b.'s of lower limb
lunate b.
malar b.
marble b.'s
b. marrow
b. marrow dose
b. marrow embolism
b. marrow transplantation
mastoid b.
b. matrix
medial cuneiform b.
membrane b.
mesethmoid b.
metacarpal b.
metatarsal b.
middle cuneiform b.
middle turbinated b.
multangular b.
nasal b.
navicular b.
navicular b. of hand
nonlamellar b.
occipital b.
orbicular b.
palatine b.
parietal b.
perichondral b.
periosteal b.
periotic b.
peroneal b.
petrosal b.
petrous b.
ping-pong b.
pipe b.
Pirie's b.
pisiform b.
b. plate
pneumatic b.
postsphenoid b.
preinterparietal b.
premaxillary b.
presphenoid b.
pubic b.
pyramidal b.
b. reflex
replacement b.
b. resorption
reticulated b.
rider's b.
Riolan's b.'s
sacred b.

scaphoid b.
b. sclerosis
scroll b.'s
second cuneiform b.
semilunar b.
b. sensibility
septal b.
sesamoid b.
shin b.
short b.
sieve b.
b.'s of skull
sphenoid b.
sphenoidal turbinated b.'s
spongy b.
b.'s of superior limb
superior turbinated b.
suprainterparietal b.
suprasternal b.
supreme turbinated b.
sutural b.'s
tail b.
tarsal b.'s
tcmporal b.
thigh b.
third cuneiform b.
three-cornered b.
b. tissue
tongue b.
trabecular b.
trapezium b.
trapezoid b.
triangular b.
triquetral b.
turbinated b.'s
tympanic b.
tympanohyal b.
unciform b.
upper jaw b.
b.'s of upper limb
Vesalius' b.
b.'s of visceral cranium
wedge b.
wormian b.'s
woven b.
yoke b.
zygomatic b.
bonelet
Bonhoeffer's sign
Bonnet's capsule
Bonney test
Bonnier's syndrome
Bonwill triangle
bony
b. ankylosis
b. crepitus
b. heart
b. labyrinth

b. nasal septum
b. palate
b. part of auditory tube
b. part of external acoustic meatus
b. part of nasal septum
b. semicircular canals
Böök syndrome
booster
b. dose
b. response
boot
Gibney's b.
Junod's b.
borborygmus, pl. **borborygmi**
Bordeau theory
border
alveolar b.
anterior b.
anterior b. of eyelids
anterior b. of fibula
anterior b. of lung
anterior b. of pancreas
anterior b. of radius
anterior b. of testis
anterior b. of tibia
anterior b. of ulna
brush b.
b. cells
ciliary b. of iris
denture b.
b.'s of eyelids
free b.
free b. of nail
free b. of ovary
frontal b.
frontal b. of parietal bone
frontal b. of sphenoid bone
inferior b.
inferior b. of liver
inferior b. of lung
inferior b. of pancreas
interosseous b.
interosseous b. of fibula
interosseous b. of radius
interosseous b. of tibia
interosseous b. of ulna
lacrimal b. of maxilla
lambdoid b. of occipital bone
lateral b.
lateral b. of foot
lateral b. of forearm
lateral b. of humerus
lateral b. of kidney
lateral b. of nail
lateral b. of scapula
mastoid b. of occipital bone
medial b.
medial b. of foot

B

border *(continued)*
    medial b. of forearm
    medial b. of humerus
    medial b. of kidney
    medial b. of scapula
    medial b. of suprarenal gland
    medial b. of tibia
    mesovarian b. of ovary
    b. molding
    b. movements
    nasal b. of frontal bone
    occipital b.
    occipital b. of parietal bone
    occipital b. of temporal bone
    occult b. of nail
    parietal b.
    parietal b. of frontal bone
    parietal b. of sphenoid bone
    parietal b. of temporal bone
    posterior b. of eyelids
    posterior b. of fibula
    posterior b. of petrous part of
      temporal bone
    posterior b. of radius
    posterior b. of testis
    posterior b. of ulna
    proximal b. of nail
    pupillary b. of iris
    radial b. of forearm
    right b. of heart
    sagittal b. of parietal bone
    b. seal
    sphenoidal b. of temporal bone
    squamous b.
    squamous b. of parietal bone
    squamous b. of sphenoid bone
    striated b.
    superior b.
    superior b. of pancreas
    superior b. of petrous part of
      temporal bone
    superior b. of scapula
    superior b. of spleen
    superior b. of suprarenal gland
    tibial b. of foot
    b. tissue movements
    b. of uterus
    ventral b.
    vermilion b.
    vertebral b. of scapula
    zygomatic b. of greater wing of
      sphenoid bone
borderline
    b. case
    b. hypertension
    b. leprosy
    b. personality

    b. personality disorder
    b. tumor
Bordetella
    B. pertussis
Bordet-Gengou
    B.-G. bacillus
    B.-G. phenomenon
    B.-G. potato blood agar
Bordet and Gengou reaction
Bordeu theory
Börjeson-Forssman-Lehmann syndrome
Borna disease virus
Bornholm
    B. disease
    B. disease virus
Born method of wax plate
    reconstruction
Borrelia
    B. anserina
    B. burgdorferi
    B. caucasica
    B. crocidurae
    B. duttonii
    B. hermsii
    B. hispanica
    B. latyschewii
    B. mazzottii
    B. parkeri
    B. persica
    B. recurrentis
    B. turicatae
    B. venezuelensis
borreliosis
    Lyme b.
Borrel's blue stain
Borst-Jadassohn type intraepidermal
    epithelioma
bosch yaws
Bosin's disease
boss
bosselated
bosselation
Boston exanthema
Botallo's
    B. duct
    B. foramen
    B. ligament
botfly
    human b.
    warble b.
bothria (*pl. of* bothrium)
bothriocephaliasis
Bothriocephalus
    B. cordatus
    B. latus
    B. mansoni
    B. mansonoides
bothrium, pl. **bothria**

botryoid
    b. odontogenic cyst
    b. sarcoma
Botryomyces
bots
    ox b.
    sheep b.
Böttcher's
    B. canal
    B. cells
    B. crystals
    B. ganglion
    B. space
bottle
    Mariotte b.
botulinogenic
botulism
    wound b.
botulogenic
boubas
Bouchard's disease
bouche de tapir
Bouchut's tube
Bouffardi's
    B. black mycetoma
    B. mycetomas
    B. white mycetoma
bougie
    b. à boule
    bulbous b.
    Eder-Pustow b.
    elastic b.
    elbowed b.
    filiform b.
    following b.
    Hurst b.'s
    Maloney b.'s
    Savary b.'s
    tapered b.
    wax-tipped b.
    whip b.
bougienage
Bouillaud's disease
Bouin's fixative
boulimia
boundary lamina
bouquet
    b. fever
    Riolan's b.
Bourdon tube
Bourgery's ligament
Bourneville-Pringle disease
Bourneville's disease
bouton
    axonal terminal b.'s
    b. de Bagdad, b. d'Orient
    b. de Biskra
    b. en chemise

    b.'s en passage
    synaptic b.'s
    terminal b.'s, b. terminaux
boutonneuse fever
boutonnière
    b. deformity
Bovero's muscle
Bovicola
Bovie
bovine
    b. colloid
    b. leukemia virus
    b. leukosis virus
    b. papular stomatitis virus
    b. rhinoviruses
    b. serum albumin
    b. virus diarrhea virus
bow
    Logan's b.
Bowditch
    B. effect
    B. law
bowel
    b. bypass
    b. bypass syndrome
    large b.
    b. movement
    small b.
    b. sounds
bowenoid
    B. cells
    b. papulosis
Bowen's
    B. disease
    B. precancerous dermatosis
Bowie's stain
bowleg, bow-leg
Bowles type stethoscope
Bowman's
    B. capsule
    B. disks
    B. gland
    B. membrane
    B. muscle
    B. probe
    B. space
    B. theory
box
    black b.
    fracture b.
    Skinner b.
    TATA b.
    view b.
boxer's
    b. ear
    b. fracture
boxing
    b. wax

B

Boyd communicating perforation veins
Boyden
  B. meal
  B. sphincter
Boyer's
  B. bursa
  B. cyst
Bozeman-Fritsch catheter
Bozeman's
  B. operation
  B. position
Bozzolo's sign
B-P fistula
Braasch catheter
brace

BPD
BRonchiAl
Pulmony-
dtstenin

  cast b.
  Taylor's back b.
bracelet
  Nussbaum's b.
braces
brachia (*pl. of* brachium)
brachial
  b. anesthesia
  b. artery
  b. birth palsy
  b. fascia
  b. gland
  b. lymph nodes
  b. muscle
  b. neuritis
  b. plexitis
  b. plexus
  b. plexus neuropathy
  b. veins
brachialgia
  b. statica paresthetica
brachialis muscle
brachiocephalic
  b. arteritis
  b. trunk
  b. veins
brachiocrural
brachiocubital
brachiogram
brachioradial
  b. muscle
  b. reflex
brachioradialis muscle
brachium, pl. brachia
  b. colliculi inferioris
  b. colliculi superioris
  b. conjunctivum cerebelli
  b. of inferior colliculus
  inferior quadrigeminal b.
  b. pontis
  b. quadrigeminum inferius
  b. quadrigeminum superius

  b. of superior colliculus
  superior quadrigeminal b.
Bracht maneuver
Bracht-Wachter lesion
brachybasia
brachybasocamptodactyly
brachybasophalangia
brachycardia
brachycephalia
brachycephalic
brachycephalism
brachycephalous
brachycephaly
brachycheilia, brachychilia
brachycnemic, brachyknemic
brachycranic
brachydactylia
brachydactylic
brachydactyly
brachyesophagus
brachyfacial
brachyglossal
brachygnathia
brachygnathous
brachykerkic
brachyknemic (*var. of* brachycnemic)
brachymelia
brachymesophalangia
brachymetacarpalia, brachymetacarpalism
brachymetacarpia
brachymetapody
brachymetatarsia
brachymorphic
brachyodont
brachyonychia
brachypellic
  b. pelvis
brachypelvic
brachyphalangia
brachypodous
brachyprosopic
brachyrhinia
brachyrhynchus
brachyskelic
brachystaphyline
brachysyndactyly
brachytelephalangia
brachytherapy
  interstitial b.
brachytype
brachyuranic
bracing
bracket
Bradford frame
bradyarrhythmia
bradyarthria
bradycardia
  central b.

essential b.
fetal b.
idiopathic b.
marked fetal b.
mild fetal b.
nodal b.
postinfectious b.
sinus b.
vagal b.
ventricular b.
bradycardiac
bradycardic
bradycinesia
bradycrotic
bradydiastole
bradyesthesia
bradyglossia
bradykinesia
bradykinetic
    b. analysis
bradylalia
bradylexia
bradylogia
bradypepsia
bradyphagia
bradyphasia
bradyphemia
bradypnea
bradypragia
bradypsychia
bradyrhythmia
bradyspermatism
bradysphygmia
bradystalsis
bradytachycardia syndrome
bradyteleocinesia
bradyteleokinesis
bradytocia
bradyuria
bradyzoite
braille
Brailsford-Morquio disease
brain
    b. cicatrix
    b. concussion
    b. congestion
    b. contusion
    b. death
    b. edema
    b. laceration
    b. mantle
    b. murmur
    b. potential
    respirator b.
    b. sand
    split b.
    b. stem
    b. swelling

visceral b.
b. wave
b. wave complex
b. wave cycle
braincase
brain-heart infusion agar
Brain's reflex
brainstem, brain stem
    b. evoked response audiometry
    b. glioma
    b. hemorrhage
brainwashing
branch
    accessory meningeal b. of middle
      meningeal artery
    acetabular b.
    acromial b. of suprascapular artery
    acromial b. of thoracoacromial
      artery
    anastomotic b.
    anastomotic b. of middle meningeal
      artery to lacrimal artery
    anterior b.
    anterior auricular b.'s of superficial
      temporal artery
    anterior basal b.
    anterior cutaneous b. of
      iliohypogastric nerve
    anterior cutaneous b.'s of
      intercostal nerves
    anterior scrotal b.'s of external
      pudendal artery
    anterior superior alveolar b.'s of
      infraorbital nerve
    anteromedial central b.'s
    apical b.
    apical b. of inferior lobar branch
      of right pulmonary artery
    apicoposterior b. of left superior
      pulmonary vein
    articular b.'s
    ascending b.
    ascending anterior b.
    ascending b. of the inferior
      mesenteric artery
    ascending posterior b.
    atrial b.'s
    atrioventricular nodal b.
    b. to atrioventricular node
    auricular b. of occipital artery
    auricular b. of vagus nerve
    b. of auriculotemporal nerve to
      tympanic membrane
    basal tentorial b. of internal
      carotid artery
    buccal b.'s of facial nerve
    calcarine b. of medial occipital
      artery

branch (*continued*)

capsular b.'s of renal artery
carotid sinus b.
caudate b.'s
cavernous b. of internal carotid
  artery
cavernous sinus b. of internal
  carotid artery
celiac b.'s of vagus nerve
cervical b. of facial nerve
choroid b.'s
circumflex b. of left coronary
  artery
clavicular b. of thoracoacromial
  artery
cochlear b. of labyrinthine artery
collateral b.'s of posterior
  intercostal arteries 3–11
communicating b.
communicating b.'s of
  auriculotemporal nerve to facial
  nerve
communicating b. of chorda
  tympani to lingual nerve
communicating b. of facial nerve
  with glossopharyngeal nerve
communicating b. of facial nerve
  with tympanic plexus
communicating b. of
  glossopharyngeal nerve with
  auricular branch of vagus nerve
communicating b. of lacrimal nerve
  with zygomatic nerve
communicating b.'s of lingual
  nerve to hypoglossal nerve
communicating b. of median nerve
  with ulnar nerve
communicating b. of otic ganglion
  to auriculotemporal nerve
communicating b. of otic ganglion
  to chorda tympani
communicating b. of otic ganglion
  with medial pterygoid nerve
communicating b. of otic ganglion
  with meningeal branch of
  mandibular nerve
communicating b. of peroneal
  artery
communicating b.'s of spinal
  nerves
communicating b. of superior
  laryngeal nerve with recurrent
  laryngeal nerve
communicating b.'s of sympathetic
  trunk
cutaneous b. of obturator nerve
deep b.

deep b. of the lateral plantar
  nerve
deep b. of the medial femoral
  circumflex artery
deep b. of the medial plantar
  artery
deep palmar b. of ulnar artery
deep plantar b. of dorsalis pedis
  artery
deep b. of the radial nerve
deep b. of the transverse cervical
  artery
deep b. of the ulnar nerve
deltoid b.
dental b.'s
descending b.
descending anterior b.
descending b. of hypoglossal nerve
descending b. of lateral circumflex
  femoral artery
descending b. of occipital artery
descending posterior b.
digastric b. of facial nerve
dorsal b., dorsal b.'s
dorsal carpal b. of radial artery
dorsal carpal b. of ulnar artery
dorsal lingual b.'s of lingual artery
dorsal b. of the lumbar artery
dorsal b. of the posterior
  intercostal arteries 3–11
dorsal b. of the posterior
  intercostal veins 4–11
dorsal b. of the subcostal artery
dorsal b. of the superior intercostal
  artery
dorsal b. of the ulnar nerve
duodoneal b.'s of superior
  pancreaticoduodenal artery
epiploic b.'s
esophageal b.'s
esophageal b.'s of the inferior
  thyroid artery
esophageal b.'s of the left gastric
  artery
esophageal b.'s of the recurrent
  laryngeal nerve
esophageal b.'s of the thoracic
  aorta
esophageal b.'s of the vagus nerve
external b. of accessory nerve
external nasal b.'s
external b. of superior laryngeal
  nerve
faucial b.'s of lingual nerve
femoral b. of genitofemoral nerve
frontal b. of superficial temporal
  artery

ganglionic b. of internal carotid artery
ganglionic b.'s of lingual nerve
ganglionic b.'s of maxillary nerve
gastric b.'s of anterior vagal trunk
gastric b.'s of posterior vagal b.
genital b. of genitofemoral nerve
genital b. of iliohypogastric nerve
glandular b.'s
glandular b.'s of anterior/lateral/posterior branches of superior thyroid artery
glandular b.'s of facial artery
glandular b.'s of inferior thyroid artery
glandular b.'s of submandibular ganglion
b. of glossopharyngeal nerve to stylopharyngeus muscle
hepatic b.'s of vagus nerve
iliac b. of iliolumbar artery
inferior b.
inferior cervical cardiac b.'s of vagus nerve
inferior dental b.'s of inferior dental plexus
inferior gingival b.'s of inferior dental plexus
inferior labial b.'s of mental nerve
inferior lingular b. of lingular branch of left pulmonary artery
inferior b. of oculomotor nerve
inferior b. of pubic bone
inferior b. of superior gluteal artery
inferior b.'s of transverse cervical nerve
infrahyoid b. of superior thyroid artery
infrapatellar b. of saphenous nerve
inguinal b.'s of external pudendal arteries
internal b. of accessory nerve
internal nasal b.'s
internal b. of superior laryngeal nerve
joint b.'s
laryngopharyngeal b.'s of superior cervical ganglion
lateral b.'s
lateral basal b.
lateral calcaneal b.'s of sural nerve
lateral costal b. of internal thoracic artery
lateral cutaneous b.
lateral cutaneous b.'s of intercostal nerves
lateral cutaneous b.'s of ventral

primary ramus of thoracic spinal nerves
lateral mammary b.'s
lateral mammary b.'s of lateral cutaneous branches of intercostal nerves
lateral mammary b.'s of lateral cutaneous branches of thoracic spinal nerves
lateral mammary b.'s of lateral thoracic artery
lateral nasal b.'s of anterior ethmoidal nerve
lateral orbitofrontal b.
left b.
lingual b.'s
lingual b. of facial nerve
lingular b.
lumbar b. of iliolumbar artery
mammary b.'s
marginal mandibular b. of facial nerve
marginal tentorial b. of internal carotid artery
mastoid b. of occipital artery
mastoid b.'s of posterior auricular artery
medial b.'s
medial basal b. of pulmonary artery
medial calcaneal b.'s of tibial nerve
medial crural cutaneous b.'s of saphenous nerve
medial cutaneous b.
medial mammary b.'s
medial nasal b.'s of anterior ethmoidal nerve
mediastinal b.'s
mediastinal b.'s of internal thoracic artery
mediastinal b.'s of thoracic aorta
meningeal b.'s
meningeal b. of internal carotid artery
meningeal b. of mandibular nerve
meningeal b. of occipital artery
meningeal b. of ophthalmic nerve
meningeal b. of spinal nerves
meningeal b. of vagus nerve
mental b.'s of mental nerve
middle lobe b.
middle meningeal b. of maxillary nerve
middle superior alveolar b. of infraorbital nerve
muscular b.'s
occipital b.

branch *(continued)*

omental b.'s
orbital b. of middle meningeal artery
orbital b.'s of pterygopalatine ganglion
ovarian b. of uterine artery
palmar carpal b. of radial artery
palmar carpal b. of ulnar artery
palmar b. of median nerve
palmar b. of ulnar nerve
palpebral b.'s of infratrochlear nerve
pancreatic b.'s
parietal b.
parietal b. of medial occipital artery
parietal b. of middle meningeal artery
parietal b. of superficial temporal artery
parotid b.'s
pectoral and abdominal anterior cutaneous b. of intercostal nerves
pectoral b.'s of thoracoacromial artery
perforating b.'s
perforating b.'s of internal thoracic artery
perforating b.'s of palmar metacarpal arteries
perforating b. of peroneal artery
perforating b.'s of plantar metatarsal arteries
pericardial b. of phrenic nerve
pericardial b.'s of thoracic aorta
perineal b.'s of posterior femoral cutaneous nerve
peroneal communicating b.
petrosal b. of middle meningeal artery
pharyngeal b.'s
pharyngeal b. of the artery of pterygoid canal
pharyngeal b. of the ascending pharyngeal artery
pharyngeal b. of descending palatine artery
pharyngeal b. of glossopharyngeal nerve
pharyngeal b. of inferior thyroid artery
pharyngeal b. of pterygopalatine ganglion
pharyngeal b. of vagus nerve
phrenicoabdominal b.'s of phrenic nerve
posterior b.'s

posterior basal b.
posterior b. of great auricular nerve
posterior inferior nasal b.'s of greater palatine nerve
posterior b. of inferior pancreaticoduodenal artery
posterior b. of lateral cerebral sulcus
posterior b. of obturator artery
posterior b. of obturator nerve
posterior b. of recurrent ulnar artery
posterior b. of renal artery
posterior b. of right branch of portal vein
posterior b. of right hepatic duct
posterior b. of right superior pulmonary vein
posterior scrotal b.'s of internal pudendal artery
posterior b. of spinal nerves
posterior superior alveolar b.'s of maxillary nerve
posterior superior lateral nasal b.'s of pterygopalatine ganglion
posterior superior medial nasal b.'s of pterygopalatine ganglion
posterior b. of superior thyroid artery
pterygoid b.'s of maxillary artery
pubic b. of inferior epigastric artery
pubic b. of obturator artery
pulmonary b.'s of autonomic nervous system
recurrent meningeal b. of spinal nerves
renal b. of lesser splanchnic b.
renal b.'s of vagus nerve
right b.
right b. of portal vein
right b. of proper hepatic artery
saphenous b. of descending genicular artery
b.'s of segmental bronchi
septal b.'s
sinuatrial nodal b. of right coronary artery
b. to sinuatrial node
splenic b.'s of splenic artery
stapedial b. of stylomastoid artery
sternal b.'s of internal thoracic artery
sternocleidomastoid b. of occipital artery
sternocleidomastoid b. of superior thyroid artery

stylohyoid b. of facial nerve
subscapular b.'s of axillary artery
superficial b.
superficial b. of the lateral plantar
  nerve
superficial b. of the medial plantar
  artery
superficial palmar b. of radial
  artery
superficial b. of the radial nerve
superficial b. of the superior
  gluteal artery
superficial temporal b.'s of
  auriculotemporal nerve
superficial b. of the transverse
  cervical artery
superficial b. of the ulnar nerve
superior b., superior b.'s
superior cervical cardiac b.'s of
  vagus nerve
superior dental b.'s of superior
  dental plexus
superior gingival b.'s of superior
  dental plexus
superior labial b.'s of infraorbital
  nerve
superior lingular b. of lingular
  branch of superior lobar left
  pulmonary artery
superior b. of the oculomotor
  nerve
superior b. of the pubic bone
superior b. of the right and left
  inferior pulmonary veins
superior b. of the superior gluteal
  artery
superior b. of the transverse
  cervical nerve
suprahyoid b. of lingual artery
sympathetic b. to submandibular
  ganglion
temporal b.'s of facial nerve
thoracic cardiac b.'s of vagus
  nerve
thymic b.'s of internal thoracic
  artery
tonsillar b. of the facial artery
tonsillar b.'s of glossopharyngeal
  nerve
tracheal b.'s
transverse b.'s
b. to trigeminal ganglion
tubal b.
tubal b. of the tympanic plexus
tubal b. of the uterine artery
ulnar communicating b. of
  superficial radial nerve

ulnar b. of medial antebrachial
  cutaneous nerve
ureteral b.'s
ureteric b.'s
ureteric b.'s of the ovarian artery
ureteric b.'s of the patent part of
  umbilical artery
ureteric b.'s of the renal artery
ureteric b.'s of the testicular artery
ventral b.
vestibular b.'s of labyrinthine
  artery
zygomatic b.'s of facial nerve
zygomaticofacial b. of zygomatic
  nerve
zygomaticotemporal b. of zygomatic
  nerve
branched
  b. calculus
  b. chain ketoaciduria
  b. chain ketonuria
brancher
  b. deficiency glycogenosis
  b. glycogen storage disease
branchial
  b. arches
  b. cartilages
  b. cleft cyst
  b. clefts
  b. cyst
  b. efferent column
  b. fissure
  b. fistula
  b. groove
  b. mesoderm
  b. pouches
branching
  false b.
branchiogenic, branchiogenous
branchioma
branchiomere
branchiomeric muscles
branchiomerism
branchiomotor
  b. nuclei
Brandt-Andrews maneuver
brandy nose
Branhamella
  B. catarrhalis
Branham's sign
branny
  b. desquamation
  b. tetter
Brasdor's method
brass
  b. founder's ague
  b. founder's fever

B

brassy
  b. body
  b. cough
Braune's
  B. canal
  B. muscle
  B. valve
Braun's anastomosis
brawny
  b. arm
  b. edema
  b. scleritis
Braxton
  B. Hicks contraction
  B. Hicks sign
  B. Hicks version
Brazelton's Neonatal Behavioral
  Assessment Scale
brazilein
Brazilian
  B. blastomycosis
  B. hemorrhagic fever
  B. pemphigus
  B. purpuric fever
  B. spotted fever
brazilin
brazing
bread-and-butter pericardium
breakaway phenomenon
breakbone fever
breakoff
  b. phenomenon
break shock
breakthrough
breast
  accessory b.
  b. bone
  caked b.
  chicken b.
  funnel b.
  irritable b.
  male b.
  b. pang
  pigeon b.
  b. pump
  supernumerary b.
breath
  b. analysis test
  liver b.
  uremic b.
breath-holding
  b.-h. test
breathing
  apneustic b.
  ataxic b.
  b. bag
  Biot's b.
  bronchial b.

continuous positive pressure b.
glossopharyngeal b.
intermittent positive pressure b.
mouth b.
positive-negative pressure b.
pursed lips b.
b. reserve
shallow b.
stertorous b.
Breda's disease
bredouillement
breech
  b. delivery
  b. extraction
  b. presentation
breeding
bregma
bregmatic
  b. fontanel
bregmatolambdoid arc
bregmocardiac reflex
bremsstrahlung
Brenner tumor
brephoplastic graft
Breschet's
  B. bones
  B. canals
  B. hiatus
  B. sinus
  B. vein
Brescia-Cimino fistula
Breslow's thickness
Breus mole
brevicollis
Brewer's infarcts
brickdust deposit
Bricker operation
brickmaker's anemia
bridge
  arteriolovenular b.
  cantilever b.
  cell b.'s
  b. corpuscle
  cytoplasmic b.'s
  dentin b.
  extension b.
  fixed b.
  Gaskell's b.
  intercellular b.'s
  myocardial b.
  removable b.
  Wheatstone's b.
bridgework
bridging hepatic necrosis
bridle
  b. of clitoris
  b. stricture
  b. suture

brief psychotherapy
brightness difference threshold
Bright's disease
brilliant
    b. cresyl blue
    b. green salt agar
    b. vital red
    b. yellow
Brill's disease
Brill-Symmers disease
Brill-Zinsser disease
brim
    pelvic b.
Brinell hardness number
Briquet's
    B. ataxia
    B. disease
    B. syndrome
brisement forcé
Brissaud-Marie syndrome
Brissaud's
    B. disease
    B. infantilism
    B. reflex
bristle cell
brittle
    b. bones
    b. diabetes
broach
    barbed b.
    smooth b.
broad
    b. fascia
    b. ligament of the uterus
Broadbent's
    B. law
    B. sign
broadest muscle of back
Broca's
    B. angles
    B. aphasia
    B. area
    B. basilar angle
    B. center
    B. diagonal band
    B. facial angle
    B. field
    B. fissure
    B. formula
    B. parolfactory area
    B. pouch
    B. visual plane
Brock
    B. operation
    B. syndrome
Brockenbrough sign
Brocq's disease
Brödel's bloodless line

Brodie
    B. abscess
    B. bursa
    B. disease
    B. fluid
    B. knee
    B. ligament
Brodmann's areas
Broesike's fossa
bromhidrosis
bromide acne
bromidrosiphobia
bromidrosis
bromocresol green
bromoderma
bromohyperhidrosis, bromohyperidrosis
bromophenol blue
bromphenol
    b. blue
    b. test
bromsulphalein test
bromthymol blue
bronchi (*pl. of* bronchus)
bronchi
bronchia
bronchial
    b. adenoma
    b. arteries
    b. arteriography
    b. asthma
    b. atresia
    b. breathing
    b. bud
    b. calculus
    b. fremitus
    b. glands
    b. pneumonia
    b. polyp
    b. respiration
    b. tubes
    b. veins
    b. voice
bronchic cells
bronchiectasia
    b. sicca
bronchiectasis
    congenital b.
    cylindrical b.
    cystic b.
    dry b.
    saccular b.
bronchiectatic
bronchiloquy
bronchiogenic
bronchiolar
    b. adenocarcinoma
    b. carcinoma
    b. exocrine cell

B

bronchiole
    respiratory b.'s
    terminal b.
bronchiolectasia
bronchiolectasis
bronchioli
bronchioli (*pl. of* bronchiolus)
bronchiolitis
    constrictive b.
    exudative b.
    b. fibrosa obliterans
    b. obliterans
    b. obliterans with organizing
        pneumonia
    proliferative b.
bronchioloalveolar adenocarcinoma
bronchiolo-alveolar carcinoma
bronchiolopulmonary
bronchiolus, pl. bronchioli
    bronchioli respiratorii
    b. terminalis
bronchiostenosis
bronchitic
    b. asthma
bronchitis
    asthmatic b.
    Castellani's b.
    chronic b.
    croupous b.
    fibrinous b.
    hemorrhagic b.
    obliterative b., b. obliterans
    plastic b.
    pseudomembranous b.
    putrid b.
bronchium
bronchoalveolar
bronchobiliary fistula
bronchocavernous
bronchocavitary fistula
bronchocele
bronchocentric granulomatosis
bronchoconstriction
bronchoedema
bronchoesophageal
    b. fistula
    b. muscle
bronchoesophagology
bronchoesophagoscopy
bronchofiberscope
bronchogenic
    b. carcinoma
    b. cyst
bronchogram
    air b.
bronchography
    tantalum b.
broncholith

broncholithiasis
bronchomalacia
bronchomediastinal trunk
bronchomycosis
bronchophony
    whispered b.
bronchoplasty
bronchopleural fistula
bronchopneumonia
    postoperative b.
    tuberculous b.
bronchopneumonic aspergillosis
bronchopulmonary
    b. aspergillosis
    b. dysplasia
    b. lymph nodes
    b. segment
    b. sequestration
    b. spirochetosis
bronchorrhaphy
bronchorrhea
bronchoscope
bronchoscopic
    b. brush
    b. smear
    b. sponge
bronchoscopy
bronchospasm
bronchospirochetosis
bronchospirography
bronchospirometer
bronchospirometry
bronchostaxis
bronchostenosis
bronchostomy
bronchotomy
bronchotracheal
bronchovesicular
    b. respiration
bronchus, pl. bronchi
    eparterial b.
    hyparterial bronchi
    intermediate b.
    b. intermedius
    left main b.
    lobar bronchi
    bronchi lobares, b. lobaris inferior,
        b. lobaris medius, b. lobaris superior
    mucoid impaction of b.
    primary b.
    b. principalis dexter
    b. principalis sinister
    right main b.
    segmental b.
    b. segmentalis
    stem b.
brontophobia

bronzed
>b. diabetes
>b. disease
>b. skin

bronze diabetes
brood
>b. capsules
>b. cell

Brooke
>B. disease
>B. ileostomy
>B. tumor

brother complex
brow
>b. presentation

browlift
brown
>b. atrophy
>b. edema
>b. induration of the lung
>b. layer
>b. lung
>b. pellicle
>b. striae
>b. tumor

Brown-Adson forceps
Brown-Brenn stain
Browning's vein
Brown-Séquard's
>B.-S. paralysis
>B.-S. syndrome

Brown's syndrome
Brucella
>*B. abortus*
>*B. melitensis*
>*B. suis*

Brucellaceae
brucellergin
brucellin
Bruch's
>B. glands
>B. membrane

Brücke-Bartley phenomenon
Brücke's
>B. muscle
>B. tunic

Bruck's disease
Brudzinski's sign
Brugia
>*B. malayi*

Brugsch's syndrome
Brug's filariasis
bruise
bruissement
bruit
>aneurysmal b.
>carotid b.
>b. de canon

>b. de claquement
>b. de cuir neuf
>b. de diable
>b. de frolement
>b. de galop
>b. de la roue de moulin
>b. de lime
>b. de rappel
>b. de Roger
>b. de scie
>b. de scie ou de rape
>b. de soufflet
>b. de tabourka
>b. de tambour
>b. de triolet
>Roger's b.
>systolic b.
>thyroid b.
>Traube's b.

Brumpt's white mycetoma
Brunn
>B. membrane
>B. nests
>B. reaction

brunneroma
brunnerosis
Brunner's glands
Bruns ataxia
Brunschwig's operation
Bruns' nystagmus
brush
>Ayre b.
>b. biopsy
>b. border
>bronchoscopic b.
>b. burn
>b. burn abrasion
>b. catheter
>denture b.
>Haidinger's b.'s
>Kruse's b.
>polishing b.

Brushfield's spots
Brushfield-Wyatt disease
bruxism
Bryant's
>B. sign
>B. traction
>B. triangle

BSER audiometry
BSP test
buaki
buba madre
bubas
>b. braziliana

bubble gum dermatitis
bubbling rale

bubo
    bullet b.
    chancroidal b.
    climatic b.
    indolent b.
    malignant b.
    parotid b.
    primary b.
    tropical b.
    venereal b.
    virulent b.
bubonalgia
bubonic
    b. plague
bubonulus
bucardia
bucca, gen. and pl. **buccae**
buccal
    b. angles
    b. artery
    b. branches of facial nerve
    b. caries
    b. cavity
    b. curve
    b. embrasure
    b. fat-pad
    b. flange
    b. gingiva
    b. glands
    b. lymph node
    b. nerve
    b. node
    b. occlusion
    b. pit
    b. region
    b. smear
    b. surface
    b. vestibule
buccinator
    b. artery
    b. crest
    b. muscle
    b. nerve
    b. node
buccoaxial
buccoaxiocervical
buccoaxiogingival
buccocervical
    b. ridge
buccoclusal
buccodistal
buccogingival
    b. ridge
buccolabial
buccolingual
    b. diameter
    b. dimension
    b. relation

buccomesial
bucconasal membrane
bucconeural duct
bucco-occlusal angle
buccopharyngeal
    b. fascia
    b. membrane
    b. part of superior pharyngeal
      constrictor
buccopulpal
buccoversion
buccula
Buchwald's atrophy
bucket-handle
    b.-h. incision
    b.-h. tear
buckled aorta
Buck's
    B. extension
    B. fascia
    B. traction
buckthorn polyneuropathy
buck tooth
Bucky diaphragm
bud
    bronchial b.
    end b.
    b. fission
    gustatory b.
    limb b.
    liver b.
    lung b.
    median tongue b.
    metanephric b.
    periosteal b.
    b. stage
    syncytial b.
    tail b.
    taste b.
    tooth b.
    ureteric b.
    vascular b.
Budd-Chiari syndrome
budding
Budd's
    B. cirrhosis
    B. syndrome
Budge's center
Budin's obstetrical joint
Buerger's disease
buffalo
    b. hump
    b. neck
    b. type
buffer
    secondary b.
buffy coat
bug

buggery
bulb
   aortic b.
   arterial b.
   carotid b.
   b. of corpus spongiosum
   dental b.
   duodenal b.
   end b.
   b. of eye
   hair b.
   b. of hair
   jugular b.
   b. of jugular vein
   Krause's end b.'s
   b. of lateral ventricle
   olfactory b.
   b. of penis
   b. of posterior horn of lateral
    ventricle of brain
   Rouget's b.
   speech b.
   taste b.
   b. of urethra
   b. of vestibule
bulbar
   b. apoplexy
   b. conjunctiva
   b. myelitis
   b. palsy
   b. paralysis
   b. pulse
   b. ridge
   b. septum
bulbi (*gen. and pl. of* bulbus)
bulbitis
bulbocavernosus
   b. muscle
   b. reflex
bulboid
   b. corpuscles
bulbomimic reflex
bulbonuclear
bulbopontine
bulbosacral
   b. system
bulbospinal
bulbourethral
   b. gland
bulbous bougie
bulboventricular
   b. loop
   b. ridge
bulbus, gen. and pl. **bulbi**
   b. aortae
   b. cordis
   b. cornus posterioris
   b. oculi

   b. olfactorius
   b. penis
   b. pili
   b. urethrae
   b. venae jugularis
   b. vestibuli vaginae
bulesis
bulimia
   b. nervosa
bulimic
Bulinus
bulk modulus
bulla, gen. and pl. **bullae**
   ethmoidal b.
   b. ethmoidalis
   intraepidermal b.
   pulmonary b.
   subepidermal b.
bulldog
   b. forceps
   b. head
bullectomy
bullet
   b. bubo
   b. forceps
bull neck
bullous
   b. congenital ichthyosiform
    erythroderma
   b. edema
   b. edema vesicae
   b. emphysema
   b. fever
   b. impetigo of newborn
   b. keratopathy
   b. myringitis
   b. pemphigoid
   b. syphilid
bull's-eye maculopathy
Bumke's pupil
bundle
   aberrant b.'s
   anterior ground b.
   Arnold's b.
   atrioventricular b.
   Bachmann's b.
   b. bone
   comma b. of Schultze
   Flechsig's ground b.'s
   Gantzer's accessory b.
   Gierke's respiratory b.
   ground b.'s
   Held's b.
   Helie's b.
   Helweg's b.
   His' b., b. of His
   Hoche's b.
   hooked b. of Russell

bundle *(continued)*
    Keith's b.
    Kent-His b.
    Kent's b.
    Killian's b.
    Krause's respiratory b.
    lateral ground b.
    lateral proprius b.
    Lissauer's b.
    Loewenthal's b.
    longitudinal pontine b.'s
    medial forebrain b.
    medial longitudinal b.
    Meynert's retroflex b.
    Monakow's b.
    muscle b.
    oblique b. of pons
    olfactory b.
    olivocochlear b.
    Pick's b.
    posterior longitudinal b.
    precommissural b.
    predorsal b.
    b. of Rasmussen
    Rathke's b.'s
    Schütz' b.
    solitary b.
    tendon b.
    Türck's b.
    uncinate b. of Russell
    Vicq d'Azyr's b.
bundle-branch block
bungpagga
bunion
bunionectomy
    Keller b.
    Mayo b.
Bunnell's suture
bunodont
bunolophodont
bunoselenodont
Bunostomum
    B. phlebotomum
    B. trigonocephalum
Bunsen-Roscoe law
Bunsen's solubility coefficient
Bunyamwera
    B. fever
    B. virus
Bunyaviridae
Bunyavirus
bur
    cross-cut b.
    b. drill
    end-cutting b.
    finishing b.
    fissure b.

    inverted cone b.
    round b.
Burdach's
    B. column
    B. fasciculus
    B. nucleus
    B. tract
burden
    body b.
    clinical b.
    genetic b.
Burdwan fever
Bürger-Grütz
    B.-G. disease
    B.-G. syndrome
Burger's triangle
buried
    b. flap
    b. penis
    b. suture
Burkitt's lymphoma
Burlew
    B. disk
    B. wheel
burn
    brush b.
    chemical b.
    first degree b.
    flash b.
    full-thickness b.
    mat b.
    partial-thickness b.
    radiation b.
    rope b.
    second degree b.
    superficial b.
    thermal b.
    third degree b.
burners
burner syndrome
Burnett's syndrome
burning
    b. drops sign
    b. vulva syndrome
burnisher
burnout
Burn and Rand theory
Burns'
    B. falciform process
    B. ligament
    B. space
Burow's
    B. operation
    B. triangle
    B. vein
burr
    b. cell
burrow

burrowing hairs
bursa, pl. **bursae**
    Achilles b.
    b. achillis
    b. of acromion
    adventitious b.
    b. anserina
    anserine b.
    anterior tibial b.
    bicipitoradial b.
    b. bicipitoradialis
    Boyer's b.
    Brodie's b.
    Calori's b.
    coracobrachial b.
    b. cubitalis interossea
    deep infrapatellar b.
    b. of extensor carpi radialis brevis
      muscle
    Fleischmann's b.
    b. of gastrocnemius
    gluteofemoral b.
    gluteus medius bursac
    gluteus minimus b.
    b. of great toe
    b. of hyoid
    iliac b.
    b. iliopectinea
    iliopectineal b.
    inferior b. of biceps femoris
    infracardiac b.
    infrahyoid b.
    b. infrahyoidea
    b. infrapatellaris profunda
    infraspinatus b.
    intermuscular gluteal b.
    b. intermuscularis musculorum
      gluteorum
    interosseous b. of elbow
    b. intratendinea olecrani
    intratendinous b. of elbow
    b. ischiadica musculi glutei maximi
    b. ischiadica musculi obturatoris
      interni
    ischial b.
    laryngeal b.
    lateral malleolar subcutaneous b.
    lateral malleolus b.
    b. of latissimus dorsi
    Luschka's b.
    medial malleolar subcutaneous b.
    b. of Monro
    b. mucosa
    b. musculi bicipitis femoris
      superior
    b. musculi coracobrachialis
    b. musculi extensoris carpi radialis
      brevis

    b. musculi piriformis
    b. musculi semimembranosi
    b. musculi tensoris veli palatini
    b. of obturator internus
    b. of olecranon
    omental b.
    b. omentalis
    ovarian b.
    b. ovarica
    b. pharyngea
    pharyngeal b.
    b. of the piriformis muscle
    b. of popliteus
    prepatellar b.
    b. quadrati femoris
    radial b.
    retrohyoid b.
    b. retrohyoidea
    rider's b.
    sartorius bursae
    b. of semimembranosus muscle
    subacromial b.
    b. subacromialis
    subcoracoid b.
    b. subcutanea acromialis
    b. subcutanea calcanea
    b. subcutanea infrapatellaris
    b. subcutanea malleoli lateralis
    b. subcutanea malleoli medialis
    b. subcutanea olecrani
    b. subcutanea prepatellaris
    b. subcutanea prominentiae
      laryngeae
    b. subcutanea trochanterica
    b. subcutanea tuberositatis tibiae
    subcutaneous acromial b.
    subcutaneous calcaneal b.
    subcutaneous infrapatellar b.
    subcutaneous b. of the laryngeal
      prominence
    subcutaneous b. of lateral malleolus
    subcutaneous b. of medial
      malleolus
    subcutaneous olecranon b.
    subcutaneous b. of tibial tuberosity
    subdeltoid b.
    b. subdeltoidea
    b. subfascialis prepatellaris
    subfascial prepatellar b.
    subhyoid b.
    sublingual b.
    b. sublingualis
    subscapular b.
    b. subtendineae musculi
      gastrocnemii
    bursae subtendineae musculi sartorii
    b. subtendinea iliaca

bursa *(continued)*
 b. subtendinea musculi bicipitis femoris inferior
 b. subtendinea musculi infraspinati
 b. subtendinea musculi latissimus dorsi
 b. subtendinea musculi obturatoris interni
 b. subtendinea musculi subscapularis
 b. subtendinea musculi teretis majoris
 b. subtendinea musculi tibialis anterioris
 b. subtendinea musculi trapezii
 b. subtendinea musculi tricipitus brachii
 b. subtendinea prepatellaris
 subtendinous b. of gastrocnemius muscle
 subtendinous iliac b.
 subtendinous prepatellar b.
 subtendinous b. of the tibialis anterior muscle
 superior b. of biceps femoris
 suprapatellar b.
 b. suprapatellaris
 synovial b.
 b. synovialis
 synovial trochlear b.
 b. tendinis calcanei
 b. of tendo calcaneus
 b. of tensor veli palatini muscle
 b. of teres major
 tibial intertendinous b.
 b. of trapezius
 triceps b.
 trochanteric b.
 bursae trochantericae musculi glutei medii
 b. trochanterica musculi glutei maximi
 b. trochanterica musculi glutei minimi
 trochlear synovial b.
 ulnar b.

bursal
 b. abscess
 b. cyst
 b. synovitis

bursectomy

bursitis
 anserine b.
 olecranon b.
 prepatellar b.
 subacromial b.
 subdeltoid b.

bursolith

bursotomy

burst
 respiratory b.
 b. size

bursula
 b. testium

Burton's line

Buruli ulcer

Bury's disease

Buschke-Löwenstein tumor

Buschke-Ollendorf syndrome

Buschke's disease

bush yaws

Busquet's disease

Busse-Buschke disease

butanol-extractable iodine test

butt

butterfly
 b. eruption
 b. fragment
 b. patch
 b. pattern
 b. rash
 b. vertebra

butter stools

butter yellow

buttocks

button
 Amboyna b.
 belly b.
 Biskra b.
 Murphy's b.
 Oriental b.
 peritoneal b.
 b. suture

buttonhole
 b. iridectomy
 b. stenosis

buttress plate

butyrous

buyo cheek cancer

Buzzard's maneuver

Bwamba
 B. fever
 B. virus

By antigen

Byler disease

bypass
 aortocoronary b.
 aortoiliac b.
 aortorenal b.
 bowel b.
 cardiopulmonary b.
 coronary b.
 extraanatomic b.
 extracranial-intracranial b.
 femoropopliteal b.
 gastric b.

jejunoileal b.
left heart b.
partial ileal b.
right heart b.

by-product material
byssinosis
byte
Byzantine arch palate

B

C

    C bile
    C carbohydrate antigen
    C fibers
    C group viruses
    C wave, c wave

C1

    C1 esterase
    C1 esterase inhibitor

C3

    C3 proactivator
    C3 proactivator convertase

CA-125
cabbage goiter
cable graft
Cabot-Locke murmur
Cabot's ring bodies
caché
cachectic

    c. diarrhea
    c. edema
    c. endocarditis
    c. fever
    c. pallor

cachexia

    c. aphthosa
    c. aquosa
    diabetic neuropathic c.
    hypophyseal c.
    c. hypophyseopriva
    hypophysial c.
    malarial c.
    pituitary c.
    c. strumipriva
    c. thyroidea
    c. thyropriva

cachinnation
cacodemonomania
cacogeusia
cacomelia
cacoplastic
cacosmia
cacumen, pl. **cacumina**
cacuminal
cadaver
cadaveric

    c. rigidity
    c. spasm

cadaverous
caddis worm
caduca
café au lait spots
cafe coronary
Caffey-Kempe syndrome

Caffey's

    C. disease
    C. syndrome

Caffey-Silverman syndrome
cage

    thoracic c.

Cagot ear
Cain complex
c-a interval
caisson

    c. disease
    c. sickness

Cajal's

    C. astrocyte stain
    C. cell

caked breast
cake kidney
Calabar swelling
calamus

    c. scriptorius

calcaneal, calcanean

    c. arterial network
    c. arteries
    c. articular surface of talus
    c. bone
    c. gait
    c. petechiae
    c. process of cuboid bone
    c. region
    c. sulcus
    c. tuber
    c. tubercle
    c. tuberosity

calcanei (*gen. and pl. of* calcaneus)
calcaneoapophysitis
calcaneoastragaloid
calcaneocavus
calcaneocuboid

    c. joint
    c. ligament

calcaneodynia
calcaneofibular ligament
calcaneonavicular

    c. ligament

calcaneoscaphoid
calcaneotibial

    c. ligament

calcaneovalgocavus
calcaneovalgus
calcaneovarus
calcaneum
calcaneus, gen. and pl. **calcanei**
calcar

    c. avis

C

131

calcar *(continued)*
  c. femorale
  c. pedis
calcareous
  c. conjunctivitis
  c. degeneration
  c. metastasis
  c. pancreatitis
calcarine
  c. artery
  c. branch of medial occipital
    artery
  c. fasciculus
  c. fissure
  c. sulcus
calcariuria
calcergy
calces
calcicosis
calcific
  c. nodular aortic stenosis
  c. pancreatitis
calcification
  dystrophic c.
  eggshell c.
  c. lines of Retzius
  metastatic c.
  Mönckeberg's c.
  Mönckeberg's medial c.
  pathologic c.
  pulp c.
calcified cartilage
calcifying
  c. epithelial odontogenic tumor
  c. and keratinizing odontogenic
    cyst
  c. odontogenic cyst
calcigerous
calcii (*gen. of* calcium)
calcinosis
  c. circumscripta
  c. cutis
  dystrophic c.
  c. intervertebralis
  reversible c.
  tumoral c.
  c. universalis
calcinuric diabetes
calciokinesis
calciokinetic
calciorrhachia
calciostat
calciotraumatic
calcipectic
calcipenia
calcipenic
calcipexic
calcipexis, calcipexy

calciphilia
calciphylaxis
calciprivia
calciprivic
calcitonin gene related peptide
calcium, gen. **calcii**
  c. gout
  milk of c.
  c. pyrophosphate deposition disease
  c. rigor
  c. sign
  c. tungstate
calciuria
calcodynia
calcospherite
calculated
  c. mean organism
  c. serum osmolality
calculi
calculosis
calculus, gen. and pl. **calculi**
  apatite c.
  arthritic c.
  biliary c.
  bladder calculi
  blood c.
  branched c.
  bronchial c.
  cerebral c.
  coral c.
  cystine c.
  dendritic c.
  dental c.
  encysted c.
  fibrin c.
  gastric c.
  hematogenetic c.
  hemic c.
  infection c.
  intestinal c.
  lacrimal c.
  mammary c.
  matrix c.
  metabolic c.
  mulberry c.
  nasal c.
  nephritic c.
  oxalate c.
  pancreatic c.
  pharyngeal c.
  pleural c.
  pocketed c.
  preputial c.
  primary renal c.
  prostatic c.
  pulp c.
  renal c.
  salivary c.

secondary renal c.
serumal c.
staghorn c.
struvite c.
subgingival c.
supragingival c.
C. Surface Index
tonsillar c.
urethral c.
urinary c.
uterine c.
vesical c.
weddellite c.
whewellite c.

Caldani's ligament
Caldwell
C. projection
C. view
Caldwell-Luc operation
Caldwell-Moloy classification
calf, pl. **calves**
c. bone
football c.
gnome's c.
c. pump
calf-bone
caliceal
calicectasis
calicectomy
calices (*pl. of* calix)
caliciform
c. cell
c. ending
calicine
Caliciviridae
Calicivirus
calicoplasty
calicotomy
caliculus, pl. **caliculi**
c. gustatorius
c. ophthalmicus
caliectasis
California
C. psychological inventory test
C. virus
calioplasty
caliorrhaphy
caliotomy
caliper micrometer
calipers
calisthenics
calix, pl. **calices**
major calices
minor calices
calices renales majores
calices renales minores
Calkins' sign
Callahan's method

Callander's amputation
Call-Exner bodies
Calliphora
Callison's fluid
callosal
c. convolution
c. gyrus
c. sulcus
callositas
callosity
callosomarginal
c. artery
c. fissure
c. sulcus
callous
callus
central c.
definitive c.
ensheathing c.
medullary c.
permanent c.
provisional c.
temporary c.
Calmette-Guérin bacillus
Calmette test
calor
caloric
c. intake
c. nystagmus
c. test
calorific
calorigenic
calorimeter
Benedict-Roth c.
Calori's bursa
caloritropic
Calot's triangle
calvaria, pl. **calvariae**
calvarial
c. hook
calvarium
Calvé-Perthes disease
calves (*pl. of* calf)
calvities
calyceal
calyces (*pl. of* calyx)
calyciform
c. ending
calycine
calycle, calyculus
Calymmatobacterium
C. granulomatis
calyx, pl. **calyces**
cambium
c. layer
cameloid anemia
camera, pl. **camerae, cameras**
Anger c.

C

camera *(continued)*
    c. anterior bulbi
    gamma c.
    multiformat c.
    c. oculi anterior
    c. oculi major
    c. oculi minor
    c. oculi posterior
    c. posterior bulbi
    retinal c.
    scintillation c.
    c. vitrea bulbi
    vitreous c.
camerostome
camisole
CAMP
    C. factor
    C. test
camp
    c. fever
    c. hospital
Campbell
    C. ligament
    C. sound
Camper's
    C. chiasm
    C. fascia
    C. ligament
    C. line
    C. plane
campi foreli
campimeter
camplodactyly
camptocormia
camptodactyly, camptodactylia
camptomelia
camptomelic
    c. dwarfism
    c. syndrome
camptospasm
Campylobacter
    C. fetus
    C. fetus subsp. *jejuni*
    C. pylori
canal
    abdominal c.
    accessory c.
    adductor c.
    Alcock's c.
    alimentary c.
    alveolar c.'s
    alveolodental c.'s
    anal c.
    anterior condyloid c. of occipital
      bone
    anterior semicircular c.'s
    archenteric c.
    Arnold's c.

arterial c.
atrioventricular c.
auditory c.
basipharyngeal c.
Bernard's c.
Bichat's c.
birth c.
blastoporic c.
bony semicircular c.'s
Böttcher's c.
Braune's c.
Breschet's c.'s
carotid c.
carpal c.
caudal c.
central c.
central c.'s of cochlea
central c. of spinal cord
central c. of the vitreous
cervical c.
cervical axillary c.
cervicoaxillary c.
ciliary c.'s
Civinini's c.
Cloquet's c.
cochlear c.
condylar c., condyloid c.
Corti's c.
Cotunnius' c.
craniopharyngeal c.
deferent c.
dental c.'s
dentinal c.'s
diploic c.'s
Dorello's c.
Dupuytren's c.
endodermal c.
facial c.
fallopian c.
femoral c.
Ferrein's c.
Fontana's c.
galactophorous c.'s
Gartner's c.
gastric c.
greater palatine c.
gubernacular c.
c. of Guyon
gynecophoric c.
Hannover's c.
haversian c.'s
Hensen's c.
c. of Hering
Hirschfeld's c.'s
Holmgrén-Golgi c.'s
Hoyer's c.'s
Huguier's c.
Hunter's c.

hyaloid c.
hypoglossal c.
incisive c., incisor c.
inferior dental c.
infraorbital c.
inguinal c.
interdental c.'s
interfacial c.'s
Jacobson's c.
Kürsteiner's c.'s, Küersteiner's c.'s
lateral c.
lateral semicircular c.'s
Laurer's c.
Lauth's c.
Leeuwenhoek's c.'s
c.'s for lesser palatine nerves
longitudinal c.'s of modiolus
Löwenberg's c.
mandibular c.
marrow c.
mental c.
musculotubal c.
nasolacrimal c.
neural c.
neurenteric c.
notochordal c.
c. of Nuck
nutrient c.
obturator c.
optic c.
palatovaginal c.
parturient c.
pelvic c.
pericardioperitoneal c.
persistent atrioventricular c.
Petit's c.'s
pharyngeal c.
pleural c.
pleuropericardial c.'s
pleuroperitoneal c.
portal c.'s
posterior semicircular c.'s
pterygoid c.
pterygopalatine c.
pudendal c.
pulp c.
pyloric c.
Rivinus' c.'s
root c. of tooth
Rosenthal's c.
sacral c.
Santorini's c.
c.'s of Scarpa
Schlemm's c.
semicircular c.'s
small c. of chorda tympani
Sondermann's c.
spinal c.

spiral c. of cochlea
spiral c. of modiolus
Stilling's c.
subsartorial c.
Sucquet-Hoyer c.'s
Sucquet's c.'s
tarsal c.
temporal c.
Theile's c.
tubotympanic c.
tympanic c.
uniting c.
urogenital c.
uterovaginal c.
van Horne's c.
Velpeau's c.
vertebral c.
vesicourethral c.
vestibular c.
vidian c.
Volkmann's c.'s
vomerine c.
vomerobasilar c.
vomerorostral c.
vomerovaginal c.
Walther's c.'s
Wirsung's c.

canales (*pl. of* canalis)
canalicular
    c. adenoma
    c. ducts
    c. sphincter
canaliculi (*pl. of* canaliculus)
canaliculitis
canaliculization
canaliculus, pl. canaliculi
    anterior c. of chorda tympani
    auricular c.
    biliary c.
    bone c.
    caroticotympanic canaliculi
    canaliculi caroticotympanici
    c. chordae tympani
    c. cochleae
    cochlear c.
    canaliculi dentales
    c. innominatus
    intercellular c.
    intracellular c.
    lacrimal c.
    c. lacrimalis
    mastoid c.
    c. mastoideus
    posterior c. of chorda tympani
    c. reuniens
    secretory c.
    Thiersch's canaliculi

C

canaliculus *(continued)*
    tympanic c.
    c. tympanicus
canalis, pl. canales
    c. adductorius
    canales alveolares
    c. analis
    c. caroticus
    c. carpi
    c. centralis medullae spinalis
    c. cervicis uteri
    c. condylaris
    canales diploici
    c. femoralis
    c. gastrici
    c. gastricus
    c. hyaloideus
    c. hypoglossalis
    c. incisivus
    c. infraorbitalis
    c. inguinalis
    canales longitudinales modioli
    c. mandibulae
    c. musculotubarius
    c. nasolacrimalis
    c. nervi facialis
    c. nervi petrosi superficialis
      minoris
    c. nutricius
    c. obturatorius
    c. opticus
    canales palatini minores
    c. palatinus major
    c. palatovaginalis
    c. pterygoideus
    c. pudendalis
    c. pyloricus
    c. radicis dentis
    c. reuniens
    c. sacralis
    canales semicirculares anterior
    canales semicirculares lateralis
    canales semicirculares ossei
    canales semicirculares posterior
    c. spiralis cochleae
    c. spiralis modioli
    c. umbilicalis
    c. vertebralis
    c. vomerorostralis
    c. vomerovaginalis
canalization
Canavan's
    C. disease
    C. sclerosis
Canavan-van Bogaert-Bertrand disease
cancellated

cancellous
    c. bone
    c. tissue
cancellus, pl. cancelli
cancer
    c. antigen 125 test
    betel c.
    c. bodies
    buyo cheek c.
    chimney sweep's c.
    colloid c.
    conjugal c.
    c. à deux
    encephaloid c.
    c. en cuirasse
    epidermoid c.
    epithelial c.
    familial c.
    c. family
    glandular c.
    green c.
    c. juice
    kang c., kangri c.
    mouse c.
    mule-spinner's c.
    paraffin c.
    pipe-smoker's c.
    pitch-worker's c.
    scar c.
    scar c. of the lungs
    spider c.
    stump c.
    telangiectatic c.
canceration
cancerophobia
cancerous
cancra *(pl. of* cancrum)
cancriform
cancroid
cancrum, pl. cancra
    c. nasi
    c. oris
candicans
Candida
    C. albicans
candidemia
candidiasis
candidosis
canefield fever
canicola fever
canine
    c. adenovirus 1
    c. distemper virus
    c. eminence
    c. fossa
    c. prominence
    c. spasm
    c. tooth

caniniform
canister
canities
    canities c.
    c. circumscripta
    rapid c.
    c. unguium
canker
    c. sores
    water c.
cannon
    c. sound
    c. wave
cannonball pulse
Cannon-Bard theory
Cannon's
    C. point
    C. ring
    C. theory
cannula
    Hasson c.
    Karman c.
    laparoscopic c.
    perfusion c.
    washout c.
cannulation, cannulization
Cantelli's sign
cantering rhythm
canthal
    c. hypertelorism
canthectomy
canthi (*pl. of* canthus)
canthitis
cantholysis
canthomeatal plane
canthoplasty
canthorrhaphy
canthotomy
canthus, pl. **canthi**
    external c.
    internal c.
    lateral c.
    medial c.
cantilever
    c. beam
    c. bridge
Cantor tube
caoutchouc pelvis
cap
    acrosomal c.
    c. of the ampullary crest
    apical c.
    cervical c.
    chin c.
    cradle c.
    duodenal c.
    enamel c.
    head c.

    metanephric c.
    phrygian c.
    pyloric c.
    c. splint
    c. stage
capacitation
capacity
    cranial c.
    diffusing c.
    forced vital c.
    functional residual c.
    inspiratory c.
    iron-binding c.
    maximum breathing c.
    oxygen c.
    residual c.
    respiratory c.
    total lung c.
    vital c.
capeline bandage
Capgras'
    C. phenomenon
    C. syndrome
capillarectasia
Capillaria
    C. philippinensis
capillariasis
    intestinal c.
capillariomotor
capillarioscopy
capillaritis
capillaron
capillaropathy
capillaroscopy
capillary
    c. angioma
    arterial c.
    c. arteriole
    c. bed
    bile c.
    blood c.
    c. circulation
    continuous c.
    c. drainage
    fenestrated c.
    c. fracture
    c. fragility
    c. fragility test
    c. hemangioma
    c. hemangioma of infancy
    c. lake
    c. loops
    lymph c.
    c. nevus
    c. pulse
    c. resistance test
    sinusoidal c.
    c. vein

C

capillary *(continued)*
    venous c.
    c. vessel
    c. zone electrophoresis
capillus, gen. and pl. **capilli**
Capim viruses
capistration
capita (*pl. of* caput)
capital operation
capitate
    c. bone
capitellum
capitis (*gen. of* caput)
capitium
capitonnage
capitopedal
capitular
    c. joint
capitulum, pl. **capitula**
    c. humeri
    c. of humerus
Caplan's
    C. nodules
    C. syndrome
Capnocytophaga
    C. canimorsus
capnogram
capnograph
capon-comb-growth test
capped uterus
capping
    direct pulp c.
    indirect pulp c.
Capps' reflex
capriloquism
Capripoxvirus
caprizant
capsid
capsomer, capsomere
capsula, gen. and pl. **capsulae**
    c. adiposa renis
    c. articularis
    c. articularis cricoarytenoidea
    c. articularis cricothyroidea
    c. bulbi
    c. cordis
    c. externa
    c. extrema
    c. fibrosa
    c. fibrosa glandulae thyroideae
    c. fibrosa perivascularis
    c. fibrosa renis
    c. glomeruli
    c. interna
    c. lentis
    c. lienis
    c. vasculosa lentis

capsular
    c. advancement
    c. antigen
    c. branches of renal artery
    c. cataract
    c. cirrhosis of liver
    c. flap pyeloplasty
    c. glaucoma
    c. ligament
    c. precipitation reaction
    c. space
capsulation
capsule
    adipose c.
    adrenal c.
    articular c.
    atrabiliary c.
    auditory c.
    bacterial c.
    Bonnet's c.
    Bowman's c.
    brood c.'s
    cartilage c.
    c. cell
    cricoarytenoid articular c.
    cricothyroid articular c.
    Crosby c.
    crystalline c.
    external c.
    extreme c.
    eye c.
    fatty renal c.
    fibrous c.
    fibrous articular c.
    fibrous c. of kidney
    fibrous c. of liver
    fibrous c. of parotid gland
    fibrous c. of spleen
    fibrous c. of thyroid gland
    c. forceps
    Gerota's c.
    Glisson's c.
    glomerular c.
    internal c.
    joint c.
    lens c.
    lenticular c.
    malpighian c.
    Müller's c.
    nasal c.
    optic c.
    otic c.
    perivascular fibrous c.
    radiotelemetering c.
    seminal c.
    suprarenal c.
    Tenon's c.
capsulectomy

capsulitis
    adhesive c.
    hepatic c.
capsulolenticular
    c. cataract
capsuloplasty
capsulorrhaphy
capsulotome
capsulotomy
    renal c.
capture
    atrial c.
    electron c.
    K c.
    ventricular c.
capture-recapture method
Capuron's points
caput, gcn. **capitis**, pl. **capita**
    c. angulare quadrati labii superioris
    c. breve
    c. breve musculi bicipitis brachii
    c. breve musculi bicipitis femoris
    c. cornus
    c. costae
    c. epididymidis
    c. epididymis
    c. femoris
    c. fibulae
    c. gallinaginis
    c. humerale
    c. humerale musculi flexoris carpi
    ulnaris
    c. humerale musculi pronatoris
    teretis
    c. humeri
    c. humeroulnare musculi flexoris
    digitorum superificialis
    c. infraorbitale quadrati labii
    superioris
    c. laterale
    c. laterale musculi gastrocnemii
    c. laterale musculi tricipitis brachii
    c. longum
    c. longum musculi bicipitis brachii
    c. longum musculi bicipitis femoris
    c. longum musculi tricipitis brachii
    c. mallei
    c. mandibulae
    c. mediale
    c. mediale musculi gastrocnemii
    c. mediale musculi tricipitis brachii
    c. medusae
    c. nuclei caudati
    c. obliquum
    c. obliquum musculi adductoris
    hallucis
    c. obliquum musculi adductoris
    pollicis

    c. ossis femoris
    c. ossis metacarpalis
    c. ossis metatarsalis
    c. pancreatis
    c. phalangis
    c. profundum musculi flexoris
    pollicis brevis
    c. quadratum
    c. radiale
    c. radii
    c. stapedis
    c. succedaneum
    c. superficiale musculi flexoris
    pollicis brevis
    c. tali
    c. transversum
    c. transversum musculi adductoris
    hallucis
    c. transversum musculi adductoris
    pollicis
    c. ulnae
    c. ulnare
    c. ulnare musculi flexoris carpi
    ulnaris
    c. ulnare musculi pronatoris teretis
    c. zygomaticum quadrati labii
    superioris
Carabelli tubercle
Caraparu virus
carate
carbaril
carbohydrate-induced hyperlipemia
carbohydrate utilization test
carbohydraturia
carbol-thionin stain
carboluria
carbometry
carbon
    c. dioxide acidosis
    c. dioxide combining power
    c. dioxide elimination
    c. monoxide poisoning
carbonometer
carbonometry
carbonuria
carboxyhemoglobinemia
carbuncle
    kidney c., renal c.
carbuncular
carbunculosis
carcinoembryonic
    c. antigen
carcinogenesis
carcinoid
    c. flush
    c. syndrome
    c. tumor
carcinoma, pl. **carcinomas, carcinomata**

C

carcinoma *(continued)*
  acinar c.
  acinic cell c.
  acinose c., acinous c.
  adenoid cystic c.
  adenoid squamous cell c.
  adenosquamous c.
  adnexal c.
  adrenal cortical carcinomas
  alveolar cell c.
  anaplastic c.
  apocrine c.
  basal cell c.
  basaloid c.
  basal squamous cell c.
  basosquamous c., basisquamous c.
  bronchiolar c.
  bronchiolo-alveolar c.
  bronchogenic c.
  clear cell c. of kidney
  colloid c.
  cylindromatous c.
  cystic c.
  duct c., ductal c.
  embryonal c.
  endometrioid c.
  epidermoid c.
  epithelial myoepithelial c.
  c. ex pleomorphic adenoma
  fibrolamellar liver cell c.
  follicular carcinomas
  giant cell c.
  giant cell c. of thyroid gland
  glandular c.
  hepatocellular c.
  Hürthle cell c.
  inflammatory c.
  intermediate c.
  intraductal c.
  intraepidermal c.
  intraepithelial c.
  invasive c.
  juvenile c.
  kangri burn c.
  large cell c.
  latent c.
  lateral aberrant thyroid c.
  leptomeningeal c.
  liver cell c.
  lobular c.
  lobular c. in situ
  medullary c.
  melanotic c.
  meningeal c.
  mesometanephric c.
  metaplastic c.
  metastatic c.
  metatypical c.

  microinvasive c.
  mucinous c.
  mucoepidermoid c.
  c. myxomatodes
  noninfiltrating lobular c.
  oat cell c.
  occult c.
  oncoplastic c.
  papillary c.
  primary c.
  primary neuroendocrine c. of the
    skin
  renal cell c.
  sarcomatoid c.
  scar c.
  scirrhous c.
  secondary c.
  secretory c.
  signet-ring cell c.
  c. simplex
  c. in situ
  small cell c.
  spindle cell c.
  sweat gland c.
  trabecular c.
  transitional cell c.
  tubular c.
  verrucous c.
  villous c.
  wolffian duct c.
  yolk sac c.
carcinomata
carcinomatosis
  leptomeningeal c.
  meningeal c.
carcinomatous
  c. encephalomyelopathy
  c. implants
  c. myelopathy
  c. myopathy
  c. neuromyopathy
  c. pericarditis
carcinophobia
carcinosarcoma
  embryonal c.
  renal c.
carcinosis
carcoma
Carden's amputation
cardia
  gastric c.
cardiac
  c. accident
  c. albuminuria
  c. alternation
  c. aneurysm
  c. arrest
  c. arrhythmia

c. asthma
c. ballet
c. catheter
c. cirrhosis
c. competence
c. contractility
c. cycle
c. decompression
c. depressor reflex
c. dropsy
c. dyspnea
c. dysrhythmia
c. edema
c. failure
c. fibrous skeleton
c. ganglia
c. gating
c. gland
c. glands of esophagus
c. hemoptysis
c. heterotaxia
c. histiocyte
c. impression of liver
c. impression of lung
c. impulse
c. incompetence
c. index
c. infarction
c. insufficiency
c. jelly
c. liver
c. lung
c. lymphatic ring
c. mapping
c. massage
c. monitor
c. murmur
c. muscle
c. muscle tissue
c. muscle wrap
c. neurosis
c. notch
c. notch of left lung
c. opening
c. orifice
c. output
c. part of stomach
c. plexus
c. polyp
c. prominence
c. reserve
c. segment
c. shock
c. skeleton
c. souffle
c. sound
c. standstill
c. symphysis

c. syncope
c. tamponade
c. telemetry
c. tube
c. valve prosthesis
c. valvular incompetence
c. veins
cardialgia
cardiataxia
cardiatelia
cardiectasia
cardiectomy
cardiectopia
cardinal
c. ligament
c. ocular movements
c. points
c. symptom
c. veins
carding
cardioaccelerator
cardioactive
cardioangiography
cardioaortic
cardioarterial
c. interval
Cardiobacterium
C. hominis
cardiocele
cardiochalasia
cardiodiaphragmatic angle
cardiodiosis
cardiodynamics
cardiodynia
cardioesophageal
c. junction
c. relaxation
cardiofacial syndrome
cardiogenesis
cardiogenic
c. plate
c. shock
cardiogram
esophageal c.
cardiograph
cardiography
ultrasonic c.
ultrasound c.
vector c.
cardiohemothrombus
cardiohepatic
c. angle
c. triangle
cardiohepatomegaly
cardioid
c. condenser
cardiokymogram
cardiokymograph

C

cardiokymography
cardiolipin
cardiologist
cardiology
cardiolysis
cardiomalacia
cardiomegaly
    glycogen c.
    glycogenic c.
cardiometry
cardiomotility
cardiomuscular
cardiomyoliposis
cardiomyopathy
    alcoholic c.
    congestive c.
    dilated c.
    familial hypertrophic c.
    hypertrophic c.
    idiopathic c.
    peripartum c.
    postpartum c.
    primary c.
    restrictive c.
    secondary c.
cardiomyoplasty
cardiomyotomy
cardionatrin
cardionecrosis
cardionector
cardionephric
cardioneural
cardioneurosis
cardio-omentopexy
cardiopaludism
cardiopath
cardiopathia nigra
cardiopathy
cardiopericardiopexy
cardiophobia
cardiophone
cardiophony
cardiophrenia
cardiophrenic angle
cardioplasty
cardioplegia
    antegrade c.
    retrograde c.
cardioplegic
    c. arrest
cardioptosia
cardiopulmonary
    c. arrest
    c. bypass
    c. murmur
    c. resuscitation
    c. splanchnic nerves
    c. transplantation

cardiopyloric
cardiorenal
cardiorespiratory murmur
cardiorrhaphy
cardiorrhexis
cardioscope
cardiospasm
cardiosphygmograph
cardiotachometer
cardiothoracic ratio
cardiothrombus
cardiothyrotoxicosis
cardiotomy
cardiotoxic myolysis
cardiovalvulitis
cardiovascular
    c. radiology
    c. syphilis
    c. system
cardiovasculorenal
cardioversion
cardiovert
cardioverter
Cardiovirus
carditis
    rheumatic c.
care
    comprehensive medical c.
    health c.
    intensive c.
    managed c.
    medical c.
    primary medical c.
    secondary medical c.
    tertiary medical c.
Carey Coombs murmur
caribi
caries
    active c.
    arrested dental c.
    buccal c.
    cemental c.
    compound c.
    dental c.
    distal c.
    fissure c.
    incipient c.
    interdental c.
    mesial c.
    nursing bottle c.
    occlusal c.
    pit c.
    pit and fissure c.
    primary c.
    proximal c.
    radiation c.
    recurrent c.
    root c.

secondary c.
senile dental c.
smooth surface c.
carina, pl. **carinae**
   c. fornicis
   c. of trachea
   c. tracheae
   c. urethralis vaginae
   urethral c. of vagina
   c. vaginae
carinal lymph nodes
carinate abdomen
cariogenesis
cariogenic
cariogenicity
cariology
cariostatic
carious
Carlen's tube
carmalum
Carman's sign
carmine
   lithium c.
   Schneider's c.
carminic acid
carminophil, carminophile,
   carminophilous
Carmody-Batson operation
carneous
   c. degeneration
   c. mole
carnes (*pl. of* caro)
carnes
Carnett's sign
carnification
carnis (*gen. of* caro)
carnosinemia
carnosity
Carnoy's fixative
caro, gen. **carnis,** pl. **carnes**
   c. quadrata sylvii
Caroli's
   C. disease
   C. syndrome
carotenemia
carotenoderma
carotenosis cutis
carotic
caroticoclinoid ligament
caroticotympanic
   c. arteries
   c. canaliculi
   c. nerve
carotid
   c. arteries
   c. body
   c. body tumor
   c. bruit

   c. bulb
   c. canal
   c. duct
   c. endarterectomy
   c. foramen
   c. ganglion
   c. groove
   c. pulse
   c. sheath
   c. shudder
   c. sinus
   c. sinus branch
   c. sinus nerve
   c. sinus reflex
   c. sinus syncope
   c. sinus syndrome
   c. sinus test
   c. sulcus
   c. triangle
   c. tubercle
   c. wall of middle ear
carotid-cavernous fistula
carotidynia
carotinemia
carotinosis cutis
carotodynia
carpal
   c. arches
   c. artery
   c. articular surface of radius
   c. articulation
   c. bones
   c. canal
   c. groove
   c. joints
   c. tunnel
   c. tunnel syndrome
carpectomy
Carpenter's syndrome
Carpentier-Edwards valve
carphologia, carphology
carpi (*gen. and pl. of* carpus)
carp mouth
carpocarpal
Carpoglyptus
carpometacarpal
   c. joints
   c. joint of thumb
   c. ligaments
carpopedal
   c. contraction
   c. spasm
carpoptosis, carpoptosia
Carpue's method
carpus, gen. and pl. **carpi**
   c. curvus
carre-four sensitif
Carrel-Lindbergh pump

C

Carrel's treatment
carrier
  amalgam c.
  c. cell
  convalescent c.
  genetic c.
  incubatory c.
  latent c.
  manifesting c.
  c. screening
  c. state
  c. strain
  translocation c.
carrier-free
Carrington's disease
Carrión's disease
Carr-Price
  C.-P. reaction
  C.-P. test
Carr-Purcell experiment
carrying angle
car sickness
Carter's
  C. black mycetoma
  C. fever
cartilage
  accessory c.
  accessory nasal c.'s
  accessory quadrate c.
  c. of acoustic meatus
  alisphenoid c.
  annular c.
  arthrodial c.
  articular c.
  arytenoid c.
  c. of auditory tube
  auricular c.
  basilar c.
  c. bone
  branchial c.'s
  calcified c.
  c. capsule
  c. cell
  cellular c.
  ciliary c.
  circumferential c.
  conchal c.
  connecting c.
  corniculate c.
  costal c.
  cricoid c.
  cuneiform c.
  diarthrodial c.
  c. of ear
  elastic c.
  ensiform c., ensisternum c.
  epiglottic c.
  epiphysial c.

falciform c.
floating c.
greater alar c.
Huschke's c.'s
hyaline c.
hypsiloid c.
interosseous c.
intervertebral c.
intra-articular c.
intrathyroid c.
investing c.
Jacobson's c.
c. knife
c. lacuna
c.'s of larynx
lateral c. of nose
lesser alar c.'s
loose c.
Luschka's c.
mandibular c.
c. matrix
meatal c.
Meckel's c.
Meyer's c.'s
Morgagni's c.
nasal septal c.
c. of nasal septum
c.'s of nose
ossifying c.
parachordal c.
paraseptal c.
parenchymatous c.
periotic c.
permanent c.
pharyngeal c.'s
c. of pharyngotympanic tube
precursory c.
primordial c.
quadrangular c.
Reichert's c.
reticular c., retiform c.
Santorini's c.
Seiler's c.
semilunar c.
septal c.
sesamoid c. of larynx
sesamoid c.'s of nose
slipping rib c.
c. space
sternal c.
supra-arytenoid c.
tarsal c.
temporary c.
thyroid c.
tracheal c.'s
triangular c.—*fibrocartilage*
triquetrous c.
triticeal c.

tubal c.
uniting c.
vomerine c., vomeronasal c.
Weitbrecht's c.
Wrisberg's c.
xiphoid c.
Y c., Y-shaped c.
yellow c.
cartilage-hair hypoplasia
cartilagines (*pl. of* cartilago)
cartilaginoid
cartilaginous
c. articulation
c. joint
c. neurocranium
c. part of auditory tube
c. part of external acoustic meatus
c. part of skeletal system
c. septum
c. tissue
c. viscerocranium
cartilago, pl. **cartilagines**
cartilagines alares minores
c. alaris major
c. articularis
c. arytenoidea
c. auriculae
c. corniculata
c. costalis
c. cricoidea
c. cuneiformis
c. epiglottica
c. epiphysialis
cartilagines laryngis
c. meatus acustici
cartilagines nasales accessoriae
cartilagines nasi
c. nasi lateralis
c. septi nasi
c. sesamoidea laryngis
c. thyroidea
cartilagines tracheales
c. triticea
c. tubae auditivae
c. vomeronasalis
caruncle
lacrimal c.
Morgagni's c.
Santorini's major c.
Santorini's minor c.
urethral c.
caruncula, pl. **carunculae**
hymenal c.
c. hymenalis, pl. carunculae
  hymenales
c. lacrimalis
c. myrtiformis, pl. carunculae
  myrtiformes

c. salivaris
sublingual c.
c. sublingualis
Carus'
C. circle
C. curve
Carvallo's sign
carver
caryotheca
Casal's necklace
cascade
c. stomach
case
borderline c.
c. control study
c. fatality ratio
index c.
trial c.
caseation
c. necrosis
caseous
c. abscess
c. degeneration
c. necrosis
c. osteitis
c. pneumonia
c. rhinitis
c. tubercle
Casoni
C. intradermal test
C. skin test
Casselberry position
Casser's
C. fontanel
C. perforated muscle
cassette
c. mutagenesis
cast
bacterial c.
blood c.
c. brace
coma c.
dental c.
diagnostic c.
epithelial c.
false c.
fatty c.
fibrinous c.
granular c.
hair c.
halo c.
hyaline c.
investment c.
master c.
mucous c.
red blood cell c.
red cell c.
refractory c.

C

145

cast *(continued)*
    renal c.
    spurious c.
    tube c.
    urinary c.'s
    waxy c.
    white blood cell c.
    white cell c.
Castellani-Low sign
Castellani's bronchitis
casting
    centrifugal c.
    ceramo-metal c.
    c. flask
    gold c.
    c. ring
    vacuum c.
    c. wax
Castleman's disease
castration
    c. anxiety
    c. cells
    c. complex
    functional c.
casualty
catabasial
catachronobiology
catacrotic
    c. pulse
catacrotism
catadicrotic
    c. pulse
catadicrotism
catadidymus
catadioptric
catagen
catagenesis
catalepsy
cataleptic
cataleptoid
catalogia
catamenia
catamenial
catamenogenic
catamnesis
catamnestic
cataphasia
cataphora
cataplasia, cataplasis
cataplectic
cataplexy
cataract
    annular c.
    arborescent c.
    atopic c.
    axial c.
    black c.
    blue c.

    capsular c.
    capsulolenticular c.
    central c.
    cerulean c.
    complete c.
    complicated c.
    concussion c.
    copper c.
    coralliform c.
    coronary c.
    cortical c.
    crystalline c.
    cuneiform c.
    cupuliform c.
    dendritic c.
    diabetic c.
    disk-shaped c.
    electric c.
    embryonic c.
    embryopathic c.
    fibroid c., fibrinous c.
    floriform c.
    furnacemen's c.
    fusiform c.
    galactose c.
    glassworker's c.
    glaucomatous c.
    gray c.
    hard c.
    hook-shaped c.
    hypermature c.
    hypocalcemic c.
    immature c.
    infantile c.
    infrared c.
    intumescent c.
    juvenile c.
    lamellar c.
    c. lens
    life-belt c.
    mature c.
    membranous c.
    Morgagni's c.
    myotonic c.
    c. needle
    nuclear c.
    overripe c.
    perinuclear c.
    peripheral c.
    pisciform c.
    polar c.
    posterior subcapsular c.
    progressive c.
    punctate c.
    pyramidal c.
    radiation c.
    reduplicated c.
    ripe c.

rubella c.
saucer-shaped c.
secondary c.
sedimentary c.
senile c.
siderotic c.
soft c.
spindle c.
c. spoon
stationary c.
stellate c.
subcapsular c.
sugar c.
sunflower c.
sutural c.
tetany c.
total c.
toxic c.
traumatic c.
umbilicated c.
vascular c.
zonular c.
cataracta
c. adiposa
c. brunescens
c. cerulea
c. electrica
c. fibrosa
c. nigra
c. ossea
cataractogenesis
cataractogenic
cataract-oligophrenia syndrome
cataractous
catarrh
nasal c.
vernal c.
catarrhal
c. asthma
c. fever
c. gastritis
c. inflammation
c. jaundice
c. ophthalmia
catastalsis
catastasis
catastrophe theory
catastrophic reaction
catatonia
excited c.
periodic c.
stuporous c.
catatonic, catatoniac
c. dementia
c. excitement
c. pupil
c. rigidity

c. schizophrenia
c. stupor
catatrichy
catatricrotic
catatricrotism
catatropic image
cat-bite
c.-b. disease
c.-b. fever
catchment area
cat-cry syndrome
categorical trait
catelectrotonus
Catenabacterium
C. *contortum*
catenoid
catenulate
caterpillar
c. cell
c. dermatitis
c. flap
c. rash
caterpillar-hair ophthalmia
catgut suture
catharsis
cathectic
catheter
acorn-tipped c.
angiography c.
balloon c.
balloon-tip c.
bicoudate c., c. bicoudé
Bozeman-Fritsch c.
Braasch c.
brush c.
cardiac c.
central venous c.
conical c.
c. coudé
c. à demeure
de Pezzer c.
double-channel c.
elbowed c.
c. embolus
eustachian c.
female c.
c. fever
Fogarty c.
Foley c.
c. gauge
Gouley's c.
c. guide
indwelling c.
intracardiac c.
Malecot c.
Nélaton's c.
olive-tipped c.
pacing c.

147

catheter (*continued*)
    Pezzer c.
    Phillips' c.
    pigtail c.
    prostatic c.
    Robinson c.
    self-retaining c.
    spiral tip c.
    Swan-Ganz c.
    two-way c.
    vertebrated c.
    whistle-tip c.
    winged c.
catheterization
catheterize
catheterostat
cathexis
cathodal
    c. closure contraction
    c. closure tetanus
    c. duration tetanus
    c. opening clonus
    c. opening contraction
    c. opening tetanus
cathode
    c. ray oscilloscope
    c. rays
    c. ray tube
catholysis
cation-anion difference
catlin, catling
catochus
catoptric
cat-scratch disease
cat's cry syndrome
cat's-eye
    c.-e. pupil
    c.-e. syndrome
Cattell Infant Intelligence Scale
cattle plague virus
Catu virus
cauda, pl. **caudae**
    c. epididymidis
    c. epididymis
    c. equina
    c. equina syndrome
    c. fasciae dentatae
    c. helicis
    c. nuclei caudati
    c. pancreatis
    c. striati
caudad
caudal
    c. anesthesia
    c. canal
    c. flexure
    c. ligament
    c. neuropore

    c. pancreatic artery
    c. pharyngeal complex
    c. retinaculum
    c. sheath
    c. transtentorial herniation
    c. transverse fissure
caudate
    c. branches
    c. lobe
    c. nucleus
    c. process
caudatolenticular
caudatum
caudolenticular
caul, cowl
cauliflower ear
caumesthesia
causal
    c. additivity
    c. independence
    c. indication
    c. treatment
causalgia
causality
cause
    constitutional c.
    exciting c.
    necessary c.
    precipitating c.
    predisposing c.
    proximate c.
    specific c.
    sufficient c.
cauterization
cauterize
cautery
    actual c.
    BICAP c.
    bipolar c.
    chemical c.
    cold c.
    c. conization
    electric c.
    galvanic c.
    gas c.
    c. knife
    monopolar c.
cava (*pl. of* cavum)
cavagram
caval
    c. fold
    c. valve
cavalry bone
cavascope
cave
    c. sickness
    trigeminal c.
caveola, pl. **caveolae**

cavern
    c.'s of corpora cavernosa
    c.'s of corpus spongiosum
caverna, pl. **cavernae**
    cavernae corporis spongiosi
    cavernae corporum cavernosorum
caverniloquy
cavernitis
    fibrous c.
cavernoscope
cavernoscopy
cavernositis
cavernostomy
cavernous
    c. angioma
    c. arteries
    c. body of clitoris
    c. body of penis
    c. branch of internal carotid artery
    c. groove
    c. hemangioma
    c. lymphangiectasis
    c. nerves of clitoris
    c. nerves of penis
    c. part of internal carotid artery
    c. plexus of clitoris
    c. plexus of conchae
    c. plexus of penis
    c. rale
    c. resonance
    c. respiration
    c. rhonchus
    c. sinus
    c. sinus branch of internal carotid
      artery
    c. sinus syndrome
    c. tissue
    c. transfer of portal vein
    c. veins of penis
    c. voice
    c. voice sound
caviar lesion
cavitary
cavitas, pl. **cavitates**
    c. abdominalis
    c. articularis
    c. coronalis
    c. dentis
    c. glenoidalis
    c. infraglotticum
    c. laryngis
    c. medullaris
    c. nasi
    c. oris
    c. oris propria
    c. pelvis
    c. pericardialis
    c. peritonealis

    c. pharyngis
    c. pleuralis
    c. thoracis
    c. tympanica
    c. uteri
cavitation
cavitis
cavity
    abdominal c.
    abdominopelvic c.
    amniotic c.
    articular c.
    axillary c.
    body c.
    buccal c.
    cleavage c.
    c. of concha
    c.'s of corpora cavernosa
    c.'s of corpus spongiosum
    cotyloid c.
    cranial c.
    crown c.
    ectoplacental c.
    ectotrophoblastic c.
    epamniotic c.
    epidural c.
    glenoid c.
    greater peritoneal c.
    head c.
    idiopathic bone c.
    inferior laryngeal c.
    infraglottic c.
    intermediate laryngeal c.
    intracranial c.
    c. of larynx
    lesser peritoneal c.
    c. line angle
    c. liner
    c. margin
    Meckel's c.
    medullary c.
    c. of middle ear
    nasal c.
    oral c.
    oral c. proper
    orbital c.
    pelvic c.
    pericardial c.
    peritoneal c.
    perivisceral c.
    pharyngonasal c.
    c. of pharynx
    pleural c.
    pleuroperitoneal c.
    c. preparation
    c. preparation base
    c. preparation form
    primitive perivisceral c.

C

C-dif

cavity *(continued)*
pulmonary c.
pulp c.
Retzius' c.
segmentation c.
c. of septum pellucidum
somite c.
splanchnic c.
subarachnoid c.
subdural c.
subgerminal c.
superior laryngeal c.
thoracic c.
c. of tooth
trigeminal c.
tympanic c.
uterine c., c. of uterus
visceral c.
c. wall

cavogram
cavography
cavopulmonary
c. anastomosis
c. shunt

cavosurface
c. angle
c. bevel

cavum, pl. **cava**
c. abdominis
c. articulare
c. conchae
c. coronale
c. dentis
c. douglasi
c. epidurale
c. infraglotticum
c. laryngis
c. mediastinale
c. medullare
c. nasi
c. oris
c. pelvis
c. pericardii
c. peritonei
c. pharyngis
c. pleurae
c. psalterii
c. retzii
c. septi pellucidi
c. subarachnoideum
c. subdurale
c. thoracis
c. trigeminale
c. tympani
c. uteri *et*
c. vergae
c. vesicouterinum

Cazenave's vitiligo

C-banding
C.-b. stain

CB lead
CD 54
CD4/CD8 count
CDE
CDE antigens
CDE blood group

ceasmic teratosis
cebocephaly
ceca (*pl. of* cecum)
cecal
c. arteries
c. folds
c. foramen of frontal bone
c. foramen of the tongue
c. hernia
c. recess
c. volvulus

cecectomy
cecil urethroplasty
cecitis
cecocentral scotoma
cecocolostomy
cecofixation
cecoileostomy
cecopexy
cecoplication
cecorrhaphy
cecosigmoidostomy
cecostomy
cecotomy
cecum, pl. **ceca**
cupular c. of the cochlear duct
c. cupulare
vestibular c. of the cochlear duct
c. vestibulare

Ceelen-Gellerstedt syndrome
cel
celectome
celenteron
celestine blue B
Celestin tube
celiac
c. artery
c. axis
c. branches of vagus nerve
c. disease
c. ganglia
c. glands
c. (lymphatic) plexus
c. lymph nodes
c. (nervous) plexus
c. plexus
c. plexus reflex
c. rickets
c. sprue

c. syndrome
c. trunk

celiagra
celiectomy
celiocentesis
celioenterotomy
celiogastrostomy
celiogastrotomy
celiohysterectomy
celiohysterotomy
celiomyalgia
celiomyomectomy
celiomyomotomy
celiomyositis
celioparacentesis
celiopathy
celiorrhaphy
celiosalpingectomy
celiosalpingotomy
celioscopy
celiotomy

c. incision
vaginal c.

celitis
cell

A c.'s
absorptive c.'s of intestine
acid c.
acidophil c.
acinar c.
acinous c.
acoustic c.
c. adhesion molecule
adipose c.
adventitial c.
air c.'s
air c.'s of auditory tube
albuminous c.
algoid c.
alpha c.'s of anterior lobe of
    hypophysis
alpha c.'s of pancreas
alveolar c.
amacrine c.
ameboid c.
amniogenic c.'s
anabiotic c.'s
anaplastic c.
angioblastic c.'s
Anitschkow c.
anterior c.'s
anterior ethmoidal air c.'s
anterior horn c.
antigen-presenting c.'s
antigen-responsive c.
antigen-sensitive c.
apolar c.
argentaffin c.'s

argyrophilic c.'s
Aschoff c.
Askanazy c.
astroglia c.
auditory receptor c.'s
B c.
balloon c.
band c.
basal c.
basaloid c.
basilar c.
basket c.
basophil c. of anterior lobe of
    hypophysis
beaker c.
Beale's c.
Berger c.'s
berry c.
beta c. of anterior lobe of
    hypophysis
beta c. of pancreas
Betz c.'s
Bevan-Lewis c.'s
bipolar c.
Bizzozero's red c.'s
blast c.
blood c.
c. body
Boll's c.'s
bone c.
border c.'s
Böttcher's c.'s
Bowenoid c.'s
c. bridges
bristle c.
bronchic c.'s
bronchiolar exocrine c.
brood c.
burr c.
Cajal's c.
caliciform c.
capsule c.
carrier c.
cartilage c.
castration c.'s
caterpillar c.
c. center
centroacinar c.
chalice c.
chief c.
chief c. of corpus pineale
chief c. of parathyroid gland
chief c. of stomach
chromaffin c.
chromophobe c.'s of anterior lobe
    of hypophysis
Clara c.
Clarke c.'s

C

cell *(continued)*
    Claudius' c.'s
    clear c.
    cleavage c.
    cleaved c.
    clonogenic c.
    cochlear hair c.'s
    column c.'s
    commissural c.
    compound granule c.
    cone c. of retina
    connective tissue c.
    contrasuppressor c.'s
    Corti's c.'s
    crescent c.
    c. culture
    cytomegalic c.'s
    cytotoxic c.
    cytotrophoblastic c.'s
    D c.
    dark c.'s
    daughter c.
    Davidoff's c.'s
    decidual c.
    decoy c.'s
    deep c.
    Deiters' c.'s
    delta c. of anterior lobe of
      hypophysis
    delta c. of pancreas
    dendritic c.'s
    c. determination
    Dogiel's c.'s
    dome c.
    Downey c.
    dust c.
    effector c.
    egg c.
    embryonic c.
    enamel c.
    end c.
    endodermal c.'s
    endothelial c.
    enterochromaffin c.'s
    enteroendocrine c.'s
    entodermal c.'s
    ependymal c.
    epidermic c.
    epithelial c.
    epithelial reticular c.
    epithelioid c.
    erythroid c.
    ethmoid air c.'s
    ethmoidal c.'s
    external pillar c.'s
    exudation c.
    Fañanás c.
    fasciculata c.

fat c.
fat-storing c.
Ferrata's c.
floor c.
foam c.'s
follicular epithelial c.
follicular ovarian c.'s
foreign body giant c.
formative c.'s
foveolar c.'s of stomach
fuchsinophil c.
fusiform c.'s of cerebral cortex
c. fusion
G c.'s
ganglion c.
ganglion c.'s of dorsal spinal root
ganglion c.'s of retina
Gaucher c.'s
gemistocytic c.
germ c.
germinal c.
ghost c.
giant c.
Gierke c.'s
gitter c.
glia c.'s
glitter c.'s
globoid c.
glomerulosa c.
goblet c.
Golgi epithelial c.
Golgi's c.'s
Goormaghtigh's c.'s
granule c.'s
granule c. of connective tissue
granulosa c.
granulosa lutein c.'s
great alveolar c.'s
guanine c.
gustatory c.'s
gyrochrome c.
hair c.'s
hairy c.'s
Haller c.
heart failure c.'s
HeLa c.'s
helmet c.
helper c.
HEMPAS c.'s
Hensen's c.
heteromeric c.
hilus c.'s
hobnail c.'s
Hofbauer c.
horizontal c. of Cajal
horizontal c.'s of retina
horny c.
Hortega c.'s

Hürthle c.
c. hybridization
I c.
immunologically activated c.
immunologically competent c.
inclusion c.
c. inclusions
indifferent c.
inducer c.
innocent bystander c.
intercapillary c.
internal pillar c.'s
interstitial c.'s
irritation c.
islet c.
Ito c.'s
juvenile c.
juxtaglomerular c.'s
K c.'s
karyochrome c.
keratinized c.
killer c.'s
Kulchitsky c.'s
Kupffer c.'s
lacis c.
Langerhans' c.'s
Langhans' c.'s
Langhans'-type giant c.'s
LE c.
Leishman's chrome c.'s
lepra c.'s
Leydig's c.'s
light c.'s of thyroid
c. line
lining c.
Lipschütz c.
littoral c.
Loevit's c.
lupus erythematosus c.
luteal c., lutein c.
lymph c.
lymphoid c.
macroglia c.
malpighian c.
Marchand's wandering c.
c. marker
marrow c.
Martinotti's c.
mast c.
mastoid c.'s
mastoid air c.'s
c. matrix
c. membrane
Merkel's tactile c.
mesangial c.
mesenchymal c.'s
mesoglial c.'s
mesothelial c.

Mexican hat c.
Meynert's c.'s
microglia c.'s, microglial c.'s
middle c.'s
middle ethmoidal air c.'s
midget bipolar c.'s
migratory c.
Mikulicz' c.'s
mirror-image c.
mitral c.'s
monocytoid c.
mossy c.
mother c.
motor c.
mucoalbuminous c.'s
mucoserous c.'s
mucous c.
mucous neck c.
Müller's radial c.'s
multipolar c.
mural c.
myeloid c.
myoepithelial c.
myoid c.'s
Nageotte c.'s
natural killer c.'s
nerve c.
c. nests
Neumann's c.'s
neurilemma c.'s
neuroendocrine c.
neuroendocrine transducer c.
neuroepithelial c.'s
neuroglia c.'s
neurolemma c.'s
neurosecretory c.'s
nevus c.
nevus c., A-type
nevus c., B-type
nevus c., C-type
Niemann-Pick c.
NK c.'s
nonclonogenic c.
null c.'s
nurse c.'s
oat c.
OKT c.'s
olfactory c.'s
olfactory receptor c.'s
oligodendroglia c.'s
Onodi c.
Opalski c.
c. organelle
osseous c.
osteochondrogenic c.
osteogenic c.
osteoprogenitor c.
oxyntic c.

C

cell *(continued)*
  oxyphil c.'s
  P c.
  pagetoid c.'s
  Paget's c.'s
  Paneth's granular c.'s
  parafollicular c.'s
  paraganglionic c.'s
  paraluteal c.
  paralutein c.
  parenchymal c.
  parenchymatous c. of corpus
    pineale
  parent c.
  parietal c.
  peptic c.
  pericapillary c.
  peripolar c.
  perithelial c.
  peritubular contractile c.'s
  pessary c.
  phalangeal c.
  pheochrome c.
  photo c.
  photoreceptor c.'s
  physaliphorous c.
  Pick c.
  pigment c.
  pigment c.'s of iris
  pigment c.'s of retina
  pigment c. of skin
  pillar c.'s
  pillar c.'s of Corti
  pineal c.'s
  plasma c.
  pluripotent c.'s
  polar c.
  polychromatic c.
  polychromatophil c.
  posterior c.'s
  posterior ethmoidal air c.'s
  pregnancy c.'s
  pregranulosa c.'s
  prickle c.
  primary embryonic c.
  primitive reticular c.
  primordial c.
  primordial germ c.
  prolactin c.
  pseudo-Gaucher c.
  pseudounipolar c.
  pseudoxanthoma c.
  pulpar c.
  Purkinje's c.'s
  pus c.
  pyramidal c.'s
  pyrrol c., pyrrhol c.
  Raji c.

reactive c.
red blood c.
Reed c.'s
Reed-Sternberg c.'s
Renshaw c.'s
resting c.
resting wandering c.
restructured c.
reticular c.
reticularis c.
reticuloendothelial c.
rhagiocrine c.
Rieder c.'s
Rindfleisch's c.'s
rod nuclear c.
rod c. of retina
Rolando's c.'s
rosette-forming c.'s
sarcogenic c.
satellite c.'s
satellite c. of skeletal muscle
scavenger c.
Schilling's band c.
Schultze's c.'s
Schwann c.'s
segmented c.
sensitized c.
sensory c.
septal c.
seromucous c.'s
serous c.
Sertoli's c.'s
sex c.
Sézary c.
shadow c.'s
sickle c.
signet ring c.'s
silver c.
skein c.
small cleaved c.
smudge c.'s
somatic c.'s
sperm c.
spindle c.
spine c.
splenic c.'s
squamous c.
squamous alveolar c.'s
stab c.
staff c.
stellate c.'s of cerebral cortex
stellate c.'s of liver
stem c.
Sternberg c.'s
Sternberg-Reed c.'s
stichochrome c.
c. strain
strap c.

supporting c.
suppressor c.'s
c. surface marker
surface mucous c.'s of stomach
sustentacular c.
sympathetic formative c.
sympathicotropic c.'s
sympathochromaffin c.
synovial c.
T c.
tactile c.
tanned red c.'s
target c.
tart c.
taste c.'s
T cytotoxic c.'s
TDTH c.'s
tendon c.'s
Tg c.'s
theca lutein c.
theca c.'s of stomach
T helper c.'s
Tm c.'s
totipotent c.
touch c.
Touton giant c.
transducer c.
c. transformation
transitional c.
tubal air c.'s
tufted c.
tunnel c.'s
Türk c.
tympanic c.'s
tympanic air c.'s
type I c.'s
type II c.'s
Tzanck c.'s
undifferentiated c.
unipolar c.
vasoformative c.
veil c.
veiled c.'s
vestibular hair c.'s
Virchow's c.'s
virus-transformed c.
visual receptor c.'s
vitreous c.
c. wall
wandering c.
Warthin-Finkeldey c.'s
wasserhelle c.
water-clear c. of parathyroid
white blood c.
WI-38 c.'s
wing c.

yolk c.'s
zymogenic c.
cella, gen. and pl. **cellae**
c. media
cell-bound antibody
cellicolous
cell-mediated
c.-m. immunity
c.-m. reaction
celloidin
cellona
cellula, gen. and pl. **cellulae**
cellulae anteriores
cellulae coli
cellulae ethmoidales
cellulae mastoideae
cellulae mediae
cellulae pneumaticae tubae auditivae
cellulae posteriores
cellulae tympanicae
cellular
c. biology
c. blue nevus
c. cartilage
c. embolism
c. immune theory
c. immunity
c. immunity deficiency syndrome
c. immunodeficiency with abnormal
immunoglobulin synthesis
c. infiltration
c. mosaicism
c. pathology
c. polyp
c. spill
c. tenacity
c. tumor
cellularity
cellule
cellulicidal
cellulifugal
cellulipetal
cellulite
cellulitic phlegmasia
cellulitis
acute scalp c.
anaerobic c.
dissecting c.
eosinophilic c.
gangrenous c.
necrotizing c.
pelvic c.
phlegmonous c.
cellulocutaneous flap
celluloid strip
cellulose tape technique
celom, celoma
extraembryonic c.

C

celomic
   c. bay
   c. metaplasia theory of
     endometriosis
celonychia
celophlebitis
celoscope
celoscopy
celosomia
CELO virus
Celovirus
celozoic
Celsus'
   C. alopecia
   C. area
   C. papules
   C. vitiligo
Celsus kerion
cement
   c. base
   composite dental c.
   copper phosphate c.
   c. corpuscle
   dental c.
   glass ionomer c.
   inorganic dental c.
   intercellular c.
   c. line
   modified zinc oxide-eugenol c.
   organic dental c.
   polycarboxylate c.
   resin c.
   silicate c.
   tooth c.
   unmodified zinc oxide-eugenol c.
   zinc phosphate c.
cemental
   c. caries
   c. dysplasia
cementation
cementicle
cementification
cementoblast
cementoblastoma
   benign c.
cementoclasia
cementoclast
cementocyte
cementodentinal
   c. junction
cementoenamel junction
cementogenesis
cementoma
   gigantiform c.
   true c.
cementum
   afibrillar c.
   c. hyperplasia

   primary c.
   secondary c.
cenesthesia
cenesthesic, cenesthetic
cenesthopathy
cenocyte
cenocytic
cenosite
cenotrope
censor
census
center
   anospinal c.
   Broca's c.
   Budge's c.
   cell c.
   chondrification c.
   ciliospinal c.
   community mental health c.
   dentary c.
   diaphysial c.
   epiotic c.
   expiratory c.
   feeding c.
   germinal c. of Flemming
   health c.
   inspiratory c.
   Kerckring's c.
   medullary c.
   motor speech c.
   ossific c.
   c. of ossification
   primary c. of ossification
   reaction c.
   respiratory c.
   c. of ridge
   c. of rotation
   satiety c.
   secondary c. of ossification
   semioval c.
   sensory speech c.
   speech c.'s
   sphenotic c.
   vasomotor c.
   vital c.
   Wernicke's c.
Centers for Disease Control
centesis
centile
centimorgan
centipede
centra (*pl. of* centrum)
centrad
centrage
central
   c. amputation
   c. angiospastic retinitis
   c. angiospastic retinopathy

c. apnea
c. apparatus
c. areolar choroidal atrophy
c. areolar choroidal sclerosis
c. artery
c. artery of retina
c. bearing
c. body
c. bone
c. bone of ankle
c. bradycardia
c. callus
c. canal
c. canals of cochlea
c. canal of spinal cord
c. canal of the vitreous
c. cataract
c. cementifying fibroma
c. chromatolysis
c. cord syndrome
c. core disease
c. deafness
c. dogma
C. European tick-borne encephalitis virus
C. European tick-borne fever
c. excitatory state
c. fibrous body
c. ganglioneuroma
c. gray substance
c. group of axillary lymph nodes
c. gyri
c. illumination
c. incisor
c. inhibition
c. lacteal
c. and lateral intermediate substance
c. lateral nucleus of thalamus
c. limit theorem
c. lobule
c. lobule of cerebellum
c. mesenteric lymph nodes
c. necrosis
c. nervous system
c. neuritis
c. ossifying fibroma
c. osteitis
c. palmar space
c. paralysis
c. pit
c. placenta previa
c. pneumonia
c. pontine myelinolysis
c. Recklinghausen's disease type II
c. retinal fovea
c. scotoma
c. serous choroidopathy

c. serous retinopathy
c. spindle
c. sulcal artery
c. sulcus
c. tegmental fasciculus
c. tegmental tract
c. tendon of diaphragm
c. tendon of perineum
c. terminal electrode
c. thalamic radiations
c. transactional core
c. type neurofibromatosis
c. vein of retina
c. veins of liver
c. vein of suprarenal gland
c. venous catheter
c. venous pressure
c. vision
central-bearing
  c.-b. device
  c.-b. point
  c.-b. tracing device
centralis
centre médian de Luys
centrencephalic
  c. epilepsy
centri-acinar emphysema
centric
  c. contact
  c. fusion
  c. interocclusal record
  c. jaw relation
  c. occlusion
  c. position
  c. relation
centriciput
centrifugal
  c. casting
  c. current
  c. nerve
centrilobular
  c. emphysema
centriole
  anterior c.
  distal c.
  posterior c.
  proximal c.
centripetal
  c. current
  c. nerve
centroacinar cell
Centrocestus
centrocyte
centrofacial lentiginosis
centrokinesia
centrokinetic
centrolecithal
  c. ovum

C

centromedian nucleus
centromere
    c. banding stain
centromeric index
centronuclear myopathy
centroplasm
centrosome
centrosphere
centrostaltic
centrum, pl. centra
    c. medianum
    c. medullare
    c. ovale
    c. semiovale
    c. tendineum diaphragmatis
    c. tendineum perinei
    c. of a vertebra
    Vicq d'Azyr's c. semiovale
    Vieussens' c.
    Willis' c. nervosum
Centruroides
cephalad
cephalalgia
    histaminic c.
    Horton's c.
cephalea
    c. agitata, c. attonita
cephaledema
cephalemia
cephalhematocele
cephalhematoma
cephalhydrocele
cephalic
    c. angle
    c. arterial rami
    c. flexure
    c. index
    c. pole
    c. presentation
    c. reflexes
    c. tetanus
    c. triangle
    c. vein
    c. version
cephaline
cephalitis
cephalization
cephalocaudal
    c. axis
cephalocele
cephalocentesis
cephalochord
cephalodactyly
    Vogt c.
cephalodidymus
cephalodiprosopus
cephalodynia
cephalogenesis

cephalogram
cephalogyric
cephalohematocele
cephalohematoma
cephalohemometer
cephalomedullary angle
cephalomegaly
cephalomelus
cephalomeningitis
cephalometer
cephalometric
    c. analysis
    c. radiograph
    c. tracing
cephalometrics
cephalometry
    ultrasonic c.
cephalomotor
Cephalomyia
cephalont
cephalo-oculocutaneous telangiectasia
cephalo-orbital index
cephalopagus
cephalopalpebral reflex
cephalopathy
cephalopelvic
cephalopelvimetry
cephalopharyngeus
cephalorrhachidian
    c. index
Cephalosporium
cephalostat
cephalothoracic
cephalothoracopagus
    c. asymmetros
    c. disymmetros
    c. monosymmetros
cephalotome
cephalotomy
cephalotribe
cephalotrigeminal angiomatosis
ceptor
    chemical c.
    contact c.
    distance c.
ceramo-metal casting
ceratocricoid
    c. ligament
    c. muscle
ceratoglossus
ceratohyal
ceratopharyngeal part of middle
    pharyngeal constrictor
Ceratophyllidae
Ceratophyllus
    C. punjatensis
cercaria, pl. cercariae
cerci (*gen. and pl. of* cercus)

cerclage
cercocystis
cercomer
cercomonad
Cercomonas
cercus, gen. and pl. **cerci**
cerea flexibilitas
cerebella (*pl. of* cerebellum)
cerebellar
    c. arteries
    c. astrocytoma
    c. ataxia
    c. atrophy
    c. cortex
    c. cyst
    c. fissures
    c. folia
    c. fossa
    c. frenulum
    c. gait
    c. hemisphere
    c. nuclei
    c. pyramid
    c. rigidity
    c. speech
    c. sulci
    c. syndrome
    c. tonsil
    c. veins
cerebellitis
cerebellohypothalamic fibers
cerebellolental
cerebellomedullary
    c. cistern
    c. malformation syndrome
cerebello-olivary
cerebellopontile angle
cerebellopontine
    c. angle
    c. angle syndrome
    c. angle tumor
    c. cisternography
    c. recess
cerebellorubral
    c. tract
cerebellospinal fibers
cerebellothalamic tract
cerebellum, pl. cerebella
cerebra
cerebra (*pl. of* cerebrum)
cerebral
    c. agraphia
    c. amyloid angiopathy
    c. angiography
    c. anthrax
    c. aqueduct
    c. arterial circle
    c. arteries

    c. arteriography
    c. calculus
    c. cladosporiosis
    c. compression
    c. cortex
    c. cranium
    c. death
    c. decompression
    c. decortication
    c. diataxia
    c. dominance
    c. dysplasia
    c. edema
    c. fissures
    c. flexure
    c. gigantism
    c. hemisphere
    c. hemorrhage
    c. hernia
    c. index
    c. lacuna
    c. layer of retina
    c. lipidosis
    c. localization
    c. malaria
    c. palsy
    c. part of arachnoid
    c. part of dura mater
    c. part of internal carotid artery
    c. peduncle
    c. porosis
    c. rheumatism
    c. sinuses
    c. sphingolipidosis
    c. sulci
    c. surface
    c. tetanus
    c. thrombosis
    c. trigone
    c. tuberculosis
    c. veins
    c. ventricles
    c. vesicle
    c. vomiting
cerebralgia
cerebration
cerebriform
cerebritis
    suppurative c.
cerebrohepatorenal syndrome
cerebroma
cerebromalacia
cerebromeningitis
cerebropathia
cerebropathy
cerebrophysiology
cerebroretinal angiomatosis
cerebrosclerosis

C

cerebroside
   c. lipidosis
   c. lipoidosis
cerebrosidosis
cerebrospinal
   c. axis
   c. fever
   c. fluid
   c. fluid otorrhea
   c. fluid rhinorrhea
   c. index
   c. meningitis
   c. pressure
   c. system
cerebrotendinous cholesterinosis
cerebrotomy
cerebrotonia
cerebrovascular
   c. accident
   c. disease
cerebrum, pl. cerebra, cerebrums
cerecloth
Cerenkov radiation
Cerithidea
ceroid
   c. lipofuscinosis
ceroplasty
certified nurse-midwife
certified registered nurse anesthetist
cerulean
   c. cataract
ceruleus nucleus
cerumen
   c. inspissatum, inspissated c.
ceruminal
ceruminoma
ceruminosis
ceruminous
   c. glands
cervical
   c. amputation
   c. anchorage
   c. anesthesia
   c. aortic knuckle
   c. auricle
   c. axillary canal
   c. branch of facial nerve
   c. canal
   c. cap
   c. compression syndrome
   c. cyst
   c. disc syndrome
   c. diverticulum
   c. duct
   c. dysplasia
   c. enlargement
   c. enlargement of spinal cord
   c. fibrositis

   c. flexure
   c. fusion syndrome
   c. glands
   c. glands of uterus
   c. hydrocele
   c. hygroma
   c. hyperesthesia
   c. iliocostal muscle
   c. interspinales muscles
   c. interspinal muscle
   c. intraepithelial neoplasia
   c. ligament of uterus
   c. line
   c. longissimus muscle
   c. loop
   c. margin
   c. margin of tooth
   c. myelogram
   c. myositis
   c. myospasm
   c. nerves
   c. nystagmus
   c. part of esophagus
   c. part of internal carotid artery
   c. part of spinal cord
   c. part of thoracic duct
   c. patagium
   c. pleura
   c. plexus
   c. pregnancy
   c. rib
   c. rib and band syndrome
   c. rib syndrome
   c. rotator muscles
   c. segments of spinal cord
   c. sinus
   c. smear
   c. splanchnic nerves
   c. spondylosis
   c. tension syndrome
   c. triangle
   c. vein
   c. vertebrae
   c. vesicle
   c. zone
   c. zone of tooth
cervicalis
   c. ascendens
cervicectomy
cervices (pl. of cervix)
cervicis (gen. of cervix)
cervicitis
cervicoaxillary canal
cervicobrachial
cervicobuccal
cervicodynia
cervicofacial
cervicography

cervicolabial
cervicolingual
cervicolinguoaxial
cervicolumbar phenomenon
cervico-occipital
cervico-oculo-acoustic syndrome
cervicoplasty
cervicothoracic
    c. ganglion
    c. transition
cervicotomy
cervicovaginal artery
cervicovesical
cervix, gen. cervicis, pl. cervices
    c. of the axon
    c. columnae posterioris
    c. dentis
    c. uteri
    c. of uterus
    c. vesicae urinariae
cesarean
    c. hysterectomy
    c. operation
    c. section
Cestan-Chenais syndrome
Cestodaria
cestode, cestoid
Cestoidea
CF
    CF antibody
    CF lead
    CF test
Chaddock
    C. reflex
    C. sign
Chadwick's sign
chaeta
chafe
Chagas-Cruz disease
Chagas' disease
chagasic myocardiopathy
chagoma
Chagres virus
chain
    behavior c.
    cold c.
    hemolytic c.
    long c.
    ossicular c.
    c. reflex
    short c.
chain-compensated spirometer
chaining
chalasia, chalasis
chalaza
chalazion, pl. chalazia
    acute c.
    collar-stud c.

chalcosis
    c. lentis
chalice cell
chalicosis
chalinoplasty
challenge diet
chamber
    altitude c.
    anechoic c.
    anterior c. of eye
    aqueous c.'s
    decompression c.
    high altitude c.
    hyperbaric c.
    ionization c.
    posterior c. of eye
    pulp c.
    relief c.
    sinuatrial c.
    vitreous c. of eye
    Zappert counting c.
Chamberlain
    C. line
    C. procedure
Chamberlen forceps
chamecephalic
chamecephalous
chameprosopic
chamfer
Champy's fixative
Chance fracture
chancre
    hard c.
    mixed c.
    monorecidive c.
    c. redux
    soft c.
    sporotrichositic c.
    tularemic c.
chancriform
    c. pyoderma
    c. syndrome
chancroid
chancroidal
    c. bubo
chancrous
chandelier sign
Chandler syndrome
change
    Armanni-Ebstein c.
    Baggenstoss c.
    Crooke's hyaline c.
    fatty c.
    c. of life
    trophic c.'s
channel
    ion c.
    ligand-gated c.

channel *(continued)*
  transnexus c.
  voltage-gated c.
Chantemesse reaction
chaos
  mathematical c.
  c. theory
chaotic heart
chappa
chapped
character
  acquired c.
  c. analysis
  c. armor
  classifiable c.
  compound c.
  denumerable c.
  discrete c.
  c. disorder
  dominant c.
  inherited c.
  mendelian c.
  c. neurosis
  primary sex c.'s
  recessive c.
  secondary sex c.'s
  sex-linked c.
  unit c.
characteristic
  c. curve
  c. emission
  c. radiation
  receiver operating c.
characterization
  denture c.
Charcot-Böttcher crystalloids
Charcot-Bouchard aneurysm
Charcot-Leyden crystals
Charcot-Marie-Tooth disease
Charcot-Neumann crystals
Charcot-Robin crystals
Charcot's
  C. arteries
  C. disease
  C. gait
  C. intermittent fever
  C. joint
  C. syndrome
  C. triad
  C. vertigo
Charcot-Weiss-Baker syndrome
charge nurse
charlatan
charlatanism
charley horse
Charlouis' disease
Charnley hip arthroplasty
Charrière scale

chart
  Amsler's c.
  isometric c.
  quality control c.
  Tanner growth c.
  Walker's c.
Charters' method
charting
Chassaignac's
  C. space
  C. tubercle
Chauffard's syndrome
Chaussier's
  C. areola
  C. line
  C. sign
Chauveau's bacterium
Chayes' method
Cheadle's disease
Cheatle slit
check
  Δ c., delta c.
  c. ligaments of eyeball, medial and
    lateral
  c. ligaments of odontoid
checkbite
Chédiak-Higashi disease
Chédiak-Steinbrinck-Higashi anomaly
cheek
  c. bone
  c. muscle
  c. tooth
cheese
  c. maggot
  c. worker's lung
cheesy
  c. abscess
  c. pus
cheilalgia, chilalgia
cheilectomy, chilectomy
cheilectropion, chilectropion
cheilion
cheilitis, chilitis
  actinic c.
  angular c.
  commissural c.
  contact c.
  c. exfoliativa
  c. glandularis
  c. granulomatosa
  impetiginous c.
  solar c.
  c. venenata
  Volkmann's c.
cheilognathoglossoschisis
cheilognathopalatoschisis
cheilognathouranoschisis
cheilophagia, chilophagia

cheiloplasty, chiloplasty
cheilorrhaphy, chilorrhaphy
cheilosis, chilosis
cheilostomatoplasty, chilostomatoplasty
cheilotomy, chilotomy
cheirarthritis, chirarthritis
cheirobrachialgia, chirobrachialgia
cheirognostic, chirognostic
cheirokinesthesia
cheirokinesthetic
cheirology, chirology
cheiromegaly, chiromegaly
cheiroplasty, chiroplasty
cheiropodalgia, chiropodalgia
cheiropompholyx, chiropompholyx
cheirospasm, chirospasm
chelicera, pl. chelicerae
chelidon
cheloid
chemexfoliation
chemical
    c. burn
    c. cautery
    c. ceptor
    c. conjunctivitis
    c. depilatory
    c. dermatitis
    c. diabetes
    c. peeling
    c. peritonitis
    c. pneumonia
    c. prophylaxis
    c. ray
    c. sampling
    c. shift
    c. shift artifact
    c. sympathectomy
chemically cured resin
"chemical" thyroidectomy
chemicocautery
chemise
chemistry
    radiopharmaceutical c.
chemoautotroph
chemoautotrophic
chemocautery
chemoceptor
chemodectoma
chemodectomatosis
chemodifferentiation
chemoheterotroph
chemoheterotrophic
chemokines
chemolithotroph
chemolithotrophic
chemonucleolysis
chemoorganotroph
chemoorganotrophic

chemopallidectomy
chemopallidothalamectomy
chemopallidotomy
chemoreceptor
    medullary c.
    peripheral c.
    c. tumor
chemoreflex
chemoresistance
chemosis
chemosurgery
    Mohs' c.
chemothalamectomy
chemothalamotomy
chemotherapeutic index
chemotherapy
    consolidation c.
    induction c.
    intensification c.
    salvage c.
chemotic
Cheney syndrome
cherry angioma
cherry-red
    c.-r. spot
    c.-r. spot myoclonus syndrome
cherubic facies
cherubism
chessboard grafts
chest
    alar c.
    barrel c.
    flail c.
    flat c.
    foveated c., funnel c.
    c. index
    keeled c.
    c. leads
    phthinoid c.
    pigeon c.
    pterygoid c.
    c. radiology
    c. wall
Chevalier-Jackson dilator
chevron incision
chewing
    c. cycle
    c. force
    c. louse
Cheyne-Stokes
    C.-S. psychosis
    C.-S. respiration
Chiari
    C. disease
    C. II syndrome
    C. net
    C. syndrome
Chiari-Budd syndrome

C

Chiari-Frommel syndrome
chiasm
    Camper's c.
    optic c.
    tendinous c. of the digital tendons
chiasma, pl. **chiasmata**
    c. opticum
    c. syndrome
    c. tendinum
chiasmapexy
chiasmatic
    c. cistern
    c. groove
    c. sulcus
Chicago disease
chicken
    c. breast
    c. embryo lethal orphan virus
    c. fat clot
chickenpox
    c. virus
Chick-Martin test
chiclero ulcer
chief
    c. agglutinin
    c. artery of thumb
    c. cell
    c. cell of corpus pineale
    c. cell of parathyroid gland
    c. cell of stomach
    c. complaint
Chievitz'
    C. layer
    C. organ
chigger
chigoe
chikungunya virus
Chilaiditi's syndrome
chilalgia (*var. of* cheilalgia)
chilblain
    c. lupus
    c. lupus erythematosus
child
    c. abuse
    c. psychology
childbearing
    c. age
childbed fever
childbirth
childhood
    c. absence epilepsy
    c. epilepsy with occipital
     paroxysms
    c. hypophosphatasia
    c. muscular dystrophy
    c. schizophrenia
    c. tuberculosis
    c. type tuberculosis

CHILD syndrome
chilectomy (*var. of* cheilectomy)
chilectropion (*var. of* cheilectropion)
chilitis (*var. of* cheilitis)
chill
    smelter's c.'s
Chilomastix
chilophagia (*var. of* cheilophagia)
chiloplasty (*var. of* cheiloplasty)
chiloplasty
Chilopoda
chilopodiasis
chilorrhaphy (*var. of* cheilorrhaphy)
chilorrhaphy
chilosis (*var. of* cheilosis)
chilostomatoplasty (*var. of*
    cheilostomatoplasty)
chilostomatoplasty
chilotomy
chilotomy (*var. of* cheilotomy)
chimera
    radiation c.
chimeric
    c. antibodies
chimerism
chimney sweep's cancer
chimpanzee coryza agent
chin
    c. cap
    double c.
    galoche c.
    c. jerk
    c. muscle
    c. reflex
Chinese restaurant syndrome
chip
    bone c.'s
    c. graft
    c. syringe
chip-blower
chirarthritis
chirarthritis (*var. of* cheirarthritis)
chirobrachialgia
chirobrachialgia (*var. of*
    cheirobrachialgia)
chirognostic (*var. of* cheirognostic)
chirognostic
chirokinesthesia
chirology (*var. of* cheirology)
chirology
chiromegaly (*var. of* cheiromegaly)
chiroplasty (*var. of* cheiroplasty)
chiroplasty
chiropodalgia
chiropodalgia (*var. of* cheiropodalgia)
chiropodist
chiropody

chiropompholyx (*var. of* cheiropompholyx)
chiropompholyx
chiropractic
chiropractor
chiroscope
chirospasm (*var. of* cheirospasm)
chirospasm
chirurgeon
chirurgery
chirurgical
chisel
    binangle c.
chi-square
    c.-s. distribution
    c.-s. test
chiufa
Chlamydia
    C. pneumoniae
chlamydia, pl. **chlamydiae**
Chlamydiaceae
chlamydial
chlamydoconidium
Chlamydophrys
Chlamydozoon
chloasma
    c. bronzinum
chloracne
chloramphenicol
    c. acetyl transferase
chlorazol black E
chloremia
chlorhydria
chloride depletion
chloridimetry
chloridometer
chloriduria
chlorine acne
chloroanemia
chloroleukemia
chloroma
chloromyeloma
chloropenia
chloropercha
    c. method
chloropsia
chlorosis
chlorotic
    c. anemia
chlorphenol red
chloruresis
chloruria
choana, pl. **choanae**
    primary c., primitive c.
    secondary c.
choanal
    c. atresia
    c. polyp

choanate
choanoflagellate
choanoid
choanomastigote
Choanotaenia infundibulum
chocolate
    c. agar
    c. cyst
Chodzko's reflex
choked disk
chokes
cholaneresis
cholangeitis
cholangiectasis
cholangiocarcinoma
cholangioenterostomy
cholangiofibrosis
cholangiogastrostomy
cholangiogram
cholangiography
    cystic duct c.
    intravenous c.
    percutaneous c.
cholangiole
cholangiolitic
    c. cirrhosis
    c. hepatitis
cholangiolitis
cholangioma
cholangiopancreatography
    endoscopic retrograde c.
cholangioscopy
cholangiostomy
cholangiotomy
cholangitic abscess
cholangitis
    ascending c.
    c. lenta
    primary sclerosing c.
    recurrent pyogenic c.
cholascos
cholecyst
cholecystatony
cholecystectasia
cholecystectomy
cholecystenterostomy
cholecystenterotomy
cholecystic
cholecystis
cholecystitis
    acute c.
    chronic c.
    emphysematous c.
    xanthogranulomatous c.
cholecystocolostomy
cholecystoduodenal fistula
cholecystoduodenostomy
cholecystogastrostomy

C

cholecystogram
cholecystography
cholecystoileostomy
cholecystojejunostomy
cholecystokinetic
cholecystolithiasis
cholecystolithotripsy
cholecystomy
cholecystopaque
cholecystopathy
cholecystopexy
cholecystorrhaphy
cholecystosonography
cholecystostomy
cholecystotomy
 laparoscopic c.
choledoch
 c. duct
choledochal
 c. cyst
 c. sphincter
choledochectomy
choledochendysis
choledochiarctia
choledochitis
choledochocholedochostomy
choledochoduodenal junction
choledochoduodenostomy
choledochoenterostomy
choledochography
choledochojejunostomy
choledocholith
choledocholithiasis
choledocholithotomy
choledocholithotripsy
choledocholithotrity
choledochoplasty
choledochorrhaphy
choledochostomy
choledochotomy
choledochous
choledochus
cholehemia
cholelith
cholelithiasis
cholelithotomy
cholelithotripsy
cholelithotrity
cholemesis
cholemia
cholemic
 c. nephrosis
cholepathia
 c. spastica
choleperitoneum
choleperitonitis
cholera
 c. agar

Asiatic c.
c. bacillus
c. infantum
c. morbus
pancreatic c.
c. sicca
typhoid c.
choleragen
choleraic diarrhea
choleraphage
cholera-red reaction
choleresis
cholerheic
choleric
cholerine
cholerrhagia
cholerrhagic
cholescintigraphy
cholestasia, cholestasis
cholestatic
 c. hepatitis
 c. jaundice
cholesteatomatous
cholesteremia
cholesterinemia
cholesterinized antigen
cholesterinosis
 cerebrotendinous c.
cholesterinuria
cholesteroderma
cholesterol
 c. cleft
 c. embolism
 c. ester storage disease
cholesterolemia
cholesterolosis
 extracellular c.
cholesteroluria
cholesterosis
 c. cutis
choleuria
cholicele
cholinergic
 c. fibers
 c. urticaria
chololith
chololithiasis
chololithic
choloplania
cholorrhea
choloscopy
cholothorax
choluria
chondral
chondralgia
chondralloplasia
chondrectomy

chondrification
    c. center
chondrify
chondrin ball
chondritis
    costal c.
chondroblast
chondroblastoma
chondrocalcinosis
    articular c.
chondroclast
chondrocostal
chondrocranium
chondrocyte
    isogenous c.'s
chondrodermatitis nodularis chronica
  helicis
chondrodynia
chondrodysplasia
    c. punctata
chondrodystrophia
    c. calcificans congenita
    c. congenita punctata
chondrodystrophic dwarfism
chondrodystrophy
    asphyxiating thoracic c.
    asymmetrical c.
    hereditary deforming c.
    hypoplastic fetal c.
chondroectodermal
    c. dysplasia
chondrofibroma
chondrogenesis
chondroglossus
    c. muscle
chondroid
    c. syringoma
    c. tissue
chondrology
chondrolysis
chondroma
    extraskeletal c.
    juxtacortical c.
    periosteal c.
chondromalacia
    c. fetalis
    generalized c.
    c. of larynx
    c. pate'llae
    systemic c.
chondromatosis
    synovial c.
chondromatous
chondromere
chondromyxoid fibroma
chondromyxoma
chondro-osseous
chondro-osteodystrophy

chondropathy
chondropharyngeal part of middle
  pharyngeal constrictor
chondropharyngeus
chondrophyte
chondroplast
chondroplasty
chondroporosis
chondrosarcoma
chondrosis
chondroskeleton
chondrosternal
chondrosternoplasty
chondrotome
chondrotomy
chondrotrophic
chondroxiphoid
    c. ligament
chonechondrosternon
Chopart's
    C. amputation
    C. joint
chorda, pl. chordae
    c. dorsalis
    c. magna
    c. obliqua
    c. saliva
    c. spermatica
    c. spinalis
    chordae tendineae
    c. tympani
    c. umbilicalis
    c. vertebralis
    c. vocalis, pl. chordae vocales
    chordae willisii
chordal
chorda-mesoderm
chordee
chorditis
    c. vocalis inferior
chordoma
chordoskeleton
chordotomy
chorea
    c.-acanthocytosis
    acanthocytosis with c.
    acute c.
    benign familial c.
    chronic progressive c.
    c. cordis
    dancing c.
    degenerative c.
    c. dimidiata
    electric c.
    fibrillary c.
    c. gravidarum
    habit c.
    hemilateral c.

C

chorea *(continued)*
    Henoch's c.
    hereditary c.
    Huntington's c.
    hysterical c.
    juvenile c.
    laryngeal c.
    c. major
    mimetic c.
    c. minor
    Morvan's c.
    posthemiplegic c.
    procursive c.
    rheumatic c.
    rhythmic c.
    saltatory c.
    senile c.
    Sydenham's c.
choreal
choreic
    c. abasia
    c. movement
choreiform
choreoathetoid
choreoathetosis
    congenital c.
choreoid
choreophrasia
chorioadenoma
    c. destruens
chorioallantoic
    c. membrane
    c. placenta
chorioallantois
chorioamnionic placenta
chorioamnionitis
chorioangioma
chorioangiomatosis
chorioangiosis
choriocapillaris
choriocapillary layer
choriocarcinoma
choriocele
chorioepithelioma
chorioma
choriomeningitis
    lymphocytic c.
chorion
    c. frondosum
    c. laeve
    previllous c.
    primitive c.
    shaggy c.
    smooth c.
chorionic
    c. ectoderm
    c. epithelioma
    c. plate

    c. sac
    c. villi
    c. villus biopsy
chorioretinal
chorioretinitis
    c. sclopetaria
chorioretinopathy
chorista
choristoblastoma
choristoma
choroid
    c. branches
    c. capillary layer
    c. fissure
    c. glomus
    c. plexus
    c. plexus of fourth ventricle
    c. plexus of lateral ventricle
    c. plexus of third ventricle
    c. skein
    c. tela of fourth ventricle
    c. tela of third ventricle
    c. vein
    c. veins of eye
choroidal
    c. fissure
    c. ring
    c. vascular atrophy
choroidea
choroideremia
choroiditis
    anterior c.
    areolar c.
    diffuse c.
    disseminated c.
    exudative c.
    juxtapupillary c.
    metastatic c.
    multifocal c.
    posterior c.
    proliferative c.
    suppurative c.
choroidocyclitis
choroidopathy
    areolar c.
    central serous c.
    Doyne's honeycomb c.
    geographic c.
    guttate c.
    helicoid c.
    myopic c.
    serpiginous c.
choroidoretinitis
choroidosis
Chotzen's syndrome
Chr^a antigens
Christchurch chromosome
Christensen-Krabbe disease

Christian's
  C. disease
  C. syndrome
Christison's formula
Christmas
  C. disease
  C. factor
Christ-Siemens-Touraine syndrome
chromaffin
  c. body
  c. cell
  c. reaction
  c. system
  c. tissue
  c. tumor
chromaffinoma
chromaffinopathy
chromaphil
chromate stain for lead
chromatic
  c. aberration
  c. apparatus
  c. audition
  c. fiber
  c. granule
  c. vision
chromatid
chromatin
  c. body
  heteropyknotic c.
  c. network
  c. nucleolus
  oxyphil c.
  c. particles
  sex c.
chromatinolysis
chromatinorrhexis
chromatism
chromatogenous
chromatography
  high-performance liquid c.
  high-pressure liquid c.
chromatoid
chromatokinesis
chromatolysis
  central c.
  retrograde c.
  transsynaptic c.
chromatolytic
chromatopectic
chromatopexis
chromatophil
chromatophilia
chromatophilic, chromatophilous
chromatophobia
chromatophorotropic
chromatoplasm
chromatopsia

chromaturia
chrome
  c. alum
  c. alum hematoxylin-phloxine stain
  c. red
  c. ulcer
  c. yellow
chrome-cobalt alloys
chromesthesia
chromhidrosis
  apocrine c.
chromic phosphate P 32 colloidal suspension
chromidia (*pl. of* chromidium)
chromidial
  c. apparatus
  c. net
  c. substance
chromidiation
chromidiosis
chromidium, pl. chromidia
chromidrosis
Chromobacterium
    C. violaceum
chromoblast
chromoblastomycosis
chromocenter
chromocystoscopy
chromocyte
chromogen
    Porter-Silber c.'s
chromolipid
chromolysis
chromomere
chromomycosis
chromonema, pl. chromonemata
chromonychia
chromopectic
chromopexis
chromophage
chromophil, chromophile
  c. adenoma
  c. granule
  c. substance
chromophilia
chromophilic, chromophilous
chromophobe
  c. adenoma
  c. cells of anterior lobe of hypophysis
  c. granules
chromophobia
chromophobic
  c. adenoma
chromophototherapy
chromoplastid
chromosomal
  c. breakage syndromes

C

chromosomal *(continued)*
    c. deletion
    c. gap
    c. instability syndromes
    c. region
    c. syndrome
    c. trait
chromosomal map
chromosome
    c. aberration
    accessory c.
    acentric c.
    acrocentric c.
    c. band
    bivalent c.
    Christchurch c.
    derivative c.
    dicentric c.
    double minute c.'s
    fragile X c.
    giant c.
    heterotypical c.
    homologous c.'s
    lampbrush c., lamp-brush c.
    late replicating c.
    c. map
    c. mapping
    marker c.
    metacentric c.
    mitochondrial c.
    c. mosaicism
    nonhomologous c.'s
    nucleolar c.
    odd c.
    c. pair
    c. pairing
    Philadelphia c.
    polytene c.
    ring c.
    c. satellite
    sex c.'s
    submetacentric c.
    telocentric c.
    translocation c.
    unpaired c.
    W c., X c., Y c., Z c.
    c. walking
chromotherapy
chromotoxic
chromotrichia
chromotrichial
chromotrope
chromotrope 2R
chronaxia
chronaxie
chronaximeter
chronaximetry
chronaxis

chronaxy
chronic
    c. abscess
    c. absorptive arthritis
    c. acholuric jaundice
    c. active inflammation
    c. active liver disease
    c. adrenocortical insufficiency
    c. African sleeping sickness
    c. alcoholism
    c. allograft rejection
    c. anaphylaxis
    c. anterior poliomyelitis
    c. appendicitis
    c. ataxia
    c. atrophic polychondritis
    c. atrophic thyroiditis
    c. atrophic vulvitis
    c. bacillary diarrhea
    c. bronchitis
    c. bullous dermatosis of childhood
    c. cholecystitis
    c. cicatrizing enteritis
    c. conjunctivitis
    c. constrictive pericarditis
    c. cutaneous leishmaniasis
    c. cystic mastitis
    c. desquamative gingivitis
    c. diffuse sclerosing osteomyelitis
    c. discoid lupus erythematosus
    c. eczema
    c. endemic fluorosis
    c. eosinophilic pneumonia
    c. familial icterus
    c. familial jaundice
    c. familial polyneuritis
    c. fibrosing alveolitis
    c. fibrosing pancreatitis
    c. fibrous thyroiditis
    c. focal sclerosing osteomyelitis
    c. follicular conjunctivitis
    c. glaucoma
    c. glomerulonephritis
    c. granulomatous disease
    c. hemorrhagic villous synovitis
    c. hepatitis
    c. hypertensive disease
    c. hypertrophic vulvitis
    c. hyperventilation syndrome
    c. idiopathic jaundice
    c. idiopathic xanthomatosis
    c. inflammation
    c. inflammatory demyelinating
      polyneuropathy
    c. interstitial hepatitis
    c. interstitial hypertrophic
      neuropathy
    c. interstitial salpingitis

c. lymphadenoid thyroiditis
c. lymphocytic thyroiditis
c. malaria
c. mountain sickness
c. nephritis
c. nonleukemic myelosis
c. obstructive pulmonary disease
c. pancreatitis
c. persistent hepatitis
c. persisting hepatitis
c. pleurisy
c. pneumonia
c. progressive chorea
c. progressive external
  ophthalmoplegia
c. progressive syphilitic
  meningoencephalitis
c. pyelonephritis
c. rejection
c. relapsing pancreatitis
c. rheumatism
c. rhinitis
c. shock
c. soroche
c. subglottic laryngitis
c. tamponade
c. trypanosomiasis
c. ulcer
c. ulcerative proctitis
c. urticaria
c. vertigo
chronicity
chronobiology
chronognosis
chronologic age
chronometry
  mental c.
chrono-oncology
chronophobia
chronophotograph
chronotaraxis
chronotropic
chronotropism
  negative c.
  positive c.
chrysiasis
chrysocyanosis
chrysoderma
Chrysomyia
Chrysops
Chrysosporium parvum
chrysotherapy
chthonophagia, chthonophagy
chunking
Churg-Strauss syndrome
chutta
Chvostek's sign
chylangioma

chylaqueous
chyle
  c. cistern
  c. corpuscle
  c. cyst
  c. peritonitis
  c. vessel
chylemia
chylidrosis
chylifaction
chylifactive
chyliferous
chylification
chyliform
  c. ascites
chylocele
  parasitic c.
chylocyst
chyloderma
chylomediastinum
chylomicronemia
chylopericarditis
chylopericardium
chyloperitoneum
chylophoric
chylopleura
chylopneumothorax
chylopoiesis
chylopoietic
chylorrhea
chylosis
chylothorax
chylous
  c. arthritis
  c. ascites
  c. hydrothorax
  c. urine
chyluria
chymification
chymopoiesis
chymorrhea
α-chymotrypsin-induced glaucoma
Ciaccio's
  C. glands
  C. stain
cibophobia
cicatrectomy
cicatrices (*pl. of* cicatrix)
cicatricial
  c. alopecia
  c. conjunctivitis
  c. ectropion
  c. entropion
  c. horn
  c. pemphigoid
cicatricotomy, cicatrisotomy
cicatrix, pl. cicatrices
  brain c.

C

cicatrix *(continued)*
    filtering c.
    meningocerebral c.
    vicious c.
cicatrization
    c. atelectasis
cigarette drain
cigarette-paper scars
cilia *(pl. of* cilium)
ciliary
    c. blepharitis
    c. body
    c. border of iris
    c. canals
    c. cartilage
    c. crown
    c. disk
    c. folds
    c. ganglion
    c. ganglionic plexus
    c. glands
    c. ligament
    c. margin of iris
    c. movement
    c. muscle
    c. part of retina
    c. poliosis
    c. process
    c. ring
    c. staphyloma
    c. veins
    c. wreath
    c. zone
    c. zonule
Ciliata
ciliated
    c. epithelium
ciliates
ciliectomy
ciliogenesis
Ciliophora
cilioretinal
cilioscleral
ciliospinal
    c. center
    c. reflex
cilium, pl. cilia
cillo
Cillobacterium
cillosis
Cimex lectularius
cimicosis
cinanesthesia
cinclisis
cincture sensation
cineangiocardiography
cinefluorography
cinefluoroscopy

cinegastroscopy
cinematic amputation
cinematics
cinephotomicrography
cineplastic amputation
cineplastics
cineradiography
cinerea
cinereal
cineritious
cineroentgenography
cineseismography
cinetoplasm, cinetoplasma
cingula *(pl. of* cingulum)
cingulate
    c. convolution
    c. gyrus
    c. herniation
    c. sulcus
cingulectomy
cingulotomy
cingulum, gen. cinguli, pl. cingula
    c. dentis
    c. membri inferioris
    c. membri superioris
    c. rest
    c. of tooth
cinocentrum
cion
circadian
    c. rhythm
circellus
    c. venosus hypoglossi
circhoral
circinate
    c. retinitis
    c. retinopathy
circle
    c. absorption anesthesia
    arterial c. of cerebrum
    articular vascular c.
    Baudelocque's uterine c.
    Carus' c.
    cerebral arterial c.
    closed c.
    defensive c.
    greater arterial c. of iris
    Haller's c.
    Huguier's c.
    least diffusion c.
    lesser arterial c. of iris
    Pagenstecher's c.
    Ridley's c.
    rolling c.
    semi-closed c.
    vascular c.
    vascular c. of optic nerve
    venous c. of mammary gland

vicious c.
c. of Willis
Zinn's vascular c.
circuit
anesthetic c.
Papez c.
reverberating c.
circular
c. amputation
c. anastomosis
c. bandage
c. dichroism
c. fibers
c. folds
c. layer of muscular coat
c. layers of muscular tunics
c. layer of tympanic membrane
c. reaction
c. sinus
c. sulcus of insula
c. sulcus of Reil
circulation
assisted c.
blood c.
capillary c.
collateral c.
compensatory c.
embryonic c.
enterohepatic c.
extracorporeal c.
fetal c.
greater c.
hypophysial portal c.
hypothalamohypophysial portal c.
lesser c.
lymph c.
placental c.
portal c.
portal hypophysial c.
pulmonary c.
Servetus' c.
systemic c.
thebesian c.
c. time
circulatory
c. arrest
c. collapse
c. system
circulus, gen. and pl. **circuli**
c. arteriosus cerebri
c. arteriosus halleri
c. arteriosus iridis major
c. arteriosus iridis minor
c. articularis vasculosus
c. vasculosus nervi optici
c. venosus halleri
c. venosus ridleyi
c. zinnii

circumalveolar fixation
circumanal
c. glands
circumarticular
circumaxillary
circumbulbar
circumcise
circumcision
circumcorneal
circumduction
c. gait
circumference
articular c. of radius
articular c. of ulna
circumferentia
c. articularis radii
c. articularis ulnae
circumferential
c. cartilage
c. clasp
c. clasp arm
c. fibrocartilage
c. lamella
c. wiring
circumflex
c. branch of left coronary artery
c. femoral arteries
c. fibular artery
c. humeral arteries
c. iliac arteries
c. nerve
c. scapular artery
c. veins
circumgemmal
circumintestinal
circumlental
circummandibular
c. fixation
circumnuclear
circumocular
circumoral
circumorbital
circumrenal
circumscribed
c. craniomalacia
c. myxedema
c. peritonitis
c. pyocephalus
circumscriptus
circumstantiality
circumvallate
c. papilla
circumvascular
circumventricular
c. organs
circumvolute
circumzygomatic fixation

C

circus
    c. movement
    c. rhythm
cirrhogenous, cirrhogenic
cirrhonosus
cirrhosis
    alcoholic c.
    biliary c.
    Budd's c.
    capsular c. of liver
    cardiac c.
    cholangiolitic c.
    congestive c.
    cryptogenic c.
    fatty c.
    Glisson's c.
    Hanot's c.
    juvenile c.
    Laënnec's c.
    necrotic c.
    periportal c.
    pigment c.
    pigmentary c.
    pipe stem c.
    portal c.
    posthepatitic c.
    postnecrotic c., post-necrotic c.
    primary biliary c.
    pulmonary c.
    stasis c.
    syphilitic c.
cirrhotic
cirrose, cirrous
cirrus, pl. **cirri**
cirsectomy
cirsocele
cirsodesis
cirsoid
    c. aneurysm
    c. varix
cirsomphalos
cirsophthalmia
cirsotome
cirsotomy
cis phase
cissa
cistern
    ambient c.
    basal c.
    cerebellomedullary c.
    c. of chiasm
    chiasmatic c.
    chyle c.
    c. of cytoplasmic reticulum
    c. of great cerebral vein
    c. of great vein of cerebrum
    interpeduncular c.
    c. of lateral fossa of cerebrum

    lumbar c.
    c. of nuclear envelope
    Pecquet's c.
    pontine c.
    subarachnoidal c.'s
    superior c.
    Sylvian c.
cisterna, gen. and pl. **cisternae**
    c. ambiens
    c. basalis
    c. caryothecae
    c. cerebellomedullaris
    c. chiasmatis
    c. chyli
    c. cruralis
    c. fossae lateralis cerebri
    c. interpeduncularis
    c. magna
    c. perilymphatica
    c. pontis
    cisternae subarachnoideales
    subsurface c.
    c. superioris
    terminal cisternae
    c. venae magnae cerebri
cisternal
    c. puncture
cisternography
    cerebellopontine c.
    radionuclide c.
cisvestism, cisvestitism
citrate intoxication
Citrobacter
    C. amalonatica
    C. diversus
    C. freundii
    C. koseri
citrullinemia
citrullinuria
citta, cittosis
Civatte
    C. bodies
    C. disease
Civinini's
    C. canal
    C. ligament
    C. process
cladiosis
Cladorchis watsoni
Clado's
    C. anastomosis
    C. band
    C. ligament
    C. point
cladosporiosis
    cerebral c.
Cladosporium
    C. bantianum

C. carrionii
C. cladosporioides
C. werneckii
Clagett procedure for empyema
clairvoyance
clamp
Cope's c.
Crafoord c.
Crile's c.
Fogarty c.
c. forceps
Gant's c.
gingival c.
Goldblatt's c.
Joseph's c.
Kelly c.
Kocher c.
liver-shod c.
Mikulicz c.
Mixter c.
Mogen c.
mosquito c.
Ochsner c.
Payr's c.
Potts' c.
Rankin's c.
right angle c.
rubber dam c.
rubber shod c., rubber-shod c.
clamp connection
clang association
clapotage, clapotement
Clapton's line
Clara cell
Clarke
C. cells
C. column
C. nucleus
Clarke-Hadfield syndrome
Clark's
C. level
C. weight rule
clasmatocyte
clasmatosis
clasp
c. arm
c. bar
bar c.
circumferential c.
continuous c.
extended c.
c. guideline
Roach c.
clasping reflex
clasp-knife
c.-k. effect
c.-k. rigidity
c.-k. spasticity

class
c. I antigens
c. II antigens
c. III antigens
c. switch
classic
c. cervical rib syndrome
c. migraine
classical
c. cesarean section
c. conditioning
c. genetics
c. hemophilia
classifiable character
classification
adansonian c.
Angle's c. of malocclusion
Arneth c.
Black's c.
Caldwell-Moloy c.
Cummer's c.
DeBakey's c.
Denver c.
Dukes' c.
Gell and Coombs C.
International Labour
  Organization C.
Jansky's c.
Kennedy c.
Kiel c.
Lancefield c.
Lennert c.
Lukes-Collins c.
multiaxial c.
New York Heart Association c.
Rappaport c.
Rye c.
Salter-Harris c. of epiphysial plate
  injuries
Tessier c.
clastic
c. anatomy
clastogen
clastogenic
clastothrix
Claude's syndrome
claudication
intermittent c.
claudicatory
Claudius'
C. cells
C. fossa
claustra (*pl. of* claustrum)
claustral
c. layer
claustrophobia
claustrophobic
claustrum, pl. **claustra**

C

claustrum *(continued)*
c. gutturis, c. oris
c. virginale
clausura
clava
claval
clavate
c. papillae
clavi (*pl. of* clavus)
Claviceps purpurea
clavicle
clavicula, pl. **claviculae**
clavicular
c. branch of thoracoacromial artery
c. facet
c. head of pectoralis major muscle
c. notch of sternum
c. part of pectoralis major muscle
c. percussion
claviculus, pl. **claviculi**
clavipectoral fascia
clavus, pl. **clavi**
clavus hystericus
claw
c. foot
c. hand
clawfoot
clawhand
Claybrook's sign
clay shoveler's fracture
cleaning
ultrasonic c.
clear
c. cell
c. cell acanthoma
c. cell adenocarcinoma
c. cell carcinoma of kidney
c. cell hidradenoma
c. layer of epidermis
c. liquid diet
clearance
p-aminohippurate c.
creatinine c.
endogenous creatinine c.
exogenous creatinine c.
free water c.
interocclusal c.
inulin c.
maximum urea c.
occlusal c.
osmolal c.
standard urea c.
urea c.
clearer
clearing
c. factors
c. medium

cleavage
abnormal c. of cardiac valve
adequal c.
c. cavity
c. cell
complete c.
determinate c.
discoidal c.
c. division
enamel c.
equal c.
equatorial c.
holoblastic c.
incomplete c.
indeterminate c.
c. lines
meridional c.
meroblastic c.
progressive c.
pudendal c.
c. spindle
subdural c.
superficial c.
total c.
unequal c.
yolk c.
cleaved cell
cleaver
enamel c.
Cleemann's sign
cleft
anal c.
branchial c.'s
cholesterol c.
facial c.
first visceral c.
gill c.'s
gingival c.
gluteal c.
c. hand
hyobranchial c.
hyomandibular c.
interneuromeric c.'s
Larrey's c.
c. lip
Maurer's c.'s
median maxillary anterior
alveolar c.
natal c.
c. nose
oblique facial c.
c. palate
pudendal c.
residual c.
Schmidt-Lanterman c.'s
c. spine
subdural c.
synaptic c.

c. tongue
urogenital c.
visceral c.
cleidagra, clidagra
cleidal
cleidocostal
cleidocranial
c. dysostosis
c. dysplasia
cleistothecium
clenched fist sign
cleoid
cleptoparasite
clerical spectacles
Clevenger's fissure
click
ejection c.
mitral c.
c. syndrome
systolic c.
clicking
c. rale
c. tinnitus
clidagra (*var. of* cleidagra)
clidal
clidocostal
clidocranial
c. dysostosis
c. dysplasia
clidoic
client-centered therapy
climacophobia
climacteric
grand c.
c. psychosis
c. syndrome
climacterium
climatic
c. bubo
c. keratopathy
climatotherapy
climax
climbing fibers
climograph
cline
clinic
clinical
c. anatomy
c. burden
c. crown
c. diagnosis
c. epidemiology
c. eruption
c. fitness
c. genetics
c. lethal
c. medicine
c. nurse specialist

c. pathology
c. psychology
c. recording
c. root
c. sensitivity
c. thermometer
c. trial
clinician
clinicopathologic
clinocephalic, clinocephalous
clinocephaly
clinodactyly
clinography
clinoid
c. process
clinoscope
clip
c. forceps
wound c.
clipped speech
clithrophobia
clition
clitoral recession
clitoridean
clitoridectomy
clitoriditis
clitoris, pl. **clitorides**
clitorism
clitoritis
clitoromegaly
clitoroplasty
clival
clivus, pl. **clivi**
Blumenbach's c.
c. ocularis
CL lead
cloaca
ectodermal c.
endodermal c.
persistent c.
cloacal
c. exstrophy
c. membrane
c. plate
c. theory
clock
lens c.
clomiphene test
clonal
c. aging
c. deletion theory
c. expansion
c. selection theory
clone
clonic
c. convulsion
c. seizure
c. spasm

C

clonicity
clonicotonic
cloning
clonism
clonogenic
    c. assay
    c. cell
clonograph
clonospasm
clonus
    ankle c.
    cathodal opening c.
    toe c.
    wrist c.
Cloquet's
    C. canal
    C. hernia
    C. septum
    C. space
close bite
closed
    c. anesthesia
    c. angiography
    c. bite
    c. chest massage
    c. circle
    c. circuit method
    c. comedo
    c. dislocation
    c. drainage
    c. fracture
    c. head injury
    c. hospital
    c. laparoscopy
    c. reduction of fractures
    c. skull fracture
    c. surgery
closed-angle glaucoma
closed-loop obstruction
closing
    c. contraction
    c. membranes
    c. snap
    c. volume
clostridia (*pl. of* clostridium)
clostridial
    c. myonecrosis
Clostridium
    C. bifermentans
    C. botulinum
    C. butyricum
    C. cadaveris
    C. carnis
    C. chauvoei
    C. cochlearium
    C. difficile
    C. fallax
    C. haemolyticum

    C. histolyticum
    C. innominatum
    C. microsporum
    C. multifermentans
    C. nigrificans
    C. novyi
    C. oedematiens
    C. parabotulinum
    C. paraputrificum
    C. perfringens
    C. ramosum
    C. septicum
    C. sphenoides
    C. sporogenes
    C. tale
    C. tertium
    C. tetani
    C. tetanoides
    C. tetanomorphum
    C. thermosaccharolyticum
    C. welchii
clostridium, pl. clostridia
closure
    flask c.
    c. principle
    velopharyngeal c.
clot
    agonal c.
    antemortem c.
    blood c.
    chicken fat c.
    currant jelly c.
    laminated c.
    passive c.
    postmortem c.
    c. retraction time
    Schede's c.
clottage
clotting
    c. factor
    c. time
clouding of consciousness
Cloudman melanoma
cloudy
    c. swelling
    c. urine
cloverleaf
    c. skull
    c. skull syndrome
club
    c. foot
    c. hair
    c. hand
clubbed
    c. digits
    c. fingers
    c. penis

clubbing
    hereditary c.
clubfoot
clubhand
    radial c.
    ulnar c.
clump
clumping
cluneal
clunes
cluster
    c. analysis
    egg c.
    c. headache
    c. sample
cluster of differentiation
    c. of d. 2
    c. of d. 3
    c. of d. 4
    c. of d. 8
cluttering
Clutton's joints
clysis
clyster
cnemial
cnemis
cnidosis
Cnidospora
Cnidosporidia
coadaptation
coagglutinin
coagulation
    disseminated intravascular c.
    c. factor
    c. necrosis
    c. time
coagulopathy
    consumption c.
coalescence
coapt
coaptation
    c. splint
    c. suture
coarct
coarctate
    c. retina
coarctation
    reversed c.
coarctectomy
coarctotomy
coarse tremor
coat
    buffy c.
    muscular c.
    muscular c. of bronchi
    muscular c. of colon
    muscular c. of ductus deferens
    muscular c. of esophagus
    muscular c. of female urethra
    muscular c. of gallbladder
    muscular c. of pharynx
    muscular c. of rectum
    muscular c. of small intestine
    muscular c. of stomach
    muscular c. of trachea
    muscular c. of ureter
    muscular c. of urinary bladder
    muscular c. of uterine tube
    muscular c. of uterus
    muscular c. of vagina
    sclerotic c.
    serous c.
coated tongue
coating
    antireflection c.
Coats' disease
cobbler's suture
Cobb syndrome
cobra
    c. hemotoxin
    c. venom cofactor
    c. venom factor
cocainization
cocarcinogen
cocarde reaction
Coccaceae
coccal
cocci (*pl. of* coccus)
Coccidia
coccidia
coccidial
Coccidiasina
coccidioidal
    c. granuloma
Coccidioides
coccidioidin test
coccidioidoma
coccidioidomycosis
    asymptomatic c.
    disseminate c.
    latent c.
    primary c.
    primary extrapulmonary c.
    secondary c.
coccinellin
coccobacillary
coccobacillus
coccoid
coccus, pl. **cocci**
    Neisser's c.
    Weichselbaum's c.
coccyalgia
coccycephaly
coccydynia
coccygalgia

coccygeal
    c. body
    c. bone
    c. cornua
    c. dimple
    c. fistula
    c. foveola
    c. ganglion
    c. gland
    c. horn
    c. joint
    c. muscle
    c. nerve
    c. part of spinal cord
    c. plexus
    c. segments of spinal cord
    c. sinus
    c. vertebrae
    c. whorl
coccygectomy
coccyges (*pl. of* coccyx)
coccygeus
    c. muscle
coccygis (*gen. of* coccyx)
coccygodynia
coccygotomy
coccyodynia
coccyx, gen. **coccygis**, pl. **coccyges**
Cochin China diarrhea
cochlea, pl. **cochleae**
    membranous c.
cochlear
    c. aqueduct
    c. area
    c. branch of labyrinthine artery
    c. canal
    c. canaliculus
    c. duct
    c. ganglion
    c. hair cells
    c. implant
    c. joint
    c. labyrinth
    c. nerve
    c. nuclei
    c. part of vestibulocochlear nerve
    c. prosthesis
    c. recess
    c. root of vestibulocochlear nerve
    c. root of VIII nerve
    c. window
cochleare
cochleariform
    c. process
cochleate
cochleo-orbicular reflex
cochleopalpebral reflex
cochleopupillary reflex

cochleosacculotomy
cochleostapedial reflex
cochleovestibular
Cochliomyia
    C. americana
cockade reaction
Cockayne's
    C. disease
    C. syndrome
Cockett communicating perforating veins
cockscomb ulcer
coconsciousness
coconut sound
code
    soundex c.
codfish vertebrae
coding
Codman's
    C. sign
    C. triangle
    C. tumor
codominant
    c. allele
    c. gene
    c. inheritance
    c. trait
codon
    initiation c.
coefficient
    biological c.
    Bunsen's solubility c.
    c. of consanguinity
    correlation c.
    extraction c.
    filtration c.
    hygienic laboratory c.
    c. of inbreeding
    isotonic c.
    c. of kinship
    lethal c.
    linear absorption c.
    Long's c.
    oxygen utilization c.
    phenol c.
    reflection c.
    c. of relationship
    reliability c.
    respiratory c.
    Rideal-Walker c.
    selection c.
    ultrafiltration c.
    c. of variation
Coelenterata
coelenterate
coelom
coelomic metaplasia
coenesthesia

coenocyte
coenocytic
coeur
    c. en sabot
Coe virus
cofactor
    cobra venom c.
    platelet c. I
    platelet c. II
coffee-ground vomit
Coffey suspension
Coffin-Lowry syndrome
Coffin-Siris syndrome
Cogan-Reese syndrome
Cogan's syndrome
cognition
cognitive
    c. development
    c. dissonance
    c. dissonance theory
    c. laterality quotient
    c. psychology
    c. therapy
cogwheel
    c. ocular movements
    c. phenomenon
    c. respiration
    c. rigidity
cohesive gold
Cohnheim's
    C. area
    C. field
    C. theory
cohort
    c. study
coil
    detector c.
    c. gland
    surface c.
coiled artery of the uterus
coin
    c. lesion of lungs
    c. test
coin-counting
coinosite
cointegrate
coital
Coiter's muscle
coition
coitophobia
coitus
    c. interruptus
    c. reservatus
col
cold
    c. abscess
    c. agglutination
    c. agglutinin

c. allergy
c. antibody
c. autoagglutinin
c. autoantibody
c. bend test
c. cautery
c. chain
c. conization
c. erythema
c. gangrene
c. in the head
c. hemagglutinin disease
c. hemolysin
c. nodule
c. pack
c. pressor test
rose c.
c. snare
c. sore
c. stage
c. ulcer
c. urticaria
c. virus
cold-reactive antibody
cold-rigor point
Cole-Cecil murmur
colectasia
colectomy
coleocele
Coleoptera
coleoptosis
coleotomy
colibacillus, pl. colibacilli
colic
    appendicular c.
    c. arteries
    biliary c.
    copper c.
    Devonshire c.
    gallstone c.
    gastric c.
    hepatic c.
    c. impression
    infantile c.
    c. intussusception
    lead c.
    c. lymph nodes
    meconial c.
    menstrual c.
    ovarian c.
    painter's c.
    pancreatic c.
    Poitou c.
    renal c.
    salivary c.
    saturnine c.
    c. sphincter
    c. surface of spleen

C

colic (continued)
    c. teniae
    tubal c.
    ureteral c.
    uterine c.
    c. veins
    vermicular c.
    zinc c.
colica
colicin
colicinogeny
colicky
colicoplegia
coliform bacilli
coliphage
coliplication
colipuncture
colitis
    amebic c.
    collagenous c.
    c. cystica profunda
    c. cystica superficialis
    granulomatous c.
    c. gravis
    hemorrhagic c.
    mucous c.
    myxomembranous c.
    pseudomembranous c.
    ulcerative c.
    uremic c.

[handwritten: C. difficile colitis]

colitose
colla (*pl. of* collum)
collacin
collagen
    c. diseases
    c. fiber
    c. fibrils
    c. injection
collagenosis
    reactive perforating c.
collagenous
    c. colitis
    c. fiber
    c. pneumoconiosis
collagen-vascular diseases
collapse
    absorption c.
    circulatory c.
    c. delirium
    c. of dental arch
    massive c.
    pressure c.
    pulmonary c.
    c. therapy
collapsing pulse
collar
    c. bone
    c. incision

    renal c.
    c. of Venus
collar-button abscess
collared flagellate
collarette
collar-stud chalazion
collastin
collateral
    c. artery
    c. branches of posterior intercostal
      arteries 3–11
    c. circulation
    c. digital artery
    c. eminence
    c. fissure
    c. hyperemia
    c. inheritance
    c. ligament
    c. sulcus
    c. trigone
    c. vessel
collecting tubule
collectins
collective unconscious
Colles'
    C. fascia
    C. fracture
    C. ligament
    C. space
Collet-Sicard syndrome
colliculectomy
colliculitis
colliculus, pl. **colliculi**
    c. of arytenoid cartilage
    c. cartilaginis arytenoideae
    facial c.
    c. facialis
    c. inferior
    inferior c.
    inferior nasal c.
    seminal c.
    c. seminalis
    superior c.
    c. superior
    c. urethralis
Collier's
    C. sign
    C. tract
    C. tucked lid sign
collier's
    c. lung
collimation
collimator
colliotomy
colliquation
colliquative
    c. albuminuria
    c. degeneration

c. diarrhea
c. necrosis
c. sweat
Collis-Belsey procedure
Collis gastroplasty
collision tumor
collodion baby
colloid
c. acne
c. adenoma
c. bath
c. bodies
bovine c.
c. cancer
c. carcinoma
c. corpuscle
c. cyst
c. degeneration
c. goiter
c. milium
c. pseudomilium
thyroid c.
colloidal
c. gold reaction
c. gold test
colloidoclasia, colloidoclasis
colloidoclastic
collum, pl. colla
c. anatomicum humeri
c. chirurgicum humeri
c. costae
c. dentis
c. distortum
c. femoris
c. fibulae
c. folliculi pili
c. glandis penis
c. humeri
c. mallei
c. mandibulae
c. ossis femoris
c. radii
c. scapulae
c. tali
c. vesicae biliaris
c. vesicae felleae
coloboma
c. of choroid
Fuchs' c.
c. iridis
c. lentis
c. lobuli
macular c.
c. of optic nerve
c. palpebrale
c. of vitreous
colocentesis
colocholecystostomy

colocolic
colocolostomy
colocutaneous fistula
colocystoplasty
coloenteritis
colohepatopexy
coloileal fistula
cololysis
colon
c. ascendens
ascending c.
c. bacillus
c. cutoff sign
c. descendens
descending c.
giant c.
iliac c.
irritable c.
lead-pipe c.
mucosa of c.
c. pelvinum
sigmoid c.
c. sigmoideum
spastic c.
transverse c.
c. transversum
colonalgia
colonic
c. diverticula
c. fistula
c. smear
colonization
genetic c.
colonogram
colonometer
colonopathy
colonorrhagia
colonorrhea
colonoscope
colonoscopy
colony
daughter c.
filamentous c.
Gheel c.
H c.
lenticular c.
mother c.
mucoid c.
O c.
rough c.
smooth c.
spheroid c.
colony-stimulating factors
colopathy
colopexostomy
colopexotomy
colopexy
coloplication

C

coloproctia
coloproctitis
coloproctostomy
coloptosis, coloptosia
colopuncture
color
    c. aberration
    c. agnosia
    c. blindness
    complementary c.'s
    confusion c.'s
    c. constancy
    extrinsic c.
    c. hearing
    incidental c.
    intrinsic c.
    opponent c.
    primary c.
    pure c.
    reflected c.'s
    saturated c.
    c. scotoma
    c. sense
    simple c.
    c. solid
    c. taste
    tone c.
    c. triangle
Colorado
    C. tick fever
    C. tick fever virus
color-contrast microscope
colorectal
colorectitis
colorectostomy
colored vision
colorimetric caries susceptibility test
color match
colorrhagia
colorrhaphy
colorrhea
coloscopy
colosigmoidostomy
colostomy
    c. bag
colostration
colostric
colostrorrhea
colostrous
colostrum corpuscle
colotomy
Colour Index
colovaginal fistula
colovesical fistula
colpatresia
colpectasis, colpectasia
colpectomy
colpocele

colpocleisis
colpocystitis
colpocystocele
colpocystoplasty
colpocystotomy
colpocystoureterotomy
colpodynia
colpohysterectomy
colpohysteropexy
colpohysterotomy
colpomicroscope
colpomicroscopy
colpomycosis
colpomyomectomy
colpopathy
colpoperineoplasty
colpoperineorrhaphy
colpopexy
colpoplasty
colpopoiesis
colpoptosis, colpoptosia
colporectopexy
colporrhagia
colporrhaphy
colporrhexis
colposcope
colposcopy
colpospasm
colpostat
colpostenosis
colpostenotomy
colpotomy
colpoureterotomy
colpoxerosis
Columbia
    C. Mental Maturity Scale
    C. S. K. virus
columella, pl. columellae
    c. cochleae
    c. nasi
column
    anal c.'s
    anterior c.
    anterior gray c.
    anterior c. of medulla oblongata
    anterolateral c. of spinal cord
    Bertin's c.'s
    branchial efferent c.
    Burdach's c.
    c. cells
    Clarke's c.
    dorsal c. of spinal cord
    c. of fornix
    general somatic afferent c.
    general somatic efferent c.
    general visceral afferent c.,
      splanchnic afferent c.

general visceral efferent c.,
  splanchnic efferent c.
Goll's c.
Gowers' c.
gray c.'s
intermediolateral cell c. of spinal
  cord
lateral c.
lateral c. of spinal cord
Lissauer's c.
Morgagni's c.'s
posterior c.
posterior c. of spinal cord
rectal c.'s
renal c.'s
Rolando's c.
rugal c.'s of vagina
Sertoli's c.'s
special somatic afferent c.
special visceral efferent c.
spinal c.
c. of Spitzka-Lissauer
splanchnic afferent c. (*var. of*
  general visceral afferent c.)
splanchnic efferent c. (*var. of*
  general visceral efferent c.)
Stilling's c.
Türck's c.
vaginal c.'s
ventral white c.
vertebral c.
columna, gen. and pl. **columnae**
columnae anales
c. anterior
columnae carneae
c. fornicis
columnae griseae
c. lateralis
c. posterior
columnae renales
columnae rugarum
c. vertebralis
columnar
c. epithelium
c. layer
columnella, pl. **columnellae**
colypeptic
coma
c. aberration
c. carcinomatosum
c. cast
delayed c. after hypoxia
diabetic c.
hepatic c.
hyperosmolar (hyperglycemic)
  nonketotic c.
hypoglycemic c.
hypoventilation c.

Kussmaul's c.
metabolic c.
c. scale
thyrotoxic c.
trance c.
uremic c.
c. vigil
comatose
combat
c. exhaustion
c. neurosis
comb-growth test
combination
c. beat
binary c.
new c.
c. restoration
combinatorial
combined
c. fat- and carbohydrate-induced
  hyperlipemia
c. glaucoma
c. immunodeficiency
c. immunodeficiency syndrome
c. pregnancy
c. sclerosis
c. system disease
c. version
combining site
comblike septum
Comby's sign
comedo, pl. **comedos, comedones**
closed c.
c. nevus
open c.
comedocarcinoma
comedogenic
comedonecrosis
comedones (*pl. of* comedo)
comedos (*pl. of* comedo)
comes, pl. **comites**
comet
c. sign
c. tail sign
comfort zone
comitance
comitant
c. strabismus
comites (*pl. of* comes)
comma
c. bacillus
c. bundle of Schultze
c. tract of Schultze
commando
c. operation
c. procedure
commemorative sign

C

commensal
   c. parasite
commensalism
   epizoic c.
comminuted
   c. fracture
   c. skull fracture
comminution
commissura, gen. and pl. **commissurae**
   c. alba
   c. anterior
   c. anterior grisea
   c. bulborum
   c. cinerea
   c. colliculorum inferiorum
   c. colliculorum superiorum
   c. fornicis
   c. grisea
   c. habenularum
   c. hippocampi
   c. labiorum
   c. labiorum anterior
   c. labiorum posterior
   c. palpebrarum lateralis
   c. palpebrarum medialis
   c. posterior cerebri
   c. posterior grisea
   commissurae supraopticae
   c. ventralis alba
commissural
   c. cell
   c. cheilitis
   c. fibers
   c. myelotomy
commissure
   anterior c.
   anterior labial c.
   anterior white c.
   c. of cerebral hemispheres
   c. of fornix
   Ganser's c.'s
   Gudden's c.'s
   c. of habenulae
   habenular c.
   hippocampal c.
   c. of inferior colliculi
   labial c.
   lateral palpebral c.
   c. of lips
   medial palpebral c.
   Meynert's c.'s
   posterior cerebral c.
   posterior labial c.
   c. of superior colliculus
   supraoptic c.'s
   c. of vestibular bulb
   Wernekinck's c.
   white c.

commissurotomy
   mitral c.
commisural pits
commitment
common
   c. antigen
   c. baldness
   c. basal vein
   c. bile duct
   c. cardinal veins
   c. carotid artery
   c. carotid plexus
   c. cold virus
   c. crus of semicircular ducts
   c. facial vein
   c. fibular nerve
   c. flexor sheath
   c. hepatic artery
   c. hepatic duct
   c. iliac artery
   c. iliac lymph nodes
   c. iliac vein
   c. interosseous artery
   c. limb of membranous
     semicircular ducts
   c. migraine
   c. opsonin
   c. palmar digital artery
   c. palmar digital nerves
   c. peroneal nerve
   c. peroneal tendon sheath
   c. plantar digital artery
   c. plantar digital nerves
   c. tendinous ring
   c. variable immunodeficiency
   c. vehicle spread
   c. wart
commotio
   c. cerebri
   c. retinae
communicable
   c. disease
communicans, pl. **communicantes**
communicating
   c. artery
   c. branch
   c. branch of chorda tympani to
     lingual nerve
   c. branches of auriculotemporal
     nerve to facial nerve
   c. branches of lingual nerve to
     hypoglossal nerve
   c. branches of spinal nerves
   c. branches of sympathetic trunk
   c. branch of facial nerve with
     glossopharyngeal nerve
   c. branch of facial nerve with
     tympanic plexus

c. branch of glossopharyngeal nerve with auricular branch of vagus nerve
c. branch of lacrimal nerve with zygomatic nerve
c. branch of median nerve with ulnar nerve
c. branch of otic ganglion to auriculotemporal nerve
c. branch of otic ganglion to chorda tympani
c. branch of otic ganglion with medial pterygoid nerve
c. branch of otic ganglion with meningeal branch of mandibular nerve
c. branch of peroneal artery
c. branch of superior laryngeal nerve with recurrent laryngeal nerve
c. hematoma
c. hydrocele
c. hydrocephalus
c. rami of spinal nerves
c. rami of sympathetic trunk

communication

community
c. dentistry
c. health nurse
c. medicine
c. mental health center
c. nurse
c. psychiatry
c. psychology
therapeutic c.

Comolli's sign

comorbidity

compact
c. bone
c. substance

compacta

compages thoracis

companion
c. artery to sciatic nerve
c. lymph nodes of accessory nerve
c. vein
c. veins

comparascope

comparative
c. medicine
c. physiology

comparator microscope

compartmental syndrome

compensated
c. acidosis
c. alkalosis
c. glaucoma
c. metabolic alkalosis

c. respiratory acidosis
c. respiratory alkalosis

compensating
c. curve
c. emphysema
c. ocular

compensation
attenuation c.
depth c.
gene dosage c.
c. neurosis
time-gain c.

compensatory
c. atrophy
c. circulation
c. emphysema
c. hypertrophy
c. hypertrophy of the heart
c. pause
c. polycythemia

competence
cardiac c.
immunological c.

competing risk

competition
antigenic c.

competitive binding assay

complaint
chief c.

complement
c. binding assay
c. chemotactic factor
c. fixation

complemental air

complementarity determining regions

complementary
c. air
c. colors
c. hypertrophy
c. role

complementation
intergenic c.
intragenic c.

complement-fixation
c.-f. reaction
c.-f. test

complement-fixing antibody

complete
c. abortion
c. achromatopsia
c. antibody
c. antigen
c. ascertainment
c. atrioventricular dissociation
c. A-V block
c. A-V dissociation
c. blood count
c. cataract

C

complete *(continued)*
    c. cleavage
    c. denture
    c. denture impression
    c. fistula
    c. hemianopia
    c. hernia
    c. iridoplegia
    c. medium
    c. metamorphosis
    c. tetanus
    c. transduction

complex
    aberrant c.
    AIDS dementia c.
    AIDS-related c.
    amygdaloid c.
    anomalous c.
    antigen-antibody c.
    antigenic c.
    apical c.
    atrial c.
    auricular c.
    brain wave c.
    brother c.
    Cain c.
    castration c.
    caudal pharyngeal c.
    Diana c.
    diphasic c.
    EAHF c.
    Eisenmenger's c.
    Electra c.
    electrocardiographic c.
    equiphasic c.
    father c.
    c. febrile convulsion
    femininity c.
    Ghon's c.
    Golgi c.
    H-2 c.
    histocompatibility c.
    HLA c.
    immune c.
    inferiority c.
    isodiphasic c.
    j-g c.
    Jocasta c.
    junctional c.
    juxtaglomerular c.
    K c.
    Lear c.
    c. learning processes
    c. locus
    MAC c.
    major histocompatibility c.
    membrane attack c.
    Meyenburg's c.

monophasic c.
mother superior c.
c. odontoma
Oedipus c.
ostiomeatal c.
c. partial seizure
persecution c.
c. precipitated epilepsy
primary c.
QRS c.
ribosome-lamella c.
Shone's c.
sicca c.
spike and wave c.
superiority c.
symptom c.
synaptinemal c.
Tacaribe c. of viruses
triple symptom c.
VATER c.
ventricular c.

complexion
complexus
compliance
    bladder c.
    c. of bladder
    detrusor c.
    dynamic c. of lung
    c. of heart
    specific c.
    static c.
    thoracic c.
    ventilatory c.
complicated
    c. cataract
    c. fracture
    c. migraine
complication
component
    anterior c. of force
    c. of complement
    c. of force
    c.'s of mastication
    c.'s of occlusion
    plasma thromboplastin c.
    secretory c.
composite
    c. dental cement
    c. flap
    c. graft
    c. joint
    c. resin
composition
    modeling c.
compos mentis
compound
    c. aneurysm
    c. articulation

c. caries
c. character
c. cyst
c. dislocation
c. flap
c. fracture
genetic c.
c. gland
c. granule cell
c. heterozygote
c. hyperopic astigmatism
impression c.
c. joint
c. lens
c. microscope
modeling c.
c. myopic astigmatism
c. nevus
c. odontoma
c. pregnancy
c. restoration
c. skull fracture
comprehension
comprehensive medical care
compress
graduated c.
wet c.
compressed sponge
compressible cavernous bodies
compression
c. anesthesia
c. of brain
cerebral c.
c. cyanosis
c. molding
c. neuropathy
c. paralysis
c. plating
c. retinopathy
c. syndrome
c. thrombosis
c. of tissue
compressive
c. myelopathy
c. nystagmus
compressor
c. muscle of lips
c. venae dorsalis penis
compressorium
Compton
C. effect
C. scatter
C. scattering
compulsion
compulsive
c. idea
c. neurosis
c. personality

computed
c. perimetry
c. radiography
c. tomography (CT)
computer
c. model
c. simulation
computerized axial tomography
CO_2 narcosis
conarium
conation
conative
conatus
concameration
concatamer
concatenate
Concato's disease
concave
c. lens
c. mirror
concavity
concavoconcave
c. lens
concavoconvex
c. lens
concealed
c. conduction
c. hemorrhage
c. hernia
c. penis
concentration
M c.
mean corpuscular hemoglobin c.
minimal alveolar c.
minimal anesthetic c.
minimal inhibitory c.
concentric
c. fibroma
c. hypertrophy
c. lamella
concept
c. formation
no-threshold c.
self c.
concepti (*pl. of* conceptus)
conception
imperative c.
conceptual
conceptus, pl. concepti
concha, pl. conchae
c. auriculae
c. bullosa
c. of ear
highest c.
inferior nasal c.
middle nasal c.
Morgagni's c.
c. nasalis inferior

C

189

concha *(continued)*
    c. nasalis media
    c. nasalis superior
    c. nasalis suprema
    Santorini's c., c. santorini
    sphenoidal conchae
    conchae sphenoidales
    superior nasal c.
    supreme c.
    supreme nasal c.

conchal
    c. cartilage
    c. crest
    c. crest of maxilla
    c. crest of palatine bone

conchoidal
    c. bodies

concomitance

concomitant
    c. immunity
    c. strabismus
    c. symptom

concordance
    c. rate

concordant
    c. alternans
    c. alternation
    c. atrioventricular connections

concrement

concrescence

concrete
    c. operations
    c. seborrhea
    c. thinking

concretio cordis

concretion

concretization

concurrent
    c. disinfection
    c. validity

concussion
    brain c.
    c. cataract
    c. myelitis
    spinal c.
    spinal cord c.

concussor

condense

condenser
    Abbé's c.
    automatic c.
    cardioid c.
    dark-field c.
    paraboloid c.

condensing osteitis

condition

conditional probability

conditioned
    c. avitaminosis
    c. hemolysis
    c. insomnia
    c. reflex
    c. response
    c. stimulus

conditioning
    assertive c.
    aversive c.
    avoidance c.
    classical c.
    escape c.
    higher order c.
    instrumental c.
    operant c.
    pavlovian c.
    respondent c.
    second-order c.
    skinnerian c.
    c. therapy
    trace c.

condom

conductance

conduct disorder

conducting
    c. airway
    c. system of heart

conduction
    aberrant ventricular c.
    accelerated c.
    air c.
    c. analgesia
    c. anesthesia
    anomalous c.
    antegrade c.
    anterograde c.
    c. aphasia
    atrioventricular c., A-V c.
    avalanche c.
    c. block
    bone c.
    concealed c.
    decremental c.
    delayed c.
    forward c.
    intra-atrial c.
    intraventricular c.
    nerve c.
    orthograde c.
    Purkinje c.
    retrograde c.
    saltatory c.
    sinoventricular c.
    supranormal c.
    synaptic c.
    ventricular c.
    ventriculoatrial c., V-A c.

conductive deafness
conductivity
    hydraulic c.
conductor
conduit
    apical-aortic c.
    ileal c.
conduplicate
conduplicato corpore
condylar
    c. articulation
    c. axis
    c. canal
    c. emissary vein
    c. fossa
    c. guidance
    c. guidance inclination
    c. guide
    c. hinge position
    c. joint
    c. process
condylarthrosis
condyle
    balancing side c.
    c. cord
    c. of humerus
    lateral c.
    lateral c. of femur
    lateral c. of tibia
    mandibular c.
    medial c.
    medial c. of femur
    medial c. of tibia
    occipital c.
    c. path
    working side c.
condylectomy
condylion
condyloid
    c. canal
    c. process
condyloma, pl. condylomata
    c. acuminatum
    flat c.
    giant c.
    c. latum
    pointed c.
condylomatous
condylotomy
condylus
    c. humeri
    c. lateralis
    c. lateralis femoris
    c. lateralis tibiae
    c. medialis
    c. medialis femoris
    c. medialis tibiae
    c. occipitalis

cone
    antipodal c.
    arterial c.
    c. cell of retina
    c. degeneration
    c. disks
    c. down
    c. dystrophy
    elastic c.
    c. fiber
    c. granule
    gutta-percha c.
    Haller's c.'s
    implantation c.
    keratosic c.'s
    c. of light
    medullary c.
    ocular c.
    Politzer's luminous c.
    pulmonary c.
    retinal c.'s
    silver c.
    theca interna c.
    twin c.
    vascular c.'s
    c. vision
conexus, pl. conexus
    c. intertendineus
confabulation
confertus
confidence interval
confidentiality
confinement
conflict
    approach-approach c.
    approach-avoidance c.
    avoidance-avoidance c.
    c. of interest
    interpersonal c.
    intrapersonal c.
    role c.
confluence
    c. of sinuses
confluens
    c. sinuum
confluent
    c. articulation
    c. and reticulate papillomatosis
    c. smallpox
conformer
confounding
confrontation
    c. method
confusion
    c. colors
confusional
congelation
    c. urticaria

C

congener
congenerous
congenic
    c. strain
congenital
    c. adrenal hyperplasia
    c. afibrinogenemia
    c. amputation
    c. anemia
    c. ankyloblepharon
    c. aplasia of thymus
    c. aplastic anemia
    c. atonic pseudoparalysis
    c. baldness
    c. bronchiectasis
    c. cerebellar atrophy
    c. cerebral aneurysm
    c. choreoathetosis
    c. conus
    c. diaphragmatic hernia
    c. dyserythropoietic anemia
    c. dysphagocytosis
    c. dysplastic angiectasia
    c. dysplastic angiomatosis
    c. ectodermal defect
    c. ectodermal dysplasia
    c. elephantiasis
    c. epulis of newborn
    c. facial diplegia
    c. fibrosis of the extraocular
       muscles
    c. generalized fibromatosis
    c. heart block
    c. hemolytic anemia
    c. hemolytic icterus
    c. hemolytic jaundice
    c. hydrocele
    c. hydrocephalus
    c. hypophosphatasia
    c. hypoplastic anemia
    c. hypothyroidism
    c. ichthyosiform erythroderma
    c. lobar emphysema
    c. lymphedema
    c. methemoglobinemia
    c. myxedema
    c. nevus
    c. nonregenerative anemia
    c. nystagmus
    c. pancytopenia
    c. paramyotonia
    c. pneumonia
    c. pulmonary arteriovenous fistula
    c. pyloric stenosis
    c. rubella syndrome
    c. sebaceous hyperplasia
    c. spastic paraplegia
    c. stridor

    c. sutural alopecia
    c. syphilis
    c. torticollis
    c. total lipodystrophy
    c. toxoplasmosis
    c. valve
    c. virilizing adrenal hyperplasia
congenitus
congested
congestion
    active c.
    brain c.
    functional c.
    hypostatic c.
    passive c.
    physiologic c.
    venous c.
congestive
    c. cardiomyopathy
    c. cirrhosis
    c. heart failure
    c. splenomegaly
conglobate
conglobation
conglomerate
conglutinant
conglutination
conglutinin
Congolian red fever
congophilic
    c. angiopathy
Congo red
    C. r. paper
congruent points
congruous hemianopia
coni (*pl. of* conus)
conic, conical
    c. papillae
conidia (*pl. of* conidium)
conidial
Conidiobolus
conidiogenous
conidiophore
    Phialophore-type c.
conidium, pl. conidia
coniofibrosis
coniolymphstasis
coniometer
coniophage
coniosis
coniotomy
conization
    cautery c.
    cold c.
conjoined
    c. anastomosis
    c. asymmetrical twins
    c. equal twins

c. nerve root
c. symmetrical twins
c. tendon
c. twins
c. unequal twins
conjoint
c. tendon
c. therapy
conjugal cancer
conjugant
conjugata
c. diagonalis
c. vera
conjugate
c. axis
c. deviation of the eyes
diagonal c.
c. diameter of pelvic inlet
c. diameter of pelvic outlet
c. division
effective c.
external c.
false c.
c. foci
c. foramen
c. gaze
internal c.
c. movement of eyes
c. nystagmus
obstetric c.
obstetric c. of pelvic outlet
c. of pelvic inlet
c. of pelvic outlet
c. point
true c.
conjugated
c. antigen
c. bilirubin
c. hapten
conjugative plasmid
conjunctiva, pl. **conjunctivae**
bulbar c.
palpebral c.
conjunctival
c. arteries
c. cul-de-sac
c. fornix
c. glands
c. layer of bulb
c. layer of eyelids
c. reflex
c. ring
c. sac
c. varix
c. veins
conjunctive
conjunctiviplasty

conjunctivitis
actinic c.
acute catarrhal c.
acute contagious c.
acute epidemic c.
acute follicular c.
acute hemorrhagic c.
acute viral c.
allergic c.
angular c.
arc-flash c.
c. arida
blennorrheal c.
calcareous c.
chemical c.
chronic c.
chronic follicular c.
cicatricial c.
diphtheritic c.
follicular c.
gonococcal c.
gonorrheal c.
granular c.
hyperacute purulent c.
inclusion c.
infantile purulent c.
lacrimal c.
larval c.
ligneous c.
c. medicamentosa
meibomian c.
membranous c.
molluscum c.
Moraxella c.
mucopurulent c.
necrotic infectious c.
neonatal c.
Parinaud's c.
Pascheff's c.
c. petrificans
phlyctenular c.
prairie c.
pseudomembranous c.
purulent c.
reflux c.
simple c.
snow c.
spring c.
squirrel plague c.
swimming pool c.
toxicogenic c.
trachomatous c.
tularemic c., c. tularensis
vernal c.
welder's c.
conjunctivodacryocystorhinostomy
conjunctivodacryocystostomy
conjunctivoplasty

C

conjunctivorhinostomy
connecting
    c. cartilage
    c. stalk
    c. tubule
connection
    ambiguous atrioventricular c.'s
    atrioventricular c.'s
    concordant atrioventricular c.'s
    discordant atrioventricular c.'s
    double inlet atrioventricular c.'s
    intertendinous c.'s
    total or partial anomalous
      pulmonary venous c.'s
    univentricular c.'s
connective
    c. tissue
    c. tissue cell
    c. tissue group
    c. tumor
connective-tissue diseases
connector
    major c.
    minor c.
Connell's suture
connexus
    c. intertendineus
Conn's syndrome
conoid
    c. ligament
    c. process
    Sturm's c.
    c. tubercle
conomyoidin
Conradi-Drigalski agar
Conradi's
    C. disease
    C. line
consanguineous
consanguinity
conscious
consciousness
    clouding of c.
    double c.
    field of c.
consecutive
    c. amputation
    c. aneurysm
    c. angiitis
    c. esotropia
consensual
    c. light reflex
    c. reaction
    c. validation
conservation
conservative
    c. treatment
consistency principle

consolidation
    c. chemotherapy
consonating rale
conspicuity
constancy
    color c.
    object c.
    c. phenomenon
constant
    Ambard's c.
    association c.
    binding c.
    c. coupling
    c. field equation
    c. infusion pump
    time c.
    transformation c.
constellation
constipate
constipated
constipation
constitutional
    c. cause
    c. hepatic dysfunction
    c. hirsutism
    c. psychology
    c. reaction
    c. symptom
    c. thrombopathy
    c. ulcer
constitutive heterochromatin
constriction
    esophageal c.'s
    c. hyperemia
    primary c.
    pyloric c.
    c. ring
    secondary c.
    c.'s of ureter
constrictive
    c. bronchiolitis
    c. endocarditis
    c. pericarditis
constrictor
construct
    c. validity
constructional
    c. agraphia
    c. apraxia
consultand
    dummy c.
consultant
consultation
consulting staff
consumption
    c. coagulopathy
    oxygen c.
consumptive

contact
  c. allergy
  c. area
  balancing c.
  centric c.
  c. ceptor
  c. cheilitis
  deflective occlusal c.
  c. dermatitis
  c. hypersensitivity
  c. illumination
  c. inhibition
  initial c.
  interceptive occlusal c.
  c. lens
  c. point
  premature c.
  proximal c., proximate c.
  c. splint
  c. surface of tooth
  c. with reality
  working c.'s
contactant
contact-type dermatitis
contagion
  immediate c.
  mediate c.
  psychic c.
contagious
  c. disease
  c. ecthyma (pustular dermatitis)
    virus of sheep
  c. pustular stomatitis virus
contagiousness
contagium
containment
content
  c. analysis
  latent c.
  manifest c.
  c. validity
contiguity
  law of c.
  solution of c.
  spatial c.
  temporal c.
contiguous
continence
continent
contingency table
continued
  c. fever
continuity
continuous
  c. ambulatory peritoneal dialysis
  c. arrhythmia
  c. bar retainer
  c. beam

  c. capillary
  c. clasp
  c. epidural anesthesia
  c. eruption
  c. loop wiring
  c. murmur
  c. passive motion
  c. positive airway pressure
  c. positive pressure breathing
  c. positive pressure ventilation
  c. random variable
  c. reinforcement schedule
  c. spinal anesthesia
  c. suture
  c. tremor
  c. variable
  c. variation
contour
  flange c.
  gingival c.
  gum c.
  height of c.
  c. lines of Owen
contra-angle
contra-aperture
contrabevel
contraception
contraceptive
  barrier c.
  c. device
  intrauterine c. device
  c. sponge
contract
contracted
  c. kidney
  c. pelvis
contractile
  c. stricture
  c. vacuole
contractility
  cardiac c.
contraction
  after-c.
  anodal closure c.
  anodal opening c.
  automatic c.
  c. band
  c. band necrosis
  Braxton Hicks c.
  carpopedal c.
  cathodal closure c.
  cathodal opening c.
  closing c.
  escape c.
  escape ventricular c.
  fibrillary c.'s
  front-tap c.
  Gowers' c.

C

contraction *(continued)*
  hourglass c.
  hunger c.'s
  idiomuscular c.
  isometric c.
  isotonic c.
  myotatic c.
  opening c.
  paradoxical c.
  postural c.
  premature c.
  reflex detrusor c.
  c. stress test
  tetanic c.
  tonic c.
  uterine c.
contractual
  c. psychiatry
  c. psychotherapy
contractural diathesis
contracture
  c. deformity
  Dupuytren's c.
  fixed c.
  functional c.
  ischemic c. of the left ventricle
  organic c.
  Volkmann's c.
contrafissura
contraindicant
contraindication
contralateral
  c. hemiplegia
  c. partner
  c. reflex
  c. sign
contrast
  c. agent
  c. bath
  c. echocardiography
  c. enema
  c. enhancement
  c. material
  c. medium
  c. sensitivity
  simultaneous c.
  c. stain
  successive c.
contrasuppressor cells
contrecoup
  c. injury of brain
contrectation
control
  c. animal
  aversive c.
  birth c.
  C. of Communicable Diseases in
  Man

  c. gene
  c. group
  idiodynamic c.
  own c.'s
  quality c.
  reflex c.
  c. release suture
  social c.
  stimulus c.
  synergic c.
  c. syringe
  time-varied gain c.
  tonic c.
  vestibulo-equilibratory c.
controlled
  c. hypotension
  c. mechanical ventilation
  c. respiration
  c. ventilation
contusion
  brain c.
  c. pneumonia
  scalp c.
conular
conus, pl. **coni**
  c. arteriosus
  congenital c.
  distraction c.
  c. elasticus
  coni epididymidis
  c. medullaris
  myopic c.
  pulmonary c.
  supertraction c.
  coni vasculosi
convalescence
convalescent
  c. carrier
  c. serum
convenience form
conventional
  c. animal
  c. signs
  c. thoracoplasty
  c. tomography
convergence
  accommodative c.
  amplitude of c.
  angle of c.
  c. excess
  far point of c.
  c. insufficiency
  near point of c.
  negative c.
  c. nucleus of Perlia
  positive c.
  range of c.
  unit of c.

convergence-retraction nystagmus
convergent
 c. evolution
 c. squint
 c. strabismus
converging meniscus
conversion
 c. disorder
 c. hysteria
 c. hysteria neurosis
 c. neurosis
 c. reaction
convertase
convertin
convex
 high c.
 c. lens
 low c.
 c. mirror
convexity
 cortical c.
convexobasia
convexoconcave
 c. lens
convexoconvex
 c. lens
convolute
convoluted
 c. bone
 c. gland
 c. part of kidney lobule
 c. seminiferous tubule
 c. tubule of kidney
convolution
 angular c.
 anterior central c.
 ascending frontal c.
 ascending parietal c.
 callosal c.
 cingulate c.
 first temporal c.
 hippocampal c.
 inferior frontal c.
 inferior temporal c.
 middle frontal c.
 middle temporal c.
 posterior central c.
 second temporal c.
 superior frontal c.
 superior temporal c.
 supramarginal c.
 third temporal c.
 transitional c.
 transverse temporal c.'s
 Zuckerkandl's c.
convulsant
 c. threshold

convulsion
 benign neonatal c.'s
 clonic c.
 complex febrile c.
 coordinate c.
 ether c.
 febrile c.
 hysterical c., hysteroid c.
 immediate posttraumatic c.
 infantile c.
 mimic c.
 puerperal c.'s
 salaam c.'s
 tetanic c.
 tonic c.
convulsive
 c. reflex
 c. seizure
 c. state
 c. therapy
 c. tic
cooing murmur
Cooke's speculum
cooled-knife method
Cooley's anemia
Coolidge tube
coolie itch
Coomassie brilliant blue R-250
Coombs'
 C. serum
 C. test
Coombs murmur
Cooperia
 C. bisonis
 C. curticei
 C. fieldingi
 C. oncophora
 C. pectinata
 C. punctata
 C. spatulata
Coopernail's sign
Cooper's
 C. fascia
 C. hernia
 C. herniotome
 C. ligaments
coordinate
 c. convulsion
coordinated reflex
coordination
co-ossification
co-ossify
cope
copepod
Cope's clamp
copia elements
coping
 transfer c.

C

copper
    c. cataract
    c. colic
    c. nose
    c. pennies
    c. phosphate cement
    c. sulfate method
copper-64
copra itch
coprecipitation
copremesis
coproantibodies
coprolagnia
coprolalia
coprolith
coprology
coproma
coprophagous
coprophagy
coprophil, coprophilic
coprophile
coprophilia
coprophilic (*var. of* coprophil)
coprophobia
coprophrasia
coproplanesia
coproporphyria
coprostasis
coprozoa
coprozoic
coptic lung
coptosis
copula
      His' c.
    c. linguae
copulation
coquille
cor, gen. **cordis**
    c. adiposum
    c. biloculare
    c. bovinum
    c. mobile
    c. pendulum
    c. pulmonale
    c. triatriatum
    c. triloculare
    c. triloculare biatriatum
    c. triloculare biventriculare
coracidium
coracoacromial
    c. arch
    c. ligament
coracobrachial
    c. bursa
    c. muscle
coracobrachialis
    c. muscle

coracoclavicular
    c. ligament
coracohumeral
    c. ligament
coracoid
    c. process
    c. tuberosity
coral calculus
coralliform cataract
corallin
    yellow c.
cord
    Bergmann's c.'s
    Billroth's c.'s
    c. blood
    condyle c.
    dental c.
    false vocal c.
    Ferrein's c.'s
    gangliated c.
    genital c.
    germinal c.'s
    gonadal c.'s
    gubernacular c.
    hepatic c.'s
    c. hydrocele
    lateral c. of brachial plexus
    lymph c.'s
    medial c. of brachial plexus
    medullary c.'s
    nephrogenic c.
    oblique c.
    omphalomesenteric c.
    posterior c. of brachial plexus
    psalterial c.
    red pulp c.'s
    rete c.'s
    sex c.'s
    spermatic c.
    spinal c.
    splenic c.'s
    tendinous c.'s
    testicular c.
    testis c.'s
    true vocal c.
    c. of tympanum
    umbilical c.
    vitelline c.
    vocal c.
    Weitbrecht's c.
    Wilde's c.'s
    Willis' c.'s
cordate
    c. pelvis
cordectomy
cordiform
    c. pelvis
    c. uterus

cordis (*gen. of* cor)
cordis
    diastasis c.
cordocentesis
cordon sanitaire
cordopexy
cordotomy
    anterolateral c.
    open c.
    posterior column c.
    spinothalamic c.
    stereotactic c.
Cordylobia
    C. anthropophaga
cordy pulse
core
    central transactional c.
    c. pneumonia
corectopia
corelysis
coremium
coreoplasty
corepexy
    purse-string c.
corepraxy
    laser c.
    mechanical c.
Cori's disease
corium, pl. coria
corn
    asbestos c.
    c. ergot
    hard c.
    seed c.
    soft c.
cornea
    conical c.
    c. farinata
    floury c.
    c. urica
    c. verticillata
corneal
    c. astigmatism
    c. corpuscles
    c. decompensation
    c. dystrophy
    c. ectasia
    c. endothelial polymorphism
    c. facet
    c. graft
    c. layer of epidermis
    c. lens
    c. margin
    c. pannus
    c. reflex
    c. space
    c. spot
    c. staphyloma

    c. transplantation
    c. trepanation
Cornelia de Lange syndrome
corneoblepharon
corneocyte
    c. envelope
corneosclera
corneoscleral
    c. part of trabecular reticulum
corneous
Corner-Allen test
Corner's tampon
corneum
corniculate
    c. cartilage
    c. tubercle
corniculopharyngeal ligament
corniculum
    c. laryngis
cornification
cornified
    c. layer of nail
cornmeal agar
cornoid lamella
corn smut
cornu, gen. cornus, pl. cornua
    c. ammonis
    c. anterius
    coccygeal cornua
    cornua coccygealia
    c. cutaneum
    cornua of falciform margin of
      saphenous opening
    cornua of hyoid bone
    c. inferius
    c. inferius cartilaginis thyroideae
    c. inferius marginalis falciformis
      hiatus sapheni
    c. inferius ventriculi lateralis
    c. laterale
    cornua of lateral ventricle
    c. majus ossis hyoidei
    c. minus ossis hyoidei
    c. posterius
    c. posterius ventriculi lateralis
    sacral cornua
    cornua sacralia
    cornua of spinal cord
    styloid c.
    c. superius cartilaginis thyroideae
    c. superius marginalis falciformis
    cornua of thyroid cartilage
    c. uteri
cornual
    c. pregnancy
corona, pl. coronae
    c. capitis
    c. ciliaris

C

corona *(continued)*
    c. clinica
    c. dentis
    c. glandis
    c. of glans penis
    c. radiata
    c. seborrheica
    c. veneris
    Zinn's c.
coronad
coronal
    c. epispadias
    c. hypospadias
    c. plane
    c. pulp
    c. section
    c. suture
coronale
coronalis
coronaria
coronarism
coronaritis
coronary
    c. angiography
    c. arteriosclerosis
    c. arteritis
    c. artery
    c. artery aneurysm
    c. atherectomy
    c. bypass
    cafe c.
    c. care unit
    c. cataract
    c. endarterectomy
    c. failure
    c. groove
    c. insufficiency
    c. ligament of knee
    c. ligament of liver
    c. nodal rhythm
    c. node
    c. occlusion
    c. ostial stenosis
    c. perfusion pressure
    c. plexus
    c. sinus
    c. sinus rhythm
    c. steal
    c. sulcus
    c. tendon
    c. thrombosis
    c. valve
    c. vein
coronary-prone behavior
Coronaviridae
Coronavirus
coronavirus
coroner

coronion
coronoid
    c. fossa of humerus
    c. process
coronoidectomy
corporeal
corpse
corps ronds
corpulence, corpulency
corpulent
corpus, gen. **corporis**, pl. **corpora**
    c. adiposum
    c. adiposum buccae
    c. adiposum fossae ischiorectalis
    c. adiposum infrapatellare
    c. adiposum orbitae
    c. albicans
    c. amygdaloideum
    c. amylaceum, pl. corpora amylacea
    c. aorticum
    c. arantii
    corpora arenacea
    atretic c. luteum
    c. atreticum
    corpora bigemina
    c. callosum
    c. candicans
    c. cavernosum clitoridis
    c. cavernosum conchae
    c. cavernosum penis
    c. cavernosum urethrae
    c. ciliare
    c. claviculae
    c. clitoridis
    c. coccygeum
    c. costae
    c. dentatum
    c. epididymidis
    c. epididymis
    c. femoris
    c. fibrosum
    c. fibulae
    c. fimbriatum
    c. fornicis
    c. gastricum [ventriculi]
    c. geniculatum externum
    c. geniculatum internum
    c. geniculatum laterale
    c. geniculatum mediale
    c. glandulae sudoriferae
    c. hemorrhagicum
    c. highmori, c. highmorianum
    c. humeri
    c. incudis
    c. linguae
    corpora lutea cysts
    c. luteum, c. luteum spurium, c. luteum verum

c. luteum deficiency syndrome
c. luteum hematoma
c. luysi
c. mamillare
c. mammae
c. mandibulae
c. maxillae
c. medullare cerebelli
c. nuclei caudati
c. olivare
c. ossis femoris
c. ossis hyoidei
c. ossis ilii
c. ossis ischii
c. ossis metacarpalis
c. ossis pubis
c. ossis sphenoidalis
c. pampiniforme
c. pancreatis
c. papillare
corpora para-aortica
c. paraterminale
c. penis
c. phalangis
c. pontobulbare
corpora quadrigemina
c. quadrigeminum anterius
c. quadrigeminum posterius
c. radii
c. restiforme
c. spongiosum penis
c. spongiosum urethrae muliebris
c. sterni
c. striatum
c. tali
c. tibiae
c. trapezoideum
c. triticeum
c. ulnae
c. unguis
c. uteri
c. vertebrae
c. vesicae biliaris
c. vesicae felleae
c. vesicae urinariae
c. vitreum

corpuscle
amniotic c.
amylaceous c., amyloid c.
articular c.'s
axis c., axile c.
basal c.
Bizzozero's c.
blood c.
bone c.
bridge c.
bulboid c.'s
cement c.

chyle c.
colloid c.
colostrum c.
corneal c.'s
Dogiel's c.
Donné's c.
dust c.'s
Eichhorst's c.'s
exudation c.
genital c.'s
ghost c.
Gluge's c.'s
Golgi c.
Golgi-Mazzoni c.
Hassall's concentric c.'s
inflammatory c.
lamellated c.'s
lymph c., lymphatic c., lymphoid c.
malpighian c.'s
Mazzoni c.
Meissner's c.
Merkel's c.
Mexican hat c.
molluscum c.
Negri c.'s
Norris' c.'s
oval c.
pacchionian c.'s
pacinian c.'s
pessary c.
phantom c.
plastic c.
Purkinje's c.'s
pus c.
Rainey's c.'s
red c.
renal c.
reticulated c.
Ruffini's c.'s
salivary c.
Schwalbe's c.
shadow c.
splenic c.'s
tactile c.
taste c.
terminal nerve c.'s
third c.
thymic c.
touch c.
Toynbee's c.'s
Traube's c.
Tröltsch's c.'s
Valentin's c.'s
Vater-Pacini c.'s
Vater's c.'s
Virchow's c.'s

C

corpuscle *(continued)*
   white c.
   Zimmermann's c.
corpuscular
   c. lymph
   c. radiation
corpusculum, pl. **corpuscula**
   corpuscula articularia
   corpuscula bulboidea
   corpuscula genitalia
   corpuscula lamellosa
   corpuscula nervosa terminalia
   c. renis, pl. corpuscula renis
   c. tactus, pl. corpuscula tactus
corralin yellow
corrected
   c. dextrocardia
   c. transposition of the great
     vessels
correction
   occlusal c.
   spontaneous c. of placenta previa
corrective emotional experience
corrector
   function c.
correlation
   c. coefficient
   product-moment c.
   rank-difference c.
correlational method
correlative differentiation
Correra's line
correspondence
   abnormal c.
   anomalous c.
   dysharmonious c.
   harmonious c.
Corrigan's
   C. disease
   C. pulse
   C. sign
corrosion preparation
corrosive ulcer
corrugator
   c. cutis muscle of anus
   c. muscle
   c. supercilii muscle
cortex, gen. **corticis**, pl. **cortices**
   adrenal c.
   agranular c.
   association c.
   auditory c.
   cerebellar c.
   c. cerebelli
   cerebral c.
   c. cerebri
   deep c.
   dysgranular c.

   fetal adrenal c.
   frontal c.
   c. glandulae suprarenalis
   granular c.
   c. of hair shaft
   heterotypic c.
   homotypic c.
   insular c.
   laminated c.
   c. of lens
   c. lentis
   c. of lymph node
   motor c.
   c. nodi lymphatici
   olfactory c.
   orbitofrontal c.
   c. ovarii
   c. of ovary
   parastriate c.
   peristriate c.
   piriform c.
   prefrontal c.
   premotor c.
   primary visual c.
   provisional c.
   renal c.
   c. renis
   secondary sensory c.
   secondary visual c.
   sensory c.
   somatic sensory c.,
     somatosensory c.
   striate c.
   supplementary motor c.
   suprarenal c.
   temporal c.
   tertiary c.
   c. of thymus
   visual c.
cortical
   c. apraxia
   c. arches of kidney
   c. arteries
   c. audiometry
   c. blindness
   c. bone
   c. cataract
   c. convexity
   c. deafness
   c. dysplasia
   c. epilepsy
   c. implantation
   c. lobules of kidney
   c. osteitis
   c. part
   c. part of middle cerebral artery
   c. sensibility
   c. substance

corticalization
corticalosteotomy
corticectomy
cortices (*pl. of* cortex)
corticifugal
corticipetal
corticis (*gen. of* cortex)
corticoafferent
corticobulbar
    c. fibers
    c. tract
corticocerebellum
corticoefferent
corticofugal
corticomedial
corticonuclear fibers
corticopontine
    c. fibers
    c. tract
corticoreticular fibers
corticorubral fibers
corticospinal
    c. fibers
    c. tract
corticosteroid-induced glaucoma
corticothalamic
    c. fibers
corticotroph
corticotropin-like intermediate-lobe
   peptide
Corticoviridae
Corti's
    C. arch
    C. auditory teeth
    C. canal
    C. cells
    C. ganglion
    C. membrane
    C. organ
    C. pillars
    C. rods
    C. tunnel
coruscation
Corvisart's facies
corymbiform
corymbose syphilid
corynebacteria (*pl. of* corynebacterium)
corynebacteriophage
    β c.
Corynebacterium
    C. acnes
    C. bovis
    C. enzymicum
    C. haemolyticum
    C. hofmannii
    C. minutissimum
    C. murisepticum
    C. parvum

    C. phocae
    C. pseudodiphtheriticum
    C. xerosis
corynebacterium, pl. corynebacteria
coryneform bacteria
coryza
    allergic c.
Coryzavirus
cosmesis
cosmetic
    c. dermatitis
    c. surgery
cosmetics
costa, gen. and pl. costae
    c. cervicalis
    costae fluctuantes
    costae fluitantes
    costae spuriae
    costae verae
costal
    c. angle
    c. arch
    c. arch reflex
    c. cartilage
    c. chondritis
    c. facets
    c. fringe
    c. groove
    c. groove for subclavian artery
    c. notch
    c. part of diaphragm
    c. pit of transverse process
    c. pleura
    c. pleurisy
    c. process
    c. respiration
    c. surface
    c. surface of lung
    c. surface of scapula
    c. tuberosity
costalgia
costectomy
Costen's syndrome
costicartilage
costiform
costive
costiveness
costoaxillary vein
costocentral
costocervical
    c. artery
    c. trunk
costochondral
    c. joint
    c. junction
    c. syndrome
costochondritis

C

costoclavicular
   c. ligament
   c. line
   c. syndrome
costocolic ligament
costocoracoid
costodiaphragmatic recess
costogenic
costoinferior
costomediastinal
   c. recess
   c. sinus
costopectoral reflex
costophrenic
   c. angle
   c. septal lines
   c. sulcus
costoscapular
costoscapularis
costosternal
costosternoplasty
costosuperior
costotome
costotomy
costotransverse
   c. foramen
   c. joint
   c. ligament
costotransversectomy
costovertebral
   c. joints
costoxiphoid
   c. ligament
Cotard's syndrome
cot death
cotranslational
cotransport
Cotte's operation
cotton-dust asthma
cotton-fiber embolism
cotton-mill fever
cottonpox
cotton-wool
   c.-w. patches
   c.-w. spots
Cotunnius'
   C. aqueduct
   C. canal
   C. liquid
   C. space
Cotunnius disease
cotyle
cotyledon
   fetal c.
   maternal c.
cotyledonary placenta
Cotylogonimus

cotyloid
   c. cavity
   c. joint
   c. ligament
   c. notch
couching
   c. needle
cough
   aneurysmal c.
   brassy c.
   c. fracture
   privet c.
   reflex c.
   c. reflex
   weaver's c.
   whooping c.
Coumel's tachycardia
Councilman
   C. body
   C. hyaline body
   C. lesion
Councilmania
counseling
   genetic c.
   marital c.
   pastoral c.
   c. psychology
count
   Addis c.
   Arneth c.
   blood c.
   c. density
   epidermal ridge c.
   filament-nonfilament c.
counter
   automated differential leukocyte c.
   electronic cell c.
   Geiger-Müller c.
   proportional c.
   scintillation c.
   c. transference
   well c.
   whole-body c.
counterbalancing
counterconditioning
countercurrent
   c. exchanger
   c. mechanism
   c. multiplier
counterdie
counterextension
counterimmunoelectrophoresis
counterincision
counterinvestment
counterirritation
counteropening
counterphobic

counterpulsation
    intra-aortic balloon c.
counterpuncture
countershock
counterstain
countertraction
countertransference
countertransport
coup
    c. de sabre
    c. injury of brain
coupled
    c. beats
    c. pulse
    c. rhythm
coupling
    constant c.
    c. defect
    fixed c.
    c. interval
    c. phase
    variable c.
Cournand's dip
Courvoisier's
    C. gallbladder
    C. law
    C. sign
couvade
Couvelaire uterus
couvercle
cove plane
cover
    c. glass
    c. test
coverage
covering
    c.'s of spermatic cord
coverslip
covert sensitization
cover-uncover test
cow
    c. face
    c. kidney
    c. milk anemia
    radioactive c.
Cowden's disease
Cowdry's
    C. type A inclusion bodies
    C. type B inclusion bodies
CO_2-withdrawal seizure test
cowl
cowl (*var. of* caul)
    c. muscle
Cowling's rule
cowperitis
Cowper's
    C. cyst

C. gland
C. ligament
cowpox virus
coxa, gen. and pl. **coxae**
    c. adducta
    false c. vara
    c. magna
    c. plana
    c. valga
    c. vara
    c. vara luxans
coxal bone
coxalgia
Coxiella
    C. burnetii
coxitic scoliosis
coxodynia
coxofemoral
coxotomy
coxotuberculosis
Coxsackie
    C. encephalitis
    C. virus
Coxsackievirus
crab
    c. hand
    c. yaws
crack
cracked heel
cracked-pot
    c.-p. resonance
    c.-p. sound
crackle
    pleural c.'s
crackling
    c. jaw
    parchment c.
    c. rale
cradle
    c. cap
Crafoord clamp
craft palsy
Craigia
Cramer wire splint
cramp
    accessory c.
    heat c.'s
    intermittent c.
    miner's c.'s
    musician's c.
    pianist's c., piano-player's c.
    seamstress's c.
    shaving c.
    stoker's c.'s
    tailor's c.
    typist's c.
    violinist's c.
    waiter's c.

C

cramp (continued)
>> watchmaker's c.
>> writer's c.

Crampton
>> C. line
>> C. muscle
>> C. test

Crandall's syndrome
crania (pl. of cranium)
crania
craniad
cranial
>> c. arteritis
>> c. base
>> c. bones
>> c. capacity
>> c. cavity
>> c. epidural space
>> c. flexure
>> c. fontanels
>> c. index
>> c. nerves
>> c. neuropore
>> c. root of accessory nerve
>> c. roots
>> c. sinuses
>> c. sutures
>> c. synchondroses
>> c. vault
>> c. vertebra

craniamphitomy
craniectomy
>> linear c.

cranio-aural
craniocardiac reflex
craniocarpotarsal
>> c. dysplasia
>> c. dystrophy

craniocele
craniocerebral
cranioclasia, cranioclasis
cranioclast
craniocleidodysostosis
craniodiaphysial dysplasia
craniodidymus
craniofacial
>> c. angle
>> c. appliance
>> c. axis
>> c. dysjunction fracture
>> c. dysostosis
>> c. fixation
>> c. notch
>> c. surgery
>> c. suspension wiring

craniofenestria
craniognomy
craniograph

craniography
craniolacunia
craniology
>> Gall's c.

craniomalacia
>> circumscribed c.

craniomeningocele
craniometaphysial dysplasia
craniometer
craniometric
>> c. points

craniometry
craniopagus
>> c. occipitalis
>> c. parasiticus

craniopathy
>> metabolic c.

craniopharyngeal
>> c. canal
>> c. duct

craniopharyngioma
>> ameloblastomatous c.
>> cystic papillomatous c.

craniophore
cranioplasty
craniopuncture
craniorrhachidian
craniorrhachischisis
craniosacral
>> c. system

cranioschisis
craniosclerosis
cranioscopy
craniospinal
>> c. ganglia

craniospinalia ganglia
craniostenosis
craniostosis
craniosynostosis
craniotabes
craniotome
craniotomy
>> attached c.
>> detached c.
>> osteoplastic c.

craniotonoscopy
craniotrypesis
craniotympanic
cranium, pl. crania
>> c. bifidum, bifid c.
>> c. cerebrale, cerebral c.
>> c. viscerale, visceral c.

crapulent, crapulous
crash cart
crater
>> c. arc

crateriform
craterization

cravat bandage
craw-craw
crazing
C-reactive protein
cream
    leukocyte c.
crease
    digital c.
    digital flexion c.
    ear lobe c.
    flexion c.
    palmar c.
    simian c.
    Sydney c.
    c. wound
creatine kinase isoenzymes
creatinemia
creatinine clearance
creatinuria
creative thinking
Credé's
    C. maneuvers
    C. methods
creep
    c. recovery
creeping
    c. eruption
    c. myiasis
    c. palsy
    c. thrombosis
    c. ulcer
cremaster
    c. muscle
cremasteric
    c. artery
    c. fascia
    c. reflex
cremnocele
cremnophobia
crena, pl. **crenae**
    c. ani
    c. clunium
    c. cordis
crenate, crenated
crenation
crenocyte
crenocytosis
Crenosoma vulpis
creola bodies
crepitant
    c. rale
crepitation
crepitus
    articular c.
    bony c.
crepuscular
crescendo
    c. angina

    c. murmur
    c. sleep
crescent
    articular c.
    c. cell
    c. cell anemia
    Giannuzzi's c.'s
    glomerular c.
    Heidenhain's c.'s
    malarial c.
    myopic c.
    sublingual c.
crescentic
    c. lobules of the cerebellum
crescograph
cresol red
crest
    acoustic c.
    acousticofacial c.
    alveolar c.
    c. of alveolar ridge
    ampullary c.
    anterior lacrimal c.
    arched c.
    arcuate c.
    arcuate c. of arytenoid cartilage
    articular c.'s
    basilar c. of cochlear duct
    buccinator c.
    c. of cochlear opening
    conchal c.
    conchal c. of maxilla
    conchal c. of palatine bone
    deltoid c.
    dental c.
    ethmoidal c.
    ethmoidal c. of maxilla
    ethmoidal c. of palatine bone
    external occipital c.
    falciform c.
    c. of fenestrae cochleae
    frontal c.
    ganglionic c.
    gingival c.
    gluteal c.
    c. of greater tubercle
    c. of head of rib
    iliac c.
    incisor c.
    infratemporal c.
    inguinal c.
    intermediate sacral c.'s
    internal occipital c.
    interosseous c.
    intertrochanteric c.
    lateral epicondylar c.
    lateral sacral c.'s
    lateral supracondylar c.

C

crest (continued)
  c. of lesser tubercle
  marginal c.
  medial epicondylar c.
  medial c. of fibula
  medial supracondylar c.
  median sacral c.
  c.'s of nail bed
  nasal c.
  c. of neck of rib
  neural c.
  obturator c.
  c. of palatine bone, palatine c.
  c. of petrous part of temporal
    bone
  posterior lacrimal c.
  pubic c.
  sacral c.
  c. of scapular spine
  sphenoid c.
  spiral c.
  supinator c., c. of supinator muscle
  supramastoid c.
  supraventricular c.
  terminal c.
  tibial c.
  transverse c.
  transverse c. of internal acoustic
    meatus
  triangular c.
  trigeminal c.
  trochanteric c.
  turbinated c.
  urethral c.
  urethral c. of female
  urethral c. of male
  vestibular c., c. of vestibule
cresta
CREST syndrome
cresyl
  c. blue, c. blue brilliant
  c. echt, c. fast violet
  c. violet acetate
cretin
cretinism
cretinistic
cretinoid
cretinous
Creutzfeldt-Jakob disease
crevice
  gingival c.
crevicular
  c. epithelium
  c. fluid
crib
  c. death
  tongue c.
cribra (pl. of cribrum)

cribrate
cribration
cribriform
  c. area of the renal papilla
  c. fascia
  c. hymen
  c. plate of ethmoid bone
cribrous lamina
cribrum, pl. cribra
Crichton-Browne's sign
cricoarytenoid
  c. articular capsule
  c. articulation
  c. joint
cricoarytenoideus
cricoesophageal tendon
cricoid
  c. cartilage
cricoidynia
cricopharyngeal
  c. ligament
  c. myotomy
  c. part of inferior pharyngeal
    constrictor
cricopharyngeus muscle
cricosantorinian ligament
cricothyroid
  c. artery
  c. articular capsule
  c. articulation
  c. joint
  c. ligament
  c. membrane
  c. muscle
cricothyroideus
cricothyroidotomy
cricothyrotomy
cricotomy
cricotracheal
  c. ligament
  c. membrane
cricovocal membrane
cri du chat syndrome
cri-du-chat syndrome
Crigler-Najjar
  C.-N. disease
  C.-N. syndrome
Crile's clamp
Crimean-Congo
  C.-C. hemorrhagic fever
  C.-C. hemorrhagic fever virus
Crimean fever
criminal
  c. abortion
  c. anthropology
  c. hygiene
  c. insanity

c. irresponsibility
c. psychology
criminology
crinis, pl. crines
crinogenic
crinophagy
crippled
crisis, pl. crises
addisonian c.
adolescent c.
adrenal c.
anaphylactoid c.
blast c.
blood c.
Dietl's c.
febrile c.
gastric c.
glaucomatocyclitic c.
identity c.
c. intervention
laryngeal c.
midlife c.
myasthenic c.
myelocytic c.
ocular c.
oculogyric crises
salt-depletion c.
sickle cell c.
tabetic c.
therapeutic c.
thyrotoxic c., thyroid c.
visceral crises
crispation
crisscross heart
crista, pl. cristae
c. ampullaris
c. arcuata cartilaginis arytenoideae
c. basilaris ductus cochlearis
c. buccinatoria
c. capitis costae
c. colli costae
c. conchalis
c. conchalis maxillae
c. conchalis ossis palatini
cristae cutis
c. dentalis
c. dividens
c. ethmoidalis
c. ethmoidalis maxillae
c. ethmoidalis ossis palatini
c. fenestrae cochleae
c. frontalis
c. galli
c. glutea
c. helicis
c. iliaca
c. infratemporalis
c. intertrochanterica

c. lacrimalis anterior
c. lacrimalis posterior
c. marginalis
cristae matricis unguis
c. medialis fibulae
cristae of mitochondria, cristae mitochondriales
c. musculi supinatoris
c. nasalis
c. obturatoria
c. occipitalis externa
c. occipitalis interna
c. palatina
c. phallica
c. pubica
c. quarta
cristae sacrales intermediae
cristae sacrales laterales
c. sacralis
c. sacralis mediana
c. sphenoidalis
c. spiralis
c. supracondylaris lateralis
c. supracondylaris medialis
c. supramastoidea
c. supraventricularis
c. terminalis
c. transversa
c. transversalis
c. triangularis
c. tuberculi majoris
c. tuberculi minoris
c. urethralis
c. urethralis femininae
c. urethralis masculinae
c. vestibuli
criterion, pl. criteria   NASCET
Spiegelberg's criteria
criterion-related validity
Crithidia
crithidia
critical
c. angle
c. care unit
c. flicker fusion frequency
c. illness polyneuropathy
c. illumination
c. organ
c. period
c. rate
CR lead
crocidismus
crocodile
c. tears
c. tears syndrome
Crocq's disease
Crohn's disease
Cronkhite-Canada syndrome

209

Crooke's
    C. granules
    C. hyaline change
    C. hyaline degeneration
Crookes' glass
Crookes-Hittorf tube
Crosby capsule
cross
    c. agglutination
    back c.
    c. birth
    double back c.
    c. flap
    hair c.'s
    c. hybridization
    c. infection
    c. mating
    Ranvier's c.'s
    c. reaction
    c. section
    test c.
crossbite
    c. teeth
crossbreed
crossbreeding
cross-cultural psychiatry
cross-cut bur
cross-dressing
crossed
    c. adductor jerk
    c. adductor reflex
    c. anesthesia
    c. aphasia
    c. cylinders
    c. diplopia
    c. embolism
    c. extension reflex
    c. eyes
    c. fixation
    c. hemianesthesia
    c. hemianopia
    c. hemiplegia
    c. immunoelectrophoresis
    c. jerk
    c. knee jerk
    c. knee reflex
    c. laterality
    c. paralysis
    c. phrenic phenomenon
    c. pyramidal tract
    c. reflex
    c. reflex of pelvis
    c. renal ectopia
    c. spino-adductor reflex
    c. testicular ectopia
cross-eye
crossing a bridge

crossing-over, crossover
    somatic c.-o.
    uneven c.-o., unequal c.-o.
cross-matching
cross-over study
cross-reacting
    c.-r. agglutinin
    c.-r. antibody
    c.-r. material
cross-section
cross-sectional
    c.-s. echocardiography
    c.-s. method
    c.-s. study
cross-table lateral projection
crossway
    sensory c.
crotaphion
croup-associated virus
croupous
    c. bronchitis
    c. laryngitis
    c. lymph
    c. membrane
croupy
Crouzon's
    C. disease
    C. syndrome
crowding
crowing inspiration
crown
    anatomical c.
    artificial c.
    bell-shaped c.
    c. cavity
    ciliary c.
    clinical c.
    c. flask
    c. glass
    c. of head
    jacket c.
    radiate c.
    c. of tooth
    c. tubercle
    c. of Venus
crown-heel length
crowning
crown-rump length
cruces (*pl. of* crux)
crucial
    c. anastomosis
    c. bandage
    c. ligament
cruciate
    c. anastomosis
    c. eminence
    c. ligament of the atlas
    c. ligament of leg

c. ligaments of knee
c. muscle

cruciform
c. eminence
c. ligament of atlas
c. loops
c. part of fibrous digital sheath
c. part of fibrous sheath
c. pulley

crude
c. death rate
c. urine

cruor
crura (*pl. of* crus)
crural
c. arch
c. fascia
c. fossa
c. hernia
c. interosseous nerve
c. ring
c. septum
c. sheath
c. triangle

cruralis posterior
crureus
crus, gen. **cruris**, pl. **crura**
ampullary crura of semicircular
ducts
anterior c. of stapes
c. anterius capsulae internae
c. anterius stapedis
c. anthelicis
c. of antihelix
crura of bony semicircular canals
c. breve incudis
c. cerebri
c. clitoridis
c. of clitoris
common c. of semicircular ducts
c. corporis cavernosi penis
c. dextrum diaphragmatis
c. dextrum fasciculi
atrioventricularis
c. fornicis
c. of fornix
c. helicis
c. of helix
c. I
c. II
lateral c.
c. laterale
c. laterale anuli inguinalis
superficialis
c. laterale cartilaginis alaris majoris
lateral c. of facial canal
lateral c. of the greater alar
cartilage of the nose

lateral c. of horizontal part of the
facial canal
lateral c. of the superficial
inguinal ring
left c. of atrioventricular bundle
left c. of diaphragm
long c. of incus
c. longum incudis
medial c.
c. mediale
c. mediale annuli inguinalis
superficialis
c. mediale cartilaginis alaris
majoris
medial c. of facial canal
medial c. of greater alar cartilage
of nose
medial c. of the horizontal part of
the facial canal
medial c. of the superficial
inguinal ring
crura membranacea ampullaria
ductus semicircularis
c. membranaceum commune ductus
semicircularis
c. membranaceum simplex ductus
semicircularis
crura ossea canalium
semicircularium
c. of penis
c. penis
posterior c. of stapes
c. posterius capsulae internae
c. posterius stapedis
right c. of atrioventricular bundle
right c. of diaphragm
short c. of incus
simple c. of semicircular duct
c. sinistrum diaphragmatis
c. sinistrum fasciculi
atrioventricularis

crush
c. kidney
c. syndrome

crusotomy
crust
milk c.

crusta, pl. **crustae**
c. inflammatoria
c. lactea
c. phlogistica

crusted
c. ringworm
c. tetter

crutch
c. palsy
c. paralysis

Cruveilhier-Baumgarten
 C.-B. disease
 C.-B. murmur
 C.-B. sign
 C.-B. syndrome
Cruveilhier's
 C. disease
 C. fascia
 C. fossa
 C. joint
 C. ligaments
 C. plexus
crux, pl. **cruces**
 c. of heart
 cruces pilorum
Cruz trypanosomiasis
cryalgesia
cryanesthesia
cryesthesia
cry for help
crymodynia
crymophilic
crymophylactic
cryoanesthesia
cryobiology
cryocautery
cryoconization
cryoextraction
cryoextractor
cryofibrinogen
cryofibrinogenemia
cryoglobulinemia
cryohypophysectomy
cryolysis
cryopallidectomy
cryopathy
cryopexy
cryophilic
cryophylactic
cryoprecipitate
cryoprecipitation
cryopreservation
cryoprobe
cryoprostatectomy
cryopulvinectomy
cryospasm
cryosurgery
cryothalamectomy
cryotherapy
cryotolerant
crypt
 c. abscesses
 anal c.'s
 dental c.
 enamel c.
 c.'s of Henle
 c.'s of iris
 Lieberkühn's c.'s

 lingual c.
 Morgagni's c.'s
 synovial c.
 tonsillar c.
crypta, pl. **cryptae**
 c. tonsillaris, pl. cryptae tonsillares
cryptectomy
cryptic
cryptitis
cryptococcoma
cryptococcosis
Cryptococcus
cryptocrystalline
Cryptocystis trichodectis
cryptodidymus
Cryptogamia
cryptogenic
 c. cirrhosis
 c. epilepsy
 c. infection
 c. pyemia
 c. septicemia
cryptolith
cryptomenorrhea
cryptophthalmus, cryptophthalmia
 c. syndrome
cryptopodia
cryptorchid
 c. testis
cryptorchidism
cryptorchidopexy
cryptorchism
cryptoscope
Cryptosporidium
Cryptostroma corticale
cryptotia
cryptozoite
cryptozygous
cry reflex
crystal
 asthma c.'s
 blood c.'s
 Böttcher's c.'s
 Charcot-Leyden c.'s
 Charcot-Neumann c.'s
 Charcot-Robin c.'s
 ear c.'s
 Florence's c.'s
 hematoidin c.'s
 knife-rest c.
 Leyden's c.'s
 Lubarsch's c.'s
 c. rash
 sperm c., spermin c.
 thorn apple c.'s
 twin c.
 Virchow's c.'s
 whetstone c.'s

crystallin
  gamma c.
crystalline
  c. capsule
  c. cataract
  c. interface
  c. lens
crystallogram
crystalloid
  Charcot-Böttcher c.'s
  Reinke c.'s
crystallophobia
crystalluria
crytotetany
C-section
Csillag's disease
"C" sliding osteotomy
CT
  computed tomography
    dynamic CT
    helical CT
    CT number
    spiral CT
    CT unit
Ctenocephalides
Cuban itch
cube pessary
cubital
  c. bone
  c. fossa
  c. joint
  c. lymph nodes
  c. nerve
cubitus, gen. and pl. **cubiti**
  c. valgus
  c. varus
cuboid, cuboidal
  c. bone
cuboideonavicular
  c. joint
  c. ligaments
cuboidodigital reflex
cue
  response-produced c.'s
cuff
  musculotendinous c.
  perivascular c.'s
  rotator c. of shoulder
cuffing
cuirass
  analgesic c.
  c. respirator
  tabetic c.
cul-de-sac, pl. **culs-de-sac**
  conjunctival c.-d.-s.
  Douglas' c.-d.-s.
  greater c.-d.-s.
  Gruber's c.-d.-s.

  lesser c.-d.-s.
  c.-d.-s. smear
culdocentesis
culdoplasty
culdoscope
culdoscopy
culdotomy
Culex
  C. pipiens
Culicidae
Culicoides
  C. austeni
  C. furens
culicosis
Culiseta melanura
Cullen's sign
culmen, pl. **culmina**
Culp pyeloplasty
culs-de-sac (*pl. of* cul-de-sac)
cult
cultivation
cultural
  c. anthropology
  c. shock
cultural diversity
culture
  cell c.
  elective c.
  enrichment c.
  hanging-block c.
  c. medium
  mixed lymphocyte c.
  needle c.
  neotype c.
  organ c.
  pure c.
  roll-tube c.
  sensitized c.
  shake c.
  slant c.
  slope c.
  smear c.
  stab c.
  stock c.
  streak c.
  tissue c.
  type c.
Cummer's
  C. classification
  C. guideline
cumulative
  c. dose
  C. Index Medicus
  c. trauma disorders
cumulus, pl. **cumuli**
  c. oöphorus
  c. ovaricus

C

cuneate
    c. fasciculus
    c. funiculus
    c. nucleus
cunei (*pl. of* cuneus)
cuneiform
    c. bone
    c. cartilage
    c. cataract
    c. lobe
    c. tubercle
cuneocerebellar tract
cuneocuboid
    c. joint
    c. ligaments
cuneometatarsal joints
cuneonavicular
    c. articulation
    c. joint
    c. ligaments
cuneoscaphoid
cuneus, pl. cunei
cuniculus, pl. cuniculi
cunnilinction, cunnilinctus
cunnilingus
cunnus
cup
    c. biopsy forceps
    Diogenes c.
    dry c.
    eye c.
    glaucomatous c.
    ocular c.
    optic c.
    c. of palm
    perilimbal suction c.
    physiologic c.
    suction c.
    wet c.
cupola
cupped
cupping
    c. glass
cupriuresis
cupula, pl. cupulae
    c. of cochlea
    c. cochleae
    c. cristae ampullaris
    c. pleurae
    pleural c.
cupular
    c. blind sac
    c. cecum of the cochlear duct
    c. part of epitympanic recess
cupulate
cupuliform
    c. cataract
cupulogram

cupulolithiasis
curage
curarization
curative
curb tenotomy
curdy pus
cure
curet
curet (*var. of* curette)
curetment
curettage
    dilation and c.
    periapical c.
    subgingival c.
curette, curet
    Hartmann's c.
curettement
curie
curing
    dental c.
curlicue ureter
Curling's ulcer
currant jelly clot
current
    action c.
    after-c.
    anodal c.
    ascending c.
    axial c.
    centrifugal c.
    centripetal c.
    d'Arsonval c.
    demarcation c.
    descending c.
    electrotonic c.
    high frequency c.
    c. of injury
    labile c.
    Tesla c.
Curschmann's
    C. disease
    C. spirals
curse
    Ondine's c.
curvatura, pl. curvaturae
    c. ventriculi major
    c. ventriculi minor
curvature
    c. aberration
    angular c.
    anterior c.
    backward c.
    gingival c.
    greater c. of stomach
    c. hyperopia
    lateral c.
    lesser c. of stomach
    c. myopia

occlusal c.
Pott's c.
spinal c.

curve
active length-tension c.
alignment c.
anti-Monson c.
Barnes' c.
buccal c.
Carus' c.
characteristic c.
compensating c.
distribution c.
dye-dilution c.
epidemic c.
flow-volume c.
force-velocity c.
Frank-Starling c.
frequency c.
Friedman c.
gaussian c.
growth c.
H and D c.
Hunter and Driffield c.
indicator-dilution c.
intracardiac pressure c.
isovolume pressure-flow c.
logistic c.
milled-in c.'s
Monson c.
muscle c.
c. of occlusion
passive length-tension c.
Pleasure c.
Price-Jones c.
probability c.
pulse c.
receiver operating characteristic c.
reverse c.
ROC c.
c. of Spee
Starling's c.
strength-duration c.
stress-strain c.
tension c.
Traube-Hering c.'s
von Spee's c.
whole-body titration c.
Curvularia
Cushing
C. basophilism
C. disease
C. effect
C. phenomenon
C. pituitary basophilism
C. response
C. suture

C. syndrome
C. syndrome medicamentosus
cushingoid
cushion
atrioventricular canal c.'s
endocardial c.'s
c. of epiglottis
eustachian c.
levator c.
Passavant's c.
pharyngoesophageal c.'s
sucking c.
cusp
c. angle
anterior c. of atrioventricular valve
c. of Carabelli
c. height
posterior c. of atrioventricular valve
semilunar c.
septal c. of tricuspid valve
talon c.
c. of tooth
cuspad
cuspal
c. interference
cuspid
c. tooth
cuspidate
c. tooth
cuspis, pl. cuspides
c. anterior valvae atrioventricularis dextrae/sinistrae
c. coronae
c. dentis
c. posterior valvae atrioventricularis dextrae/sinistrae
c. septalis valvae atrioventricularis dextrae
cuspless tooth
cusum
cutaneomeningospinal angiomatosis
cutaneomucosal
cutaneomucous muscle
cutaneomucouveal syndrome
cutaneous
c. absorption
c. albinism
c. ancylostomiasis
c. anthrax
c. apoplexy
c. blastomycosis
c. branch of obturator nerve
c. cervical nerve
c. diphtheria
c. emphysema
c. focal mucinosis
c. gangrene

C

cutaneous (continued)
    c. glands
    c. graft versus host reaction
    c. hemorrhoids
    c. horn
    c. larva migrans
    c. layer of tympanic membrane
    c. leishmaniasis
    c. loop ureterostomy
    c. lupus erythematosus
    c. meningioma
    c. muscle
    c. nerve
    c. pupil reflex
    c. reaction
    c. reflex
    c. schistosomiasis japonica
    c. test
    c. tuberculin test
    c. tuberculosis
    c. ureterostomy
    c. vasculitis
    c. vein
cutaneous-pupillary reflex
cutdown
Cuterebra
cuticle
    acquired c., acquired enamel c.
    dental c.
    enamel c.
    c. of hair
    c. of nail
    Nasmyth's c.
    posteruption c.
    c. of root sheath
cuticula, pl. cuticulae
    c. dentis
    c. pili
    c. vaginae folliculi pili
cuticularization
cutin
cutireaction
    c. test
cutis
    c. anserina
    c. graft
    c. laxa
    c. marmorata
    c. plate
    c. rhomboidalis nuchae
    c. unctuosa
    c. vera
    c. verticis gyrata
cutisector
cutization
cutting
    c. edge
    c. forceps

    c. needle
    c. teeth
cuttlefish disk
cuvette oximeter
Cuvier's
    C. ducts
    C. veins
c wave (var. of C wave)
cyanemia
cyanide-nitroprusside test
Cyanobacteria
cyanobacterium-like bodies
cyanochroic, cyanochrous
cyanophil, cyanophile
cyanophilous
Cyanophyceae
cyanopia
cyanopsia
cyanosed
cyanose tardive
cyanosis
    compression c.
    enterogenous c.
    false c.
    hereditary methemoglobinemic c.
    late c.
    c. retinae
    shunt c.
    tardive c.
cyanotic
    c. asphyxia
    c. atrophy
    c. atrophy of the liver
    c. induration
cyanuria
Cyathostoma
    C. bronchialis
Cyathostomum
cybernetics
cybrid
cyclarthrodial
cyclarthrosis
cycle
    anovulatory c.
    brain wave c.
    cardiac c.
    chewing c.
    endogenous c.
    exoerythrocytic c.
    exogenous c.
    forced c.
    genesial c.
    gonadotrophic c.
    hair c.
    life c.
    masticating c.'s
    menstrual c.
    ovarian c.

reproductive c.
restored c.
returning c.
cyclectomy
cyclencephaly, cyclencephalia
cycles per second
cyclic
    c. albuminuria
    c. esotropia
    c. neutropenia
    c. strabismus
cyclitis
    Fuchs' heterochromic c.
    heterochromic c.
    plastic c.
    purulent c.
cyclocephaly, cyclocephalia
cyclochoroiditis
cyclocryotherapy
cyclodestructive
cyclodialysis
cyclodiathermy
cycloduction
cycloelectrolysis
cycloid
cyclopea
cyclopean
    c. eye
cyclophoria
cyclophotocoagulation
cyclophrenia
Cyclophyllidae
cyclopia
cyclopian
    c. eye
cycloplegia
cyclops
cyclosis
Cyclospora
cyclothymia
cyclothymiac, cyclothymic
cyclotomy
cyclotorsion
cyclotropia
cylinder
    axis c.
    Bence Jones c.'s
    crossed c.'s
    Külz's c.
    c. retinoscopy
cylindraxis
cylindrical
    c. bronchiectasis
    c. epithelium
    c. lens
cylindroadenoma
cylindroid
    c. aneurysm

cylindroma
cylindromatous carcinoma
cylindrosarcoma
cylindruria
cyllosoma
cymba conchae
cymbocephalic, cymbocephalous
cymbocephaly
cynanthropy
cynic
    c. spasm
cynocephaly
cynodont
cynophobia
Cyon's nerve
cypridophobia
cyst
    adventitious c.
    allantoic c.
    alveolar hydatid c.
    aneurysmal bone c.
    angioblastic c.
    apical periodontal c.
    apoplectic c.
    arachnoid c.
    Baker's c.
    Bartholin's c.
    bile c.
    blood c.
    blue dome c.
    bone c.
    botryoid odontogenic c.
    Boyer's c.
    branchial c.
    branchial cleft c.
    bronchogenic c.
    bursal c.
    calcifying and keratinizing
      odontogenic c.
    calcifying odontogenic c.
    cerebellar c.
    cervical c.
    chocolate c.
    choledochal c.
    chyle c.
    colloid c.
    compound c.
    corpora lutea c.'s
    Cowper's c.
    daughter c.
    dental lamina c.
    dentigerous c.
    dermoid c.
    dermoid c. of ovary
    distention c.
    duplication c.
    echinococcus c.
    endometrial c.

217

cyst *(continued)*

endothelial c.
enterogenous c.'s
ependymal c.
epidermal c.
epidermoid c.
epithelial c.
eruption c.
extravasation c.
exudation c.
false c.
fissural c.
follicular c.
Gartner's c.
gas c.
gingival c.
globulomaxillary c.
glomerular c.'s
Gorlin c.
granddaughter c.
hemorrhagic c.
hepatic c.'s
heterotrophic oral gastrointestinal c.
hydatid c.
implantation c.
incisive canal c.
inclusion c.
involution c. *involuting cyst*
iodine c.'s
junctional c.
keratinous c.
Klestadt's c.
lacteal c.
lateral periodontal c.
leptomeningeal c.
lymphoepithelial c.
median anterior maxillary c.
median palatal c.
median raphe c. of the penis
meibomian c.
milk c.
morgagnian c.
mother c.
mucous c.
multilocular c.
multilocular hydatid c.,
  multiloculate hydatid c.
myxoid c.
nabothian c.
nasoalveolar c.
nasolabial c.
nasopalatine duct c.
necrotic c.
neural c.
neurenteric c.'s
odontogenic c.
oil c.
omphalomesenteric c.

omphalomesenteric duct c.
oophoritic c.
osseous hydatid c.
ovarian c.
paraphysial c.'s
parasitic c.
parent c.
paroophoritic c.
parvilocular c.
pearl c.
periapical c.
phaeomycotic c.
pilar c.
piliferous c.
pilonidal c.
pineal c.
posttraumatic leptomeningeal c.
primordial c.
proliferating tricholemmal c.
proliferation c., proliferative c.,
  proliferous c.
protozoan c.
pseudomucinous c.
radicular c.
Rathke's cleft c.
residual c.
retention c.
rete c. of ovary
root end c.
sanguineous c.
sebaceous c.
secretory c.
seminal vesical c.
sequestration c.
serous c.
simple bone c.
solitary bone c.
Stafne bone c.
static bone c.
sterile c.
sublingual c.
suprasellar c.
surgical ciliated c.
synovial c.
Tarlov's c.
tarry c.
tarsal c.
teratomatous c.
thyroglossal duct c., thyrolingual c.
Tornwaldt's c.
traumatic bone c.
trichilemmal c.
tubular c.
umbilical c.
unicameral c.
unicameral bone c.
unilocular c.
unilocular hydatid c.

urachal c.
urinary c.
utricular c.
vitellointestinal c.
wolffian c.
cystacanth
cystadenocarcinoma
cystadenoma
  papillary c. lymphomatosum
cystalgia
cystathioninuria
cystectasia, cystectasy
cystectomy
  Bartholin's c.
  partial c.
  radical c.
  salvage c.
  total c.
  vulvovaginal c.
cystic
  c. acne
  c. adenomatoid malformation
  c. artery
  c. bronchiectasis
  c. carcinoma
  c. diathesis
  c. disease of the breast
  c. disease of renal medulla
  c. duct
  c. duct cholangiography
  c. fibrosis
  c. fibrosis of the pancreas
  c. gall duct
  c. goiter
  c. hygroma
  c. hyperplasia
  c. hyperplasia of the breast
  c. kidney
  c. lymphangiectasis
  c. lymph node
  c. medial necrosis
  c. mole
  c. node
  c. papillomatous craniopharyngioma
  c. polyp
  c. vein
cysticerci (*pl. of* cysticercus)
cysticercoid
Cysticercus
  C. cellulosae
cysticercus, pl. **cysticerci**
  c. disease
cystides (*pl. of* cystis)
cystifelleotomy
cystiform
cystigerous
cystine
  c. calculus

c. disease
c. storage disease
cystinemia
cystinosis
cystinotic leukocyte
cystinuria
cystiphorous
cystis, pl. **cystides**
  c. fellea
  c. urinaria
cystistaxis
cystitis
  bacterial c.
  c. colli
  c. cystica
  emphysematous c.
  eosinophilic c.
  follicular c.
  c. glandularis
  hemorrhagic c.
  incrusted c.
  interstitial c.
  viral c.
cystoadenoma
cystocarcinoma
cystocele
cystochromoscopy
cystocolostomy
cystoduodenal ligament
cystoduodenostomy
  pancreatic c.
cystoenterocele
cystoenterostomy
cystoepiplocele
cystoepithelioma
cystofibroma
cystogastrostomy
cystogram
  voiding c.
cystography
  antegrade c.
cystoid
  c. macular edema
  c. maculopathy
cystojejunostomy
cystolith
cystolithalopaxy
cystolithiasis
cystolithic
cystolithotomy
cystoma
cystometer
cystometrogram
cystometrography
cystometry
cystomorphous
cystomyoma
cystomyxoadenoma

C

cystomyxoma
cystopanendoscopy
cystoparalysis
cystopexy
cystopherous
cystophotography
cystoplasty
cystoplegia
cystoprostatectomy
cystopyelitis
cystopyelonephritis
cystoradiogram
cystoradiography
cystorrhaphy
cystorrhea
cystosarcoma
    c. phyllodes
cystoscope
cystoscopic urography
cystoscopy
cystospasm
cystostomy
cystotome
cystotomy
    suprapubic c.
cystoureteritis
cystoureterogram
cystoureterography
cystourethritis
cystourethrocele
cystourethrogram
cystourethrography
cystourethroscope
cystous
Cystoviridae
cytapheresis
cytase
Cytauxzoon
    C. felis
cythemolytic icterus
cytoanalyzer
cytoarchitectonics
cytoarchitectural
cytoarchitecture
cytobiology
cytobiotaxis
cytocentrum
cytochylema
cytocidal
cytocide
cytoclasis
cytoclastic
cytoclesis
cytocrine secretion
cytocyst
cytodiagnosis
cytodieresis
cytogene

cytogenesis
cytogeneticist
cytogenetics
cytogenic
    c. reproduction
cytogenous
cytoglucopenia
cytohyaloplasm
cytoid
    c. bodies
cytokeratin filaments
cytokine
    c. network
cytokinesis
cytolemma
cytologic
    c. examination
    c. filter preparation
    c. screening
    c. smear
    c. specimen
cytologist
cytology
    exfoliative c.
cytolymph
cytolysin
cytolysis
cytolysosome
cytolytic
cytoma
cytomatrix
cytomegalic
    c. cells
    c. inclusion disease
cytomegalovirus
    c. disease
cytomembrane
cytomere
cytometaplasia
cytometer
cytometry
    flow c.
cytomicrosome
cytomorphology
cytomorphosis
cyton
cytopathic
    c. effect
cytopathogenic
    c. virus
cytopathologic, cytopathological
cytopathologist
cytopathology
cytopathy
cytopempsis
cytopenia
cytophagic histiocytic panniculitis
cytophagous

cytophagy
cytophanere
cytopharynx
cytophil group
cytophilic
    c. antibody
cytophotometry
    flow c.
cytophylactic
cytophylaxis
cytophyletic
cytopipette
cytoplasm
    ground-glass c.
cytoplasmic
    c. bridges
    c. inclusion bodies
    c. matrix
cytoplast
cytopoiesis
cytopreparation
cytopyge
cytoreductive therapy
cytoryctes, cytorrhyctes
cytosis
cytoskeleton
cytosmear
cytosome
cytostasis
cytostatic

cytostome
cytotactic
cytotaxis, cytotaxia
    negative c.
    positive c.
cytothesis
cytotonic enterotoxin
cytotoxic
    c. cell
    c. reaction
cytotoxicity
    antibody-dependent cell-mediated c.
    lymphocyte-mediated c.
cytotoxin
cytotrophoblast
cytotrophoblastic
    c. cells
    c. shell
cytotropic
    c. antibody
    c. antibody test
cytotropism
cytozoic
cytozoon
cytozyme
cyturia
Czapek-Dox medium
Czapek's solution agar
Czerny-Lembert suture
Czerny's suture

C

Δ

    Δ check, delta check

D

    D antigen
    D cell
    D loop
    D wave

Da

    D. Fano's stain

Daae's disease
DaCosta's syndrome
dacryadenitis
dacryoadenitis
dacryoblennorrhea
dacryocele
dacryocyst
dacryocystalgia
dacryocystectomy
dacryocystitis
dacryocystocele
dacryocystogram
dacryocystorhinostomy
dacryocystotomy
dacryohemorrhea
dacryolith

    Desmarres' d.'s
    Nocardia d.'s

dacryolithiasis
dacryon
dacryops
dacryopyorrhea
dacryorrhea
dacryostenosis
dactyl
dactylagra
dactylalgia
Dactylaria
dactyledema
dactyli (*pl. of* dactylus)
dactylitis

    blistering distal d.
    sickle cell d.

dactylocampsis
dactylocampsodynia
dactylodynia
dactylogryposis
dactylology
dactylomegaly
dactyloscopy
dactylospasm
dactylus, pl. **dactyli**
dahlia
daily dose
daisy
Dakin-Carrel treatment

Dale-Feldberg law
Dalen-Fuchs nodules
Dale reaction
Dalrymple's sign
daltonian
daltonism
dam

    d. methylase
    post d.
    rubber d.

Damalinia
damping
Damus-Kaye-Stancel procedure
Damus-Stancel-Kaye anastomosis
Dana's operation
dance

    hilar d.
    Saint Anthony's d., Saint John's d.,
      Saint Vitus d.

Dance's sign
dancing

    d. chorea
    d. spasm

dandruff
dandy

    d. fever

Dandy operation
Dandy-Walker syndrome
Dane

    D. particles
    D. stain

Danforth's sign
Danielssen-Boeck disease
Danielssen's disease
Danubian endemic familial nephropathy
Danysz phenomenon
DAPI stain
DA pregnancy test
dapsone neuropathy
d'Arcet's metal
Darier's

    D. disease
    D. sign

dark

    d. adaptation
    d. cells

dark-adapted eye
dark-field

    d.-f. condenser
    d.-f. illumination
    d.-f. microscope

dark-ground illumination
Darling's disease
Darrow red

D

d'Arsonval
    d. current
    d. galvanometer
dartoic, dartoid
    d. tissue
dartos
    d. fascia
    d. muliebris
    d. muscle
darwinian
    d. ear
    D. evolution
    d. reflex
    d. tubercle
data
    objective assessment d.
    d. processing
    subjective assessment d.
date
    d. boil
    d. fever
datum
    d. plane
Daubenton's
    D. angle
    D. line
    D. plane
Dauerschlaf
daughter
    d. cell
    d. colony
    d. cyst
    d. isotope
    d. star
Davidoff's cells
Davidson syringe
Daviel's
    D. operation
    D. spoon
Davies' disease
Davis
    D. grafts
    D. interlocking sound
Davis-Crowe mouth gag
Davis interlocking sound
Dawbarn's sign
dawn phenomenon
Dawson's encephalitis
day
    d. blindness
    d. hospital
    d. residue
    d. sight
dazzling
    d. glare
d-dimer test
de
    d. Bordeau theory

    d. Clerambault syndrome
    d. Lange syndrome
    D. Morgan's spots
    d. Morsier's syndrome
    d. Musset's sign
    d. Pezzer catheter
    d. Quervain's disease
    d. Quervain's fracture
    d. Quervain's thyroiditis
    D. Sanctis-Cacchione syndrome
    D. Toni-Fanconi syndrome
    d. Wecker's scissors
dead
    d. fetus syndrome
    d. fingers
    d. nerve
    d. pulp
    d. space
    d. tooth
    d. tracts
dead-end host
deaf
deafferentation
deaf-mute
deafmutism
    endemic d.
deafness
    acoustic trauma d.
    Alexander's d.
    boilermaker's d.
    central d.
    conductive d.
    cortical d.
    functional d.
    high frequency d.
    hysterical d.
    industrial d.
    low tone d.
    Mondini d.
    nerve d., neural d.
    noise–induced d.
    occupational d.
    organic d.
    perceptive d.
    postlingual d.
    prelingual d.
    psychogenic d.
    retrocochlear d.
    Scheibe's d.
    sensorineural d.
    word d.
dealbation
dealcoholization
deallergize
Dean's fluorosis index
dearterialization
death
    black d.

brain d.
cerebral d.
d. certificate
cot d.
crib d.
crude d. rate
early neonatal d. (*var. of*
  neonatal d.)
fetal d.
genetic d.
infant d.
d. instinct
local d.
maternal d., direct maternal d.,
  indirect maternal d.
neonatal d., early neonatal d., late
  neonatal d.
perinatal d.
d. rate
somatic d., systemic d.
sudden d.
d. trance
death-rattle
Deaver's incision
DeBakey
    D. classification
    D. forceps
debanding
debilitating
debility
debouch
débouchement
debrancher deficiency
debranching deficiency limit dextrinosis
Debré phenomenon
Debré-Sémélaigne syndrome
débridement
debt
    alactic oxygen d.
    lactacid oxygen d.
    oxygen d.
debulking operation
decalvant
decant
decantation
decapacitation
    d. factor
decapitate
decapitation
decapsulation
    d. of kidney
decarbonization
decay
    free induction d.
    d. theory
deceleration
    early d.

late d.
variable d.
decentered lens
decentration
decerebrate
    d. rigidity
    d. state
decerebration
    bloodless d.
decerebrize
dechloridation
dechlorination
dechloruration
decholesterolization
decibel
decidua
    d. basalis
    d. capsularis
    ectopic d.
    d. menstrualis
    d. parietalis
    d. polyposa
    d. reflexa
    d. serotina
    d. spongiosa
    d. vera
decidual
    d. cell
    d. endometritis
    d. fissure
    d. reaction
deciduate placenta
deciduation
deciduitis
deciduoma
    Loeb's d.
deciduous
    d. dentition
    d. membrane
    d. skin
    d. tooth
decimorgan
decision analysis
decision tree
declamping
    d. phenomenon
    d. shock
declination
declinator
declive
declivis
décollement
decompensation
    corneal d.
decomposition of movement
decompression
    cardiac d.
    cerebral d.

D

decompression *(continued)*
    d. chamber
    d. disease
    explosive d.
    internal d.
    nerve d.
    d. operations
    optic nerve sheath d.
    orbital d.
    pericardial d.
    rapid d.
    d. sickness
    spinal d.
    suboccipital d.
    subtemporal d.
    trigeminal d.
deconvolution
decorticate
    d. rigidity
    d. state
decortication
    cerebral d.
    reversible d.
decoy cells
decrement
decremental conduction
decrudescence
decubation
decubital
    d. gangrene
decubitus
    Andral's d.
    d. film
    d. radiograph
    d. ulcer
    ventral d.
decurrent
decussate
decussatio, pl. decussationes
    d. brachii conjunctivi
    d. fontinalis
    d. lemniscorum
    d. motoria
    d. nervorum trochlearium
    d. pedunculorum cerebellarium
      superiorum
    d. pyramidum
    d. sensoria
    decussationes tegmenti
decussation
    d. of brachia conjunctiva
    dorsal tegmental d.
    d. of the fillet
    Forel's d.
    fountain d.
    Held's d.
    d. of medial lemniscus
    Meynert's d.

    motor d.
    optic d.
    pyramidal d.
    rubrospinal d.
    sensory d. of medulla oblongata
    d. of superior cerebellar peduncles
    tectospinal d.
    tegmental d.'s
    d. of trochlear nerves
    ventral tegmental d.
    Wernekinck's d.
dedentition
dedifferentiation
dedolation
de-efferentation
deep
    d. abdominal reflexes
    d. artery of clitoris
    d. artery of penis
    d. artery of thigh
    d. artery of tongue
    d. auricular artery
    d. bite
    d. brachial artery
    d. branch
    d. branch of the lateral plantar
      nerve
    d. branch of the medial femoral
      circumflex artery
    d. branch of the medial plantar
      artery
    d. branch of the radial nerve
    d. branch of the transverse
      cervical artery
    d. branch of the ulnar nerve
    d. cardiac plexus
    d. cell
    d. cerebral veins
    d. cervical artery
    d. cervical fascia
    d. cervical vein
    d. circumflex iliac artery
    d. circumflex iliac vein
    d. cortex
    d. crural arch
    d. dorsal sacrococcygeal ligament
    d. dorsal vein of clitoris
    d. dorsal vein of penis
    d. epigastric artery
    d. epigastric vein
    d. facial vein
    d. fascia
    d. fascia of arm
    d. fascia of forearm
    d. fascia of leg
    d. fascia of neck
    d. fascia of penis
    d. fascia of thigh

d. femoral vein
d. fibular nerve
d. flexor muscle of fingers
d. gray layer of superior colliculus
d. head of flexor pollicis brevis
d. hypothermic arrest
d. infrapatellar bursa
d. inguinal lymph nodes
d. inguinal ring
d. lamina
d. layer
d. layer of levator palpebrae superioris muscle
d. layer of temporalis fascia
d. lingual artery
d. lingual vein
d. lymphatic vessel
d. middle cerebral vein
d. muscles of back
d. origin
d. palmar (arterial) arch
d. palmar branch of ulnar artery
d. palmar venous arch
d. parotid lymph nodes
d. part of external anal sphincter
d. part of flexor retinaculum
d. part of masseter muscle
d. part of parotid gland
d. percussion
d. perineal pouch
d. perineal space
d. peroneal nerve
d. petrosal nerve
d. places
d. plantar branch of dorsalis pedis artery
d. posterior sacrococcygeal ligament
d. punctate keratitis
d. reflex
d. scleritis
d. sensibility
d. temporal artery
d. temporal nerves
d. temporal veins
d. transitional gyrus
d. transverse metacarpal ligament
d. transverse metatarsal ligament
d. transverse muscle of perineum
d. transverse perineal muscle
d. vein of penis
d. veins of clitoris
d. white layer of superior colliculus
de-epicardialization
deer-fly
d.-f. disease
d.-f. fever
Deetjen's bodies

DEF
D. caries index
defatigation
def caries index
defecate
defecation
defecography
defect
aortic septal d., aorticopulmonary septal d.
atrial septal d.
atrial ventricular canal d.
birth d.
congenital ectodermal d.
coupling d.
Eisenmenger's d.
endocardial cushion d.
fibrous cortical d.
filling d.
Gerbode d.
iodide transport d.
iodotyrosine deiodinase d.
luteal phase d.
metaphysial fibrous cortical d.
organification d.
osteoporotic marrow d.
postinfarction ventricular septal d.
relative afferent pupillary d.
salt-losing d.
ventricular septal d.
defective
d. bacteriophage
d. interfering particle
d. phage
d. probacteriophage
d. prophage
d. virus
defemination
defense
d. mechanism
d. reflex
screen d.
ur-d.'s
defensive
d. circle
d. medicine
deferent
d. canal
d. duct
deferentectomy
deferential
d. artery
d. plexus
deferentitis
deferred shock
defervescence
defervescent stage
defibrillation

D

defibrillator
    external d.
defibrination
deficiency
    adult lactase d.
    d. anemia
    antitrypsin d.
    arch length d.
    debrancher d.
    d. disease
    familial high density lipoprotein d.
    galactokinase d.
    glucose-6-phosphate
      dehydrogenase d.
    glucosephosphate isomerase d.
    β-*d*-glucuronidase d.
    glutathione synthetase d.
    hypoxanthine guanine
      phosphoribosyltransferase d.
    immune d.
    immunity d.
    immunological d.
    LCAT d.
    luteal phase d.
    mental d.
    muscle phosphorylase d.
    phosphohexose isomerase d.
    placental sulfatase d.
    α-1-proteinase d.
    proximal femoral focal d.
    pseudocholinesterase d.
    pyruvate kinase d.
    riboflavin d.
    secondary antibody d.
    d. symptom
    taste d.
deficit
    base d.
    oxygen d.
    pulse d.
definition
definitive
    d. callus
    d. host
    d. lysosomes
    d. method
    d. prosthesis
deflection
    intrinsic d.
    intrinsicoid d.
deflective occlusal contact
deflexion
deflorescence
defluvium
    d. capillorum
    d. unguium
defluxion
deformability

deformation
deforming
deformity
    Åkerlund d.
    Arnold-Chiari d.
    bell clapper d.
    boutonnière d.
    contracture d.
    Erlenmeyer flask d.
    gunstock d.
    Haglund's d.
    J-sella d.
    keyhole d.
    lobster-claw d.
    Madelung's d.
    mermaid d.
    parachute d.
    reduction d.
    seal-fin d.
    silver-fork d.
    Sprengel's d.
    swan-neck d.
    torsional d.
    whistling d.
    Whitehead d.
defurfuration
deganglionate
degeneracy
degenerate
degeneratio
degeneration
    adipose d.
    adiposogenital d.
    age-related macular d.
    albuminoid d., albuminous d.
    amyloid d.
    angiolithic d.
    ascending d.
    atheromatous d.
    axon d.
    axonal d.
    ballooning d.
    basophilic d.
    calcareous d.
    carneous d.
    caseous d.
    colliquative d.
    colloid d.
    cone d.
    Crooke's hyaline d.
    descending d.
    disciform d.
    disciform macular d.
    ectatic marginal d. of cornea
    elastoid d.
    elastotic d.
    familial pseudoinflammatory
      macular d.

(handwritten annotations: "(ALL CAPS) SLACK wrist deformity" and "neurAl (2 woRds) deficit")

fascicular d.
fatty d.
fibrinoid d., fibrinous d.
fibrous d.
granular d.
granulovacuolar d.
gray d.
hepatolenticular d.
hyaline d.
hyaloideoretinal d.
hydropic d.
infantile neuronal d.
Kuhnt-Junius d.
lenticular progressive d.
liquefaction d.
macular d.
marginal corneal d.
Mönckeberg's d.
mucinoid d.
mucoid d.
mucoid medial d.
myelinic d.
myopic d.
myxoid d., myxomatous d.
ncurofibrillary d.
Nissl d.
olivopontocerebellar d.
orthograde d.
parenchymatous d.
primary neuronal d.
primary pigmentary d. of retina
primary progressive cerebellar d.
pseudotubular d.
red d.
reticular d.
retrograde d.
Salzmann's nodular corneal d.
secondary d.
senile d.
Sorsby's macular d.
spongy d. of infancy
subacute combined d. of the spinal
  cord
tapetoretinal d.
Terrien's marginal d.
transsynaptic d.
Türck's d.
vacuolar d.
vitelliform d.
vitelliruptive d.
wallerian d.
waxy d.
xerotic d.
Zenker's d.
degenerative
  d. arthritis
  d. chorea
  d. index

  d. inflammation
  d. joint disease
  d. myopia
degloving
  d. injury
deglutition
  d. apnea
  d. pneumonia
  d. reflex
deglutitive
Degos'
  D. acanthoma
  D. disease
  D. syndrome
degranulation
degree
  d.'s of freedom
  d. of kindred
degustation
Dehio's test
dehiscence
  iris d.
  root d.
  wound d.
dehumanization
dehydration
  d. fever
  voluntary d.
dehydrocholate test
dehypnotize
deinstitutionalization
deionization
deiterospinal tract
Deiters'
  D. cells
  D. nucleus
  D. terminal frames
déjà
  déjà vu
  déjà vu phenomenon
  d. voulu
dejecta
dejection
Dejerine-Klumpke
  D.-K. palsy
  D.-K. syndrome
Dejerine-Lichtheim phenomenon
Dejerine-Roussy syndrome
Dejerine's
  D. disease
  D. hand phenomenon
  D. reflex
  D. sign
Dejerine-Sottas disease
Delafield's hematoxylin
delamination
delayed
  d. allergy

D

delayed *(continued)*
    d. coma after hypoxia
    d. conduction
    d. dentition
    d. eruption
    d. flap
    d. graft
    d. hypersensitivity
    d. reaction
    d. reaction experiment
    d. reflex
    d. sensation
    d. shock
    d. suture
Delbet's sign
Del Castillo syndrome
DeLee's maneuver
deleterious
deletion
    chromosomal d.
    gene d.
    interstitial d.
    nucleotide d.
    point d.
    terminal d.
Delhi
    D. boil
    D. sore
delicate
delimitation
delimiting keratotomy
delirious
    d. shock
delirium, pl. **deliria**
    acute d.
    alcohol withdrawal d.
    anxious d.
    collapse d.
    d. cordis
    low d.
    d. mussitans, muttering d.
    posttraumatic d.
    senile d.
    toxic d.
    d. tremens
delitescence
deliver
delivery
    assisted cephalic d.
    breech d.
    forceps d.
    high forceps d.
    low forceps d.
    midforceps d.
    outlet forceps d.
    perimortem d.
    postmortem d.

    premature d.
    spontaneous cephalic d.
delle
dellen
delomorphous
delphian node
delta
    d. agent
    d. alcoholism
    d. antigen
    d. cell of anterior lobe of
      hypophysis
    d. cell of pancreas
    d. fornicis
    Galton's d.
    d. granule
    d. hepatitis
    d. mesoscapulae
    d. rhythm
    d. virus
    d. wave
deltoid
    d. branch
    d. crest
    d. eminence
    d. impression
    d. ligament
    d. muscle
    d. region
    d. tuberosity
deltoideopectoral
    d. triangle
    d. trigone
deltopectoral flap
delusion
    d. of control, d. of being controlled
    encapsulated d.
    expansive d.
    d. of grandeur
    grandiose d.
    d. of negation
    nihilistic d.
    organic d.'s
    d. of passivity
    d. of persecution, persecutory d.
    d. of reference
    somatic d.
    systematized d.
    unsystematized d.
delusional
    d. disorder
demand
    d. pacemaker
    d. pulse generator
demarcation
    d. current
    d. line of retina
    d. potential

Demarquay's symptom
demasculinizing
Dematiaceae
dematiaceous
    d. fungi
deme
demented
dementia
    AIDS d.
    Alzheimer's d.
    catatonic d.
    dialysis d.
    epileptic d.
    hebephrenic d.
    multi-infarct d.
    paralytic d.
    d. paralytica
    d. paranoides
    posttraumatic d.
    d. praecox
    presenile d., d. presenilis
    primary d.
    primary senile d.
    secondary d.
    senile d.
    toxic d.
    transmissible d.
    vascular d.
demethylation
demigauntlet
    d. bandage
demilune
    d. body
    Giannuzzi's d.'s
    Heidenhain's d.'s
    serous d.'s
demipenniform
demodectic
    d. acariasis
    d. blepharitis
demography
    dynamic d.
Demoivre's formula
demoniac
demonstration ophthalmoscope
demonstrator
demucosation
demyelinated myelitis
demyelinating
    d. disease
    d. encephalopathy
    d. polyneuropathy
demyelination, demyelinization
dendraxon
dendriform
    d. keratitis
dendrite
    apical d.

dendritic
    d. calculus
    d. cataract
    d. cells
    d. corneal ulcer
    d. depolarization
    d. keratitis
    d. process
    d. spines
    d. thorns
dendrogram
dendroid
dendron
denervate
denervation
dengue
    d. fever
    hemorrhagic d.
    d. hemorrhagic fever
    d. shock syndrome
    d. virus
denial
denidation
Denis
    D. Browne splint
    D. Browne's pouch
denitrogenation
Denman's spontaneous evolution
Dennie's
    D. infraorbital fold
    D. line
denominator
Denonvilliers'
    D. aponeurosis
    D. ligament
dens, pl. dentes
    dentes acustici
    d. angularis
    d. bicuspidus, pl. dentes bicuspidi
    d. caninus, pl. dentes canini
    d. cuspidatus, pl. dentes cuspidati
    d. deciduus, pl. dentes decidui
    d. in dente
    d. incisivus, pl. dentes incisivi
    d. invaginatus
    d. lacteus
    d. molaris, pl. dentes molares
    d. permanens, pl. dentes permanentes
    d. premolaris, pl. dentes premolares
    d. sapientiae
    d. serotinus
    d. succedaneus
dense-deposit disease
density
    count d.
    incidence d.
    photon d.

D

density (*continued*)
    spin d.
    vapor d.
dental
    d. abscess
    d. anatomy
    d. anesthesia
    d. ankylosis
    d. apparatus
    d. arch
    d. articulation
    d. biomechanics
    d. biophysics
    d. branches
    d. bulb
    d. calculus
    d. canals
    d. caries
    d. cast
    d. cement
    d. cord
    d. crest
    d. crypt
    d. curing
    d. cuticle
    d. drill
    d. dysfunction
    d. engine
    d. engineering
    d. fibers
    d. fistula
    d. floss
    d. follicle
    d. forceps
    d. formula
    d. furnace
    d. geriatrics
    d. germ
    d. granuloma
    d. groove
    d. hygienist
    d. impaction
    d. implants
    d. index
    d. jurisprudence
    d. lamina
    d. lamina cyst
    d. ledge
    d. lever
    d. lymph
    d. material
    d. neck
    d. nerve
    d. orthopedics
    d. osteoma
    d. papilla
    d. pathology
    d. plaque

    d. polyp
    d. process
    d. prophylaxis
    d. prosthesis
    d. prosthetics
    d. pulp
    d. pump
    d. rami
    d. ridge
    d. sac
    d. sealant
    d. senescence
    d. shelf
    d. surgeon
    d. syringe
    d. tubercle
    d. tubules
    d. ulcer
    d. wedge
dentalgia
dentary center
dentate
    d. fascia
    d. fissure
    d. fracture
    d. gyrus
    d. ligament of spinal cord
    d. line
    d. nucleus of cerebellum
    d. suture
dentatectomy
dentatorubral
    d. cerebellar atrophy with
      polymyoclonus
    d. fibers
dentatothalamic
    d. fibers
    d. tract
dentatum
dentes (*pl. of* dens)
dentia
    d. praecox
    d. tarda
denticle
denticulate, denticulated
    d. hymen
    d. ligament
dentiform
dentigerous
    d. cyst
dentilabial
dentilingual
dentin
    d. bridge
    d. dysplasia
    d. globule
    hereditary opalescent d.
    hypersensitive d.

interglobular d.
irregular d., irritation d.
opalescent d.
peritubular d.
primary d.
reparative d.
sclerotic d.
secondary d.
tertiary d.
transparent d.
vascular d.

dentinal
    d. canals
    d. fibers
    d. fluid
    d. papilla
    d. pulp
    d. sheath
    d. tubules
dentinalgia
dentine
dentinocemental
    d. junction
dentinoenamel
    d. junction
dentinogenesis
    d. imperfecta
dentinoid
dentinoma
dentinum
dentiparous
dentist
dentistry
    community d.
    esthetic d.
    forensic d.
    legal d.
    operative d.
    pediatric d.
    preventive d.
    prosthetic d.
    public health d.
    restorative d.
dentition
    artificial d.
    deciduous d.
    delayed d.
    first d.
    mandibular d.
    maxillary d.
    natural d.
    primary d.
    retarded d.
    secondary d.
    succedaneous d.
dentoalveolar
    d. abscess
    d. joint

dentode
dentogingival lamina
dentoid
dentolegal
dentoliva
dentulous
denture
    bar joint d.
    d. basal surface
    d. base
    d. border
    d. brush
    d. characterization
    complete d.
    design d.
    d. edge
    d. esthetics
    fixed partial d.
    d. flange
    d. flask
    d. foundation
    d. foundation area
    d. foundation surface
    full d.
    d. hyperplasia
    immediate d.
    immediate insertion d.
    implant d.
    d. impression surface
    interim d.
    d. occlusal surface
    overlay d.
    d. packing
    partial d.
    partial d., distal extension
    d. polished surface
    d. prognosis
    provisional d.
    removable partial d.
    d. retention
    d. service
    d. sore mouth
    d. space
    d. stability
    telescopic d.
    temporary d.
    transitional d.
    treatment d.
    trial d.
    wax model d.
denture-bearing area
denture-supporting
    d.-s. area
    d.-s. structures
denturist
Denucé's ligament
denucleated
denudation

D

hydroxyapatite deposition

denude
denumerable character
Denver
    D. classification
    D. Developmental Screening Test
    D. shunt
Denys-Leclef phenomenon
deontology
deorsumduction
deoxyadenosine methylase
deoxyribonucleic acid
    A-DNA
    B-DNA
    linker DNA
    Z-DNA
deoxyvirus
deozonize
dependence
    substance d.
dependent
    d. beat
    d. drainage
    d. edema
    d. personality
    d. personality disorder
    d. variable
Dependovirus
depersonalization
    d. disorder
    d. syndrome
dephasing
depigmentation
depilate
depilation
depilatory
    chemical d.
depletion
    chloride d.
    d. response
    salt d.
    water d.
depletional hyponatremia
depolarization
    dendritic d.
depolarize
depolarizing block
deposit
    brickdust d.
depot
    d. injection
    d. reaction
    d. therapy
depravation
depraved
depravity
depressed
    d. fracture
    d. skull fracture

depression
    agitated d.
    anaclitic d.
    endogenous d., endogenomorphic d.
    exogenous d.
    involutional d.
    lingual salivary gland d.
    major d.
    nonreactive d.
    d. of optic disk
    pacchionian d.'s
    postdrive d.
    pterygoid d.
    reactive d.
    spreading d.
depressive
    d. neurosis
    d. psychosis
    d. reaction
    d. stupor
    d. syndrome
depressor
    d. anguli oris muscle
    d. fibers
    d. labii inferioris muscle
    d. muscle of epiglottis
    d. muscle of eyebrow
    d. muscle of lower lip
    d. muscle of septum
    d. nerve of Ludwig
    d. reflex
    d. septi muscle
    d. supercilii muscle
    tongue d.
deprivation
    d. amblyopia
    emotional d.
    sensory d.
depth
    anesthetic d.
    d. compensation
    d. dose
    focal d., d. of focus
    d. perception
    d. psychology
    d. recording
depulization
deradelphus
derailment
deranencephaly, deranencephalia
derangement
    Hey's internal d.
derby hat fracture
Dercum's disease
derealization
dereism
dereistic
derencephalia

derencephalocele
derencephaly
derivation
derivative chromosome
dermabrader
dermabrasion
Dermacentor
    D. andersoni
    D. variabilis
dermad
dermagraphy
dermahemia
dermal
    d. bone
    d. duct tumor
    d. graft
    d. leishmanoid
    d. papillae
    d. sinus
    d. system
    d. tuberculosis
dermalaxia
dermal-fat graft
dermametropathism
Dermanyssus gallinae
dermatalgia
dermatic
dermatitis, pl. **dermatitides**
    actinic d.
    d. aestivalis
    allergic contact d.
    d. ambustionis
    ancylostoma d.
    d. artefacta
    atopic d.
    d. atrophicans
    d. autophytica
    berloque d., berlock d.
    blastomycetic d., d. blastomycotica
    bubble gum d.
    d. calorica
    caterpillar d.
    chemical d.
    d. combustionis
    d. congelationis
    contact d.
    contact-type d.
    cosmetic d.
    dhobie mark d.
    diaper d.
    d. exfoliativa
    d. exfoliativa infantum, d.
      exfoliativa neonatorum
    exfoliative d.
    exudative discoid and lichenoid d.
    factitial d.
    d. gangrenosa infantum
    d. herpetiformis

    d. hiemalis
    infectious eczematoid d.
    irritant contact d.
    livedoid d.
    mango d.
    meadow d., meadow grass d.
    d. medicamentosa
    d. multiformis
    nickel d.
    d. nodosa
    d. nodularis necrotica
    nummular d.
    d. papillaris capillitii
    papular d. of pregnancy
    d. pediculoides ventricosus
    plant d.
    primary irritant d.
    rat mite d.
    d. repens
    rhus d.
    sandal strap d.
    Schamberg's d.
    schistosomal d.
    seborrheic d., d. seborrheica
    d. simplex
    solar d.
    stasis d.
    subcorneal pustular d.
    traumatic d.
    d. vegetans
    d. venenata
    d. verrucosa
dermatitis-arthritis-tenosynovitis
  syndrome
dermatoalloplasty
dermatoarthritis
    lipoid d.
dermatoautoplasty
Dermatobia
    D. cyaniventris
dermatocellulitis
dermatochalasis
dermatoconiosis
dermatocyst
dermatodynia
dermatofibroma
dermatofibrosarcoma protuberans
    pigmented d. p.
dermatofibrosis lenticularis disseminata
dermatogenic torticollis
dermatoglyphics
dermatograph
dermatographism
dermatography
dermatoheteroplasty
dermatohomoplasty
dermatoid
dermatologist

D

dermatology
dermatolysis
dermatoma
dermatomal distribution
dermatome
    electric d.
dermatomegaly
dermatomere
dermatomic area
dermatomycosis
    d. pedis
dermatomyoma
dermatomyositis
dermatoneurosis
dermatonosology
dermatopathia
    d. pigmentosa reticularis
dermatopathic
    d. lymphadenitis
    d. lymphadenopathy
dermatopathology
dermatopathy
Dermatophagoides pteronyssinus
Dermatophilus congolensis
dermatophobia
dermatophone
dermatophylaxis
dermatophyte
dermatophytid
dermatophytosis
dermatoplastic
dermatoplasty
dermatopolyneuritis
dermatorrhagia
dermatorrhea
dermatorrhexis
dermatosclerosis
dermatoscopy
dermatosis, pl. dermatoses
    acarine d.
    acute febrile neutrophilic d.
    ashy d.
    Bowen's precancerous d.
    chronic bullous d. of childhood
    dermolytic bullous d.
    digitate d.
    lichenoid d.
    d. medicamentosa
    d. papulosa nigra
    pigmented purpuric lichenoid d.
    progressive pigmentary d.
    radiation d.
    seborrheic d.
    subcorneal pustular d.
    transient acantholytic d.
dermatotherapy
dermatothlasia
dermatoxenoplasty

dermatozoiasis
dermatozoon
dermatozoonosis
dermatrophia, dermatrophy
dermenchysis
dermic
dermis
dermoblast
dermocyma
dermoepidermal interface
dermographia, dermographism,
    dermography
dermoid
    d. cyst
    d. cyst of ovary
    inclusion d.
    sequestration d.
    d. system
    d. tumor
dermoidectomy
dermolysis
dermolytic bullous dermatosis
dermonecrotic
dermoneurosis
dermonosology
dermopathy
    diabetic d.
dermophlebitis
dermoplasty
dermoskeleton
dermostenosis
dermostosis
dermosyphilopathy
dermotoxin
dermotuberculin reaction
dermovascular
derodidymus
derotation
Desault's bandage
Descartes' law
descemetitis
descemetocele
Descemet's membrane
descendens
    d. cervicalis
    d. hypoglossi
descending
    d. anterior branch
    d. aorta
    d. artery of knee
    d. branch
    d. branch of hypoglossal nerve
    d. branch of lateral circumflex
      femoral artery
    d. branch of occipital artery
    d. colon
    d. current
    d. degeneration

d. genicular artery
d. neuritis
d. nucleus of the trigeminus
d. palatine artery
d. part of aorta
d. part of duodenum
d. part of facial canal
d. posterior branch
d. scapular artery
d. tract of trigeminal nerve

descensus
d. testis
d. uteri
d. ventriculi

descent
Deschamps needle
descriptive
d. anatomy
d. myology
d. psychiatry
d. statistics

desensitization
heterologous d.
homologous d.
systematic d.

desensitize
desert
d. fever
d. sore

deserted places
desetope
desflurane
deshydremia
design denture
Desmarres' dacryoliths
desmectasis, desmectasia
desmitis
desmocranium
desmodynia
desmogenous
desmography
desmoid
extra-abdominal d.
d. tumor

desmology
desmon
desmopathy
desmoplasia
desmoplastic
d. cerebral astrocytoma
d. fibroma
d. malignant melanoma
d. medulloblastoma
d. trichoepithelioma

desmosome
desmoteric medicine
despeciation
D'Espine's sign

despumation
desquamate
desquamation
branny d.

desquamative
d. inflammatory vaginitis
d. interstitial pneumonia
d. pneumonia

destrudo
Desulfotomaculum
D. nigrificans

desynchronous
detachable balloon
detached
d. cranial section
d. craniotomy
d. retina

detachment
exudative retinal d.
retinal d., d. of retina
rhegmatogenous retinal d.
vitreous d.

detector
d. coil
solid-state d.

deterioration
alcoholic d.
senile d.

determinant
allotypic d.'s
antigenic d.
genetic d.
d. group
idiotypic antigenic d.
isoallotypic d.'s
mathematical d.

determinate cleavage
determination
cell d.
sex d.

determinism
psychic d.

detrition
detritus
detrusor
d. areflexia
d. compliance
d. hyperreflexia
d. instability
d. muscle of urinary bladder
d. pressure
d. sphincter dyssynergia
d. stability

detumescence
deturgescence
deutencephalon
deuteranomaly
deuteranope

D

deuteranopia
deuteromycetes
Deuteromycota
deuteropathic
deuteropathy
deuteroplasm
deuterosome
deuterotocia
deuterotoky
deutogenic
deutomerite
deutoplasm
deutoplasmic
deutoplasmigenon
deutoplasmolysis
Deutschländer's disease
devascularization
develop
development
    cognitive d.
    life-span d.
    psychosexual d.
developmental
    d. age
    d. anomaly
    d. disability
    d. grooves
    d. lines
    d. psychology
Deventer's pelvis
deviance
deviant
deviation
    axis d.
    conjugate d. of the eyes
    immune d.
    d. to the left
    left axis d.
    primary d.
    d. to the right
    right axis d.
    secondary d.
    sexual d.
    skew d.
    standard d.
deviational nystagmus
device
    central-bearing d.
    central-bearing tracing d.
    contraceptive d.
    intra-aortic d.
    intrauterine d.'s
    intrauterine contraceptive d.'s
    left-ventricular assist d.
    ventricular assist d.
Devic's disease
devil's grip
Devine exclusion

deviometer
devitalization
devitalize
devitalized
    d. tooth
devolution
Devonshire colic
Dewar flask
dew itch
dexamethasone suppression test
dexiocardia
dexter
dextrad
dextral
dextrality
dextrinosis
    debranching deficiency limit d.,
      limit d.
dextrinuria
dextrocardia
    corrected d.
    false d.
    isolated d.
    mirror image d.
    secondary d.
    type 1 d.
    type 2 d.
    type 3 d.
    type 4 d.
    d. with situs inversus
dextrocardiogram
dextrocerebral
dextroclination
dextrocular
dextrocycloduction
dextroduction
dextrogastria
dextrogram
dextrogyration
dextromanual
dextropedal
dextroposition
    d. of the heart
dextrosinistral
dextrosuria
dextrotorsion
dextrotropic
dextroversion
    d. of the heart
DF, df
    DF caries index
df caries index
Dharmendra antigen
d'Herelle phenomenon
dhobie
    d. itch
    d. mark
    d. mark dermatitis

Di
    D. antigen
    D. Guglielmo's disease
    D. Guglielmo's syndrome
diabetes
    adult-onset d.
    alimentary d.
    brittle d.
    bronze d.
    bronzed d.
    calcinuric d.
    chemical d.
    galactose d.
    gestational d.
    growth-onset d.
    d. innocens
    d. insipidus
    insulin-dependent d. mellitus
    insulinopenic d.
    d. intermittens
    juvenile d.
    juvenile-onset d.
    ketosis-prone d.
    ketosis-resistant d.
    latent d.
    lipoatrophic d.
    lipogenous d.
    maturity-onset d.
    maturity onset d. of youth
    d. mellitus
    metahypophysial d.
    Mosler's d.
    nephrogenic d. insipidus
    non-insulin-dependent d. mellitus
    phlorizin d.
    phosphate d.
    pregnancy d.
    renal d.
    starvation d.
    steroid d.
    steroidogenic d.
    subclinical d.
    thiazide d.
    type I d.
    type II d.
    type I d. mellitus
    vasopressin-resistant d.
diabetic
    d. acidosis
    d. amyotrophy
    d. arthropathy
    d. cataract
    d. coma
    d. dermopathy
    d. diet
    d. fetopathy
    d. gangrene

    d. gingivitis
    d. glomerulosclerosis
    d. lipemia
    d. myelopathy
    d. neuropathic cachexia
    d. neuropathy
    d. polyneuropathy
    d. polyradiculopathy
    d. puncture
    d. retinitis
    d. retinopathy
    d. thoracic radiculopathy
diabetogenic
diabetogenous
diabetology
diacele
diacetemia
diacetonuria
diaceturia
diachronic
    d. study
diaclasis, diaclasia
diacrinous
diacrisis
diacritic, diacritical
diadermic
diadochocinesia
diadochokinesia, diadochokinesis
diadochokinetic
diagnose
diagnosis
    antenatal d.
    clinical d.
    differential d.
    d. by exclusion
    laboratory d.
    neonatal d.
    pathologic d.
    physical d.
    prenatal d.
    d. related group
diagnosis-related group
diagnostic
    d. anesthesia
    d. audiometry
    d. cast
    DNA d.'s
    d. sensitivity
    d. specificity
    D. and Statistical Manual
    d. ultrasound
diagnostician
diagonal
    d. conjugate
    d. conjugate diameter
    d. section
diagonalis stria

D

diagram
  Dieuaide d.
  Venn d.
diakinesis
dial
  astigmatic d.
  d. manometer
Dialister
dialysance
dialysis
  continuous ambulatory peritoneal d.
  d. dementia
  d. disequilibrium syndrome
  d. encephalopathy syndrome
  equilibrium d.
  extracorporeal d.
  peritoneal d.
  d. retinae
  d. shunt
di-amelia
diameter
  anteroposterior d. of the pelvic inlet
  Baudelocque's d.
  biparietal d.
  buccolingual d.
  conjugate d. of pelvic inlet
  conjugate d. of pelvic outlet
  diagonal conjugate d.
  external conjugate d.
  d. mediana
  d. obliqua
  oblique d.
  obstetric conjugate d.
  occipitofrontal d.
  occipitomental d.
  posterior sagittal d.
  suboccipitobregmatic d.
  total end-diastolic d.
  total end-systolic d.
  trachelobregmatic d.
  d. transversa
  transverse d.
  zygomatic d.
diamniotic
diamond
  d. cutting instruments
  d. disk
  d. fuchsin
  d. skin
Diamond-Blackfan
  D.-B. anemia
  D.-B. syndrome
diamond-shaped murmur
Diana complex
diandry, diandria
dianoetic

diapause
  embryonic d.
diapedesis
diaper
  d. dermatitis
  d. rash
diaphanography
diaphanoscope
diaphanoscopy
diaphemetric
diaphoresis
diaphragm
  aperture d.
  Bucky d.
  pelvic d., d. of pelvis
  d. pessary
  Potter-Bucky d.
  d. of sella
  d. sellae
  urogenital d.
diaphragma, pl. **diaphragmata**
  d. pelvis
  d. sellae
  d. urogenitale
diaphragmalgia
diaphragmatic
  d. flutter
  d. hernia
  d. ligament of the mesonephros
  d. myocardial infarction
  d. nodes
  d. pacemaker
  d. peritonitis
  d. pleura
  d. pleurisy
  d. surface
diaphragmatocele
diaphragmodynia
diaphyseal
diaphysectomy
diaphysial
  d. aclasis
  d. center
  d. dysplasia
diaphysis, pl. **diaphyses**
diaphysitis
diapiresis
diaplacental
diaplasis
diaplastic
diaplexus
diapophysis
Diaptomus
diarrhea
  cachectic d.
  choleraic d.
  chronic bacillary d.
  Cochin China d.

colliquative d.
dientamoeba d.
dysenteric d.
fatty d.
flagellate d.
gastrogenous d.
lienteric d.
morning d.
mucous d.
nocturnal d.
pancreatic d.
d. pancreatica
pancreatogenous d.
serous d.
summer d.
traveler's d.
tropical d.
diarrheal, diarrheic
diarthric
diarthrodial
    d. cartilage
    d. joint
diarthrosis, pl. **diarthroses**
diarticular
diaschisis
diascope
diascopy
diastalsis
diastaltic
diastasis
    d. cordis
    d. recti
diastasuria
diastatic
    d. skull fracture
diastematocrania
diastematomyelia
diaster
diastole
    atrial d.
    electrical d.
    gastric d.
    late d.
    ventricular d.
diastolic
    d. afterpotential
    d. murmur
    d. pressure
    d. shock
    d. thrill
diastrophic dwarfism
diastrophism
diataxia
    cerebral d.
diatela
diathermal
diathermancy
diathermanous

diathermic
    d. therapy
diathermocoagulation
diathermy
    medical d.
    short wave d.
    surgical d.
    ultrashortwave d.
diathesis
    contractural d.
    cystic d.
    gouty d.
    hemorrhagic d.
    spasmophilic d.
diathetic
diatom
diatomaceous
diatoric
diazo
    d. reaction
    d. stain for argentaffin granules
diazonium salts
Di blood group (*var. of* Diego blood
    group)
Dibothriocephalus
    D. latus
dicelous
dicentric
    d. chromosome
dicephalous
dicephalus
    d. diauchenos
    d. dipus dibrachius
    d. dipus tetrabrachius
    d. dipus tribrachius
    d. dipygus
    d. monauchenos
dicheilia, dichilia
dicheiria, dichiria
Dichelobacter nodosus
dichilia (*var. of* dicheilia)
dichorial, dichorionic
    d. twins
dichotic
dichotomous
dichotomy
dichroic
dichroism
    circular d.
dichromat
dichromatic
dichromatism
dichromatopsia
dichromic
dichromophil, dichromophile
Dick
    D. method
    D. test

D

dicoria
dicrotic
    d. notch
    d. pulse
    d. wave
dicrotism
dictyoma
dictyotene
dicumarol resistance
didactic
    d. analysis
didactylism
didelphic
dideoxy procedure
didymus
die
Dieffenbach's method
Diego blood group, Di blood group, Di
  blood group
diel
dielectrography
diencephala (*pl. of* diencephalon)
diencephalic
    d. epilepsy
    d. syndrome of infancy
diencephalohypophysial
diencephalon, pl. diencephala
diener
dientamoeba diarrhea
Dientamoeba fragilis
dieresis
dieretic
diet
    acid-ash d.
    alkaline-ash d.
    balanced d.
    basal d.
    basic d.
    bland d.
    challenge d.
    clear liquid d.
    diabetic d.
    elimination d.
    full liquid d.
    Giordano-Giovannetti d.
    Giovannetti d.
    gluten-free d.
    gout d.
    high-calorie d.
    high-fat d.
    high-fiber d.
    Kempner d.
    ketogenic d.
    low-calorie d.
    low-fat d.
    low purine d.
    low residue d.
    low salt d.

    macrobiotic d.
    Meulengracht's d.
    Minot-Murphy d.
    Ornish prevention d.'s
    Ornish reversal d.
    purine-free d.
    purine-restricted d.
    rachitic d.
    reducing d.
    rice d.
    Schmidt d.
    Schmidt-Strassburger d.
    sippy d.
    smooth d.
    soft d.
    subsistence d.
    Wilder's d.
dietary
    d. amenorrhea
    d. fiber
Dieterle's stain
dietetic
    d. albuminuria
    d. treatment
dietetics
dietitian
Dietl's crisis
Dieuaide diagram
Dieulafoy's
    D. erosion
    D. theory
difference
    alveolar-arterial oxygen d.
    arteriovenous carbon dioxide d.
    arteriovenous oxygen d.
    cation-anion d.
    individual d.'s
    light d.
    standard error of d.
differential
    d. blood pressure
    d. diagnosis
    d. growth
    d. renal function test
    d. spinal anesthesia
    d. stain
    d. stethoscope
    threshold d.
    d. threshold
    d. ureteral catheterization test
    d. white blood count
differentiated
differentiation
    correlative d.
    echocardiographic d.
    invisible d.
diffraction
diffraction grating

diffuse
- d. abscess
- d. aneurysm
- d. angiokeratoma
- d. arterial ectasia
- d. choroiditis
- d. cutaneous leishmaniasis
- d. cutaneous mastocytosis
- d. deep keratitis
- d. emphysema
- d. esophageal spasm
- d. ganglion
- d. glomerulonephritis
- d. goiter
- d. idiopathic skeletal hyperostosis
- d. infantile familial sclerosis
- d. leishmaniasis
- d. mastocytosis
- d. mesangial proliferation
- d. obstructive emphysema
- d. panbronchiolitis
- d. peritonitis
- d. phlegmon
- d. small cleaved cell lymphoma
- d. waxy spleen

diffused
- d. psoriasis
- d. reflex

diffusing capacity

diffusion
- d. anoxia
- gel d.
- d. hypoxia
- d. method
- d. respiration
- d. shell

digametic

digastric
- d. branch of facial nerve
- d. fossa
- d. groove
- d. muscle
- d. notch
- d. triangle

digastricus

Digenea

digenesis

digenetic

DiGeorge syndrome

digestive
- d. albuminuria
- d. apparatus
- d. fever
- d. glycosuria
- d. leukocytosis
- d. system
- d. tract
- d. tube

digit
- binary d.
- clubbed d.'s

digital
- d. collateral artery
- d. crease
- d. dilatation
- d. flexion crease
- d. fossa
- d. furrow
- d. gray scale
- d. joints
- d. plethysmograph
- d. pulp
- d. radiography
- d. reflex
- d. subtraction angiography
- d. veins
- d. whorl

digitalization

digitate
- d. dermatosis
- d. impressions
- d. wart

digitation

digitationes hippocampi

digiti

digitus, pl. **digiti**
- d. annularis
- d. auricularis
- digiti hippocratici
- d. manus
- d. medius
- d. minimus
- d. pedis
- d. primus
- d. quintus
- d. secundus
- d. tertius
- d. valgus
- d. varus

diglossia

dignathus

digyny, digynia

diheterozygote

dihybrid

diiodotyrosine

diisopropyl iminodiacetic acid

dilaceration

dilantin gingivitis

dilatancy

dilatation
- digital d.

dilate

dilated
- d. cardiomyopathy
- d. pore

D

dilation
d. and curettage
d. and evacuation
post-stenotic d.
d. thrombosis
urethral d.

dilator
Chevalier-Jackson d.
Goodell's d.
Hanks d.'s
Hegar's d.'s
hydrostatic d.
d. iridis
Kollmann's d.
d. muscle
d. muscle of ileocecal sphincter
d. muscle of pylorus
Plummer's d.
Pratt d.'s
d. of pupil
d. pupillae muscle
d. tubae
Walther's d.

dildo, dildoe
dilution anemia
dimelia
dimension
buccolingual d.
occlusal vertical d.
rest vertical d.
vertical d.

dimensional stability
dimethylaminoazobenzene
dimethyl iminodiacetic acid
dimethyl sulfate
dimetria
dimidiate hermaphroditism
Dimmer's keratitis
dimorphic anemia
dimorphism
sexual d.

dimorphous leprosy
dimple
coccygeal d.
d. sign

dimpling
dinitrophenylhydrazine test
dinner pad
dinoflagellate
dinormocytosis
Dioctophyma
D. renale

Diogenes cup
diopter
prism d.

dioptric aberration
dioptrics
diorthosis

diovular
d. twins

diovulatory
DIP
D. joints

dip
Cournand's d.
d. phenomenon
type I d.
type II d.

D.I. particle
Dipetalonema
D. reconditum
D. streptocerca

diphallus
diphasic
d. complex
d. milk fever

diphenylhydantoin gingivitis
diphenylmethane dyes
diphtheria
cutaneous d.
false d.
faucial d.
laryngeal d.
laryngotracheal d.

diphtherial, diphtheritic
diphtheric
diphtheritis
diphtheroid
diphtherotoxin
diphyllobothriasis
Diphyllobothrium
D. cordatum
D. latum
D. linguloides
D. mansoni
D. mansonoides

diphyllobothrium anemia
diphyodont
diplacusis
d. binauralis
d. dysharmonica
d. echoica
d. monauralis

diplegia
congenital facial d.
facial d.
infantile d.
masticatory d.
spastic d.

diploalbuminuria
diplobacillus
Morax-Axenfeld d.

diplobacteria
diploblastic
diplocardia
diplocephalus

diplocheiria, diplochiria
diplococcemia
diplococci (*pl. of* diplococcus)
diplococcin
Diplococcus
diplococcus, pl. **diplococci**
diplocoria
diploë
diplogenesis
Diplogonoporus
diploic
     d. canals
     d. vein
diploid
     d. nucleus
diplokaryon
diplomelituria
diplomyelia
diplonema
diploneural
diplopagus
diplopia
     crossed d.
     heteronymous d.
     homonymous d.
     monocular d.
     simple d.
     uncrossed d.
diplopodia
diplosome
diplosomia
diplotene
diploteratology
dipodia
dipole theory
diprosopus
dipsesis
dipsomania
dipsosis
dipsotherapy
Diptera
dipteran
dipterous
Dipus sagitta
dipygus
Dipylidium caninum
direct
     d. acrylic restoration
     d. auscultation
     d. bone impression
     d. composite resin restoration
     d. Coombs' test
     d. embolism
     d. filling resin
     d. flap
     d. fluorescent antibody test
     d. fracture
     d. fulguration

     d. illumination
     d. image
     d. inguinal hernia
     d. laryngoscopy
     d. lead
     d. maternal death
     d. method for making inlays
     d. nuclear division
     d. ophthalmoscope
     d. ophthalmoscopy
     d. ovular transmigration
     d. percussion
     d. pulp capping
     d. pyramidal tract
     d. rays
     d. reacting bilirubin
     d. resin restoration
     d. retainer
     d. retention
     d. technique
     d. transfusion
     d. vision
directional atherectomy
directive psychotherapy
director
dirigation
dirigomotor
Dirofilaria
     D. conjunctivae
     D. immitis
dirt-eating
disability
     developmental d.
     learning d.
disaggregation
disappearing bone disease
disarticulation
disassimilation
disassociation
disc
     articular d.
     articular d. of acromioclavicular
      joint
     articular d. of distal radioulnar
      joint
     articular d. of sternoclavicular joint
     interpubic d.
     intervertebral d.
     sacrococcygeal d.
discectomy
discharge
     after-d.
discharging tubule
dischronation
disci (*pl. of* discus)
disciform
     d. degeneration

D

disciform *(continued)*
    d. keratitis
    d. macular degeneration
discission
discitis
disclosing solution
discoblastic
discoblastula
discogastrula
discogenic
discoid
    d. lupus erythematosus
discoidal cleavage
disconjugate
    d. movement of eyes
disconnection syndrome
discontinuous sterilization
discopathy
    traumatic cervical d.
discoplacenta
discordance
discordant
    d. alternans
    d. alternation
    d. atrioventricular connections
discotomy
discrete
    d. character
    d. random variable
    d. smallpox
    d. variable
discriminant
    d. analysis
    d. function
    d. stimulus
discrimination
discus, pl. **disci**
    d. articularis
    d. articularis acromioclavicularis
    d. articularis radioulnaris
    d. articularis sternoclavicularis
    d. articularis temporomandibularis
    d. interpubicus
    d. intervertebralis
    d. lentiformis
    d. nervi optici
    d. proligerus
disdiaclast
disease
    ABO hemolytic d. of the newborn
    accumulation d.
    Acosta's d.
    Adams-Stokes d.
    adaptation d.'s
    Addison-Biermer d.
    Addison's d.
    akamushi d.
    Akureyri d.

Albers-Schönberg d.
Albert's d.
Albright's d.
Alexander's d.
Almeida's d.
Alpers d.
altitude d.
Alzheimer's d.
anarthritic rheumatoid d.
Anders' d.
Andersen's d.
antibody deficiency d.
aortoiliac occlusive d.
Aran-Duchenne d.
Australian X d.
autoimmune d.
aviator's d.
Ayerza's d.
Azorean d.
Baelz' d.
Baló's d.
Baltic myoclonus d.
Bamberger-Marie d.
Bamberger's d.
Bannister's d.
Banti's d.
Barclay-Baron d.
Barlow's d.
Barraquer's d.
Basedow's d.
Batten d.
Batten-Mayou d.
Bayle's d.
Bazin's d.
Bechterew's d.
Becker's d.
Begbie's d.
Béguez César d.
Behçet's d.
Behr's d.
Berger's d.
Bernhardt's d.
Besnier-Boeck-Schaumann d.
Best's d.
Bielschowsky's d.
Biermer's d.
Binswanger's d.
bird-breeder's d.
blinding d.
Bloch-Sulzberger d.
Blocq's d.
Blount-Barber d.
Blount's d.
blue d.
Boeck's d.
Bornholm d.
Bosin's d.
Bouchard's d.

Bouillaud's d.
Bourneville-Pringle d.
Bourneville's d.
Bowen's d.
Brailsford-Morquio d.
brancher glycogen storage d.
Breda's d.
Bright's d.
Brill's d.
Brill-Symmers d.
Brill-Zinsser d.
Briquet's d.
Brissaud's d.
Brocq's d.
Brodie's d.
bronzed d.
Brooke's d.
Bruck's d.
Brushfield-Wyatt d.
Buerger's d.
Bürger-Grütz d.
Bury's d.
Buschke's d.
Busquet's d.
Busse-Buschke d.
Byler d.
Caffey's d.
caisson d.
calcium pyrophosphate deposition d.
Calvé-Perthes d.
Canavan's d.
Canavan-van Bogaert-Bertrand d.
Caroli's d.
Carrington's d.
Carrión's d.
Castleman's d.
cat-bite d.
cat-scratch d.
celiac d.
central core d.
central Recklinghausen's d. type II
cerebrovascular d.
Chagas' d.
Chagas-Cruz d.
α chain d.
Charcot-Marie-Tooth d.
Charcot's d.
Charlouis' d.
Cheadle's d.
Chédiak-Higashi d.
Chiari's d.
Chicago d.
cholesterol ester storage d.
Christensen-Krabbe d.
Christian's d.
Christmas d.
chronic active liver d.
chronic granulomatous d.

chronic hypertensive d.
chronic obstructive pulmonary d.
Civatte's d.
Coats' d.
Cockayne's d.
cold hemagglutinin d.
collagen d.'s, collagen-vascular d.'s
combined system d.
communicable d.
Concato's d.
connective-tissue d.'s
Conradi's d.
contagious d.
Cori's d.
Corrigan's d.
Cotunnius d.
Cowden's d.
Creutzfeldt-Jakob d.
Crigler-Najjar d.
Crocq's d.
Crohn's d.
Crouzon's d.
Cruveilhier-Baumgarten d.
Cruveilhier's d.
Csillag's d.
Curschmann's d.
Cushing's d.
cystic d. of the breast
cysticercus d.
cystic d. of renal medulla
cystine d.
cystine storage d.
cytomegalic inclusion d.
cytomegalovirus d.
Daae's d.
Danielssen-Boeck d.
Danielssen's d.
Darier's d.
Darling's d.
Davies' d.
decompression d.
deer-fly d.
deficiency d.
degenerative joint d.
Degos' d.
Dejerine's d.
Dejerine-Sottas d.
demyelinating d.
dense-deposit d.
de Quervain's d.
Dercum's d.
Deutschländer's d.
Devic's d.
Di Guglielmo's d.
disappearing bone d.
diverticular d.
dog d.
dominantly inherited Lévi's d.

D

disease *(continued)*
    Donohue's d.
    drug-induced d.
    Dubois' d.
    Duchenne-Aran d.
    Duchenne's d.
    Duhring's d.
    Dukes' d.
    Duncan's d.
    Duplay's d.
    Dupuytren's d. of the foot
    Duroziez' d.
    Dutton's d.
    dynamic d.
    Eales' d.
    Ebstein's d.
    echinococcus d.
    Eisenmenger's d.
    elevator d.
    emotional d.
    endemic d.
    Engelmann's d.
    English d.
    English sweating d.
    eosinophilic endomyocardial d.
    epidemic d.
    Epstein's d.
    Erb d.
    Erb-Charcot d.
    Erdheim d.
    ergot alkaloid-associated heart d.
    Eulenburg's d.
    exanthematous d.
    extramammary Paget d.
    extrapyramidal d.
    extrapyramidal motor system d.
    Fabry's d.
    Fahr's d.
    Farber's d.
    Favre-Durand-Nicholas d.
    Favre-Racouchet's d.
    Feer's d.
    femoropopliteal occlusive d.
    Fenwick's d.
    fibrocystic d. of the breast
    fibrocystic d. of the pancreas
    fifth d.
    Filatov Dukes' d.
    Filatov's d.
    Flatau-Schilder d.
    flax-dresser's d.
    Flegel's d.
    flint d.
    focal metastatic d.
    Folling's d.
    Forbes' d.
    Fordyce's d.
    Forestier's d.

    Fothergill's d.
    Fournier's d.
    fourth d.
    Fox-Fordyce d.
    Franklin's d.
    Freiberg's d.
    Friend d.
    functional d.
    functional cardiovascular d.
    fusospirochetal d.
    Gairdner's d.
    Gamna's d.
    Gandy-Nanta d.
    garapata d.
    Garré's d.
    Gaucher's d.
    Gerhardt-Mitchell d.
    Gerhardt's d.
    Gerlier's d.
    Gierke's d.
    Gilbert's d.
    Gilchrist's d.
    Gilles de la Tourette's d.
    Glanzmann's d.
    glycogen-storage d.
    Goldflam d.
    Gorham's d.
    Gougerot and Blum d.
    Gougerot-Sjögren d.
    Gowers d.
    graft versus host d.
    granulomatous d.
    Graves' d.
    Greenhow's d.
    Griesinger's d.
    Grover's d.
    GVH d.
    Haff d.
    Haglund's d.
    Hailey-Hailey d.
    Hallervorden-Spatz d.
    Hallopeau's d.
    Hamman's d.
    Hammond's d.
    hand-foot-and-mouth d.
    Hand-Schüller-Christian d.
    Hansen's d.
    Harada's d.
    Hartnup d.
    Hashimoto's d.
    heavy chain d.
    α-heavy-chain d.
    γ-heavy-chain d.
    μ-heavy-chain d.
    Hebra's d.
    Heck's d.
    Heerfordt's d.
    hemoglobin C d.

hemoglobin H d.
hemolytic d. of newborn
hemorrhagic d. of the newborn
hepatolenticular d.
herring-worm d.
Hers' d.
hidebound d.
Hirschsprung's d.
Hodgson's d.   *Hodgkin's*
holoendemic d.
hookworm d.
Huntington's d.
Hurler's d.
Hutchinson-Gilford d.
hyaline membrane d. of the
  newborn
Hyde's d.
hyperendemic d.
Iceland d., Icelandic d.
I-cell d.
idiopathic d.
immune complex d.
immunoproliferative small
  intestinal d.
inborn lysosomal d.
inclusion body d.
inclusion cell d.
industrial d.
infantile celiac d.
infectious d., infective d.
intercurrent d.
interstitial d.
iron-storage d.
island d.
Jaffe-Lichtenstein d.
Jakob-Creutzfeldt d.
Jansky-Bielschowsky d.
Jensen's d.
jumping d., jumper d.
jumping Frenchmen of Maine d.,
  jumper d. of Maine
Jüngling's d.
Kashin-Bek d.
Katayama d.
Kawasaki's d.
Kennedy's d.
Kienböck's d.
Kimmelstiel-Wilson d.
Kimura's d.
kinky-hair d., kinky hair d.
Köhler's d.
Krabbe's d.
Kufs d.
Kugelberg-Welander d.
Kuhnt-Junius d.
Kussmaul's d.
Kyasanur Forest d.
Kyrle's d.

Lafora body d.
Lafora's d.
Lane's d.
Larrey-Weil d.
Lasègue's d.
laughing d.
L-chain d.
Legg-Calvé-Perthes d., Legg-
  Perthes d., Legg's d.
Legionnaire's d.
Leigh's d.
Leiner's d.
Lenègre's d.
Leri-Weill d.
Letterer-Siwe d.
Lev's d.
Lindau's d.
linear IgA bullous d. in children
Little's d.
Lobo's d.
Löffler's d.
Lorain's d.   *Lyme disease*
Lou Gehrig's d.
Luft's d.
lung fluke d.
Lutz-Splendore-Almeida d.
Lyell's d.
lysosomal d.
Machado-Joseph
Madelung's d.
Majocchi's d.
Manson's d.
maple bark d.
marble bone d.
Marburg d.   *McCune-Albright Disease (syndrome)*
Marburg virus d.
Marchiafava-Bignami d.
Marfan's d.
margarine d.
Marie-Strümpell d.
Marion's d.
Martin's d.
McArdle's d.
McArdle-Schmid-Pearson d.
mechanobullous d.
Meige's d.
Ménétrier's d.
Ménière's d.
mental d.
Merzbacher-Pelizaeus d.
metabolic d.
Meyenburg's d.
Meyer-Betz d.
mianeh d.
Mibelli's d.
microcystic d. of renal medulla
micrometastatic d.
Mikulicz' d.

D

disease *(continued)*

Milian's d.
Milroy's d.
Milton's d.
Minamata d.
miner's d.
minimal-change d.
Mitchell's d.
mixed connective-tissue d.
molecular d.
Mondor's d.
Monge's d.
Morgagni's d.
Morquio's d.
Morquio-Ullrich d.
Morvan's d.
Moschcowitz' d.
motor neuron d.
motor system d.
mountain d.
moyamoya d.
Mucha-Habermann d.
multicore d.
Neftel's d.
Neumann's d.
neutral lipid storage d.
Nicolas-Favre d.
Niemann d.
Niemann-Pick d.
nil d.
Norrie's d.
oasthouse urine d.
occupational d.
Ofuji's d.
Oguchi's d.
Ollier's d.
Oppenheim's d.
organic d.
Ormond's d.
orphan d.
Osgood-Schlatter d.
Osler's d.
Osler-Vaquez d.
Otto's d.
Owren's d.
Paas' d.
Paget's d.
Panner's d.
paper mill worker's d.
parasitic d.
Parkinson's d.
Parrot's d.
Parry's d.
Pauzat's d.
Pavy's d.
Paxton's d.
pearl-worker's d.
Pel-Ebstein d.

Pelizaeus-Merzbacher d.
Pellegrini's d.
Pellegrini-Stieda d.
pelvic inflammatory d.
periodic d.
perna d.
Perthes d.
Pette-Döring d.
Peyronie's d.
Pick's d.
pink d.
plaster of Paris d.
Plummer's d.
polycystic d. of kidneys
polycystic liver d.
Pompe's d.
Portuguese-Azorean d.
Posadas d.
Potter's d.
Pott's d.
poultry handler's d.
primary d.
Pringle's d.
pseudo-Hurler d.
pulseless d.
Purtscher's d.
quiet hip d.
Quincke's d.
ragpicker's d.
ragsorter's d., ragsorter's d.
railroad d.
rat-bite d.
Raussly d.
Rayer's d.
Raynaud's d.
Recklinghausen's d. of bone
Recklinghausen's d. type I
Refsum's d.
Reiter's d.
rhesus d.
rheumatic d.
rheumatic heart d.
rheumatoid d.
Ribas-Torres d.
rice d.
Riedel's d.
Riga-Fede d.
Robinson's d.
Roger's d.
Rokitansky's d.
Romberg's d.
Rosai-Dorman d.
Rosenbach's d.
Roth-Bernhardt d.
Roth's d.
Rougnon-Heberden d.
Roussy-Lévy d.
runt d.

Rust's d.
salivary gland d.
salivary gland virus d.
Sandhoff's d.
sandworm d.
San Joaquin Valley d.
Schenck's d.
Scheuermann's d.
Schilder's d.
Schlatter's d., Schlatter-Osgood d.
Scholz' d.
Schönlein's d.
Schottmueller's d.
Schüller's d.
sclerocystic d. of the ovary
sea-blue histiocyte d.
secondary d.
self-limited d.
Senear-Usher d.
senile hip d.
serum d.
sexually transmitted d.
Shaver's d.
shimamushi d.
sickle cell d.
sickle cell C d.
sickle cell-thalassemia d.
silo-filler's d.
Simmonds' d.
Simons' d.
sixth d.
sixth venereal d.
Sjögren's d.
skinbound d.
Sneddon-Wilkinson d.
social d.'s
specific d.
Spielmeyer-Sjögren d.
Spielmeyer-Stock d.
Spielmeyer-Vogt d.
Stargardt's d.
Steele-Richardson-Olszewski d.
Steinert's d.
Sticker's d.
Still's d.
Stokes-Adams d.
stone-mason's d.
storage d.
Strümpell-Marie d.
Strümpell's d.
Strümpell-Westphal d.
Sturge-Weber d.
Sulzberger-Garbe d.
Sutton's d.
Swediauer's d.
Sweet's d.
Swift's d.
swineherd's d.

swollen belly d.
Sydenham's d.
Sylvest's d.
systemic autoimmune d.'s
systemic febrile d.'s
Takahara's d.
Takayasu's d.
Tangier d.
Taussig-Bing d.
Taylor's d.
Tay-Sachs d.
Thiemann's d.
third d.
Thomsen's d.
Thygeson's d.
thyrocardiac d.
thyrotoxic heart d.
Tommaselli's d.
Tornwaldt's d.
torsion d. of childhood
Tourette's d.
Trevor's d.
tropical d.'s
tsutsugamushi d.
Underwood's d.
Unna's d.
Unverricht's d.
Urbach-Wiethe d.
vagabond's d.
vagrant's d.
van Buren's d.
Vaquez' d.
venereal d.
veno-occlusive d. of the liver
Vidal's d.
Vincent's d.
Virchow's d.
virus X d.
Vogt-Spielmeyer d.
Voltolini's d.
von Economo's d.
von Gierke's d.
von Meyenburg's d.
von Recklinghausen d.
von Willebrand's d.
Voorhoeve's d.
Wagner's d.
Wardrop's d.
wasting d.
Weber-Christian d.
Wegner's d.
Weil's d.
Weir Mitchell's d.
Werdnig-Hoffmann d.
Werlhof's d.
Wernicke's d.
Werther's d.
Westphal's d.

D

disease *(continued)*
    Whipple's d.
    white spot d.
    Wilkie's d.
    Wilson's d.
    Winiwarter-Buerger d.
    Winkler's d.
    Wohlfart-Kugelberg-Welander d.
    Wolman's d.
    woolsorter's d., woolsorter's d.
    Woringer-Kolopp d.
    yellow d.
    Ziehen-Oppenheim d.
disengagement
disequilibrium
    genetic d.
    linkage d.
disgerminoma
dish
    d. face
    Petri d.
    Stender d.
disharmony
    occlusal d.
dishpan fracture
disimpaction
disinfect
disinfection
    concurrent d.
    terminal d.
disinfestation
disinhibition
disinsection, disinsectization
disinvagination
disjoined pyeloplasty
disjunction
disjunctive absorption
disk
    A d.'s
    acromioclavicular d.
    anisotropic d.'s
    articular d.
    articular d. of temporomandibular
      joint
    blastodermic d.
    blood d.
    Bowman's d.'s
    Burlew d.
    choked d.
    ciliary d.
    cone d.'s
    cuttlefish d.
    diamond d.
    embryonic d.
    emery d.'s
    germinal d., germ d.
    H d.
    hair d.

    Hensen's d.
    herniated d.
    I d.
    intercalated d.
    intermediate d.
    interpubic d.
    intervertebral d.
    isotropic d.
    d. kidney
    mandibular d.
    Merkel's tactile d.
    Newton's d.
    optic d.
    Placido da Costa's d.
    proligerous d.
    protruded d.
    Q d.'s
    radioulnar d., radioulnar articular d.
    Ranvier's d.'s
    rod d.'s
    ruptured d.
    sandpaper d.'s
    d. sensitivity method
    d. space
    stenopeic d., stenopaic d.
    sternoclavicular d., sternoclavicular
      articular d.
    stroboscopic d.
    d. syndrome
    tactile d.
    temporomandibular articular d.
    transverse d.
    triangular d. of wrist
    Z d.
diskitis
diskogram
diskography
disk-shaped cataract
dislocate
dislocatio
    d. erecta
dislocation
    d. of articular processes
    closed d.
    compound d.
    fracture d.
    d. fracture
    Kienböck's d.
    d. of lens
    Nélaton's d.
    open d.
    perilunar d.
    simple d.
dismember
dismembered pyeloplasty
disobliteration
disofenin
disomic

disomy
disorder
    adjustment d.'s
    affective d.'s
    affective personality d.
    antisocial personality d.
    anxiety d.'s
    asthenic personality d.
    attention deficit d.
    attention deficit hyperactivity d.
    autistic d.
    autonomic d.
    avoidant d. of adolescence
    avoidant d. of childhood
    avoidant personality d.
    behavior d.
    bipolar d.
    body dysmorphic d.
    borderline personality d.
    character d.
    conduct d.
    conversion d.
    cumulative trauma d.'s
    cyclothymic d.
    cyclothymic personality d.
    delusional d.
    dependent personality d.
    depersonalization d.
    dissociative d.'s
    dysthymic d.
    eating d.'s
    emotional d.
    erotomanic type of paranoid d.
    factitious d.
    familial bipolar mood d.
    functional d.
    Gaucher d.
    gender identity d.'s
    generalized anxiety d.
    grandiose type of paranoid d.
    histrionic personality d.
    identity d.
    immune complex d.
    immunoproliferative d.'s
    impulse control d.
    induced psychotic d.
    intermittent explosive d.
    isolated explosive d.
    jealous type of paranoid d.
    kinky-hair d.
    late luteal phase dysphoric d.
    LDL receptor d.
    major mood d.
    manic-depressive d.
    mental d.
    mood d.'s
    multiple personality d.
    narcissistic personality d.
    neuropsychologic d.
    obsessive-compulsive d.
    obsessive-compulsive personality d.
    oppositional d.
    organic mental d.
    overanxious d.
    panic d.
    paranoid d.
    paranoid personality d.
    persecutory type of paranoid d.
    personality d.
    pervasive developmental d.
    plasma iodoprotein d.
    posttraumatic stress d.
    psychogenic pain d.
    psychosomatic d.,
      psychophysiologic d.
    reactive attachment d.
    REM behavior d.
    rumination d.
    schizophreniform d.
    separation anxiety d.
    shared psychotic d.
    sleep terror d.
    somatization d.
    somatoform d.
    substance abuse d.'s
    substance-induced organic
      mental d.'s
    thought process d.
    visceral d.
disorganization
disorganized schizophrenia
disorientation
disparate
disparity
    d. angle
    fixation d.
    retinal d.
dispermy, dispermia
disperse placenta
dispersing electrode
dispersion
    temporal d.
dispireme
displaceability
    tissue d.
displacement
    affect d.
    d. analysis
    d. loop
    mesial d.
    d. threshold
    tissue d.
disproportionate dwarfism
disputed neurogenic thoracic outlet
    syndrome
dissect

D

dissecting cellulitis
dissection
    aortic d.
    d. tubercle
disseminate coccidioidomycosis
disseminated
    d. aspergillosis
    d. choroiditis
    d. cutaneous gangrene
    d. cutaneous leishmaniasis
    d. gonococcal infection
    d. intravascular coagulation
    d. lupus erythematosus
    d. recurrent infundibulofolliculitis
    d. sclerosis
    d. tuberculosis
dissepiment
Disse's space
dissimilation
dissimulation
dissociated
    d. anesthesia
    d. nystagmus
dissociation
    albuminocytologic d.
    atrial d.
    atrioventricular d., A-V d.
    complete atrioventricular d.,
      complete A-V d.
    electromechanical d.
    incomplete atrioventricular d.,
      incomplete A-V d.
    interference d.
    d. by interference
    isorhythmic d.
    light-near d.
    longitudinal d.
    pupillary light-near d.
    d. sensibility
    sleep d.
    syringomyelic d.
    tabetic d.
dissociative
    d. anesthesia
    d. disorders
    d. hysteria
    d. reaction
dissonance
    cognitive d.
dissymmetry
distad
distal
    d. caries
    d. centriole
    d. end
    d. ileitis
    d. interphalangeal joints
    d. myopathy

    d. occlusion
    d. part of anterior lobe of
      hypophysis
    d. radioulnar articulation
    d. radioulnar joint
    d. spiral septum
    d. splenorenal shunt
    d. surface of tooth
    d. tibiofibular joint
    d. tingling on percussion
distalis
distance
    d. ceptor
    focal d.
    infinite d.
    interarch d.
    interocclusal d.
    interridge d.
    large interarch d.
    map d.
    pupillary d.
    reduced interarch d.
    small interarch d.
    sociometric d.
distant flap
distemper virus
distensibility
distention, distension
    d. cyst
    d. ulcer
distichiasis
distobuccal
distobucco-occlusal
distobuccopulpal
distocervical
distoclusal
distoclusion
distogingival
distoincisal
distolabial
distolabiopulpal
distolingual
distolinguo-occlusal
Distoma
distomiasis, distomatosis
    hemic d.
    pulmonary d.
distomolar
Distomum
disto-occlusal
disto-occlusion
distoplacement
distopulpal
distortion
    d. aberration
    parataxic d.
distoversion
distractibility

distraction
    d. conus
distress
    fetal d.
distributed effort
distributing artery
distribution
    Bernoulli d.
    binomial d.
    chi-square d.
    d. curve
    dermatomal d.
    epidemiological d.
    exponential d.
    f d.
    frequency d.
    gaussian d.
    d. leukocytosis
    lognormal d.
    multinomial d.
    normal d.
    Poisson d.
    skew d.
    t d.
    d. volume
distributive analysis
districhiasis
distrix
disturbance
    emotional d., mental d.
disuse atrophy
Dittrich's
    D. plugs
    D. stenosis
diuresis
    alcohol d.
    osmotic d.
    water d.
diurnal
    d. enuresis
    d. periodicity
    d. rhythm
divarication
divergence
    d. excess exotropia
    d. insufficiency
    d. insufficiency exotropia
divergent
    d. squint
    d. strabismus
diverging meniscus
diver's
    d. palsy
    d. paralysis
divers' spectacles
diverticula (*pl. of* diverticulum)
diverticular
    d. disease

diverticulectomy
diverticulitis
diverticuloma
diverticulopexy
diverticulosis
diverticulum, pl. **diverticula**
    allantoenteric d.
    allantoic d.
    diverticula ampullae ductus
      deferentis
    cervical d.
    diverticula of colon
    colonic diverticula
    diverticula of ampulla of ductus
      deferens
    duodenal d.
    epiphrenic d.
    false d.
    Heister's d.   < Hutch
    hypopharyngeal d.
    Kommerell's d.
    laryngotracheal d.
    Meckel's d.
    metanephric d.
    Nuck's d.
    pancreatic diverticula
    Pertik's d.
    pharyngoesophageal d.
    pituitary d.
    pulsion d.
    Rathke's d.
    thyroid d., thyroglossal d.
    tracheobronchial d.
    traction d.
    true d.
    urethral d.
    ventricular d.
    vesical d.
    Zenker's d.
divided
    d. dose
    d. spectacles
diving
    d. goiter
    d. reflex
division
    anterior primary d.
    cleavage d.
    conjugate d.
    direct nuclear d.
    equatorial d.
    indirect nuclear d.
    meiotic d.
    mitotic d.
    multiplicative d.
    posterior primary d.
    reduction d.
    Remak's nuclear d.

D

divulse
divulsion
divulsor
dizygotic, dizygous
    d. twins
dizziness
DMFS
    D. caries index
dmfs caries index
DNA
    DNA diagnostics
    DNA markers
    DNA profiling
    DNA typing
DNA virus
d'Ocagne nomogram
docking protein
doctor
doctrine
    humoral d.
    Monro-Kellie d.
    Monro's d.
Döderlein's bacillus
Doerfler-Stewart test
dog
    d. disease
    d. distemper virus
    d. ear
    d. nose
Dogiel's
    D. cells
    D. corpuscle
dogma
    central d.
Döhle
    D. bodies
    D. inclusions
dol
dolichocephalic, dolichocephalous
dolichocephaly, dolichocephalism
dolichocolon
dolichocranial
dolichoectatic artery
dolichofacial
dolichopellic, dolichopelvic
    d. pelvis
dolichoprosopic, dolichoprosopous
dolichostenomelia
dolichouranic, dolichuranic
doll's eye sign
dolor
    d. capitis
dolorific
dolorimetry
dolorogenic zone
dolorology
Dombrock blood group
dome cell

domestic violence
domiciliated
dominance
    cerebral d.
    false d.
    genetic d.
    d. hierarchy
    d. of traits
dominant
    d. character
    d. eye
    d. frequency
    d. gene
    d. hemisphere
    d. idea
    d. inheritance
    d. lethal trait
    d. trait
dominantly inherited Lévi's disease
Donath-Landsteiner
    D.-L. cold autoantibody
    D.-L. phenomenon
Donders'
    D. glaucoma
    D. law
    D. pressure
    D. rings
Don Juan
Don Juanism
Donné's corpuscle
Donohue's
    D. disease
    D. syndrome
donor
    d. insemination
    universal d.
donovanosis
Donovan's bodies
Doose syndrome
dopaminergic
Doppler
    D. color flow
    D. echocardiography
    D. effect
    D. phenomenon
    D. shift
    D. ultrasonography
doraphobia
Dorello's canal
Dorendorf's sign
Dorfman-Chanarin syndrome
Dorno rays
doromania
Dor procedure
dorsa (*pl. of* dorsum)
dorsabdominal
dorsad

dorsal
d. accessory olivary nucleus
d. artery of clitoris
d. artery of foot
d. artery of nose
d. artery of penis
d. branch
d. branches
d. branch of the lumbar artery
d. branch of the posterior
  intercostal arteries 3–11
d. branch of the posterior
  intercostal veins 4–11
d. branch of the subcostal artery
d. branch of the superior
  intercostal artery
d. branch of the ulnar nerve
d. calcaneocuboid ligament
d. callosal vein
d. carpal branch of radial artery
d. carpal branch of ulnar artery
d. carpal ligament
d. carpal network
d. carpometacarpal ligaments
d. column of spinal cord
d. column stimulation
d. cuboideonavicular ligament
d. cuneocuboid ligament
d. cuneonavicular ligaments
d. digital artery
d. digital nerves
d. digital nerves of foot
d. digital nerves of hand
d. digital veins of foot
d. digital veins of toes
d. fascia of foot
d. fascia of hand
d. flexure
d. funiculus
d. hood
d. hypothalamic region
d. interosseous artery
d. interosseous muscles of foot
d. interosseous muscles of hand
d. interosseous nerve
d. lateral cutaneous nerve
d. lingual branches of lingual
  artery
d. lingual vein
d. longitudinal fasciculus
d. medial cutaneous nerve
d. mesocardium
d. mesogastrium
d. metacarpal artery
d. metacarpal ligaments
d. metacarpal veins
d. metatarsal artery
d. metatarsal ligaments
d. metatarsal veins
d. motor nucleus of vagus
d. muscles
d. nasal artery
d. nerve of clitoris
d. nerve of penis
d. nerve of scapula
d. nerves of toes
d. nucleus
d. nucleus of trapezoid body
d. nucleus of vagus
d. nucleus of vagus nerve
d. pancreas
d. pancreatic artery
d. part of pons
d. plate of neural tube
d. position
d. primary ramus of spinal nerve
d. radiocarpal ligament
d. reflex
d. root
d. root ganglion
d. sacrococcygeal muscle
d. sacrococcygeus muscle
d. sacroiliac ligaments
d. scapular artery
d. scapular nerve
d. scapular vein
d. spine
d. surface
d. surface of digit
d. surface of sacrum
d. surface of scapula
d. talonavicular bone
d. talonavicular ligament
d. tegmental decussation
d. thalamus
d. thoracic artery
d. tubercle of radius
d. vagal nucleus
d. vein of corpus callosum
d. veins of clitoris
d. veins of penis
d. venous arch of foot
d. venous network of foot
d. venous network of hand
d. vertebrae
dorsalgia
dorsalis
d. pedis artery
Dorset's culture egg medium
dorsi (*gen. of* dorsum)
dorsiduct
dorsiflexion
dorsiscapular
dorsispinal
d. veins
dorsocephalad

dorsodynia
dorsolateral
    d. fasciculus
    d. plate of neural tube
    d. tract
dorsolumbar
dorsomedial
    d. hypothalamic nucleus
    d. nucleus
    d. nucleus of hypothalamus
dorsosacral position
dorsoventrad
dorsum, gen. **dorsi**, pl. **dorsa**
    d. ephippii
    d. of foot
    d. of foot reflex
    d. linguae
    d. manus
    d. nasi
    d. of nose
    d. pedis
    d. pedis reflex
    d. penis
    d. of penis
    d. scapulae
    d. sellae
    d. of tongue
dose
    absorbed d.
    air d.
    bone marrow d.
    booster d.
    cumulative d.
    daily d.
    depth d.
    divided d.
    epilation d.
    equivalent d.
    erythema d.
    exit d.
    exposure d.
    fractional d.
    gonad d.
    gonadal d.
    initial d.
    integral d.
    L d.'s
    L^+ d., L_+ d.
    Lf d., L_f d.
    Lo d., L_o d.
    loading d.
    Lr d., L_r d.
    maintenance d.
    maximal d.
    maximal permissible d.
    maximum permissible d.
    minimal d.
    minimal infecting d.

    minimal reacting d.
    optimum d.
    preventive d.
    sensitizing d.
    shocking d.
    skin d.
    tissue culture infectious d.
    tolerance d.
dose-response relationship
dosimeter
dosimetry
    thermoluminescence d.
    x-ray d.
dot
    Gunn's d.'s
    Horner-Trantas d.'s
    Maurer's d.'s
    Schüffner's d.'s
    Trantas' d.'s
    Ziemann's d.'s
dotage
dotardness
dotted tongue
double
    d. antibody immunoassay
    d. antibody method
    d. antibody precipitation
    d. antibody sandwich assay
    d. aortic arch
    d. aortic stenosis
    d. athetosis
    d. back cross
    d. bind
    d. blind study
    d. bubble sign
    d. chin
    d. compartment hydrocephalus
    d. concave lens
    d. congenital athetosis
    d. consciousness
    d. contrast enema
    d. convex lens
    d. enterostomy
    d. flap amputation
    d. fracture
    d. (gel) diffusion precipitin test in one dimension
    d. (gel) diffusion precipitin test in two dimensions
    d. hemiplegia
    d. immunodiffusion
    d. inlet atrioventricular connections
    d. intussusception
    d. lip
    d. loop hernia
    d. minute chromosomes
    d. outlet right ventricle
    d. pedicle flap

d. pleurisy
d. pneumonia
d. product
d. protrusion
d. quartan
d. quotidian fever
d. refraction
d. stain
d. tachycardia
d. tertian
d. tertian malaria
d. track sign
d. vision
double-channel catheter
double-mouthed uterus
double-point threshold
double-shock sound
doublet
Wollaston's d.
doubly
d. armed suture
d. heterozygous
douche
d. bath
Douglas
D. abscess
D. bag
D. cul-de-sac
D. fold
D. graft
D. line
D. mechanism
D. pouch
D. spontaneous evolution
dousing bath
dovetail
dowager's hump
dowel
downbeat nystagmus
Downey cell
Downs' analysis
Down's syndrome
downward drainage
doxacurium chloride
Doyère's eminence
Doyle's operation
Doyne's honeycomb choroidopathy
DPT
Drabkin's reagent
dracontiasis
dracunculiasis, dracunculosis
Dracunculus
D. lova
D. medinensis
D. oculi
D. persarum
drag
solvent d.

Dragendorff's test
Dräger respirometer
drain
cigarette d.
Mikulicz' d.
Penrose d.
stab d.
sump d.
drainage
capillary d.
closed d.
dependent d.
downward d.
infusion-aspiration d.
open d.
postural d.
suction d.
through d.
tidal d.
d. tube
Wangensteen d.
drain-trap stomach
drape
drapetomania
drawer
d. sign
d. test
draw-sheet
dream
anxiety d.
d. associations
d. pain
wet d.
dream-work
dreamy state
Drechslera
drepanidium
drepanocyte
drepanocytic
d. anemia
dresser
dressing
adhesive absorbent d.
antiseptic d.
bolus d.
dry d.
fixed d.
d. forceps
Lister's d.
occlusive d.
pressure d.
tie-over d.
water d.
Dressler
D. beat
D. syndrome
Dreulofoy's lesion
Dreyer's formula

D

dribble
drift
    antigenic d.
    genetic d.
    d. movements
    pure random d.
drifting
drifts
Drigalski-Conradi agar
drill
    bur d.
    dental d.
Drinker respirator
drip
    intravenous d.
    Murphy d.
    d. phleboclysis
    postnasal d.
    d. transfusion
drip-suck irrigation
drive
    acquired d.'s
    exploratory d.
    learned d.
    meiotic d.
    physiological d.'s
    primary d.'s
    secondary d.'s
driver's thigh
driving
    photic d.
dromic
dromograph
dromomania
dromotropic
    negatively d.
    positively d.
drooping lily sign
drop
    d. attack
    enamel d.
    d. finger
    d. foot
    d. hand
    hanging d.
    d. heart
droplet
    d. infection
    d. nuclei
dropped beat
dropsical
dropsy
    abdominal d.
    cardiac d.
    epidemic d.
    famine d.
    nutritional d.
    d. of pericardium

drowning
    dry d.
    near d.
    secondary d.
drowsiness
drug
    d. eruption
    d. fever
    orphan d.'s
    d. psychosis
    d. rash
drug-fast
drug-induced
    d.-i. disease
    d.-i. lupus
drum, drumhead
    d. membrane
Drummond's sign
drumstick appendage
drunkenness
    sleep d.
drusen
    giant d.
    intrapapillary d.
    d. of the macula
    macular d.
    optic nerve d.
    d. of the optic nerve head
dry
    d. abscess
    d. amputation
    d. beriberi
    d. bronchiectasis
    d. cup
    d. cutaneous leishmaniasis
    d. dressing
    d. drowning
    d. eye syndrome
    d. gangrene
    d. hernia
    d. labor
    d. leprosy
    d. nurse
    d. pack
    d. pericarditis
    d. pleurisy
    d. rale
    d. socket
    d. synovitis
    d. tetter
    d. vomiting
D-S test
dual
    d. personality
    d. relationships
dual-cure resin
Duane's syndrome
Dubin-Johnson syndrome

Dubois'
    D. abscesses
    D. disease
DuBois' formula
Du Bois-Reymond's law
Dubowitz score
Dubreuil-Chambardel syndrome
Duchenne
    D. disease
    D. dystrophy
    D. sign
    D. syndrome
Duchenne-Aran disease
Duchenne-Erb paralysis
duck
    d. hepatitis virus
    d. influenza virus
    d. plague virus
duckbill speculum
Duckworth's phenomenon
Ducrey's bacillus
Ducrey test
duct
    aberrant d.'s
    aberrant bile d.'s
    accessory pancreatic d.
    alveolar d.
    amniotic d.
    anal d.'s
    arterial d.
    Bartholin's d.
    Bellini's d.'s
    Bernard's d.
    bile d.
    biliary d.
    Blasius' d.
    Botallo's d.
    bucconeural d.
    d. of bulbourethral gland
    canalicular d.'s
    d. carcinoma
    carotid d.
    cervical d.
    choledoch d.
    cochlear d.
    common bile d.
    common hepatic d.
    craniopharyngeal d.
    Cuvier's d.'s
    cystic d., cystic gall d.
    deferent d.
    efferent d.
    ejaculatory d.
    endolymphatic d.
    d. of epididymis
    excretory d.
    excretory d.'s of lacrimal gland
    excretory d. of seminal vesicle

frontonasal d.
galactophorous d.'s
gall d.
Gartner's d.
genital d.
guttural d.
hemithoracic d.
Hensen's d.
hepatic d.
hepatocystic d.
Hoffmann's d.
hypophysial d.
incisive d.
intercalated d.'s
interlobar d.
interlobular d.
intralobular d.
jugular d.
lactiferous d.'s
left d. of caudate lobe
left hepatic d.
longitudinal d. of epoöphoron
Luschka's d.'s
lymphatic d.
major sublingual d.
mamillary d.'s
mammary d.'s
mesonephric d.
metanephric d.
milk d.'s
minor sublingual d.'s
Müller's d., müllerian d.
nasal d.
nasolacrimal d.
nephric d.
omphalomesenteric d.
pancreatic d.
papillary d.'s
d. papilloma
paramesonephric d.
paraurethral d.'s
parotid d.
Pecquet's d.
perilymphatic d.
pharyngobranchial d.'s
pronephric d.
prostatic d.'s
right d. of caudate lobe
right hepatic d.
right lymphatic d.
Rivinus' d.'s
salivary d.
Santorini's d.
Schüller's d.'s
secretory d.
semicircular d.'s
seminal d.
d.'s of Skene's glands

D

duct *(continued)*
  spermatic d.
  Stensen's d., Steno's d.
  striated d.
  subclavian d.
  submandibular d.
  submaxillary d.
  sudoriferous d.
  sweat d.
  d. of sweat glands
  testicular d.
  thoracic d.
  thyroglossal d.
  thyrolingual d.
  umbilical d.
  uniting d.
  utriculosaccular d.
  vitelline d., vitellointestinal d.
  Walther's d.'s
  Wharton's d.
  Wirsung's d.
  wolffian d.
ductal
  d. aneurysm
  d. carcinoma
  d. hyperplasia
duction
  F d.
  forced d.
  passive d.
ductless
  d. glands
ductular
ductule
  aberrant d.'s
  biliary d.'s
  efferent d.'s of testis
  excretory d.'s of lacrimal gland
  inferior aberrant d.
  interlobular d.'s
  prostatic d.'s
  superior aberrant d.
  transverse d.'s of epoöphoron
ductulus, pl. **ductuli**
  d. aberrans inferior
  d. aberrans superior
  ductuli aberrantes
  d. alveolaris, pl. ductuli alveolares
  ductuli biliferi
  d. efferens testis, pl. ductuli
    efferentes testis
  ductuli excretorii glandulae
    lacrimalis
  ductuli interlobulares
  ductuli paroöphori
  ductuli prostatici
  ductuli transversi epoöphori
ductus, gen. and pl. **ductus**

  d. aberrantes
  d. arteriosus
  d. biliferi
  d. caroticus
  d. choledochus
  d. cochlearis
  d. cysticus
  d. deferens
  d. deferens vestigialis
  d. dorsopancreaticus
  d. ejaculatorius
  d. endolymphaticus
  d. epididymidis
  d. epoöphori longitudinalis
  d. excretorius
  d. excretorius vesiculae seminalis
  d. glandulae bulbourethralis
  d. hemithoracicus
  d. hepaticus communis
  d. hepaticus dexter
  d. hepaticus sinister
  d. incisivus
  d. lactiferi
  d. lingualis
  d. lobi caudati dexter
  d. lobi caudati sinister
  d. lymphaticus dexter
  d. mesonephricus
  d. nasolacrimalis
  d. pancreaticus
  d. pancreaticus accessorius
  d. paramesonephricus
  d. paraurethrales
  d. parotideus
  patent d. arteriosus
  d. perilymphaticus
  d. pharyngobranchialis III
  d. pharyngobranchialis IV
  d. prostatici
  d. reuniens
  d. semicirculares, d. semicircularis
    anterior, d. semicircularis lateralis,
    d. semicircularis posterior
  d. sublinguales minores
  d. sublingualis major
  d. submandibularis
  d. submaxillaris
  d. sudoriferus
  d. thoracicus
  d. thoracicus dexter
  d. thyroglossus
  d. utriculosaccularis
  d. venosus
  d. venosus arantii
Duddell's membrane
Duffy
  D. antigens
  D. blood group

Dugas' test
Duhring's disease
Dührssen's incisions
Duke bleeding time test
Dukes'
  D. classification
  D. disease
dull
dullness, dulness
  shifting d.
dumas
dumbbell ganglioneuroma
Dumdum fever
dummy
  d. consultand
Dumontpallier's pessary
dumping
  d. syndrome
Duncan's
  D. disease
  D. folds
  D. mechanism
  D. ventricle
duodena (pl. of duodenum)
duodenal
  d. ampulla
  d. bulb
  d. cap
  d. diverticulum
  d. fistula
  d. fossae
  d. glands
  d. impression
  d. smear
  d. sphincter
duodenectomy
duodeni (gen. of duodenum)
duodenitis
duodenocholangitis
duodenocholecystostomy
duodenocholedochotomy
duodenocystostomy
duodenoenterostomy
duodenojejunal
  d. angle
  d. flexure
  d. fold
  d. fossa
  d. hernia
  d. junction
  d. recess
  d. sphincter
duodenojejunostomy
duodenolysis
duodenomesocolic fold
duodenorenal ligament
duodenorrhaphy

duodenoscopy
duodenostomy
duodenotomy
duodenum, gen. duodeni, pl. duodena
duodoneal branches of superior
  pancreaticoduodenal artery
duovirus
Duplay's disease
duplex
  d. Doppler scan
  d. echocardiography
  d. kidney
  d. transmission
  d. ultrasonography
  d. uterus
duplication
  d. of chromosomes
  d. cyst
duplicitas
  d. anterior
  d. posterior
duplicity theory of vision
Dupré's muscle
Dupuy-Dutemps operation
Dupuytren's
  D. amputation
  D. canal
  D. contracture
  D. disease of the foot
  D. fascia
  D. fracture
  D. hydrocele
  D. sign
  D. suture
  D. tourniquet
duraencephalosynangiosis
dural
  d. sheath
  d. sheath of optic nerve
  d. venous sinuses
duralumin
dura mater
  d. m. of brain
  d. m. cranialis
  d. m. encephali
  d. m. of spinal cord
  d. m. spinalis
duramatral
duraplasty
duration
  half amplitude pulse d.
  pulse d.
  d. tetany
Dürck's nodes
Duret's
  D. hemorrhage
  D. lesion

D

Durham
    D. rule
    D. tube
Duroziez'
    D. disease
    D. murmur
    D. sign
dust
    d. asthma
    blood d.
    d. cell
    d. corpuscles
Dutton's
    D. disease
    D. relapsing fever
Duverney's
    D. fissures
    D. foramen
    D. gland
    D. muscle
dwarf
    hypophysial d.
    hypothyroid d.
    d. pelvis
    pituitary d.
dwarfed enamel
dwarfishness
dwarfism
    achondroplastic d.
    acromelic d.
    aortic d.
    asexual d.
    ateliotic d.
    camptomelic d.
    chondrodystrophic d.
    diastrophic d.
    disproportionate d.
    Fröhlich's d.
    hypothyroid d.
    infantile d.
    Laron type d.
    lethal d.
    Lorain-Lévi d.
    mesomelic d.
    metatropic d.
    micromelic d.
    phocomelic d.
    physiologic d.
    pituitary d.
    polydystrophic d.
    primordial d.
    Robinow d.
    Seckel d.
    senile d.
    sexual d.
    Silver-Russell d.
    snub-nose d.

    thanatophoric d.
    true d.
dyadic
    d. psychotherapy
    d. symbiosis
dye
    acidic d.'s
    acridine d.'s
    azin d.'s
    azocarmine d.'s
    basic d.'s
    diphenylmethane d.'s
    d. exclusion test
    ketonimine d.'s
    natural d.'s
    nitro d.'s
    oxazin d.'s
    rosanilin d.'s
    salt d.
    synthetic d.'s
    thiazin d.'s
    triphenylmethane d.'s
    xanthene d.'s
dye-dilution curve
Dyggve-Melchior-Clausen syndrome
dynamic
    d. aorta
    d. compliance of lung
    d. computed tomography
    d. CT
    d. demography
    d. disease
    d. friction
    group d.'s
    d. ileus
    d. murmur
    d. platform posturography
    d. psychiatry
    d. psychology
    d. psychotherapy
    d. refraction
    d. relations
    d. splint
    d. viscosity
dynamogenesis
dynamogenic
dynamogeny
dynamograph
dynamometer
dynamoscope
dynamoscopy
dynatherm
dynein arm
dysacousia, dysacusia
dysacusis
dysadaptation
dysantigraphia
dysaphia

dysaphic
dysarteriotony
dysarthria
    ataxic d.
    hyperkinetic d.
    hypokinetic d.
    d. literalis
    lower motor neuron d.
    rigid d.
    spastic d.
    d. syllabaris spasmodica
dysarthric
dysarthrosis
dysautonomia
    familial d.
dysbarism
dysbasia
    d. angiosclerotica, d. angiospastica
    d. lordotica progressiva
dysbolism
dysbulia
dysbulic
dyscalculia
dyscephalia
    d. mandibulo-oculofacialis
dyscephaly
dyscheiral, dyschiral
dyscheiria, dyschiria
dyschezia
dyschiral (var. of dyscheiral)
dyschondrogenesis
dyschondroplasia
    d. with hemangiomas
dyschondrosteosis
dyschroia, dyschroa
dyschromatopsia
dyschromatosis
dyschromia
dyscinesia
dyscoimesis
dysconjugate gaze
dyscontrol
dyscoria
dyscrasia
    blood d.
    plasma cell d.
dyscrasic, dyscratic
    d. fracture
dysdiadochokinesia, dysdiadochocinesia
dysdiadochokinesis
dysembryoma
dysembryoplasia
dysembryoplastic neuroepithelial tumor
dysemia
dysencephalia splanchnocystica
dysenteric
    d. algid malaria
    d. diarrhea

dysentery
    amebic d.
    bacillary d.
    d. bacillus
    balantidial d.
    bilharzial d.
    fulminating d.
    helminthic d.
    Japanese d.
    malignant d.
    Sonne d.
    spirillar d.
    viral d.
dyserethism
dysergia
dysesthesia
dysfibrinogenemia
dysfunction
    constitutional hepatic d.
    dental d.
    Le Fort III craniofacial d.
    minimal brain d.
    papillary muscle d.
    phagocyte d.
    placental d.
    psychosexual d., sexual d.
    sphincter of Oddi d.
    temporomandibular joint d.
dysfunctional uterine bleeding
dysgammaglobulinemia
dysgenesis
    gonadal d., XO gonadal d., XX
      gonadal d., XY gonadal d.
    iridocorneal mesodermal d.
    seminiferous tubule d.
    testicular d.
dysgenic
dysgerminoma
dysgeusia
dysgnathia
dysgnathic
dysgnosia
dysgonic
dysgranular cortex
dysgraphia
dysharmonious correspondence
dyshematopoiesis
dyshematopoietic
dyshemopoiesis
dyshemopoietic
    d. anemia
dyshidria
dyshidrosis
dysidria
dysidrosis
dysjunctive nystagmus
dyskaryosis
dyskaryotic

D

dyskeratoma
    warty d.
dyskeratosis
    benign d.
    d. congenita
    hereditary benign intraepithelial d.
    intraepithelial d.
    isolated d. follicularis
    malignant d.
dyskeratotic
dyskinesia
    d. algera
    biliary d.
    extrapyramidal d.'s
    d. intermittens
    lingual-facial-buccal d.
    tardive d.
    tracheobronchial d.
dyskinetic
dyslexia
dyslexic
dyslogia
dysmasesis
dysmature
    placental d.
dysmaturity
dysmelia
dysmenorrhea
    essential d.
    functional d.
    intrinsic d.
    mechanical d.
    membranous d.
    obstructive d.
    ovarian d.
    primary d.
    secondary d.
    spasmodic d.
    tubal d.
    ureteric d.
    uterine d.
    vaginal d.
dysmenorrheal membrane
dysmetria
    ocular d.
dysmimia
dysmnesia
dysmnesic
    d. psychosis
    d. syndrome
dysmorphia
dysmorphism
dysmorphogenesis
dysmorphology
dysmorphophobia
dysmyelination
dysmyotonia
dysnystaxis

dysodontiasis
dysontogenesis
dysontogenetic
dysorexia
dysosmia
dysosteogenesis
dysostosis
    acrofacial d.
    cleidocranial d., clidocranial d.
    craniofacial d.
    mandibuloacral d.
    mandibulofacial d.
    metaphysial d.
    d. multiplex
    orodigitofacial d.
    otomandibular d.
    peripheral d.
dyspallia
dyspareunia
dyspepsia
    acid d.
    adhesion d.
    atonic d.
    fermentative d.
    flatulent d.
    functional d.
    nervous d.
    reflex d.
dyspeptic
dysphagia, dysphagy
    d. lusoria
    d. nervosa, nervous d.
    sideropenic d.
    vallecular d.
dysphagocytosis
    congenital d.
dysphasia
dysphemia
dysphonia
    d. plicae ventricularis
    spastic d.
    d. spastica
dysphoria
dysphrasia
dysphylaxia
dyspigmentation
dyspinealism
dyspituitarism
dysplasia
    anhidrotic ectodermal d.
    anterofacial d., anteroposterior d.,
      anteroposterior facial d.
    asphyxiating thoracic d.
    bronchopulmonary d.
    cemental d. (*var. of* florid
      osseous d.)
    cerebral d.
    cervical d.

chondroectodermal d.
cleidocranial d., clidocranial d.
congenital ectodermal d.
cortical d.
craniocarpotarsal d.
craniodiaphysial d.
craniometaphysial d.
dentin d.
diaphysial d.
ectodermal d.
enamel d.
d. epiphysialis hemimelia
d. epiphysialis multiplex
d. epiphysialis punctata
epithelial d.
faciodigitogenital d.
familial white folded d.
fibromuscular d.
fibrous d. of bone
fibrous d. of jaws
florid osseous d., cemental d.
hidrotic ectodermal d.
hypohidrotic ectodermal d.
lymphopenic thymic d.
mammary d.
mandibulofacial d.
metaphysial d.
Mondini d.
monostotic fibrous d.
mucoepithelial d.
multiple epiphysial d.
neuronal intestinal d.
oculoauriculovertebral d., OAV d.
oculodentodigital d.
oculovertebral d.
odontogenic d.
ophthalmomandibulomelic d.
periapical cemental d.
polyostotic fibrous d.
pseudoachondroplastic
  spondyloepiphysial d.
retinal d.
septo-optic d.
spondyloepiphysial d.
ventriculoradial d.
dysplastic
d. nevus
d. nevus syndrome
dyspnea
cardiac d.
exertional d.
expiratory d.
functional d.
nocturnal d.
paroxysmal nocturnal d.
Traube's d.
dyspneic
dyspraxia

dysproteinemia
dysproteinemic
d. retinopathy
dysraphism, dysraphia
dysrhythmia
cardiac d.
electroencephalographic d.
esophageal d.
paroxysmal cerebral d.
dyssebacia, dyssebacea
dyssomnia
dysspermatogenic sterility
dysspondylism
dysstasia
dysstatic
dyssyllabia
dyssynergia
d. cerebellaris myoclonica
detrusor sphincter d.
dystasia
hereditary areflexic d.
dystelephalangy
dysthymia
dysthymic
d. disorder
dysthyroidal infantilism
dystocia
fetal d.
maternal d.
placental d.
dystonia
d. lenticularis
d. musculorum deformans
torsion d.
dystonic
d. reaction
d. torticollis
dystopia
dystopic
dystrophia
d. adiposogenitalis
d. brevicollis
d. myotonica
d. unguium
dystrophic
d. calcification
d. calcinosis
dystrophy
adiposogenital d.
adult pseudohypertrophic
  muscular d.
Barnes' d.
Becker type muscular d.
Becker type tardive muscular d.
childhood muscular d.
cone d.
corneal d.
craniocarpotarsal d.

D

267

dystrophy *(continued)*
   Duchenne d.
   endothelial d. of cornea
   epithelial d.
   facioscapulohumeral muscular d.
   Favre's d.
   fingerprint d.
   fleck d. of cornea
   Fuchs' epithelial d.
   Groenouw's corneal d.
   gutter d. of cornea
   hypertrophic d.
   infantile neuroaxonal d.
   juvenile epithelial corneal d.
   Landouzy-Dejerine d.
   lattice corneal d.
   Leyden-Möbius muscular d.
   limb-girdle muscular d.
   macular d.
   map-dot-fingerprint d.
   Meesman d.
   microcystic epithelial d.
   mucopolysaccharide keratin d.

   muscular d.
   myotonic d.
   neuroaxonal d.
   oculopharyngeal d.
   pelvofemoral muscular d.
   progressive muscular d.
   progressive tapetochoroidal d.
   pseudohypertrophic muscular d.
   reflex sympathetic d.
   reticular d. of cornea
   ring-like corneal d.
   scapulohumeral muscular d.
   sympathetic reflex d.
   thoracic-pelvic-phalangeal d.
   twenty-nail d.
   vitreo-tapetoretinal d.
   vulvar d.
dystropy
dysuria
dysuric
dysury
dysversion

EAC
> EAC rosette
> EAC rosette assay

Eagle
> E. basal medium
> E. minimum essential medium
> E. syndrome

Eagle-Barrett syndrome
EAHF complex
Eales' disease
ear
> aviator's e.
> Aztec e.
> bat e.
> Blainville e.'s
> e. bones
> boxer's e.
> Cagot e.
> cauliflower e.
> e. crystals
> darwinian e.
> dog e.
> external e.
> glue e.
> inner e.
> internal e.
> e. lobe
> e. lobe crease
> lop e.
> middle e.
> Morel's e.
> Mozart e.
> scroll e.
> Stahl's e.
> swimmer's e.
> e. wax
> Wildermuth's e.

earache
eardrum
Earle
> E. L fibrosarcoma
> E. solution

early
> e. deceleration
> e. diastolic murmur
> e. infantile autism
> e. juvenile type
> e. latent syphilis
> e. neonatal death
> e. posttraumatic epilepsy
> e. reaction
> e. receptor potential
> e. seizure
> e. syphilis

early-phase response

earth-eating
earwax
East
> E. African sleeping sickness
> E. African trypanosomiasis

eastern equine encephalomyelitis virus
eat
eating
> e. disorders
> e. epilepsy

Eaton
> E. agent
> E. agent pneumonia

Eaton-Lambert syndrome
Ebbinghaus test
Eberth's
> E. bacillus
> E. lines
> E. perithelium

Ebner's
> E. glands
> E. reticulum

Ebola
> E. hemorrhagic fever
> E. virus

ebonation
ébranlement
Ebstein's
> E. anomaly
> E. disease
> E. sign

ebullism
ebur
> e. dentis

eburnation
> e. of dentin

eburneous
eburnitis
EB virus
écarteur
eccentric
> e. amputation
> e. fixation
> e. hypertrophy
> e. interocclusal record
> e. occlusion
> e. position
> e. relation

eccentrochondroplasia
eccentropiesis
ecchondroma
ecchondrosis
ecchondrotome
ecchordosis physaliformis, ecchordosis
> **physaliphora**

E

ecchymoma
ecchymosed
ecchymosis
    bilateral medial orbital e.'s
    Tardieu's e.'s
ecchymotic
    e. mask
eccrine
    e. acrospiroma
    e. gland
    e. poroma
    e. spiradenoma
eccrinology
eccrisis
eccyesis
ecdemic
ecdysial glands
ecdysiasm
ECG trigger
echeosis
echinate
Echinochasmus
echinococciasis
Echinococcus
    E. vogeli
echinococcus
    e. cyst
    e. disease
echinocyte
Echinorhynchus
echinosis
Echinostoma
    E. ilocanum
    E. malayanum
echinulate
echo
    atrial e.
    e. beat
    nodus sinuatrialis e., NS e.
    e. planar
    e. reaction
    e. speech
    spin e.
echoacousia
echoaortography
echocardiogram
echocardiographic differentiation
echocardiography
    B-mode e.
    contrast e.
    cross-sectional e.
    Doppler e.
    duplex e.
    stress e.
    transesophageal e.
    transthoracic e.
    two-dimensional e.
echoencephalography

echo-free
echogenic
echogram
echographer
echographia
echography
echokinesis, echokinesia
echolalia
echomatism
echomimia
echomotism
echopathy
echophony, echophonia
echophotony
echophrasia
echopraxia
echoscope
ECHO virus
echovirus
    E. 28
Ecker's fissure
Eck fistula
eclabium
eclampsia
    puerperal e.
    superimposed e.
eclamptic
    e. retinopathy
eclamptogenic, eclamptogenous
eclectic
eclipse
    e. blindness
    e. period
    e. phase
ecmnesia
ECMO virus
ecoid
ecological fallacy
ecological system
ecology
    human e.
ecomania
economy
ecophobia
ecosystem
    parasite-host e.
ecotaxis
ecotropic virus
écouteur
écouvillon
ecphoria
ecphorize
ecphyma
écraseur
ECSO virus
ecstasy
ecstatic
ecstrophe

ectacolia
ectad
ectal
    e. origin
ectasia, ectasis
    annuloaortic e.
    aortoannular e.
    e. cordis
    corneal e.
    diffuse arterial e.
    familial aortic e.
    hypostatic e.
    mammary duct e.
    papillary e.   *Telangiectasia*
    scleral e.
    senile e.
    e. ventriculi paradoxa
ectatic
    e. aneurysm
    e. emphysema
    e. marginal degeneration of cornea
ectental
ectethmoid
ecthyma
    e. gangrenosum
ecthymatiform, ecthymiform
ecthymatous syphilid
ectiris
ectoantigen
ectoblast
ectocardia
ectocervical
    e. smear
ectochoroidea
ectocornea
ectocyst
ectoderm
    amniotic e.
    blastodermic e.
    chorionic e.
    epithelial e.
    extraembryonic e.
    superficial e.
ectodermal
    e. cloaca
    e. dysplasia
ectodermatosis
ectodermic
ectodermosis
    e. erosiva pluriorificialis
ectoentad
ectoental
ectoethmoid
ectogenic teratosis
ectogenous
ectoglobular
ectomere
ectomerogony

ectomesenchyme
ectomorph
ectomorphic
ectopagus
ectoparasite
ectoparasitism
ectoperitonitis
ectophyte
ectopia   *crossed fused ectopia*
    e. cloacae
    e. cordis
    crossed renal e.
    crossed testicular e.
    e. lentis
    e. maculae
    e. pupillae congenita
    e. renis
    e. testis
    testis e.
    e. vesicae
ectopic
    e. ACTH syndrome
    e. beat
    e. decidua
    e. eyelash
    e. hormone
    e. impulse
    e. pacemaker
    e. pinealoma
    e. pregnancy
    e. rhythm
    e. schistosomiasis
    e. tachycardia
    e. teratosis
    e. testis
    e. ureter
ectoplacental cavity
ectoplasm
ectoplasmatic, ektoplasmic, ektoplastic
ectopy
ectoretina
ectosarc
ectoscopy
ectosteal
ectostosis
ectothrix
ectotrophoblastic cavity
ectozoon
ectrocheiry, ectrochiry
ectrodactyly, ectrodactylia, ectrodactylism
ectrogenic
ectrogeny
ectromelia virus
ectromelic
ectropion, ectropium
    atonic e.
    cicatricial e.
    flaccid e.

E

271

ectropion *(continued)*
 paralytic e.
 spastic e.
 e. uveae
ectropody
ectrosyndactyly
ectype
ecuresis
eczema
 allergic e.
 atopic e.
 baker's e.
 chronic e.
 e. craquelé
 e. diabeticorum
 e. epilans
 e. erythematosum
 flexural e.
 hand e.
 e. herpeticum
 e. hypertrophicum
 infantile e.
 e. intertrigo
 lichenoid e.
 e. marginatum
 nummular e.
 e. nummulare
 e. papulosum
 e. parasiticum
 e. pustulosum
 e. rubrum
 seborrheic e.
 e. squamosum
 stasis e.
 tropical e.
 e. tyloticum
 e. vaccinatum
 varicose e.
 e. verrucosum
 e. vesiculosum
 weeping e.
 winter e.
eczematization
eczematoid
 e. seborrhea
eczematous
eddy sounds
edea
edema
 ambulant e.
 angioneurotic e.
 Berlin's e.
 blue e.
 brain e.
 brawny e.
 brown e.
 bullous e.
 bullous e. vesicae

cachectic e.
cardiac e.
cerebral e.
cystoid macular e.
dependent e.
gestational e.
e. glottidis
heat e.
hereditary angioneurotic e.
hydremic e.
infantile acute hemorrhagic e. of
 the skin
inflammatory e.
lymphatic e.
marantic e.
menstrual e.
e. neonatorum
nephrotic e.
noninflammatory e.
nonpitting e.
nutritional e.
periodic e.
pitting e.
premenstrual e.
pulmonary e.
Quincke's e.
salt e.
solid e.
Yangtze e.
edematization
edematous
Eder-Pustow bougie
edge
 cutting e.
 denture e.
 e. enhancement
 incisal e.
 leading e.
 shearing e.
edge-to-edge
 e.-t.-e. bite
 e.-t.-e. occlusion
edgewise appliance
Edinger-Westphal nucleus
Edridge-Green lamp
education
 health e.
educational psychology
Edwardsiella
Edwards' syndrome
EEE virus
EEG activation
effect
 abscopal e.
 after-e.
 Anrep e.
 Arias-Stella e.
 autokinetic e.

Bowditch e.
clasp-knife e.
Compton e.
Cushing e.
cytopathic e.
Doppler e.
electrophonic e.
experimenter e.'s
Fahraeus-Lindqvist e.
Fenn e.
founder e.
gene dosage e.
generation e.
Haldane e.
halo e.
Hawthorne e.
healthy worker e.
Mach e.
e. modifier
Orbeli e.
oxygen e.
photechic e.
piezoelectric e.
position e.
Rivero-Carvallo e.
Russell e.
second gas e.
sigma e.
Somogyi e.
Staub-Traugott e.
Stiles-Crawford e.
Venturi e.
Wedensky e.
Wolff-Chaikoff e.
Zeeman e.

effective
e. conjugate
e. half-life
e. refractory period
e. renal blood flow
e. renal plasma flow
e. temperature index
effectiveness
relative biological e.
effector cell
effemination
efferent
e. duct
e. ductules of testis
e. fibers
gamma e.
e. glomerular arteriole
e. lymphatic
e. nerve
e. vessel
efficacy
efficiency
visual e.

effleurage
effluvium, pl. **effluvia**
anagen e.
telogen e.
effort
distributed e.
e. syndrome
effort-induced thrombosis
effuse
effusion
joint e.
pericardial e.
pleural e.
subpulmonic e.
egersis
egesta
egg
e. cell
e. cluster
e. membrane
e. shell nail
Egger's line
Eggleston method
eggshell calcification
egg-white
e.-w. injury
e.-w. syndrome
Eglis' glands
ego
e. analysis
e. ideal
e. identity
e. instincts
ego-alien
egobronchophony
egocentric
egocentricity
ego-dystonic
e.-d. homosexuality
ego-ideal
egomania
egophonic
egophony
ego-syntonic
egotropic
Egyptian
E. hematuria
E. ophthalmia
E. splenomegaly
Ehlers-Danlos syndrome
Ehrenritter's ganglion
Ehret's phenomenon
Ehrlichia
E. canis
E. chaffeensis
E. risticii
E. sennetsu
Ehrlichieae

E

ehrlichiosis
    human e.
    human granulocytic e.
Ehrlich's
    E. acid hematoxylin stain
    E. anemia
    E. aniline crystal violet stain
    E. benzaldehyde reaction
    E. diazo reaction
    E. inner body
    E. phenomenon
    E. side-chain theory
    E. triacid stain
    E. triple stain
Ehrlich-Türk line
Eichhorst's
    E. corpuscles
    E. neuritis
Eicken's method
eidetic
    e. image
eighth
    e. cranial nerve
    e. nerve
    e. nerve tumor
Eikenella corrodens
eikonometer
eiloid
Eimeria
    E. sardinae
Eimeriidae
Einarson's gallocyanin-chrome alum stain
Einthoven's
    E. equation
    E. law
    E. string galvanometer
    E. triangle
Eisenlohr's syndrome
Eisenmenger's
    E. complex
    E. defect
    E. disease
    E. syndrome
    E. tetralogy
eisodic
ejaculate
ejaculatio
    e. deficiens
    e. praecox
    e. retardata
ejaculation
    premature e.
ejaculatory
    e. duct
ejecta
ejection
    e. click

    e. fraction
    e. murmur
    e. period
    e. sounds
ejector
    saliva e.
Ejrup maneuver
Ekbom syndrome
EKG trigger
ekiri
ektoplasmic (*var. of* ectoplasmatic)
ektoplastic (*var. of* ectoplasmatic)
elaboration
    secondary e.
Elaeophora schneideri
elaiopathia
elastance
elastic
    e. artery
    e. bandage
    e. band fixation
    e. bougie
    e. cartilage
    e. cone
    e. fibers
    intermaxillary e.
    e. lamella
    e. laminae of arteries
    e. layers of arteries
    e. layers of cornea
    e. ligature
    e. membrane
    e. skin
    vertical e.
elastica
elasticity
    physical e. of muscle
    physiologic e. of muscle
    total e. of muscle
elastofibroma
elastoid degeneration
elastolysis
    generalized e.
elastoma
    juvenile e.
    Miescher's e.
elastometer
elastorrhexis
elastosis
    e. colloidalis conglomerata
    e. dystrophica
    e. perforans serpiginosa
    solar e.
elastotic degeneration
elation
Elaut's triangle
elbow
    e. bone

e. jerk
e. joint
Little Leaguer's e.
miner's e.
nursemaid's e.
e. reflex
tennis e.
elbowed
e. bougie
e. catheter
elder abuse
elective
e. abortion
e. culture
e. mutism
Electra complex
electric
e. anesthesia
e. bath
e. cardiac pacemaker
e. cataract
e. cautery
e. chorea
e. dermatome
e. irritability
e. retinopathy
e. shock
e. sleep
electrical
e. alternans
e. alternation of heart
e. axis
e. diastole
e. failure
e. formula
e. heart position
e. systole
electroanalgesia
electroanesthesia
electroaxonography
electrobasograph
electrobasography
electrobioscopy
electrocardiogram
scalar e.
unipolar e.
electrocardiograph
electrocardiographic
e. complex
e. wave
electrocardiography
fetal e.
precordial e.
electrocardiophonogram
electrocardiophonography
electrocauterization
electrocautery

electrocerebral inactivity
electrocerebral silence
electrocholecystectomy
electrocholecystocausis
electrocoagulation
electrocochleogram
electrocochleography
electrocontractility
electroconvulsive
e. therapy
electrocorticogram
electrocorticography
electrocute
electrocution
electrocystography
electrode
active e.
e. catheter ablation
central terminal e.
dispersing e.
exciting e.
exploring e.
indifferent e.
ion-selective e.'s
e. knife
localizing e.
silent e.
therapeutic e.
electrodermal
e. audiometry
electrodermatome
electrodesiccation
electrodiagnosis
electroencephalogram
flat e.
isoelectric e.
electroencephalograph
electroencephalographic dysrhythmia
electroencephalography
electrogastrogram
electrogastrograph
electrogastrography
electrogram
His bundle e.
electrographic seizure
electrohemostasis
electrohydraulic shock wave lithotripsy
electrohysterograph
electroimmunodiffusion
electrokymogram
electrokymograph
electrolyzer
electromagnetic
e. flowmeter
e. induction
e. radiation
electromassage

E

electromechanical
    e. dissociation
    e. systole
electromicturation
electromotive force
electromuscular sensibility
electromyogram
electromyograph
electromyography
electron
    e. beam
    e. capture
    e. interferometer
    e. interferometry
    e. micrograph
    e. microscope
    e. microscopy
    e. radiography
    transition e.
electronarcosis
electroneurography
electroneurolysis
electroneuromyography
electronic
    e. cell counter
    e. fetal monitor
    e. pacemaker
    e. pacemaker load
electronystagmography
electro-oculogram
electro-oculography
electro-olfactogram
electroparacentesis
electropathology
electrophobia
electrophonic effect
electrophoresis
    capillary zone e.
    isoenzyme e.
    lipoprotein e.
    pulsed-field gel e.
electrophototherapy
electrophrenic
    e. respiration
electrophysiologic audiometry
electrophysiology
electropneumograph
electropuncture
electroradiology
electroradiometer
electroretinogram
electroretinography
electroscission
electroshock
    e. therapy
electrospectrography
electrospinogram
electrospinography

electrostenolysis
electrostethograph
electrosurgery
electrotaxis
    negative e.
    positive e.
electrothanasia
electrotherapeutic
    e. bath
    e. sleep
    e. sleep therapy
electrotherapeutics, electrotherapy
electrotherm
electrotome
electrotomy
electrotonic
    e. current
    e. junction
    e. synapse
electrotonus
electrotropism
eleidin
element
    anatomical e.
    copia e.'s
    extrachromosomal e.,
        extrachromosomal genetic e.
    fold-back e.'s
    labile e.'s
    morphologic e.
    P e.'s
    picture e.
    volume e.
elementary
    e. bodies
    e. granule
    e. particle
eleoma
eleopathy
eleotherapy
elephantiac, elephantiasic
elephantiasis
    congenital e.
    gingival e.
    e. neuromatosa
    nevoid e.
    e. scroti
    e. telangiectodes
    e. vulvae
elephant leg
elephantoid fever
eleutheromania
elevation
    tactile e.'s
elevator
    e. disease
    e. muscle of anus
    e. muscle of prostate

e. muscle of rib
e. muscle of scapula
e. muscle of soft palate
e. muscle of thyroid gland
e. muscle of upper eyelid
e. muscle of upper lip
e. muscle of upper lip and wing
   of nose
periosteal e.
screw e.
eleventh cranial nerve
elfin facies
elimination
carbon dioxide e.
e. diet
elinguation
elinin
Ellik evacuator
Elliot's
E. operation
E. position
Elliott's law
ellipsis
ellipsoid
ellipsoidal joint
elliptical
e. amputation
e. anastomosis
e. recess
elliptocytary anemia
elliptocytic anemia
elliptocytosis
elliptocytotic anemia
Ellis
E. type 1 glomerulonephritis
E. type 2 glomerulonephritis
E. type 1 nephritis
Ellis-van Creveld syndrome
Ellsworth-Howard test
Eloesser procedure
Elschnig
E. pearls
E. spots
El Tor vibrio
elusive ulcer
emaciation
emaculation
emanation
actinium e.
radium e.
thorium e.
emanatorium
emancipation
emanon
emanotherapy
emarginate
emargination

emasculation
EMB
E. agar
Embadomonas
embalm
embed
embedding agents
embolalia
embole
embolectomy
embolemia
emboli (*pl. of* embolus)
embolia
embolic
e. abscess
e. gangrene
e. infarct
e. pneumonia
emboliform
e. nucleus
embolism
air e.
amniotic fluid e.
atheroma e.
bland e.
bone marrow e.
cellular e.
cholesterol e.
cotton-fiber e.
crossed e.
direct e.
fat e.
gas e.
hematogenous e.
infective e.
lymph e., lymphogenous e.
miliary e.
multiple e.
obturating e.
oil e.
pantaloon e.
paradoxical e.
pulmonary e.
pyemic e.
retinal e.
retrograde e.
riding e.
saddle e.
straddling e.
tumor e.
venous e.
embolization
embololalia
embolomycotic
e. aneurysm
embolophasia
embolophrasia

E

embolotherapy
embolus, pl. **emboli**
    catheter e.
emboly
embouchement
embrasure
    buccal e.
    gingival e.
    incisal e.
    labial e.
    lingual e.
    occlusal e.
embryatrics
embryo
    heterogametic e.
    hexacanth e.
    homogametic e.
    oncosphere e.
    presomite e.
    e. transfer
embryoblast
embryocardia
    jugular e.
embryogenesis
embryogenic, embryogenetic
embryogeny
embryoid
embryologist
embryology
embryoma
    e. of the kidney
embryomorphous
embryonal
    e. adenoma
    e. area
    e. carcinoma
    e. carcinosarcoma
    e. leukemia
    e. medulloepithelioma
    e. rhabdomyosarcomas
    e. tumor
    e. tumor of ciliary body
embryonate
embryonic
    e. anideus
    e. area
    e. axis
    e. blastoderm
    e. cataract
    e. cell
    e. circulation
    e. diapause
    e. disk
    e. membrane
    e. shield
    e. tumor
embryoniform
embryonization

Embospheres

embryonoid
embryony
embryopathic cataract
embryopathy
embryophore
embryoplastic
embryotomy
embryotoxicity
embryotoxon
    anterior e.
    posterior e.
embryotrophic
embryotrophy
EMC virus
emedullate
emeiocytosis
emergence
    property e.
emergency
    e. theory
emergent
    e. evolution
emerging viruses
emery disks
emesis
    e. basin
EMG
    EMG biofeedback
    EMG examination
    EMG syndrome
emiction
emigration
    e. theory
eminence
    abducens e.
    arcuate e.
    articular e. of temporal bone
    canine e.
    collateral e.
    e. of concha
    cruciate e.
    cruciform e.
    deltoid e.
    Doyère's e.
    facial e.
    forebrain e.
    frontal e.
    genital e.
    hypobranchial e.
    hypoglossal e.
    hypothenar e.
    ileocecal e.
    iliopectineal e.
    iliopubic e.
    intercondylar e., intercondyloid e.
    maxillary e.
    medial e.
    median e.

olivary e.
orbital e. of zygomatic bone
parietal e.
pyramidal e.
radial e. of wrist
restiform e.
round e.
e. of scapha
thenar e.
thyroid e.
e. of triangular fossa of auricle
ulnar e. of wrist
eminentia, pl. **eminentiae**
    e. abducentis
    e. arcuata
    e. articularis ossis temporalis
    e. carpi radialis
    e. carpi ulnaris
    e. collateralis
    e. conchae
    e. cruciformis
    e. facialis
    e. fossae triangularis auricularis
    e. frontalis
    e. hypoglossi
    e. hypothenaris
    e. iliopubica
    e. intercondylaris
    e. intercondyloidea
    e. maxillae
    e. medialis
    e. mediana
    e. orbitalis ossis zygomatici
    e. parietalis
    e. pyramidalis
    e. restiformis
    e. scaphae
    e. symphysis
    e. teres
    e. thena'ris
    e. triangularis
    vagi e.
emiocytosis
EMI scan
emissarium
    e. condyloideum
    e. mastoideum
    e. occipitale
    e. parietale
emissary
    e. sphenoidal foramen
    e. vein
emission
    characteristic e.
    nocturnal e.
emmenia
emmenic
emmeniopathy

emmenology
emmetropia
emmetropic
emmetropization
Emmet's
    E. needle
    E. operation
Emmonsiella capsulata
emotion
emotional
    e. age
    e. amenorrhea
    e. amnesia
    e. attitudes
    e. deprivation
    e. disease
    e. disorder
    e. disturbance
    e. leukocytosis
    e. overlay
    e. tone
emotiovascular
empathic
    e. index
empathize
empathy
    generative e.
emperipolesis
emphlysis
emphractic
emphraxis
emphysema
    alveolar duct e.
    bullous e.
    centri-acinar e.
    centrilobular e.
    compensating e., compensatory e.
    congenital lobar e.
    cutaneous e.
    diffuse e.
    diffuse obstructive e.
    ectatic e.
    familial e.
    gangrenous e.
    generalized e.
    increased markings e.
    interlobular e.
    interstitial e.
    intestinal e.
    irregular e.
    mediastinal e.
    panacinar e.
    panlobular e.
    paraseptal e.
    pulmonary e.
    senile e.
    subcutaneous e.
    subgaleal e.

E

emphysema *(continued)*
    surgical e.
    unilateral lobar e.
emphysematous
    e. cholecystitis
    e. cystitis
    e. gangrene
    e. phlegmon
empiric
    e. risk
    e. treatment
empiricism
emprosthotonos
empty sella
empyectomy
empyema
    e. articuli
    e. benignum
    e. of gallbladder
    latent e.
    loculated e.
    mastoid e.
    e. necessitatis
    e. of the pericardium
    pneumococcal e.
    pulsating e.
    streptococcal e.
    e. tube
empyemic
    e. scoliosis
empyesis
empyocele
E-M syndrome
emuresis
enamel
    e. cap
    e. cell
    e. cleavage
    e. cleaver
    e. crypt
    e. cuticle
    e. drop
    dwarfed e.
    e. dysplasia
    e. epithelium
    e. fibers
    e. fissure
    e. germ
    e. hypocalcification
    e. hypoplasia
    e. lamella
    e. layer
    e. ledge
    e. membrane
    mottled e.
    nanoid e.
    e. niche
    e. nodule

    e. organ
    e. pearl
    e. prisms
    e. projection
    e. pulp
    e. rod inclination
    e. rods
    e. rod sheath
    e. tuft
    e. wall
    whorled e.
enameloblast
enamelogenesis
    e. imperfecta
enameloma
enamelum
enanthem, enanthema
enanthematous
enanthesis
enarthrodial
    e. joint
enarthrosis
en bloc
encapsulated
    e. delusion
encapsulation
encapsuled
encarditis
encatarrhaphy
encelitis, enceliitis
encephala (*pl. of* encephalon)
encephalalgia
encephalatrophic
encephalatrophy
encephalauxe
encephalemia
encephalic
    e. vesicle
encephalitic
encephalitis, pl. encephalitides
    acute hemorrhagic e.
    acute inclusion body e.
    acute necrotizing e.
    Australian X e.
    bacterial e.
    Coxsackie e.
    Dawson's e.
    epidemic e.
    experimental allergic e.
    Far East Russian e.
    e. hemorrhagica
    herpes e.
    herpes simplex e.
    hyperergic e.
    Ilhéus e.
    inclusion body e.
    Japanese B e.
    e. japonica

lead e.
e. lethargica
Mengo e.
Murray Valley e.
necrotizing e.
e. neonatorum
e. periaxialis concentrica
e. periaxialis diffusa
postvaccinal e.
Powassan e.
purulent e.
e. pyogenica
Russian autumn e.
Russian spring-summer e. (Eastern subtype)
Russian spring-summer e. (Western subtype)
Russian tick-borne e.
secondary e.
subacute inclusion body e.
e. subcorticalis chronica
suppurative e.
tick-borne e. (Central European subtype)
tick-borne e. (Eastern subtype)
van Bogaert e.
varicella e.
vernal e.
e. virus
woodcutter's e.
encephalitogen
encephalitogenic
Encephalitozoon
E. cuniculi
E. hellum
encephalization
encephalocele
encephaloclastic microcephaly
encephalocraniocutaneous lipomatosis
encephalocystocele
encephaloduroarteriosynangios
encephalodynia
encephalodysplasia
encephalogram
encephalography
gamma e.
encephaloid
e. cancer
encephalolith
encephalology
encephaloma
encephalomalacia
encephalomeningitis
encephalomeningocele
encephalomeningopathy
encephalomere
encephalometer

encephalomyelitis
acute disseminated e.
acute necrotizing hemorrhagic e.
e. associated with carcinoma
benign myalgic e.
epidemic myalgic e.
experimental allergic e.
granulomatous e.
herpes B e.
postvaccinal e.
viral e., virus e.
zoster e.
encephalomyelocele
encephalomyeloneuropathy
encephalomyelonic axis
encephalomyelopathy
carcinomatous e.
epidemic myalgic e.
necrotizing e.
paracarcinomatous e.
paraneoplastic e.
subacute necrotizing e.
encephalomyeloradiculitis
encephalomyeloradiculopathy
encephalomyocarditis
e. virus
encephalon, pl. **encephala**
encephalonarcosis
encephalopathia
e. addisonia
encephalopathy
bilirubin e.
Binswanger's e.
demyelinating e.
hepatic e.
HIV e.
hypernatremic e.
hypertensive e.
hypoxic-hypercarbic e.
lead e.
metabolic e.
necrotizing e.
palindromic e.
pancreatic e.
portal-systemic e.
progressive subcortical e.
pulmonary e.
recurrent e.
saturnine e.
severe postanoxic e.
spongiform e.
subacute spongiform e.
subcortical arteriosclerotic e.
thyrotoxic e.
traumatic e.
traumatic progressive e.
Wernicke-Korsakoff e.
Wernicke's e.

E

encephalopsy
encephalopyosis
encephalorrhachidian
encephalorrhagia
encephaloschisis
encephalosclerosis
encephaloscope
encephaloscopy
encephalospinal
encephalothlipsis
encephalotome
encephalotomy
encephalotrigeminal
    e. angiomatosis
    e. vascular syndrome
enchondral
enchondroma
enchondromatosis
enchondromatous
enchondrosarcoma
enclave
enclosed space
encoding
encopresis
encounter group
encranial
encranius
encu method
encysted
    e. calculus
    e. pleurisy
encystment
end
    acromial e. of clavicle
    e. artery
    e. bud
    e. bulb
    e. cell
    distal e.
    e. organ
    e. piece
    e. plate
    e. stage
    sternal e. of clavicle
endadelphos
Endamoeba
endangiitis, endangeitis
    e. obliterans
endaortitis
endarterectomy
    carotid e.
    coronary e.
endarteritis
    bacterial e.
    e. deformans
    e. obliterans, obliterating e.
    e. proliferans, proliferating e.

endaural
    e. incision
endbrain
end-brush
end-bulb
end-cutting bur
end-diastolic
    e.-d. volume
endemia
endemic
    e. deafmutism
    e. disease
    e. funiculitis
    e. goiter
    e. hematuria
    e. hemoptysis
    e. hypertrophy
    e. index
    e. influenza
    e. neuritis
    e. nonbacterial infantile gastroenteritis
    e. paralytic vertigo
    e. syphilis
    e. typhus
endemoepidemic
endermic, endermatic
endermism
endermosis
end-feet
endgut
ending
    annulospiral e.
    calyciform e., caliciform e.
    epilemmal e.
    flower-spray e.
    free nerve e.'s
    grape e.'s
    hederiform e.
    nerve e.
    sole-plate e.
    synaptic e.'s
endoabdominal
Endo agar
endoaneurysmoplasty
endoaneurysmorrhaphy
endoangiitis
endo-aortitis
endoappendicitis
endoarteritis
endoauscultation
endobag
endobasion
endobiotic
endoblast
endobronchial
    e. tube
endocardia (*pl. of* endocardium)

endocardiac, endocardial
endocardiography
endocarditic
endocarditis
    abacterial thrombotic e.
    acute bacterial e.
    atypical verrucous e.
    bacteria-free stage of bacterial e.
    bacterial e.
    cachectic e.
    e. chordalis
    constrictive e.
    infectious e., infective e.
    isolated parietal e.
    Libman-Sacks e.
    Löffler's e., Löffler's fibroplastic e.
    Loffler's parietal fibroplastic e.
    malignant e.
    marantic e.
    mural e.
    mycotic e.
    nonbacterial thrombotic e.
    nonbacterial verrucous e.
    polypous e.
    rheumatic e.
    septic e.
    subacute bacterial e.
    terminal e.
    valvular e.
    vegetative e., verrucous e.
endocardium, pl. **endocardia**
endoceliac
endocervical
    e. sinus tumor
    e. smear
endocervicitis
endocervix
endochondral
    e. bone
    e. ossification
endocolitis
endocolpitis
endocranial
endocranium
endocrine
    e. exophthalmos
    e. glands
    e. ophthalmopathy
    e. part of pancreas
    e. system
endocrinologist
endocrinology
endocrinoma
endocrinopathic
endocrinopathy
endocrinotherapy
endocyst
endocystitis

endocytosis
endoderm
endodermal
    e. canal
    e. cells
    e. cloaca
    e. pouches
    e. sinus tumor
Endodermophyton
endodiascope
endodiascopy
endodontia
endodontic
    e. stabilizer
    e. treatment
endodontics
endodontist
endodontologist
endodontology
endodyocyte
endodyogeny
endoenteritis
endoesophagitis
endofaradism
endogalvanism
endogamy
endogastric
endogastritis
endogenic
endogenomorphic depression
endogenote
endogenous
    e. creatinine clearance
    e. cycle
    e. depression
    e. fibers
    e. hyperglyceridemia
    e. infection
    e. pyrogens
endoglobular, endoglobar
endognathion
endoherniotomy
endointoxication
endolaryngeal
Endolimax
endolith
endolymph
endolympha
endolymphatic
    e. duct
    e. hydrops
    e. sac
endolymphic
endomerogony
endometria (*pl. of* endometrium)
endometrial
    e. cyst
    e. implants

E

endometrial *(continued)*
    e. smear
    e. stromal sarcoma
endometrioid
    e. carcinoma
    e. tumor
endometrioma
endometriosis
endometritis
    decidual e.
    e. dissecans
endometrium, pl. **endometria**
    Swiss cheese e.
endometropic
endomitosis
endomorph
endomorphic
endomotorsonde
Endomyces geotrichum
Endomycetales
endomyocardial
    e. fibroelastosis
    e. fibrosis
endomyocarditis
endomyometritis
endomysium
endoneuritis
endoneurium
end-on mattress suture
endonucleolus
endo-osseous implant
endoparasite
endoparasitism
endopelvic fascia
endoperiarteritis
endopericardiac
endopericarditis
endoperimyocarditis
endoperineuritis
endoperitonitis
endophlebitis
endophthalmitis
    granulomatous e.
    e. ophthalmia nodosa
    e. phacoanaphylactica
endophthalmodonesis
endophyte
endophytic
endoplasm
endoplast
endoplastic
endopolygeny
endopolyploid
endopolyploidy
endorectal pull-through procedure
endoreduplication
endorphinergic
endorrhachis

Endo's
    E. fuchsin agar
    E. medium
endosac
endosalpingiosis
endosalpingitis
endosalpinx
endosarc
endoscope
endoscopic
    e. biopsy
    e. retrograde
        cholangiopancreatography
endoscopist
endoscopy
    peroral e.
endoskeleton
endosome
endosonography
endosonoscopy
endosperm
endospore
endosteal
    e. implant
endosteitis, endostitis
endosteoma
endostethoscope
endosteum
endostitis *(var. of* endosteitis)
endostoma
endotendineum
endoteric bacterium
endothelia *(pl. of* endothelium)
endothelial
    e. cell
    e. cyst
    e. dystrophy of cornea
    e. leukocyte
    e. myeloma
    e. relaxing factor
endothelial-leukocyte adhesion molecule
endothelin
endotheliochorial placenta
endotheliocyte
endothelio-endothelial placenta
endothelioid
endothelioma
endotheliosis
endothelium, pl. **endothelia**
    e. of anterior chamber
    e. camerae anterioris
endothoracic fascia
endothrix
endotoxemia
endotoxic
endotoxicosis
endotoxin
    e. shock

endotracheal
  e. anesthesia
  e. intubation
  e. stylet
  e. tube
endotrachelitis
endourology
endovaccination
endovaginal ultrasonography
endovasculitis
  hemorrhagic e.
endovenous
  e. septum
end-piece
endplate, end-plate
  motor e.
end-point nystagmus
endstage lung
end-systolic volume
end-tidal
  e.-t. sample
end-to-end
  e.-t.-e. bite
  e.-t.-e. occlusion
endyma
enema
  air contrast e.
  air contrast barium e.
  analeptic e.
  barium e.
  blind e.
  contrast e.
  double contrast e.
  flatus e.
  high e.
  Hypaque e.
  nutrient e.
  oil retention e.
  small bowel e.
  soapsuds e.
  turpentine e.
enemator
enemiasis
energometer
energy
  kinetic e.
  latent e.
  e. of position
  potential e.
  psychic e.
  total e.
enervation
engagement
engastrius
Engelmann's
  E. basal knobs
  E. disease

engine
  dental e.
  e. reamer
engineering
  biomedical e.
  dental e.
Englisch's sinus
English
  E. disease
  E. position
  E. rhinoplasty
  E. sweating disease
englobe
englobement
engorged
engorgement
engram
engraphia
en grappe
enhancement
  acoustic e.
  contrast e.
  edge e.
  immunological e.
  ring e.
enhancers
enhematospore, enhemospore
enkephalinergic
enlargement
  cervical e.
  cervical e. of spinal cord
  gingival e.
  lumbar e.
  lumbar e. of spinal cord
  tympanic e.
enophthalmia
enophthalmos
enorganic
enosimania
enostosis
enrichment culture
ensheathing callus
ensiform
  e. cartilage
  e. process
ensisternum
  e. cartilage
enstrophe
ensu method
entad
ental
  e. origin
entamebiasis
Entamoeba
  E. buccalis
  E. coli
  E. gingivalis
  E. hartmanni

E

Entamoeba (*continued*)
    E. *histolytica*
    E. *moshkovskii*
Entemopoxvirus
enteral
enteralgia
enterdynia
enterectasis
enterectomy
enterelcosis
enteric
    e. cytopathogenic bovine orphan virus
    e. cytopathogenic human orphan virus
    e. cytopathogenic monkey orphan virus
    e. cytopathogenic swine orphan virus
    e. fever
    e. orphan viruses
    e. plexus
    e. tuberculosis
    e. viruses
entericoid fever
enteritis
    e. anaphylactica
    chronic cicatrizing e.
    diphtheritic e.
    granulomatous e.
    mucomembranous e.
    e. necroticans
    phlegmonous e.
    e. polyposa
    pseudomembranous e.
    regional e.
    tuberculous e.
enteroanastomosis
enteroapocleisis
Enterobacter
    E. *aerogenes*
    E. *cloacae*
Enterobacteriaceae
enterobacterium, pl. **enterobacteria**
enterobiasis
Enterobius
enterobrosis, enterobrosia
enterocele
    partial e.
enterocentesis
enterocholecystostomy
enterocholecystotomy
enterochromaffin cells
enterocleisis
    omental e.
enteroclysis
    radiological e.
enterococcemia

Enterococcus
enterococcus, pl. **enterococci**
enterocolitis
    antibiotic e.
    necrotizing e.
    pseudomembranous e.
    regional e.
enterocolostomy
enterocutaneous fistula
enterocyst
enterocystocele
enterocystoma
Enterocytozoon
    E. *bieneusi*
enterodynia
enteroendocrine cells
enteroenterostomy
enterogastric reflex
enterogastritis
enterogenous
    e. cyanosis
    e. cysts
    e. methemoglobinemia
enterograph
enterography
enterohemorrhagic *Escherichia coli*
enterohepatic circulation
enterohepatitis
enterohepatocele
enteroidea
enteroinvasive *Escherichia coli*
enterokinesis
enterokinetic
enterolith
enterolithiasis
enterology
enterolysis
enteromegaly, enteromegalia
enteromenia
enteromerocele
enterometer
Enteromonas
enteromycosis
enteroparesis
enteropathic arthritis
enteropathogen
enteropathogenic
    e. *Escherichia coli*
enteropathy
    gluten e.
    protein-losing e.
enteropexy
enteroplasty
enteroplegia
enteroplex
enteroplexy
enteroproctia
enteroptosis, enteroptosia

enteroptotic
enterorenal
enterorrhagia
enterorrhaphy
enterorrhexis
enteroscope
enterosepsis
enterospasm
enterostasis
enterostaxis
enterostenosis
enterostomy
    double e.
enterotome
enterotomy
enterotoxigenic
    e. *Escherichia coli*
enterotoxin
    cytotonic e.
    Escherichia coli e.
    staphylococcal e.
enterotoxism
enterotropic
enterovaginal fistula
enterovesical fistula
Enterovirus
enterozoic
enterozoon
enthesis
enthesitis
enthesopathic
enthesopathy
enthetic
enthlasis
en thyrse
entire
entity
entoblast
entocele
entochoroidea
entocone
entoconid
entocornea
entocranial
entocranium
entoderm
entodermal cells
entoectad
Entoloma sinuatum
entomion
entomology
entomophobia
entomophthoramycosis
    e. basidiobolae
entopic
entoplasm
entoptic
    e. pulse

entoretina
entorhinal area
entosarc
Entozoa
entozoal
entozoon, pl. entozoa
entrance block
entrapment neuropathy
entropion, entropium
    atonic e.
    cicatricial e.
    spastic e.
entropionize
entry zone
entypy
enucleate
enucleation
enuresis
    diurnal e.
    nocturnal e.
envelope
    corneocyte e.
    e. flap
    nuclear e.
    viral e.
environment
environmental
    e. illness
    e. psychology
envy
    penis e.
enzootic encephalomyelitis virus
enzygotic
    e. twins
enzyme immunoassay
enzyme-linked immunosorbent assay
enzyme-multiplied immunoassay
  technique
enzymopathy
eosin
    alcohol-soluble e.
    e. B
    ethyl e.
    e. I bluish
    e. y, e. Ys
    e. yellowish
eosin-methylene blue agar
eosinocyte
eosinopenia
eosinophil, eosinophile
    e. adenoma
    e. chemotactic factor of
      anaphylaxis
    e. granule
eosinophilia
    simple pulmonary e.
    tropical e.
eosinophilia-myalgia syndrome

E

eosinophilic
    e. cellulitis
    e. cystitis
    e. endomyocardial disease
    e. fasciitis
    e. gastritis
    e. gastroenteritis
    e. granuloma
    e. leukemia
    e. leukocyte
    e. leukocytosis
    e. leukopenia
    e. meningoencephalitis
    e. pneumonia
    e. pneumonopathy
    e. pustular folliculitis
eosinophilocytic leukemia
eosinophiluria
eosinotactic
eosinotaxis
eosophobia
epactal
    e. bones
    e. ossicles
epamniotic
    e. cavity
eparsalgia
eparterial
    e. bronchus
epaxial
ependyma
ependymal
    e. cell
    e. cyst
    e. layer
    e. zone
ependymitis
ependymoblast
ependymoblastoma
ependymocyte
ependymoma
    myxopapillary e.
epersalgia
ephapse
ephaptic
ephebic
ephebology
ephelis, pl. **ephelides**
ephemeral
    e. fever
    e. fever virus
epiblast
epiblastic
epiblepharon
epiboly, epibole
epibranchial placodes
epibulbar
epicanthal fold

epicanthus
    e. inversus
    e. palpebralis
    e. supraciliaris
    e. tarsalis
epicardia
epicardial
epicardium
epichordal
epicomus
epicondylalgia
    e. externa
epicondyle
    lateral e. of femur
    lateral e. of humerus
    medial e. of femur
    medial e. of humerus
epicondyli (*pl. of* epicondylus)
epicondylian
epicondylic
epicondylitis
    lateral humeral e.
epicondylus, pl. **epicondyli**
    e. lateralis humeri
    e. lateralis ossis femoris
    e. medialis humeri
    e. medialis ossis femoris
epicoracoid
epicranial
    e. aponeurosis
    e. muscle
epicranium
epicranius muscle
epicrisis
epicritic
    e. sensibility
epicystitis
epicyte
epidemic
    behavioral e.
    e. benign dry pleurisy
    e. cerebrospinal meningitis
    e. curve
    e. diaphragmatic pleurisy
    e. disease
    e. dropsy
    e. encephalitis
    e. exanthema
    e. gangrenous proctitis
    e. gastroenteritis virus
    e. hemoglobinuria
    e. hemorrhagic fever
    e. hepatitis
    e. hiccup
    e. hysteria
    e. keratoconjunctivitis
    e. keratoconjunctivitis virus
    e. myalgia

e. myalgia virus
e. myalgic encephalomyelitis
e. myalgic encephalomyelopathy
e. myositis
e. nausea
e. neuromyasthenia
e. nonbacterial gastroenteritis
outbreak e.
e. parotiditis
e. parotitis virus
e. pleurodynia
e. pleurodynia virus
e. polyarthritis
e. roseola
e. stomatitis
e. tetany
e. transient diaphragmatic spasm
e. typhus
e. vertigo
e. vomiting
epidemicity
epidemiography
epidemiological
e. distribution
e. genetics
epidemiologist
epidemiology
clinical e.
epiderm, epiderma
epidermal, epidermatic
e. cyst
e. ridge count
e. ridges
epidermalization
epidermatoplasty
epidermic
e. cell
e. graft
epidermic-dermic nevus
epidermidosis
epidermis, pl. **epidermides**
epidermitis
epidermization
epidermodysplasia
e. verruciformis
epidermoid
e. cancer
e. carcinoma
e. cyst
epidermolysis
e. bullosa
e. bullosa, dermal type
e. bullosa dystrophica
e. bullosa, epidermal type
e. bullosa, junctional type
e. bullosa lethalis
e. bullosa simplex
epidermolytic hyperkeratosis

Epidermophyton
epidermosis
epidermotropism
epidialysis
epidiascope
epididymal
epididymectomy
epididymis, gen. **epididymidis**,
pl. **epididymides**
caput e.
cauda e.
corpus e.
epididymitis
epididymo-orchitis
epididymoplasty
epididymotomy
epididymovasectomy
epididymovasostomy
epidural
e. anesthesia
e. block
e. cavity
e. hematoma
e. meningitis
e. space
epidurography
epifascial
epifascicular epineurium
epigastralgia
epigastric
e. angle
e. fold
e. fossa
e. hernia
e. reflex
e. region
e. veins
e. voice
epigastrium
epigastrius
epigastrocele
epiglottic, epiglottidean
e. cartilage
e. folds
e. tubercle
e. vallecula
epiglottidectomy
epiglottiditis
epiglottis
epiglottitis
epignathus
epihyal
e. bone
e. ligament
epihyoid
epikeratophakia
epikeratophakic keratoplasty
epikeratoprosthesis

E

epilamellar
epilate
epilation
    e. dose
epilemma
epilemmal ending
epilepidoma
epilepsia
    e. partialis continua
epilepsy
    anosognosic e.
    automatic e.
    autonomic e.
    benign childhood e. with
      centrotemporal spikes
    centrencephalic e.
    childhood absence e.
    childhood e. with occipital
      paroxysms
    complex precipitated e.
    cortical e.
    cryptogenic e.
    diencephalic e.
    early posttraumatic e.
    eating e.
    focal e.
    frontal lobe e.
    generalized e.
    generalized tonic-clonic e.
    grand mal e.
    idiopathic e.
    intractable e.
    jacksonian e.
    juvenile absence e.
    juvenile myoclonic e.
    Kojewnikoff's e.
    laryngeal e.
    local e.
    localization related e.
    major e.
    masked e.
    matutinal e.
    myoclonic astatic e.
    myoclonus e.
    nocturnal e.
    occipital lobe e.
    parietal lobe e.
    partial e.
    pattern sensitive e.
    petit mal e.
    pharmacoresistent e.
    photogenic e.
    posttraumatic e.
    primary generalized e.
    procursive e.
    psychomotor e.
    reflex e.
    rolandic e.

    secondary generalized e.
    sensory e.
    sensory precipitated e.
    sleep e.
    somnambulic e.
    startle e.
    supplementary motor area e.
    symptomatic e.
    temporal lobe e.
    tonic e.
    tornado e.
    uncinate e.
    vasomotor e.
    vasovagal e.
    visceral e.
    e. with grand mal seizures on
      awakening
    e. with myoclonic absences
epileptic
    e. dementia
    e. seizure
epileptiform
    e. neuralgia
epileptogenic, epileptogenous
    e. zone
epileptoid
epiloia
epimandibular
epimastical
    e. fever
epimastigote
epimenorrhagia
epimenorrhea
epimere
epimerite
epimicroscope
epimorphosis
epimyoepithelial islands
epimysiotomy
epimysium
epinephros
epineural
epineurial
epineurium
    epifascicular e.
epinosic
epinosis
epionychium
epiotic center
epipapillary membrane
epipericardial
    e. ridge
epipharynx
epiphenomenon
epiphora
    atonic e.
epiphrenic, epiphrenal
    e. diverticulum

epiphyses (*pl. of* epiphysis)
epiphysial, epiphyseal
    e. arrest
    e. aseptic necrosis
    e. cartilage
    e. eye
    e. fracture
    e. line
    e. plate
epiphysiodesis
epiphysiolysis
epiphysiopathy
epiphysis, pl. **epiphyses**
    atavistic e.
    e. cerebri
    pressure e.
    stippled e.
    traction e.
epiphysitis
epipial
epiplocele
epiploic
    e. appendage
    e. appendix
    e. branches
    e. foramen
    e. tags
epiploon
epiplopexy
epipteric
    e. bone
epipygus
epiretinal membrane
episclera
episcleral
    e. artery
    e. lamina
    e. space
    e. veins
episcleritis
    e. multinodularis
    nodular e.
    e. periodica fugax
episioperineorrhaphy
episioplasty
episiorrhaphy
episiostenosis
episiotomy
episode
    acute schizophrenic e.
    manic e.
episodic dyscontrol syndrome
episome
    resistance-transferring e.'s
epispadias
    balanitic e.
    coronal e.

    penile e.
    penopubic e.
epispinal
episplenitis
epistasis
epistasy
epistatic
epistaxis
    renal e.
epistemology
epistemophilia
episternal
    e. bone
episternum
epistropheus
epitarsus
epitaxy
epitendineum
epitenon
epithalamus
epithalaxia
epithelia (*pl. of* epithelium)
epithelial
    e. attachment
    e. body
    e. cancer
    e. cast
    e. cell
    e. choroid layer
    e. cyst
    e. dysplasia
    e. dystrophy
    e. ectoderm
    e. inlay
    e. lamina
    e. layers
    e. migration
    e. myoepithelial carcinoma
    e. nest
    e. pearl
    e. plug
    e. reticular cell
    e. tissue
epithelialization
epitheliochorial placenta
epitheliocyte
epitheliofibril
epithelioglandular
epithelioid
    e. cell
    e. cell nevus
epitheliolytic
epithelioma
    e. adenoides cysticum
    basal cell e.
    Borst-Jadassohn type
     intraepidermal e.
    chorionic e.

E

epithelioma *(continued)*
    e. cuniculatum
    Malherbe's calcifying e.
    malignant ciliary e.
    multiple self-healing squamous e.
    sebaceous e.
epitheliomatous
epitheliopathy
    pigment e.
epitheliosis
epithelite
epithelium, pl. **epithelia**
    anterior e. of cornea
    e. anterius corneae
    Barrett's e.
    ciliated e.
    columnar e.
    crevicular e.
    cuboidal e.
    cylindrical e.
    e. ductus semicircularis
    enamel e.
    external dental e., external
      enamel e.
    germinal e.
    gingival e.
    glandular e.
    inner dental e., inner enamel e.
    junctional e.
    laminated e.
    e. of lens
    e. lentis
    mesenchymal e.
    muscle e.
    olfactory e.
    pavement e.
    pigment e.
    pigment e. of optic retina
    pseudostratified e.
    reduced enamel e.
    respiratory e.
    e. of semicircular duct
    seminiferous e.
    simple e.
    simple squamous e.
    stratified e.
    stratified ciliated columnar e.
    stratified squamous e.
    sulcular e.
    surface e.
    transitional e.
epithelization
epithesis
epithet
    specific e.
epitope
epitoxoid

epitrichial
    e. layer
epitrichium
epitrochlea
epitrochlear
    e. nodes
epituberculosis
epituberculous infiltration
epitympanic
    e. recess
    e. space
epitympanum
epityphlitis
epizoic
    e. commensalism
epizoon, pl. **epizoa**
épluchage
eponychia
eponychium
epoophorectomy
epoöphoron
epornitic
epoxy resin
epsilon alcoholism
Epstein-Barr virus
Epstein's
    E. disease
    E. pearls
    E. sign
    E. symptom
epulis
    congenital e. of newborn
    e. fissuratum
    giant cell e.
    e. gravidarum
    pigmented e.
epuloid
equal cleavage
equation
    alveolar gas e.
    Bohr's e.
    constant field e.
    Einthoven's e.
    Goldman e.
    Goldman-Hodgkin-Katz e., GHK e.
    Hüfner's e.
    Nernst's e.
    personal e.
    Rayleigh e.
equator
    e. bulbi oculi
    e. of eyeball
    e. of lens
    e. lentis
equatorial
    e. cleavage
    e. division
    e. plane

e. plate
e. staphyloma
equiaxial
equilibrium
e. dialysis
genetic e.
Hardy-Weinberg e.
nitrogenous e.
nutritive e.
physiologic e.
random mating e.
secular e.
stable e.
transient e.
unstable e.
equine
e. abortion virus
e. arteritis virus
e. gait
e. influenza viruses
e. rhinopneumonitis virus
e. rhinoviruses
equinovalgus
equinovarus
equiphasic complex
equivalence zone
equivalent
e. dose
e. form reliability
lethal e.
metabolic e.
nitrogen e.
e. power
starch e.
equivocal symptom
eradication
Eranko's fluorescence stain
erasion
Erb
E. atrophy
E. disease
E. palsy
E. paralysis
E. sign
E. spinal paralysis
Erb-Charcot disease
Erb-Westphal sign
Erdheim
E. disease
E. tumor
erectile
e. tissue
erect illumination
erection
erector
e. muscles of hairs
e. muscle of spine
e. spinae muscles

erector-spinal reflex
eremophilia
eremophobia
erethism
erethismic, erethistic, erethitic
ereuthophobia
ergasia
ergasiomania
ergasiophobia
ergasthenia
ergastoplasm
ergodynamograph
ergoesthesiograph
ergogenic
ergograph
Mosso's e.
ergographic
ergometer
ergonomics
ergostat
ergot
e. alkaloid-associated heart disease
corn e.
ergotherapy
ergotropic
Erichsen's sign
erisophake
Erlenmeyer
E. flask
E. flask deformity
erogenous
e. zone
eros
erose
E rosette
E-rosette test
erosion
Dieulafoy's e.
recurrent corneal e.
erosive adenomatosis of nipple
erotic
e. zoophilism
erotism, eroticism
anal e.
erotization
erotogenesis
erotogenic
e. zone
erotomania
erotomanic type of paranoid disorder
erotopathic
erotopathy
erotophobia
erratic
erroneous projection
error
alpha e.
beta e.

E

293

error *(continued)*
    experimental e.
    e. of the first kind
    inborn e.'s of metabolism
    interobserver e.
    intraobserver e.
    residual e.
    e. of the second kind
    technical e.
    type I e.
    type II e.
error-prone repair
erubescence
erubescent
eructation
eruption
    accelerated e.
    butterfly e.
    clinical e.
    continuous e.
    creeping e.
    e. cyst
    delayed e.
    drug e.
    feigned e.
    fixed drug e.
    iodine e.
    Kaposi's varicelliform e.
    medicinal e.
    passive e.
    polymorphous light e.
    e. sequestrum
    serum e.
    surgical e.
eruptive
    e. fever
    e. phase
    e. stage
    e. xanthoma
erysipelas
    ambulant e.
    e. internum
    e. migrans
    e. perstans faciei
    phlegmonous e.
    e. pustulosum
    surgical e.
    e. verrucosum
    wandering e.
erysipelatous
erysipeloid
Erysipelothrix
erysipelotoxin
erythema
    e. ab igne
    acrodynic e.
    e. annulare
    e. annulare centrifugum

    e. annulare rheumaticum
    e. arthriticum epidemicum
    e. bullosum
    e. caloricum
    e. chronicum migrans
    e. circinatum
    cold e.
    e. dose
    e. dyschromicum perstans
    e. elevatum diutinum
    e. exfoliativa
    e. figuratum perstans
    e. fugax
    e. gyratum
    hemorrhagic exudative e.
    e. induratum
    e. infectiosum
    e. intertrigo
    e. iris
    Jacquet's e.
    e. keratodes
    macular e.
    e. marginatum
    e. migrans, e. migrans linguae
    Milian's e.
    e. multiforme
    e. multiforme bullosum
    e. multiforme exudativum
    e. multiforme major
    necrolytic migratory e.
    e. neonatorum
    ninth-day e.
    e. nodosum
    e. nodosum leprosum
    e. nodosum migrans
    e. palmare hereditarium
    e. papulatum
    e. paratrimma
    e. pernio
    e. perstans
    e. polymorphe
    scarlatiniform e., e. scarlatinoides
    e. simplex
    e. solare
    symptomatic e.
    e. threshold
    e. toxicum
    e. toxicum neonatorum
    e. tuberculatum
erythematous
    e. syphilid
erythematovesicular
erythermalgia
erythralgia
erythrasma
erythredema
erythremia
    altitude e.

erythremic myelosis
erythrism
erythristic
erythroblast
erythroblastemia
erythroblastic anemia
erythroblastopenia
erythroblastosis
erythroblastotic
erythrocatalysis
erythrochromia
erythroclasis
erythroclastic
erythrocyanosis
erythrocyte
    e. adherence phenomenon
    e. adherence test
    e. fragility test
    e. indices
    e. sedimentation rate
erythrocythemia
erythrocytic
    e. scries
erythrocytoblast
erythrocytolysin
crythrocytolysis
erythrocytometer
erythrocytopenia
erythrocytopoiesis
erythrocytorrhexis
erythrocytoschisis
erythrocytosis
erythrocyturia
erythrodegenerative
erythroderma
    bullous congenital ichthyosiform e.
    congenital ichthyosiform e.
    e. desquamativum
    e. exfoliativa
    ichthyosiform e.
    nonbullous congenital
      ichthyosiform e.
    e. psoriaticum
    Sézary e.
erythrodermatitis
erythrodontia
erythrodysesthesia syndrome
erythrogenesis imperfecta
erythrogenic
erythrogonium, pl. erythrogonia
erythroid
    e. cell
erythrokeratodermia
    e. variabilis
erythrokinetics
erythroleukemia
erythroleukosis
erythrolysin

erythrolysis
erythromelalgia
erythromelia
erythron
erythroneocytosis
erythronormoblastic anemia
erythropenia
erythrophagia
erythrophagocytosis
erythrophil
erythrophilic
erythrophore
erythroplakia
erythroplasia
    e. of Queyrat
    Zoon's e.
erythropoiesis
erythropoietic
    e. porphyria
    e. protoporphyria
erythroprosopalgia
erythropsia
erythropyknosis
erythrorrhcxis
erythrosin B
erythruria
Esbach's reagent
escape
    e. beat
    e. conditioning
    e. contraction
    e. impulse
    e. interval
    junctional e.
    e. phenomenon
    e. rhythm
    e. training
    ventricular e.
    e. ventricular contraction
escape-capture bigeminy
escaped beat
eschar
escharectomy
escharotomy
Escherichia
    E. coli
    E. coli enterotoxin
    enterohemorrhagic *E. coli*
    enteroinvasive *E. coli*
    enteropathogenic *E. coli*
    enterotoxigenic *E. coli*
    E. freundii
Escherich's sign
esculent
Esmarch
    E. bandage
    E. tourniquet
esodeviation

E

esodic
> e. nerve

esoethmoiditis

esogastritis

esophagalgia

esophageal
> e. achalasia
> e. arteries
> e. atresia
> e. branches
> e. branches of the inferior thyroid artery
> e. branches of the left gastric artery
> e. branches of the recurrent laryngeal nerve
> e. branches of the thoracic aorta
> e. branches of the vagus nerve
> e. cardiogram
> e. constrictions
> e. dysrhythmia
> e. glands
> e. hiatus
> e. impression
> e. lead
> e. manometry
> e. mucosa
> e. opening
> e. plexus
> e. reflux
> e. smear
> e. spasm
> e. speech
> e. varices
> e. veins
> e. web

esophagectasis, esophagectasia

esophagectomy
> transhiatal e.
> transthoracic e.

esophagi (*pl. of* esophagus)

esophagism

esophagitis
> peptic e.
> reflux e.

esophagocardioplasty

esophagocele

esophagodynia

esophagoenterostomy

esophagogastrectomy

esophagogastric
> e. junction
> e. orifice
> e. vestibule

esophagogastroanastomosis

esophagogastroduodenoscopy

esophagogastromyotomy

esophagogastroplasty

esophagogastrostomy

esophagogram

esophagography

esophagology

esophagomalacia

esophagomycosis

esophagomyotomy

esophagoplasty

esophagoplication

esophagoptosis, esophagoptosia

esophagosalivary reflex

esophagoscope

esophagoscopy

esophagospasm

esophagostenosis

esophagostomy

esophagotomy

esophagram

esophagus, pl. **esophagi**
> Barrett's e.

esophoria

esophoric

esosphenoiditis

esotropia
> A-e.
> basic e.
> consecutive e.
> cyclic e.
> mixed e.
> nonaccommodative e.
> nonrefractive accommodative e.
> refractive accommodative e.
> V-e.
> X-e.

esotropic

espundia

esquinancea

essential
> e. albuminuria
> e. anemia
> e. anisocoria
> e. bradycardia
> e. dysmenorrhea
> e. fever
> e. fructosuria
> e. hypertension
> e. nutrients
> e. phthisis bulbi
> e. progressive atrophy of iris
> e. pruritus
> e. tachycardia
> e. telangiectasia
> e. thrombocytopenia
> e. tremor

Esser
> E. graft
> E. operation

Essick's cell bands

Essig splint
established cell line
esterase
    C1 e.
Estes operation
esthematology
esthesia
esthesic
esthesiodic
    e. system
esthesiogenesis
esthesiogenic
esthesiography
esthesiology
esthesiometer
esthesiometry
esthesioneuroblastoma
    olfactory e.
esthesioneurocytoma
esthesiophysiology
esthesioscopy
esthesodic
esthetic
    e. dentistry
    e. surgery
esthetics
    denture e.
estimate
estimation
estimator
    least squares e.
    maximum likelihood e.
estival
estivoautumnal
Estlander
    E. flap
    E. operation
estrogenic
état
    e. criblé
    e. mamelonné
ether
    e. convulsion
    e. test
etherization
ethical
ethics
    medical e.
ethidium bromide
ethmocranial
ethmofrontal
ethmoid
    e. air cells
    e. angle
    e. bone
    e. infundibulum
ethmoidal
    e. bulla

e. cells
e. crest
e. crest of maxilla
e. crest of palatine bone
e. foramen
e. groove
e. infundibulum
e. labyrinth
e. notch
e. process
e. sinuses
e. veins
ethmoidale
ethmoidal-lacrimal fistula
ethmoidectomy
ethmoiditis
ethmoidolacrimal suture
ethmoidomaxillary suture
ethmolacrimal
ethmomaxillary
ethmonasal
ethmopalatal
ethmosphenoid
ethmoturbinals
ethmovomerine
    e. plate
ethnic group
ethnocentrism
ethnology
ethyl
    e. eosin
    e. green
etiogenic
etiologic
etiology
etiopathic
etiopathology
etiotropic
eualleles
Eubacteriales
Eubacterium
    E. aerofaciens
    E. biforme
    E. combesi
    E. contortum
    E. crispatum
    E. disciformans
    E. ethylicum
    E. filamentosum
    E. lentum
    E. limosum
    E. minutum
    E. moniliforme
    E. multiforme
    E. niosii
    E. parvum
    E. plauti
    E. poeciloides

E

[handwritten: et vergae]

[handwritten: ethylene glycol]

Eubacterium *(continued)*
    E. *pseudotortuosum*
    E. *quartum*
    E. *quintum*
    E. *rectale*
    E. *tenue*
    E. *tortuosum*
eubiotics
eubolism
eucapnia
Eucaryotae *(var. of* Eukaryotae)
eucaryote
eucaryotic
euchlorhydria
eucholia
euchromatic
euchromatin
euchromosome
eucorticalism
eucrasia
eudemonia
eudiaphoresis
eudipsia
Euflagellata
eugenic
eugenics
eugenism
Euglena
    E. *gracilis*
    E. *viridis*
Euglenidae
euglobulin clot lysis time
euglycemia
euglycemic
eugnathia
eugnathic anomaly
eugnosia
eugonic
Eugregarinida
euhydration
Eukaryotae, Eucaryotae
eukaryote
eukaryotic
eukinesia
Eulenburg's disease
eumelanosome
eumetria
eumorphism
eumycetes
Eumycetozoea
eunoia
eunuch
eunuchism
eunuchoid
    e. gigantism
    e. state
    e. voice

eunuchoidism
    hypergonadotropic e.
    hypogonadotropic e.
euosmia
eupancreatism
euparal
Euparyphium
eupepsia
eupeptic
euphenics
euphoria
euplasia
euplastic
    e. lymph
euploid
euploidy
eupnea
eupraxia
eurhythmia
European
    E. tarantula
    E. typhus
euroxenous parasite
eurycephalic, eurycephalous
eurygnathic
eurygnathism
eurygnathous
euryon
euryopic
eurysomatic
euscope
Eusimulium
eustachian
    e. catheter
    e. cushion
    e. tonsil
    e. tube
    e. tuber
    e. valve
eustachitis
eusthenia
Eustrongylus
eusystole
eusystolic
eutectic alloy
euthanasia
euthenics
eutherapeutic
euthermic
euthymia
euthymic
euthyroid
    e. hypometabolism
    e. sick syndrome
euthyroidism
euthyscope
euthyscopy
eutonic

eutrichosis
eutrophia
eutrophic
eutrophy
euvolia
evacuant
evacuate
evacuation
    dilation and e.
evacuator
    Ellik e.
evagination
evaluation
evanescent
Evans
    E. blue
    E. forceps
    E. syndrome
evasion
    macular e.
event
    life e.'s
eventration
    e. of the diaphragm
eversion
evert
evidement
evil
    king's e.
eviration
evisceration
evisceroneurotomy
evocation
evocator
evoked
    e. potential
    e. response
    e. response audiometry
evolution
    biologic e.
    convergent e.
    Darwinian e.
    Denman's spontaneous e.
    Douglas' spontaneous e.
    emergent e.
    organic e.
    saltatory e.
    spontaneous e.
evolutionary fitness
evulsion
Ewart's
    E. procedure
    E. sign
Ewingella
Ewing's
    E. sarcoma
    E. sign
    E. tumor

exacerbation
exaltation
examination
    cytologic e.
    EMG e.
    Papanicolaou e.
    physical e.
    postmortem e.
examiner
    medical e.
examining table
exanthem
exanthema
    Boston e.
    epidemic e.
    keratoid e.
    e. subitum
exanthematous
    e. disease
    e. fever
    e. typhus
exanthesis
    e. arthrosia
exanthrope
exanthropic
exarteritis
exarticulation
excalation
excavatio
    e. disci
    e. papillae
    e. rectouterina
    e. rectovesicalis
    e. vesicouterina
excavation
    atrophic e.
    glaucomatous e.
    e. of optic disc
    physiologic e.
excavator
    hatchet e.
    hoe e.
excementosis
excentric
    e. amputation
excess
    antibody e.
    antigen e.
    base e.
    convergence e.
    e. lactate
    negative base e.
exchange
    sister chromatid e.
    e. transfusion
exchanger
    countercurrent e.
excise

E

excision
> e. biopsy
> loop e.

excitability
> supranormal e.

excitable
> e. area
> e. gap

excitation
> anomalous atrioventricular e.
> ventricular pre-e.
> e. wave

excitatory
> e. junction potential
> e. postsynaptic potential

excited catatonia

excitement
> catatonic e.
> manic e.

exciting
> e. cause
> e. electrode
> e. eye

excitomotor

excitomuscular

excitoreflex nerve

excitor nerve

exclamation point hair

exclave

exclusion
> allelic e.
> Devine e.
> e. of pupil

exconjugant

excoriate

excoriation
> neurotic e.

excrement

excrementitious

excrescence
> Lambl's e.'s

excreta

excrete

excretion

excretory
> e. duct
> e. duct of seminal vesicle
> e. ducts of lacrimal gland
> e. ductules of lacrimal gland
> e. gland
> e. urography

excursion
> lateral e.
> protrusive e.
> retrusive e.

excycloduction

excyclophoria

excyclotorsion

excyclotropia

excyclovergence

excystation

exduction

exemia

exencephalia

exencephalic

exencephalocele

exencephalous

exencephaly

exenteration
> anterior pelvic e.
> orbital e.
> pelvic e.
> posterior pelvic e.
> total pelvic e.

exenteritis

exercise
> e. bone
> e. imaging
> isometric e.
> isotonic e.
> Kegel's e.'s
> e. radionuclide angiocardiography
> e. test

exercise-induced amenorrhea

exeresis

exertional
> e. dyspnea
> e. rhabdomyolysis

exflagellation

exfoliation
> e. of lens
> e. syndrome

exfoliative
> e. cytology
> e. dermatitis
> e. gastritis

exhalation

exhale

exhaustion
> e. atrophy
> combat e.
> heat e.
> e. psychosis

exhibitionism

exhibitionist

exhilarant

existential
> e. psychiatry
> e. psychology
> e. psychotherapy

exit
> e. block
> e. dose

exitus

Exner's plexus

exoantigen

exocardia
exoccipital bone
exocelomic membrane
exocrine
    e. gland
    e. pancreatic insufficiency
    e. part of pancreas
exocytosis
exodeviation
exodic nerve
exodontia
exodontist
exoerythrocytic
    e. cycle
    e. stage
exogamy
exogastrula
exogenetic
exogenote
exogenous
    e. creatinine clearance
    e. cycle
    e. depression
    e. fibers
    e. hemochromatosis
    e. hyperglyceridemia
    e. ochronosis
    e. pigmentation
    e. pyrogens
exolever
exomphalos
exon shuffle
Exophiala
    E. jeanselmei
    E. werneckii
exophoria
exophoric
exophthalmic
    e. goiter
    e. ophthalmoplegia
exophthalmometer
exophthalmos, exophthalmus
    endocrine e.
    malignant e.
exophyte
exophytic
exoplasm
exoserosis
exoskeleton
exospore
exosporium
exostectomy
exostosectomy
exostosis, pl. **exostoses**
    e. bursata
    e. cartilaginea
    hereditary multiple exostoses
    ivory e.

    multiple e.
    solitary osteocartilaginous e.
    subungual e.
exoteric
    e. bacterium
exotropia
    A-e.
    basic e.
    divergence excess e.
    divergence insufficiency e.
    V-e.
    X-e.
expansion
    e. arch
    clonal e.
    extensor e.
    extensor digital e.
    hygroscopic e.
    perceptual e.
    setting e.
    wax e.
expansive delusion
expansiveness
expectation
    e. neurosis
expectation of life
    e. o. l. at age x
    e. o. l. at birth
expected
expectorate
expectoration
    prune-juice e.
experience
    corrective emotional e.
experiment
    Carr-Purcell e.
    delayed reaction e.
    factorial e.'s
    hertzian e.'s
    Mariotte's e.
    Nussbaum's e.
    Scheiner's e.
    Stensen's e.
    Weber's e.
experimental
    e. allergic encephalitis
    e. allergic encephalomyelitis
    e. error
    e. group
    e. medicine
    e. method
    e. neurosis
    e. psychology
experimenter effects
expiration
expiratory
    e. center
    e. dyspnea

E

expiratory *(continued)*
    e. reserve volume
    e. resistance
    e. stridor
expire
expired gas
explant
explantation
exploration
exploratory
    e. drive
explorer
exploring
    e. electrode
    e. needle
explosive
    e. decompression
    e. speech
exponential distribution
expose
exposed pulp
exposure
    e. dose
    e. keratitis
express
expressed skull fracture
expression
    e. library
expressive aphasia
expressivity
expulsive
    e. pains
exquisite
exsanguinate
exsanguination
    e. transfusion
exsanguine
exsect
exsection
exsiccation fever
exsomatize
exsorption
exstrophy
    e. of the bladder
    e. of the cloaca
    cloacal e.
extend
extended
    e. clasp
    e. family
    e. family therapy
    e. pyelotomy
    e. radical mastectomy
extension
    e. bridge
    Buck's e.
    e. form
    nail e.

    primer e.
    ridge e.
    skeletal e.
extensor
    e. aponeurosis
    e. carpi radialis brevis muscle
    e. carpi radialis longus muscle
    e. carpi ulnaris muscle
    e. digital expansion
    e. digiti minimi muscle
    e. digitorum brevis muscle
    e. digitorum brevis muscle of hand
    e. digitorum longus muscle
    e. digitorum muscle
    e. expansion
    e. hallucis brevis muscle
    e. hallucis longus muscle
    e. indicis muscle
    e. muscle of fingers
    e. muscle of little finger
    e. pollicis brevis muscle
    e. pollicis longus muscle
    e. retinaculum
exterior
exteriorize
extern
external
    e. absorption
    e. acoustic foramen
    e. acoustic meatus
    e. acoustic pore
    e. anal sphincter
    e. aperture of cochlear canaliculus
    e. aperture of vestibular aqueduct
    e. arcuate fibers
    e. artery of nose
    e. auditory foramen
    e. auditory meatus
    e. auditory pore
    e. axis of eye
    e. base of skull
    e. branch of accessory nerve
    e. branch of superior laryngeal
      nerve
    e. canthus
    e. capsule
    e. cardiac massage
    e. carotid artery
    e. carotid nerves
    e. carotid plexus
    e. cephalic version
    e. collateral ligament of wrist
    e. conjugate
    e. conjugate diameter
    e. cuneate nucleus
    e. defibrillator
    e. dental epithelium
    e. ear

e. enamel epithelium
e. exudative retinopathy
e. female genital organs
e. fistula
e. fixation
e. genitalia
e. hemorrhoid
e. hemorrhoids
e. hydrocephalus
e. iliac artery
e. iliac lymph nodes
e. iliac plexus
e. iliac vein
e. inguinal ring
e. intercostal membrane
e. intercostal muscles
e. jugular vein
e. lip of iliac crest
e. male genital organs
e. malleolar sign
e. malleolus
e. mammary artery
e. maxillary artery
e. maxillary plexus
e. meningitis
e. naris
e. nasal branches
e. nasal veins
e. nose
e. nuclear layer of retina
e. oblique muscle
e. oblique reflex
e. oblique ridge
e. obturator muscle
e. occipital crest
e. occipital protuberance
e. opening of urethra
e. ophthalmopathy
e. ophthalmoplegia
e. os of uterus
e. ovular transmigration
e. pacemaker
e. pillar cells
e. pin fixation
e. pin fixation, biphase
e. pterygoid muscle
e. pudendal arteries
e. pudendal veins
e. pyocephalus
e. respiration
e. respiratory nerve of Bell
e. root sheath
e. salivary gland
e. saphenous nerve
e. secretion
e. semilunar fibrocartilage
e. sheath of optic nerve
e. spermatic artery

e. spermatic fascia
e. spermatic nerve
e. sphincter muscle of anus
e. sphincterotomy
e. spiral sulcus
e. squint
e. strabismus
e. surface
e. surface of frontal bone
e. surface of parietal bone
e. traction
e. urethral orifice
e. urethral sphincter
e. urethrotomy
e. wall of cochlear duct
externus
exteroceptive
exteroceptor
exterofective
   e. system
extinction
   visual e.
extinguish
extirpation
extorsion
extortor
extra-abdominal desmoid
extraamniotic pregnancy
extraanatomic bypass
extra-articular
extra-axial
extrabuccal
extrabulbar
extracaliceal
extracapsular
   e. ankylosis
   e. fracture
   e. ligaments
extracardiac murmur
extracarpal
extracellular
   e. cholesterolosis
   e. fluid
   e. fluid volume
extrachorial pregnancy
extrachromosomal
   e. element
   e. genetic element
   e. inheritance
extracoronal retainer
extracorporeal
   e. circulation
   e. dialysis
   e. photophoresis
   e. shock wave lithotripsy
extracorpuscular
extracranial
   e. arteritis

E

extracranial *(continued)*
    e. ganglia
    e. pneumatocele
    e. pneumocele
extracranial-intracranial bypass
extract
    allergenic e.
    allergic e.
extracting forceps
extraction
    Baker's pyridine e.
    breech e.
    e. coefficient
    partial breech e.
    podalic e.
    e. ratio
    serial e.
    spontaneous breech e.
    total breech e.
extractor
    vacuum e.
extracystic
extradural
    e. anesthesia
    e. hematorrhachis
    e. hemorrhage
extraembryonic
    e. blastoderm
    e. celom
    e. ectoderm
    e. membrane
    e. mesoderm
extraepiphysial
extragenital
extraglomerular mesangium
extrahepatic
extrajection
extraligamentous
extramalleolus
extramammary Paget disease
extramedullary
extramembranous pregnancy
extramural
    e. practice
extraneous
extranuclear
    e. inheritance
extraocular
    e. muscles
extraoral
    e. anchorage
    e. fracture appliance
extraovular
extrapapillary
extraparenchymal
extraperineal
extraperiosteal

extraperitoneal
    e. fascia
extraphysiologic
extrapineal pinealoma
extraplacental
extrapleural pneumothorax
extraprostatic
extrapsychic
extrapulmonary
extrapyramidal
    e. cerebral palsy
    e. disease
    e. dyskinesias
    e. motor system
    e. motor system disease
    e. syndrome
extrasaccular hernia
extrasensory
    e. perception
    e. thought transference
extraserous
extraskeletal chondroma
extrasomatic
extrasystole
    atrial e.
    atrioventricular e., A-V e.
    atrioventricular nodal e., A-V
      nodal e.
    auricular e.
    infranodal e.
    interpolated e.
    junctional e.
    lower nodal e.
    midnodal e.
    return e.
    supraventricular e.
    upper nodal e.
    ventricular e.
extratarsal
extrathyroidal hypermetabolism
extratracheal
extratubal
extrauterine
    e. pregnancy
extravaginal
    e. torsion
extravasate
extravasation
    e. cyst
extravascular
    e. fluid
extraventricular
extraversion
extravert
extravisual
extravital ultraviolet
extreme capsule

extremis
    in e.
extremital
extremitas
    e. acromialis claviculae
    e. anterior
    e. inferior
    e. inferior renis
    e. inferior testis
    e. posterior
    e. sternalis claviculae
    e. superior
    e. superior renis
    e. superior testis
    e. tubaria ovarii
    e. uterina ovarii
extremity
    acromial e. of clavicle
    anterior e.
    anterior e. of caudate nucleus
    inferior e.
    lower e.
    posterior e.
    sternal e. of clavicle
    superior e.
    tubal e. of ovary
    upper e.
    upper e. of fibula
    uterine e. of ovary
extrinsic
    e. allergic alveolitis
    e. asthma
    e. color
    e. incubation period
    e. motivation
    e. muscles
    e. sphincter
extrogastrulation
extrospection
extroversion
extrovert
extrude
extruded teeth
extrusion
    e. of a tooth
extubate
extubation
exuberant
exudate
exudation
    e. cell
    e. corpuscle
    e. cyst
exudative
    e. bronchiolitis
    e. choroiditis
    e. discoid and lichenoid dermatitis
    e. glomerulonephritis

    e. inflammation
    e. retinal detachment
    e. retinitis
    e. tuberculosis
    e. vitreoretinopathy
exude
exulcerans
exumbilication
exuviae
eye
    amaurotic cat's e.
    aphakic e.
    artificial e.
    e. bank
    black e.
    blear e.
    bleary e.
    e. capsule
    crossed e.'s
    e. cup
    cyclopian e., cyclopean e.
    dark-adapted e.
    dominant e.
    epiphysial e.
    exciting e.
    fixing e.
    hare's e.
    e. lens
    light-adapted e.
    Listing's reduced e.
    master e.
    parietal e.
    phakic e.
    photopic e.
    pineal e.
    raccoon e.'s
    reduced e.
    e. reflex
    schematic e.
    scotopic e.
    e. socket
    e. speculum
    squinting e.
    sympathizing e.
    e. tooth
    watery e.
    web e.
eyeball
    e. compression reflex
eyeball-heart reflex
eyebrow
eye-closure
    e.-c. pupil reaction
    e.-c. reflex
eye-ear plane
eyeglasses
eyegrounds

E

eyelash
>ectopic e.
>piebald e.
>e. sign

eyelid
>lower e.
>upper e.

eyepiece
eyespot
eyestone
eyestrain

F

F agent
F duction
F factor
F genote
F pili
F pilus
F plasmid
F thalassemia
F waves

f̂

f distribution

Fab

F. fragment
F. piece

fabella

Faber's

F. anemia
F. syndrome

fabism

fabrication

Fabricius' ship

Fabry's disease

fabulation

face

bird f.
cow f.
dish f.
f. form
frog f.
hippocratic f.
masklike f.
moon f.
moon shaped f.
f. peel
f. presentation
f. validity

face-bow

adjustable axis f.
f. fork
kinematic f.
f. record

face-lift

facet, facette

articular f.
f. of atlas for dens
clavicular f.
corneal f.
costal f.'s
inferior articular f. of atlas
inferior costal f.
f. joints
Lenoir's f.
locked f.'s
f. rhizotomy

superior articular f. of atlas
superior costal f.
transverse costal f.

facetectomy

facial

f. angle
f. artery
f. axis
f. bones
f. canal
f. cleft
f. colliculus
f. diplegia
f. eminence
f. height
f. hemiatrophy
f. hemiatrophy of Romberg
f. hemiplegia
f. hillock
f. index
f. lymph nodes
f. motor nucleus
f. muscles
f. myokymia
f. nerve
f. neuralgia
f. nucleus
f. palsy
f. paralysis
f. plane
f. plexus
f. profile
f. reflex
f. root
f. spasm
f. surface of tooth
f. tic
f. triangle
f. trophoneurosis
f. vein
f. vision

facialis

f. phenomenon

facies, pl. **facies**

acromial articular f. of clavicle
adenoid f.
f. antebrachialis anterior
f. antebrachialis posterior
f. anterior
f. anterior antebrachii
f. anterior brachii
f. anterior corneae
f. anterior corporis maxillae
f. anterior cruris
f. anterior glandulae suprarenalis

F

facies *(continued)*
f. anterior iridis
f. anterior lateralis corporis humeri
f. anterior lentis
f. anterior medialis corporis humeri
f. anterior membri inferioris
f. anterior palpebrarum
f. anterior pancreatis
f. anterior partis petrosae ossis
  temporalis
f. anterior patellae
f. anterior prostatae
f. anterior radii
f. anterior renis
f. anterior ulnae
f. anterolateralis corporis humeri
f. anteromedialis corporis humeri
f. antonina
aortic f.
f. approximalis dentis
f. articularis
f. articularis acromialis claviculae
f. articularis acromii
f. articularis anterior dentis
f. articularis arytenoidea cricoideae
f. articularis calcanea tali
f. articularis capitis costae
f. articularis capitis fibulae
f. articularis carpi radii
f. articularis cartilaginis
  arytenoideae
f. articularis cuboidea calcanei
f. articularis fibularis tibiae
f. articularis inferior atlantis
f. articularis inferior tibiae
f. articularis malleoli fibulae
f. articularis malleoli tibiae
f. articularis navicularis tali
f. articularis ossis temporalis
f. articularis patellae
f. articularis posterior dentis
f. articularis sternalis claviculae
f. articularis superior atlantis
f. articularis superior tibiae
f. articularis talaris anterior
  calcanei
f. articularis talaris calcanei
f. articularis talaris media calcanei
f. articularis talaris posterior
  calcanei
f. articularis thyroidea cricoideae
f. articularis tuberculi costae
f. auricularis ossis ilii
f. auricularis ossis sacri
f. bovina
f. brachialis anterior
f. brachialis posterior
f. buccalis

f. cerebralis
cherubic f.
f. colica splenis
f. contactus dentis
Corvisart's f.
f. costalis
f. costalis pulmonis
f. costalis scapulae
f. cruralis anterior
f. cruralis posterior
f. cubitalis anterior
f. cubitalis posterior
f. diaphragmatica
f. digitalis dorsalis
f. digitalis palmaris
f. digitalis plantaris
f. digitalis ventralis
f. distalis dentis
f. dolorosa
f. dorsalis
f. dorsalis ossis sacri
f. dorsalis scapulae
elfin f.
f. externa
f. externa ossis frontalis
f. externa ossis parietalis
f. facialis dentis
f. femoralis anterior
f. femoralis posterior
f. gastrica splenis
f. glutea ossis ilii
hippocratic f., f. hippocratica
hound-dog f.
Hutchinson's f.
f. inferior cerebri
f. inferior hemispherii cerebelli
f. inferior linguae
f. inferior pancreatis
f. inferior partis petrosae ossis
  temporalis
f. inferolateralis prostatae
f. infratemporalis maxillae
f. interlobares pulmonis
f. interna
f. interna ossis frontalis
f. interna ossis parietalis
f. intestinalis uteri
f. labialis
f. lateralis
f. lateralis brachii
f. lateralis cruris
f. lateralis digiti manus
f. lateralis digiti pedis
f. lateralis fibulae
f. lateralis membri inferioris
f. lateralis ossis zygomatici
f. lateralis ovarii
f. lateralis testis

f. lateralis tibiae
leonine f.
f. lingualis dentis
f. lunata acetabuli
f. malleolaris lateralis tali
f. malleolaris medialis tali
f. masticatoria
f. maxillaris alae majoris
f. maxillaris ossis palatini
f. medialis
f. medialis cartilaginis arytenoideae
f. medialis cerebri
f. medialis digiti pedis
f. medialis fibulae
f. medialis ovarii
f. medialis pulmonis
f. medialis testis
f. medialis tibiae
f. medialis ulnae
f. mediastinalis pulmonis
f. mesialis dentis
mitral f.
moon f.
myasthenic f.
myopathic f.
f. nasalis maxillae
f. nasalis ossis palatini
f. occlusalis dentis
f. orbitalis
f. palatina laminae horizontalis
ossis palatini
Parkinson's f.
f. patellaris femoris
f. pelvina ossis sacri
f. poplitea femoris
f. posterior
f. posterior cartilaginis arytenoideae
f. posterior corneae
f. posterior corporis humeri
f. posterior cruris
f. posterior fibulae
f. posterior glandulae suprarenalis
f. posterior iridis
f. posterior lentis
f. posterior membri inferioris
f. posterior palpebrarum
f. posterior pancreatis
f. posterior partis petrosae ossis
temporalis
f. posterior prostatae
f. posterior radii
f. posterior renis
f. posterior tibiae
f. posterior ulnae
Potter's f.
f. pulmonalis cordis
f. renalis glandulae suprarenalis
f. renalis lienis

f. renalis splenis
f. sacropelvina ossis ilii
f. scaphoidea
f. sternocostalis cordis
f. superior hemispherii cerebelli
f. superior tali
f. superolateralis cerebri
f. symphysialis
f. temporalis
f. urethralis penis
f. vesicalis uteri
f. vestibularis dentis
f. visceralis hepatis
f. visceralis splenis
facilitation
Wedensky f.
facing
faciodigitogenital dysplasia
faciolingual
facioplasty
facioplegia
facioscapulohumeral
f. atrophy
f. muscular dystrophy
factitial dermatitis
factitious
f. disorder
f. purpura
f. urticaria
factor
f. 3
f. A
ABO f.'s
accelerator f.
adrenal weight f.
adrenocorticotropic releasing f.
angiogenesis f.
antihemophilic f. A
antihemophilic f. B
antinuclear f.
atrial natriuretic f.
f. B
bacteriocin f.'s
B-cell differentiating f.
B cell differentiation/growth f.'s
B-cell stimulatory f. 2
bifidus f.
biotic f.'s
Bittner's milk f.
CAMP f.
Christmas f.
clearing f.'s
clotting f.
coagulation f.
cobra venom f.
colony-stimulating f.'s
complement chemotactic f.
f. D

F

factor *(continued)*
 decapacitation f.
 f. E
 endothelial relaxing f.
 eosinophil chemotactic f. of
  anaphylaxis
 F f.
 fertility f.
 fibrin-stabilizing f.
 Fletcher f.
 glass f.
 f. Gm
 granulocyte colony-stimulating f.
 granulocyte-macrophage colony-
  stimulating f.
 growth f.'s
 Hageman f.
 f. I
 f. III
 inhibition f.
 insulin-like growth f.'s
 ischemia-modifying f.'s
 f. IV
 f. IX
 labile f.
 Laki-Lorand f.
 LE f.'s
 lethal f.
 leukocytosis-promoting f.
 leukopenic f.
 L-L f.
 lymph node permeability f.
 macrophage-activating f.
 macrophage colony-stimulating f.
 migration-inhibitory f.
 milk f.
 müllerian inhibiting f.
 müllerian regression f., müllerian
  duct inhibitory f.
 multi-colony-stimulating f.
 myocardial depressant f.
 natural killer cell stimulating f.
 nephritic f.
 neutrophil activating f.
 neutrophil chemotactant f.
 osteoclast activating f.
 P f.
 plasma labile f.
 plasma thromboplastin f.
 plasma thromboplastin f. B
 plasma f. X
 plasmin prothrombins conversion f.
 platelet f. 3
 platelet-activating f.
 platelet-aggregating f.
 platelet tissue f.
 predisposing f.'s
 properdin f. A

 properdin f. B
 properdin f. D
 properdin f. E
 quality f.
 R f.'s
 radiation weighting f.
 recognition f.'s
 resistance f.'s
 resistance-inducing f.
 resistance-transfer f.
 rheumatoid f.'s
 risk f.
 S f.
 secretor f.
 sex f.
 slow-reacting f. of anaphylaxis
 stable f.
 Stuart f., Stuart-Prower f.
 T-cell growth f.
 T-cell growth f.-1
 T-cell growth f.-2
 thyrotoxic complement-fixation f.
 tissue weighting f.
 transforming growth f. α
 transforming growth f. β
 tumor angiogenic f.
 tumor necrosis f.-beta
 uterine relaxing f.
 f. V
 f. VII
 f. VIII, F. VIII:C, f. VIIIR
 von Willebrand f.
 f. X
 f. XI
 f. XII
 f. XIII
factorial experiments
facultative
 f. anaerobe
 f. heterochromatin
 f. hyperopia
 f. parasite
 f. saprophyte
faculty
Faden suture
fading time
Faget's sign
Fahraeus-Lindqvist effect
Fahr's disease
failure
 acute respiratory f.
 backward heart f.
 cardiac f.
 congestive heart f.
 coronary f.
 electrical f.
 forward heart f.
 heart f.

high output f.
left-sided heart f.
left ventricular f.
low output f.
pacemaker f.
power f.
pump f.
renal f.
right ventricular f.
f. to thrive

faint
faith healing
falcate
falces (*pl. of* falx)
falcial
falciform
f. cartilage
f. crest
f. ligament
f. ligament of liver
f. lobe
f. margin
f. process
f. retinal fold

falcine
falciparum
f. fever
f. malaria

falcula
falcular
fallen arches
falling
f. palate
f. sickness
f. of the womb

fallopian
f. aqueduct
f. arch
f. canal
f. hiatus
f. ligament
f. neuritis
f. pregnancy
f. tube

Fallot's
F. tetrad
F. triad

false
f. agglutination
f. albuminuria
f. anemia
f. aneurysm
f. angina
f. ankylosis
f. blepharoptosis
f. branching
f. cast
f. conjugate

f. coxa vara
f. cyanosis
f. cyst
f. dextrocardia
f. diphtheria
f. diverticulum
f. dominance
f. glottis
f. hematuria
f. hermaphroditism
f. hypertrophy
f. image
f. joint
f. knots
f. knots of umbilical cord
f. labor
f. macula
f. masturbation
f. membrane
f. mole
f. negative
f. neuroma
f. nucleolus
f. pains
f. paracusis
f. pelvis
f. positive
f. pregnancy
f. projection
f. ribs
f. suture
f. thirst
f. vertebrae
f. vocal cord
f. waters

false-negative reaction
false-positive reaction
falsification
retrospective f.

falx, pl. **falces**
f. aponeurotica
f. cerebelli
f. cerebri
f. inguinalis
f. septi

familial
f. aggregation
f. amyloid neuropathy
f. amyloidosis
f. aortic ectasia
f. aortic ectasia syndrome
f. bipolar mood disorder
f. cancer
f. dysautonomia
f. emphysema
f. erythroblastic anemia
f. fat-induced hyperlipemia
f. glycinuria

F

familial *(continued)*
    f. high density lipoprotein
      deficiency
    f. hyperbetalipoproteinemia
    f. hyperbetalipoproteinemia and
      hyperprebetalipoproteinemia
    f. hypercholesteremic xanthomatosis
    f. hypercholesterolemia
    f. hypercholesterolemia with
      hyperlipemia
    f. hyperchylomicronemia
    f. hyperchylomicronemia with
      hyperprebetalipoproteinemia
    f. hyperlipoproteinemia
    f. hyperprebetalipoproteinemia
    f. hypertriglyceridemia
    f. hypertrophic cardiomyopathy
    f. hypogonadotropic hypogonadism
    f. hypoparathyroidism
    f. hypoplastic anemia
    f. intestinal polyposis
    f. juvenile nephrophthisis
    f. lipodystrophy
    f. Mediterranean fever
    f. microcytic anemia
    f. multiple endocrine adenomatosis
    f. nephrosis
    f. paroxysmal polyserositis
    f. paroxysmal rhabdomyolysis
    f. periodic paralysis
    f. pseudoinflammatory macular
      degeneration
    f. pseudoinflammatory maculopathy
    f. pyridoxine-responsive anemia
    f. recurrent polyserositis
    f. screening
    f. spinal muscular atrophy
    f. splenic anemia
    f. tremor
    f. white folded dysplasia
familial neuroviscerolipidosis
family
    cancer f.
    extended f.
    f. medicine
    nuclear f.
    f. physician
    f. practice
    f. therapy
famine
    f. dropsy
    f. fever
Fañanás cell
FANA test
Fanconi's
    F. anemia
    F. pancytopenia
    F. syndrome

Fannia
fan sign
fantasy
far
    F. East hemorrhagic fever
    F. East Russian encephalitis
    f. point
    f. point of convergence
    f. sight
Farabeuf's
    F. amputation
    F. triangle
faradization
faradocontractility
faradomuscular
faradopalpation
faradotherapy
far-and-near suture
Farber's
    F. disease
    F. syndrome
fardel
farina
    f. avenae
    f. tritici
farmer's
    f. lung
    f. skin
Farnsworth-Munsell color test
Farrant's mounting fluid
Farre's line
Farr's law
farsightedness
fascia, fascias, pl. **fasciae, fascias**
    Abernethy's f.
    f. adherens
    anal f.
    antebrachial f.
    f. antebrachii
    f. axillaris
    axillary f.
    bicipital f.
    brachial f.
    f. brachii
    broad f.
    f. buccopharyngea
    buccopharyngeal f.
    Buck's f.
    f. bulbi
    Camper's f.
    f. cervicalis
    f. cervicalis profunda
    f. cinerea
    clavipectoral f.
    f. clavipectoralis
    f. clitoridis
    f. of clitoris
    Colles' f.

Cooper's f.
cremasteric f.
f. cremasterica
cribriform f.
f. cribrosa
crural f.
f. cruris
Cruveilhier's f.
dartos f.
deep f.
deep f. of arm
deep cervical f.
deep f. of forearm
deep f. of leg
deep f. of neck
deep f. of penis
deep f. of thigh
f. dentata hippocampi
dentate f.
f. diaphragmatis pelvis inferior
f. diaphragmatis pelvis superior
f. diaphragmatis urogenitalis inferior
f. diaphragmatis urogenitalis
  superior
dorsal f. of foot
dorsal f. of hand
f. dorsalis manus
f. dorsalis pedis
Dupuytren's f.
endopelvic f.
endothoracic f.
f. endothoracica
external spermatic f.
f. of extraocular muscles
extraperitoneal f.
f. of forearm
Gerota's f.
Godman's f.
f. graft
Hesselbach's f.
iliac f.
f. iliaca
iliopectineal f.
inferior f. of pelvic diaphragm
inferior f. of urogenital diaphragm
infraspinatus f., f. infraspinata
infundibuliform f.
intercolumnar fasciae
internal spermatic f.
interosseous f.
investing f.
lacrimal f.
f. lata
f. of leg
lumbodorsal f.
masseteric f.
f. masseterica
middle cervical f.

muscular f. of extraocular muscle
f. muscularis musculorum bulbi
f. nuchae
nuchal f.
obturator f.
f. obturatoria
orbital fasciae
fasciae orbitales
palmar f.
parietal pelvic f.
parotid f.
f. parotidea
parotideomasseteric f.
f. parotideomasseterica
pectoral f.
f. pectoralis
pelvic f.
f. pelvis
f. pelvis parietalis
f. pelvis visceralis
f. penis
f. of penis
f. penis profunda
f. penis superficialis
f. perinei superficialis
perirenal f.
pharyngobasilar f.
f. pharyngobasilaris
phrenicopleural f.
f. phrenicopleuralis
plantar f.
popliteal f.
Porter's f.
pretracheal f.
prevertebral f.
f. profunda
f. prostatae
f. of prostate
rectovesical f.
renal f.
f. renalis
Scarpa's f.
semilunar f.
Sibson's f.
f. spermatica externa
f. spermatica interna
subperitoneal f.
f. subperitonealis
subsartorial f.
superficial f.
f. superficialis
superficial f. of penis
superficial f. of perineum
superior f. of pelvic diaphragm
superior f. of urogenital diaphragm
temporal f.
f. temporalis
f. thoracolumbalis

F

fascia *(continued)*
    thoracolumbar f.
    Toldt's f.
    transversalis f.
    f. transversalis
    Treitz's f.
    triangular f.
    f. triangularis abdominis
    Tyrrell's f.
    umbilical prevesical f.
    umbilicovesical f.
    vastoadductor f.
    visceral pelvic f.
    Zuckerkandl's f.
fascial
    f. hernia
    f. sheath of eyeball
    f. sheaths of extraocular muscles
fascicle
    muscle f.
    nerve f.
fascicular
    f. block
    f. degeneration
    f. graft
    f. keratitis
    f. ophthalmoplegia
    f. sarcoma
    f. ulcer
fasciculata cell
fasciculate, fasciculated
fasciculation
fasciculus, gen. and pl. **fasciculi**
    f. anterior proprius
    anterior pyramidal f.
    arcuate f.
    f. atrioventricularis
    Burdach's f.
    calcarine f.
    central tegmental f.
    f. circumolivaris pyramidis
    f. corticospinalis anterior
    f. corticospinalis lateralis
    cuneate f.
    f. cuneatus
    dorsal longitudinal f.
    dorsolateral f.
    f. dorsolateralis
    Flechsig's fasciculi
    Foville's f.
    fronto-occipital f.
    gracile f.
    f. gracilis
    hooked f.
    inferior longitudinal f.
    interfascicular f.
    f. interfascicularis
    intersegmental fasciculi

    f. lateralis plexus brachialis
    f. lateralis proprius
    lateral pyramidal f.
    lenticular f.
    f. lenticularis
    Lissauer's f.
    fasciculi longitudinales ligamenti cruciformis atlantis
    fasciculi longitudinales pontis
    f. longitudinalis dorsalis
    f. longitudinalis inferior
    f. longitudinalis medialis
    f. longitudinalis superior
    longitudinal pontine fasciculi
    macular f.
    f. macularis
    mamillotegmental f.
    f. mamillotegmentalis
    mamillothalamic f.
    f. mamillothalamicus
    marginal f.
    f. marginalis
    f. medialis plexus brachialis
    medial longitudinal f.
    Meynert's f.
    oblique pontine f.
    f. obliquus pontis
    occipitofrontal f.
    f. occipitofrontalis
    oval f.
    f. pedunculomamillaris
    pedunculomamillary f.
    perpendicular f.
    f. posterior plexus brachialis
    proper fasciculi
    fasciculi proprii
    f. pyramidalis anterior
    f. pyramidalis lateralis
    retroflex f.
    f. retroflexus
    f. rotundus
    round f.
    rubroreticular fasciculi
    fasciculi rubroreticulares
    semilunar f.
    f. semilunaris
    septomarginal f.
    f. septomarginalis
    slender f.
    f. solitarius
    solitary f.
    subcallosal f.
    f. subcallosus
    subthalamic f.
    superior longitudinal f.
    thalamic f.
    f. thalamicus
    f. thalamomamillaris

transverse fasciculi
fasciculi transversi
unciform f., uncinate f.
uncinate f. of Russell
f. uncinatus
wedge-shaped f.
fasciectomy
fasciitis
    eosinophilic f.
    group A streptococcal
      necrotizing f.
    necrotizing f.
    nodular f.
    parosteal f.
    proliferative f.
    pseudosarcomatous f.
fasciodesis
Fasciola
    F. gigantica
fasciola, pl. **fasciolae**
    f. cinerea
fasciolar
    f. gyrus
fasciolid
fasciolopsiasis
Fasciolopsis
    F. buski
    F. rathouisi
fascioplasty
fasciorrhaphy
fasciotomy
fascitis
fast
    f. green FCF
    f. smear
fastidious
    f. organism
fastidium cibi
fastigatum
fastigial nucleus
fastigiobulbar
    f. fibers
    f. tract
fastigiospinal fibers
fastigium
fasting hypoglycemia
fastness
fat
    f. body of cheek
    f. body of ischiorectal fossa
    f. body of orbit
    f. cell
    f. embolism
    f. graft
    f. hernia
    f. indigestion
    f. necrosis
    f. pad

    f. tide
    unilocular f.
    white f.
fatal
fatality
    f. rate
fate
    f. map
    prospective f.
father complex
fatigability
fatigable
fatigue
    auditory f.
    battle f.
    f. fever
    f. fracture
    functional vocal f.
    f. strength
fat-pad
    Bichat's f.-p.
    buccal f.-p.
    Imlach's f.-p.
    infrapatellar f.-p.
    ischiorectal f.-p.
    orbital f.-p.
fat-storing cell
fatty
    f. ascites
    f. atrophy
    f. cast
    f. change
    f. cirrhosis
    f. degeneration
    f. diarrhea
    f. heart
    f. hernia
    f. infiltration
    f. kidney
    f. layer of superficial fascia
    f. liver
    f. metamorphosis
    f. phanerosis
    f. renal capsule
    f. stool
    f. tissue
fatty acid
    unesterified free f. a.
fauces, gen. **faucium**
faucial
    f. branches of lingual nerve
    f. diphtheria
    f. paralysis
    f. reflex
    f. tonsil
faulty union
faun tail nevus

F

faveolate
faveolus, pl. faveoli
favic chandeliers
favid
FA virus
favism
Favre-Durand-Nicholas disease
Favre-Racouchet's disease
Favre-Racouchot syndrome
Favre's dystrophy
favus
Fc
    F. fragment
    F. piece
    F. receptor

FDC concentration

fear
feather louse
featural surgery
features
febricula
febrile
    f. albuminuria
    f. convulsion
    f. crisis
    f. psychosis
    f. seizure
    f. urine
    f. urticaria
febris
    f. melitensis
    f. undulans
fecal
    f. abscess
    f. fistula
    f. impaction
    f. incontinence
    f. tumor
    f. vomiting
fecalith
fecaloid
fecaloma
fecaluria
feces
Fechner-Weber law
feculent
fecund
fecundate
fecundation
fecundity
feedback
    negative f.
    positive f.
    f. system
feeding
    f. center
    fictitious f.
    forced f., forcible f.
    gastric f.

    nasal f.
    sham f.
    f. tube
feeling
    f. tone
Feer's disease
feigned eruption
Feiss line
feline
    f. panleukopenia virus
    f. rhinotracheitis virus
fellatio
fellation
fellatorism
fellatrix
felon
Felson
feltwork
Felty's syndrome
female
    f. catheter
    genetic f.
    f. genital tract cytologic smear
    f. gonad
    f. hermaphroditism
    f. homosexuality
    f. pattern alopecia
    f. pronucleus
    f. prostate
    f. pseudohermaphroditism
    f. sterility
    f. urethra
    f. urethral syndrome
    XO f.
    XXX f.
femininity complex
feminization
    testicular f.
femora (*pl. of* femur)
femoral
    f. arch
    f. artery
    f. branch of genitofemoral nerve
    f. canal
    f. fossa
    f. hernia
    f. muscle
    f. nerve
    f. opening
    f. plexus
    f. reflex
    f. region
    f. ring
    f. septum
    f. sheath
    f. triangle
    f. vein
femoris (*gen. of* femur)

femoroabdominal reflex
femorocele
femoropopliteal
    f. bypass
    f. occlusive disease
femorotibial
femur, gen. **femoris**, pl. **femora**
fenestra, pl. **fenestrae**
    f. of the cochlea
    f. cochleae
    f. nov-ovalis
    f. ovalis
    f. rotunda
    f. of the vestibule
    f. vestibuli
fenestrated
    f. capillary
    f. membrane
    f. sheath
fenestration
    f. operation
    optic nerve sheath f.
    tracheal f.
Fenn effect
Fenwick-Hunner ulcer
Fenwick's disease
Fergusson's incision
fermentative dyspepsia
Fernandez reaction
Fernbach flask
ferning
fern test
Ferrata's cell
Ferrein's
    F. canal
    F. cords
    F. foramen
    F. ligament
    F. pyramid
    F. tube
    F. vasa aberrantia
ferric chloride test
ferrokinetics
ferrotherapy
ferrugination
ferruginous bodies
ferrule
Ferry-Porter law
fertile
    f. period
fertility
    f. agent
    f. factor
    f. ratio
fertilization
    f. membrane
    in vitro f.
    in vivo f.

fertilized ovum
fervescence
fester
festinant
festinating gait
festination
festoon
    gingival f.
festooning
fetal
    f. adrenal cortex
    f. age
    f. aspiration syndrome
    f. attitude
    f. bradycardia
    f. circulation
    f. cotyledon
    f. death
    f. death rate
    f. distress
    f. dystocia
    f. electrocardiography
    f. face syndrome
    f. fracture
    f. gigantism
    f. habitus
    f. heart rate
    f. hydantoin syndrome
    f. hydrops
    f. inclusion
    f. medicine
    f. membrane
    f. movement
    f. ovoid
    f. placenta
    f. reticularis
    f. souffle
    f. tachycardia
    f. trimethadione syndrome
    f. zone
fetalism
feticide
fetid
fetish
fetishism
fetography
fetology
fetomaternal transfusion
fetometry
fetopathy
    diabetic f.
fetoplacental
    f. anasarca
fetoproteins, α-fetoproteins, β-fetoproteins, γ-fetoproteins
    α f.

F

317

fetor
  f. hepaticus
  f. oris
fetoscope
fetoscopy
fetus, pl. **fetuses**
  f. in fetu
  harlequin f.
  impacted f.
  f. papyraceus
  f. sanguinolentis
Feulgen
  F. reaction
  F. stain
fever
  absorption f.
  acclimating f.
  Aden f.
  aestivoautumnal f.
  African hemorrhagic f.
  African tick f.
  algid pernicious f.
  ardent f.
  Argentinean hemorrhagic f.
  artificial f.
  aseptic f.
  Assam f.
  Australian Q f.
  autumn f.
  bilious remittent f.
  black f.
  blackwater f.
  f. blister
  blue f.
  Bolivian hemorrhagic f.
  bouquet f.
  boutonneuse f.
  brass founder's f.
  Brazilian hemorrhagic f.
  Brazilian purpuric f.
  Brazilian spotted f.
  breakbone f.
  bullous f.
  Bunyamwera f.
  Burdwan f.
  Bwamba f.
  cachectic f.
  camp f.
  canefield f.
  canicola f.
  Carter's f.
  catarrhal f.
  cat-bite f.
  catheter f.
  Central European tick-borne f.
  cerebrospinal f.
  Charcot's intermittent f.
  childbed f.

  Colorado tick f.
  Congolian red f.
  continued f.
  cotton-mill f.
  Crimean f.
  Crimean-Congo hemorrhagic f.
  dandy f.
  date f.
  deer-fly f.
  dehydration f.
  dengue f.
  dengue hemorrhagic f.
  desert f.
  digestive f.
  diphasic milk f.
  double quotidian f.
  drug f.
  Dumdum f.
  Dutton's relapsing f.
  Ebola hemorrhagic f.
  elephantoid f.
  enteric f.
  entericoid f.
  ephemeral f.
  epidemic hemorrhagic f.
  epimastical f.
  eruptive f.
  essential f.
  exanthematous f.
  exsiccation f.
  falciparum f.
  familial Mediterranean f.
  famine f.
  Far East hemorrhagic f.
  fatigue f.
  field f.
  five-day f.
  flood f.
  food f.
  Fort Bragg f.
  foundryman's f.
  Gambian f.
  glandular f.
  Haverhill f.
  hay f.
  hematuric bilious f.
  hemoglobinuric f.
  hemorrhagic f.
  hemorrhagic f. with renal syndrome
  hepatic intermittent f.
  herpetic f.
  hospital f.
  icterohemorrhagic f.
  Ilhéus f.
  inanition f.
  induced f.
  intermittent malarial f.
  inundation f.

island f.
jail f.
Japanese river f.
jungle f.
jungle yellow f.
Katayama f.
kedani f.
Kenya f.
Kew Gardens f.
Kinkiang f.
Korean hemorrhagic f.
Lassa f.
Lassa hemorrhagic f.
laurel f.
malarial f.
malignant tertian f.
Manchurian f.
Manchurian hemorrhagic f.
Marseilles f.
marsh f.
Mediterranean exanthematous f.
meningotyphoid f.
metal fume f.
Mexican spotted f.
mianeh f.
miliary f.
mill f.
miniature scarlet f.
monoleptic f.
Mossman f.
mumu f.
nanukayami f.
nodal f.
North Queensland tick f.
Omsk hemorrhagic f.
o'nyong-nyong f.
Oroya f.
Pahvant Valley f.
paludal f.
pappataci f.
papular f.
paratyphoid f.
parenteric f.
Pel-Ebstein f.
periodic f.
Persian relapsing f.
pharyngoconjunctival f.
Philippine hemorrhagic f.
phlebotomus f.
pinta f.
polka f.
polyleptic f.
pretibial f.
protein f.
puerperal f.
Pym's f.
pyogenic f.
quartan f.

quintan f.
quotidian f.
rabbit f.
rat-bite f.
recrudescent typhus f.
recurrent f.
red f., red f. of the Congo
relapsing f.
remittent f.
remittent malarial f.
rheumatic f.
rice-field f.
Rocky Mountain spotted f.
Roman f.
Ross River f.
sakushu f.
Salinem f.
salt f.
sandfly f.
San Joaquin f.
San Joaquin Valley f.
São Paulo f.
scarlet f.
septic f.
seven-day f.
shin bone f.
ship f.
shoddy f.
Sindbis f.
slime f.
slow f.
smelter's f.
snail f.
solar f.
Songo f.
South African tick-bite f.
spirillum f.
spotted f.
steroid f.
symptomatic f.
syphilitic f.
tertian f.
therapeutic f.
f. therapy
thermic f.
thirst f.
three-day f.
Tobia f.
traumatic f.
trench f.
trypanosome f.
tsutsugamushi f.
typhoid f.
undifferentiated type f.'s
undulating f.
urethral f.
urinary f.
urticarial f.

F

fever *(continued)*
    uveoparotid f.
    Uzbekistan hemorrhagic f.
    valley f.
    viral hemorrhagic f.
    vivax f.
    West African f.
    West Nile f.
    wound f.
    Yangtze Valley f.
    yellow f.
    Zika f.
    zinc fume f.
feverish
    f. urine
Fevold test
ff waves
FGT cytologic smear
fiber
    A f.'s
    accelerator f.'s
    adrenergic f.'s
    afferent f.'s
    alpha f.'s
    anastomosing f.'s, anastomotic f.'s
    arcuate f.'s
    arcuate f.'s of cerebrum
    argyrophilic f.'s
    association f.'s
    augmentor f.'s
    B f.'s
    Bergmann's f.'s
    beta f.'s
    C f.'s
    cerebellohypothalamic f.'s
    cerebellospinal f.'s
    cholinergic f.'s
    chromatic f.
    circular f.'s
    climbing f.'s
    collagen f., collagenous f.
    commissural f.'s
    cone f., inner cone f., outer cone f.
    corticobulbar f.'s
    corticonuclear f.'s
    corticopontine f.'s
    corticoreticular f.'s
    corticorubral f.'s
    corticospinal f.'s
    corticothalamic f.'s
    dentatorubral f.'s
    dentatothalamic f.'s
    dentinal f.'s, dental f.'s
    depressor f.'s
    dietary f.
    efferent f.'s
    elastic f.'s
    enamel f.'s

    endogenous f.'s
    exogenous f.'s
    external arcuate f.'s
    fastigiobulbar f.'s
    fastigiospinal f.'s
    gamma f.'s
    Gerdy's f.'s
    Gratiolet's f.'s
    gray f.'s
    hypothalamocerebellar f.'s
    inhibitory f.'s
    inner cone f. (*var. of* cone f.)
    intercolumnar f.'s
    intercrural f.'s
    internal arcuate f.'s
    intrafusal f.'s
    intrinsic f.'s
    James f.'s
    Korff's f.'s
    Kühne's f.
    f.'s of lens
    Mahaim f.'s
    medullated nerve f.
    meridional f.'s
    mossy f.'s
    motor f.'s
    Müller's f.'s
    myelinated nerve f.
    Nélaton's f.'s
    nerve f.
    nodoventricular f.'s
    nonmedullated f.'s
    nuclear bag f.
    nuclear chain f.
    nucleocortical f.'s
    oblique f.'s of stomach
    olivocochlear f.'s
    osteocollagenous f.'s
    osteogenetic f.'s
    outer cone f. (*var. of* cone f.)
    pectinate f.'s
    perforating f.'s
    periodontal ligament f.'s
    periventricular f.'s
    pilomotor f.'s
    postganglionic f.'s
    precollagenous f.'s
    preganglionic f.'s
    pressor f.'s
    projection f.'s
    Prussak's f.'s
    Purkinje's f.'s
    pyramidal f.'s
    raphespinal f.'s
    red f.'s
    Reissner's f.
    Remak's f.'s
    reticular f.'s

Retzius' f.'s
rod f.
Rosenthal f.
Sappey's f.'s
Sharpey's f.'s
skeletal muscle f.'s
spindle f.
spinoreticular f.'s
striatonigral f.'s
strionigral f.'s
sudomotor f.'s
sustentacular f.'s of retina
T f.
tautomeric f.s
thalamocortical f.'s
Tomes' f.'s
transseptal f.'s
transverse pontine f.'s
unmyelinated f.'s
vasomotor f.'s
Weitbrecht's f.'s
white f.
yellow f.'s
zonular f.'s

fiberoptic
f. gastroscope
fiberoptics
fiberscope
fibra, pl. **fibrae**
fibrae arcuatae cerebri
fibrae arcuatae externae
fibrae arcuatae internae
fibrae circulares
fibrae corticonucleares
fibrae corticopontinae
fibrae corticoreticulares
fibrae corticospinales
fibrae dentatorubrales
fibrae intercrurales
fibrae lentis
fibrae meridionales
fibrae obliquae gastrici
fibrae periventriculares
fibrae pontis transversae
fibrae pyramidales
fibrae zonulares
fibre
fibremia
fibril
collagen f.'s
muscular f.
subpellicular f.
unit f.'s
fibrilla, pl. **fibrillae**
fibrillar, fibrillary
f. baskets
fibrillate
fibrillated

fibrillation
atrial f., auricular f.
f. threshold
ventricular f.
fibrillatory waves
fibrillin
fibrilloflutter
fibrillogenesis
fibrin
f. calculus
f. thrombus
fibrin/fibrinogen degradation products
fibrinocellular
fibrinogen
fibrinogenemia
fibrinogen-fibrin conversion syndrome
fibrinogenic, fibrinogenous
fibrinogenolysis
fibrinogenopenia
fibrinogenous (*var. of* fibrinogenic)
fibrinoid
f. degeneration
f. necrosis
fibrinolytic purpura
fibrinopurulent
f. inflammation
fibrinoscopy
fibrinous
f. adhesion
f. bronchitis
f. cast
f. cataract
f. degeneration
f. inflammation
f. iritis
f. lymph
f. pericarditis
f. pleurisy
f. polyp
fibrin-stabilizing factor
fibrinuria
fibroadenoma
giant f.
intracanalicular f.
pericanalicular f.
fibroadipose
fibroareolar
fibroblast
f. interferon
fibroblastic
fibrocarcinoma
fibrocartilage
basilar f.
circumferential f.
external semilunar f.
interarticular f.
internal semilunar f. of knee joint

F

fibrocartilage *(continued)*
    semilunar f.
    stratiform f.
fibrocartilaginous
    f. ring of tympanic membrane
fibrocartilago
    f. basalis
    f. interarticularis
    f. intervertebralis
fibrocaseous peritonitis
fibrocellular
fibrochondritis
fibrochondroma
fibrocongestive
fibrocyst
fibrocystic
    f. condition of the breast
    f. disease of the pancreas
fibrocystoma
fibrocyte
fibrodysplasia
    f. ossificans progressiva
fibroelastic
    f. membrane of larynx
fibroelastosis
    endocardial f., endomyocardial f.
fibroenchondroma
fibroepithelial polyp
fibroepithelioma
fibrofatty
fibrofolliculoma
fibrogenesis
fibrogliosis
fibrohyaline tissue
fibroid
    f. adenoma
    f. cataract
    f. inflammation
    f. lung
    f. tumor
fibroidectomy
fibrokeratoma
fibrolamellar liver cell carcinoma
fibroleiomyoma
fibrolipoma
fibroma
    ameloblastic f.
    aponeurotic f.
    central cementifying f.
    central ossifying f.
    chondromyxoid f.
    concentric f.
    desmoplastic f.
    giant cell f.
    irritation f.
    f. molle
    f. molle gravidarum
    f. myxomatodes

    nonossifying f.
    nonosteogenic f.
    odontogenic f.
    peripheral ossifying f.
    periungual f.
    rabbit f.
    recurring digital f.'s of childhood
    senile f.
    Shope f.
    telangiectatic f.
fibromatoid
fibromatosis
    abdominal f.
    aggressive infantile f.
    f. colli
    congenital generalized f.
    gingival f.
    infantile digital f.
    juvenile hyalin f.
    juvenile palmo-plantar f.
    palmar f.
    penile f.
    plantar f.
    f. virus of rabbits
fibromatous
fibromectomy
fibrometer
fibromuscular
    f. dysplasia
    f. hyperplasia
fibromyectomy
fibromyoma
fibromyositis
fibromyxoma
fibronectins
    plasma f.
fibroneuroma
fibro-osteoma
fibropapilloma
fibroplasia
    retrolental f.
fibroplastic
fibroplate
fibropolypus
fibroreticulate
fibrosarcoma
    ameloblastic f.
    Earle L f.
    infantile f.
fibrose
fibroserous
fibrosing
    f. adenomatosis
    f. adenosis
    f. alveolitis
    f. mediastinitis
fibrosis
    African endomyocardial f.

congenital f. of the extraocular
   muscles
cystic f., cystic f. of the pancreas
endocardial f.
endomyocardial f.
idiopathic interstitial f.
idiopathic pulmonary f.
interstitial pulmonary f.
leptomeningeal f.
mediastinal f.
nodular subepidermal f.
oral submucous f.
pericentral f.
perimuscular f.
pipestem f.
replacement f.
retroperitoneal f.
subadventitial f.
Symmers' clay pipestem f.,
   Symmers' f.

fibrositic headache
fibrositis
   cervical f.
fibrothorax
fibrotic
   f. ophthalmoplegia
fibrous
   f. adhesion
   f. ankylosis
   f. appendix of liver
   f. articular capsule
   f. astrocyte
   f. bacterial viruses
   f. capsule
   f. capsule of kidney
   f. capsule of liver
   f. capsule of parotid gland
   f. capsule of spleen
   f. capsule of thyroid gland
   f. cavernitis
   f. cortical defect
   f. degeneration
   f. digital sheaths of foot
   f. digital sheaths of hand
   f. dysplasia of bone
   f. dysplasia of jaws
   f. goiter
   f. hamartoma of infancy
   f. histiocytoma
   f. joint
   f. layer
   f. mediastinitis
   f. membrane
   f. pericarditis
   f. pericardium
   f. pneumonia
   f. polyp
   f. ring

f. ring of heart
f. ring of intervertebral disc
f. sheaths
f. skeleton of heart
f. tendon sheath
f. tissue
f. trigones of heart
f. tubercle
f. tunic of corpus spongiosum
f. tunic of eye
f. union
f. xanthoma
fibroxanthoma
   atypical f.
fibula
fibular
   f. artery
   f. articular surface of tibia
   f. collateral ligament
   f. collateral ligament of ankle
   f. lymph node
   f. margin of foot
   f. node
   f. notch
   f. veins
fibularis
fibulocalcaneal
Fick
   F. method
   F. principle
Ficoll-Hypaque technique
ficosis
fictitious feeding
Fiedler's myocarditis
field
   auditory f.
   f. block
   f. block anesthesia
   Broca's f.
   Cohnheim's f.
   f. of consciousness
   f. emission tube
   f. fever
   f. of fixation
   f.'s of Forel
   free f.
   f. gradient
   H f.'s
   individuation f.
   f. lens
   magnetic f.
   microscopic f.
   nerve f.
   prerubral f.
   f. survey
   tegmental f.'s of Forel
   visual f.
   Wernicke's f.

F

Fielding's membrane
Field's rapid stain
field-vole
Fiessinger-Leroy-Reiter syndrome
fièvre
    f. boutonneuse
fifth
    f. cranial nerve
    f. disease
    f. finger
    f. ventricle
fight or flight reaction
Figueira's syndrome
figuratus
figure
    authority f.
    flame f.
    fortification f.'s
    mitotic f.
    myelin f.
    Purkinje's f.'s
figure and ground
figure-of-8
    f.-o. abnormality
    f.-o. bandage
    f.-o. suture
fig wart
fila (*pl. of* filum)
fila
filaceous
filament
    actin f.
    axial f.
    cytokeratin f.'s
    intermediate f.'s
    keratin f.'s
    myosin f.
    parabasal f.
    f. polymorphonuclear leukocyte
    root f.'s
    spermatic f.
    Z f.
filamenta (*pl. of* filamentum)
filamentary
    f. keratitis
    f. keratopathy
filament-nonfilament count
filamentous
    f. bacterial viruses
    f. bacteriophage
    f. colony
filamentum, pl. filamenta
filar
    f. mass
    f. micrometer
    f. substance
Filaria
filaria, pl. filariae

filarial
    f. arthritis
    f. funiculitis
    f. hydrocele
    f. periodicity
    f. synovitis
filariasis
    bancroftian f.
    Brug's f.
    periodic f.
filariform
    f. larva
Filariicae
Filarioidea
Filatov
    F. disease
    F. Dukcs' disease
    F. flap
    F. operation
    F. spots
Filatov-Gillies
    F.-G. flap
    F.-G. tubed pedicle
file
    Hedström f.
    periodontal f.
    root canal f.
filial
    f. generation
filiform
    f. adnatum
    f. bougie
    f. nucleus
    f. papillae
    f. pulse
    f. wart
filioparental
filler graft
fillet
    lateral f.
    f. layer
    medial f.
filling
    f. defect
film
    absorbable gelatin f.
    bitewing f.
    decubitus f.
    horizontal beam f.
    latitude f.
    panoramic x-ray f.
    plain f.
    precorneal f.
    right or left lateral decubitus f.
    scout f.
    f. speed
    spot f.

tear f.
wide-latitude f.

film changer
rapid f. c.
serial f. c.

filopodium, pl. filopodia
filopressure
filovaricosis
Filoviridae
Filovirus
filter
bandpass f.
Berkefeld f.
bird's nest f.
Greenfield f.
high-pass f.
low-pass f.
nitinol f.
vena cava f.
venocaval f.

filtering
f. cicatrix
f. operation

filtrable, filterable
f. virus

filtration
f. angle
f. coefficient
f. fraction
f. slits
f. space

filtrum
Merkel's f. ventriculi
f. ventriculi

filum, pl. fila
f. durae matris spinalis
fila olfactoria
olfactory fila
radicular fila
fila radicularia
f. of spinal dura mater
terminal f.
f. terminale

fimbria, pl. fimbriae
f. hippocampi
ovarian f.
f. ovarica
fimbriae tubae uterinae
fimbriae of uterine tube

fimbriate, fimbriated
fimbriectomy
fimbriocele
fimbriodentate sulcus
fimbrioplasty
final
f. host
f. impression

Finckh test

finding
fine
f. needle biopsy
f. structure
f. tremor

fineness
finger
f. agnosia
baseball f.
blubber f.
bolster f.
clubbed f.'s
dead f.'s
drop f.
fifth f.
first f.
fourth f.
hammer f.
hippocratic f.'s
index f.
jerk f.
little f.
lock f.
mallet f.
middle f.
f. percussion
f. phenomenon
ring f.
sausage f.'s
seal f.'s
second f.
snap f.
spade f.'s
speck f.
spider f.
spring f.
stuck f.
third f.
trigger f.
waxy f.'s
webbed f.'s
whale f.'s
white f.'s

fingernail
finger-nose test
fingerprint
f. dystrophy
Galton's system of classification
of f.'s
genetic f.

finger-thumb reflex
finger-to-finger test
finishing bur
Fink-Heimer stain
Finney
F. operation
F. pyloroplasty

fire

F

325

first
- f. aid
- f. arch syndrome
- f. cranial nerve
- f. cuneiform bone
- f. degree A-V block
- f. degree burn
- f. degree prolapse
- f. dentition
- f. duodenal sphincter
- f. finger
- f. heart sound
- f. molar
- f. parallel pelvic plane
- f. permanent molar
- f. rank symptoms
- f. temporal convolution
- f. visceral cleft

first-set rejection

Fischer's
- F. sign
- F. symptom

fish
- f. skin
- f. tapeworm anemia

Fishberg concentration test

Fisher's
- F. exact test
- F. syndrome

Fishman-Lerner unit

fish-mouth
- f.-m. meatus
- f.-m. mitral stenosis

fission
- binary f.
- bud f.
- f. fungi
- multiple f.
- simple f.

fissiparity

fissiparous

fissura, pl. **fissurae**
- f. antitragohelicina
- f. calcarina
- fissurae cerebelli
- f. cerebri lateralis
- f. choroidea
- f. collateralis
- f. dentata
- f. hippocampi
- f. horizontalis cerebelli
- f. horizontalis pulmonis dextri
- f. ligamenti teretis
- f. ligamenti venosi
- f. longitudinalis cerebri
- f. mediana anterior medullae oblongatae

- f. mediana anterior medullae spinalis
- f. obliqua pulmonis
- f. orbitalis inferior
- f. orbitalis superior
- f. parietooccipitalis
- f. petro-occipitalis
- f. petrosquamosa
- f. petrotympanica
- f. posterolateralis
- f. prima cerebelli
- f. pterygoidea
- f. pterygomaxillaris
- f. pterygopalatina
- f. pudendi
- f. secunda cerebelli
- f. sphenopetrosa
- f. transversa cerebelli
- f. transversa cerebri
- f. tympanomastoidea
- f. tympanosquamosa

fissural
- f. cyst

fissuration

fissure
- abdominal f.
- Ammon's f.
- anal f.
- anterior median f. of medulla oblongata
- anterior median f. of spinal cord
- antitragohelicine f.
- auricular f.
- azygos f.
- Bichat's f.
- branchial f.
- Broca's f.
- f. bur
- calcarine f.
- callosomarginal f.
- f. caries
- caudal transverse f.
- cerebellar f.'s
- cerebral f.'s
- choroid f.
- choroidal f.
- Clevenger's f.
- collateral f.
- decidual f.
- dentate f.
- Duverney's f.'s
- Ecker's f.
- enamel f.
- glaserian f.
- great horizontal f.
- great longitudinal f.
- Henle's f.'s
- hippocampal f.

horizontal f. of cerebellum
horizontal f. of right lung
inferior accessory f.
inferior orbital f.
lateral cerebral f.
left sagittal f.
f. for ligamentum teres
f. of ligamentum venosum
linguogingival f.
f.'s of liver
longitudinal f. of cerebrum
f.'s of lung
major f.
minor f.
oblique f.
oblique f. of lung
optic f.
oral f.
palpebral f.
Pansch's f.
paracentral f.
parieto-occipital f.
petro-occipital f.
petrosquamous f.
petrotympanic f.
portal f.
postcentral f.
posterior median f. of the medulla
  oblongata
posterior median f. of spinal cord
posterolateral f.
posthippocampal f.
postlingual f.
postlunate f.
postpyramidal f.
postrhinal f.
prenodular f.
primary f. of cerebellum
pterygoid f.
pterygomaxillary f.
rhinal f.
right sagittal f.
f. of Rolando
f. of round ligament of liver
Santorini's f.'s
f. sealant
secondary f. of cerebellum
f. sign
sphenoidal f.
sphenomaxillary f.
sphenopetrosal f.
squamotympanic f.
superior orbital f.
superior temporal f.
sylvian f., f. of Sylvius
transverse f. of cerebellum
transverse f. of cerebrum
transverse f. of the lung

tympanomastoid f.
tympanosquamous f.
umbilical f.
f. of venous ligament
vestibular f. of cochlea
zygal f.

fissured
  f. fracture
  f. tongue

fistula, pl. **fistulae, fistulas**
  abdominal f.
  amphibolic f., amphibolous f.
  anal f.
  arteriovenous f.
  f. auris congenita
  biliary f.
  f. bimucosa
  blind f.
  B-P f.
  branchial f.
  Brescia-Cimino f.
  bronchobiliary f.
  bronchocavitary f.
  bronchoesophageal f.
  bronchopleural f.
  carotid-cavernous f.
  cholecystoduodenal f.
  coccygeal f.
  f. colli congenita
  colocutaneous f.
  coloileal f.
  colonic f.
  colovaginal f.
  colovesical f.
  complete f.
  congenital pulmonary
    arteriovenous f.
  dental f.
  duodenal f.
  Eck f.
  enterocutaneous f.
  enterovaginal f.
  enterovesical f.
  ethmoidal-lacrimal f.
  external f.
  fecal f.
  gastric f.
  gastrocolic f.
  gastrocutaneous f.
  gastroduodenal f.
  gastrointestinal f.
  genitourinary f.
  gingival f.
  hepatic f.
  hepatopleural f.
  horseshoe f.
  H-type f.
  H-type tracheoesophageal f.

F

fistula *(continued)*
    incomplete f.
    internal f.
    internal lacrimal f.
    intestinal f.
    f. knife
    lacrimal f., f. lacrimalis
    lacteal f.
    lymphatic f.
    mammary f.
    Mann-Bollman f.
    metroperitoneal f.
    oroantral f.
    orofacial f.
    oronasal f.
    parietal f.
    perineovaginal f.
    pharyngeal f.
    pilonidal f.
    pulmonary f.
    rectolabial f.
    rectourethral f.
    rectovaginal f.
    rectovesical f.
    rectovestibular f.
    rectovulvar f.
    reverse Eck f.
    salivary f.
    sigmoidovesical f.
    spermatic f.
    T-E f.
    f. test
    Thiry's f.
    Thiry-Vella f.
    thoracic f.
    tracheal f.
    tracheobiliary f.
    tracheoesophageal f.
    umbilical f.
    urachal f.
    ureterocutaneous f.
    ureterovaginal f.
    urethrovaginal f.
    urinary f.
    urogenital f.
    uteroperitoneal f.
    Vella's f.
    vesical f.
    vesicocolic f.
    vesicocutaneous f.
    vesicointestinal f.
    vesicouterine f.
    vesicovaginal f.
    vesicovaginorectal f.
    vitelline f.
fistulation, fistulization
fistulatome
fistulectomy

fistulization *(var. of* fistulation)
fistuloenterostomy
fistulotomy
fistulous
fit
    uncinate f.
fitness
    clinical f.
    evolutionary f.
    genetic f.
    physical f.
FIT test
Fitz-Hugh and Curtis syndrome
five-day fever
five year survival rate
fixation
    bifoveal f.
    binocular f.
    circumalveolar f.
    circummandibular f.
    circumzygomatic f.
    complement f.
    craniofacial f.
    crossed f.
    f. disparity
    eccentric f.
    elastic band f.
    external f.
    external pin f.
    external pin f., biphase
    freudian f.
    genetic f.
    intermaxillary f.
    internal f.
    intraosseous f.
    mandibulomaxillary f.
    maxillomandibular f.
    nasomandibular f.
    f. nystagmus
    f. reaction
fixational ocular movement
fixative
    acetone f.
    Altmann's f.
    Bouin's f.
    Carnoy's f.
    Champy's f.
    Flemming's f.
    formaldehyde f.
    formol-calcium f.
    formol-Müller f.
    formol-saline f.
    formol-Zenker f.
    glutaraldehyde f.
    Golgi's osmiobichromate f.
    Helly's f.
    Hermann's f.
    Kaiserling's f.

Luft's potassium permanganate f.
Marchi's f.
methanol f.
Müller's f.
neutral buffered formalin f.
Newcomer's f.
Orth's f.
osmic acid f.
Park-Williams f.
picroformol f.
Regaud's f.
Schaudinn's f.
Thoma's f.
Zenker's f.

fixator
    f. muscle

fixed
    f. bridge
    f. contracture
    f. coupling
    f. dressing
    f. drug eruption
    f. idea
    f. macrophage
    f. partial denture
    f. pupil
    f. rate pulse generator
    f. torticollis
    f. virus

fixed-interval reinforcement schedule
fixed-rate pacemaker
fixed-ratio reinforcement schedule
fixing
    f. eye

flaccid
    f. ectropion
    f. membrane
    f. paralysis
    f. part of tympanic membrane

flaccidity
Flack's node
flag
    f. flap
    f. sign

flagella (*pl. of* flagellum)
flagellar
    f. agglutinin
    f. antigen

Flagellata
flagellate
    collared f.
    f. diarrhea

flagellated
flagellation
flagellosis
flagellum, pl. **flagella**

flail
    f. chest
    f. joint

flame
    f. arc
    f. figure
    f. nevus
    f. photometer
    f. spots

flammable anesthetic
flange
    buccal f.
    f. contour
    denture f.
    labial f.
    lingual f.

flank
    f. bone
    f. incision
    f. position

flap
    Abbe f.
    advancement f.
    f. amputation
    arterial f.
    axial pattern f.
    bilobed f.
    bipedicle f.
    bone f.
    buried f.
    caterpillar f.
    cellulocutaneous f.
    composite f., compound f.
    cross f.
    delayed f.
    deltopectoral f.
    direct f.
    distant f.
    double pedicle f.
    envelope f.
    Estlander f.
    Filatov f.
    Filatov-Gillies f.
    flag f.
    flat f.
    free f.
    free bone f.
    French f.
    full-thickness f.
    gingival f.
    hinged f.
    immediate f.
    Indian f.
    interpolated f.
    island f.
    Italian f.
    jump f.
    lined f.

F

flap *(continued)*
    lingual f.
    liver f.
    local f.
    mucoperichondrial f.
    mucoperiosteal f.
    musculocutaneous f.
    myocutaneous f.
    myodermal f.
    neurovascular f.
    open f.
    f. operation
    parabiotic f.
    partial-thickness f.
    pedicle f.
    pericoronal f.
    permanent pedicle f.
    pharyngeal f.
    random pattern f.
    rope f.
    rotation f.
    sickle f.
    skin f.
    sliding f.
    split-thickness f.
    subcutaneous f.
    tongue f.
    tubed f.
    tubed pedicle f.
    turnover f.
    von Langenbeck's bipedicle
      mucoperiosteal f.
    V-Y f.
    waltzed f.
    Zimany's bilobed f.
flapless amputation
flapping tremor
flare
    aqueous f.
flarimeter
flash
    f. blindness
    f. burn
    hot f.
    f. keratoconjunctivitis
flashback
flashing pain syndrome
flask
    casting f.
    f. closure
    crown f.
    denture f.
    Dewar f.
    Erlenmeyer f.
    Fernbach f.
    Florence f.
    injection f.
    refractory f.

    vacuum f.
    volumetric f.
flasking
flat
    f. affect
    f. bone
    f. chest
    f. condyloma
    f. electroencephalogram
    f. flap
    f. hand
    f. papular syphilid
    f. pelvis
    f. plate
    f. top waves
    f. wart
Flatau-Schilder disease
Flatau's law
flatfoot
flatulence
flatulent
    f. dyspepsia
flatus
    f. enema
    f. vaginalis
flatworm
flavedo
flavianic acid
Flaviviridae
Flavivirus
Flavobacterium
    F. aquatile
    F. breve
    F. piscicida
flavus
flax-dresser's disease
flea
flea-bitten kidney
flea-borne typhus
Flechsig's
    F. areas
    F. fasciculi
    F. ground bundles
    F. tract
fleck
    f. dystrophy of cornea
    f. retina of Kandori
flecked
    f. retina
    f. retina syndrome
flection
fleece worm
Flegel's disease
Fleischer's
    F. ring
    F. vortex
Fleischer-Strumpell ring
Fleischmann's bursa

Fleischner lines
Fleisch pneumotachograph
Fleitmann's test
Flemming's
    F. fixative
    F. triple stain
Flesch formula
flesh
    goose f.
    proud f.
fleshflies
fleshy
    f. mole
    f. polyp
Fletcher factor
flex
flexibilitas cerea
fleximeter
flexion
    f. crease
    palmar f.
    plantar f.
Flexner's bacillus
flexor
    f. carpi radialis muscle
    f. carpi ulnaris muscle
    f. digiti minimi brevis muscle of foot
    f. digiti minimi brevis muscle of hand
    f. digitorum brevis muscle
    f. digitorum longus muscle
    f. digitorum profundus muscle
    f. digitorum superficialis muscle
    f. hallucis brevis muscle
    f. hallucis longus muscle
    f. pollicis brevis muscle
    f. pollicis longus muscle
    f. reflex
    f. retinaculum
    f. retinaculum of forearm
    f. retinaculum of lower limb
flexura, pl. flexurae
    f. coli dextra
    f. coli sinistra
    f. duodeni inferior
    f. duodeni superior
    f. duodenojejunalis
    f. perinealis recti
    f. sacralis recti
    f. sigmoidea
flexural
    f. eczema
flexure
    anorectal f.
    basicranial f.
    caudal f.
    cephalic f.

    cerebral f.
    cervical f.
    cranial f.
    dorsal f.
    duodenojejunal f.
    hepatic f.
    inferior f. of duodenum
    left colic f.
    lumbar f.
    mesencephalic f.
    perineal f. of rectum
    pontine f.
    right colic f.
    sacral f.
    sacral f. of rectum
    sigmoid f.
    splenic f.
    superior f. of duodenum
    telencephalic f.
    transverse rhombencephalic f.
flicker
    f. fusion
    f. fusion frequency technique
    f. perimetry
    f. photometer
flick movements
flicks
Flieringa's ring
flight
    f. blindness
    f. or fight response
    f. of ideas
    f. nurse
flight into disease
flight into health
flint
    f. disease
    f. glass
Flint's
    F. arcade
    F. murmur
flip
    f. angle
flittering scotoma
floater
floating
    f. cartilage
    f. kidney
    f. organ
    f. patella
    f. ribs
    f. spleen
    f. villus
floc
floccillation
floccose
flocculable

F

floccular
    f. fossa
flocculate
flocculation
    f. reaction
    f. test
floccule
flocculence
flocculent
flocculonodular
    f. lobe
flocculus, pl. flocculi
    accessory f.
flood
    f. fever
flooding
Flood's ligament
floor
    f. cell
    f. of orbit
    f. plate
    f. of tympanic cavity
floppy valve syndrome
Florence flask
Florence's crystals
florid
    f. oral papillomatosis
    f. osseous dysplasia
floriform cataract
Florschütz' formula
floss
    dental f.
    f. silk
flotation method
Flourens' theory
floury cornea
flow
    Bingham f.
    f. cytometry
    f. cytophotometry
    Doppler color f.
    effective renal blood f.
    effective renal plasma f.
    forced expiratory f.
    gene f.
    laminar f.
    newtonian f.
    peak expiratory f.
    shear f.
    f. void
flower basket of Bochdalek
Flower's
    F. bone
    F. dental index
flower-spray
    f.-s. ending
    f.-s. organ of Ruffini
flowing hyperostosis

flowmeter
    electromagnetic f.
flow-over vaporizer
flow-volume curve
flu
fluctuate
fluctuation
fluence
fluent aphasia
fluid
    allantoic f.
    amniotic f.
    Brodie f.
    Callison's f.
    cerebrospinal f.
    crevicular f.
    dentinal f.
    extracellular f.
    extravascular f.
    Farrant's mounting f.
    gingival f.
    interstitial f.
    intracellular f.
    intraocular f.
    newtonian f.
    non-newtonian f.
    pleural f.
    prostatic f.
    pseudoplastic f.
    Rees-Ecker f.
    f. retinopexy
    Scarpa's f.
    seminal f.
    sulcular f.
    synovial f.
    tissue f.
    transcellular f.'s
    ventricular f.
    f. wave
fluidity
fluke
flumen, pl. flumina
    flumina pilorum
fluorescein
    f. angiography
    f. instillation test
    f. isothiocyanate
    f. sodium
    f. string test
fluorescence
    f. microscope
    f. microscopy
    f. plus Giemsa stain
    f. quenching
fluorescence-activated cell sorter
fluorescent
    f. antibody
    f. antibody technique

f. antinuclear antibody test
f. screen
f. stain
f. treponemal antibody-absorption
  test
fluoridated teeth
fluoridization
fluorochrome
fluorochroming
fluorocyte
fluorography
fluorophotometry
fluororoentgenography
fluoroscope
fluoroscopic
fluoroscopy
  video f.
fluorosis
  chronic endemic f.
fluosol-DA
Flury strain rabies virus
flush
  carcinoid f.
  hectic f.
  histamine f.
  hot f.
  malar f.
  f. technique
flutter
  atrial f., auricular f.
  diaphragmatic f.
  impure f.
  ocular f.
  pure f.
  ventricular f.
flutter-fibrillation
  f.-f. waves
flux
  luminous f.
  net f.
  f. ratio
  unidirectional f.
fluxionary hyperemia
fly
  f. blister
  heel f.
  louse f.'s
  mangrove f.
flying
  f. blister
  f. spot microscope
Flynn-Aird syndrome
Flynn phenomenon
FMD virus
foam
  f. cells
  f. stability test

foamy
  f. agents
  f. viruses
focal
  f. amyloidosis
  f. appendicitis
  f. condensing osteitis
  f. depth
  f. dermal hypoplasia
  f. distance
  f. embolic glomerulonephritis
  f. epilepsy
  f. epithelial hyperplasia
  f. glomerulonephritis
  f. illumination
  f. infection
  f. interval
  f. lymphocytic thyroiditis
  f. metastatic disease
  f. motor seizure
  f. necrosis
  f. nephritis
  f. point
  f. reaction
  f. sclerosing glomerulopathy
  f. sclerosis
  f. segmental glomerulosclerosis
  f. spot
  f. spot size
focimeter
focus, pl. **foci**
  conjugate foci
  Ghon's f.
  natural f. of infection
  principal f.
  real f.
  virtual f.
focused grid
Fogarty
  F. catheter
  F. clamp
fogging
  f. retinoscopy
fogo selvagem
foil
  gold f.
  platinum f.
Foix-Alajouanine
  F.-A. myelitis
  F.-A. syndrome
Foix-Cavany-Marie syndrome
fold
  adipose f.'s of the pleura
  alar f.'s
  ampullary f.'s of uterine tube
  anterior axillary f.
  aryepiglottic f.,
    arytenoepiglottidean f.

F

fold *(continued)*
    axillary f.
    caval f.
    cecal f.'s
    f. of chorda tympani
    ciliary f.'s
    circular f.'s
    Dennie's infraorbital f.
    Douglas' f.
    Duncan's f.'s
    duodenojejunal f.
    duodenomesocolic f.
    epicanthal f.
    epigastric f.
    epiglottic f.'s
    falciform retinal f.
    fimbriated f.
    gastric f.'s
    gastropancreatic f.'s
    genital f.
    giant gastric f.'s
    glossopalatine f.
    gluteal f.
    Guérin's f.
    Hasner's f.
    head f.
    Houston's f.'s
    ileocecal f.
    incudal f.
    inferior duodenal f.
    infrapatellar synovial f.
    inguinal f.
    inguinal aponeurotic f.
    interdigital f.'s
    interureteric f.
    f.'s of iris
    Kerckring's f.'s
    labioscrotal f.'s
    lacrimal f.
    f. of laryngeal nerve
    lateral f.'s
    lateral glossoepiglottic f.
    lateral nasal f.
    lateral umbilical f.
    f. of left vena cava
    longitudinal f. of duodenum
    malar f.
    mallear f.
    mammary f.
    Marshall's vestigial f.
    medial nasal f.
    medial umbilical f.
    median glossoepiglottic f.
    median umbilical f.
    medullary f.'s
    mesonephric f.
    middle glossoepiglottic f.
    middle transverse rectal f.

middle umbilical f.
mongolian f.
Morgan's f.
mucobuccal f.
mucosal f.'s of gallbladder
nail f.
nasojugal f.
Nêlaton's f.
neural f.'s
opercular f.
palmate f.'s
palpebronasal f.
paraduodenal f.
pharyngoepiglottic f.
pleuropericardial f.
pleuroperitoneal f.
posterior axillary f.
presplenic f.
rectal f.'s
rectouterine f.
rectovesical f.
retinal f.
retrotarsal f.
Rindfleisch's f.'s
sacrogenital f.'s
sacrouterine f.
sacrovaginal f.
sacrovesical f.
salpingopalatine f.
salpingopharyngeal f.
semilunar f.
semilunar f. of colon
spiral f. of cystic duct
stapedial f.
sublingual f.
superior duodenal f.
f. of superior laryngeal nerve
synovial f.
tail f.
tarsal f.
transverse palatine f.
transverse rectal f.'s
transverse vesical f.
Treves' f.
triangular f.
Tröltsch's f.
tubal f.'s of uterine tubes
urachal f.
ureteric f.
urorectal f.
uterovesical f.
vascular f. of the cecum
Vater's f.
ventricular f.
vestibular f.
vestigial f.
vocal f.
fold-back elements

folded-lung syndrome
folding fracture
Foley
    F. catheter
    F. operation
    F. Y-plasty pyeloplasty
folia (*pl. of* folium)
foliaceous
foliar
foliate
    f. papillae
    f. papillitis
folic acid deficiency anemia
folie
    f. à deux
    f. du doute
    f. du pourquoi
    f. gémellaire
Folin-Looney test
Folin's test
foliose
folium, pl. **folia**
    cerebellar folia
    folia cerebelli
    folia linguae
    f. vermis
    vermis f.
folk medicine
follian process
follicle
    aggregated lymphatic f.'s
    aggregated lymphatic f.'s of
      vermiform appendix
    anovular ovarian f.
    atretic ovarian f.
    dental f.
    gastric f.'s
    gastric lymphatic f.'s
    graafian f.
    growing ovarian f.
    hair f.
    intestinal f.'s
    laryngeal lymphatic f.'s
    Lieberkühn's f.'s
    lingual f.'s
    lymph f., lymphatic f.
    lymphatic f.'s of larynx
    lymphatic f.'s of rectum
    mature ovarian f.
    Montgomery's f.'s
    nabothian f.
    ovarian f.
    polyovular ovarian f.
    primary ovarian f.
    primordial ovarian f.
    sebaceous f.'s
    secondary f.
    solitary f.'s

    solitary lymphatic f.'s
    splenic lymph f.'s
    f.'s of thyroid gland
    vesicular ovarian f.
follicular
    f. abscess
    f. adenoma
    f. antrum
    f. carcinomas
    f. conjunctivitis
    f. cyst
    f. cystitis
    f. epithelial cell
    f. gland
    f. goiter
    f. impetigo
    f. iritis
    f. lymphoma
    f. mucinosis
    f. ovarian cells
    f. papule
    f. predominantly large cell
      lymphoma
    f. predominantly small cleaved cell
      lymphoma
    f. stigma
    f. syphilid
    f. trachoma
    f. urethritis
    f. vulvitis
folliculi (*pl. of* folliculus)
folliculitis
    f. abscedens et suffodiens
    f. barbae
    f. decalvans
    eosinophilic pustular f.
    f. keloidalis
    f. nares perforans
    perforating f.
    f. ulerythematosa reticulata
folliculoma
folliculosis
folliculus, pl. **folliculi**
    folliculi glandulae thyroideae
    folliculi linguales
    folliculi lymphatici aggregati
    folliculi lymphatici aggregati
      appendicis vermiformis
    folliculi lymphatici gastrici
    folliculi lymphatici laryngei
    folliculi lymphatici lienales
    folliculi lymphatici recti
    folliculi lymphatici solitarii
    f. lymphaticus
    f. ovaricus primarius
    f. ovaricus vesiculosus
    f. pili
Folling's disease

F

Folli's process
following bougie
follow-up study
Foltz' valvule
fomes, pl. **fomites**
fomite
Fonio's solution
Fonsecaea
Fontan
    F. operation
    F. procedure
Fontana-Masson silver stain
Fontana's
    F. canal
    F. spaces
    F. stain
fontanel, fontanelle
    anterior f.
    anterolateral f.
    bregmatic f.
    Casser's f.
    cranial f.'s
    frontal f.
    Gerdy's f.
    mastoid f.
    occipital f.
    posterior f.
    posterolateral f.
    sagittal f.
    sphenoidal f.
fonticulus, pl. **fonticuli**
    f. anterior
    f. anterolateralis
    fonticuli cranii
    f. mastoideus
    f. posterior
    f. posterolateralis
    f. sphenoidalis
food
    f. asthma
    f. fever
    f. impaction
foot
    athlete's f.
    claw f.
    club f.
    drop f.
    fungous f.
    f. of hippocampus
    Hong Kong f.
    immersion f.
    Madura f.
    Morand's f.
    mossy f.
    f. plate
    f. plugger
    f. presentation
    f. process

    reel f.
    sandal f.
    spastic flat f.
    trench f.
    f. yaws
foot-and-mouth disease virus
football calf
foot-drop
footling presentation
footplate, foot-plate
footprinting
Foot's reticulin impregnation stain
forage
foramen, pl. **foramina**
    alveolar foramina
    foramina alveolaria
    anterior condyloid f.
    anterior palatine f.
    aortic f.
    apical dental f.
    apical f. of tooth
    f. apicis dentis
    arachnoid f.
    f. of Arnold
    Bichat's f.
    blind f. of frontal bone
    blind f. of the tongue
    Bochdalek's f.
    Botallo's f.
    f. bursae omentalis majoris
    carotid f.
    cecal f. of frontal bone
    cecal f. of the tongue
    f. cecum of frontal bone
    f. cecum linguae
    f. cecum medullae oblongatae
    f. cecum ossis frontalis
    f. cecum posterius
    f. cecum of tongue
    conjugate f.
    f. costotransversarium
    costotransverse f.
    f. diaphragmatis sellae
    Duverney's f.
    emissary sphenoidal f.
    epiploic f.
    f. epiploicum
    ethmoidal f.
    f. ethmoidale, f. ethmoidale anterius,
      f. ethmoidale posterius
    external acoustic f.
    external auditory f.
    Ferrein's f.
    frontal f.
    f. frontale
    great f.
    greater palatine f.
    Huschke's f.

Hyrtl's f.
incisive f.
f. incisivum
incisor f.
inferior dental f.
infraorbital f.
f. infraorbitale
interatrial f. primum
interatrial f. secundum
internal acoustic f.
internal auditory f.
interventricular f.
f. interventriculare
intervertebral f.
f. intervertebrale
f. ischiadicum, f. ischiadicum majus,
  f. ischiadicum minus
jugular f.
f. jugulare
f. of Key-Retzius
lacerated f.
f. lacerum
f. lacerum anterius
f. lacerum medium
f. lacerum posterius
Lannelongue's foramina
f. lateralis ventriculi quarti
lesser palatine foramina
f. of Luschka
Magendie's f.
f. magnum
malar f.
f. mandibulae
mandibular f.
mastoid f.
f. mastoideum
mental f.
f. mentale
Monro's f.
Morgagni's f.
nasal f.
foramina nervosa
f. nutricium
nutrient f.
obturator f.
f. obturatum
olfactory f.
f. omentale
optic f.
f. opticum
f. ovale, oval f.
foramina palatina minora
f. palatinum majus
foramina papillaria renis
papillary foramina of kidney
parietal f.
f. parietale
petrosal f.

f. petrosum
pleuroperitoneal f.
posterior condyloid f.
posterior palatine foramina
postglenoid f.
primary interatrial f.
f. processus transversi
f. quadratum
Retzius' f.
root f.
f. rotundum
round f.
sacral f.
f. sacrale, foramina sacralia dorsalia,
  foramina sacralia pelvina
Scarpa's foramina
sciatic f.
secondary interatrial f.
f. singulare
foramina of the smallest veins of
  heart
solitary f.
sphenopalatine f.
f. sphenopalatinum
sphenotic f.
f. spinosum
Stensen's f.
stylomastoid f.
f. stylomastoideum
f. subseptale
supraorbital f.
f. supraorbitale
thebesian foramina
thyroid f.
f. thyroideum
f. transversarium
transverse f.
f. of transverse process
f. of vena cava
vena caval f.
f. venae cavae
foramina of the venae minimae
foramina venarum minimarum
  cordis
f. venosum
venous f.
vertebral f.
f. vertebrale
vertebroarterial f.
f. vertebroarterialis
Vesalius' f.
Vicq d'Azyr's f.
Vieussens' foramina
Weitbrecht's f.
Winslow's f.
zygomaticofacial f.
f. zygomaticofaciale
zygomatico-orbital f.

F

foramen *(continued)*
    f. zygomatico-orbitale
    zygomaticotemporal f.
    f. zygomaticotemporale
foraminal
    f. herniation
    f. lymph node
    f. node
Foraminifera
foraminiferous
foraminotomy
foraminulum, pl. **foraminula**
Forbes-Albright syndrome
Forbes' disease
force
    animal f.
    chewing f.
    electromotive f.
    f. of mastication
    masticatory f.
    nerve f., nervous f.
    occlusal f.
    psychic f.
    reciprocal f.'s
    reserve f.
    vital f.
forced
    f. alimentation
    f. beat
    f. cycle
    f. duction
    f. expiratory flow
    f. expiratory time
    f. expiratory volume
    f. feeding
    f. grasping reflex
    f. respiration
    f. vital capacity
force platform
forceps
    Adson f.
    alligator f.
    Allis f.
    f. anterior
    Arruga's f.
    arterial f.
    axis-traction f.
    Barton's f.
    bayonet f.
    bone f.
    Brown-Adson f.
    bulldog f.
    bullet f.
    capsule f.
    Chamberlen f.
    clamp f.
    clip f.
    cup biopsy f.

    cutting f.
    DeBakey f.
    f. delivery
    dental f.
    dressing f.
    Evans f.
    extracting f.
    Graefe f.
    hemostatic f.
    jeweller's f.
    Kjelland's f.
    Lahey f.
    Laplace's f.
    Levret's f.
    lion-jaw bone-holding f.
    Löwenberg's f.
    f. major
    major f.
    minor f.
    f. minor
    mosquito f.
    mouse-tooth f.
    needle f.
    nonfenestrated f.
    obstetrical f.
    O'Hara f.
    Piper's f.
    f. posterior
    Randall stone f.
    rubber dam clamp f.
    Simpson's f.
    speculum f.
    Tarnier's f.
    tenaculum f.
    thumb f.
    tubular f.
    Tucker-McLean f.
    vulsella f., vulsellum f.
    Willett's f.
force-velocity curve
Forchheimer's sign
forcible feeding
forcipate
forcipressure
Fordyce's
    F. angiokeratoma
    F. disease
    F. granules
    F. spots
forearm
forebrain
    f. eminence
    f. prominence
    f. vesicle
foreconscious
forefinger
foregut

forehead
  olympian f.
foreign
  f. body
  f. body giant cell
  f. body granuloma
  f. body salpingitis
  f. body tumorigenesis
  f. protein therapy
  f. serum
foreign-body appendicitis
forekidney
forelock
  white f.
Forel's decussation
forensic
  f. dentistry
  f. medicine
  f. odontology
  f. psychiatry
  f. psychology
foreplay
forepleasure
forequarter amputation
foreskin
Forestier's disease
forestomach
forest yaws
forewaters
forgetting
fork
  bite f.
  face-bow f.
  tuning f.
form
  accolé f.'s
  appliqué f.'s
  arch f.
  cavity preparation f.
  convenience f.
  extension f.
  face f.
  involution f.
  L f.
  occlusal f.
  outline f.
  posterior tooth f.
  resistance f.
  retention f.
  sickle f.
  tooth f.
  wave f.
  wax f.
Formad's kidney
formaldehyde fixative
formalin pigment
formal operations
formatio, pl. formationes

f. hippocampalis
f. reticularis
formation
  concept f.
  personality f.
  reaction f.
  reticular f.
  rouleaux f.
  symptom f.
formative cells
formazan
formboard
formed visual hallucination
forme fruste, pl. formes frustes
formication
formol-calcium fixative
formol-Müller fixative
formol-saline fixative
formol-Zenker fixative
formula, pl. formulas, formulae
  Arneth f.
  Bazett's f.
  Bernhardt's f.
  Black's f.
  Broca's f.
  Christison's f.
  Demoivre's f.
  dental f.
  Dreyer's f.
  DuBois' f.
  electrical f.
  Flesch f.
  Florschütz' f.
  Gorlin f.
  Hamilton-Stewart f.
  Häser's f.
  Jellinek f.
  Ledermann f.
  Long's f.
  Mall's f.
  Meeh f.
  Meeh-Dubois f.
  Pignet's f.
  Poisson-Pearson f.
  Ranke's f.
  Reuss' f.
  Runeberg's f.
  Toronto f. for pulmonary artery
    banding
  Trapp-Häser f.
  Trapp's f.
  Van Slyke's f.
  vertebral f.
formulation
  American Law Institute f.
N-formylmethionine
fornicate
  f. gyrus

F

fornication
fornix, gen. **fornicis**, pl. **fornices**
    f. conjunctivae, f. conjunctivae
      inferior, f. conjunctivae superior
    conjunctival f.
    f. of the lacrimal sac
    pharyngeal f.
    f. pharyngis
    f. sacci lacrimalis
    transverse f.
    f. uteri
    f. vaginae
    vaginal f.
Forssman
    F. antibody
    F. antigen
    F. antigen-antibody reaction
    F. reaction
Förster's uveitis
Fort Bragg fever
fortification
    f. figures
    f. spectrum
fortified milk
forward
    f. conduction
    f. heart failure
Fosdick-Hansen-Epple test
Foshay test
fossa, gen. and pl. **fossae**
    acetabular f.
    f. acetabuli
    adipose fossae
    amygdaloid f.
    anconal f.
    anterior cranial f.
    f. anthelicis
    f. of anthelix
    articular f. of temporal bone
    f. axillaris
    axillary f.
    Bichat's f.
    Biesiadecki's f.
    Broesike's f.
    f. canina
    canine f.
    f. carotica
    cerebellar f.
    Claudius' f.
    condylar f.
    f. condylaris
    f. coronoidea humeri
    coronoid f. of humerus
    f. cranii anterior
    f. cranii media
    f. cranii posterior
    crural f.
    Cruveilhier's f.

cubital f.
f. cubitalis
digastric f.
f. digastrica
digital f.
f. ductus venosi
f. of ductus venosus
duodenal fossae
duodenojejunal f.
epigastric f.
f. epigastrica
femoral f.
floccular f.
f. for gallbladder
gallbladder f.
Gerdy's hyoid f.
f. glandulae lacrimalis
glenoid f.
greater supraclavicular f.
Gruber-Landzert f.
f. of helix
hyaloid f.
f. hyaloidea
hypophysial f.
f. hypophysialis
iliac f.
f. iliaca
iliacosubfascial f.
f. iliacosubfascialis
iliopectineal f.
f. incisiva
incisive f.
incudal f.
f. incudis
f. for incus
inferior duodenal f.
infraclavicular f.
f. infraclavicularis
infraduodenal f.
f. infraspinata
infraspinous f.
infratemporal f.
f. infratemporalis
inguinal f.
f. inguinalis lateralis
f. inguinalis medialis
f. innominata
innominate f.
intercondylar f.
f. intercondylaris
intercondyloid f., intercondylic f.
f. intermesocolica transversa
interpeduncular f.
f. interpeduncularis
intrabulbar f.
ischioanal f.
ischiorectal f.
f. ischiorectalis

Jobert de Lamballe's f.
Jonnesco's f.
jugular f.
f. jugularis
lacrimal f.
f. of lacrimal gland
f. of lacrimal sac
Landzert's f.
lateral f. of brain
lateral cerebral f.
lateral inguinal f.
f. lateralis cerebri
f. of lateral malleolus
lenticular f.
lesser supraclavicular f.
little f. of the cochlear window
little f. of the vestibular window,
  little f. of the vestibular round
  window
Malgaigne's f.
f. malleoli fibulae
f. malleoli lateralis
mandibular f.
f. mandibularis
mastoid f., f. mastoidea
medial inguinal f.
Merkel's f.
mesentericoparietal f.
middle cranial f.
Mohrenheim's f.
Morgagni's f.
mylohyoid f.
f. navicularis auriculae
f. navicularis auris
f. navicularis Cruveilhier
f. navicularis urethrae
f. navicularis vestibulae vaginae
navicular f. of urethra
f. olecrani
olecranon f.
oval f.
f. ovalis
ovarian f.
f. ovarica
paraduodenal f.
parajejunal f.
f. parajejunalis
pararectal f.
paravesical f.
f. paravesicalis
patellar f. of vitreous
peritoneal fossae
petrosal f.
piriform f.
pituitary f.
f. poplitea
popliteal f.
posterior cranial f.

f. provesicalis
pterygoid f.
f. pterygoidea
pterygomaxillary f.
f. pterygopalatina
pterygopalatine f.
radial f. of humerus
f. radialis humeri
retroduodenal f.
retromandibular f.
f. retromandibularis
retromolar f.
rhomboid f.
f. rhomboidea
Rosenmüller's f.
f. sacci lacrimalis
scaphoid f.
f. scaphoidea ossis sphenoidalis
scaphoid f. of sphenoid bone
f. scarpae major
sigmoid f.
sphenomaxillary f.
f. subarcuata
subarcuate f.
subcecal f.
subinguinal f.
sublingual f.
submandibular f.
f. submandibularis
submaxillary f.
subscapular f.
f. subscapularis
superior duodenal f.
f. supraclavicularis major
f. supraclavicularis minor
supramastoid f.
f. supraspinata
supraspinous f.
supratonsillar f.
f. supratonsillaris
supravesical f.
f. supravesicalis
f. of Sylvius
temporal f.
f. temporalis
f. terminalis urethrae
tonsillar f.
f. tonsillaris
Treitz's f.
triangular f.
f. triangularis
trochanteric f.
f. trochanterica
trochlear f.
f. trochlearis
umbilical f.
Velpeau's f.
f. venae cavae

F

fossa (*continued*)
 f. venae umbilicalis
 f. venosa
 vermian f.
 f. vesicae biliaris [felleae]
 vestibular f.
 f. of vestibule of vagina
 f. vestibuli vaginae
 Waldeyer's fossae
 zygomatic f.
fossette
fossula, pl. **fossulae**
 f. fenestrae cochleae
 f. fenestrae vestibuli
 f. petrosa
 petrosal f.
 f. rotunda
 tonsillar fossulae
 fossulae tonsillares
fossulate
Foster
 F. frame
 F. Kennedy's syndrome
Fothergill's
 F. disease
 F. neuralgia
 F. operation
 F. sign
Fouchet's stain
foulage
foundation
 denture f.
founder
 f. effect
 f. principle
foundryman's fever
fountain
 f. decussation
 f. syringe
fourchette
Fourier
 F. analysis
 F. transfer
 F. transform
Fournier's
 F. disease
 F. gangrene
four-tailed bandage
fourth
 f. cranial nerve
 f. disease
 f. finger
 f. heart sound
 f. lumbar nerve
 f. parallel pelvic plane
 f. turbinated bone
 f. ventricle
fovea, pl. **foveae**

f. anterior
anterior f.
f. articularis capitis radii
f. articularis inferior atlantis
f. articularis superior atlantis
f. capitis ossis femoris
f. cardiaca
f. centralis retinae
central retinal f.
f. coccygis
f. costalis inferior
f. costalis processus transversi
f. costalis superior
f. dentis atlantis
f. elliptica
f. ethmoidalis
f. of the femoral head
f. femoralis
f. hemielliptica
f. hemispherica
f. inferior
inferior f.
f. inguinalis interna
Morgagni's f.
f. oblonga cartilaginis arytenoideae
oblong f. of arytenoid cartilage
pterygoid f.
f. pterygoidea
f. of the radial head
f. spherica
f. sublingualis
f. submandibularis
f. submaxillaris
f. superior
superior f.
f. supravesicalis
triangular f. of arytenoid cartilage
f. triangularis cartilaginis
 arytenoideae
trochlear f.
f. trochlearis
foveate, foveated
foveation
foveola, pl. **foveolae**
 f. coccygea
 coccygeal f.
 f. gastrica
 foveolae granulares
 f. ocularis
 f. papillaris
 f. retinae
 f. suprameatica
foveolar
 f. cells of stomach
foveolate
Foville's
 F. fasciculus
 F. syndrome

fowl
- f. erythroblastosis virus
- f. lymphomatosis virus
- f. myeloblastosis virus
- f. neurolymphomatosis virus
- f. plague virus

Fowler's position
fowlpox virus
fox encephalitis virus
Fox-Fordyce disease
fraction
- blood plasma f.'s
- ejection f., systolic ejection f.
- filtration f.
- recombination f.
- regurgitant f.

fractional
- f. dose
- f. epidural anesthesia
- f. spinal anesthesia
- f. sterilization

fracture
- apophysial f.
- articular f.
- avulsion f.
- Barton's f.
- basal skull f.
- f. bed
- bending f.
- Bennett's f.
- birth f.
- blow-out f. *burst*
- f. box
- boxer's f.
- capillary f.
- Chance f.
- clay shoveler's f.
- closed f.
- closed skull f.
- Colles' f.
- comminuted f.
- comminuted skull f.
- complicated f.
- compound f.
- compound skull f.
- f. by contrecoup
- cough f.
- craniofacial dysjunction f.
- dentate f.
- depressed f.
- depressed skull f.
- de Quervain's f.
- derby hat f.
- diastatic skull f.
- direct f.
- dishpan f.
- f. dislocation
- dislocation f.

- double f.
- Dupuytren's f.
- dyscrasic f.
- epiphysial f., epiphyseal f.
- expressed skull f.
- extracapsular f.
- fatigue f.
- fetal f.
- fissured f.   *flail-type (tsatalis)*
- folding f.
- Galeazzi's f.
- Gosselin's f.
- greenstick f.
- growing f.
- Guérin's f.
- gutter f.
- hairline f.
- hangman's f.
- horizontal f.
- impacted f.
- incomplete f.
- indirect f.
- intra-articular f.   *Jones fx*
- intracapsular f.
- intraperiosteal f.
- intrauterine f.
- Le Fort I f.   *Lisfranc*
- Le Fort II f.
- Le Fort III f.
- linear f.
- linear skull f.
- longitudinal f.
- march f.
- Monteggia's f.
- multiple f.
- neurogenic f.
- oblique f.
- occult f.
- open f.
- open skull f.
- parry f.
- pathologic f.
- pertrochanteric f.
- pilon f.
- ping-pong f.
- pond f.
- Pott's f.
- pyramidal f.
- segmental f.
- sentinel spinous process f.
- Shepherd's f.
- silver-fork f.
- simple f.
- simple skull f.
- Skillern's f.
- skull f.
- Smith's f.
- spiral f.

F

343

fracture *(continued)*
    splintered f.
    spontaneous f.
    sprain f.
    stable f.
    stellate f.
    stellate skull f.
    strain f.
    stress f.
    subcapital f.
    subperiosteal f.
    supracondylar f.
    torsion f.
    torus f.
    transcervical f.
    transcondylar f.
    transverse f.
    transverse facial f.
    trimalleolar f.
    tripod f.
    unstable f.
    ununited f.
    Wagstaffe's f.
Fraenkel's pneumococcus
Fraenkel-Weichselbaum pneumococcus
fragile
    f. site
    f. X chromosome
    f. X syndrome
fragilitas
    f. crinium
    f. sanguinis
fragility
    f. of the blood
    capillary f.
    osmotic f.
    f. test
fragilocyte
fragilocytosis
fragment
    butterfly f.
    Fab f.
    Fc f.
    Klenow f.
fragmentation
    f. myocarditis
    f. of the myocardium
fraise
Fraley syndrome
frambesia tropica
frambesiform
    f. syphilid
frambesioma
frame
    Balkan f.
    Bradford f.
    Deiters' terminal f.'s
    Foster f.

    occluding f.
    Stryker f.
    trial f.
    Whitman's f.
frameshift
framework
Framingham Heart study
Franceschetti-Jadassohn syndrome
Franceschetti's syndrome
Francisella
    F. novicida
    F. tularensis
Francke's needle
frank
    f. breech presentation
Frankenhäuser's ganglion
Frankfort
    F. horizontal plane
    F. plane
Frankfort-mandibular incisor angle
Franklin
    F. disease
    F. spectacles
franklinic taste
Frank-Starling curve
Fräntzel's murmur
Fraser-Lendrum stain for fibrin
Fraser's syndrome
fraternal twins
Fraunhofer's lines
Frazier's needle
Frazier-Spiller operation
freckle
    Hutchinson's f.
    iris f.'s
    melanotic f.
Fredet-Ramstedt operation
free
    f. association
    f. bone flap
    f. border
    f. border of nail
    f. border of ovary
    f. field
    f. flap
    f. gingiva
    f. graft
    f. induction decay
    f. macrophage
    f. mandibular movements
    f. margin
    f. margin of eyelids
    f. nerve endings
    f. tenia
    f. thyroxine index
    f. villus
    f. water clearance
free-floating anxiety

free-hand knife
Freeman-Sheldon syndrome
freeway space
freezing
    gastric f.
Freiberg's disease *infraction*
Frei-Hoffmann reaction
Frei test
Frejka pillow splint
frémissement cattaire
fremitus
    bronchial f.
    hydatid f.
    pericardial f.
    pleural f.
    rhonchal f.
    subjective f.
    tactile f.
    tussive f.
    vocal f.
frena (*pl. of* frenum)
frenal
French
    f. flap
    f. polio
    f. proof agar
    f. scale
frenectomy
Frenkel's
    F. anterior ocular traumatic
      syndrome
    F. symptom
frenoplasty
frenotomy
frenulum, pl. frenula
    cerebellar f.
    f. cerebelli
    f. clitoridis
    f. of clitoris
    f. epiglottidis
    f. of Giacomini
    f. of ileocecal valve
    f. of the labia minora
    f. labii inferioris, f. labii superioris
    f. labiorum minorum
    f. labiorum pudendi
    f. linguae
    lingual f.
    f. of lower lip, f. of upper lip
    f. of M'Dowel
    f. of Morgagni
    f. of prepuce
    f. preputii
    f. preputii clitoridis
    f. of pudendal lips
    f. pudendi
    f. of superior medullary velum
    synovial frenula

    f. of tongue
    f. of upper lip (*var. of* f. of lower
      lip)
    f. valvae ileocecalis
    f. veli medullaris superioris
frenum, pl. frena, frenums
    Morgagni's f.
    synovial frena
frenzy
frequency
    critical flicker fusion f.
    f. curve
    f. distribution
    f. domain
    dominant f.
    f. encoding
    fundamental f.
    gene f.
    Larmor f.
    f. of micturition
    resonant f.
    respiratory f.
    f. spectrum
Frerichs' theory
Fresnel
    F. lens
    F. prism
fressreflex
fretting
fretum, pl. freta
freudian
    f. fixation
    f. psychoanalysis
    f. slip
Freud's theory
Freund's
    F. adjuvant
    F. anomaly
    F. incomplete adjuvant
    F. operation
Frey's
    F. hairs
    F. syndrome
fricative
friction
    dynamic f.
    f. murmur
    f. rub
    f. sound
    starting f.
    static f.
frictional attachment
Fridenberg's stigometric card test
Friderichsen-Waterhouse syndrome
Friedländer's
    F. bacillus
    F. bacillus pneumonia

F

Friedländer's *(continued)*
    F. pneumonia
    F. stain for capsules
Friedman curve
Friedreich's
    F. ataxia
    F. phenomenon
    F. sign
Friend
    F. disease
    F. leukemia virus
    F. virus
fright reaction
frigid
frigidity
frigorism
frill, pl. **irides**
    iris f., pl. irides
fringe
    costal f.
    Richard's f.'s
    synovial f.
frit
frog face
frog-leg lateral projection
Fröhlich's
    F. dwarfism
    F. syndrome
Frohn's reagent
Froin's syndrome
frôlement
Froment's sign
frons, gen. **frontis**
frontad
frontal
    f. angle of parietal bone
    f. area
    f. artery
    f. belly of occipitofrontalis muscle
    f. bone
    f. border
    f. border of parietal bone
    f. border of sphenoid bone
    f. branch of superficial temporal
      artery
    f. cortex
    f. crest
    f. eminence
    f. fontanel
    f. foramen
    f. grooves
    f. horn
    f. lobe
    f. lobe of cerebrum
    f. lobe epilepsy
    f. margin
    f. nerve
    f. notch

    f. part of corpus callosum
    f. plane
    f. plate
    f. pole
    f. pole of cerebrum
    f. process of maxilla
    f. process of zygomatic bone
    f. region of head
    f. section
    f. sinus
    f. sinus aperture
    f. sinusitis
    f. squama
    f. suture
    f. triangle
    f. tuber
    f. veins
frontalis
    f. muscle
frontis (*gen. of* frons)
frontoanterior position
frontoethmoidal suture
frontolacrimal suture
frontomalar
frontomaxillary
    f. suture
frontonasal
    f. duct
    f. primordium
    f. process
    f. prominence
    f. suture
fronto-occipital
    f.-o. fasciculus
fronto-orbital area
frontoparietal
frontopontine tract
frontoposterior position
frontosphenoidal process
frontotemporal
    f. tract
frontotemporale
frontotransverse position
frontozygomatic
    f. suture
front-tap
    f.-t. contraction
    f.-t. reflex
Froriep's
    F. ganglion
    F. induration
frost
    f. itch
    urea f., uremic f.
frostbite
frosted
    f. heart
    f. liver

Frost suture
frottage
frotteur
frozen
    f. pelvis
    f. section
    f. shoulder
fructosemia
fructosuria
    essential f.
fruiting body
frustration
    f. tolerance
frustration-aggression hypothesis
FTA-ABS
    FTA-ABS test
Fuchs'
    F. adenoma
    F. black spot
    F. coloboma
    F. epithelial dystrophy
    F. heterochromic cyclitis
    F. spur
    F. stomas
    F. syndrome
    F. uveitis
fuchsin
    acid f.
    f. agar
    aldehyde f.
    aniline f.
    basic f.
    f. bodies
    diamond f.
fuchsinophil
    f. cell
    f. granule
    f. reaction
fuchsinophilia
fuchsinophilic
fucosidosis
fugacity
fugitive
    f. swelling
    f. wart
fugue
fulcrum, pl. **fulcra, fulcrums**
    f. line
fulgurant
fulgurating
    f. migraine
fulguration
    direct f.
    indirect f.
full
    f. breech presentation
    f. denture
    f. liquid diet

full-thickness
    f.-t. burn
    f.-t. flap
    f.-t. graft
fulminant
    f. hepatitis
    f. hyperpyrexia
fulminating
    f. dysentery
    f. smallpox
fumigate
fumigation
functio laesa
function
    allomeric f.
    arousal f.
    atrial transport f.
    f. corrector
    discriminant f.
    isomeric f.
    line spread f.
    maping f.
    modulation transfer f.
functional
    f. albuminuria
    f. anatomy
    f. aphasia
    f. apoplexy
    f. asplenia
    f. autonomy
    f. blindness
    f. cardiovascular disease
    f. castration
    f. chew-in record
    f. congestion
    f. contracture
    f. deafness
    f. disease
    f. disorder
    f. dysmenorrhea
    f. dyspepsia
    f. dyspnea
    f. hypertrophy
    f. illness
    f. jaw orthopedics
    f. mandibular movements
    f. murmur
    f. neurosurgery
    f. occlusal harmony
    f. occlusion
    f. orthodontic therapy
    f. pathology
    f. pleiotropy
    f. prepubertal castration syndrome
    f. psychosis
    f. refractory period
    f. residual air
    f. residual capacity

F

functional *(continued)*
    f. spasm
    f. sphincter
    f. splint
    f. stricture
    f. terminal innervation ratio
    f. visual loss
    f. vocal fatigue
functionalism
fundament
fundamental
    f. frequency
    f. tone
fundectomy
fundi *(pl. of* fundus)
fundic
fundiform
    f. ligament of foot
    f. ligament of penis
fundoplication
fundus, pl. fundi
    f. albipunctatus
    f. diabeticus
    f. flavimaculatus
    f. of gallbladder
    f. gastricus
    f. glands
    f. of internal acoustic meatus
    f. of internal auditory meatus
    leopard f.
    f. meatus acustici interni
    mosaic f.
    f. oculi
    pepper and salt f.
    f. polycythemicus
    f. reflex
    f. of stomach
    tessellated f.
    f. tigré
    tigroid f.
    f. tympani
    f. of urinary bladder
    f. uteri
    f. of uterus
    f. ventriculi
    f. vesicae biliaris (felleae)
    f. vesicae urinariae
funduscope
funduscopy
fundusectomy
fungal
fungate
fungating sore
fungemia
fungi *(pl. of* fungus)
fungiform
    f. papillae
Fungi Imperfecti

fungilliform
fungoid
fungosity
fungous
    f. foot
fungus, pl. fungi
    f. ball
    f. cerebri
    dematiaceous fungi
    fission fungi
    imperfect f.
    perfect f.
    ray f.
    thrush f.
    umbilical f.
    yeast f.
funic
    f. souffle
funicle
funicular
    f. graft
    f. hydrocele
    f. myelitis
    f. myelosis
    f. process
    f. souffle
funiculi *(pl. of* funiculus)
funiculitis
    endemic f.
    filarial f.
funiculopexy
funiculus, pl. funiculi
    anterior f.
    f. anterior
    cuneate f.
    dorsal f.
    f. dorsalis
    f. gracilis
    lateral f.
    f. lateralis
    lateral f. of spinal cord
    funiculi medullae spinalis
    posterior f.
    f. posterior
    f. separans
    f. solitarius
    f. spermaticus
    f. teres
    f. umbilicalis
funiform
funipuncture
funis
funnel
    f. breast
    f. chest
    Martegiani's f.
    pial f.
funnel-shaped pelvis

fura-2
furcal
    f. nerve
furcation
furfur, pl. **furfures**
furfuraceous
furfurol reaction
furnace
    dental f.
    muffle f.
furnacemen's cataract
furor epilepticus
furred tongue
furrow
    digital f.
    genital f.
    gluteal f.
    mentolabial f.
    primitive f.
    skin f.'s
furuncle
furuncular
furunculi (*pl. of* furunculus)
furunculoid
furunculosis
    f. orientalis
furunculous
furunculus, pl. **furunculi**
Fusarium
fuseau
fused
    f. kidney
    f. teeth
fusiform
    f. aneurysm

    f. cataract
    f. cells of cerebral cortex
    f. gyrus
    f. layer
    f. muscle
Fusiformis
fusimotor
fusion
    f. area
    f. beat
    cell f.
    centric f.
    flicker f.
    spinal f., spine f.
    splenogonadal f.
    vertebral f.
fusional movement
fusion-inferred threshold test
Fusobacterium
    F. mortiferum
    F. nucleatum
    F. plauti
fusocellular
fusospirochetal
    f. disease
    f. gingivitis
    f. stomatitis
fustic
fustigation
Futcher's line
Fy
    Fy antigens
    Fy blood group

F

G

G antigen
G cells
G syndrome
Gaboon ulcer
Gaddum and Schild test
gadfly
gadodiamide
gadopentetate
gadoteridol
Gaenslen's sign
Gaffky

G. scale
G. table
gag

Davis-Crowe mouth g.
g. reflex
gain

primary g.
secondary g.
time-compensated g.
time compensation g.
time-varied g.
Gairdner's disease
Gaisböck's syndrome
gait

antalgic g.
g. apraxia
ataxic g.
calcaneal g.
cerebellar g.
Charcot's g.
circumduction g.
equine g.
festinating g.
gluteus maximus g.
gluteus medius g.
helicopod g.
hemiplegic g.
high steppage g.
hysterical g.
scissor g.
spastic g.
steppage g.
toppling g.
waddling g.
galactacrasia
galactidrosis
galactoblast
galactobolic
galactocele
galactokinase deficiency
galactophagous
galactophore
galactophoritis

galactophorous
g. canals
g. ducts
galactopoiesis
galactopoietic
galactorrhea
galactose
g. cataract
g. diabetes
g. tolerance test
galactosemia
β **galactosidase**
galactosis
galactosuria
galactosylceramide lipoidosis
galactotherapy
Galant's reflex
Galassi's pupillary phenomenon
galea
g. aponeurotica
Galeati's glands
galeatomy
Galeazzi's fracture
Galen's
G. anastomosis
G. nerve
gall
g. bladder
g. duct
Gallavardin's phenomenon
gallbladder
Courvoisier's g.
g. fossa
porcelain g.
sandpaper g.
strawberry g.
Gallego's differentiating solution
Gallie's transplant
gallocyanin, gallocyanine
gallop
atrial g.
presystolic g.
protodiastolic g.
g. rhythm
S_7 g.
g. sound
summation g.
systolic g.
Gall's craniology
gallstone
g. colic
g. ileus
opacifying g.'s
silent g.'s
gallus adeno-like virus

G

galoche chin
galtonian
    g. genetics
    g. inheritance
    g. trait
Galtonian-Fisher genetics
Galton's
    G. delta
    G. law
    G. system of classification of
      fingerprints
    G. whistle
galvanic
    g. cautery
    g. nystagmus
    g. skin reaction
    g. skin reflex
    g. skin response
    g. threshold
galvanocaustic snare
galvanocautery
galvanocontractility
galvanofaradization
galvanometer
    d'Arsonval g.
    Einthoven's string g.
galvanomuscular
galvanopalpation
galvanoscope
galvanosurgery
galvanotaxis
galvanotherapy
galvanotonus
galvanotropism
GAL virus
Gambian
    G. fever
    G. trypanosomiasis
game
    language g.
    model g.
    g. theory
gamekeeper's thumb
gametangium
gamete
    joint g.
gametic nucleus
gametocyst
gametocyte
gametogenesis
gametogonia
gametogony
gametoid
gametokinetic
gametophagia
Gamgee tissue
gamic

gamma
    g. alcoholism
    g. angle
    g. camera
    g. crystallin
    g. efferent
    g. encephalography
    g. fibers
    g. loop
    g. motor neurons
    g. motor system
    g. radiation
    g. ray knife
    g. rays
gammacism
gammagram
gammopathy
    biclonal g.
    monoclonal g.
    polyclonal g.
Gamna-Favre bodies
Gamna-Gandy
    G.-G. bodies
    G.-G. nodules
Gamna's disease
gamogenesis
gamogony
gamont
gamophagia
gamophobia
Gandy-Gamna bodies
Gandy-Nanta disease
ganglia (*pl. of* ganglion)
ganglial
gangliate, gangliated
gangliectomy
gangliform
gangliitis
ganglioblast
gangliocyte
gangliocytoma
ganglioform
ganglioglioma
gangliolysis
    percutaneous radiofrequency g.
ganglioma
ganglion, pl. **ganglia, ganglions**
    aberrant g.
    acousticofacial g.
    Acrel's g.
    Andersch's g.
    aorticorenal ganglia
    ganglia aorticorenalia
    Arnold's g.
    auditory g.
    Auerbach's ganglia
    auricular g.
    autonomic ganglia

ganglia of autonomic plexuses
basal ganglia
Bezold's g.
Bochdalek's g.
Bock's g.
Böttcher's g.
cardiac ganglia
ganglia cardiaca
carotid g.
celiac ganglia
ganglia celiaca
g. cell
g. cells of dorsal spinal root
g. cells of retina
g. cervicale inferius
g. cervicale medium
g. cervicale superius
cervicothoracic g.
g. cervicothoracicum
g. ciliare
ciliary g.
coccygeal g.
cochlear g.
Corti's g.
craniospinal ganglia
craniospinalia ganglia
diffuse g.
dorsal root g.
Ehrenritter's g.
extracranial ganglia
g. extracraniale
g. of facial nerve
Frankenhäuser's g.
Froriep's g.
gasserian g.
geniculate g.
g. geniculi
Gudden's g.
g. habenulae
hypogastric ganglia
g. impar
inferior cervical g.
inferior g. of glossopharyngeal
   nerve
inferior mesenteric g.
inferior g. of vagus nerve
g. inferius nervi glossopharyngei
g. inferius nervi vagi
intercrural g.
ganglia intermedia
intermediate ganglia
g. of intermediate nerve
interpeduncular g.
intervertebral g.
intracranial g.
g. isthmi
jugular g.
Laumonier's g.

Lee's g.
lenticular g.
Lobstein's g.
Ludwig's g.
ganglia lumbalia
lumbar ganglia
Meckel's g.
g. mesentericum inferius
g. mesentericum superius
middle cervical g.
nasal g.
nerve g., neural g.
g. of nervus intermedius
nodose g.
otic g.
g. oticum
parasympathetic ganglia
paravertebral ganglia
pelvic ganglia
ganglia pelvina
periosteal g.
petrosal g., petrous g.
phrenic ganglia
ganglia phrenica
ganglia plexuum autonomicorum
prevertebral ganglia
pterygopalatine g.
g. pterygopalatinum
Remak's ganglia
renal ganglia
ganglia renalia
Ribes' g.
g. ridge
sacral ganglia
ganglia sacralia
Scarpa's g.
Schacher's g.
semilunar g.
sensory g.
Soemmerring's g.
solar ganglia
sphenopalatine g.
spinal g.
g. spinale
spiral g. of cochlea
spiral cochlear g.
g. spirale cochleae
splanchnic g.
g. splanchnicum
stellate g.
g. stellatum
sublingual g.
g. sublinguale
submandibular g.
g. submandibulare
submaxillary g.
superior cervical g.

G

ganglion *(continued)*
    superior g. of glossopharyngeal nerve
    superior mesenteric g.
    superior g. of vagus nerve
    g. superius nervi glossopharyngei
    g. superius nervi vagi
    sympathetic ganglia
    ganglia of sympathetic trunk
    terminal g.
    g. terminale
    thoracic ganglia
    ganglia thoracica
    trigeminal g.
    g. trigeminale
    Troisier's g.
    ganglia trunci sympathici
    g. of trunk of vagus
    tympanic g.
    g. tympanicum
    Valentin's g.
    vertebral g.
    g. vertebrale
    vestibular g.
    g. vestibulare
    Vieussens' ganglia
    Walther's g.
    Wrisberg's ganglia
ganglionated
ganglionectomy
ganglioneuroma
    central g.
    dumbbell g.
ganglioneuromatosis
ganglionic
    g. branches of lingual nerve
    g. branches of maxillary nerve
    g. branch of internal carotid artery
    g. crest
    g. layer of cerebellar cortex
    g. layer of cerebral cortex
    g. layer of optic nerve
    g. layer of retina
    g. motor neuron
    g. saliva
ganglionitis
ganglionostomy
ganglions (*pl. of* ganglion)
ganglioside lipidosis
gangliosidosis
    G_{M2} g.
    generalized g.
    infantile G_{M2} g.
    infantile, generalized G_{M1} g.
    Type 1 G_{M1} g.
gangosa
gangrene
    arteriosclerotic g.

    cold g.
    cutaneous g.
    decubital g.
    diabetic g.
    disseminated cutaneous g.
    dry g.
    embolic g.
    emphysematous g.
    Fournier's g.
    gas g.
    hemorrhagic g.
    hospital g.
    hot g.
    Meleney's g.
    moist g.
    nosocomial g.
    Pott's g.
    presenile spontaneous g.
    pressure g.
    progressive bacterial synergistic g.
    senile g.
    spontaneous g. of newborn
    static g.
    symmetrical g.
    thrombotic g.
    trophic g.
    venous g.
    wet g.
    white g.
gangrenous
    g. appendicitis
    g. cellulitis
    g. emphysema
    g. pharyngitis
    g. pneumonia
    g. rhinitis
    g. stomatitis
ganoblast
Ganser's
    G. commissures
    G. syndrome
gantry
Gant's clamp
Gantzer's
    G. accessory bundle
    G. muscle
Ganzfeld stimulation
gap
    g. 1
    g. 2
    air-bone g.
    anion g.
    g. arthroplasty
    auscultatory g.
    Bochdalek's g.
    chromosomal g.
    excitable g.
    interocclusal g.

g. junction
g. phenomenon
silent g.
garapata disease
Gardner-Diamond syndrome
Gardnerella
   G. vaginalis
Gardnerella **vaginitis**
Gardner's syndrome
gargantuan mastitis
Gariel's pessary
Garland's triangle
garment
pneumatic antishock g.
Garré's
   G. disease
   G. osteomyelitis
Gartner's
   G. canal
   G. cyst
   G. duct
Gärtner's
   G. bacillus
   G. method
   G. tonometer
   G. vein phenomenon
gas
g. abscess
alveolar g.
anesthetic g.
g. bacillus
blood g.'s
g. cautery
g. cyst
g. embolism
expired g.
g. gangrene
ideal alveolar g.
inspired g.
mixed expired g.
g. peritonitis
g. phlegmon
g. retinopexy
gaseous
g. mediastinography
g. pulse
Gaskell's bridge
gasometer
gasometric
gasometry
gasserian ganglion
gaster
Gasterophilidae
gastradenitis
gastralgia
gastral mesoderm
gastrea theory
gastrectasis, gastrectasia

gastrectomy
Hofmeister g.
Pólya g.
gastric
g. algid malaria
g. analysis
g. area
g. arteries
g. branches of anterior vagal trunk
g. branches of posterior vagal trunk
g. bypass
g. calculus
g. canal
g. cardia
g. colic
g. crisis
g. diastole
g. feeding
g. fistula
g. folds
g. follicles
g. freezing
g. glands
g. hemorrhage
g. hypersecretion
g. impression
g. indigestion
g. lymphatic follicles
g. mucosa
g. neurasthenia
g. pit
g. plexuses of autonomic system
g. smear
g. stapling
g. surface of spleen
g. tetany
g. ulcer
g. veins
g. vertigo
g. volvulus
gastricus
gastrinoma
gastritis
alkaline reflux g.
atrophic g.
bile g.
catarrhal g.
g. cystica polyposa
eosinophilic g.
exfoliative g.
g. fibroplastica
hypertrophic g.
interstitial g.
phlegmonous g.
polypous g.
pseudomembranous g.
sclerotic g.

G

gastroacephalus
gastroadenitis
gastroalbumorrhea
gastroamorphus
gastroanastomosis
gastroatonia
gastroblennorrhea
gastrocardiac
    g. syndrome
gastrocele
gastrochronorrhea
gastrocnemius
    g. muscle
gastrocolic
    g. fistula
    g. ligament
    g. omentum
    g. reflex
gastrocolitis
gastrocoloptosis
gastrocolostomy
gastrocutaneous fistula
gastrocystoplasty
gastrodialysis
gastrodiaphragmatic ligament
Gastrodiscoides hominis
Gastrodiscus hominis
gastroduodenal
    g. artery
    g. fistula
    g. lymph nodes
    g. orifice
gastroduodenitis
gastroduodenoscopy
gastroduodenostomy
gastrodynia
gastroenteric
gastroenteritis
    acute infectious nonbacterial g.
    endemic nonbacterial infantile g.
    eosinophilic g.
    epidemic nonbacterial g.
    infantile g.
    viral g.
    g. virus type A
    g. virus type B
gastroenteroanastomosis
gastroenterocolitis
gastroenterocolostomy
gastroenterologist
gastroenterology
gastroenteropathy
gastroenteroplasty
gastroenteroptosis
gastroenterostomy
gastroenterotomy

gastroepiploic
    g. arteries
    g. veins
gastroesophageal
    g. hernia
    g. reflux
    g. vestibule
gastroesophagitis
gastroesophagostomy
gastrogastrostomy
gastrogavage
gastrogenic
gastrogenous diarrhea
gastrografin swallow
gastrograph
gastrohepatic
    g. omentum
gastrohydrorrhea
gastroileac reflex
gastroileitis
gastroileostomy
gastrointestinal
    g. fistula
    g. tract
gastrojejunal loop obstruction syndrome
gastrojejunocolic
gastrojejunostomy
gastrokinesograph
gastrolavage
gastrolienal
    g. ligament
gastrolith
gastrolithiasis
gastrologist
gastrology
gastrolysis
gastromalacia
gastromegaly
gastromelus
gastromyxorrhea
gastronesteostomy
gastro-omental arteries
gastropagus
gastropancreatic folds
gastroparalysis
gastroparasitus
gastroparesis
    g. diabeticorum
gastropathic
gastropathy
    hypertrophic hypersecretory g.
gastropexy
Gastrophilidae
Gastrophilus
gastrophrenic
    g. ligament

gastroplasty
Collis g.
vertical banded g.
gastroplication
gastropneumonic
gastropod
Gastropoda
gastroptosis, gastroptosia
gastroptyxis
gastropulmonary
gastropylorectomy
gastropyloric
gastrorrhagia
gastrorrhaphy
gastrorrhea
gastrorrhexis
gastroschisis
gastroscope
fiberoptic g.
gastroscopic
gastroscopy
gastrospasm
gastrosplenic
g. ligament
g. omentum
gastrostaxis
gastrostenosis
gastrostogavage
gastrostolavage
gastrostomy
percutaneous endoscopic g.
gastrothoracopagus
gastrotome
gastrotomy
gastrotonometer
gastrotonometry
gastrotoxic
gastrotoxin
gastrotropic
gastroxia
gastroxynsis
gastrula
gastrulation
Gatch bed
gate
gate-control
g.-c. hypothesis
g.-c. theory
gated radionuclide angiocardiography
gatekeeper
gating
cardiac g.
g. mechanism
Gaucher
G. cells
G. disease
G. disorder

gauge
bite g.
Boley g.
catheter g.
strain g.
undercut g.
gauntlet
g. bandage
gaussian
g. curve
g. distribution
Gauss' sign
gauze bandage
gavage
Gavard's muscle
gay
g. bowel syndrome
Gay's glands
gaze
conjugate g.
dysconjugate g.
g. paretic nystagmus
G-banding
G. b. stain
Ge antigen
Gedoelstia
Geigel's reflex
Geiger-Müller
G.-M. counter
G.-M. tube
gel
g. diffusion
g. diffusion precipitin tests
g. diffusion precipitin tests in one
dimension
g. diffusion precipitin tests in two
dimensions
g. diffusion reactions
gelasmus
gelastic seizure
gelatinoid
gelatinous
g. ascites
g. infiltration
g. nucleus
g. polyp
g. scleritis
g. substance
g. tissue
g. varix
Gélineau's syndrome
Gell
G. and Coombs Classification
G. and Coombs reactions
Gellé test
gelosis
gelotripsy
Gély's suture

G

Gemella
gemellipara
gemellology
gemellus
geminate
geminated teeth
gemination
geminous
gemistocyte
gemistocytic
    g. astrocyte
    g. astrocytoma
    g. cell
    g. reaction
gemistocytoma
gemma
gemmation
gemmule
    Hoboken's g.'s
gena
genal
    g. glands
gender
    g. dysphoria syndrome
    g. identity
    g. identity disorders
    g. role
gene
    allelic g.
    autosomal g.
    codominant g.
    control g.
    g. deletion
    dominant g.
    g. dosage compensation
    g. dosage effect
    g. flow
    g. frequency
    H g.
    histocompatibility g.
    holandric g.
    homeotic g.'s
    housekeeping g.'s
    immune response g.'s
    jumping g.
    lethal g.
    g. library
    g. mapping
    mimic g.'s
    mitochondrial g.
    modifier g.
    g. mosaicism
    mutant g.
    pleiotropic g.
    polyphenic g.
    g. pool
    repressor g.
    SOS g.'s

    split g.'s
    g. therapy
    transfer g.'s
    transforming g.
    X-linked g.
    Y-linked g.
genealogy
genera (*pl. of* genus)
general
    g. adaptation reaction
    g. adaptation syndrome
    g. anatomy
    g. anesthesia
    g. anesthetic
    g. bloodletting
    g. duty nurse
    g. fertility rate
    g. hospital
    g. immunity
    g. paresis
    g. peritonitis
    g. physiology
    g. practice
    g. sensation
    g. somatic afferent column
    g. somatic efferent column
    g. transduction
    g. tuberculosis
    g. visceral afferent column
    g. visceral efferent column
generalist
generalization
    stimulus g.
generalized
    g. anaphylaxis
    g. anxiety disorder
    g. chondromalacia
    g. cortical hyperostosis
    g. elastolysis
    g. emphysema
    g. epidermolytic hyperkeratosis
    g. epilepsy
    g. eruptive histiocytoma
    g. gangliosidosis
    g. glycogenosis
    g. lentiginosis
    g. myokymia
    g. paralysis
    g. pustular psoriasis of Zambusch
    g. seizures
    g. Shwartzman phenomenon
    g. tetanus
    g. tonic-clonic epilepsy
    g. tonic-clonic seizure
    g. vaccinia
    g. xanthelasma
generate
generated occlusal path

generation
    asexual g.
    g. effect
    filial g.
    nonsexual g.
    parental g.
    sexual g.
    skipped g.
    virgin g.
generational
generative
    g. empathy
generator
    asynchronous pulse g.
    atrial synchronous pulse g.
    atrial triggered pulse g.
    demand pulse g.
    fixed rate pulse g.
    g. potential
    pulse g.
    radionuclide g.
    standby pulse g.
    ventricular inhibited pulse g.
    ventricular synchronous pulse g.
    ventricular triggered pulse g.
    x-ray g.
genesial
    g. cycle
genesiology
genesis
genetic
    g. amplification
    g. association
    g. burden
    g. carrier
    g. colonization
    g. compound
    g. counseling
    g. death
    g. determinant
    g. disequilibrium
    g. dominance
    g. drift
    g. equilibrium
    g. female
    g. fingerprint
    g. fitness
    g. fixation
    g. heterogeneity
    g. homeostasis
    g. human male
    g. isolate
    g. lethal
    g. linkage
    g. load
    g. locus
    g. map
    g. marker

    g. model
    g. penetrance
    g. polymorphism
    g. psychology
    g. recombination
    g. testing
geneticist
genetics
    behavioral g.
    classical g.
    clinical g.
    epidemiological g.
    galtonian g.
    Galtonian-Fisher g.
    human g.
    mathematical g.
    medical g.
    mendelian g.
    microbial g.
    modern g.
    molecular g.
    multilocal g.
    population g.
    quantitative g.
    reverse g.
    somatic cell g.
    statistical g.
    transplantation g.
genetotrophic
Geneva lens measure
Gengou phenomenon
genial, genian
    g. tubercle
genicula (*pl. of* geniculum)
genicular
    g. arteries
geniculate
    g. body
    g. ganglion
    g. neuralgia
    g. otalgia
    g. zoster
geniculated
geniculatus lateralis nucleus
geniculocalcarine
    g. radiation
    g. tract
geniculum, pl. **genicula**
    g. canalis facialis
    g. of facial canal
    g. of facial nerve
    g. nervi facialis
genioglossal muscle
genioglossus
    g. muscle
geniohyoid
    g. muscle
geniohyoideus

G

genion
genioplasty
genital
  g. branch of genitofemoral nerve
  g. branch of iliohypogastric nerve
  g. cord
  g. corpuscles
  g. duct
  g. eminence
  g. fold
  g. furrow
  g. gland
  g. herpes
  g. ligament
  g. organs
  g. phase
  g. primacy
  g. ridge
  g. stage
  g. swellings
  g. system
  g. tract
  g. tubercle
  g. wart
genitalia
  ambiguous external g.
  external g.
  indifferent g.
genitality
genitals
genitocrural
  g. nerve
genitofemoral
  g. nerve
genitoinguinal ligament
genitourinary
  g. apparatus
  g. fistula
  g. system
genius
Gennari's
  G. band
  G. stria
genoblast
genocopy
genodermatology
genodermatosis
genomic
genospecies
genote
  F g., F-g.
genotype
genotypic
genotypical
gentian aniline water
gentianophil, gentianophile
gentianophilous
gentianophobic

gentian violet
genu, gen. **genus**, pl. **genua**
  g. capsulae internae
  g. corporis callosi
  g. of corpus callosum
  g. of facial canal
  g. of facial nerve
  g. of internal capsule
  g. nervi facialis
  g. recurvatum
  g. valgum
  g. varum
genual
genucubital position
genupectoral position
genus, pl. **genera**
genus (*gen. of* genu)
genyantrum
geode
geographic
  g. choroidopathy
  g. keratitis
  g. stippling of nails
  g. tongue
geomedicine
geometrical sense
geometric mean
geopathology
geophagia, geophagism, geophagy
geophilic
Geophilus
geotaxis
geotrichosis
Geotrichum
geotropism
gephyrophobia
Geraghty's test
geratology
Gerbode defect
Gerdy's
  G. fibers
  G. fontanel
  G. hyoid fossa
  G. interatrial loop
  G. ligament
  G. tubercle
Gerhardt-Mitchell disease
Gerhardt's
  G. disease
  G. reaction
  G. sign
  G. test for urobilin in the urine
Gerhardt-Semon law
geriatric
  g. medicine
  g. therapy
geriatrics
  dental g.

Gerlach's
G. annular tendon
G. tonsil
G. valve
G. valvula
Gerlier's disease
germ
g. cell
dental g.
g. disk
enamel g.
g. layer
g. layer theory
g. line
g. membrane
g. nucleus
reserve tooth g.
g. theory
tooth g.
g. tube
g. tube test
wheat g.
German
G. measles
G. measles virus
germinal
g. aplasia
g. area
g. cell
g. center of Flemming
g. cords
g. disk
g. epithelium
g. localization
g. membrane
g. mosaicism
g. pole
g. rod
g. streak
g. vesicle
germinative
g. layer
g. layer of nail
germinoma
Germiston virus
geroderma
gerodontics, gerodontology
geromarasmus
gerontal
gerontologist
gerontology
gerontophilia
gerontophobia
gerontotherapeutics
gerontotherapy
gerontoxon
Gerota's
G. capsule

G. fascia
G. method
Gerstmann-Sträussler syndrome
Gerstmann syndrome
gestalt
g. phenomenon
g. psychology
g. theory
g. therapy
gestaltism
gestational
g. age
g. diabetes
g. edema
g. proteinuria
g. psychosis
gestosis, pl. **gestoses**
gesture
suicide g.
G_{M2} gangliosidosis
Gheel colony
GHK equation
Ghon's
G. complex
G. focus
G. primary lesion
G. tubercle
Ghon-Sachs bacillus
ghost
g. cell
g. cell glaucoma
g. corpuscle
g. tooth
ghoul hand
Giannuzzi's
G. crescents
G. demilunes
Gianotti-Crosti syndrome
giant
g. axonal neuropathy
g. cell
g. cell aortitis
g. cell arteritis
g. cell carcinoma
g. cell carcinoma of thyroid gland
g. cell epulis
g. cell fibroma
g. cell granuloma
g. cell hepatitis
g. cell hyaline angiopathy
g. cell monstrocellular sarcoma of Zülch
g. cell myeloma
g. cell myocarditis
g. cell pneumonia
g. cell sarcoma
g. cell thyroiditis
g. cell tumor of bone

G

giant *(continued)*
 g. cell tumor of tendon sheath
 g. chromosome
 g. colon
 g. condyloma
 g. drusen
 g. fibroadenoma
 g. follicular lymphoblastoma
 g. follicular thyroiditis
 g. gastric folds
 g. hives
 g. hypertrophy of gastric mucosa
 g. melanosome
 g. osteoid osteoma
 g. pigmented nevus
 g. urticaria
giantism
Giardia
 G. intestinalis
 G. lamblia
gibbous
gibbus
Gibney's
 G. boot
 G. fixation bandage
Gibson
 G. bandage
 G. murmur
Giemsa
 G. chromosome banding stain
 G. stain
Gierke
 G. cells
 G. disease
 G. respiratory bundle
Gifford's reflex
gigantiform cementoma
gigantism
 acromegalic g.
 cerebral g.
 eunuchoid g.
 fetal g.
 pituitary g.
 primordial g.
gigantocellular
 g. glioma
 g. nucleus of medulla oblongata
gigantomastia
Gigantorhynchus
Gigli's
 G. operation
 G. saw
gilbert
Gilbert's
 G. disease
 G. syndrome

Gilchrist's
 G. disease
 G. mycosis
gill
 g. arch skeleton
 g. clefts
Gilles
 G. de la Tourette's disease
 G. de la Tourette's syndrome
Gillette's suspensory ligament
Gilliam's operation
Gillies' operation
Gillmore needle
Gilmer wiring
Gil-Vernet operation
Gimbernat's ligament
ginger paralysis
gingiva, gen. and pl. **gingivae**
 alveolar g.
 attached g.
 buccal g.
 free g.
 labial g.
 lingual g.
 septal g.
gingival
 g. abrasion
 g. abscess
 g. atrophy
 g. clamp
 g. cleft
 g. contour
 g. crest
 g. crevice
 g. curvature
 g. cyst
 g. elephantiasis
 g. embrasure
 g. enlargement
 g. epithelium
 g. festoon
 g. fibromatosis
 g. fistula
 g. flap
 g. fluid
 g. hyperplasia
 G. Index
 g. margin
 g. massage
 g. mucosa
 g. pocket
 g. proliferation
 g. recession
 g. repositioning
 g. resorption
 g. retraction
 g. septum
 g. space

g. sulcus
g. tissues
g. trough
g. zone
Gingival-Periodontal Index
gingivectomy
gingivitis
    acute necrotizing ulcerative g.
    atypical g.
    chronic desquamative g.
    diabetic g.
    dilantin g.
    diphenylhydantoin g.
    fusospirochetal g.
    hormonal g.
    hyperplastic g.
    leukemic hyperplastic g.
    marginal g.
    necrotizing ulcerative g.
    plasma cell g.
    proliferative g.
    suppurative g.
    ulceromembranous g.
gingivoaxial
gingivobuccal
    g. groove
    g. sulcus
gingivodental ligament
gingivoglossitis
gingivolabial
    g. groove
    g. sulcus
gingivolingual
    g. groove
    g. sulcus
gingivolinguoaxial
gingivo-osseous
gingivoplasty
gingivosis
gingivostomatitis
ginglyform
ginglymoarthrodial
ginglymoid
    g. joint
ginglymus
    helicoid g.
    lateral g.
Giordano-Giovannetti diet
Giovannetti diet
Girard's reagent
girdle
    g. anesthesia
    Hitzig's g.
    Neptune's g.
    g. pain
    pectoral g.
    pelvic g.
    g. sensation

    shoulder g.
    thoracic g.
Girdlestone procedure
gitter cell
gitterzelle
glabella
glabellad
glabrous, glabrate
    g. skin
gladiate
gladiolus
glairy mucus
glancing wound
gland
    accessory g.
    accessory lacrimal g.'s
    accessory parotid g.
    accessory suprarenal g.'s
    accessory thyroid g.
    acid g.
    acinotubular g.
    acinous g.
    admaxillary g.
    adrenal g.
    aggregate g.'s
    agminate g.'s, agminated g.'s
    Albarran's g.'s
    albuminous g.
    alveolar g.
    anterior lingual g.
    apical g.
    apocrine g.
    apocrine sweat g.'s
    areolar g.'s
    arteriococcygeal g.
    arytenoid g.'s
    g.'s of auditory tube
    axillary g.'s
    axillary sweat g.'s
    Bartholin's g.
    basal g.
    Bauhin's g.
    Baumgarten's g.'s
    g.'s of biliary mucosa
    Blandin's g.
    Boerhaave's g.'s
    Bowman's g.
    brachial g.
    bronchial g.'s
    Bruch's g.'s
    Brunner's g.'s
    buccal g.'s
    bulbourethral g.
    cardiac g.
    cardiac g.'s of esophagus
    celiac g.'s
    ceruminous g.'s
    cervical g.'s

G

gland *(continued)*
cervical g.'s of uterus
Ciaccio's g.'s
ciliary g.'s
circumanal g.'s
coccygeal g.
coil g.
compound g.
conjunctival g.'s
convoluted g.
Cowper's g.
cutaneous g.'s
ductless g.'s
duodenal g.'s
Duverney's g.
Ebner's g.'s
eccrine g.
ecdysial g.'s
Eglis' g.'s
endocrine g.'s
esophageal g.'s
g.'s of eustachian tube
excretory g.
exocrine g.
external salivary g.
g.'s of the female urethra
follicular g.
fundus g.'s
Galeati's g.'s
gastric g.'s
Gay's g.'s
genal g.'s
genital g.
Gley's g.'s
glomiform g.'s
greater vestibular g.
Guérin's g.'s
Havers' g.'s
hemal g.
hematopoietic g.
hemolymph g.
Henle's g.'s
holocrine g.
inguinal g.'s
internal salivary g.
g.'s of internal secretion
interstitial g.
intestinal g.'s
intraepithelial g.'s
jugular g.
Knoll's g.'s
Krause's g.'s
labial g.'s
lacrimal g.
lactiferous g.
laryngeal g.'s
lesser vestibular g.'s
Lieberkühn's g.'s

Littré's g.'s
Luschka's g.
Luschka's cystic g.'s
lymph g.
major salivary g.'s
g.'s of the male urethra
malpighian g.'s
mammary g.
marrow-lymph g.
master g.
maxillary g.
meibomian g.'s
merocrine g.
Méry's g.
mesenteric g.'s
milk g.
minor salivary g.'s
mixed g.
molar g.'s
Moll's g.'s
Montgomery's g.'s
g.'s of mouth
mucilaginous g.
muciparous g.
mucous g.
mucous g.'s of auditory tube
nasal g.'s
Nuhn's g.
olfactory g.'s
oxyntic g.
pacchionian g.'s
palatine g.'s
palpebral g.'s
parathyroid g.
paraurethral g.'s
parotid g.
pectoral g.'s
peptic g.
peritracheal g.'s
perspiratory g.'s
Peyer's g.'s
pharyngeal g.'s
Philip's g.'s
pileous g.
pineal g.
pituitary g.
Poirier's g.
prehyoid g.
preputial g.'s
prostate g.
prothoracic g.'s
pyloric g.'s
racemose g.
Rivinus' g.
Rosenmüller's g.
saccular g.
salivary g.
sebaceous g.'s

seminal g.
sentinel g.
seromucous g.
serous g.
Serres' g.'s
sexual g.
Skene's g.'s
solitary g.'s
sublingual g.
submandibular g.
submaxillary g.
sudoriferous g.'s
suprahyoid g.
suprarenal g.
Suzanne's g.
sweat g.'s
synovial g.'s
target g.
tarsal g.'s
Terson's g.'s
Theile's g.'s
thoracic g.'s
thymus g.
thyroid g.
Tiedemann's g.
tracheal g.'s
trachoma g.'s
tubular g.
tubuloacinar g.
tubuloalveolar g.
tympanic g.
Tyson's g.'s
unicellular g.
urethral g.'s
uterine g.'s
vaginal g.
vascular g.
ventral g.'s
vesical g.
vestibular g.'s
vulvovaginal g.
Waldeyer's g.'s
Wasmann's g.'s
Weber's g.'s
Wepfer's g.'s
Wölfler's g.
Wolfring's g.'s
Zeis' g.'s
glanders bacillus
glandes (*pl. of* glans)
glandilemma
glandula, pl. **glandulae**
   glandulae areolares
   g. atrabiliaris
   g. basilaris
   glandulae bronchiales
   glandulae buccales
   g. bulbourethralis

glandulae ceruminosae
glandulae cervicales uteri
glandulae ciliares
glandulae circumanales
glandulae conjunctivales
glandulae cutis
glandulae duodenales
glandulae endocrinae
glandulae esophageae
glandulae gastricae
glandulae glomiformes
glandulae intestinales
glandulae labiales
glandulae lacrimales accessoriae
g. lacrimalis
glandulae laryngeae
g. lingualis anterior
g. mammaria
glandulae molares
g. mucosa
glandulae mucosae biliosae
glandulae nasales
glandulae olfactoriae
glandulae oris
glandulae palatinae
g. parathyroidea
g. parotidea
g. parotidea accessoria
g. parotis
g. parotis accessoria
glandulae pharyngeae
g. pituitaria
glandulae preputiales
glandulae propriae
g. prostatica
glandulae pyloricae
g. salivaria
glandulae sebaceae
g. seminalis
g. seromucosa
g. serosa
glandulae sine ductibus
g. sublingualis
g. submandibularis
glandulae sudoriferae
glandulae suprarenales accessoriae
g. suprarenalis
glandulae tarsales
g. thyroidea
g. thyroidea accessoria,
  pl. glandulae thyroideae accessoriae
glandulae tracheales
glandulae tubariae
glandulae urethrales femininae
glandulae urethrales masculinae
glandulae uterinae
glandulae vestibulares minores
g. vestibularis major

G

glandular
 g. branches
 g. branches of
 anterior/lateral/posterior branches
 of superior thyroid artery
 g. branches of facial artery
 g. branches of inferior thyroid
 artery
 g. branches of submandibular
 ganglion
 g. cancer
 g. carcinoma
 g. epithelium
 g. fever
 g. lobe of hypophysis
 g. mastitis
 g. plague
 g. substance of prostate
 g. system
 g. tularemia
glandule
glandulopreputial lamella
glandulous
glans, pl. **glandes**
 g. clitoridis
 g. of clitoris
 g. penis
glanular hypospadias
Glanzmann's disease
glare
 blinding g.
 dazzling g.
 g. of light
 peripheral g.
 specular g.
 veiling g.
glarometer
glaserian
 g. artery
 g. fissure
Glasgow
 G. coma scale
 G. sign
glass
 g. bead sterilizer
 g. body
 cover g.
 Crookes' g.
 crown g.
 cupping g.
 g. factor
 flint g.
 g. ionomer cement
 object g.
 quartz g.
 g. rays
 vita g.
 Wood's g.

glasses
glassworker's cataract
glassy membrane
glaucoma
 absolute g.
 acute g.
 angle-closure g.
 aphakic g.
 capsular g.
 chronic g.
 α-chymotrypsin-induced g.
 closed-angle g.
 combined g.
 compensated g.
 corticosteroid-induced g.
 Donders' g.
 g. fulminans
 ghost cell g.
 hemorrhagic g.
 hypersecretion g.
 low tension g.
 malignant g.
 narrow-angle g.
 neovascular g.
 open-angle g.
 phacogenic g.
 phacolytic g.
 phacomorphic g.
 pigmentary g.
 pseudoexfoliative capsular g.
 pupillary block g.
 secondary g.
 simple g., g. simplex
glaucomatocyclitic
 g. crisis
glaucomatous
 g. cataract
 g. cup
 g. excavation
 g. halo
 g. nerve-fiber bundle scotoma
 g. ring
glaucosuria
Gleason's
 G. score
 G. tumor grade
gleet
Glenn
 G. operation
 G. shunt
Glenner-Lillie stain for pituitary
glenohumeral
 g. articulation
 g. ligaments
glenoid
 g. cavity
 g. fossa
 g. labrum

g. ligament
g. surface
glenoidal lip
Gley's glands
glia
g. cells
gliacyte
glial
g. limiting membrane
glide
mandibular g.
gliding
g. joint
g. occlusion
glioblast
glioblastoma multiforme
glioblastosis cerebri
glioma
brainstem g.
gigantocellular g.
mixed g.
nasal g.
g. of optic chiasm
optic nerve g.
g. of the spinal cord
telangicctatic g., g. telangiectodes
gliomatosis
g. cerebri
gliomatous
gliomyxoma
glioneuroma
gliosarcoma
gliosis
isomorphous g.
piloid g.
g. uteri
glissonitis
Glisson's
G. capsule
G. cirrhosis
G. sphincter
glitter cells
global
g. aphasia
g. paralysis
globe
g. cell anemia
g. of eye
pale g.
globi (*pl. of* globus)
Globocephalus
globoid cell
globosus nucleus
globular
g. heart
g. leukocyte
g. process

g. sputum
g. thrombus
globule
dentin g.
Morgagni's g.'s
polar g.
globuliferous
globulin
accelerator g.
antihemophilic g. A
antihemophilic g. B
antihuman g.
β_{1C} g.
β_{1E} g.
β_{1F} g.
gonadal steroid-binding g.
plasma accelerator g.
β_{1E} **globulin**
β_{1C} **globulin**
β_{1F} **globulin**
globulinuria
globulomaxillary cyst
globulus
globus, pl. **globi**
g. hystericus
g. major
g. minor
g. pallidus
glomal
glomangioma
glomangiosis
pulmonary g.
glome
glomectomy
glomera (*pl. of* glomus)
glomerular
g. capsule
g. crescent
g. cysts
g. filtration rate
g. layer of olfactory bulb
g. nephritis
g. sclerosis
glomerule
glomeruli (*pl. of* glomerulus)
glomerulitis
glomerulonephritis
acute g.
acute crescentic g.
acute hemorrhagic g.
acute post-streptococcal g.
anti-basement membrane g.
Berger's focal g.
chronic g.
diffuse g.
Ellis type 1 g.
Ellis type 2 g.
exudative g.

G

glomerulonephritis *(continued)*
    focal g.
    focal embolic g.
    hypocomplementemic g.
    immune complex g.
    lobular g.
    local g.
    membranoproliferative g.
    membranous g.
    mesangial proliferative g.
    mesangiocapillary g.
    proliferative g.
    rapidly progressive g.
    segmental g.
    subacute g.
glomerulopathy
    focal sclerosing g.
glomerulosa cell
glomerulosclerosis
    diabetic g.
    focal segmental g.
    intercapillary g.
glomerulose
glomerulus, pl. **glomeruli**
    malpighian g.
    g. of mesonephros
    olfactory g.
    g. of pronephros
glomiform glands
glomus, pl. **glomera**
    glomera aortica, gen. corporis,
      pl. corpora
    g. body
    g. caroticum
    choroid g.
    g. choroideum
    g. coccygeum
    intravagal g.
    g. intravagale
    jugular g.
    g. jugulare
    g. jugulare tumor
    g. pulmonale
    pulmonary g.
    g. tumor
glossa
glossagra
glossal
glossalgia
glossectomy
Glossina
    G. morsitans
    G. pallidipes
    G. palpalis
glossitis
    g. areata exfoliativa
    atrophic g.
    benign migratory g.

    g. desiccans
    Hunter's g.
    median rhomboid g.
    Moeller's g.
glossocele
glossocinesthetic
glossodontotropism
glossodynamometer
glossodynia
glossodyniotropism
glossoepiglottic, glossoepiglottidean
    g. ligament
glossograph
glossohyal
glossokinesthetic
glossolabiolaryngeal paralysis
glossolabiopharyngeal paralysis
glossolalia
glossology
glossolysis
glossoncus
glossopalatine
    g. arch
    g. fold
glossopalatinus
glossopalatolabial paralysis
glossopathy
glossopharyngeal
    g. breathing
    g. nerve
    g. neuralgia
    g. part of superior pharyngeal
      constrictor
    g. tic
glossopharyngeolabial paralysis
glossopharyngeus
glossoplasty
glossoplegia
glossoptosis, glossoptosia
glossopyrosis
glossorrhaphy
glossospasm
glossosteresis
glossotomy
glossotrichia
glossy skin
glottal
glottic
glottidospasm
glottis, pl. **glottides**
    false g.
    g. respiratoria
    g. spuria
    true g.
    g. vera
    g. vocalis
glottitis
glottology

glove anesthesia
gloved-finger sign
Glover
    G. phenomenon
glover's suture
glucagon
    gut g.
glucagonoma
    g. syndrome
glucemia
glucohemia
glucokinetic
glucopenia
glucose
    g. oxidase method
    g. oxidase paper strip test
    g. tolerance test
    g. transport maximum
glucose-6-phosphatase hepatorenal
    glycogenosis
glucose-6-phosphate dehydrogenase
    deficiency
glucosephosphate isomerase deficiency
glucosuria
β-d-glucuronidase deficiency
glue ear
Gluge's corpuscles
glutaraldehyde fixative
glutathione synthetase deficiency
gluteal
    g. cleft
    g. crest
    g. fold
    g. furrow
    g. hernia
    g. line
    g. lymph nodes
    g. reflex
    g. region
    g. ridge
    g. surface of ilium
    g. tuberosity
    g. veins
gluten enteropathy
gluten-free diet
gluteofemoral
    g. bursa
gluteoinguinal
gluteus
    g. maximus gait
    g. maximus muscle
    g. medius bursae
    g. medius gait
    g. medius muscle
    g. minimus bursa
    g. minimus muscle
glutitis
glycemia

L-glyceric aciduria
glycine-rich β-glycoprotein
glycine-rich β-glycoproteinase
glycinuria
    familial g.
glycocalyx
glycogen
    g. cardiomegaly
    g. granule
glycogenic
    g. acanthosis
    g. cardiomegaly
glycogenosis
    brancher deficiency g.
    generalized g.
    glucose-6-phosphatase hepatorenal g.
    hepatophosphorylase deficiency g.
    myophosphorylase deficiency g.
    type 1 g.
    type 2 g.
    type 3 g.
    type 4 g.
    type 5 g.
    type 6 g.
    type 7 g.
glycogen-storage disease
glycogeusia
glycoglycinuria
glycolic aciduria
glycolipid lipidosis
glycopenia
Glycophagus
glycophilia
β_2-glycoprotein II
glycoptyalism
glycorrhachia
glycorrhea
glycosecretory
glycosialia
glycosialorrhea
glycostatic
glycosuria
    alimentary g.
    benign g.
    digestive g.
    nondiabetic g.
    nonhyperglycemic g.
    normoglycemic g.
    orthoglycemic g.
    pathologic g.
    phlorizin g., phloridzin g.
    renal g.
glycuresis
glycuronuria
Gm
    G. allotypes
    G. antigens
Gmelin's test

G

GMS stain
gnashing
gnat
gnathic
    g. index
gnathion
gnathocephalus
gnathodynamics
gnathodynamometer
gnathography
gnathological
gnathology
gnathoplasty
gnathoschisis
gnathostatics
Gnathostoma
    G. siamense
    G. spinigerum
gnathostomiasis
gnome's calf
gnosia
gnotobiota
gnotobiote
gnotobiotic
goal
goatpox virus
goat's milk anemia
goblet cell
Godélier's law
Godman's fascia
Godwin tumor
Goeckerman treatment
Goethe's bone
Gofman test
Goggia's sign
goggle
    plethysmographic g.
goiter
    aberrant g.
    acute g.
    adenomatous g.
    Basedow's g.
    cabbage g.
    colloid g.
    cystic g.
    diffuse g.
    diving g.
    endemic g.
    exophthalmic g.
    fibrous g.
    follicular g.
    lingual g.
    lymphadenoid g.
    microfollicular g.
    multinodular g.
    nontoxic g.
    parenchymatous g.
    simple g.

    substernal g.
    suffocative g.
    thoracic g.
    toxic g.
    wandering g.
goitrous
gold
    g. alloy
    g. casting
    cohesive g.
    g. foil
    g. inlay
    mat g.
    noncohesive g.
    powdered g.
    g. sol test
    g. standard
Goldblatt
    G. clamp
    G. hypertension
    G. kidney
    G. phenomenon
Goldenhar's syndrome
Goldflam disease
Goldman equation
Goldman-Fox knives
Goldman-Hodgkin-Katz equation
Goldmann
    G. applanation tonometer
    G. perimeter
gold-myokymia syndrome
Goldscheider's test
Goldstein's toe sign
Goldthwait's sign
golfer's skin
golf-hole ureteral orifice
Golgi
    G. apparatus
    G. cells
    G. complex
    G. corpuscle
    G. epithelial cell
    G. internal reticulum
    G. osmiobichromate fixative
    G. stain
    G. tendon organ
    G. type II neuron
    G. type I neuron
    G. zone
Golgi-Mazzoni corpuscle
golgiokinesis
Goll's column
Goltz syndrome
Gombault's triangle
gomitoli
Gomori-Jones periodic acid-methenamine-silver stain

Gomori's
G. aldehyde fuchsin stain
G. chrome alum hematoxylin-phloxine stain
G. methenamine-silver stain
G. nonspecific acid phosphatase stain
G. nonspecific alkaline phosphatase stain
G. one-step trichrome stain
G. silver impregnation stain
Gompertz'
G. hypothesis
G. law
gompholic joint
gomphosis
gonad
g. dose
female g.
indifferent g.
male g.
g. nucleus
streak g.
gonadal
g. agenesis
g. aplasia
g. cords
g. dose
g. dysgenesis
g. mosaicism
g. ridge
g. steroid-binding globulin
g. streak
gonadectomy
gonadopathy
gonadotroph
gonadotrophic cycle
gonadotropin-producing adenoma
gonaduct
gonalgia
gonarthritis
gonarthrotomy
gonatagra
gonatocele
gonecyst, gonecystis
gonecystolith
gonia (*pl. of* gonion)
goniocraniometry
goniodysgenesis
gonion, pl. **gonia**
goniopuncture
gonioscope
gonioscopy
goniosynechia
goniotomy
gonitis
gonocele
gonochorism, gonochorismus

gonococcal
g. arthritis
g. conjunctivitis
g. stomatitis
gonococcemia
gonococcic
gonococcus, pl. **gonococci**
gonocyte
gonohemia
gono-opsonin
gonophage
gonophore, gonophorus
gonorrhea
gonorrheal
g. arthritis
g. conjunctivitis
g. ophthalmia
g. rheumatism
g. salpingitis
g. urethritis
gonosome
gonotoxemia
gonotoxin
gonotyl
Gonyaulax catanella
gonycampsis
Good
G. antigen
Goodell's
G. dilator
G. sign
Goodenough draw-a-man test
Goodman's syndrome
goodness of fit
goodness of fit test
good object
Goodpasture's
G. stain
G. syndrome
Goormaghtigh's cells
gooseflesh, goose flesh
Gopalan's syndrome
Gordius
Gordon
G. reflex
G. sign
G. and Sweet stain
G. symptom
gorget
probe g.
Gorham's disease
Goriaew's rule
Gorlin
G. cyst
G. formula
G. sign
G. syndrome
Gorlin-Chaudhry-Moss syndrome

G

Gorman's syndrome
gorondou
Gosselin's fracture
Gothic
    G. arch
    G. arch tracing
    G. palate
Göthlin's test
gouge
Gougerot and Blum disease
Gougerot-Carteaud syndrome
Gougerot-Sjögren disease
Gould's suture
Gouley's catheter
goundou
gout
    abarticular g.
    articular g.
    calcium g.
    g. diet
    idiopathic g.
    interval g.
    latent g.
    lead g.
    masked g.
    primary g.
    retrocedent g.
    saturnine g.
    secondary g.
    tophaceous g.
gouty
    g. arthritis
    g. diathesis
    g. pearl
    g. tophus
    g. urine
government hospital
Gowers'
    G. column
    G. contraction
    G. syndrome
    G. tract
Gowers disease
graafian follicle
gracile
    g. fasciculus
    g. habitus
    g. lobule
    g. nucleus
    g. tubercle
gracilis
    g. muscle
    g. syndrome
grade
    Gleason's tumor g.
    Heath-Edwards g.'s
    g. I astrocytoma
    g. II astrocytoma

    g. III astrocytoma
    g. IV astrocytoma
Gradenigo's syndrome
gradient
    atrioventricular g.
    g. encoding
    field g.
    magnetic field g.
    mitral g.
    systolic g.
    ventricular g.
graduated
    g. compress
    g. pipette
    g. tenotomy
graduate nurse
Graefe
    G. forceps
    G. knife
    G. operation
    G. sign
    G. spots
Graefenberg ring
Graffi's virus
graft
    accordion g.
    adipodermal g.
    allogeneic g.
    anastomosed g.
    animal g.
    augmentation g.
    autodermic g.
    autogeneic g.
    autologous g.
    autoplastic g.
    Blair-Brown g.
    bone g.
    brephoplastic g.
    cable g.
    chessboard g.'s
    chip g.
    composite g.
    corneal g.
    cutis g.
    Davis g.'s
    delayed g.
    dermal g.
    dermal-fat g.
    Douglas g.
    epidermic g.
    Esser g.
    fascia g.
    fascicular g.
    fat g.
    filler g.
    free g.
    full-thickness g.
    funicular g.

H g.
heterologous g.
heteroplastic g.
heterospecific g.
heterotopic g.
homologous g.
homoplastic g.
hyperplastic g.
implantation g.
infusion g.
inlay g.
interspecific g.
isogeneic g.
isologous g.
isoplastic g.
Krause g.
Krause-Wolfe g.
mesh g.
mucosal g.
nerve g.
Ollier g.
Ollier-Thiersch g.
omental g.
onlay g.
orthotopic g.
osteoperiosteal g.
partial-thickness g.
pedicle g.
periosteal g.
Phemister g.
pinch g.
porcine g.
postage stamp g.'s
primary skin g.
punch g.'s
Reverdin g.
sieve g.
skin g.
sleeve g.
split-skin g.
split-thickness g.
Stent g.
syngeneic g.
tendon g.
Thiersch g.
vascularized g.
g. versus host disease
g. versus host reaction
white g.
Wolfe g.
Wolfe-Krause g.
zooplastic g.
grafting
Graham
    G. Little syndrome
    G. Steell's murmur
Graham-Cole test
Grahamella

grain itch
grains
Gram-negative
Gram-positive
Gram's
    G. iodine
    G. stain
grana
grand
    g. climacteric
    g. mal
    g. mal epilepsy
    g. mal seizure
    g. multipara
granddaughter cyst
grandiose
    g. delusion
    g. type of paranoid disorder
Granger
    G. line
    G. projection
Granit's loop
granny knot
Gr antigen
granular
    g. cast
    g. cell myoblastoma
    g. cell tumor
    g. conjunctivitis
    g. cortex
    g. degeneration
    g. endoplasmic reticulum
    g. kidney
    g. layer of cerebellar cortex
    g. layer of cerebellum
    g. layer of epidermis
    g. layers of cerebral cortex
    g. layers of retina
    g. layer of a vesicular ovarian follicle
    g. leukoblast
    g. leukocyte
    g. lids
    g. ophthalmia
    g. pits
    g. pneumonocytes
    g. trachoma
    g. urethritis
granulatio, pl. **granulationes**
    granulationes arachnoideales
granulation
    arachnoid g.'s
    arachnoidal g.'s
    pacchionian g.'s
    g. tissue
granule
    α g.'s
    acidophil g.

G

373

granule *(continued)*
    acrosomal g.
    alpha g.
    Altmann's g.
    amphophil g.
    argentaffin g.'s
    azurophil g.
    basal g.
    basophil g.
    Bensley's specific g.'s
    beta g.
    Birbeck's g.
    g. cell of connective tissue
    g. cells
    chromatic g.
    chromophil g.
    chromophobe g.'s
    cone g.
    Crooke's g.'s
    delta g.
    elementary g.
    eosinophil g.
    Fordyce's g.'s
    fuchsinophil g.
    glycogen g.
    iodophil g.
    juxtaglomerular g.'s
    kappa g.
    keratohyalin g.'s
    lamellar g.
    Langerhans' g.
    Langley's g.'s
    membrane-coating g.
    metachromatic g.'s
    mucinogen g.'s
    Neusser's g.'s
    neutrophil g.
    Nissl g.'s
    oxyphil g.
    proacrosomal g.'s
    prosecretion g.'s
    rod g.
    Schüffner's g.'s
    secretory g.
    seminal g.
    volutin g.'s
    Zimmermann's g.
granuloblast
granulocyte
    g. colony-stimulating factor
    immature g.
granulocyte-macrophage colony-stimulating factor
granulocytic
    g. leukemia
    g. sarcoma
    g. series
granulocytopenia

granulocytopoiesis
granulocytopoietic
granulocytosis
granuloma
    actinic g.
    amebic g.
    g. annulare
    apical g.
    beryllium g.
    bilharzial g.
    coccidioidal g.
    dental g.
    g. endemicum
    eosinophilic g.
    g. faciale
    foreign body g.
    g. gangrenescens
    giant cell g.
    g. gravidarum
    infectious g.
    g. inguinale
    g. inguinale tropicum
    laryngeal g.
    lethal midline g.
    lipoid g.
    lipophagic g.
    Majocchi g.'s
    malignant g.
    Miescher's g.
    g. multiforme
    oily g.
    paracoccidioidal g.
    parasitic g.
    periapical g.
    g. pudendi
    pulse g.
    pyogenic g., g. pyogenicum
    reparative giant cell g.
    reticulohistiocytic g.
    root end g.
    sarcoidal g.
    schistosome g.
    sea urchin g.
    silica g.
    silicotic g.
    swimming pool g.
    g. telangiectaticum
    g. tropicum
    ulcerating g. of pudenda
    g. venereum
    zirconium g.
granulomatosis
    allergic g.
    bronchocentric g.
    lipid g., lipoid g.
    lipophagic intestinal g.
    lymphomatoid g.

g. siderotica
Wegener's g.
granulomatous
g. arteritis
g. colitis
g. disease
g. encephalomyelitis
g. endophthalmitis
g. enteritis
g. inflammation
g. mastitis
g. nocardiosis
g. rosacea
granulomere
granulopenia
granuloplasm
granuloplastic
granulopoiesis
granulopoietic
granulosa
g. cell
g. cell tumor
g. lutein cells
granulosis
g. rubra nasi
granulosity
granulovacuolar degeneration
granum
granzymes
grape
g. endings
g. mole
graph
graphanesthesia
graphesthesia
graphic aphasia
graphology
graphomania
graphomotor
g. aphasia
graphopathology
graphophobia
graphorrhea
graphospasm
grasp
palm g.
pen g.
g. reflex
grasping reflex
grass bacillus
Grasset-Gaussel phenomenon
Grasset's
G. law
G. phenomenon
G. sign
Gratiolet's
G. fibers
G. radiation

grattage
Gräupner's method
grave
g. wax
gravel
Graves'
G. disease
G. ophthalmopathy
G. optic neuropathy
G. orbitopathy
gravid
g. uterus
gravida, gravida I, gravida II
gravidic
g. retinitis
g. retinopathy
gravidism
graviditas
g. examnialis
g. exochorialis
gravidity
gravireceptors
gravitation abscess
gravitational ulcer
gravity
zero g.
Grawitz'
G. basophilia
G. tumor
gray
g. baby syndrome
g. cataract
g. columns
g. degeneration
g. fibers
g. hepatization
g. induration
g. infiltration
g. layer of superior colliculus
g. matter, grey matter
g. rami communicantes
g. scale
g. substance
g. syndrome
g. tuber
g. tubercle
g. wing
gray-scale ultrasonography
great
g. adductor muscle
g. alveolar cells
g. anastomotic artery
g. auricular nerve
g. cardiac vein
g. cerebral vein
g. cerebral vein of Galen
g. foramen
g. horizontal fissure

G

great *(continued)*
   g. longitudinal fissure
   g. pancreatic artery
   g. radicular artery
   g. saphenous vein
   g. sciatic nerve
   g. superior pancreatic artery
   g. toe
   g. vein of Galen
greater
   g. alar cartilage
   g. arterial circle of iris
   g. circulation
   g. cul-de-sac
   g. curvature of stomach
   g. horn of hyoid bone
   g. multangular bone
   g. occipital nerve
   g. omentum
   g. palatine artery
   g. palatine canal
   g. palatine foramen
   g. palatine groove
   g. palatine nerve
   g. pectoral muscle
   g. pelvis
   g. peritoneal cavity
   g. petrosal nerve
   g. posterior rectus muscle of head
   g. psoas muscle
   g. rhomboid muscle
   g. ring of iris
   g. sciatic notch
   g. splanchnic nerve
   g. superficial petrosal nerve
   g. supraclavicular fossa
   g. trochanter
   g. tubercle of humerus
   g. tuberosity of humerus
   g. tympanic spine
   g. vestibular gland
   g. wing of sphenoid bone
   g. zygomatic muscle
greatest length
great-toe reflex
green
   g. cancer
   g. monkey virus
   g. pus
   g. sickness
   g. sputum
   g. stain
   g. tobacco sickness
   g. tooth
   g. vision
Greenfield
   G. filter
Greenhow's disease

greenstick fracture
greffotome
gregaloid
Gregarina
gregarine
Gregarinia
gregarinosis
Greig's syndrome
grenz
   g. ray
   g. zone
gression
Greville bath
grey matter *(var. of* gray matter)
Grey Turner's sign
grid
   focused g.
   g. ratio
   Wetzel g.
Gridley's
   G. stain
   G. stain for fungi
grief
Griesinger's
   G. disease
   G. sign
   G. symptom
grinding
   selective g.
   g. surface
grinding-in
grip
   devil's g.
grippe
griseus
Grisolle's sign
Grisonella ratellina
gristle
Gritti's operation
Gritti-Stokes amputation
Grocco's
   G. sign
   G. triangle
grocer's itch
Grocott-Gomori methenamine-silver stain
Groenouw's corneal dystrophy
groin
   g. ulcer
Grönblad-Strandberg syndrome
groove
   alveolobuccal g.
   alveololabial g.
   alveololingual g.
   anterior auricular g.
   anterior intermediate g.
   anterior interventricular g.
   anterolateral g.
   anteromedian g.

g. for arch of aorta
arterial g.'s
atrioventricular g.
g. for auditory tube
auriculoventricular g.
bicipital g.
branchial g.
carotid g.
carpal g.
cavernous g.
chiasmatic g.
coronary g.
costal g.
costal g. for subclavian artery
g. of crus of the helix
dental g.
g. for the descending aorta
developmental g.'s
digastric g.
ethmoidal g.
frontal g.'s
gingivobuccal g.
gingivolabial g.
gingivolingual g.
greater palatine g.
g. of greater petrosal nerve
Harrison's g.
inferior petrosal g.
g. for inferior petrosal sinus
g. for inferior venae cava
infraorbital g.
interosseous g.
interosseous g. of calcaneus
interosseous g. of talus
intertubercular g.
interventricular g.'s
lacrimal g.
laryngotracheal g.
lateral bicipital g.
g. of lesser petrosal nerve
linguogingival g.
Lucas' g.
g. of lung for subclavian artery
major g.
mastoid g.
medial bicipital g.
median g. of tongue
medullary g.
middle meningeal artery g.
g. for middle temporal artery
minor g.
musculospiral g.
mylohyoid g.
g. of nail matrix
nasolabial g.
nasopalatine g.
nasopharyngeal g.
neural g.

obturator g.
occipital g.
olfactory g.
optic g.
palatine g.
palatovaginal g.
paraglenoid g.
pharyngeal g.'s
pharyngotympanic g.
pontomedullary g.
popliteal g.
posterior auricular g.
posterior intermediate g.
posterior interventricular g.
posterolateral g.
preauricular g.
primary labial g.
primitive g.
g. of pterygoid hamulus
pterygopalatine g.
g. for radial nerve
retention g.
rhombic g.'s
sagittal g.
Sibson's g.
sigmoid g.
g. for sigmoid sinus
g. sign
skin g.'s
g. for spinal nerve
spiral g.
subclavian g.
g. for subclavian vein
subcostal g.
g. for superior petrosal sinus
g. for superior sagittal sinus
g. for superior vena cava
supplemental g.
supra-acetabular g.
g. for tendon of flexor hallucis
  longus
g. for tendon of peroneus longus
  muscle
g. for tibialis posterior tendon
tracheobronchial g.
transverse anthelicine g.
transverse nasal g.
g. for transverse sinus
tympanic g.
g. for ulnar nerve
urethral g.
venous g.'s
vertebral g.
g. for vertebral artery
vomeral g.
vomerovaginal g.
grooved tongue

G

Gross'
    G. leukemia virus
    G. virus
gross
    g. anatomy
    g. hematuria
    g. lesion
    g. reproduction rate
ground
    g. bundles
    g. itch
    g. itch anemia
    g. lamella
ground-glass
    g.-g. cytoplasm
    g.-g. pattern
group
    g. agglutination
    g. agglutinin
    g. antigens
    g. A streptococcal necrotizing
      fasciitis
    g. A streptococci
    blood g.
    g. B streptococci
    connective tissue g.
    control g.
    cytophil g.
    determinant g.
    diagnosis related g.
    g. dynamics
    encounter g.
    experimental g.
    HACEK g.
    g. hospital
    g. III mycobacteria
    g. II mycobacteria
    g. immunity
    g. I mycobacteria
    g. IV mycobacteria
    linkage g.
    matched g.'s
    g. practice
    g. psychotherapy
    g. reaction
    sensitivity training g.
    symptom g.
    g. test
    therapeutic g.
    training g.
grouping
    blood g.
Grover's disease
growing
    g. fracture
    g. ovarian follicle
    g. pains

growth
    accretionary g.
    appositional g.
    g. arrest lines
    auxetic g.
    g. curve
    differential g.
    g. factors
    g. hormone inhibiting hormone
    g. hormone-producing adenoma
    interstitial g.
    intussusceptive g.
    multiplicative g.
    new g.
    g. phase
    g. rate
    g. rate of population
growth-onset diabetes
grub
Gruber-Landzert fossa
Gruber's
    G. cul-de-sac
    G. method
    G. reaction
Gruber-Widal reaction
grumous
Grunert's spur
Grunstein-Hogness assay
Grynfeltt's triangle
gryochrome
gryposis
    g. penis
    g. unguium
g-tolerance
guaiacin
guaiac test
Guama virus
guanine cell
guarding
    abdominal g.
    involuntary g.
    voluntary g.
Guarnieri
    G. bodies
    G. gelatin agar
Guaroa virus
gubernacular
    g. canal
    g. cord
gubernaculum
    g. dentis
    Hunter's g.
    g. testis
Gubler's
    G. line
    G. paralysis
    G. syndrome
    G. tumor

Gudden's
    G. commissures
    G. ganglion
    G. tegmental nuclei
Guéneau de Mussy's point
Guérin's
    G. fold
    G. fracture
    G. glands
    G. sinus
    G. valve
guidance
    condylar g.
    incisal g.
guide
    anterior g.
    catheter g.
    condylar g.
    incisal g.
    mold g.
    g. plane
    g. wire
guideline
    clasp g.
    Cummer's g.
guidewire
Guillain-Barré
    G.-B. reflex
    G.-B. syndrome
guillotine
    g. amputation
guinea
    g. corn yaws
    g. green B
Gulf War syndrome
gullet
gum
    g. contour
    g. lancet
    g. line
    g. resection
gumboil
gumma, pl. **gummata, gummas**
gummatous
    g. abscess
    g. syphilid
    g. ulcer
Gumprecht's shadows
Gunn
    G. crossing sign
    G. dots
    G. phenomenon
    G. pupil
    G. sign
    G. syndrome
Gunning splint
gunshot wound
gunstock deformity

Günz' ligament
gurgling rale
gurney
Gussenbauer's suture
gustation
gustatory
    g. anesthesia
    g. bud
    g. cells
    g. hallucination
    g. hyperesthesia
    g. hyperhidrosis
    g. lemniscus
    g. nucleus
    g. organ
    g. pore
    g. rhinorrhea
    g. sweating syndrome
gustatory-sudorific reflex
gut
    blind g.
    g. glucagon
    postanal g.
    postcloacal g.
    preoral g.
    primitive g.
gut-associated lymphoid tissue
Guthrie
    G. muscle
    G. test
gutta, pl. **guttae**
    g. serena
gutta-percha
    g.-p. cone
    g.-p. points
    g.-p. spreader
guttate
    g. choroidopathy
gutter
    g. dystrophy of cornea
    g. fracture
    paracolic g.'s
    paravertebral g.
    g. wound
guttural
    g. duct
    g. pulse
    g. rale
gutturotetany
Gutzeit's test
Guyon's
    G. amputation
    G. isthmus
    G. sign
GVH disease
Gymnamoebida
gymnastics
    Swedish g.

G

379

Gymnoascaceae
gymnophobia
gymnothecium
gynandrism
gynandroblastoma
gynandroid
gynandromorphism
gynandromorphous
gynatresia
gynecic
gynecogenic
gynecography
gynecoid
    g. pelvis
gynecologic, gynecological
gynecologist
gynecology
gynecomania
gynecomastia, gynecomasty
    refeeding g.
gynecophoric canal
gynephobia
gyniatrics
gyniatry
gynogenesis
gynopathy
gynoplasty, gynoplastics
gyrase
gyrate
gyration
gyrectomy
gyrencephalic
gyri (*gen. and pl. of* gyrus)
gyrochrome
    g. cell
gyromagnetic ratio
Gyromitra esculenta
gyrosa
gyrose
gyrospasm
gyrus, gen. and pl. gyri
    angular g.
    g. angularis
    annectent g.
    anterior central g.
    anterior piriform g.
    ascending frontal g.
    ascending parietal g.
    gyri breves insulae
    callosal g.
    central gyri
    gyri cerebri, gyri of cerebrum
    cingulate g.
    g. cinguli
    deep transitional g.
    dentate g.
    g. dentatus
    fasciolar g.

g. fasciolaris
fornicate g.
g. fornicatus
g. frontalis inferior
g. frontalis medius
g. frontalis superior
fusiform g.
g. fusiformis
Heschl's gyri
hippocampal g.
inferior frontal g.
inferior occipital g.
inferior parietal g.
inferior temporal g.
gyri insulae
insular gyri
interlocking gyri
lateral occipitotemporal g.
lingual g.
g. lingualis
long g. of insula
g. longus insulae
marginal g.
medial occipitotemporal g.
middle frontal g.
middle temporal g.
occipital gyri
g. occipitotemporalis lateralis
g. occipitotemporalis medialis
orbital gyri
gyri orbitales
parahippocampal g.
g. parahippocampalis
paraterminal g.
g. paraterminalis
postcentral g.
g. postcentralis
posterior central g.
precentral g.
g. precentralis
prepiriform g.
g. rectus
Retzius' g.
short gyri of insula
splenial g.
straight g.
subcallosal g.
g. subcallosus
superior frontal g.
superior occipital g.
superior parietal g.
superior temporal g.
supracallosal g.
supramarginal g.
g. supramarginalis
gyri temporales transversi
g. temporalis inferior
g. temporalis medius

g. temporalis superior
transitional g.

transverse temporal gyri
uncinate g.

G

H

H agglutinin
H antigen
H band
H colony
H and D curve
H disk
H fields
H gene
H graft
H rays
H reflex
H shunt

H-2

H-2 antigens
H-2 complex

HA1 virus
HA2 virus
haarscheibe tumor
Haase's rule
habena, pl. **habenae**
habenal, habenar
habenula, pl. **habenulae**
h. of cecum
Haller's h.
habenulae perforata
pineal h.
Scarpa's h.
h. urethralis
habenular
h. commissure
h. nucleus
h. sulcus
h. trigone
habenulointerpeduncular tract
habenulopeduncular tract
Haber's syndrome
habit
h. chorea
h. scoliosis
h. spasm
h. tic
habitual abortion
habituation
habitus
fetal h.
gracile h.
habromania
Habronema
H. majus
H. megastoma
H. microstoma
H. muscae
HACEK group
hacking

Hadrurus
Haeckel's
H. gastrea theory
H. law
Haemadipsa ceylonica
Haemamoeba
Haematopinus
Haemobartonella
H. muris
Haemococcidium
Haemodipsus ventricosus
Haemogregarina
Haemophilus
H. actinomycetemcomitans
H. aegypticus
H. aphrophilus
H. ducreyi
H. gallinarum
H. haemolyticus
H. influenzae
H. influenzae type B vaccine
H. parahaemolyticus
H. parainfluenzae
Haemoproteus
Haemosporina
Haemostrongylus vasorum
Haenel's symptom
Haff disease
Hafnia
hafussi bath
Hagedorn needle
Hageman factor
hagiotherapy
Haglund's
H. deformity
H. disease
Hahn's oxine reagent
Haidinger's brushes
Hailey-Hailey disease
hair
auditory h.'s
axillary h.
bamboo h.
bayonet h.
beaded h.
h. bulb
burrowing h.'s
h. cast
h. cells
club h.
h. crosses
h. cycle
h. disk
exclamation point h.
h. follicle

H

hair *(continued)*
>Frey's h.'s
>ingrown h.'s
>kinky h.
>lanugo h.
>moniliform h.
>nettling h.'s
>h. papilla
>ringed h.
>h. root
>scalp h.
>Schridde's cancer h.'s
>h. shaft
>stellate h.
>h. streams
>taste h.'s
>terminal h.
>h. transplant
>twisted h.'s
>vellus h.
>h. whorls
>woolly h.

hairline fracture
hairpin loops
hairworm
hairy
>h. cell leukemia
>h. cells
>h. heart
>h. leukoplakia
>h. mole
>h. tongue

halation
Halberstaedter-Prowazek bodies
Haldane
>H.'s apparatus
>H. effect
>H. transformation
>H. tube

Haldane-Priestley sample
Hale's colloidal iron stain
Hales' piesimeter
half
>h. amplitude pulse duration
>h. axial view
>h. and half nail

half-axial projection
half-glass spectacles
half-life
>biological h.-l.
>effective h.-l.
>physical h.-l.

half-moon
>red h.-m.

half-value layer
halfway house
haliphagia
halisteresis

halisteretic
halitosis
halitus
Haller cell
Hallermann-Streiff-François syndrome
Hallermann-Streiff syndrome
Haller's
>H. annulus
>H. ansa
>H. arches
>H. circle
>H. cones
>H. habenula
>H. insula
>H. line
>H. plexus
>H. rete
>H. tripod
>H. tunica vasculosa
>H. unguis
>H. vas aberrans
>H. vascular tissue

Hallervorden-Spatz
>H.-S. disease
>H.-S. syndrome

Hallervorden syndrome
Hallé's point
hallex, pl. **hallices**
Hallgren's syndrome
Hallopeau's disease
hallucal
halluces (*pl. of* hallux)
hallucination
>auditory h.
>formed visual h.
>gustatory h.
>haptic h.
>hypnagogic h.
>hypnopompic h.
>lilliputian h.
>mood-congruent h.
>mood-incongruent h.
>olfactory h.
>stump h.
>tactile h.
>unformed visual h.

hallucinatory neuralgia
hallucinogenesis
hallucinosis
>organic h.

hallus
hallux, pl. **halluces**
>h. dolorosus
>h. extensus
>h. flexus
>h. malleus
>h. rigidus

h. valgus
h. varus
halo
anemic h.
h. cast
h. effect
glaucomatous h.
h. melanoma
h. nevus
senile h.
h. sign
h. sign of hydrops
h. traction
h. vision
Halococcus
H. morrhuae
halogen acne
halogenoderma
halometer
halophil, halophile
halophilic
halosteresis
halothane hepatitis
Halstead-Reitan battery
Halsted's
H. law
H. operation
H. suture
Halteridium
halzoun
ham
hamartia
hamartoblastoma
hamartochondromatosis
hamartoma
fibrous h. of infancy
pulmonary h.
hamartomatous
hamartophobia
hamate bone
hamatum
hamaxophobia
Hamburger's law
Hamilton's pseudophlegmon
Hamilton-Stewart
H.-S. formula
H.-S. method
Hamman-Rich syndrome
Hamman's
H. disease
H. murmur
H. sign
H. syndrome
hammer
h. finger
h. nose
h. toe
Hammerschlag's method

hammock
h. bandage
h. ligament
Hammond's disease
Hampton
H. hump
H. line
H. maneuver
H. technique
Ham's test
hamstring
h. muscles
h. tendon
hamular
h. notch
h. process of lacrimal bone
h. process of sphenoid bone
hamulus, gen. and pl. **hamuli**
h. cochleae
lacrimal h.
h. lacrimalis
h. laminae spiralis
h. ossis hamati
pterygoid h.
h. pterygoideus
h. of spiral lamina
Hancock's amputation
hand
accoucheur's h.
ape h.
claw h.
cleft h.
club h.
crab h.
drop h.
h. eczema
flat h.
ghoul h.
h. of hand
Marinesco's succulent h.
monkey h.
obstetrical h.
opera-glass h.
h. ratio
simian h.
skeleton h.
spade h.
split h.
trench h.
trident h.
writing h.
hand-and-foot syndrome
handedness
hand-foot-and-mouth
h.-f.-a.-m. disease
h.-f.-a.-m. disease virus
handicap
handpiece

H

Hand-Schüller-Christian disease
hanging
    h. drop
    h. septum
hanging-block culture
hangman's fracture
hangnail
Hanhart's syndrome
Hanks dilators
Hannover's canal
Hanot's cirrhosis
Hansemann macrophage
Hansen's
    H. bacillus
    H. disease
Hantaan virus
Hantavirus
hapalonychia
haphalgesia
haphazard
    h. sampling
haphephobia
haploid
    h. set
haplology
haploscope
    mirror h.
haploscopic
    h. vision
Haplosporidia
haplotype
happy puppet syndrome
Hapsburg
    H. jaw
    H. lip
hapten
    conjugated h.
    h. inhibition of precipitation
haptic hallucination
haptics
haptodysphoria
haptoglobin
haptometer
Harada's
    H. disease
    H. syndrome
hard
    h. cataract
    h. chancre
    h. corn
    h. pad virus
    h. palate
    h. papilloma
    h. pulse
    h. rays
    h. sore
    h. tissue

    h. tubercle
    h. ulcer
hardened pelvis
hardiness
Harding-Passey melanoma
hardness
    indentation h.
hardware
Hardy-Rand-Ritter test
Hardy-Weinberg
    H.-W. equilibrium
    H.-W. law
harelip
hare's eye
harlequin
    h. fetus
    h. ichthyosis
    h. reaction
harmonia
harmonic
    h. mean
    h. suture
harmonious correspondence
harmony
    functional occlusal h.
    occlusal h.
harpaxophobia
harpoon
Harrington-Flocks test
Harris
    H. and Ray test
    H. syndrome
    H. test
Harris'
    H. hematoxylin
    H. lines
    H. migraine
Harrison's groove
Hartel technique
Hartmannella
Hartmann's
    H. curette
    H. operation
    H. pouch
Hartman's solution
Hartnup
    H. disease
    H. syndrome
harvest bug
harvester ant
hasamiyami
Häser's formula
Hashimoto's
    H. disease
    H. struma
    H. thyroiditis

Hasner's
    H. fold
    H. valve
Hassall-Henle bodies
Hassall's
    H. bodies
    H. concentric corpuscle
Hasson
    H. cannula
    H. trocar
hatchet
    h. excavator
Haubenfelder
Hauch
Haudek's niche
haustorium, pl. **haustoria**
haustra (*pl. of* haustrum)
haustral
haustration
    h.'s of colon
haustrum, pl. **haustra**
    haustra coli
    haustra of colon
Haverhill fever
Haverhillia multiformis
Havers' glands
haversian
    h. canals
    h. lamella
    h. spaces
    h. system
Hawley
    H. appliance
    H. retainer
Hawthorne effect
hay
    h. asthma
    h. bacillus
    h. fever
Hayem's
    H. hematoblast
    H. solution
Hayem-Widal syndrome
Hayflick's limit
Haygarth's
    H. nodes
    H. nodosities
hazard rate
head
    bulldog h.
    h. cap
    h. of the caudate nucleus
    h. cavity
    clavicular h. of pectoralis major
      muscle
    deep h. of flexor pollicis brevis
    h. of epididymis
    h. of femur

    h. of fibula
    h. fold
    hourglass h.
    humeral h.
    humeroulnar h. of flexor digitorum
      superficialis muscle
    h. of humerus
    lateral h.
    little h. of humerus
    long h.
    h. of malleus
    h. of mandible
    medial h.
    Medusa h.
    h. of metacarpal bone
    h. of metatarsal bone
    h. mirror
    h. nurse
    oblique h.
    optic nerve h.
    h. of pancreas
    h. of phalanx
    h. presentation
    h. process
    radial h.
    h. of radius
    h. of rib
    saddle h.
    short h.
    short h. of biceps brachii muscle
    short h. of biceps femoris muscle
    h. of stapes
    sternocostal h. of pectoralis major
      muscle
    superficial h. of flexor pollicis
      brevis muscle
    h. of talus
    h. tetanus
    h. of thigh bone
    transverse h.
    h. tremors
    h. of ulna
    ulnar h.
headache
    bilious h.
    blind h.
    cluster h.
    fibrositic h.
    histaminic h.
    Horton's h.
    migraine h.
    nodular h.
    organic h.
    reflex h.
    sick h.
    spinal h.
    symptomatic h.
    tension h.

H

headache *(continued)*
    vacuum h.
    vascular h.
head-bobbing doll syndrome
head-dropping test
headgear
headgut
head-nodding
Head's
    H. areas
    H. lines
    H. zones
head-tilt
heal
healed
    h. tuberculosis
    h. ulcer
healer
healing
    faith h.
    h. by first intention
    h. by second intention
    h. by third intention
health
    h. behavior
    behavioral h.
    h. care
    H. Care Financing Administration
    h. center
    h. education
    h. indicator
    h. maintenance organization
    mental h.
    h. promotion
    h. psychology
    public h.
    h. risk h.
    h. status index
healthy
    h. worker effect
Heaney's operation
He antigens
hear
hearing
    h. aid
    color h.
    h. impairment
    h. level
    h. loss
    normal h.
heart
    h. antigen
    armor h.
    armored h.
    h. arrest
    artificial h.
    athlete's h.
    athletic h.

    h. beat
    beer h.
    beriberi h.
    h. block
    bony h.
    chaotic h.
    crisscross h.
    h. disease
    drop h.
    h. failure
    h. failure cells
    fatty h.
    frosted h.
    globular h.
    hairy h.
    Holmes h.
    horizontal h.
    hyperthyroid h.
    hypoplastic h.
    icing h.
    intermediate h.
    irritable h.
    Jarvik artificial h.
    left h.
    h. massage
    mechanical h.
    movable h.
    myxedema h.
    ox h.
    parchment h.
    pendulous h.
    h. position
    pulmonary h.
    h. rate
    right h.
    round h.
    sabot h.
    h. sac
    semihorizontal h.
    semivertical h.
    soldier's h.
    h. sounds
    stone h.
    h. stroke
    systemic h.
    h. tamponade
    three-chambered h.
    tiger h.
    tobacco h.
    h. tones
    h. transplantation
    univentricular h.
    h. valve prosthesis
    venous h.
    vertical h.
    wooden-shoe h.
heartbeat
heartburn

heart-lung
    h.-l. machine
    h.-l. preparation
    h.-l. transplantation
heart-shaped
    h.-s. pelvis
    h.-s. uterus
heartworm
heat
    h. apoplexy
    h. coagulation test
    h. cramps
    h. edema
    h. exhaustion
    h. hyperpyrexia
    initial h.
    h. instability test
    h. lamp
    prickly h.
    h. prostration
    h. rash
    h. shock proteins
    h. stroke
    h. treatment
    h. urticaria
Heath-Edwards grades
heat-rigor point
heatstroke
heavy
    h. chain disease
    h. metal neuropathy
γ-heavy-chain disease
μ-heavy-chain disease
α-heavy-chain disease
Hebeloma
hebephrenia
hebephrenic
    h. dementia
    h. schizophrenia
Heberden's
    H. angina
    H. nodes
    H. nodosities
hebetic
hebetude
hebiatrics
Hebra's
    H. disease
    H. prurigo
hecateromeric
hecatomeral, hecatomeric
Hecht's pneumonia
Heck's disease
hectic
    h. flush
hederiform
    h. ending

hedonophobia
hedrocele
Hedström file
heel
    black h.
    h. bone
    cracked h.
    h. fly
    h. jar
    painful h.
    prominent h.
    h. tap
    h. tendon
heel-tap
    h.-t. reaction
    h.-t. test
heel-to-knee-to-toe test
heel-to-shin test
Heerfordt's disease
Hegar's
    H. dilators
    H. sign
Hegglin's
    H. anomaly
    H. syndrome
Heidenhain pouch
Heidenhain's
    H. azan stain
    H. crescents
    H. demilunes
    H. iron hematoxylin stain
    H. law
height
    anterior facial h.
    h. of contour
    cusp h.
    facial h.
    nasal h.
    orbital h.
    h. vertigo
height-length index
Heilbronner's thigh
Heim-Kreysig sign
Heimlich maneuver
Heineke-Mikulicz pyloroplasty
Heinz
    H. bodies
    H. body anemia
    H. body test
Heinz-Ehrlich body
Heister's
    H. diverticulum
    H. valve
HeLa cells
Helbings' sign
helcomenia
helcoplasty

H

Held's
    H. bundle
    H. decussation
helical
    h. computed tomography
    h. CT
helicine arteries of the penis
helicis
    h. major muscle
    h. minor muscle
Helicobacter
    H. pylori
helicoid
    h. choroidopathy
    h. ginglymus
helicopod gait
helicopodia
helicotrema
heliencephalitis
Helie's bundle
helioaerotherapy
heliopathy
heliophobia
heliosis
heliotaxis
heliotropism
Heliozoea
helium speech
Heller
    H. myotomy
    H. operation
    H. plexus
Hellin's law
HELLP syndrome
Helly's fixative
helmet
    neurasthenic h.
helmet cell
Helmholtz
    H. theory of accommodation
    H. theory of color vision
    H. theory of hearing
Helmholtz' axis ligament
helminth
helminthemesis
helminthiasis
helminthic dysentery
helminthism
helminthoid
helminthology
helminthoma
helminthophobia
Helminthosporium
heloma
    h. durum
    h. molle
helosis
helotomy

helper
    h. cell
    h. virus
helplessness
    learned h.
Helvella esculenta
Helweg-Larssen syndrome
Helweg's bundle
hemachrome
hemachrosis
hemacytometer
hemacytozoon
hemadostenosis
hemadrometer
hemadromograph
hemadromometer
hemadsorption
    h. virus test
    h. virus type 1
    h. virus type 2
hemadynamometer
hemafacient
hemagglutinating cold autoantibody
hemagglutination
    h. inhibition
    passive h.
    reverse passive h.
    h. test
    viral h.
hemagglutinin
hemagogic
hemal
    h. arches
    h. gland
hemalum
hemamebiasis
hemanalysis
hemangiectasis, hemangiectasia
hemangiectatic hypertrophy
hemangioblast
hemangioblastoma
hemangioendothelioblastoma
hemangioendothelioma
    h. tuberosum multiplex
hemangiofibroma
    juvenile h.
hemangioma
    capillary h.
    capillary h. of infancy
    cavernous h.
    h. planum extensum
    racemose h.
    sclerosing h.
    senile h.
    spider h.
    strawberry h.
    verrucous h.
hemangioma-thrombocytopenia syndrome

hemangiomatosis
hemangiopericytoma
hemangiosarcoma
hemapheic
hemaphein
hemapheism
hemarthron, hemarthros
hemarthrosis
hemastrontium
hematachometer
hematapostema
hematein
 Baker's acid h.
hematemesis
hematencephalon
hematherapy
hemathidrosis
hemathorax
hematid
hematidrosis
hematimeter
hematinemia
hematobilia
hematobium
hematoblast
 Hayem's h.
hematocele
 pelvic h.
 pudendal h.
hematocephaly
hematochezia
hematochlorin
hematochyluria
hematocolpometra
hematocolpos
hematocrit
hematocyst
hematocystis
hematocyte
hematocytoblast
hematocytolysis
hematocytometer
hematocytozoon
hematodyscrasia
hematodystrophy
hematogenesis
hematogenetic calculus
hematogenic, hematogenous
hematohistioblast
hematoid
hematoidin
 h. crystals
hematologist
hematology
hematolymphangioma
hematolysis
hematolytic

hematoma
 communicating h.
 corpus luteum h.
 epidural h.
 intracranial h.
 intramural h.
 pulsatile h.
 subdural h.
hematomanometer
hematometra
hematometry
hematomphalocele
hematomyelia
hematomyelopore
hematopathology
hematopathy
hematopenia
hematophagia
hematophagous
hematophagus
hematoplastic
hematopoiesis
hematopoietic
 h. gland
 h. system
hematoporphyria
hematoporphyrinemia
hematoporphyrinuria
hematopsia
hematorrhachis
 h. externa
 extradural h.
 h. interna
 subdural h.
hematosalpinx
hematosepsis
hematosis
hematospectroscope
hematospectroscopy
hematospermatocele
hematospermia
hematostaxis
hematosteon
hematotoxic (*var. of* hemotoxic)
hematotoxin
hematotrachelos
hematotropic
hematotympanum
hematoxic (*var. of* hemotoxic)
hematoxin
hematoxylin
 h. bodies
 Boehmer's h.
 Delafield's h.
 h. and eosin stain
 Harris' h.
 iron h.
 phosphotungstic acid h.

H

391

hematoxylin-malachite green-basic
  fuchsin stain
hematoxylin-phloxine B stain
hematoxyphil bodies
hematozoic
hematozoon
hematuria
    Egyptian h.
    endemic h.
    false h.
    gross h.
    initial h.
    microscopic h.
    painful h.
    painless h.
    renal h.
    terminal h.
    total h.
    urethral h.
    vesical h.
hematuric bilious fever
hemendothelioma
hemeralopia
hemeranopia
hemiacardius
hemiacrosomia
hemiageusia
hemiageustia
hemialgia
hemianalgesia
hemianencephaly
hemianesthesia
    alternate h.
    crossed h.
hemianopia
    absolute h.
    altitudinal h.
    binasal h.
    bitemporal h.
    complete h.
    congruous h.
    crossed h.
    heteronymous h.
    homonymous h.
    incomplete h.
    incongruous h.
    pseudo-h.
    quadrantic h.
    unilateral h., uniocular h.
hemianopic
    h. scotoma
    h. spectacles
hemianopsia
hemianosmia
hemiaplasia
hemiapraxia
hemiarthroplasty
hemiasynergia

hemiataxia
hemiathetosis
hemiatrophy
    facial h.
    facial h. of Romberg
    lingual h.
hemiazygos vein
hemiballism
hemiballismus
hemiblock
hemic
    h. calculus
    h. distomiasis
    h. murmur
hemicardia
    h. dextra
    h. sinistra
hemicentrum
hemicephalalgia
hemicephalia
hemicerebrum
hemichorea
hemicolectomy
hemicorporectomy
hemicrania
hemicraniectomy
hemicraniosis
hemicraniotomy
hemidesmosomes
hemidiaphoresis
hemidrosis
hemidysesthesia
hemidystrophy
hemiectromelia
hemifacial
hemigastrectomy
hemigeusia
hemiglossal
hemiglossectomy
hemiglossitis
hemignathia
hemihepatectomy
hemihidrosis
hemihydranencephaly
hemihypalgesia
hemihyperesthesia
hemihyperhidrosis
hemihyperidrosis
hemihypertonia
hemihypertrophy
hemihypesthesia
hemihypoesthesia
hemihypotonia
hemikaryon
hemilaminectomy
hemilaryngectomy
hemilateral
    h. chorea

hemilesion
hemilingual
hemimacroglossia
hemimandibulectomy
hemimetabolous
hemiopalgia
hemipagus
hemipancreatectomy
hemiparesis
hemipelvectomy
hemiplegia
    alternating h.
    contralateral h.
    crossed h.
    double h.
    facial h.
    infantile h.
    spastic h.
hemiplegic
    h. amyotrophy
    h. gait
    h. migraine
Hemiptera
hemisection
hemisensory
hemiseptum
hemispasm
hemisphere
    h. of bulb of penis
    cerebellar h.
    cerebral h.
    dominant h.
hemispherectomy
hemispherium
    h. bulbi urethrae
    h. cerebelli
    h. cerebri
Hemispora
hemistrumectomy
hemisyndrome
hemisystole
hemithermoanesthesia
hemithoracic duct
hemithorax
hemitonia
hemitremor
hemitruncus
hemivertebra
hemizona assay
hemizygosity
hemizygote
hemizygotic
hemizygous
hemoagglutination
hemoagglutinin
hemoantitoxin
Hemobartonella
hemobilia

hemoblast
    lymphoid h. of Pappenheim
hemoblastosis
hemocatharsis
hemocatheresis
hemocatheretic
hemoccult test
hemocele
hemocholecyst
hemocholecystitis
hemochorial placenta
hemochromatosis
    exogenous h.
    primary h.
    secondary h.
hemoclasis, hemoclasia
hemoclastic
    h. reaction
hemoconcentration
hemoconia
hemoconiosis
hemocryoscopy
hemocyte
hemocytoblast
hemocytocatheresis
hemocytolysis
hemocytometer
hemocytometry
hemocytotripsis
hemocytozoon
hemodiagnosis
hemodialysis
hemodialyzer
    ultrafiltration h.
hemodilution
hemodromograph
hemodromometer
hemodynamic
hemodynamics
hemodynamometer
hemodyscrasia
hemodystrophy
hemoendothelial placenta
hemofiltration
hemoflagellates
hemogenesis
hemogenic
hemoglobin
    aberrant h.
    h. C disease
    h. F (hereditary persistence of)
    h. H disease
    mean corpuscular h.
    variant h.
hemoglobinemia
hemoglobinocholia
hemoglobinopathy
hemoglobinophilic

H

hemoglobinuria
    epidemic h.
    intermittent h.
    malarial h.
    march h.
    paroxysmal cold h.
    paroxysmal nocturnal h.
    toxic h.
hemoglobinuric
    h. fever
    h. nephrosis
hemogram
hemohistioblast
hemolamella
hemoleukocyte
hemolith
hemology
hemolymph
    h. gland
    h. node
hemolysate
hemolysin
    α h.
    β h.
    bacterial h.
    cold h.
    heterophil h.
    immune h.
    natural h.
    specific h.
    warm-cold h.
hemolysinogen
hemolysis
    α′ h.
    β h.
    biologic h.
    conditioned h.
    γ h.
    immune h.
    phenylhydrazine h.
    venom h.
    viridans h.
γ hemolysis
hemolytic
    h. anemia
    h. chain
    h. disease of newborn
    h. jaundice
    h. splenomegaly
    h. streptococci
    h. uremic syndrome
β-hemolytic streptococci
hemolyzation
hemolyze
hemomanometer
hemomediastinum
hemometra
hemometry

hemonephrosis
hemopathology
hemopathy
hemoperfusion
hemopericardium
hemoperitoneum
hemophagia
hemophagocytosis
hemophil, hemophile
hemophilia
    h. C
    classical h.
hemophiliac
hemophilic
    h. arthritis
    h. joint
hemophobia
hemophoresis
hemophthalmia, hemophthalmus
hemophthisis
hemoplastic
hemoplasty
hemopneumopericardium
hemopneumothorax
hemopoiesis
hemopoietic
    h. tissue
hemoprecipitin
hemoptysis
    cardiac h.
    endemic h.
    parasitic h.
hemopyelectasis, hemopyelectasia
hemorheology
hemorrhachis
hemorrhage
    brainstem h.
    cerebral h.
    concealed h.
    Duret's h.
    extradural h.
    gastric h.
    intermediate h.
    internal h.
    intracerebral h.
    intracranial h.
    intrapartum h.
    intraventricular h.
    nasal h.
    parenchymatous h.
    h. per rhexis
    petechial h.
    pontine h.
    postpartum h.
    primary h.
    punctate h.
    renal h.
    secondary h.

[handwritten note: Labyrinthine hemmorage]

serous h.
splinter h.'s
subarachnoid h.
subdural h.
subgaleal h.
syringomyelic h.
unavoidable h.
hemorrhagic
h. anemia
h. ascites
h. bronchitis
h. colitis
h. cyst
h. cystitis
h. dengue
h. diathesis
h. disease of the newborn
h. endovasculitis
h. exudative erythema
h. fever
h. fever with renal syndrome
h. gangrene
h. glaucoma
h. infarct
h. iritis
h. measles
h. nephritis
h. pachymeningitis
h. pericarditis
h. pian
h. plague
h. pleurisy
h. rickets
h. scurvy
h. shock
h. smallpox
hemorrhagins
hemorrhoid
external h.
hemorrhoidal
h. nerves
h. plexus
h. veins
h. zone
hemorrhoidectomy
hemorrhoids
cutaneous h.
external h.
internal h.
hemosalpinx
hemosialemesis
hemosiderosis
idiopathic pulmonary h.
nutritional h.
pulmonary h.
hemospermia
h. spuria
h. vera

hemosporidium
hemosporines
hemostasia
hemostasis
hemostat
hemostatic forceps
hemosuccus pancreaticus
hemotachogram
hemotachometer
hemotherapy, hemotherapeutics
hemothorax
hemothymia
hemotoxic, hematotoxic, hematoxic
hemotoxin
cobra h.
hemotroph, hemotrophe
hemotropic
hemotympanum
hemozoic
hemozoon
HEMPAS cells
hen-cluck stertor
Hendersonula toruloidea
Henke's space
Henle's
H. ampulla
H. ansa
H. fenestrated elastic membrane
H. fiber layer
H. fissures
H. glands
H. layer
H. loop
H. membrane
H. nervous layer
H. reaction
H. sheath
H. spine
H. tubules
H. warts
Hennebert
Hennebert's sign
Henoch's
H. chorea
H. purpura
Henoch-Schönlein
H.-S. purpura
H.-S. syndrome
henpuye
Henry-Gauer response
Hensen's
H. canal
H. cell
H. disk
H. duct
H. knot
H. line

H

Hensen's *(continued)*
    H. node
    H. stripe
Hensing's ligament
Hepadnaviridae
hepar, gen. **hepatis**
    h. lobatum
heparinemia
heparinize
hepatatrophia, hepatatrophy
hepatectomy
hepatic
    h. adenoma
    h. amebiasis
    h. arteries
    h. branches of vagus nerve
    h. capsulitis
    h. colic
    h. coma
    h. cords
    h. cysts
    h. duct
    h. encephalopathy
    h. fistula
    h. flexure
    h. infantilism
    h. insufficiency
    h. intermittent fever
    h. laminae
    h. lobule
    h. lymph nodes
    h. plexus
    h. porphyria
    h. portal system
    h. portal vein
    h. prominence
    h. segments
    h. steatosis
    h. triad
    h. veins
    h. venous segments
hepaticodochotomy
hepaticoduodenostomy
hepaticoenterostomy
hepaticogastrostomy
hepaticolithotomy
hepaticolithotripsy
hepaticopulmonary
hepaticostomy
hepaticotomy
hepatis (*gen. of* hepar)
hepatitic
hepatitis
    h. A
    active chronic h.
    acute parenchymatous h.
    anicteric h.
    anicteric virus h.

    h. A virus
    h. B
    h. B core antigen
    h. B e antigen
    h. B surface antigen
    h. B virus
    h. C
    cholangiolitic h.
    cholestatic h.
    chronic h.
    chronic interstitial h.
    chronic persistent h.
    chronic persisting h.
    h. C virus
    h. D
    delta h.
    h. delta virus
    h. E
    epidemic h.
    h. E virus
    h. externa
    fulminant h.
    giant cell h.
    halothane h.
    infectious h.
    long incubation h.
    lupoid h.
    MS-1 h.
    NANB h.
    neonatal h.
    non-A, non-B h.
    non-A, non-B, non-C h.
    peliosis h.
    persistent chronic h.
    plasma cell h.
    serum h.
    short incubation h.
    subacute h.
    suppurative h.
    transfusion h.
    viral h.
    viral h. type A
    viral h. type B
    viral h. type C
    viral h. type D
    viral h. type E
    virus h.
    virus A h.
    virus B h.
    virus C h.
hepatitis-associated antigen
hepatization
    gray h.
    red h.
    yellow h.
hepatoblastoma
hepatocarcinoma
hepatocele

hepatocellular
   h. adenoma
   h. carcinoma
   h. jaundice
hepatocholangioenterostomy
hepatocholangiojejunostomy
hepatocholangiostomy
hepatocholangitis
hepatocolic ligament
hepatocystic
   h. duct
Hepatocystis
hepatocyte
hepatoduodenal ligament
hepatoduodenostomy
hepatodysentery
hepatoenteric
   h. recess
hepatoesophageal ligament
hepatofugal
hepatogastric
   h. ligament
hepatogenic, hepatogenous
hepatography
hepatohemia
hepatoid
hepatojugular
   h. reflex
   h. reflux
hepatojugularometer
hepatolenticular
   h. degeneration
   h. disease
hepatolienography
hepatolienomegaly
hepatolith
hepatolithectomy
hepatolithiasis
hepatologist
hepatology
hepatolysin
hepatoma
   malignant h.
hepatomalacia
hepatomegaly, hepatomegalia
hepatomelanosis
hepatomphalocele
hepatomphalos
hepatonecrosis
hepatonephoric syndrome
hepatonephric
hepatonephromegaly
hepatopancreatic
   h. ampulla
   h. sphincter
hepatopathic
hepatopathy
hepatoperitonitis

hepatopetal
hepatopexy
hepatophosphorylase deficiency
  glycogenosis
hepatophyma
hepatopleural fistula
hepatopneumonic
hepatoportal
hepatoptosis
hepatopulmonary
hepatorenal
   h. ligament
   h. pouch
   h. recess
   h. syndrome
hepatorrhagia
hepatorrhaphy
hepatorrhexis
hepatoscopy
hepatosplenitis
hepatosplenography
hepatosplenomegaly
hepatosplenopathy
hepatostomy
hepatotherapy
hepatotomy
hepatotoxemia
hepatotoxin
Hepatozoon
herald patch
herd
   h. immunity
   h. instinct
hereditary
   h. angioedema
   h. angioneurotic edema
   h. areflexic dystasia
   h. benign intraepithelial dyskeratosis
   h. cerebellar ataxia
   h. chorea
   h. clubbing
   h. deforming chondrodystrophy
   h. hemorrhagic telangiectasia
   h. hemorrhagic thrombasthenia
   h. hypertrophic neuropathy
   h. lymphedema
   h. methemoglobinemia
   h. methemoglobinemic cyanosis
   h. multiple exostoses
   h. multiple trichoepithelioma
   h. myokymia
   h. nephritis
   h. opalescent dentin
   h. photomyoclonus
   h. progressive arthro-ophthalmopathy
   h. sensory radicular neuropathy
   h. spherocytosis

H

hereditary *(continued)*
    h. spinal ataxia
    h. syphilis
heredity
heredofamilial tremor
heredopathia atactica polyneuritiformis
heredotaxia
Herellea
Hering-Breuer reflex
Hering's
    H. sinus nerve
    H. test
    H. theory of color vision
heritability
    h. in the broad sense
    h. in the narrow sense
heritage
Herlitz syndrome
Hermann's fixative
Hermansky-Pudlak syndrome type VI
hermaphrodism
hermaphrodite
hermaphroditism
    adrenal h.
    bilateral h.
    dimidiate h.
    false h.
    female h.
    lateral h.
    male h.
    transverse h.
    true h.
    unilateral h.
hernia
    abdominal h.
    Barth's h.
    Béclard's h.
    bilocular femoral h.
    Bochdalek's h.
    h. of the broad ligament of the
      uterus
    cecal h.
    cerebral h.
    Cloquet's h.
    complete h.
    concealed h.
    congenital diaphragmatic h.
    Cooper's h.
    crural h.
    diaphragmatic h.
    direct inguinal h.
    double loop h.
    dry h.
    duodenojejunal h.
    h. en bissac
    epigastric h.
    extrasaccular h.
    fascial h.

fat h.
fatty h.
femoral h.
gastroesophageal h.
gluteal h.
Hesselbach's h.
Hey's h.
hiatal h., hiatus h.
Holthouse's h.
iliacosubfascial h.
incarcerated h.
incisional h.
indirect inguinal h.
infantile h.
inguinal h., indirect inguinal h.
inguinocrural h., inguinofemoral h.
inguinolabial h.
inguinoscrotal h.
inguinosuperficial h.
internal h.
intersigmoid h.
interstitial h.
intraepiploic h.
intrailiac h.
intrapelvic h.
irreducible h.
ischiatic h.
h. knife
Krönlein's h.
labial h.
lateral ventral h.
Laugier's h.
levator h.
Littré's h.
lumbar h.
Malgaigne's h.
meningeal h.
mesenteric h.
obturator h.
orbital h.
pannicular h.
pantaloon h.
paraduodenal h.
paraesophageal h.
parahiatal h.
paraperitoneal h.
parasaccular h.
parasternal h.
parietal h.
perineal h.
Petit's h.
posterior vaginal h.
properitoneal inguinal h.
pudendal h.
reducible h.
retrograde h.
retroperitoneal h.
retropubic h.

retrosternal h.
Richter's h.
Rokitansky's h.
sciatic h.
scrotal h.
sliding h.
sliding esophageal hiatal h.
sliding hiatal h.
slipped h.
spigelian h.
strangulated h.
synovial h.
Treitz's h.
umbilical h.
h. uteri inguinale
Velpeau's h.
ventral h.
vesicle h.
vitreous h.
"w" h.

hernial
h. aneurysm
h. sac

herniated
h. disk

herniation
caudal transtentorial h.
cingulate h.
foraminal h.
rostral transtentorial h.
sphenoidal h.
subfalcial h.
tonsillar h.
transtentorial h.
uncal h.

hernioenterotomy
herniography
hernioid
herniolaparotomy
hernioplasty
herniopuncture
herniorrhaphy
herniotome
Cooper's h.
herniotomy
Petit's h.
heroic
herpangina
herpes
h. B encephalomyelitis
h. catarrhalis
h. circinatus bullosus
h. corneae
h. desquamans
h. digitalis
h. encephalitis
h. facialis
h. febrilis

h. generalisatus
h. genitalis, genital h.
h. gestationis
h. gladiatorum
h. iris
h. labialis
neonatal h.
h. progenitalis
h. simplex
h. simplex encephalitis
h. simplex virus
traumatic h.
h. virus
h. whitlow
h. zoster
h. zoster ophthalmicus
h. zoster oticus
h. zoster varicellosus
h. zoster virus

Herpesviridae
herpesvirus
human h. 1
human h. 2
human h. 3
human h. 4
human h. 5
human h. 6
human h. 7
suid h.

herpetic
h. fever
h. keratitis
h. keratoconjunctivitis
h. meningoencephalitis
h. ulcer
h. whitlow

herpetiform
h. aphthae

Herpetomonas
Herpetoviridae
Herpetovirus
herpetovirus
Herring bodies
herring-worm disease
Herrmann's syndrome
hersage
Hers' disease
Hertwig's sheath
hertzian experiments
Herxheimer's reaction
herzstoss
Heschl's gyri
hesitancy
Hesselbach's
H. fascia
H. hernia
H. ligament
H. triangle

H

Hess screen
Hess' test
heteradelphus
heterakid
heteralius
heteraxial
heterecious
heterecism
heteresthesia
heteroagglutinin
heteroalleles
heteroantibody
heteroantiserum
heteroblastic
heterocellular
heterocentric
heterocephalus
heterocheiral, heterochiral
heterochromatic
heterochromatin
    constitutive h.
    facultative h.
    satellite-rich h.
heterochromia
    atrophic h.
    binocular h.
    h. iridis, h. of iris
    monocular h.
    simple h.
    sympathetic h.
heterochromic
    h. cyclitis
    h. uveitis
heterochromosome
heterochromous
heterochron
heterochronia
heterochronic
heterochronous
heterocladic
heterocrine
heterocrisis
heterocytotropic
    h. antibody
heterodermic
heterodont
Heterodoxus spiniger
heterodromous
heterodymus
heteroerotic
heteroeroticism
heteroerotism
heterogametic
    h. embryo
heterogamous
heterogamy
heterogeneic (*var. of* heterogenic)
    h. antigen

heterogeneity
    genetic h.
heterogeneous
    h. radiation
heterogenetic
    h. antibody
    h. antigen
    h. parasite
heterogenic, heterogeneic
    h. enterobacterial antigen
heterogenote
heterogenous
    h. keratoplasty
heterograft
heterohypnosis
heterokaryon
heterokaryotic
heterokeratoplasty
heterokinesia
heterokinesis
heterolalia
heterolateral
heteroliteral
heterologous
    h. antiserum
    h. desensitization
    h. graft
    h. insemination
    h. serotype
    h. stimulus
    h. tumor
    h. twins
heterology
heterolysin
heterolysis
heterolytic
heteromastigote
heteromeral
heteromeric cell
heteromerous
heterometabolous
    h. metamorphosis
heterometaplasia
heterometric
    h. autoregulation
heterometropia
heteromorphism
heteromorphosis
heteromorphous
heteronomous
    h. psychotherapy
heteronomy
heteronuclear
heteronymous
    h. diplopia
    h. hemianopia
    h. image
    h. parallax

hetero-osteoplasty
heteropagus
heteropathy
heterophagy
heterophasia
heterophemia, heterophemy
heterophil, heterophile
  h. antibody
  h. antigen
  h. hemolysin
heterophonia
heterophoria
heterophthalmus
heterophthongia
Heterophyes
  H. brevicaeca
  H. heterophyes
  H. katsuradai
heterophyiasis
heterophyid
Heterophyidae
heterophyidiasis
heteroplasia
heteroplastic
  h. graft
heteroplastid
heteroplasty
heteroploid
heteroploidy
heteropsychologic
heteropyknosis
  negative h.
  positive h.
heteropyknotic
  h. chromatin
heteroscedasticity
heterosexual
heterosexuality
heterosmia
heterosome
heterospecific
  h. graft
heterosuggestion
heterotaxia
  cardiac h.
heterotaxic
heterotaxis, heterotaxy
heterothallic
heterotonia
heterotopia
  h. maculae
heterotopic
  h. graft
  h. pregnancy
  h. stimulus
heterotopous
heterotransplantation
heterotrichosis

heterotroph
heterotrophic oral gastrointestinal cyst
heterotropia, heterotropy
heterotype mitosis
heterotypic
  h. cortex
heterotypical chromosome
heterovaccine therapy
heteroxenous
  h. parasite
heterozygosity, heterozygosis
heterozygote
  compound h.
  manifesting h.
heterozygous
  doubly h.
Heubner's arteritis
Heuser's membrane
hexacanth
  h. embryo
hexadactyly, hexadactylism
Hexadnovirus
hexametazime
hexamethylpropyleneamine oxime
hexaploidy
Hexapoda
hexaxial reference system
hexazonium salts
hexokinase method
hexon
  h. antigen
Heyer-Pudenz valve
Heyns' abdominal decompression
  apparatus
Hey's
  H. amputation
  H. hernia
  H. internal derangement
  H. ligament
Hfr
  Hfr strain
HFR strain
hiatal
  h. hernia
hiatus, pl. hiatus
  adductor h.
  h. adductorius
  aortic h.
  h. aorticus
  Breschet's h.
  h. of canal for greater petrosal
    nerve
  h. canalis facialis
  h. canalis nervi petrosi majoris
  h. canalis nervi petrosi minoris
  h. of canal of lesser petrosal
    nerve
  esophageal h.

H

hiatus *(continued)*
    h. esophageus
    h. ethmoidalis
    h. of facial canal
    fallopian h.
    h. maxillaris
    maxillary h.
    pleuropericardial h.
    pleuroperitoneal h.
    sacral h.
    h. sacralis
    saphenous h.
    h. saphenus
    scalene h.
    Scarpa's h.
    semilunar h.
    h. semilunaris
    h. subarcuatus
    h. tendineus
    h. totalis sacralis
hibernating myocardium
hibernoma
hiccup, hiccough
    epidemic h.
hidden
    h. nail skin
    h. part
hidebound disease
hidradenitis
    h. axillaris of Verneuil
    h. suppurativa
hidradenoma
    clear cell h.
    nodular h.
    papillary h.
    h. papilliferum
hidroa
hidrocystoma
hidromeiosis
hidropoiesis
hidrosadenitis
hidroschesis
hidrosis
hidrotic
    h. ectodermal dysplasia
hierarchy
    dominance h.
    Maslow's h.
    response h.
    h. of terms
hieromania
hierophobia
hierotherapy
high
    h. altitude chamber
    h. convex
    h. dose tolerance
    h. endothelial postcapillary venules

    h. enema
    h. forceps delivery
    h. frequency current
    h. frequency deafness
    h. frequency transduction
    h. lip line
    h. lithotomy
    h. molecular weight kininogen
    h. osmolar contrast agent
    h. osmolar contrast medium
    h. output failure
    h. pressure oxygen
    h. resolution computed tomography
    h. spinal anesthesia
    h. steppage gait
high-calorie diet
higher order conditioning
highest
    h. concha
    h. intercostal artery
    h. intercostal vein
    h. nuchal line
    h. thoracic artery
    h. turbinated bone
high-fat diet
high-fiber diet
high-kV technique
Highmore's body
high-pass filter
high-performance liquid chromatography
high-pressure liquid chromatography
high-resolution banding
Higoumenakia sign
hila (*pl. of* hilum)
hila
hilar
    h. cell tumor of ovary
    h. dance
    h. lymph nodes
    h. shadow
hilitis
Hill
    H. operation
    H. phenomenon
    H. sign
Hillis-Müller maneuver
hillock
    axon h.
    facial h.
    seminal h.
Hill-Sachs lesion
Hilton's
    H. law
    H. method
    H. sac
    H. white line
hilum, pl. **hila**
    h. of dentate nucleus

h. of kidney
h. lienis
h. of lung
h. of lymph node
h. nodi lymphatici
h. nuclei dentati
h. nuclei olivaris
h. of olivary nucleus
h. ovarii
h. of ovary
h. pulmonis
h. renalis
h. of spleen
h. splenicum

hilus
h. cells

himantosis
hindbrain
h. vesicle

hindgut
hind kidney
hindquarter amputation
hindwater
Hines-Brown test
hinge
h. axis
h. joint
h. movement
h. position

hinge-bow
hinged flap
Hinman syndrome
Hinton test
hip
h. bone
h. joint
h. phenomenon
snapping h.

hip-flexion phenomenon
Hippobosca
hippocampal
h. commissure
h. convolution
h. fissure
h. gyrus
h. sclerosis
h. sulcus

hippocampus
h. major
major h.
h. minor
minor h.

hippocratic
h. face
h. facies
h. fingers
h. nails

h. succussion
h. succussion sound

hippuria
hippus
respiratory h.

hirci
hircismus
hircus, gen. and pl. **hirci**
Hirschberg's method
Hirschfeld's canals
Hirschowitz syndrome
Hirsch-Peiffer stain
Hirschsprung's disease
hirsute
hirsuties
hirsutism
Apert's h.
constitutional h.
idiopathic h.

hirtellous
hirudin
Hirudinea
hirudinization
Hirudo
His'
H. band
H. bundle
H. copula
H. line
H. perivascular space
H. rule
H. spindle

His bundle electrogram
Hiss' stain
Histalog test
histamine
h. flush
h. test

histamine-fast
histaminemia
histaminic
h. cephalalgia
h. headache

histaminuria
histangic
His-Tawara system
histidinemia
histidinuria
histioblast
histiocyte
cardiac h.
sea-blue h.

histiocytic
h. lymphoma
h. medullary reticulosis

histiocytoma
fibrous h.

H

histiocytoma *(continued)*
    generalized eruptive h.
    malignant fibrous h.
histiocytosis
    lipid h.
    malignant h.
    nodular non-X h.
    nonlipid h.
    regressing atypical h.
    sinus h. with massive
      lymphadenopathy
    h. X
    h. Y
histiogenic
histioid
histioma
histionic
histoangic
histoblast
histocompatibility
    h. antigen
    h. complex
    h. gene
    h. testing
histocyte
histocytosis
histodifferentiation
histofluorescence
histogenesis
histogenetic
histogenous
histogeny
histogram
histoid
    h. leprosy
    h. neoplasm
    h. tumor
histoincompatibility
histologic, histological
    h. accommodation
histologist
histology
    pathologic h.
histolysis
histoma
histometaplastic
histomorphometry
histonectomy
histoneurology
histonomy
histonuria
histopathogenesis
histopathology
histophysiology
Histoplasma capsulatum
histoplasmin-latex test
histoplasmoma

histoplasmosis
    African h.
    presumed ocular h.
historadiography
historrhexis
histotome
histotomy
histotope
histotoxic
    h. anoxia
histotroph
histotrophic
histozoic
histrionic
    h. personality
    h. personality disorder
    h. spasm
hitchhiker
    h. thumbs
Hitzig's girdle
HIV-1
HIV-2
HIV encephalopathy
hives
    giant h.
HLA
    HLA complex
    HLA typing
HL-A antigens
Hoagland's sign
Ho antigen
hoarse
hoarseness
hobnail
    h. cells
    h. liver
    h. tongue
Hoboken's
    H. gemmules
    H. nodules
    H. valves
Hoche's
    H. bundle
    H. tract
Hodgen splint
Hodge's pessary
Hodgkin-Key murmur
Hodgkin's lymphoma
Hodgson's disease
hodoneuromere
hodophobia
hoe
    h. excavator
    h. scaler
HOECHST 33258
hof
Hofbauer cell
Hoffa's operation

Hoffmann's
   H. duct
   H. muscular atrophy
   H. phenomenon
   H. reflex
   H. sign
   H. violet
Hofmann's bacillus
Hofmeister gastrectomy
Hofmeister-Pólya anastomosis
Hofmeister's operation
Hogben number
hog cholera virus
holandric
   h. gene
   h. inheritance
holarthritic
holarthritis
Holden's line
hole in retina
holiday
   h. heart syndrome
   h. syndrome
holism
holistic
   h. medicine
   h. psychology
Hollander test
Hollenhorst plaques
hollow
   h. back
   h. bone
   Sebileau's h.
Holl's ligament
Holmes-Adie
   H.-A. pupil
   H.-A. syndrome
Holmes heart
Holmes-Rahe questionnaire
Holmes' stain
Holmgrén-Golgi canals
Holmgren's wool test
holoacardius
   h. acephalus
   h. amorphus
holoacrania
holoanencephaly
holoblastic
   h. cleavage
holocephalic
holocord
holocrine
   h. gland
holodiastolic
holoendemic
   h. disease
hologastroschisis
hologram

holography
hologynic
   h. inheritance
holomastigote
holometabolous
   h. metamorphosis
holomiantic (infection)
holomorphosis
holophytic
holoprosencephaly
holorachischisis
holosystolic
   h. murmur
holotelencephaly
holotrichous
holozoic
Holter monitor
Holthouse's hernia
Holt-Oram syndrome
Holzknecht unit
homalocephalous
homaluria
Homans' sign
homaxial
home health nurse
homeometric
   h. autoregulation
homeomorphous
homeopath
homeopathist
homeopathy
homeoplasia
homeoplastic
homeorrhesis
homeosis
homeostasis
   genetic h.
   Lerner h.
   ontogenic h.
   waddingtonian h.
homeostatic lag
homeotherapeutic
homeotherapy, homeotherapeutics
homeotic
   h. genes
homeotypical
home, returning to
homergy
Homer-Wright rosettes
Home's lobe
homicidal
homicide
hominal physiology
homing value
Homo
   H. sapiens
homoblastic
homocentric

homochronous
homocladic
homocystinemia
homocystinuria
homocytotropic
    h. antibody
homodont
homodromous
homoerotism, homoeroticism
homogametic
    h. embryo
homogamy
homogeneous
    h. immersion
    h. radiation
homogenesis
homogenous
    h. keratoplasty
homogeny
homograft
    h. reaction
homoioplasia
homokaryon
homokaryotic
homokeratoplasty
homolateral
homologous
    h. antigen
    h. antiserum
    h. chromosomes
    h. desensitization
    h. graft
    h. insemination
    h. serotype
    h. serum jaundice
    h. stimulus
    h. tumor
homolysin
homolysis
homomorphic
homonomous
homonomy
homonuclear
homonymous
    h. diplopia
    h. hemianopia
    h. images
    h. parallax
homophenes
homophil
homoplastic
    h. graft
homoplasty
homorganic
homoscedasticity
homosexual
    h. panic

homosexuality
    ego-dystonic h.
    female h.
    latent h.
    male h.
    overt h.
    unconscious h.
homothallic
homotonic
homotopic
homotransplantation
homotype
homotypic, homotypical
    h. cortex
homovanillic acid test
homozygosity, homozygosis
homozygote
homozygous
    h. achondroplasia
homozygous by descent
honeycomb
    h. lung
    h. macula
    h. pattern
    h. ringworm
    h. tetter
honey urine
Hong Kong
    H. K. foot
    H. K. influenza
    H. K. toe
honk
    systolic h.
hood
    dorsal h.
hooded prepuce
hook
    calvarial h.
    h. of hamate bone
    palate h.
    sliding h.
    h. of spiral lamina
    squint h.
    tracheotomy h.
hookean behavior
hooked
    h. bone
    h. bundle of Russell
    h. fasciculus
Hooker-Forbes test
Hooke's law
hooklets
hook-shaped cataract
hookworm
    h. anemia
    h. disease
Hoover's signs
Hoplopsyllus anomalus

Hopmann's
    H. papilloma
    H. polyp
hoquet diabolique
hordeolum
    h. externum
    h. internum
    h. meibomianum
horizontal
    h. atrophy
    h. beam film
    h. cell of Cajal
    h. cells of retina
    h. fissure of cerebellum
    h. fissure of right lung
    h. fracture
    h. growth phase
    h. heart
    h. osteotomy
    h. overlap
    h. part of duodenum
    h. part of facial canal
    h. plane
    h. plate of palatine bone
    h. resorption
    h. transmission
    h. vertigo
horizontalis
hormion
hormonal gingivitis
hormone
    adrenal androgen-stimulating h.
    adrenomedullary h.'s
    ectopic h.
    growth hormone inhibiting h.
    inappropriate h.
    lactation h.
    local h.
    h. replacement therapy
hormonogenesis
hormonogenic
hormonopoiesis
hormonopoietic
hormonoprivia
hormonotherapy
horn
    Ammon's h.
    anterior h.
    cicatricial h.
    coccygeal h.
    cutaneous h.
    frontal h.
    greater h. of hyoid bone
    h.'s of hyoid bone
    iliac h.
    inferior h.
    inferior h. of falciform margin of
      saphenous opening

    inferior h. of lateral ventricle
    inferior h. of thyroid cartilage
    lateral h.
    lesser h. of hyoid bone
    nail h.
    occipital h.
    posterior h.
    pulp h.
    sacral h.'s
    h.'s of saphenous opening
    sebaceous h.
    superior h. of falciform margin of
      saphenous opening
    superior h. of thyroid cartilage
    temporal h.
    h.'s of thyroid cartilage
    uterine h., h. of uterus
    ventral h.
    warty h.
Horner's
    H. muscle
    H. pupil
    H. syndrome
    H. teeth
Horner-Trantas dots
hornification
horny
    h. cell
    h. layer of epidermis
    h. layer of nail
horopter
horripilation
horror
    h. autotoxicus
    h. fusionis
horsepox virus
horseshoe
    h. fistula
    h. kidney
    h. placenta
Hortega
    H. cells
    H. neuroglia stain
Horton's
    H. arteritis
    H. cephalalgia
    H. headache
hospice
hospital
    base h.
    camp h.
    closed h.
    day h.
    h. fever
    h. gangrene
    general h.
    government h.
    group h.

H

hospital *(continued)*
    maternity h.
    mental h.
    municipal h.
    night h.
    h. nurse
    open h.
    philanthropic h.
    private h.
    proprietary h.
    public h.
    h. record
    special h.
    state h.
    teaching h.
    Veterans Administration h.
    voluntary h.
    weekend h.
hospitalism
hospitalization
host
    accidental h.
    amplifier h.
    dead-end h.
    definitive h.
    final h.
    intermediate h., intermediary h.
    paratenic h.
    reservoir h.
    secondary h.
    transport h.
hot
    h. abscess
    h. flash
    h. flush
    h. gangrene
    h. nodule
    h. pack
    h. salt sterilizer
    h. snare
    h. spot
hotfoot
hottentotism
hound-dog facies
Hounsfield
    H. number
    H. unit
hourglass
    h. contraction
    h. head
    h. murmur
    h. pattern
    h. stomach
    h. vertebrae
house
    h. officer
    h. staff
    h. surgeon

housefly
housekeeping genes
housemaid's knee
Houssay
    H. animal
    H. syndrome
Houston's
    H. folds
    H. muscle
    H. valves
Howard test
Howell-Jolly bodies
Howship's lacunae
Hoyer's
    H. anastomoses
    H. canals
H-R conduction time
H-shape vertebrae
H-tetanase
H-type
    H.-t. fistula
    H.-t. tracheoesophageal fistula
Hu antigens
Hubbard tank
Hubrecht's protochordal knot
Hucker-Conn stain
Hudson-Stähli line
hue
Hueck's ligament
Hueter's
    H. maneuver
    H. sign
Hüfner's equation
Huggins' operation
Hughes-Stovin syndrome
Huguier's
    H. canal
    H. circle
    H. sinus
Huhner test
Hull's triad
hum
    venous h.
human
    h. botfly
    h. companionship
    h. diploid cell vaccine
    h. ecology
    h. ehrlichiosis
    h. genetics
    H. Genome Initiative
    H. Genome Project
    h. granulocytic ehrlichiosis
    h. herpesvirus 1
    h. herpesvirus 2
    h. herpesvirus 3
    h. herpesvirus 4
    h. herpesvirus 5

h. herpesvirus 6
h. herpesvirus 7
h. immunodeficiency virus
h. leukemia-associated antigens
h. lymphocyte antigens
h. measles immune serum
h. papilloma virus
h. pertussis immune serum
h. scarlet fever immune serum
h. serum jaundice
h. T-cell lymphoma/leukemia virus
h. T-cell lymphotropic virus
h. T lymphotrophic virus
humanistic psychology
Humby knife
humeral
h. artery
h. articulation
h. head
humeri (*gen. and pl. of* humerus)
humeroradial
h. articulation
h. joint
humeroscapular
humeroulnar
h. head of flexor digitorum
superficialis muscle
h. joint
humerus, gen. and pl. **humeri**
humidity
absolute h.
relative h.
humid tetter
Hummelsheim's operation
humor, gen. **humoris**
aqueous h.
h. aquosus
Morgagni's h.
ocular h.
peccant humors
vitreous h.
h. vitreus
humoral
h. doctrine
h. immunity
h. pathology
hump
buffalo h. *dromedARY*
dowager's h.
Hampton's h.
humpback
Humphry's ligament
hunchback
hunger
affect h.
h. contractions
narcotic h.

h. pain
h. swelling
Hung's method
Hunner's
H. stricture
H. ulcer
Hunter
H. canal
H. and Driffield curve
H. glossitis
H. gubernaculum
H. ligament
H. line
H. membrane
H. operation
H. syndrome
Hunter-Schreger
H.-S. bands
H.-S. lines
hunting
h. phenomenon
h. reaction
Huntington's
H. chorea
H. disease
Hunt's
H. atrophy
H. neuralgia
H. paradoxical phenomenon
H. syndrome
Hurler's
H. disease
H. syndrome
Hurst bougies
Hürthle
H. cell
H. cell adenoma
H. cell carcinoma
H. cell tumor
Huschke's
H. auditory teeth
H. cartilages
H. foramen
H. valve
Hutchinson-Gilford
H.-G. disease
H.-G. syndrome
Hutchinson's
H. crescentic notch
H. facies
H. freckle
H. mask
H. patch
H. pupil
H. teeth
H. triad
Hutchison syndrome

H

Huxley's
    H. layer
    H. membrane
    H. sheath
Huygens'
    H. ocular
    H. principle
H-V
    H-V conduction time
    H-V interval
HVA test
hyalin
    alcoholic h.
hyalinasis cutis et mucosae
hyaline
    h. bodies
    h. bodies of pituitary
    h. cartilage
    h. cast
    h. degeneration
    h. leukocyte
    h. membrane
    h. membrane disease of the
    newborn
    h. membrane syndrome
    h. thrombus
    h. tubercle
hyalinization
hyalinosis
    systemic h.
hyalinuria
hyalitis
    suppurative h.
hyalocapsular ligament
hyalocyte
hyalohyphomycosis
hyaloid
    h. artery
    h. body
    h. canal
    h. fossa
    h. membrane
hyaloideoretinal degeneration
hyalomere
Hyalomma
    H. marginatum
    H. variegatum
hyalophagia, hyalophagy
hyalophobia
hyaloplasm, hyaloplasma
    nuclear h.
hyaloserositis
hyalosis
    asteroid h.
    punctate h.
hyalosome
H-Y antigen
hybaroxia

hybrid
    h. prosthesis
    SV40-adenovirus h.
hybridism
hybridization
    cell h.
    cross h.
    overlap h.
    in situ h.
    in situ nucleic acid h.
    somatic cell h.
hybridoma
hydatid
    h. cyst
    h. fremitus
    h. mole
    Morgagni's h.
    nonpedunculated h.
    pedunculated h.
    h. polyp
    h. pregnancy
    h. rash
    h. resonance
    h. sand
    sessile h.
    stalked h.
    h. thrill
hydatidiform
    h. mole
hydatidocele
hydatidoma
hydatidosis
hydatidostomy
Hydatigera taeniaeformis
hydatoid
Hyde's disease
hydradenitis
hydradenoma
hydralazine syndrome
hydramnion, hydramnios
hydranencephaly
hydrarthrodial
hydrarthron
hydrarthrosis
    intermittent h.
hydrarthrus
hydraulic conductivity
hydrazine yellow
hydremia
hydremic edema
hydrencephalocele
hydrencephalomeningocele
hydrencephalus
hydriatric, hydriatic
hydroa
    h. aestivale
    h. febrile
    h. gestationis

h. herpetiforme
h. puerorum
h. vacciniforme
h. vesiculosum
hydroadipsia
hydroappendix
hydrocalycosis
hydrocele
cervical h.
h. colli
communicating h.
congenital h.
cord h.
Dupuytren's h.
h. feminae
filarial h.
funicular h.
h. muliebris
noncommunicating h.
Nuck's h.
h. spinalis
hydrocelectomy
hydrocephalic
hydrocephalocele
hydrocephaloid
hydrocephalus
communicating h.
congenital h.
double compartment h.
external h.
h. ex vacuo
noncommunicating h.
normal pressure h.
obstructive h.
occult h.
otitic h.
postmeningitic h.
posttraumatic h.
primary h.
secondary h.
thrombotic h.
toxic h.
hydrocephaly
hydrocholecystis
hydrocholeresis
hydrocholeretic
hydrocolpocele, hydrocolpos
hydrocyst
hydrocystoma
hydrodipsomania
hydrodiuresis
hydrodynamics
hydroelectric bath
hydroencephalocele
hydrogen pump
hydrokinetic
hydrokinetics
hydrolability

hydroma
hydromassage
hydromeningocele
hydrometra
hydrometrocolpos
hydromicrocephaly
hydromphalus
hydromyelia
hydromyelocele
hydromyoma
hydronephrosis
hydronephrotic
hydroparasalpinx
hydropathic
hydropathy
hydropenia
hydropenic
hydropericarditis
hydropericardium
hydroperitoneum, hydroperitonia
hydrophilia
hydrophobia
hydrophobic tetanus
hydrophorograph
hydrophthalmia, hydrophthalmos, hydrophthalmus
hydropic
h. degeneration
hydropneumatosis
hydropneumogony
hydropneumopericardium
hydropneumoperitoneum
hydropneumothorax
hydrops
h. articuli
endolymphatic h.
fetal h., h. fetalis
h. folliculi
h. of gallbladder
immune fetal h.
nonimmune fetal h.
h. ovarii
h. pericardii
h. tubae
h. tubae profluens
hydropyonephrosis
hydrorchis
hydrorrhea
h. gravidae, h. gravidarum
hydrosalpinx
intermittent h.
hydrosarca
hydrosarcocele
hydrosphygmograph
hydrostat
hydrostatic
h. dilator
hydrosudopathy

H

411

hydrosudotherapy
hydrosyringomyelia
hydrotaxis
hydrotherapeutic
hydrotherapeutics
hydrotherapy
hydrothermal
hydrothionemia
hydrothionuria
hydrothorax
  chylous h.
hydrotomy
hydrotropism, negative hydrotropism,
  positive hydrotropism
hydrotubation
hydroureter
hydrovarium
17-hydroxycorticosteroid test
hydroxykynureninuria
17-hydroxylase deficiency syndrome
hydroxyphenyluria
hydroxyprolinemia
hygieiolatry
hygieiology
hygieist
hygiene
  criminal h.
  industrial h.
  mental h.
  oral h.
hygienic
  h. laboratory coefficient
hygienist
  dental h.
hygroma
  h. axillare
  cervical h.
  h. colli cysticum
  cystic h.
  subdural h.
hygrophobia
hygroscopic expansion
hygrostomia
hyla
hylephobia
hylic
  h. tumor
hyloma
  mesenchymal h.
  mesothelial h.
hymen
  h. bifenestratus, h. biforis
  cribriform h.
  denticulate h.
  imperforate h.
  infundibuliform h.
  h. sculptatus
  septate h.

  h. subseptus
  vertical h.
hymenal
  h. caruncula
hymenectomy
hymenitis
hymenoid
hymenolepidid
Hymenolepididae
Hymenolepis
  H. diminuta
  H. lanceolata
  H. nana
  H. nana, var. *fraterna*
hymenology
Hymenoptera
hymenorrhaphy
hymenotomy
Hynes pharyngoplasty
hyobranchial cleft
hyoepiglottic
  h. ligament
hyoepiglottidean
hyoglossal
  h. membrane
  h. muscle
hyoglossus
  h. muscle
hyoid arch
hyomandibular cleft
hyopharyngeus
hyothyroid
hypacusia
hypacusis
hypalbuminemia
hypalgesia
hypalgesic, hypalgetic
hypalgia
hypamnion, hypamnios
hypanakinesia, hypanakinesis
Hypaque
  H. enema
hypaque swallow
hyparterial
  h. bronchi
hypaxial
hypazoturia
hypencephalon
hypengyophobia
hyperabduction syndrome
hyperacanthosis
hyperacidity
hyperactive child syndrome
hyperactivity
hyperacusis, hyperacusia
hyperacute
  h. purulent conjunctivitis
  h. rejection

hyperadenosis
hyperadiposis, hyperadiposity
hyperadrenalcorticalism
hyperadrenocorticalism
hyperaldosteronism
hyperalgesia
hyperalgesic, hyperalgetic
hyperalgia
hyperalimentation
    parenteral h.
hyperallantoinuria
hyperaminoaciduria
hyperammonemia
hyperamylasemia
hyperanacinesia, hyperanacinesis
hyperanakinesia, hyperanakinesis
hyperaphia
hyperaphic
hyperbaric
    h. anesthesia
    h. chamber
    h. medicine
    h. oxygen
    h. oxygenation
    h. oxygen therapy
    h. spinal anesthesia
hyperbarism
hyperbetalipoproteinemia
    familial h.
    familial h. and
        hyperprebetalipoproteinemia
hyperbilirubinemia
    neonatal h.
hyperbrachycephaly
hypercalcemia
hypercalcemic
    h. sarcoidosis
    h. uremia
hypercalcinuria
hypercalcuria
hypercapnia
hypercarbia
hypercardia
hypercatabolic
hypercatharsis
hypercathexis
hypercementosis
hyperchloremia
hyperchloremic acidosis
hyperchlorhydria
hyperchloruria
hypercholesteremia
hypercholesterinemia
hypercholesterolemia
    familial h.
    familial h. with hyperlipemia
hypercholesterolia
hypercholia

hyperchromaffinism
hyperchromasia
hyperchromatic
    h. anemia
    h. macrocythemia
hyperchromatism
hyperchromia
    macrocytic h.
hyperchromic anemia
hyperchylia
hyperchylomicronemia
    familial h.
    familial h. with
        hyperprebetalipoproteinemia
hypercinesis, hypercinesia
hypercoagulability
hypercoagulable
hypercorticoidism
hypercortisolism
hypercryalgesia
hypercryesthesia
hypercupremia
hypercyanotic
    h. angina
hypercyesis, hypercyesia
hypercythemia
hypercytochromia
hypercytosis
hyperdicrotic
hyperdicrotism
hyperdiploid
hyperdipsia
hyperdistention
hyperdynamia
    h. uteri
hyperdynamic
hyperechoic
hyperemesis
    h. gravidarum
    h. lactentium
hyperemetic
hyperemia
    active h.
    arterial h.
    Bier's h.
    collateral h.
    constriction h.
    fluxionary h.
    passive h.
    peristatic h.
    reactive h.
    venous h.
hyperemic
hyperencephaly
hyperendemic disease
hypereosinophilia
hypereosinophilic syndrome
hyperephidrosis

H

413

hyperepithymia
hyperergasia
hyperergia
hyperergic
    h. encephalitis
hypererythrocythemia
hyperesophoria
hyperesthesia
    auditory h.
    cervical h.
    gustatory h.
    muscular h.
    olfactory h., h. olfactoria
    h. optica
    tactile h.
hyperesthetic
hypereuryprosopic
hyperexophoria
hyperextension
hyperextension-hyperflexion injury
hyperferremia
hyperfibrinogenemia
hyperfibrinolysis
hyperflexion
hyperfolliculoidism
hyperfunctional occlusion
hypergalactosis
hypergammaglobulinemia
hyperganglionosis
hypergasia
hypergenesis
hypergenetic
hypergenic teratosis
hypergenitalism
hypergeusia
hypergia
hypergic
hyperglandular
hyperglobulia, hyperglobulism
hyperglobulinemia
hyperglobulinemic purpura
hyperglobulism (var. of hyperglobulia)
hyperglycemia
    ketotic h.
    nonketotic h.
    posthypoglycemic h.
hyperglyceridemia
    endogenous h.
    exogenous h.
hyperglycinemia
    ketotic h.
    nonketotic h.
hyperglycinuria
hyperglycogenolysis
hyperglycorrhachia
hyperglycosemia
hyperglycosuria
hyperglyoxylemia

hypergnosis
hypergonadism
hypergonadotropic
    h. eunuchoidism
    h. hypogonadism
hypergranulosis
hyperguanidinemia
hypergynecosmia
hyperhedonia, hyperhedonism
hyperhemoglobinemia
hyperheparinemia
hyperhidrosis
    gustatory h.
    h. oleosa
hyperhydration
hyperhydrochloria
hyperhydrochloridia
hyperhydropexy, hyperhydropexis
hyperidrosis
hyperimmune
    h. serum
hyperimmunity
hyperimmunization
hyperimmunoglobulin E syndrome
hyperindicanemia
hyperinfection
hyperinosemia
hyperinosis
hyperinsulinemia
hyperinsulinism
    alimentary h.
hyperinvolution
hyperkalemia
hyperkalemic periodic paralysis
hyperkaliemia
hyperkaluresis
hyperkeratinization
hyperkeratomycosis
hyperkeratosis
    h. congenita
    h. eccentrica
    epidermolytic h.
    h. figurata centrifuga atrophica
    h. follicularis et parafollicularis
    generalized epidermolytic h.
    h. lenticularis perstans
    h. penetrans
    h. subungualis
hyperketonemia
hyperketonuria
hyperkinemia
hyperkinesis, hyperkinesia
hyperkinetic
    h. dysarthria
    h. heart syndrome
    h. syndrome
hyperlactation
hyperleukocytosis

hyperlexia
hyperlipemia
    carbohydrate-induced h.
    combined fat- and carbohydrate-
      induced h.
    familial fat-induced h.
    idiopathic h.
    mixed h.
hyperlipidemia
    mixed h.
    mixed hyperlipoproteinemia familial,
      type 5 h.
hyperlipoidemia
hyperlipoproteinemia
    acquired h.
    familial h.
    type II familial h.
    type III familial h.
    type IV familial h.
    type V familial h.
hyperliposis
hyperlithuria
hyperlogia
hyperlordosis
hyperlucent
    h. lung
hyperlysinemia
hyperlysinuria
hypermagnesemia
hypermastia
hypermature cataract
hypermenorrhea
hypermetabolism
    extrathyroidal h.
hypermetamorphosis
hypermetria
hypermetrope
hypermetropia
    index h.
hypermnesia
hypermobility
hypermorph
hypermyotonia
hypermyotrophy
hypernatremia
hypernatremic encephalopathy
hyperneocytosis
hypernephroid
hypernephroma
hypernephronia
hypernoia
hypernomic
hypernutrition
hyperoncotic
hyperonychia
hyperope
hyperopia
    absolute h.

    axial h.
    curvature h.
    facultative h.
    latent h.
    manifest h.
    total h.
hyperopic
    h. astigmatism
hyperorality
hyperorchidism
hyperorexia
hyperorthocytosis
hyperosmia
hyperosmolar (hyperglycemic) nonketotic
  coma
hyperosphresia, hyperosphresis
hyperosteoidosis
hyperostosis
    ankylosing h.
    h. corticalis deformans
    diffuse idiopathic skeletal h.
    flowing h.
    h. frontalis interna
    generalized cortical h.
    infantile cortical h.
    streak h.
hyperostotic spondylosis
hyperovarianism
hyperoxaluria
    primary h. and oxalosis
hyperoxia
hyperpancreatism
hyperparasite
hyperparasitism
hyperparathyroidism
    primary h.
    secondary h.
hyperparotidism
hyperpathia
hyperpepsia
hyperpepsinia
hyperperistalsis
hyperphagia
hyperphalangism
hyperphenylalaninemia
hyperphonesis
hyperphonia
hyperphoria
hyperphosphatasemia
hyperphosphatasia
hyperphosphatemia
hyperphosphaturia
hyperphrenia
hyperpiesis, hyperpiesia
hyperpietic
hyperpigmentation
hyperpipecolatemia
hyperpituitarism

H

hyperplasia
    angiofollicular mediastinal lymph
      node h.
    angiolymphoid h. with eosinophilia
    atypical melanocytic h.
    basal cell h.
    benign giant lymph node h.
    cementum h.
    congenital adrenal h.
    congenital sebaceous h.
    congenital virilizing adrenal h.
    cystic h.
    cystic h. of the breast
    denture h.
    ductal h.
    fibromuscular h.
    focal epithelial h.
    gingival h.
    inflammatory fibrous h.
    inflammatory papillary h.
    intravascular papillary endothelial h.
    neuronal h.
    nodular h. of prostate
    nodular regenerative h.
    pseudoepitheliomatous h.,
      pseudocarcinomatous h.
    senile sebaceous h.
    squamous cell h.
    verrucous h.
hyperplastic
    h. arteriosclerosis
    h. gingivitis
    h. graft
    h. inflammation
    h. polyp
    h. pulpitis
hyperpnea
hyperpolarization
hyperponesis
hyperpotassemia
hyperpragia
hyperpraxia
hyperprebetalipoproteinemia
    familial h.
hyperprochoresis
hyperproinsulinemia
hyperprolactinemia
hyperprolactinemic amenorrhea
hyperprolinemia
hyperprosexia
hyperproteinemia
hyperproteosis
hyperpyretic
hyperpyrexia
    fulminant h.
    heat h.
    malignant h.
hyperpyrexial

hyperquantivalent idea
hyperreactive malarious splenomegaly
hyperreflexia
    detrusor h.
hyperreflexic bladder
hyperresonance
hypersalemia
hypersalivation
hypersarcosinemia
hypersecretion
    gastric h.
hypersecretion glaucoma
hypersegmented neutrophil
hypersensitive
    h. dentin
    h. xiphoid syndrome
hypersensitiveness
hypersensitivity
    h. angiitis
    contact h.
    delayed h.
    immediate h.
    h. pneumonitis
    h. reaction
    tuberculin-type h.
    h. vasculitis
hypersensitization
hyperserotonemia
hyperskeocytosis
hypersomatotropism
hypersomnia
hypersonic
hypersphyxia
hypersplenism
hypersteatosis
hypersthenia
hypersthenic
hypersthenuria
hypersusceptibility
hypersystole
hypersystolic
hypertelorism
    Bixler type h.
    canthal h.
    ocular h.
hypertension
    accelerated h.
    adrenal h.
    benign h.
    borderline h.
    essential h.
    Goldblatt h.
    idiopathic h.
    labile h.
    malignant h.
    pale h.
    portal h.
    postpartum h.

primary h.
pulmonary h.
renal h.
renovascular h.
secondary h.
systemic venous h.
hypertensive
    h. arteriopathy
    h. arteriosclerosis
    h. encephalopathy
    h. retinopathy
hypertensor
hypertestoidism
hyperthecosis
    stromal h.
    testoid h.
hyperthelia
hyperthermalgesia
hyperthermia
hyperthermoesthesia
hyperthrombinemia
hyperthymia
hyperthymic
hyperthymism
hyperthymization
hyperthyrea
hyperthyroid heart
hyperthyroidism
    iodine-induced h.
    masked h.
    ophthalmic h.
    primary h.
    secondary h.
hyperthyroxinemia
hypertonia
    h. polycythemica
    sympathetic h.
hypertonic bladder
hypertonicity
hypertrichiasis
hypertrichophrydia
hypertrichosis
    h. lanuginosa
    nevoid h.
    h. partialis
    h. universalis
hypertriglyceridemia
    familial h.
hypertroph
hypertrophia
hypertrophic
    h. arthritis
    h. cardiomyopathy
    h. cervical pachymeningitis
    h. dystrophy
    h. gastritis
    h. hypersecretory gastropathy
    h. interstitial neuropathy

h. pulpitis
h. pyloric stenosis
h. rhinitis
h. rosacea
h. scar
hypertrophy
    adaptive h.
    benign prostatic h.
    compensatory h.
    compensatory h. of the heart
    complementary h.
    concentric h.
    eccentric h.
    endemic h.
    false h.
    functional h.
    giant h. of gastric mucosa
    hemangiectatic h.
    lipomatous h.
    numerical h.
    physiologic h.
    quantitative h.
    simple h.
    simulated h.
    true h.
    vicarious h.
hypertropia
hypertyrosinemia
hyperuresis
hyperuricemia
hyperuricemic
hyperuricuria
hypervaccination
hypervalinemia
hypervariable regions
hypervascular
hyperventilation
    h. syndrome
    h. test
    h. tetany
hyperviscosity syndrome
hypervolemia
hypervolemic
hypervolia
hypesthesia
    olfactory h.
hypha, pl. **hyphae**
    racquet h.
    spiral hyphae
hyphedonia
hyphema
hyphemia
    intertropical h., tropical h.
Hyphomyces destruens
Hyphomycetes
hypnagogic
    h. hallucination
    h. image

H

hypnalgia
hypnapagogic
hypnesthesia
hypnic
hypnoanalysis
hypnoanalytic
hypnocatharsis
hypnocinematograph
hypnocyst
hypnodontics
hypnogenesis
hypnogenic, hypnogenous
    h. spot
hypnoidal
hypnoid state
hypnologist
hypnology
hypnophobia
hypnopompic
    h. hallucination
    h. image
hypnosis
    lethargic h.
    major h.
    minor h.
hypnotherapy
hypnotic
    h. psychotherapy
    h. relationship
    h. sleep
    h. state
    h. suggestion
hypnotism
hypnotist
hypnotize
hypnotoid
hypnozoite
hypoacidity
hypoacusis
hypoadenia
hypoadrenalism
hypoalbuminemia
hypoaldosteronism
    hyporeninemic h.
    selective h., isolated h.
hypoaldosteronuria
hypoalgesia
hypoalimentation
hypoazoturia
hypobaria
hypobaric
    h. spinal anesthesia
hypobarism
hypobaropathy
hypobetalipoproteinemia
hypoblast
hypoblastic

hypobranchial
    h. eminence
hypocalcemia
hypocalcemic cataract
hypocalcification
    enamel h.
hypocapnia
hypocarbia
hypocelom
hypochloremia
hypochloremic
hypochlorhydria
hypochloruria
hypocholesteremia
hypocholesterinemia
hypocholesterolemia
hypocholia
hypochondria (*pl. of* hypochondrium)
hypochondriac
    h. region
hypochondriacal
    h. melancholia
    h. neurosis
hypochondrial reflex
hypochondriasis
hypochondrium, pl. hypochondria
hypochondroplasia
hypochordal
hypochromasia
hypochromatic
hypochromatism
hypochromia
hypochromic
    h. anemia
    h. microcytic anemia
hypochrosis
hypochylia
hypocinesis, hypocinesia
hypocitraturia
hypocomplementemia
hypocomplementemic
    h. glomerulonephritis
    h. vasculitis
hypocone
hypoconid
hypoconule
hypoconulid
hypocorticoidism
hypocupremia
hypocycloidal
    h. tomography
hypocystotomy
hypocythemia
hypocytosis
hypodactyly, hypodactylia, hypodactylism
hypoderm
Hypoderma
hypodermatic

hypodermatoclysis
hypodermatomy
hypodermic
    h. injection
    h. needle
    h. syringe
hypodermis
hypodermoclysis
hypodermolithiasis
hypodiploid
hypodipsia
hypodontia
hypodynamia
    h. cordis
hypodynamic
hypoeccrisis
hypoeccritic
hypoechoic
hypoeosinophilia
hypoesophoria
hypoesthesia
hypoexophoria
hypoferremia
hypoferric anemia
hypofibrinogenemia
hypofunction
hypogalactia
hypogalactous
hypogammaglobinemia
hypogammaglobulinemia
    acquired h.
    primary h.
    secondary h.
    transient h. of infancy
    X-linked h., X-linked infantile h.
hypoganglionosis
hypogastric
    h. artery
    h. ganglia
    h. nerve
    h. reflex
    h. vein
hypogastrium
hypogastrocele
hypogastropagus
hypogastroschisis
hypogenesis
    polar h.
hypogenetic
hypogenitalism
hypogeusia
hypoglobulia
hypoglossal
    h. canal
    h. eminence
    h. nerve
    h. nucleus
    h. trigone

hypoglossis
hypoglossus
hypoglottis
hypoglycemia
    fasting h.
    leucine h.
    leucine-induced h.
    mixed h.
    neonatal h.
hypoglycemic
    h. coma
hypoglycogenolysis
hypoglycorrhachia
hypognathous
hypognathus
hypogonadism
    familial hypogonadotropic h.
    hypergonadotropic h.
    hypogonadotropic h.
    male h.
    primary h.
    secondary h.
    h. with anosmia
hypogonadotropic
    h. eunuchoidism
    h. hypogonadism
hypogranulocytosis
hypohepatia
hypohidrosis
hypohidrotic
    h. ectodermal dysplasia
hypohydremia
hypohydrochloria
hypohyloma
hypohypnotic
hypokalemia
hypokalemic
    h. nephropathy
    h. periodic paralysis
hypokinemia
hypokinesis, hypokinesia
hypokinetic
    h. dysarthria
hypolepidoma
hypoleukemia
hypoleydigism
hypoliposis
hypologia
hypolymphemia
hypomagnesemia
hypomania
hypomastia
hypomazia
hypomelancholia
hypomelanosis
    h. of Ito
hypomelia
hypomenorrhea

H

hypomere
hypometabolic
    h. state
    h. syndrome
hypometabolism
    euthyroid h.
hypometria
hypomnesia
hypomorph
hypomotility
hypomyelination, hypomyelinogenesis
hypomyotonia
hypomyxia
hyponatremia
    depletional h.
hyponeocytosis
hyponoia
hyponychial
hyponychium
hyponychon
hypooncotic
hypoorthocytosis
hypoovarianism
hypopancreatism
hypopancreorrhea
hypoparathyroidism
    familial h.
    h. syndrome
hypoparathyroid tetany
hypopepsia
hypoperistalsis
hypophalangism
hypopharyngeal diverticulum
hypopharynx
hypophonesis
hypophonia
hypophoria
hypophosphatasemia
hypophosphatasia
    adult h.
    childhood h.
    congenital h.
hypophosphatemia
hypophosphaturia
hypophrasia
hypophyseal
    h. cachexia
    h. pouch
hypophysectomize
hypophysectomy
hypophyseoportal system
hypophyseoprivic
hypophyseotropic
hypophysial
    h. amenorrhea
    h. cachexia
    h. duct
    h. dwarf

    h. fossa
    h. infantilism
    h. portal circulation
    h. portal system
    h. syndrome
hypophysioportal system
hypophysioprivic
hypophysio-sphenoidal syndrome
hypophysiotropic
hypophysis
    h. cerebri
    pharyngeal h.
hypophysitis
    lymphocytic h.
    lymphoid h.
hypopiesis
    orthostatic h.
hypopituitarism
hypoplasia
    cartilage-hair h.
    enamel h.
    focal dermal h.
    optic nerve h.
    renal h.
    h. of right ventricle
    right ventricular h.
    thymic h.
hypoplastic
    h. anemia
    h. fetal chondrodystrophy
    h. heart
    h. left heart syndrome
hypopnea
hypoposia
hypopotassemia
hypopraxia
hypoproaccelerinemia
hypoproconvertinemia
hypoproteinemia
hypoproteinosis
hypoprothrombinemia
hypoptyalism
hypopyon
    recurrent h.
    h. ulcer
hyporeflexia
hyporeninemia
hyporeninemic
    h. hypoaldosteronism
hyporiboflavinosis
hyposalemia
hyposalivation
hyposarca
hyposcheotomy
hyposcleral
hyposensitivity
hyposensitization
hyposkeocytosis

hyposmia
hyposmosis
hyposomatotropism
hyposomia
hyposomniac
hypospadiac
hypospadias
    balanic h.
    coronal h.
    glanular h.
    penile h.
    penoscrotal h.
    perineal h.
    subcoronal h.
hyposphresia
hyposphyxia
hyposplenism
hypostasis
    postmortem h.
    pulmonary h.
hypostatic
    h. abscess
    h. congestion
    h. ectasia
    h. pneumonia
hyposthenia
hyposthenic
hyposthenuria
hypostome
hypostomia
hypostosis
hyposupradrenalism
hyposystole
hypotaxia
hypotelorism
hypotension
    arterial h.
    idiopathic orthostatic h.
    induced h., controlled h.
    intracranial h.
    orthostatic h.
    postural h.
hypotensive
    h. anesthesia
hypothalamic
    h. amenorrhea
    h. infundibulum
    h. obesity
    h. obesity with hypogonadism
    h. sulcus
hypothalamocerebellar fibers
hypothalamohypophysial
    h. portal circulation
    h. portal system
    h. tract
hypothalamus

hypothenar
    h. eminence
    h. prominence
hypothermal
hypothermia
    accidental h.
    moderate h.
    profound h.
    regional h.
    total body h.
hypothermic anesthesia
hypothesis
    alternative h.
    autocrine h.
    Bayesian h.
    frustration-aggression h.
    gate-control h.
    Gompertz' h.
    insular h.
    Lyon h.
    Makeham's h.
    mnemic h.
    Neyman-Pearson statistical h.
    null h.
    sliding filament h.
    Starling's h.
hypothetical
    h. mean organism
    h. mean strain
hypothrombinemia
hypothromboplastinemia
hypothymia
hypothymic
hypothymism
hypothyroid
    h. dwarf
    h. dwarfism
    h. infantilism
hypothyroidism
    congenital h.
    infantile h.
    secondary h.
hypothyroxinemia
hypotonia
hypotonus, hypotony
hypotrichiasis
hypotrichosis
hypotropia
hypotympanotomy
hypotympanum
hypouresis
hypouricemia
hypouricuria
hypovarianism
hypoventilation
    h. coma
hypovolemia

H

hypovolemic
   h. shock
hypovolia
hypoxanthine guanine
  phosphoribosyltransferase deficiency
hypoxemia
   h. test
hypoxia
   anemic h.
   diffusion h.
   hypoxic h.
   ischemic h.
   oxygen affinity h.
   stagnant h.
   h. warning system
hypoxic
   h. hypoxia
   h. nephrosis
hypoxic-hypercarbic encephalopathy
hypsarhythmia, hypsarrhythmia
hypsibrachycephalic
hypsicephaly
hypsiconchous
hypsiloid
   h. angle
   h. cartilage
   h. ligament
hypsistaphylia
hypsistenocephalic
hypsocephaly
hypsodont
hypurgia
Hyrtl's
   H. anastomosis
   H. epitympanic recess
   H. foramen
   H. loop
   H. sphincter
hysteralgia
hysteratresia
hysterectomy
   abdominal h.
   abdominovaginal h.
   cesarean h.
   modified radical h.
   paravaginal h.
   Porro h.
   radical h.
   subtotal h.
   supracervical h.
   vaginal h.
hysteresis
   static h.
hystereurysis
hysteria
   anxiety h.
   conversion h.
   dissociative h.

epidemic h.
major h.
mass h.
minor h.
hysterical, hysteric
   h. amblyopia
   h. anesthesia
   h. aphonia
   h. ataxia
   h. blindness
   h. chorea
   h. convulsion
   h. deafness
   h. gait
   h. joint
   h. neurosis
   h. paralysis
   h. personality
   h. polydipsia
   h. pregnancy
   h. psychosis
   h. syncope
   h. torticollis
   h. tremor
   h. vertigo
hystericoneuralgic
hysterics
hysterocatalepsy
hysterocele
hysterocleisis
hysterocolposcope
hysterocystopexy
hysterodynia
hysteroepilepsy
hysterogenic, hysterogenous
hysterogram
hysterograph
hysterography
hysteroid
   h. convulsion
hysterolith
hysterolysis
hysterometer
hysteromyoma
hysteromyomectomy
hysteromyotomy
hysteronarcolepsy
hystero-oophorectomy
hysteropathy
hysteropexy
   abdominal h.
hysterophore
hysteroplasty
hysterorrhaphy
hysterorrhexis
hysterosalpingectomy
hysterosalpingography
hysterosalpingo-oophorectomy

hysterosalpingostomy
hysteroscope
hysteroscopy
    laparoscopic-assisted vaginal h.
hysterospasm
hysterosystole
hysterothermometry
hysterotomy
    abdominal h.
    vaginal h.

hysterotonin
hysterotrachelectomy
hysterotracheloplasty
hysterotrachelorrhaphy
hysterotrachelotomy
hysterotrismus
hysterotubography

H

I
    I antigens
    I band
    I cell
    I disk
    I pili
    I region
iatraliptic
iatraliptics
iatric
iatrogenic
    i. transmission
iatrology
iatromathematical school
iatrophysics
iatrotechnique
IBR virus
ICAO standard atmosphere
Iceland disease
Icelandic disease
I-cell disease
ichnogram
ichor
ichoremia
ichoroid
ichorous
    i. pus
ichorrhea
ichorrhemia
ichthyismus
    i. exanthematicus
    i. hystrix
ichthyophobia
ichthyosiform erythroderma
ichthyosis
    acquired i.
    i. congenita neonatorum
    i. corneae
    i. follicularis
    harlequin i.
    i. hystrix
    i. intrauterina
    lamellar i.
    i. linearis circumflexa
    nacreous i.
    i. palmaris et plantaris
    i. scutulata
    i. sebacea
    i. sebacea cornea
    i. simplex
    i. spinosa
    i. uteri
    i. vulgaris
ichthyotic
ichthyotoxin

icing
    i. heart
    i. liver
iconic signs
iconomania
icosahedral
ictal
icteric
    i. index
icteroanemia
icterogenic
icterohematuric
icterohemoglobinuria
icterohemolytic anemia
icterohemorrhagic fever
icterohepatitis
icteroid
icterus
    acquired hemolytic i.
    benign familial i.
    chronic familial i.
    congenital hemolytic i.
    cythemolytic i.
    i. gravis
    i. index
    infectious i.
    i. melas
    i. neonatorum
    physiologic i.
    i. praecox
ictometer
ictus
    i. cordis
    i. epilepticus
    i. paralyticus
    i. solis
ICU psychosis
id
    i. reaction
idea
    autochthonous i.'s
    compulsive i.
    dominant i.
    fixed i.
    flight of i.'s
    hyperquantivalent i.
    overvalued i.
    permanent dominant i.
    i. of reference
ideal
    i. alveolar gas
    ego i.
ideation
ideational
    i. apraxia

ideatory apraxia
idée fixe
identical twins
identification
identity
    i. crisis
    i. disorder
    ego i.
    gender i.
    i. matrix
    sense of i.
ideokinetic
    i. apraxia
ideology
ideomotion
ideomotor
    i. apraxia
ideophobia
ideoplastia
idioagglutinin
idiodynamic
    i. control
idiogamist
idiogenesis
idioglossia
idioglottic
idiogram
idiographic
    i. approach
idioheteroagglutinin
idioheterolysin
idiohypnotism
idioisoagglutinin
idioisolysin
idiojunctional rhythm
idiolalia
idiolysin
idiomuscular
    i. contraction
idionodal
    i. rhythm
idiopathetic
idiopathic
    i. aldosteronism
    i. bilateral vestibulopathy
    i. bone cavity
    i. bradycardia
    i. cardiomyopathy
    i. disease
    i. epilepsy
    i. fibrous mediastinitis
    i. fibrous retroperitonitis
    i. gout
    i. hirsutism
    i. hypercalcemic sclerosis of infants
    i. hyperlipemia
    i. hypertension
    i. hypertrophic osteoarthropathy

    i. hypertrophic subaortic stenosis
    i. infantilism
    i. interstitial fibrosis
    i. megacolon
    i. muscular atrophy
    i. myocarditis
    i. neuralgia
    i. orthostatic hypotension
    i. paroxysmal rhabdomyolysis
    i. proctitis
    i. pulmonary fibrosis
    i. pulmonary hemosiderosis
    i. roseola
    i. thrombocytopenic purpura
idiopathy
idiophrenic
idiopsychologic
idioreflex
idiosome
idiospasm
idiosyncrasy
idiosyncratic
    i. sensitivity
idiotope
idiot-prodigy
idiotrophic
idiotropic
idiot-savant
idiotype
    i. antibody
    i. autoantibody
    set of i.'s
idiotypic antigenic determinant
idioventricular
    i. kick
    i. rhythm
idrosis
IgA nephropathy
IgM nephropathy
ignipedites
ignipuncture
ikota
ileac
ileadelphus
ileal
    i. arteries
    i. bladder
    i. conduit
    i. intussusception
    i. sphincter
    i. veins
ileectomy
ileitis
    backwash i.
    distal i.
    regional i.
    terminal i.
ileoanal pouch

ileocecal
    i. eminence
    i. fold
    i. intussusception
    i. junction
    i. opening
    i. orifice
    i. valve
ileocecocolic sphincter
ileocecocystoplasty
ileocecostomy
ileocecum
ileocolic
    i. artery
    i. intussusception
    i. lymph nodes
    i. valve
    i. vein
ileocolitis
ileocolonic
ileocolostomy
ileocystoplasty
ileoentectropy
ileoileostomy
ileojejunitis
ileopexy
ileoproctostomy
ileorectostomy
ileorrhaphy
ileosigmoidostomy
ileostomy
    Brooke i.
    Kock i.
ileotomy
ileotransversostomy
ileum
    i. duplex
ileus
    adynamic i.
    dynamic i.
    gallstone i.
    mechanical i.
    meconium i.
    occlusive i.
    paralytic i.
    spastic i.
    i. subparta
    terminal i.
    verminous i.
Ilhéus
    I. encephalitis
    I. fever
    I. virus
ilia (*pl. of* ilium)
iliac
    i. arteries
    i. bone
    i. branch of iliolumbar artery

    i. bursa
    i. colon
    i. crest
    i. fascia
    i. fossa
    i. horn
    i. muscle
    i. plexus
    i. region
    i. roll
    i. spine
    i. steal
    i. tubercle
    i. tuberosity
    i. veins
iliacosubfascial
    i. fossa
    i. hernia
iliacus
    i. minor muscle
    i. muscle
iliadelphus
iliococcygeal
    i. muscle
iliococcygeus muscle
iliocolotomy
iliocostal
    i. muscle
iliocostalis
    i. cervicis muscle
    i. lumborum muscle
    i. muscle
    i. thoracis muscle
iliofemoral
    i. ligament
    i. triangle
iliofemoroplasty
iliohypogastric
    i. nerve
ilioinguinal
    i. nerve
iliolumbar
    i. artery
    i. ligament
    i. vein
iliometer
iliopagus
iliopectineal
    i. arch
    i. bursa
    i. eminence
    i. fascia
    i. fossa
    i. ligament
    i. line
iliopelvic
    i. sphincter
iliopsoas muscle

iliopubic
>i. eminence
>i. tract

iliosacral

iliosciatic
>i. notch

iliospinal

iliothoracopagus

iliotibial
>i. band
>i. tract

iliotrochanteric
>i. ligament

ilioxiphopagus

ilium, pl. **ilia**

illegal abortion

illinition

illness
>environmental i.
>functional i.
>manic-depressive i.
>mental i.

illumination
>axial i.
>central i.
>contact i.
>critical i.
>dark-field i.
>dark-ground i.
>direct i.
>erect i.
>focal i.
>Köhler i.
>lateral i.
>oblique i.
>vertical i.

illuminism

illusion
>i. of doubles
>i. of movement
>oculogravic i.
>oculogyral i.
>optical i.

illusional

Ilosvay reagent

ima

image
>accidental i.
>i. amplifier
>body i.
>catatropic i.
>direct i.
>eidetic i.
>false i.
>heteronymous i.
>homonymous i.'s
>hypnagogic i.
>hypnopompic i.

(handwritten: Ilizarov / Ilizarof device)

>inverted i.
>mental i.
>mirror i.
>motor i.
>negative i.
>optical i.
>phase i.
>Purkinje i.'s
>Purkinje-Sanson i.'s
>real i.
>retinal i.
>Sanson's i.'s
>sensory i.
>specular i.
>tactile i.
>unequal retinal i.
>virtual i.
>visual i.

image intensifier

imagery

imaginal

imagines (*pl. of* imago)

imaging
>blood pool i.
>exercise i.
>nuclear magnetic resonance i.,
>   NMR i.
>pharmacologic stress i.
>through transfer i.
>transfer i.

imaging department

imago, pl. **imagines**

imbalance
>autonomic i.
>occlusal i.
>sex chromosome i.
>sympathetic i.
>vasomotor i.

imbecile

imbed

imbricate, imbricated

imbrication
>i. lines of von Ebner

imitative tetanus

IML

Imlach's
>I. fat-pad
>I. ring

immature
>i. cataract
>i. granulocyte
>i. neutrophil

immediate
>i. allergy
>i. amputation
>i. auscultation
>i. contagion
>i. denture

i. flap
i. hypersensitivity
i. hypersensitivity reaction
i. insertion denture
i. percussion
i. posttraumatic automatism
i. posttraumatic convulsion
i. reaction
i. transfusion
immedicable
immersion
i. bath
i. foot
homogeneous i.
i. lens
i. microscopy
i. objective
oil i., water i.
imminent abortion
immittance
immobilization
immobilize
immobilizing antibody
immortalization
immotile cilia syndrome
immovable
i. bandage
i. joint
immune
i. adherence
i. adherence phenomenon
i. adhesion test
i. adsorption
i. agglutination
i. agglutinin
i. complex
i. complex disease
i. complex disorder
i. complex glomerulonephritis
i. complex nephritis
i. deficiency
i. deviation
i. electron microscopy
i. fetal hydrops
i. hemolysin
i. hemolysis
i. inflammation
i. interferon
i. opsonin
i. paralysis
i. precipitation
i. protein
i. reaction
i. response
i. response genes
i. serum
i. surveillance
i. system

i. thrombocytopenia
i. thrombocytopenic purpura
immunifacient
immunity
acquired i.
active i.
adoptive i.
antiviral i.
artificial active i.
artificial passive i.
bacteriophage i.
cell-mediated i., cellular i.
concomitant i.
i. deficiency
general i.
group i.
herd i.
humoral i.
infection i.
innate i.
local i.
maternal i.
natural i., nonspecific i.
passive i.
relative i.
specific i.
specific active i.
specific passive i.
stress i.
immunization
active i.
passive i.
immunize
immunoadjuvant
immunoagglutination
immunoassay
double antibody i.
enzyme i.
enzyme-multiplied i. technique
solid phase i.
thin-layer i.
immunobiology
immunoblast
immunoblastic
i. lymphadenopathy
i. lymphoma
i. sarcoma
immunoblot, immunoblotting
immunoblotting
immunochemical assay
immunocompetence
immunocompetent
immunocomplex
immunocompromised
immunoconglutinin
immunocyte
immunocytoadherence
immunocytochemistry

immunodeficiency
    cellular i. with abnormal
      immunoglobulin synthesis
    combined i.
    common variable i.
    phagocytic dysfunction i.
    phagocytic dysfunction disorders i.
    secondary i.
    severe combined i.
    i. syndrome
    i. with hypoparathyroidism
immunodeficient
immunodepressant
immunodepressor
immunodiagnosis
immunodiffusion
    double i.
    radial i.
    single i.
immunoelectrophoresis
    crossed i.
    rocket i.
    two-dimensional i.
immunoenhancement
immunoenhancer
immunoferritin
immunofluorescence
    i. method
    i. microscopy
immunofluorescent stain
immunogen
    behavioral i.
immunogenetics
immunogenic
immunogenicity
immunoglobulin
    i. domains
    monoclonal i.
    secretory i.
    secretory i. A
    thyroid-stimulating i.'s
immunohematology
immunohistochemistry
immunolocalization
immunologic
    i. high dose tolerance
    i. pregnancy test
    i. tolerance
immunological
    i. competence
    i. deficiency
    i. enhancement
    i. mechanism
    i. paralysis
    i. surveillance
    i. tolerance
immunologically
    i. activated cell

    i. competent cell
    i. privileged sites
immunologist
immunology
immunopathology
immunoperoxidase technique
immunopotentiation
immunopotentiator
immunoprecipitation
immunoproliferative
    i. disorders
    i. small intestinal disease
immunoradiometric assay
immunoreaction
immunoreactive
    i. insulin
immunoselection
immunosorbent
immunosuppression
immunosurveillance
immunosympathectomy
immunotherapy
    adoptive i.
    biological i.
immunotolerance
immunotransfusion
impact
    i. resistance
impacted
    i. fetus
    i. fracture
    i. tooth
impaction
    dental i.
    fecal i.
    food i.
    mucus i.
impaired glucose tolerance
impairment
    hearing i.
    mental i.
imparidigitate
impatent
impedance
    acoustic i.
    i. angle
    i. method
    i. plethysmography
imperative conception
imperception
imperfect
    i. fungus
    i. stage
    i. state
imperforate
    i. anus
    i. hymen
imperforation

impersistence
    motor i.
impetiginization
impetiginous
    i. cheilitis
    i. syphilid
impetigo
    Bockhart's i.
    i. bullosa
    bullous i. of newborn
    i. circinata
    i. contagiosa
    i. contagiosa bullosa
    i. eczematodes
    follicular i.
    i. herpetiformis
    i. neonatorum
    i. vulgaris
impetus
implant
    bag-gel i.
    carcinomatous i.'s
    cochlear i.
    dental i.'s
    i. denture
    i. denture substructure
    i. denture superstructure
    endometrial i.'s
    endo-osseous i.
    endosteal i.
    inflatable i.
    intraocular i.
    magnetic i.
    orbital i.
    penile i.
    pin i.
    post i.
    silicone i.
    submucosal i.
    subperiosteal i.
    supraperiosteal i.
    testicular i.
    triplant i.
implantation
    i. cone
    cortical i.
    i. cyst
    i. graft
    nerve i.
    periosteal i.
    subcutaneous i.
    i. theory of the production of
        endometriosis
implanted suture
implosive therapy
impotence, impotency
    paretic i.
    psychic i.

    symptomatic i.
    vasculogenic i.
impregnation
    silver i.
impressio, pl. **impressiones**
    i. cardiaca hepatis
    i. cardiaca pulmonis
    i. colica
    impressiones digitatae
    i. duodenalis
    i. esophagea
    i. gastrica
    i. ligamenti costoclavicularis
    i. petrosa pallii
    i. renalis
    i. suprarenalis
    i. trigeminalis
impression
    i. area
    basilar i.
    cardiac i. of liver
    cardiac i. of lung
    i. for cerebral gyri
    colic i.
    complete denture i.
    i. compound
    i. for costoclavicular ligament
    deltoid i.
    digitate i.'s
    direct bone i.
    duodenal i.
    esophageal i.
    i.'s of esophagus
    final i.
    gastric i.
    i. material
    mental i.
    partial denture i.
    petrosal i. of the pallium
    preliminary i., primary i.
    renal i.
    rhomboid i.
    sectional i.
    suprarenal i.
    i. tray
    trigeminal i.
impressive aphasia
imprinting
impulse
    apex i.
    cardiac i.
    i. control disorder
    ectopic i.
    escape i.
    irresistible i.
    morbid i.
    right parasternal i.'s
impulsion

impulsive
 i. obsession
impure flutter
imus
in situ
 i. s. hybridization
 i. s. nucleic acid hybridization
inaction
inactivate
inactivated serum
inactivation
inactive
 i. mutant
 i. tuberculosis
inadequate
 i. personality
 i. stimulus
inanimate
inanition
 i. fever
inapparent
 i. infection
inappetence
inappropriate
 i. affect
 i. hormone
inarticulate
inassimilable
inattention
 selective i.
 sensory i.
 visual i.
inborn
 i. error of metabolism
 i. errors of metabolism
 i. lysosomal disease
 i. reflex
inbred
incarcerated
 i. hernia
 i. placenta
incarceration symptom
incarial bone
incarnant
incarnative
incasement theory
incendiarism
incentive
inception rate
incertae sedis
incest
 i. barrier
incestuous
incidence
 i. density
 i. rate
incident
 i. angle

 i. point
 i. ray
incidental
 i. color
 i. learning
 i. parasite
incidentaloma
incipient
 i. abortion
 i. caries
incisal
 i. edge
 i. embrasure
 i. guidance
 i. guide
 i. guide angle
 i. margin
 i. path
 i. point
 i. rest
 i. surface
incise
incised wound
incision
 i. biopsy
 bucket-handle i.
 celiotomy i.
 chevron i.
 collar i.
 Deaver's i.
 Dührssen's i.'s
 endaural i.
 Fergusson's i.
 flank i.
 Kocher's i.
 McBurney's i.
 midline i.
 paramedian i.
 Pfannenstiel's i.
 transverse abdominal i.
incisional hernia
incisive
 i. bone
 i. canal
 i. canal cyst
 i. duct
 i. foramen
 i. fossa
 i. papilla
 i. suture
incisor
 i. canal
 central i.
 i. crest
 i. foramen
 lateral i.

second i.
i. tooth
incisura, pl. **incisurae**
   i. acetabuli
   i. angularis
   i. anterior auris
   i. apicis cordis
   i. cardiaca
   i. cardiaca pulmonis` sinistri
   incisurae cartilaginis meatus acustici externi
   i. cerebelli anterior
   i. cerebelli posterior
   i. clavicularis
   i. costalis
   i. ethmoidalis
   i. fibularis
   i. frontalis
   i. interarytenoidea
   i. intertragica
   i. ischiadica major
   i. ischiadica minor
   i. jugularis ossis occipitalis
   i. jugularis ossis temporalis
   i. jugularis sternalis
   i. lacrimalis
   i. ligamenti teretis hepatis
   i. mandibulae
   i. mastoidea
   i. nasalis
   i. pancreatis
   i. parietalis
   i. preoccipitalis
   i. pterygoidea
   i. radialis
   i. rivini
   incisurae santorini
   i. scapulae
   i. semilunaris ulnae
   i. sphenopalatina
   i. supraorbitalis
   i. tentorii
   i. terminalis auris
   i. thyroidea inferior
   i. thyroidea superior
   i. tragica
   i. trochlearis
   i. tympanica
   i. ulnaris
   i. umbilicalis
   i. vertebralis
incisure
   Lanterman's i.'s
   Rivinus' i.
   Santorini's i.'s

Schmidt-Lanterman i.'s
   tympanic i.
inclinatio, pl. **inclinationes**
   i. pelvis
inclination
   condylar guidance i.
   enamel rod i.
   lateral condylar i.
   i. of pelvis
inclinometer
inclusion
   i. blennorrhea
   i. bodies
   i. body disease
   i. body encephalitis
   i. cell
   cell i.'s
   i. cell disease
   i. conjunctivitis
   i. conjunctivitis viruses
   i. cyst
   i. dermoid
   Döhle i.'s
   fetal i.
   leukocyte i.'s
incoherent
incomitant strabismus
incompatible blood transfusion reaction
incompetence, incompetency
   aortic i.
   cardiac i.
   cardiac valvular i.
   mitral i.
   muscular i.
   pulmonary i., pulmonic i.
   pyloric i.
   relative i.
   tricuspid i.
   valvular i.
incompetent cervical os
incomplete
   i. abortion
   i. achromatopsia
   i. agglutinin
   i. alexia
   i. antibody
   i. antigen
   i. ascertainment
   i. atrioventricular block
   i. atrioventricular dissociation
   i. A-V dissociation
   i. cleavage
   i. conjoined twins
   i. fistula
   i. foot presentation
   i. fracture
   i. hemianopia
   i. knee presentation

incomplete *(continued)*
    i. metamorphosis
    i. neurofibromatosis
    i. tetanus
incongruent nystagmus
incongruous hemianopia
inconstant
incontinence
    fecal i.
    i. of feces
    i. of milk
    overflow i.
    paradoxical i.
    passive i.
    i. of pigment
    reflex i.
    stress urinary i.
    urge i., urgency i.
    urinary exertional i.
    i. of urine
incontinent
incontinentia
    i. pigmenti
    i. pigmenti achromians
incoordination
incorporation
increase
    absolute cell i.
increased markings emphysema
increment
incremental
    i. lines
    i. lines of von Ebner
incretion
incrustation
incrusted cystitis
incubation
    i. period
incubative stage
incubator
incubatory carrier
incubus
incudal
    i. fold
    i. fossa
incudectomy
incudes (*pl. of* incus)
incudiform
    i. uterus
incudis (*gen. of* incus)
incudomallealar
incudomalleolar
    i. articulation
    i. joint
incudostapedial
    i. articulation
    i. joint
incurable

incurvation
incus, gen. **incudis,** pl. **incudes**
incycloduction
incyclophoria
incyclotropia
indenization
indentation
    i. hardness
independence
    causal i.
    stochastic i.
independent
    i. assortment
    i. variable
indeterminate
    i. cleavage
    i. leprosy
index, gen. **indicis,** pl. **indices, indexes**
    alveolar i.
    i. ametropia
    anesthetic i.
    antitryptic i.
    Arneth i.
    auricular i.
    Ayala's i.
    basilar i.
    Bödecker i.
    body mass i.
    Calculus Surface I.
    cardiac i.
    i. case
    centromeric i.
    cephalic i.
    cephalo-orbital i.
    cephalorrhachidian i.
    cerebral i.
    cerebrospinal i.
    chemotherapeutic i.
    chest i.
    cranial i.
    Cumulative I. Medicus
    Dean's fluorosis i.
    def caries i., DEF caries i.
    degenerative i.
    dental i.
    df caries i., DF caries i.
    dmfs caries i., DMFS caries i.
    effective temperature i.
    empathic i.
    endemic i.
    erythrocyte indices
    i. extensor muscle
    facial i., superior facial i., total
      facial i.
    i. finger
    Flower's dental i.
    free thyroxine i.
    Gingival I.

gnathic i.
health status i.
height-length i.
i. hypermetropia
icteric i.
icterus i.
iron i.
karyopyknotic i.
length-breadth i.
length-height i.
leukopenic i.
Marginal Line Calculus I.
maturation i.
metacarpal i.
mitotic i.
i. myopia
nasal i.
nucleoplasmic i.
obesity i.
opsonic i.
Oral Hygiene I.
orbital i.
orbitonasal i.
palatal i., palatine i.
palatomaxillary i.
pelvic i.
Periodontal I.
Periodontal Disease I.
phagocytic i.
Pirquet's i.
Plaque I.
PMA i.
ponderal i.
pressure-volume i.
pulsatility i.
refractive i.
Robinson i.
Röhrer's i.
root caries i.
Russell's Periodontal I.
sacral i.
saturation i.
Schilling's i.
shock i.
small increment sensitivity i.
spiro-i.
splenic i.
staphylo-opsonic i.
stroke work i.
superior facial i. (*var. of*
  facial i.)
thoracic i.
tibiofemoral i.
total facial i. (*var. of* facial i.)
transversovertical i.
tuberculo-opsonic i.
uricolytic i.
vertical i.

vital i.
Volpe-Manhold i.
volume i.
zygomaticoauricular i.
indexical signs
India ink capsule stain
Indian
  I. flap
  I. method
  I. operation
  I. rhinoplasty
  I. sickness
  I. tick typhus
indicanidrosis
indicant
indicanuria
indication
  causal i.
  specific i.
  symptomatic i.
indicator
  alizarin i.
  i. dilution method
  health i.
  i. system
indicator-dilution curve
indices (*pl. of* index)
indicis (*gen. of* index)
Indiella
indifference to pain syndrome
indifferent
  i. cell
  i. electrode
  i. genitalia
  i. gonad
  i. tissue
indifferent neutrotaxis (*var. of*
  neutrotaxis)
indigenous
indigestion
  acid i.
  fat i.
  gastric i.
  nervous i.
indigouria, indiguria
indirect
  i. agglutination
  i. assay
  i. Coombs' test
  i. fluorescent antibody test
  i. fracture
  i. fulguration
  i. hemagglutination test
  i. inguinal hernia
  i. laryngoscopy
  i. lead
  i. maternal death
  i. method for making inlays

indirect (*continued*)
   i. nuclear division
   i. ophthalmoscope
   i. ophthalmoscopy
   i. ovular transmigration
   i. placentography
   i. pulp capping
   i. pupillary reaction
   i. rays
   i. reacting bilirubin
   i. retainer
   i. retention
   i. technique
   i. test
   i. transfusion
   i. vision
indisposition
indium-111
   i. chloride, i. trichloride
individual
   i. differences
   i. psychology
   i. therapy
individuation
   i. field
indocyanine green
indolaceturia
indolent
   i. bubo
   i. ulcer
indole test
indoluria
indoxyluria
induce
induced
   i. abortion
   i. apnea
   i. fever
   i. hypotension
   i. malaria
   i. mutation
   i. phagocytosis
   i. psychotic disorder
   i. radioactivity
   i. sensitivity
   i. symptom
   i. trance
inducer cell
inductance
induction
   i. chemotherapy
   electromagnetic i.
   lysogenic i.
   i. period
   spinal i.
inductor
inductorium
inductotherm

inductothermy
indulin
indulinophil, indulinophile
indurated
induration
   brown i. of the lung
   cyanotic i.
   Froriep's i.
   gray i.
   pigment i. of the lung
   plastic i.
   red i.
indurative
   i. myocarditis
indusium, pl. **indusia**
   i. griseum
industrial
   i. deafness
   i. disease
   i. hygiene
   i. psychiatry
   i. psychology
indwelling catheter
inebriation
inebriety
inertia
   psychic i.
   i. time
   uterine i., primary uterine i.,
     secondary uterine i., true uterine i.
inevitable abortion
infancy
infant
   i. death
   i. Hercules
   liveborn i.
   i. mortality rate
   postmature i.
   post-term i.
   preterm i.
   stillborn i.
   term i.
infanticide
infantile
   i. acropustulosis
   i. acute hemorrhagic edema of the
     skin
   i. autism
   i. beriberi
   i. cataract
   i. celiac disease
   i. colic
   i. convulsion
   i. cortical hyperostosis
   i. digital fibromatosis
   i. diplegia
   i. dwarfism
   i. eczema

i. fibrosarcoma
i. gastroenteritis
i. gastroenteritis virus
i., generalized G$_{M1}$ gangliosidosis
i. G$_{M2}$ gangliosidosis
i. hemiplegia
i. hernia
i. hypothyroidism
i. leishmaniasis
i. muscular atrophy
i. myofibromatosis
i. myxedema
i. neuroaxonal dystrophy
i. neuronal degeneration
i. osteomalacia
i. pellagra
i. progressive spinal muscular atrophy
i. purulent conjunctivitis
i. scurvy
i. sexuality
i. spasm
i. spastic paraplegia
i. spinal muscular atrophy
i. tetany
i. type
infantilism
Brissaud's i.
dysthyroidal i.
hepatic i.
hypophysial i.
hypothyroid i.
idiopathic i.
Lorain-Lévi i.
myxedematous i.
pancreatic i.
pituitary i.
proportionate i.
renal i.
sexual i.
static i.
tubal i.
universal i.
infarct
anemic i.
bland i.
bone i.
Brewer's i.'s
embolic i.
hemorrhagic i.
pale i.
red i.
Roesler-Bressler i.
septic i.
thrombotic i.
uric acid i.
white i.
Zahn's i.

infarction
anterior myocardial i.
anteroinferior myocardial i.
anterolateral myocardial i.
anteroseptal myocardial i.
cardiac i.
diaphragmatic myocardial i.
inferior myocardial i.
inferolateral myocardial i.
lateral myocardial i.
myocardial i.
myocardial i. in dumbbell form
nontransmural myocardial i.
posterior myocardial i.
silent myocardial i.
subendocardial myocardial i.
through-and-through myocardial i.
transmural myocardial i.
watershed i.
infect
infected abortion
infection
agonal i.
airborne i.
apical i.
i. calculus
i. control nurse
cross i.
cryptogenic i.
disseminated gonococcal i.
droplet i.
endogenous i.
focal i.
i. immunity
inapparent i.
latent i.
mass i.
mixed i.
pyogenic i.
Salinem i.
scalp i.
secondary i.
terminal i.
urinary tract i.
Vincent's i.
infection-exhaustion psychosis
infection-immunity
infectiosity
infectious
i. anemia
i. arteritis virus of horses
i. bronchitis virus
i. disease
i. ectromelia virus
i. eczematoid dermatitis
i. endocarditis
i. granuloma
i. hepatitis

infectious (*continued*)
  i. hepatitis virus
  i. icterus
  i. jaundice
  i. mononucleosis
  i. myositis
  i. papilloma virus
  i. plasmid
  i. polyneuritis
  i. porcine encephalomyelitis virus
  i. warts
infectiousness
infective
  i. disease
  i. embolism
  i. endocarditis
  i. jaundice
  i. thrombus
infectivity
infecundity
inference
inferential statistics
inferior
  i. aberrant ductule
  i. accessory fissure
  i. alveolar artery
  i. alveolar nerve
  i. anastomotic vein
  i. angle of scapula
  i. articular facet of atlas
  i. articular pit of atlas
  i. articular surface of tibia
  i. basal vein
  i. belly of omohyoid muscle
  i. border
  i. border of liver
  i. border of lung
  i. border of pancreas
  i. branch
  i. branches of transverse cervical nerve
  i. branch of oculomotor nerve
  i. branch of pubic bone
  i. branch of superior gluteal artery
  i. bursa of biceps femoris
  i. calcaneonavicular ligament
  i. cardiac vein
  i. carotid triangle
  i. cerebellar peduncle
  i. cerebral surface
  i. cerebral veins
  i. cervical cardiac branches of vagus nerve
  i. cervical cardiac nerve
  i. cervical ganglion
  i. choroid vein
  i. cluneal nerves
  i. colliculus

i. constrictor muscle of pharynx
i. costal facet
i. costal pit
i. dental arch
i. dental artery
i. dental branches of inferior dental plexus
i. dental canal
i. dental foramen
i. dental nerve
i. dental plexus
i. dental rami
i. duodenal fold
i. duodenal fossa
i. duodenal recess
i. epigastric artery
i. epigastric lymph nodes
i. epigastric vein
i. esophageal sphincter
i. extensor retinaculum
i. extremity
i. fascia of pelvic diaphragm
i. fascia of urogenital diaphragm
i. flexure of duodenum
i. fovea
i. frontal convolution
i. frontal gyrus
i. frontal sulcus
i. ganglion of glossopharyngeal nerve
i. ganglion of vagus nerve
i. gemellus muscle
i. gingival branches of inferior dental plexus
i. gluteal artery
i. gluteal nerve
i. gluteal veins
i. hemorrhoidal artery
i. hemorrhoidal nerves
i. hemorrhoidal plexuses
i. hemorrhoidal veins
i. horn
i. horn of falciform margin of saphenous opening
i. horn of lateral ventricle
i. horn of thyroid cartilage
i. hypogastric plexus
i. hypophysial artery
i. ileocecal recess
i. internal parietal artery
i. labial artery
i. labial branches of mental nerve
i. labial vein
i. laryngeal artery
i. laryngeal cavity
i. laryngeal nerve
i. laryngeal vein
i. laryngotomy

i. lateral brachial cutaneous nerve
i. lateral genicular artery
i. ligament of epididymis
i. limb
i. lingual muscle
i. lingular branch of lingular branch of left pulmonary artery
i. lingular segment
i. lobe of lung
i. longitudinal fasciculus
i. longitudinal muscle of tongue
i. longitudinal sinus
i. macular arteriole
i. macular venule
i. margin
i. maxillary nerve
i. medial genicular artery
i. mediastinum
i. medullary velum
i. mesenteric artery
i. mesenteric ganglion
i. mesenteric lymph nodes
i. mesenteric plexus
i. mesenteric vein
i. myocardial infarction
i. nasal arteriole of retina
i. nasal colliculus
i. nasal concha
i. nasal venule of retina
i. nuchal line
i. oblique muscle
i. oblique muscle of head
i. occipital gyrus
i. occipital triangle
i. olivary nucleus
i. olive
i. omental recess
i. ophthalmic vein
i. orbital fissure
i. palpebral veins
i. pancreatic artery
i. pancreaticoduodenal artery
i. parietal gyrus
i. parietal lobule
i. part
i. part of duodenum
i. part of lingular branch of left pulmonary vein
i. part of vestibular ganglion
i. part of vestibulocochlear nerve
i. pelvic aperture
i. petrosal groove
i. petrosal sinus
i. petrosal sulcus
i. phrenic artery
i. phrenic lymph nodes
i. phrenic vein
i. pole

i. pole of kidney
i. pole of testis
i. polioencephalitis
i. posterior serratus muscle
i. pubic ligament
i. quadrigeminal brachium
i. radioulnar joint
i. rectal artery
i. rectal nerves
i. rectal plexuses
i. rectal veins
i. rectus muscle
i. retinaculum of extensor muscles
i. root of ansa cervicalis
i. root of vestibulocochlear nerve
i. sagittal sinus
i. salivary nucleus
i. salivatory nucleus
i. segment
i. segmental artery of kidney
i. semilunar lobule
i. strait
i. suprarenal artery
i. surface of cerebellar hemisphere
i. surface of pancreas
i. surface of petrous part of temporal bone
i. surface of tongue
i. tarsal muscle
i. tarsus
i. temporal arteriole of retina
i. temporal convolution
i. temporal gyrus
i. temporal line
i. temporal sulcus
i. temporal venule of retina
i. thalamic peduncle
i. thalamostriate veins
i. thoracic aperture
i. thyroid artery
i. thyroid notch
i. thyroid plexus
i. thyroid tubercle
i. thyroid vein
i. tibiofibular joint
i. tracheobronchial lymph nodes
i. transverse scapular ligament
i. triangle sign
i. trunk of brachial plexus
i. turbinated bone
i. tympanic artery
i. ulnar collateral artery
i. veins of cerebellar hemisphere
i. vein of vermis
i. vena cava
i. ventricular vein
i. vesical artery
i. vesical nerves

inferior *(continued)*
   i. vesical plexus
   i. vestibular area
   i. vestibular nucleus
   i. wall of orbit
   i. wall of tympanic cavity
inferiority
   i. complex
inferolateral
   i. margin
   i. myocardial infarction
   i. surface of prostate
inferomedial margin
infertility
infest
infestation
infiltrate
   Assmann's tuberculous i.
   infraclavicular i.
infiltrating lipoma
infiltration
   adipose i.
   i. anesthesia
   cellular i.
   epituberculous i.
   fatty i.
   gelatinous i.
   gray i.
   lipomatous i.
   paraneural i.
   perineural i.
infinite distance
infinity
infirm
infirmary
infirmity
inflamed ulcer
inflammation
   active i.
   acute i.
   adhesive i.
   allergic i.
   alterative i.
   atrophic i.
   catarrhal i.
   chronic i.
   chronic active i.
   degenerative i.
   exudative i.
   fibrinopurulent i.
   fibrinous i.
   fibroid i.
   granulomatous i.
   hyperplastic i.
   immune i.
   interstitial i.
   necrotic i., necrotizing i.
   productive i.

   proliferative i.
   pseudomembranous i.
   purulent i.
   sclerosing i.
   serofibrinous i.
   serous i.
   subacute i.
   suppurative i.
inflammatory
   i. carcinoma
   i. corpuscle
   i. edema
   i. fibrous hyperplasia
   i. lymph
   i. macrophage
   i. papillary hyperplasia
   i. polyp
   i. pseudotumor
   i. rheumatism
inflatable
   i. implant
   i. splint
inflation
inflator
inflection, inflexion
influenza
   i. A
   Asian i.
   i. B
   i. bacillus
   i. C
   endemic i.
   Hong Kong i.
   i. nostras
   Russian i.
   Spanish i.
   i. viruses
influenzal
   i. pneumonia
   i. virus pneumonia
Influenzavirus
infold
information
   i. system
   i. theory
informed consent
infra-auricular
   i.-a. deep parotid lymph nodes
   i.-a. subfascial parotid lymph nodes
infra-axillary
infrabony pocket
infrabulge
infracardiac
   i. bursa
infracerebral
infraclavicular
   i. fossa
   i. infiltrate

i. part of brachial plexus
i. triangle
infraclinoid aneurysm
infraclusion
infracortical
infracostal
i. line
infracotyloid
infracristal
infraction — *Freiberg's*
infracture
infradentale
infradian
infradiaphragmatic
infraduction
infraduodenal fossa
infraglenoid
i. tubercle
i. tuberosity
infraglottic
i. cavity
i. space
infragranular layer
infrahepatic
infrahyoid
i. branch of superior thyroid artery
i. bursa
i. muscles
infralobar part of posterior branch of right pulmonary vein
inframamillary
inframammary
i. region
inframandibular
inframarginal
inframaxillary
infranodal extrasystole
infraocclusion
infraorbital
i. artery
i. canal
i. foramen
i. groove
i. margin
i. nerve
i. region
i. suture
infraorbitomeatal plane
infrapalpebral sulcus
infrapatellar
i. branch of saphenous nerve
i. fat body
i. fat-pad
i. synovial fold
infrapsychic
infrared
i. cataract
i. light

i. microscope
i. ray
i. spectrum
i. thermography
infrascapular
i. artery
i. region
infrasegmental
i. part
i. veins
infrasonic
infraspinatus
i. bursa
i. fascia
i. muscle
infraspinous
i. fossa
infrasplenic
infrasternal
i. angle
infratemporal
i. crest
i. fossa
i. surface of maxilla
infrathoracic
infratonsillar
infratrochlear
i. nerve
infraumbilical
infraversion
infriction
infundibula (*pl. of* infundibulum)
infundibular
i. part
i. recess
i. stalk
i. stem
i. stenosis
infundibulectomy
infundibuliform
i. fascia
i. hymen
i. sheath
infundibulofolliculitis
disseminated recurrent i.
infundibuloma
infundibulo-ovarian
i.-o. ligament
infundibulopelvic
i. ligament
infundibulum, pl. **infundibula**
ethmoid i.
ethmoidal i.
i. ethmoidale
i. hypothalami
hypothalamic i.
i. of lungs

infundibulum *(continued)*
    i. tubae uterinae
    i. of uterine tube
infusion-aspiration drainage
infusion graft
Infusoria
infusorian
ingesta
ingestion
ingestive
Ingrassia's
    I. apophysis
    I. wing
ingravescent
ingrowing toenail
ingrown
    i. hairs
    i. nail
inguen
inguinal
    i. aponeurotic fold
    i. branches of external pudendal
       arteries
    i. canal
    i. crest
    i. fold
    i. fossa
    i. glands
    i. hernia
    i. ligament
    i. ligament of the kidney
    i. plexus
    i. region
    i. triangle
    i. trigone
inguinocrural
    i. hernia
inguinodynia
inguinofemoral hernia
inguinolabial
    i. hernia
inguinoperitoneal
inguinoscrotal
    i. hernia
inguinosuperficial hernia
inhalation
    i. analgesia
    i. anesthesia
    i. anesthetic
inhale
inherent
inheritance
    alternative i.
    blending i.
    codominant i.
    collateral i.
    dominant i.
    extrachromosomal i.

    extranuclear i.
    galtonian i.
    holandric i.
    hologynic i.
    maternal i.
    mendelian i.
    mosaic i.
    multifactorial i.
    polygenic i.
    recessive i.
    sex-influenced i.
    sex-limited i.
    sex-linked i.
    X-linked i.
    Y-linked i.
inherited
    i. albumin variants
    i. character
inhibit
inhibiting antibody
inhibition
    allogeneic i.
    central i.
    contact i.
    i. factor
    hapten i. of precipitation
    hemagglutination i.
    potassium i.
    proactive i.
    reciprocal i.
    reflex i.
    residual i.
    retroactive i.
    Wedensky i.
inhibitor
    C1 esterase i.
    residual i.
inhibitory
    i. fibers
    i. junction potential
    i. nerve
    i. obsession
    i. postsynaptic potential
iniac
iniad
inial
iniencephaly
inion
iniopagus
iniops
initial
    i. contact
    i. dose
    i. heat
    i. hematuria
initiating agent
initiation codon
initis

inject
injected
injection
    adrenal cortex i.
    collagen i.
    depot i.
    i. flask
    hypodermic i.
    intrathecal i.
    intraventricular i.
    jet i.
    i. mass
    i. molding
    selective i.
    test i.
    Z-tract i.
injector
    jet i.
    power i.
injure
injury
    blast i.
    closed head i.
    contrecoup i. of brain
    coup i. of brain
    current of i.
    degloving i.
    egg-white i.
    hyperextension-hyperflexion i.
    i. of intervertebral disk
    open head i.
    pneumatic tire i.
    i. potential
    reperfusion i.
    steering wheel i.
    whiplash i.
inkblot test
inlay
    epithelial i.
    gold i.
    i. graft
    porcelain i.
    i. wax
inlet
    i. of larynx
    pelvic i.
innate
    i. immunity
    i. reflex
inner
    i. cell mass
    i. cone fiber
    i. dental epithelium
    i. ear
    i. enamel epithelium
    i. malleolus
    i. table of skull
innermost intercostal muscle

innervation
    i. apraxia
    reciprocal i.
innidiation
innocent
    i. bystander cell
    i. murmur
    i. tumor
innominatal
innominate
    i. artery
    i. bone
    i. cardiac veins
    i. fossa
    i. substance
    i. veins
inoculability
inoculable
inoculate
inoculation
    stress i.
inoculum
Inocybe
inopectic
inosemia
inosituria
inosuria
inotropic
    negatively i.
    positively i.
Inoviridae
inquest
inquiline
    i. parasite
insalubrious
insane
insanitary
insanity
    criminal i.
    i. defense
inscriptio
    i. tendinea
inscription
    tendinous i.
Insecta
insectarium
insect viruses
insecurity
insemination
    artificial i.
    donor i.

insemination *(continued)*
  heterologous i.
  homologous i.
insenescence
insensible
  i. perspiration
  i. thirst
insertion
  parasol i.
  thought i.
  velamentous i.
insertional mutagenesis
insheathed
insidious
insight
  i. learning
insolation
insomnia
  conditioned i.
  subjective i.
insomniac
inspectionism
inspiration
  crowing i.
inspiratory
  i. capacity
  i. center
  i. reserve volume
  i. stridor
inspire
inspired gas
inspirometer
inspissated cerumen
instability
  detrusor i.
  spinal i.
instantaneous
  i. electrical axis
  i. vector
instar
instep
instinct
  aggressive i.
  death i.
  ego i.'s
  herd i.
  life i.
  sexual i.
  social i.
instructive theory
instrument
  diamond cutting i.'s
  Krueger i. stop
  plugging i.
  purse-string i.
  Sabouraud-Noiré i.
  stereotactic i., stereotaxic i.
  test handle i.

instrumental
  i. amusia
  i. conditioning
instrumentarium
instrumentation
insudate
insufficiency
  acute adrenocortical i.
  adrenocortical i.
  aortic i.
  cardiac i.
  chronic adrenocortical i.
  convergence i.
  coronary i.
  divergence i.
  exocrine pancreatic i.
  hepatic i.
  latent adrenocortical i.
  mitral i.
  muscular i.
  myocardial i.
  parathyroid i.
  partial adrenocortical i.
  primary adrenocortical i.
  pulmonary i.
  pyloric i.
  renal i.
  respiratory i.
  secondary adrenocortical i.
  thyroid i.
  tricuspid i.
  uterine i.
  valvular i.
  velopharyngeal i.
  venous i.
insufflation
  i. anesthesia
  perirenal i.
insula, gen. and pl. **insulae**
  Haller's i.
insular
  i. area
  i. arteries
  i. cortex
  i. gyri
  i. hypothesis
  i. part
  i. part of middle cerebral artery
  i. sclerosis
  i. veins
insulin
  i. coma therapy
  i. coma treatment
  i. hypoglycemia test
  immunoreactive i.
  i. lipoatrophy
  i. lipodystrophy
  i. resistance

i. shock
i. shock treatment
insulin-dependent diabetes mellitus
insulinemia
insulin-like growth factors
insulinogenesis
insulinogenic, insulogenic
insulinoma
insulinopenic diabetes
insulitis
insulogenic (*var. of* insulinogenic)
insuloma
insult
insusceptibility
integral dose
integration
personality i.
integrity
marginal i. of amalgam
integument
integumentary
i. system
integumentum commune
intellectual aura
intellectualization
intelligence
abstract i.
artificial i.
measured i.
mechanical i.
i. quotient
social i.
i. test
intemperance
intensification chemotherapy
intensifying screen
intensity
i. of sound
intensive
i. care
i. care unit
i. psychotherapy
intention
i. spasm
i. tremor
intentional replantation
interacinar
interacinous
interaction
i. process analysis
interalveolar
i. pores
i. septum
i. space
interannular
i. segment
interarch
i. distance

interarticular
i. fibrocartilage
i. joints
interarytenoid
i. notch
interasteric
interatrial
i. foramen primum
i. foramen secundum
i. septum
interauricular
i. arc
interbody
intercadence
intercadent
intercalary
i. neuron
i. staphyloma
intercalated
i. disk
i. ducts
i. nucleus
intercanalicular
intercapillary
i. cell
i. glomerulosclerosis
intercapitular veins
intercarotic, intercarotid
intercarpal
i. joints
i. ligaments
intercartilaginous
i. part of glottic opening
i. part of rima glottidis
intercavernous
i. sinuses
intercellular
i. adhesion molecule-1
i. bridges
i. canaliculus
i. cement
i. junctions
i. lymph
intercentral
interceptive occlusal contact
intercerebral
interchondral
i. articulations
i. joints
intercilium
interclavicular
i. ligament
i. notch
interclinoid ligament
intercoccygeal
intercolumnar
i. fasciae

intercolumnar *(continued)*
  i. fibers
  i. tubercle
intercondylar, intercondylic, intercondyloid
  i. eminence
  i. fossa
  i. line of femur
  i. tubercle
intercornual ligament
intercostal
  i. anesthesia
  i. arteries
  i. ligaments
  i. lymph nodes
  i. membranes
  i. nerves
  i. neuralgia
  i. space
  i. veins
intercostobrachial nerves
intercostohumeral
  i. nerves
intercostohumeralis
intercourse
intercricothyrotomy
intercristal
intercross
intercrural
  i. fibers
  i. ganglion
intercuneiform
  i. joints
  i. ligaments
intercurrent
  i. disease
intercuspal position
intercuspation
intercusping
intercutaneomucous
interdeferential
interdental
  i. canals
  i. caries
  i. papilla
  i. septum
  i. splint
interdentium
interdigit
interdigital
  i. folds
interdigitation
interdisciplinary
interectopic interval
interface
  crystalline i.
  dermoepidermal i.

  metal i.
  structural i.
interfacial
  i. canals
  i. surface tension
interfascial space
interfascicular
  i. fasciculus
interfemoral
interference
  bacterial i.
  i. beat
  cuspal i.
  i. dissociation
  i. microscope
interferometer
  electron i.
interferometry
  electron i.
interferon
  antigen i.
  i. beta
  fibroblast i.
  i. gamma
  immune i.
  leukocyte i.
interferon-β2
interfibrillar, interfibrillary
interfibrous
interfilamentous
interfoveolar ligament
interfrontal
interganglionic
  i. rami
intergemmal
intergenic
  i. complementation
  i. suppression
interglobular
  i. dentin
  i. space
  i. space of Owen
intergluteal
intergonial
intergyral
interhemicerebral
interictal
interiliac lymph nodes
interilioabdominal amputation
interim denture
interior
interischiadic
interjudge reliability
interkinesis
interlamellar
interlaminar jelly
interleukin
interleukin-3

interleukin-4
interleukin-5
interleukin-6
interleukin-7
interleukin-8
interleukin-9
interleukin-10
interleukin-11
interleukin-12
interleukin-13
interleukin-14
interleukin-15
interlobar
 i. arteries of kidney
 i. artery
 i. duct
 i. surfaces of lung
 i. veins of kidney
interlobitis
interlobular
 i. arteries
 i. arteries of kidney
 i. arteries of liver
 i. duct
 i. ductules
 i. emphysema
 i. pleurisy
 i. septum
 i. veins of kidney
 i. veins of liver
interlocal additivity
interlocking gyri
intermalleolar
intermammary
intermammillary
intermarriage
intermaxilla
intermaxillary
 i. anchorage
 i. bone
 i. elastic
 i. fixation
 i. relation
 i. segment
 i. suture
 i. traction
intermediary
 i. host
 i. movements
 i. nerve
 i. system
intermediate
 i. abutment
 i. amputation
 i. antebrachial vein
 i. basilic vein
 i. body of Flemming
 i. bronchus

 i. carcinoma
 i. cephalic vein
 i. cervical septum
 i. cubital vein
 i. cuneiform bone
 i. disk
 i. dorsal cutaneous nerve
 i. filaments
 i. ganglia
 i. great muscle
 i. heart
 i. hemorrhage
 i. host
 i. hypothalamic region
 i. junction
 i. lacunar lymph node
 i. lacunar node
 i. lamella
 i. laryngeal cavity
 i. layer
 i. layer of the transversospinalis
  muscles
 i. line of iliac crest
 i. lumbar lymph nodes
 i. mass
 i. mesoderm
 i. nerve
 i. part
 i. part of adenohypophysis
 i. part of vestibular bulb
 i. rays
replicative i.
 i. sacral crests
 i. supraclavicular nerve
 i. temporal artery
 i. trait
 i. uveitis
 i. variable
 i. vastus muscle
 i. vein of forearm
intermediolateral
 i. cell column of spinal cord
 i. nucleus
intermediomedial nucleus
intermedius
intermembranous
 i. part of glottic opening
 i. part of rima glottidis
intermeningeal
intermenstrual
 i. pain
intermesenteric
 i. arterial anastomosis
 i. plexus
intermetacarpal
 i. joints
intermetameric

intermetatarsal
  i. articulations
  i. joints
intermetatarseum
intermission
intermit
intermittence, intermittency
intermittent
  i. acute porphyria
  i. albuminuria
  i. arthralgia
  i. claudication
  i. cramp
  i. explosive disorder
  i. hemoglobinuria
  i. hydrarthrosis
  i. hydrosalpinx
  i. malaria
  i. malarial fever
  i. mandatory ventilation
  i. positive pressure breathing
  i. positive pressure ventilation
  i. pulse
  i. reinforcement schedule
  i. self-obturation
  i. sterilization
  i. tetanus
  i. torticollis
intermuscular
  i. gluteal bursa
  i. septum
intern
internal
  i. acoustic foramen
  i. acoustic meatus
  i. acoustic pore
  i. adhesive pericarditis
  i. anal sphincter
  i. arcuate fibers
  i. attachment
  i. auditory artery
  i. auditory foramen
  i. auditory meatus
  i. auditory veins
  i. axis of eye
  i. base of skull
  i. branch of accessory nerve
  i. branch of superior laryngeal
    nerve
  i. canthus
  i. capsule
  i. capsule syndrome
  i. carotid artery
  i. carotid nerve
  i. carotid (nervous) plexus
  i. carotid venous plexus
  i. cephalic version
  i. cerebral veins

  i. collateral ligament of the wrist
  i. conjugate
  i. decompression
  i. ear
  i. female genital organs
  i. fistula
  i. fixation
  i. hemorrhage
  i. hemorrhoids
  i. hernia
  i. iliac artery
  i. iliac lymph nodes
  i. iliac vein
  i. inguinal ring
  i. intercostal membrane
  i. intercostal muscle
  i. jugular vein
  i. lacrimal fistula
  i. limiting membrane
  i. lip of iliac crest
  i. male genital organs
  i. malleolus
  i. mammary artery
  i. mammary plexus
  i. maxillary artery
  i. maxillary plexus
  i. medicine
  i. medullary lamina
  i. meningitis
  i. naris
  i. nasal branches
  i. nostril
  i. nuclear layer of retina
  i. oblique line
  i. oblique muscle
  i. obturator muscle
  i. occipital crest
  i. occipital protuberance
  i. ophthalmopathy
  i. ophthalmoplegia
  i. ovular transmigration
  i. pillar cells
  i. pterygoid muscle
  i. pudendal artery
  i. pudendal vein
  i. pyocephalus
  i. ramus of accessory nerve
  i. resorption
  i. respiration
  i. root sheath
  i. salivary gland
  i. saphenous nerve
  i. semilunar fibrocartilage of knee
    joint
  i. sheath of optic nerve
  i. spermatic artery
  i. spermatic fascia
  i. sphincter muscle of anus

i. spiral sulcus
i. squint
i. strabismus
i. surface
i. surface of frontal bone
i. surface of parietal bone
i. thoracic artery
i. thoracic lymphatic plexus
i. thoracic plexus
i. thoracic vein
i. traction
i. urethral opening
i. urethral orifice
i. urethral sphincter
i. urethrotomy
internalization
internarial
internasal
i. suture
International
I. Classification of Disease
I. Classification of Health Problems
in Primary Care
I. Classification of Impairments,
Disabilities and Handicaps
I. Committee of the Red Cross
I. Labour Organization
Classification
interne
interneuromeric
i. clefts
interneurons
internist
internodal
i. segment
internode
internuclear
internuncial
i. neuron
internus
interobserver error
interocclusal
i. clearance
i. distance
i. gap
i. record
i. rest space
interoceptive
interoceptor
interofective system
interolivary
interorbital
interosseal
interosseous
i. border
i. border of fibula
i. border of radius

i. border of tibia
i. border of ulna
i. bursa of elbow
i. cartilage
i. crest
i. cuneocuboid ligament
i. cuneometatarsal ligaments
i. fascia
i. groove
i. groove of calcaneus
i. groove of talus
i. margin
i. membrane of forearm
i. membrane of leg
i. metacarpal ligaments
i. metacarpal spaces
i. metatarsal ligaments
i. metatarsal spaces
i. muscles
i. nerve of leg
i. sacroiliac ligaments
i. talocalcaneal ligament
i. tibiofibular ligament
interosseus, pl. interossei
interpalpebral
i. zone
interpapillary ridges
interparietal
i. bone
i. sulcus
i. suture
interparoxysmal
interpectoral lymph nodes
interpediculate
interpeduncular
i. cistern
i. fossa
i. ganglion
i. nucleus
interpelviabdominal amputation
interpersonal
i. conflict
interphalangeal
i. articulations
i. joints of foot
i. joints of hand
interphase
interphyletic
interplant
interplanting
interpleural space
interpolated
i. extrasystole
i. flap
interposition arthroplasty
interpositus nucleus
interpretation

interproximal
   i. papilla
   i. space
interpubic
   i. disc
   i. disk
interpulmonary septum
interpupillary
interradial
interradicular
   i. alveoloplasty
   i. septa
   i. space
interrater reliability
interrenal
interridge distance
interrupted
   i. respiration
   i. suture
interscalene triangle
interscapular
   i. reflex
interscapulothoracic amputation
interscapulum
intersciatic
intersectio, pl. intersectiones
   i. tendinea
intersection
   tendinous i.
intersegmental
   i. fasciculi
   i. part of pulmonary vein
   i. veins
interseptal
interseptovalvular
   i. space
interseptum
intersexual
intersexuality
intersheath spaces of optic nerve
intersigmoid
   i. hernia
   i. recess
interspace
interspecific graft
interspinal
   i. line
   i. muscles
   i. plane
interspinales muscles
interspinalis
interspinous
   i. ligament
interspongioplastic substance
interstice, pl. interstices
interstitial
   i. absorption
   i. brachytherapy

   i. cells
   i. cell tumor of testis
   i. cystitis
   i. deletion
   i. disease
   i. emphysema
   i. fluid
   i. gastritis
   i. giant cell pneumonia
   i. gland
   i. growth
   i. hernia
   i. inflammation
   i. keratitis
   i. lamella
   i. mastitis
   i. myositis
   i. nephritis
   i. neuritis
   i. nucleus
   i. nucleus of Cajal
   i. pattern
   i. plasma cell pneumonia
   i. pregnancy
   i. pulmonary fibrosis
   i. therapy
   i. tissue
interstitium
intersystole
intertarsal
   i. articulations
   i. joints
intertendinous connections
interthalamic
   i. adhesion
intertragic notch
intertransversalis
intertransversarii muscles
intertransverse
   i. ligament
   i. muscles
intertriginous
intertrigo
intertrochanteric
   i. crest
   i. line
intertropical
   i. anemia
   i. hyphemia
intertubercular
   i. groove
   i. line
   i. plane
   i. sheath
   i. sulcus
intertubular
   i. zone
interureteral

interureteric
    i. fold
intervaginal space of optic nerve
interval
    A-H i.
    A-N i.
    atriocarotid i., a-c i.
    atrioventricular i.
    auriculoventricular i.
    A-V i.
    BH i.
    cardioarterial i., c-a i.
    confidence i.
    coupling i.
    escape i.
    focal i.
    i. gout
    H-V i.
    interectopic i.
    isovolumic i.
    lucid i.
    i. operation
    P-A i.
    P-J i.
    P-P i.
    P-Q i.
    P-R i.
    Q-R i.
    Q-RB i.
    QRS i.
    $Q-S_2$ i.
    Q-T i.
    R-R i.
    i. scale
    sphygmic i.
    Sturm's i.
    systolic time i.'s
intervascular
intervening variable
intervenous tubercle
intervention
    crisis i.
interventional
    i. angiography
    i. radiology
interventricular
    i. foramen
    i. grooves
    i. septum
intervertebral
    i. cartilage
    i. disc
    i. disk
    i. foramen
    i. ganglion
    i. notch
    i. symphysis
    i. vein

intervillous
    i. lacuna
    i. spaces
interzonal mesenchyme
intestina (*pl. of* intestinum)
intestinal
    i. anastomosis
    i. angina
    i. anthrax
    i. arterial arcades
    i. arteries
    i. atresia
    i. calculus
    i. capillariasis
    i. emphysema
    i. fistula
    i. follicles
    i. glands
    i. lipodystrophy
    i. lymphangiectasis
    i. metaplasia
    i. myiasis
    i. pseudo-obstruction
    i. rotation
    i. sand
    i. schistosomiasis
    i. sepsis
    i. stasis
    i. steatorrhea
    i. surface of uterus
    i. trunks
    i. villi
intestine
    large i.
    small i.
intestinotoxin
intestinum, pl. intestina
    i. cecum
    i. crassum
    i. ileum
    i. jejunum
    i. rectum
    i. tenue
    i. tenue mesenteriale
intima
intimal
intimitis
    proliferative i.
intoe
intolerance
    lactose i.
intorsion
intortor
intoxication
    acid i.
    anaphylactic i.
    citrate i.

intoxication *(continued)*
    septic i.
    water i.
intra-abdominal
intra-acinous
intra-adenoidal
intra-alveolar septa
intra-aortic
    i.-a. balloon
    i.-a. balloon counterpulsation
    i.-a. balloon pump
intra-arterial
intra-articular
    i.-a. cartilage
    i.-a. fracture
    i.-a. ligament of costal head
    i.-a. sternocostal ligament
intra-atrial
    i.-a. block
    i.-a. conduction
    i.-a. conduction time
intra-aural
intra-auricular
intrabony pocket
intrabronchial
intrabuccal
intrabulbar fossa
intracanalicular
    i. fibroadenoma
intracanicular part of optic nerve
intracapsular
    i. ankylosis
    i. fracture
    i. ligaments
    i. temporomandibular joint
      arthroplasty
intracardiac
    i. catheter
    i. lead
    i. pressure curve
intracarpal
intracartilaginous
intracatheter
intracavernous
    i. aneurysm
    i. plexus
intracavitary
intracelial
intracellular
    i. canaliculus
    i. fluid
    i. toxin
intracerebellar
intracerebral
    i. hemorrhage
intracervical
intracisternal
intracolic

intracordal
intracoronal
    i. retainer
intracorporeal
intracorpuscular
intracostal
intracranial
    i. aneurysm
    i. cavity
    i. ganglion
    i. granulomatous arteritis
    i. hematoma
    i. hemorrhage
    i. hypotension
    i. part of optic nerve
    i. part of vertebral artery
    i. pneumatocele
    i. pneumocele
    i. pressure
intractable
    i. epilepsy
    i. pain
intracutaneous
    i. reaction
intracystic
    i. papilloma
intrad
intradermal, intradermic
    i. nevus
    i. reaction
intraduct
intraductal
    i. carcinoma
    i. papilloma
intradural
intraembryonic
    i. mesoderm
intraepidermal
    i. bulla
    i. carcinoma
intraepiphysial
intraepiploic hernia
intraepithelial
    i. carcinoma
    i. dyskeratosis
    i. glands
intrafaradization
intrafascicular
intrafebrile
intrafilar
intrafusal
    i. fibers
intragalvanization
intragastric
intragemmal
intragenic
    i. complementation
    i. suppression

intraglandular
    i. deep parotid lymph nodes
    i. parotid lymph nodes
intraglobular
intragracile sulcus
intragyral
intrahepatic
intrahyoid
intrailiac hernia
intrajugular process
intralaminar
    i. nuclei of thalamus
    i. part of optic nerve
intralaryngeal
intralesional therapy
intraligamentary pregnancy
intraligamentous
intralobar
    i. part of the right superior
       pulmonary vein
intralobular
    i. duct
intralocal additivity
intralocular
intraluminal
intramaxillary anchorage
intramedullary
    i. anesthesia
    i. reamer
    i. tractotomy
intramembranous
    i. ossification
intrameningeal
intramural
    i. hematoma
    i. practice
    i. pregnancy
intramuscular
intramyocardial
intramyometrial
intranasal
    i. anesthesia
intranatal
intraneural
intranuclear
intraobserver error
intraocular
    i. fluid
    i. implant
    i. neuritis
    i. part of optic nerve
    i. pressure
intraoral
    i. anchorage
    i. anesthesia
    i. antrostomy
    i. fracture appliance
intraorbital

intraosseous
    i. anesthesia
    i. fixation
intraosteal
intraovarian
intraovular
intrapapillary drusen
intraparietal
    i. sulcus
    i. sulcus of Turner
intraparotid plexus of facial nerve
intrapartum
    i. hemorrhage
    i. period
intrapelvic
    i. hernia
intrapericardiac, intrapericardial
intraperiosteal fracture
intraperitoneal
    i. pregnancy
intrapersonal
    i. conflict
intrapial
intrapleural
intrapontine
intraprostatic
intraprotoplasmic
intrapsychic
intrapulmonary
intrapyretic
    i. amputation
intrarachidian (*var. of* intrarrhachidian)
intrarectal
intrarenal
    i. reflux
intraretinal
    i. space
intrarrhachidian, intrarachidian
intrascrotal
intrasegmental
    i. part
    i. veins
intraseptal alveoloplasty
intraspinal
    i. anesthesia
intrasplenic
intrastromal
intrasynovial
intratarsal
intratendinous bursa of elbow
intrathecal
    i. injection
intrathoracic
intrathyroid cartilage
intratonsillar
intratracheal
    i. anesthesia

I

intratracheal *(continued)*
  i. intubation
  i. tube
intratubal
intratubular
intratympanic
intrauterine
  i. amputation
  i. contraceptive device
  i. contraceptive devices
  i. devices
  i. fracture
  i. pneumonia
  i. transfusion
intravagal glomus
intravaginal torsion
intravascular
  i. ligature
  i. lymph
  i. papillary endothelial hyperplasia
intravenous
  i. anesthesia
  i. anesthetic
  i. cholangiography
  i. drip
  i. narcosis
  i. pyelography
  i. regional anesthesia
  i. urography
intraventricular
  i. block
  i. conduction
  i. hemorrhage
  i. injection
intravesical
intravital
  i. stain
  i. ultraviolet
intra vitam
intravitelline
intravitreous
intrinsic
  i. asthma
  i. color
  i. deflection
  i. dysmenorrhea
  i. fibers
  i. motivation
  i. muscles
  i. muscles of foot
  i. reflex
  i. sphincter
intrinsicoid deflection
introducer
introflection, introflexion
introgastric
introitus
  i. canalis

  i. of facial canal
  vaginal i.
introjection
intromission
intromittent
  i. organ
introspection
introspective
  i. method
introsusception
introversion
introvert
intubate
intubation
  altercursive i.
  aqueductal i.
  blind nasotracheal i.
  endotracheal i.
  intratracheal i.
  nasotracheal i.
  orotracheal i.
  tracheal i.
intubator
intuitive stage
intumesce
intumescence
  tympanic i.
intumescent
  i. cataract
intumescentia
  i. cervicalis
  i. ganglioformis
  i. lumbalis
  i. tympanica
intussusception
  colic i.
  double i.
  ileal i.
  ileocecal i.
  ileocolic i.
  jejunogastric i.
  retrograde i.
intussusceptive
  i. growth
intussusceptum
intussuscipiens
inulin clearance
inundation fever
InV
  I. allotypes
  I. group antigen
invaccination
invaginate
  i. planula
invagination
  basilar i.
invaginator
invalid

invalidism
invasion
invasive
    i. aspergillosis
    i. carcinoma
    i. mole
inventory
    Millon clinical multiaxial i.
    Minnesota Multiphasic Personality i.
    personality i.
invermination
inverse
    i. anaphylaxis
    i. ocular bobbing
    i. square law
    i. symmetry
    i. syntropy
inversed jaw-winking syndrome
inversion
    i. of chromosomes
    paracentric i.
    pericentric i.
    i. recovery
    i. of the uterus
    visceral i.
inverted
    i. cone bur
    i. follicular keratosis
    i. image
    i. papilloma
    i. pelvis
    i. radial reflex
    i. reflex
inverted repeat
invertor
investigatory reflex
investing
    i. cartilage
    i. fascia
    i. layer of deep cervical fascia
    i. tissues
    vacuum i.
investment
    i. cast
    refractory i.
inveterate
inviscation
invisible
    i. differentiation
    i. light
    i. spectrum
involucra (*pl. of* involucrum)
involucre
involucrin
involucrum, pl. **involucra**
involuntary
    i. guarding

    i. muscles
    i. nervous system
involution
    i. cyst
    i. form
    senile i.
    i. of the uterus
involutional
    i. depression
    i. melancholia
    i. psychosis
Iodamoeba
    I. bütschlii
iodate reaction of epinephrine
iodic purpura
iodide
    i. acne
    i. transport defect
iodine
    i. cysts
    i. eruption
    Gram's i.
    i. reaction of epinephrine
    i. stain
    i. test
iodine-fast
iodine-induced hyperthyroidism
iodinophil, iodinophile
iodinophilous
iodixanol
iodophil granule
iodophilia
iodotherapy
iodotyrosine deiodinase defect
ioduria
ion channel
ionic medication
ionium
ionization chamber
ionizing radiation
ion-selective electrodes
iontophoresis
iontophoretic
iontotherapy
iopentol
iophenoic acid
iophobia
iopromide
iotacism
iotrol
iotrolan
ioversol
ioxilan
ioxithalamate
ipodate
ipsefact
ipsilateral
    i. reflex

iridal
iridectomy
    buttonhole i.
    optical i.
    peripheral i.
    sector i.
    stenopeic i.
    therapeutic i.
iridencleisis
irideremia
iridescent
    i. virus
iridesis
iridial, iridian, iridic
    i. part of retina
iridoavulsion
iridocele
iridochoroiditis
iridocoloboma
iridocorneal
    i. angle
    i. endothelial syndrome
    i. mesodermal dysgenesis
    i. syndrome
iridocyclectomy
iridocyclitis
    i. septica
iridocyclochoroiditis
iridocystectomy
iridodiagnosis
iridodialysis
iridodilator
iridodonesis
iridokinetic
iridology
iridomalacia
iridomesodialysis
iridomotor
iridoparalysis
iridopathy
iridoplegia
    complete i.
    reflex i.
    sympathetic i.
iridoptosis
iridopupillary lamina
iridorrhexis
iridoschisis
iridosclerotomy
iridotomy
    laser i.
Iridoviridae
Iridovirus
IRI/G ratio
iris, pl. **irides**
    i. bicolor
    i. bombé
    i. dehiscence

    i. freckles
    i. frill
    i. pits
    plateau i.
    tremulous i.
iris-nevus syndrome
iritic
iritis
    fibrinous i.
    follicular i.
    i. glaucomatosa
    hemorrhagic i.
    nodular i.
    plastic i.
    quiet i.
    serous i.
    sympathetic i.
iron
    i. deficiency anemia
    i. hematoxylin
    i. index
    i. lung
iron-binding capacity
iron-storage disease
irradiate
irradiation
irrational
irreducible hernia
irregular
    i. astigmatism
    i. bone
    i. dentin
    i. emphysema
    i. nystagmus
    i. pulse
irresistible impulse
irresponsibility
    criminal i.
irresuscitable
irreversible
    i. pulpitis
    i. reaction
    i. shock
irrigate
irrigation
    drip-suck i.
irrigator
irritability
    electric i.
    myotatic i.
irritable
    i. breast
    i. colon
    i. heart
irritant
    i. contact dermatitis
    primary i.

irritation
    i. cell
    i. dentin
    i. fibroma
irrumation
irruption
irruptive
Irvine-Gass syndrome
Isaac's syndrome
Isamine blue
isauxesis
ischemia
    myocardial i.
    postural i.
    i. retinae
    silent i.
ischemia-modifying factors
ischemic
    i. contracture of the left ventricle
    i. hypoxia
    i. lumbago
    i. mitral regurgitation
    i. muscular atrophy
    i. necrosis
    i. neuropathy
    i. optic neuropathy
ischesis
ischia (*pl. of* ischium)
ischiadic
    i. plexus
    i. spine
ischiadicus
ischial
    i. bone
    i. bursa
    i. ramus
    i. spine
    i. tuberosity
ischialgia
ischiatic
    i. hernia
    i. notch
ischidrosis
ischii (*gen. of* ischium)
ischioanal
    i. fossa
ischiobulbar
ischiocapsular
    i. ligament
ischiocavernosus
ischiocavernous
    i. muscle
ischiocele
ischiococcygeal
ischiococcygeus
ischiodynia
ischiofemoral
    i. ligament

ischiofibular
ischiomelus
ischioneuralgia
ischionitis
ischiopagus
ischioperineal
ischiopubic
    i. ramus
ischiorectal
    i. abscess
    i. fat-pad
    i. fossa
ischiosacral
ischiothoracopagus
ischiotibial
ischiovaginal
ischiovertebral
ischium, gen. **ischii,** pl. **ischia**
ischochymia
ischuria
Ishihara test
island
    blood i.
    bone i.
    i.'s of Calleja
    i. disease
    epimyoepithelial i.'s
    i. fever
    i. flap
    Langerhans' i.'s
    pancreatic i.'s
    i. of Reil
islet
    blood i.
    i. cell
    i. cell adenoma
    i.'s of Langerhans
    pancreatic i.'s
    i. tissue
isoacceptor tRNA
isoagglutination
isoagglutinin
isoagglutinogen
isoallele
isoallotypic determinants
isoantibody
isoantigen
isobaric spinal anesthesia
isobestic
isocellular
isochoric
isochromatic
isochromatophil, isochromatophile
isochromic anemia
isochromosome
isochronia
isochronous
isochroous

I

isocline
isocoria
isocortex
isocytolysin
isodactylism
isodense
isodiphasic complex
isoelectric
    i. electroencephalogram
    i. line
    i. period
isoenzyme
    creatine kinase i.'s
    i. electrophoresis
isoerythrolysis
isogamete
isogamy
isogeneic, isogenic
    i. graft
isogenous
    i. chondrocytes
    i. nest
isognathous
isograft
isohemagglutination
isohemagglutinin
isohemolysin
isohemolysis
isohydruria
isohypercytosis
isohypocytosis
isoimmune neonatal thrombocytopenia
isoimmunization
isolate
    genetic i.
    mating i.
isolated
    i. abutment
    i. dextrocardia
    i. dyskeratosis follicularis
    i. explosive disorder
    i. hypoaldosteronism
    i. parietal endocarditis
    i. proteinuria
isolation
isolecithal
    i. ovum
isoleukoagglutinin
isologous
    i. graft
isolysin
isolysis
isolytic
isomastigote
isomeric function
isometric
    i. chart
    i. contraction

    i. contraction period
    i. exercise
    i. period of cardiac cycle
    i. relaxation
    i. relaxation period
    i. traction
isometropia
isomorphic
    i. response
isomorphism
isomorphous
    i. gliosis
isoncotic
isoniazid
    i. neuropathy
    i. polyneuropathy
isonormocytosis
isopathy
isoperistaltic anastomosis
isoplassonts
isoplastic
    i. graft
isopleth
isoprecipitin
isopropanol precipitation test
isopter
isorhythmic dissociation
isorrhea
isosbestic
isoschizomer
isosensitize
isoserum treatment
isosexual
Isospora
    I. belli
    I. bigemina
    I. canis
    I. felis
    I. rivolta
    I. suis
isosporiasis
isosthenuria
isothermal
isothiocyanate
    fluorescenin i
isotonic
    i. coefficient
    i. contraction
    i. exercise
    i. traction
isotope
    daughter i.
isotransplantation
isotropic disk
isotype
isotypic
isovolume
    i. pressure-flow curve

isovolumetric
    i. relaxation

Isovue (handwritten)

isovolumic
    i. interval
    i. relaxation

issue
    nature-nurture i.

isthmectomy

isthmi (*pl. of* isthmus)

isthmic, isthmian

isthmoparalysis

isthmoplegia

isthmus, pl. isthmi, isthmuses
    i. of aorta
    i. aortae
    i. of auditory tube
    i. of cartilage of ear
    i. cartilaginis auris
    i. of cingulate gyrus
    i. of eustachian tube
    i. of external acoustic meatus
    i. of fauces
    i. faucium
    i. glandulae thyroideae
    Guyon's i.
    i. gyri cinguli
    i. of gyrus fornicatus
    i. of His
    Krönig's i.
    i. of limbic lobe
    i. meatus acustici externi
    pharyngeal i.
    i. pharyngonasalis
    i. prostatae
    i. of prostate
    i. rhombencephali
    rhombencephalic i.
    i. of thyroid
    i. tubae auditivae
    i. tubae uterinae
    i. uteri
    i. of uterine tube
    i. of uterus
    Vieussens' i.

Italian
    I. flap
    I. method
    I. operation
    I. rhinoplasty

itch
    azo i.
    baker's i.
    barber's i.
    bath i.
    coolie i.
    copra i.
    Cuban i.

    dew i.
    dhobie i.
    frost i.
    grain i.
    grocer's i.
    ground i.
    jock i.
    kabure i.
    lumberman's i.
    Malabar i.
    Norway i.
    poultryman's i.
    prairie i.
    rice i.
    Saint Ignatius' i.
    straw i., straw-bed i.
    summer i.
    swamp i.
    swimmer's i.
    toe i.
    warehouseman's i.
    washerwoman's i.
    water i.
    winter i.

itching

iter
    i. chordae anterius
    i. chordae posterius
    i. dentis
    i. dentium
    i. a tertio ad quartum ventriculum

iteral

ithykyphosis, ithycyphosis

ithylordosis

Ito
    I. cells
    I. nevus

ITO method

Ito-Reenstierna test

^{131}I uptake test

I-V block

Ivemark's syndrome

IVF-ET

ivory
    i. exostosis
    i. membrane
    i. vertebra

Ivy
    I. bleeding time test
    I. loop wiring

Ixodes
    I. cookei
    I. dammini
    I. spinipalpis

ixodic

ixodid

Ixodoidea

Jaboulay
J. amputation
J. pyloroplasty
Jaccoud's
J. arthritis
J. arthropathy
jacket
j. crown
Minerva j.
Sayre's j.
straight j.
jackscrew
jacksonian
j. epilepsy
j. seizure
Jackson's
J. law
J. membrane
J. rule
J. sign
J. veil
Jacobaeus operation
Jacobson's
J. anastomosis
J. canal
J. cartilage
J. nerve
J. organ
J. plexus
J. reflex
Jacquart's facial angle
Jacquemet's recess
Jacques' plexus
Jacquet's erythema
jactitation
Jadassohn-Lewandowski syndrome
Jadassohn-Pellizzari anetoderma
Jadassohn's nevus
Jadassohn-Tièche nevus
Jaeger's test types
Jaffe
J. reaction
J. test
Jaffe-Lichtenstein disease
Jahnke's syndrome
jail fever
jake paralysis
Jakob-Creutzfeldt disease
Jamaican vomiting sickness
James
J. fibers
J. tracts
James-Lange theory
Jamestown Canyon virus
Janet's test

Janeway lesion
janiceps
j. asymmetrus
j. parasiticus
Jansen's operation
Jansky-Bielschowsky disease
Jansky's classification
Janus green B
Japanese
J. B encephalitis
J. B encephalitis virus
J. dysentery
J. river fever
J. schistosomiasis
jar
heel j.
jargon
j. aphasia
Jarisch-Herxheimer reaction
Jarjavay's ligament
Jarvik
J. artificial heart
Jatene procedure
jaundice
acholuric j.
anhepatic j.
anhepatogenous j.
catarrhal j.
cholestatic j.
chronic acholuric j.
chronic familial j.
chronic idiopathic j.
congenital hemolytic j.
hematogenous j.
hemolytic j.
hepatocellular j.
hepatogenous j.
homologous serum j.
human serum j.
infectious j.
infective j.
leptospiral j.
malignant j.
mechanical j.
j. of the newborn
nonobstructive j.
nuclear j.
obstructive j.
painless j.
physiologic j.
postarsphenamine j.
regurgitation j.
retention j.
Schmorl's j.
spherocytic j.

J

jaundice *(continued)*
    spirochetal j.
    toxemic j.
jaw
    j. bone
    crackling j.
    Hapsburg j.
    j. jerk
    j. joint
    lock-j.
    lower j.
    parrot j.
    j. reflex
    j. repositioning
    j. separation
    j. skeleton
    upper j.
    j. winking
Jaworski's bodies
jaw-winking
    j.-w. phenomenon
    j.-w. syndrome
jaw-working reflex
JC virus
jealous type of paranoid disorder
Jeanselme's nodules
Jeghers-Peutz syndrome
jejunal
    j. arteries
    j. and ileal veins
jejunectomy
jejunitis
jejunocolostomy
jejunogastric intussusception
jejunoileal
    j. bypass
    j. shunt
jejunoileitis
jejunoileostomy
jejunojejunostomy
jejunoplasty
jejunostomy
jejunotomy
jejunum
Jellinek formula
jelly
    cardiac j.
    interlaminar j.
    Wharton's j.
Jendrassik's maneuver
Jenner's stain
Jensen's
    J. disease
    J. sarcoma
Jericho boil
jerk
    ankle j.
    chin j.

    crossed j.
    crossed adductor j.
    crossed knee j.
    elbow j.
    j. finger
    jaw j.
    knee j.
    supinator j.
jerks
jerky
    j. nystagmus
    j. respiration
Jerne technique
Jervell and Lange-Nielsen syndrome
jet
    j. ejector pump
    j. injection
    j. injector
    j. lag
Jeune's syndrome
jeweller's forceps
Jewett
    J. sound
    J. and Strong staging
j-g complex
JH virus
Jk antigens
Jk blood group
Jobbins antigen
Jobert
    J. de Lamballe's fossa
    J. de Lamballe's suture
Job syndrome
Jocasta complex
jock itch
Jod-Basedow phenomenon
Joffroy's
    J. reflex
    J. sign
Johne's bacillus
johnin
Johnson's method
joint
    acromioclavicular j.
    ankle j.
    anterior intraoccipital j.
    arthrodial j.
    atlantoaxial j.
    atlanto-occipital j.
    j.'s of auditory ossicles
    ball-and-socket j.
    biaxial j.
    bicondylar j
    bilocular j.
    j. branches
    Budin's obstetrical j.
    calcaneocuboid j.
    capitular j.

j. capsule
carpal j.'s
carpometacarpal j.'s
carpometacarpal j. of thumb
cartilaginous j.
Charcot's j.
Chopart's j.
Clutton's j.'s
coccygeal j.
cochlear j.
composite j.
compound j.
condylar j.
costochondral j.
costotransverse j.
costovertebral j.'s
cotyloid j.
cricoarytenoid j.
cricothyroid j.
Cruveilhier's j.
cubital j.
cuboideonavicular j.
cuneocuboid j.
cuneometatarsal j.'s
cuneonavicular j.
dentoalveolar j.
diarthrodial j.
digital j.'s
DIP j.'s
distal interphalangeal j.'s
distal radioulnar j.
distal tibiofibular j.
j.'s of ear bones
j. effusion
elbow j.
ellipsoidal j.
enarthrodial j.
facet j.'s
false j.
fibrous j.
flail j.
j.'s of foot
j.'s of free inferior limb
j.'s of free lower limb
j.'s of free superior limb
j.'s of free upper limb
j. gamete
ginglymoid j.
gliding j.
gompholic j.
j.'s of hand
j. of head of rib
hemophilic j.
hinge j.
hip j.
humeroradial j.
humeroulnar j.
hysterical j.

immovable j.
incudomalleolar j.
incudostapedial j.
j.'s of inferior limb girdle
inferior radioulnar j.
inferior tibiofibular j.
interarticular j.'s
intercarpal j.'s
interchondral j.'s
intercuneiform j.'s
intermetacarpal j.'s
intermetatarsal j.'s
interphalangeal j.'s of foot
interphalangeal j.'s of hand
intertarsal j.'s
jaw j.
knee j.
lateral atlantoaxial j.
lateral atlantoepistrophic j.
Lisfranc's j.'s
lumbosacral j.
Luschka's j.'s
mandibular j.
manubriosternal j.
median atlantoaxial j.
metacarpophalangeal j.'s _—wrist—finger_
metatarsophalangeal j.'s _arch of foot—toes_
j. mice
midcarpal j.
middle atlantoepistrophic j.
middle carpal j.
middle radioulnar j.
midtarsal j.
mortise j.
movable j.
MP j.'s
multiaxial j.
neurocentral j.
neuropathic j.
j. oil
j.'s of pectoral girdle
peg-and-socket j.
j.'s of pelvic girdle
petro-occipital j.
phalangeal j.'s
PIP j.'s
pisotriquetral j.
pivot j.
plane j.
polyaxial j.
posterior intraoccipital j.
j. probability
proximal interphalangeal j.'s
proximal radioulnar j.
proximal tibiofibular j.
radiocarpal j.
rotary j., rotatory j.
sacrococcygeal j.

J

joint · junction

joint (*continued*)
  sacroiliac j.
  saddle j.
  schindyletic j.
  screw j.
  j. sense
  shoulder j.
  simple j.
  socket j.
  spheno-occipital j.
  spheroid j.
  spiral j.
  sternal j.'s
  sternoclavicular j.
  sternocostal j.'s
  subtalar j.
  j.'s of superior limb girdle
  superior radioulnar j.
  superior tibiofibular j.
  suture j.
  synarthrodial j.
  synchondrodial j.
  syndesmodial j., syndesmotic j.
  synovial j.
  talocalcaneal j.
  talocalcaneonavicular j.
  talocrural j.
  talonavicular j.
  tarsal j.'s
  tarsometatarsal j.'s
  temporomandibular j.
  thigh j.
  transverse tarsal j.
  trochoid j.
  uncovertebral j.'s
  uniaxial j.
  unilocular j.
  wedge-and-groove j.
  wrist j.
  xiphisternal j.
  zygapophyseal j.'s
Jolles' test
Jolly
  J. bodies
  J. reaction
Jones' test
Jonnesco's fossa
Jonston's
  J. alopecia
  J. area
Joseph
  J. clamp
  J. knife
  J. rhinoplasty
Joubert's syndrome
J point
Js antigen
J-sella deformity

juccuya
Judkins technique
juga (*pl. of* jugum)
jugal
  j. bone
  j. ligament
  j. point
jugale
jugomaxillary
jugular
  j. bulb
  j. duct
  j. embryocardia
  j. foramen
  j. foramen syndrome
  j. fossa
  j. ganglion
  j. gland
  j. glomus
  j. lymphatic trunk
  j. nerve
  j. notch of occipital bone
  j. notch of temporal bone
  j. plexus
  j. process
  j. pulse
  j. sinus
  j. tubercle
  j. veins
  j. venous arch
  j. wall of middle ear
jugulo-digastric lymph node
jugulodigastric node
jugulo-omohyoid
  j.-o. lymph node
  j.-o. node
jugulum
jugum, pl. juga
  j. alveolare, pl. juga alveolaria
  j. sphenoidale
juice
  appetite j.
  cancer j.
Jukes
jumper
  j. disease
  j. disease of Maine
jump flap
jumping
  j. the bite
  j. disease
  j. Frenchmen of Maine disease
  j. gene
junction
  amelodental j., amelodentinal j.
  amnioembryonic j.
  anorectal j.
  A-V j.

cardioesophageal j.
cementodentinal j.
cementoenamel j.
choledochoduodenal j.
costochondral j.
dentinocemental j.
dentinoenamel j.
duodenojejunal j.
electrotonic j.
esophagogastric j.
gap j.
ileocecal j.
intercellular j.'s
intermediate j.
j. of lips
manubriosternal j.
mucocutaneous j.
muscle-tendon j.
myoneural j.
neuroectodermal j.
neuromuscular j.
neurosomatic j.
j. nevus
rectosigmoid j.
sacrococcygeal j.
sclerocorneal j.
squamocolumnar j.
ST j.
sternomanubrial j.
tight j.
tympanostapedial j.
ureteropelvic j.

junctional
j. complex
j. cyst
j. epithelium
j. escape
j. extrasystole
j. rhythm
j. tachycardia

junctura, pl. **juncturae**
j. cartilaginea
juncturae cinguli membri superioris
j. fibrosa
j. lumbosacralis
juncturae membri inferioris liberi
juncturae membri superioris liberi
j. sacrococcygea
j. synovialis
juncturae tendinum
juncturae zygapophyseales

juncture
jungian psychoanalysis
jungle
j. fever
j. yellow fever
Jüngling's disease
Jung's muscle

Junin virus
Junod's boot
jurisprudence
dental j.
medical j.
justice
justo
j. major
j. minor
juvenile
j. absence epilepsy
j. angiofibroma
j. arrhythmia
j. arthritis
j. carcinoma
j. cataract
j. cell
j. cerebellar astrocytoma
j. chorea
j. chronic arthritis
j. cirrhosis
j. delinquent
j. diabetes
j. elastoma
j. epithelial corneal dystrophy
j. hemangiofibroma
j. hyalin fibromatosis
j. kyphosis
j. muscular atrophy
j. myoclonic epilepsy
j. neutrophil
j. osteomalacia
j. osteoporosis
j. palmo-plantar fibromatosis
j. papillomatosis
j. pattern
j. pelvis
j. periodontitis
j. polyp
j. retinoschisis
j. rheumatoid arthritis
j. spinal muscular atrophy
j. xanthogranuloma
juvenile-onset diabetes
juxta-articular nodules
juxtacortical
j. chondroma
j. osteogenic sarcoma
juxtacrine
juxtaepiphysial
juxta-esophageal
j.-e. lymph nodes
j.-e. pulmonary lymph nodes
juxtaglomerular
j. apparatus
j. body
j. cells

J

juxtaglomerular *(continued)*
   j. complex
   j. granules
juxta-intestinal lymph nodes
juxtallocortex

juxtaphrenic peak
juxtaposition
juxtapupillary choroiditis
juxtarestiform body

K

K antigens
K capture
K cells
K complex
K shell
K virus
kabure
k. itch
Kaffir pox
kafindo
Kaiserling's fixative
kakké
kala azar
kalemia
kaliopenia
kaliopenic
kaliuresis
kaliuretic
kallak
Kallikak
kallikrein system
Kallmann's syndrome
kaluresis
kaluretic
kang cancer
kangri
k. burn carcinoma
k. cancer
Kanner's syndrome
kanyemba
kaodzera
kaolinosis
Kaposi's
K. sarcoma
K. varicelliform eruption
kappa
k. angle
k. granule
k. particles
kappacism
Karman cannula
Karmen unit
Karnofsky scale
Kartagener's
K. syndrome
K. triad
karyochrome
k. cell
karyoclasis
karyocyte
karyogamic
karyogamy
karyogenesis
karyogenic

karyogonad
karyogram
karyology
karyolymph
karyolysis
karyolytic
karyomere
karyomicrosome
karyomitome
karyomorphism
karyon
karyophage
karyoplasm
karyoplasmolysis
karyoplast
karyoplastin
karyopyknosis
karyopyknotic
k. index
karyorrhexis
karyosome
karyostasis
karyotheca
karyotype
karyozoic
Kasabach-Merritt syndrome
kasai
Kasai operation
Kashin-Bek disease
Kasten's
K. fluorescent Feulgen stain
K. fluorescent PAS stain
K. fluorescent Schiff reagents
Katayama
K. disease
K. fever
K. syndrome
K. test
Kawasaki's
K. disease
K. syndrome
Kayser-Fleischer ring
Kazanjian's operation
K blood group, k blood group
Kearns-Sayre syndrome
Keating-Hart's method
ked
kedani fever
keeled chest
Keen's
K. operation
K. sign
Kegel's exercises
Kehr's sign
keirospasm

K

Keith
    K. bundle
    K. and Flack node
    K. node
kelectome
Kelev strain rabies virus
Kell blood group
Keller bunionectomy
Keller-Madlener operation
Kelly
    K. clamp
    K. operation
    K. rectal speculum
keloid
    acne k.
keloidosis
keloplasty
kelosomia
Kempner diet
Kennedy
    K. classification
    K. disease
    K. syndrome
Kenny's treatment
Kent-His bundle
Kent's bundle
Kenya fever
Kerandel's symptom
keratectasia
keratectomy
    photorefractive k.
keratiasis
keratic
    k. precipitates
keratin
    k. filaments
    k. pearl
keratinization
keratinized
    k. cell
keratinocyte
keratinophilic
keratinosome
keratinous
    k. cyst
keratitis
    actinic k.
    deep punctate k.
    dendriform k., dendritic k.
    diffuse deep k.
    Dimmer's k.
    disciform k.
    k. disciformis
    exposure k.
    fascicular k.
    filamentary k.
    k. filamentosa
    geographic k.
    herpetic k.
    interstitial k.
    lagophthalmic k.
    k. linearis migrans
    marginal k.
    metaherpetic k.
    mycotic k.
    neuroparalytic k.
    neurotrophic k.
    k. nummularis
    phlyctenular k.
    pneumococcal/suppurative k.
    polymorphic superficial k.
    k. profunda
    punctate k., k. punctata
    sclerosing k.
    scrofulous k.
    serpiginous k.
    k. sicca
    superficial linear k.
    superficial punctate k.
    trachomatous k.
    vascular k.
    vesicular k.
    xerotic k.
keratoacanthoma
keratoangioma
keratoatrophoderma
keratocele
keratoconjunctivitis
    atopic k.
    epidemic k.
    flash k.
    herpetic k.
    microsporidian k.
    k. sicca
    superior limbic k.
    ultraviolet k.
    vernal k.
    virus k.
keratoconus
keratocricoid
keratocyst
    odontogenic k.
keratocyte
keratoderma
    k. blennorrhagica
    k. blennorrhagicum
    k. eccentrica
    lymphedematous k.
    mutilating k.
    k. palmaris et plantaris
    palmoplantar k.
    k. plantare sulcatum
    punctate k.
    senile k.
    k. symmetrica
keratodermatitis

keratoectasia
keratoelastoidosis
    k. marginalis
keratoepithelioplasty
keratogenesis
keratogenetic
keratogenous
    k. membrane
keratoglobus
keratoglossus
keratography
keratohyal
keratohyalin
    k. granules
keratoid
    k. exanthema
keratoleptynsis
keratoleukoma
keratolysis
    k. exfoliativa
    pitted k.
    k. plantare sulcatum
keratolytic
keratoma
    k. disseminatum
    k. hereditarium mutilans
    k. malignum
    k. plantare sulcatum
    senile k.
keratomalacia
keratome
keratometer
keratometry
keratomileusis
keratomycosis
keratonosis
keratopachyderma
keratopathy
    band-shaped k.
    bullous k.
    climatic k.
    filamentary k.
    Labrador k.
    lipid k.
    neuroparalytic k.
    striate k.
    vesicular k.
keratophakia
keratophakic keratoplasty
keratoplasia
keratoplasty
    allopathic k.
    autogenous k.
    epikeratophakic k.
    heterogenous k.
    homogenous k.
    keratophakic k.
    lamellar k., layered k.

    nonpenetrating k.
    optical k.
    penetrating k.
    perforating k.
    refractive k.
    tectonic k.
    total k.
keratoprosthesis
keratorefractive surgery
keratorhexis, keratorrhexis
keratorus
keratoscleritis
keratoscope
keratoscopy
keratose
keratosic cones
keratosis, pl. keratoses
    actinic k.
    arsenical k.
    k. blennorrhagica
    k. diffusa fetalis
    k. follicularis
    k. follicularis contagiosa
    inverted follicular k.
    k. labialis
    lichenoid k.
    lichen planus-like k.
    k. nigricans
    k. obturans
    k. palmaris et plantaris
    k. pilaris atrophicans faciei
    k. punctata
    k. rubra figurata
    seborrheic k., k. seborrheica
    senile k., k. senilis
    solar k.
    tar k.
    k. vegetans
keratotome
keratotomy
    delimiting k.
    radial k.
    refractive k.
keraunophobia
Kerckring's
    K. center
    K. folds
    K. ossicle
    K. valves
kerion
    Celsus k.
Kerley
    K. A lines
    K. B lines
    K. C lines
kernel
kernicterus
Kernig's sign

K

Kernohan's notch
kern-plasma relation theory
keroid
kerotherapy
Kestenbaum
    K. number
    K. sign
ketoacidosis
ketoaciduria
    branched chain k.
ketogenic
    k. corticoids test
    k. diet
17-ketogenic steroid assay test
ketonemia
ketonimine dyes
ketonuria
    branched chain k.
ketosis
ketosis-prone diabetes
ketosis-resistant diabetes
ketosuria
ketotic
    k. hyperglycemia
    k. hyperglycinemia
Kety-Schmidt method
keV
Kew Gardens fever
key
    k. attachment
    k. ridge
    k. vein
keyhole
    k. deformity
    k. pupil
key-in-lock maneuver
keyway
    k. attachment
Ki-1+ lymphoma
kick
    atrial k.
    idioventricular k.
Kidd blood group
kidney
    amyloid k.
    Armanni-Ebstein k.
    arteriolosclerotic k.
    arteriosclerotic k.
    artificial k.
    Ask-Upmark k.
    atrophic k.
    k. basin
    cake k.
    k. carbuncle
    contracted k.
    cow k.
    crush k.
    cystic k.

    disk k.
    duplex k.
    fatty k.
    flea-bitten k.
    floating k.
    Formad's k.
    fused k.
    Goldblatt k.
    granular k.
    hind k.
    horseshoe k.
    medullary sponge k.
    middle k.
    mortar k.
    movable k.
    pancake k.
    pelvic k.
    polycystic k.
    putty k.
    pyelonephritic k.
    Rose-Bradford k.
    sclerotic k.
    sigmoid k.
    supernumerary k.
    thoracic k.
    wandering k.
    waxy k.
Kiel classification
Kienböck's
    K. atrophy
    K. disease
    K. dislocation
    K. unit
Kiernan's space
Kiesselbach's area
Kilham rat virus
Kilian's line
killer cells
Killian's
    K. bundle
    K. operation
    K. triangle
kilohertz
kilohm
kilojoule
kiloroentgen
kilovolt
Kimmelstiel-Wilson
    K.-W. disease
    K.-W. syndrome
Kimura's disease
kinanesthesia
kindling
kindred
    degree of k.
kinematic
    k. face-bow
    k. viscosity

kinematics
kinemometer
kineplastic amputation
kineplastics
kinesalgia
kinescope
kinesia
kinesialgia
kinesiatrics
kinesics
kinesimeter
kinesiology
kinesiometer
kinesioneurosis
kinesipathist
kinesipathy
kinesis
kinesitherapy
kinesophobia
kinesthesia
    kinesthesia k.
kinesthesiometer
kinesthesis
kinesthetic
    k. aura
    k. sense
kinetic
    k. ataxia
    k. energy
    k. perimetry
    k. strabismus
    k. system
    k. tremor
kinetocardiogram
kinetocardiograph
kinetochores
kinetogenic
kinetoplasm
kinetoplast
kinetoscope
kinetosome
kingdom
Kingella
    K. indologenes
    K. kingae
king's evil
Kingsley splint
kininogen
    high molecular weight k.
kink
    Lane's k.
kinked aorta
Kinkiang fever
kinky
    k. hair
    k. hair disease

kinky-hair
    k.-h. disease
    k.-h. disorder
kinocentrum
kinocilium
kinohapt
kinomometer
kinoplasm
kinoplasmic
kinship
Kinyoun stain
kion
Kirby-Bauer test
Kirkland knife
Kirk's amputation
Kirschner's
    K. apparatus
    K. wire
Kisch's reflex
Kisenyi sheep disease virus
Kjelland's forceps
Klapp's method
Klebsiella
    K. mobilis
    K. ozaenae
    K. pneumoniae
    K. pneumoniae subsp. ozaenae
    K. rhinoscleromatis
Klebs-Loeffler bacillus
kleeblattschädel
Kleihauer's stain
Kleine-Levin syndrome
Klein-Gumprecht shadow nuclei
Klein's muscle
Klenow fragment
kleptolagnia
kleptomania
kleptomaniac
kleptophobia
Klestadt's cyst
Klinger-Ludwig acid-thionin stain for
    sex chromatin
Klippel-Feil syndrome
Klippel-Trenaunay-Weber syndrome
Klumpke palsy
Klumpke's paralysis
Klüver-Barrera Luxol fast blue stain
Klüver-Bucy syndrome
Kluyvera
Km
    K. allotypes
    K. antigen
Knapp's
    K. streaks
    K. striae
knee
    Brodie's k.
    housemaid's k.

K

knee *(continued)*
    k. jerk
    k. joint
    locked k.
    k. phenomenon
    k. presentation
    k. reflex
kneecap
knee-chest position
knee-elbow position
knee-jerk reflex
Knemidokoptes
Kniest syndrome
knife, pl. **knives**
    amputation k.
    Beer's k.
    cartilage k.
    cautery k.
    electrode k.
    fistula k.
    free-hand k.
    gamma ray k.
    Goldman-Fox knives
    Graefe's k.
    hernia k.
    Humby k.
    Joseph k.
    Kirkland k.
    lenticular k.
    Liston's knives
    Merrifield k.
    k. needle
    valvotomy k.
knife-rest crystal
knismogenic
knismolagnia
knitting
knives (*pl. of* knife)
knob
    aortic k.
    Engelmann's basal k.'s
    malarial k.'s
knock
    pericardial k.
knock-knee
Knoll's glands
Knoop
    K. hardness number
    K. hardness test
Knoop hardness number
knot
    false k.'s, false k.'s of umbilical
      cord
    granny k.
    Hensen's k.
    Hubrecht's protochordal k.
    laparoscopic k.
    net k.

    primitive k.
    protochordal k.
    surgeon's k.
    syncytial k.
    true k., true k. of umbilical cord
    vital k.
knuckle
    aortic k.
    cervical aortic k.
    k. pads
Kobelt's tubules
Kober test
Köbner's phenomenon
Kocher
    K. clamp
    K. incision
    K. sign
Kocher-Debré-Sémélaigne syndrome
Koch's
    K. bacillus
    K. law
    K. node
    K. phenomenon
    K. postulates
    K. triangle
Koch-Weeks bacillus
Kock
    K. ileostomy
    K. pouch
Koenen's tumor
Koenig's syndrome
Koerber-Salus-Elschnig syndrome
Koerte-Ballance operation
Köhler
    K. disease
    K. illumination
Kohlmeier-Degos syndrome
Kohlrausch's
    K. muscle
    K. valves
Kohn's pores
Kohnstamm's phenomenon
koilocyte
koilocytosis
koilonychia
koilosternia
Kojewnikoff's epilepsy
kokoi venom
Kölliker's
    K. layer
    K. reticulum
Kollmann's dilator
Kolmer test
kolytic
Kommerell's diverticulum
Kondoleon operation
koniocortex
Konno procedure

Konno-Rastan procedure
Koongol viruses
Koplik's spots
kopophobia
Korean
    K. hemorrhagic fever
    K. hemorrhagic fever virus
Korff's fibers
koro
koronion
Korotkoff
    K. sounds
    K. test
Korsakoff's
    K. psychosis
    K. syndrome
Kossa stain
Kostmann syndrome
Krabbe's disease
kra-kra
Kraske's operation
kraurosis vulvae
Krause
    K. bone
    K. end bulbs
    K. glands
    K. graft
    K. ligament
    K. method
    K. muscle
    K. respiratory bundle
    K. valve
Krause-Wolfe graft
Kretschmann's space
Kreysig's sign
Krogh spirometer
Kromayer's lamp
Kronecker's stain
Krönig's
    K. isthmus
    K. steps
Krönlein
    K. hernia
    K. operation
Krueger instrument stop
Krukenberg's
    K. amputation
    K. spindle
    K. tumor
    K. veins
Kruse's brush
KUB
kubisagari, kubisagaru
Küersteiner's canals
Kufs disease
Kugelberg-Welander disease
Kugel's anastomotic artery

Kühne's
    K. fiber
    K. methylene blue
    K. phenomenon
    K. plate
    K. spindle
Kuhnt-Junius
    K.-J. degeneration
    K.-J. disease
Kuhnt's spaces
Kulchitsky cells
Külz's cylinder
Kümmell's spondylitis
Küntscher nail
Kupffer cells
Kürsteiner's canals
kurtosis
kuru
Kurunegala ulcers
Kurzrok-Ratner test
Kuskokwim syndrome
Kussmaul
    K. aphasia
    K. coma
    K. disease
    K. paradoxical pulse
    K. pulse
    K. respiration
    K. sign
    K. symptom
Kussmaul-Kien respiration
Kveim
    K. antigen
    K. test
Kveim-Stilzbach
    K.-S. antigen
    K.-S. test
kwashiorkor
    marasmic k.
Kyasanur
    K. Forest disease
    K. Forest disease virus
kyllosis
kymatism
kymogram
kymograph
kymography
kymoscope
kyphos
kyphoscoliosis
kyphoscoliotic pelvis
kyphosis
    juvenile k.
kyphotic
    k. pelvis
kyphotone
Kyrle's disease

K

L
    L doses
    L form
L_f (*var. of* Lf)
    L. dose
L_o (*var. of* Lo)
    L. dose
Laband's syndrome
Labbé's
    L. neurocirculatory syndrome
    L. triangle
    L. vein
label
la belle indifférence
labia (*pl. of* labium)
labial
    l. arch
    l. bar
    l. commissure
    l. embrasure
    l. flange
    l. gingiva
    l. glands
    l. hernia
    l. occlusion
    l. part of orbicularis oris muscle
    l. splint
    l. sulcus
    l. surface
    l. swelling
    l. tubercle
    l. veins
    l. vestibule
labialism
labially
labii (*gen. of* labium)
labile
    l. affect
    l. current
    l. elements
    l. factor
    l. hypertension
    l. pulse
labiocervical
labiochorea
labioclination
labiodental
    l. sulcus
labiogingival
    l. lamina
labioglossolaryngeal
labioglossopharyngeal
labiograph

labiolingual
    l. appliance
    l. plane
labiomental
labionasal
labiopalatine
labioplacement
labioplasty
labioscrotal
    l. folds
    l. swellings
labioversion
labitome
labium, gen. **labii**, pl. **labia**
    l. anterius ostii uteri
    l. externum cristae iliacae
    l. inferius oris
    l. internum cristae iliacae
    l. laterale lineae asperae
    l. limbi tympanicum laminae spiralis
    l. limbi vestibulare laminae spiralis
    l. majus
    l. majus pudendi, pl. labia majora
    l. mediale lineae asperae
    l. minus
    l. minus pudendi, pl. labia minora
    labia oris
    l. posterius ostii uteri
    l. superius oris
    tympanic l. of limbus of spiral lamina
    l. urethrae
    labia uteri
    vestibular l. of limbus of spiral lamina
    l. vocale, pl. labia vocalia
labor, third s
    active l.
    dry l.
    false l.
    missed l.
    l. pains
    precipitate l.
    premature l.
    stages of l.
laboratorian
laboratory
    l. diagnosis
    personal growth l.
labored respiration
labra (*pl. of* labrum)
Labrador keratopathy
labrale inferius
labrale superius

L

labrocyte
labrum, pl. **labra**
    acetabular l.
    l. acetabulare
    articular l.
    l. articulare
    glenoid l.
    l. glenoidale
labyrinth
    bony l.
    cochlear l.
    ethmoidal l.
    Ludwig's l.
    membranous l.
    osseous l.
    renal l.
    Santorini's l.
    vestibular l.
labyrinthectomy
labyrinthine
    l. angiospasm
    l. apoplexy
    l. artery
    l. nystagmus
    l. placenta
    l. reflexes
    l. righting reflexes
    l. torticollis
    l. veins
    l. vertigo
    l. wall of middle ear
labyrinthitis
labyrinthotomy
labyrinthus
    l. cochlearis
    l. ethmoidalis
    l. membranaceus
    l. osseus
    l. vestibularis
lacerable
lacerated
    l. foramen
laceration
    brain l.
    scalp l.
    through-and-through l.
    vaginal l.
lacertus
    l. cordis
    l. fibrosus
    l. of lateral rectus muscle
    l. medius
    l. musculi recti lateralis
Lachman test
lachrymal
laciniae tubae
laciniate ligament
lacis cell

Lac operon
lacrimal
    l. apparatus
    l. artery
    l. bay
    l. bone
    l. border of maxilla
    l. calculus
    l. canaliculus
    l. caruncle
    l. conjunctivitis
    l. fascia
    l. fistula
    l. fold
    l. fossa
    l. gland
    l. groove
    l. hamulus
    l. lake
    l. margin of maxilla
    l. nerve
    l. notch
    l. opening
    l. papilla
    l. part of orbicularis oculi muscle
    l. process
    l. punctum
    l. reflex
    l. sac
    l. vein
lacrimation
lacrimatory
lacrimoconchal suture
lacrimo-gustatory reflex
lacrimomaxillary suture
lacrimotomy
La Crosse virus
lactacidemia
lactacidosis
lactacid oxygen debt
lactate
    l. dehydrogenase virus
    excess l.
lactating adenoma
lactation
    l. amenorrhea
    l. hormone
lactational
    l. mastitis
lacteal
    central l.
    l. cyst
    l. fistula
    l. vessel
lactenin
lactic
    l. acid bacillus

l. acidemia
l. acidosis
lactiferous
l. ampulla
l. ducts
l. gland
l. sinus
lactigenous
lactigerous
Lactobacillaceae
lactobacillary milk
lactobacilli
Lactobacillus
L. acidophilus
L. bifidus
L. bifidus subsp. *pennsylvanicus*
L. brevis
L. buchneri
L. bulgaricus
L. casei
L. catenaformis
L. cellobiosus
L. confusus
L. coprophilus
L. coryniformis
L. crispatus
L. curvatus
L. delbrueckii
L. fermentum
L. fructivorans
L. helveticus
L. heterohiochi
L. hilgardii
L. homohiochii
L. jensenii
L. lactis
L. leichmannii
L. plantarum
L. salivarius
L. trichodes
L. viridescens
lactobacillus
lactocele
lactogenesis
lactogenic
lactorrhea
lactose intolerance
lactose-litmus agar
lactosuria
lactotherapy
lactovegetarian
lacuna, pl. **lacunae**
cartilage l.
cerebral l.
l. cerebri
Howship's lacunae
intervillous l.
lateral lacunae

lacunae laterales
lateral venous lacunae
l. magna
Morgagni's l.
muscular l.
l. musculorum
osseous l.
l. pharyngis
resorption lacunae
trophoblastic l.
urethral l.
l. urethralis, pl. lacunae urethrales
vascular l.
l. vasorum
lacunar
l. abscess
l. amnesia
l. ligament
l. state
l. tonsillitis
lacunule
lacus, pl. **lacus**
l. lacrimalis
l. seminalis
ladder splint
Ladd-Franklin theory
Ladd's
L. band
L. operation
Laelaps echidninus
Laënnec's
L. cirrhosis
L. pearls
Lafora
L. body
L. body disease
L. disease
lag
anaphase l.
homeostatic l.
jet l.
l. phase
lagging
lagophthalmia
lagophthalmic keratitis
lagophthalmos, lagophthalmia
Lahey forceps
Lahore sore
laimer triangle
lake
capillary l.
lacrimal l.
lateral l.'s
seminal l.
subchorial l.
venous l.'s
Laki-Lorand factor

L

laky
 l. blood
laliatry
laliophobia
Lallemand's bodies
lalling
Lallouette's pyramid
lalochezia
lalognosis
laloplegia
Lamaze method
Lam B
lambdacism
Lambda phage
lambdoid
 l. border of occipital bone
 l. margin of occipital bone
 l. suture
lambert
Lambert-Eaton syndrome
Lambert's syndrome
Lamblia intestinalis
Lambl's excrescences
lambo lambo
Lambrinudi operation
LAMB syndrome
lamella, pl. lamellae
 annulate lamellae
 articular l.
 l. of bone
 circumferential l.
 concentric l.
 cornoid l.
 elastic l.
 enamel l.
 glandulopreputial l.
 ground l.
 haversian l.
 intermediate l.
 interstitial l.
 triangular l.
 vitreous l.
lamellar
 l. bone
 l. cataract
 l. granule
 l. ichthyosis
 l. keratoplasty
lamellate, lamellated
lamellipodium, pl. lamellipodia
lamina, pl. laminae
 l. affixa
 l. alaris
 alar l. of neural tube
 laminae albae cerebelli
 l. anterior vaginae musculi recti
  abdominis
 l. arcus vertebrae

basal l.
basal l. of choroid
basal l. of ciliary body
basal l. of cochlear
l. basalis
l. basalis choroideae
l. basalis corporis ciliaris
basal l. of neural tube
basal l. of semicircular duct
basement l.
basilar l.
l. basilaris cochleae
boundary l.
l. cartilaginis cricoideae
l. cartilaginis lateralis tubae
 auditivae
l. cartilaginis medialis tubae
 auditivae
l. cartilaginis thyroideae
l. choriocapillaris
l. choroidea
l. choroidea epithelialis
l. choroidocapillaris
l. cinerea
l. cribrosa ossis ethmoidalis
l. cribrosa sclerae
cribrous l.
l. of cricoid cartilage
deep l.
l. densa
dental l.
l. dentata
dentogingival l.
l. dorsalis
l. dura
l. elastica anterior
l. elastica posterior
elastic laminae of arteries
episcleral l.
l. episcleralis
epithelial l.
l. epithelialis
l. externa cranii
l. fibrocartilaginea interpubica
l. fibroreticularis
l. fusca of sclera
l. fusca sclerae
hepatic laminae
l. horizontalis ossis palatini
l. interna cranii
internal medullary l.
l. internal ossium cranii
iridopupillary l.
labiogingival l.
lamina l.
lamina l. of semicircular duct
lateral l. of cartilaginous auditory
 tube

l. lateralis cartilaginis tubae
  auditivae
l. lateralis processus pterygoidei
lateral medullary l. of corpus
  striatum
l. of lens
l. limitans anterior corneae
l. limitans posterior corneae
l. lucida
medial l. of cartilaginous auditory
  tube
l. medialis cartilaginis tubae
  auditivae
l. medialis processus pterygoidei
medial medullary l. of corpus
  striatum
laminae medullares cerebelli
laminae medullares thalami
l. medullaris lateralis corporis
  striati
l. medullaris medialis corporis
  striati
medullary laminae of thalamus
l. membranacea cartilaginis tubae
  auditivae
membranous l. of cartilaginous
  auditory tube
l. of mesencephalic tectum
l. modioli
l. muscularis mucosae
orbital l. of ethmoid bone
l. orbitalis ossis ethmoidalis
osseous spiral l.
l. papyracea
l. parietalis
l. parietalis pericardii
l. parietalis tunicae vaginalis testis
periclaustral l.
l. perpendicularis
l. perpendicularis ossis ethmoidalis
l. perpendicularis ossis palatini
l. posterior vaginae musculi recti
  abdominis
l. pretrachealis
l. prevertebralis
primary dental l.
l. profunda
l. profunda fasciae temporalis
l. profunda musculi levatoris
  palpebrae superioris
l. propria mucosae
pterygoid laminae
l. quadrigemina
quadrigeminal l.
l. rara
reticular l.
l. of Rexed
rostral l.

l. rostralis
secondary spiral l.
l. septi pellucidi
l. of septum pellucidum
l. spiralis ossea
l. spiralis secundaria
substantia l. of cornea
superficial l.
l. superficialis
l. superficialis fasciae cervicalis
l. superficialis fasciae temporalis
l. superficialis musculi levatoris
  palpebrae superioris
suprachoroid l.
l. suprachoroidea
l. supraneuroporica
l. tecti mesencephali
l. terminalis cerebri
l. terminalis of cerebrum
l. of thyroid cartilage
l. tragi
l. of tragus
vascular l. of choroid
l. vasculosa choroideae
l. ventralis
l. of vertebral arch
l. visceralis
l. visceralis pericardii
l. visceralis tunicae vaginalis testis
l. vitrea
laminagram
laminagraph
laminagraphy, laminography
laminar
l. cortical necrosis
l. cortical sclerosis
l. flow
laminaria
laminated
l. clot
l. cortex
l. epithelial plug
l. epithelium
l. thrombus
lamination
laminectomy
laminography
laminography (*var. of* laminagraphy)
laminotomy
lamins
lamp
annealing l.
Edridge-Green l.
heat l.
Kromayer's l.
mercury vapor l.
mignon l.
slit l.

L

479

lamp (*continued*)
    spirit l.
    tungsten arc l.
    ultraviolet l.
    uviol l.
    Wood's l.
lampbrush chromosome
lamp-brush chromosome
Lan antigen
lance
Lancefield classification
lancet
    gum l.
    spring l.
    thumb l.
lancinating
Lancisi's sign
Landau-Kleffner syndrome
Landolfi's sign
Landouzy-Dejerine dystrophy
Landouzy-Grasset law
Landry
    L. paralysis
    L. syndrome
Landry-Guillain-Barré syndrome
Landschutz tumor
land scurvy
Landsteiner-Donath test
Landström's muscle
Landzert's fossa
Lane's
    L. band
    L. disease
    L. kink
    L. plates
Langenbeck's triangle
Langendorff's method
Langerhans'
    L. cells
    L. granule
    L. islands
Langer's
    L. arch
    L. lines
    L. muscle
Lange's
    L. solution
    L. test
Langhans'
    L. cells
    L. layer
    L. stria
Langhans'-type giant cells
Langley's granules
Langmuir trough
language
    body l.

    l. game
    l. zone
laniary
Lannelongue's
    L. foramina
    L. ligaments
Lanterman's
    L. incisures
    L. segments
lanthanic
lanthanum
    l. nitrate
lanuginous
lanugo
    l. hair
Lanz's line
laparectomy
laparocele
laparogastroscopy
laparohysterectomy
laparohystero-oophorectomy
laparohysteropexy
laparohysterosalpingo-oophorectomy
laparohysterotomy
laparomyomectomy
laparomyositis
laparorrhaphy
laparosalpingectomy
laparosalpingo-oophorectomy
laparosalpingotomy
laparoscope
laparoscopic
    l. cannula
    l. cholecystotomy
    l. knot
    l. surgery
laparoscopically assisted surgery
laparoscopic-assisted vaginal
    hysteroscopy
laparoscopy
    closed l.
    open l.
laparotomy
    l. pad
laparotrachelotomy
laparouterotomy
Lapicque's law
lapinization
lapinized
Laplace's
    L. forceps
    L. law
Laquer's stain for alcoholic hyalin
larbish
lardaceous
    l. liver
    l. spleen

large
l. bowel
l. cell carcinoma
l. cell lymphoma
l. interarch distance
l. intestine
l. muscle of helix
l. pelvis
l. pudendal lip
l. saphenous vein
l. vein
Larmor frequency
Laron type dwarfism
Laroyenne's operation
Larrey's
L. amputation
L. cleft
Larrey-Weil disease
Larsen's syndrome
larva, pl. **larvae**
l. currens
filariform l.
rhabditiform l.
larvaceous
larval
l. conjunctivitis
l. plague
larva migrans
cutaneous l. m.
ocular l. m.
spiruroid l. m.
visceral l. m.
larvate
larvicidal
larviparous
laryngeal
l. aperture
l. atresia
l. bursa
l. chorea
l. crisis
l. diphtheria
l. epilepsy
l. glands
l. granuloma
l. lymphatic follicles
l. mask
l. mucosa
l. papillomatosis
l. part of pharynx
l. pharynx
l. polyp
l. pouch
l. prominence
l. reflex
l. sinus
l. stenosis
l. stridor

l. syncope
l. tonsils
l. veins
l. ventricle
l. vertigo
laryngectomy
larynges (*pl. of* larynx)
laryngismus
l. stridulus
laryngitic
laryngitis
chronic subglottic l.
croupous l.
membranous l.
spasmodic l.
l. stridulosa
laryngocele
laryngofissure
laryngograph
laryngography
laryngology
laryngomalacia
laryngoparalysis
laryngopharyngeal
l. branches of superior cervical ganglion
laryngopharyngectomy
laryngopharyngeus
laryngopharyngitis
laryngopharynx
laryngophthisis
laryngoplasty
laryngoplegia
laryngoptosis
laryngoscope
laryngoscopic
laryngoscopist
laryngoscopy
direct l.
indirect l.
suspension l.
laryngospasm
laryngospastic reflex
laryngostenosis
laryngostomy
laryngostroboscope
laryngotomy
inferior l.
median l.
superior l.
laryngotracheal
l. diphtheria
l. diverticulum
l. groove
laryngotracheitis
laryngotracheobronchitis
larynx, pl. **larynges**
lase

L

Lasègue's
 L. disease
 L. sign
 L. syndrome
laser
 l. corepraxy
 l. iridotomy
 l. microscope
 l. photocoagulator
 pulsed dye l.
 l. trabeculoplasty
lasering
lash
Lash's operation
Lasiohelea
Lassa
 L. fever
 L. hemorrhagic fever
 L. virus
lassitude
latah
Latarget's
 L. nerve
 L. vein
late
 l. apical systolic murmur
 l. benign syphilis
 l. cyanosis
 l. deceleration
 l. diastole
 l. diastolic murmur
 l. juvenile type
 l. latent syphilis
 l. luteal phase dysphoric disorder
 l. neonatal death
 l. reaction
 l. replicating chromosome
 l. rickets
 l. seizure
 l. syphilis
 l. systole
latebra
latency
 l. period
 l. phase
latent
 l. adrenocortical insufficiency
 l. allergy
 l. carcinoma
 l. carrier
 l. coccidioidomycosis
 l. content
 l. diabetes
 l. empyema
 l. energy
 l. gout
 l. homosexuality
 l. hyperopia

 l. infection
 l. learning
 l. microbism
 l. nystagmus
 l. period
 l. rat virus
 l. reflex
 l. scarlatina
 l. schizophrenia
 l. stage
 l. syphilis
 l. tetany
 l. typhoid
 l. zone
late-phase response
latera (*pl. of* latus)
laterad
lateral
 l. aberrant thyroid carcinoma
 l. aberration
 l. alveolar abscess
 l. ampullar nerve
 l. angle of eye
 l. angle of scapula
 l. angle of uterus
 l. antebrachial cutaneous nerve
 l. anterior thoracic nerve
 l. aperture of the fourth ventricle
 l. arcuate ligament
 l. atlantoaxial joint
 l. atlantoepistrophic joint
 l. atrial vein
 l. basal branch
 l. basal segment
 l. bicipital groove
 l. border
 l. border of foot
 l. border of forearm
 l. border of humerus
 l. border of kidney
 l. border of nail
 l. border of scapula
 l. branches
 l. calcaneal branches of sural
  nerve
 l. canal
 l. canthus
 l. cartilage of nose
 l. cartilaginous layer
 l. central palmar space
 l. cerebral fissure
 l. cerebral fossa
 l. cerebral sulcus
 l. cervical nuclei
 l. circumflex artery of thigh
 l. circumflex femoral artery
 l. circumflex femoral veins
 l. collateral ligament of ankle

l. column
l. column of spinal cord
l. condylar inclination
l. condyle
l. condyle of femur
l. condyle of tibia
l. cord of brachial plexus
l. corticospinal tract
l. costal branch of internal thoracic artery
l. costotransverse ligament
l. cricoarytenoid muscle
l. crus
l. crus of facial canal
l. crus of the greater alar cartilage of the nose
l. crus of horizontal part of the facial canal
l. crus of the superficial inguinal ring
l. cuneate nucleus
l. cuneiform bone
l. curvature
l. cutaneous branch
l. cutaneous branches of intercostal nerves
l. cutaneous branches of ventral primary ramus of thoracic spinal nerves
l. cutaneous nerve of calf
l. cutaneous nerve of forearm
l. cutaneous nerve of thigh
l. decubitus radiograph
l. deep cervical lymph nodes
l. direct veins
l. dorsal cutaneous nerve
l. epicondylar crest
l. epicondylar ridge
l. epicondyle of femur
l. epicondyle of humerus
l. excursion
l. femoral circumflex artery
l. femoral cutaneous nerve
l. femoral tuberosity
l. fillet
l. folds
l. fossa of brain
l. frontobasal artery
l. funiculus
l. funiculus of spinal cord
l. geniculate body
l. ginglymus
l. glossoepiglottic fold
l. great muscle
l. ground bundle
l. group of axillary lymph nodes
l. head
l. hermaphroditism

l. horn
l. humeral epicondylitis
l. hypothalamic area
l. hypothalamic region
l. illumination
l. incisor
l. inferior genicular artery
l. inguinal fossa
l. interocclusal record
l. jugular lymph nodes
l. lacunae
l. lacunar lymph node
l. lacunar node
l. lakes
l. lamina of cartilaginous auditory tube
l. layer of cartilaginous auditory tube
l. lemniscus
l. ligament of elbow
l. ligament of knee
l. ligament of malleus
l. ligaments of the bladder
l. ligament of temporomandibular joint
l. ligament of wrist
l. limb
l. lingual swellings
l. lip of linea aspera
l. lithotomy
l. longitudinal arch of foot
l. longitudinal stria
l. lumbar intertransversarii muscles
l. lumbar intertransverse muscles
l. lumbocostal arch
l. malleolar arteries
l. malleolar ligament
l. malleolar network
l. malleolar subcutaneous bursa
l. malleolar surface of talus
l. malleolus
l. malleolus bursa
l. mammary branches
l. mammary branches of lateral cutaneous branches of intercostal nerves
l. mammary branches of lateral cutaneous branches of thoracic spinal nerves
l. mammary branches of lateral thoracic artery
l. margin
l. mass of atlas
l. mass of ethmoid bone
l. medullary lamina of corpus striatum
l. medullary syndrome
l. meniscus

L

lateral (*continued*)
l. mesoderm
l. midpalmar space
l. movement
l. myocardial infarction
l. nasal artery
l. nasal branches of anterior ethmoidal nerve
l. nasal fold
l. nasal primordium
l. nasal process
l. nasal prominence
l. nucleus of medulla oblongata
l. nucleus of thalamus
l. oblique radiograph
l. occipital artery
l. occipital sulcus
l. occipitotemporal gyrus
l. occlusion
l. orbitofrontal branch
l. palpebral commissure
l. palpebral ligament
l. palpebral raphe
l. part of longitudinal arch of foot
l. part of middle lobar branch of right superior pulmonary vein
l. part of occipital bone
l. part of posterior cervical intertransversarii muscles
l. part of sacrum
l. part of vaginal fornix
l. patellar retinaculum
l. pectoral nerve
l. pericardiac lymph nodes
l. periodontal abscess
l. periodontal cyst
l. pharyngeal space
l. plantar artery
l. plantar nerve
l. plate
l. plate mesoderm
l. plate of pterygoid process
l. pole
l. popliteal nerve
l. preoptic nucleus
l. process of calcaneal tuberosity
l. process of malleus
l. process of talus
l. projection
l. proprius bundle
l. pterygoid muscle
l. pterygoid plate
l. puboprostatic ligament
l. pyramidal fasciculus
l. pyramidal tract
l. ramus radiograph
l. recess of fourth ventricle
l. rectus muscle

l. rectus muscle of the head
l. recumbent position
l. region
l. region of neck
l. reticular nucleus
l. root of median nerve
l. root of optic tract
l. sacral artery
l. sacral crests
l. sacral veins
l. sacrococcygeal ligament
l. segment
l. semicircular canals
l. sinus
l. skull radiograph
l. spinal sclerosis
l. spinothalamic tract
l. splanchnic arteries
l. striate arteries
l. superficial cervical lymph nodes
l. superior genicular artery
l. supraclavicular nerve
l. supracondylar crest
l. supracondylar ridge
l. sural cutaneous nerve
l. surface
l. surface of arm
l. surface of fibula
l. surface of finger
l. surface of leg
l. surface of lower limb
l. surface of ovary
l. surface of testis
l. surface of tibia
l. surface of toe
l. surface of zygomatic bone
l. talocalcaneal ligament
l. tarsal artery
l. temporomandibular ligament
l. thalamic peduncle
l. thoracic artery
l. thoracic vein
l. thyrohyoid ligament
l. tuberal nuclei
l. tubercle of posterior process of talus
l. umbilical fold
l. umbilical ligament
l. vaginal wall smear
l. vastus muscle
l. vein of lateral ventricle
l. venous lacunae
l. ventral hernia
l. ventricle
l. vertigo
l. vestibular nucleus
l. wall of middle ear

l. wall of orbit
l. wall of tympanic cavity
lateralis
laterality
    crossed l.
lateralization
lateriflexion, lateriflection
lateris (*gen. of* latus)
lateroabdominal
laterodeviation
lateroduction
lateroflexion, lateroflection
lateroposition
lateropulsion
laterotorsion
laterotrusion
lateroversion
latex
    l. agglutination test
    l. fixation test
lathe
Latin square
latissimus dorsi muscle
latitude
    l. film
Latrodectus
    L. mactans
lattice corneal dystrophy
latticed layer
latus, gen. **lateris**, pl. **latera**
Latzko's cesarean section
laudable
    l. pus
laughing
    l. disease
    l. sickness
laughter reflex
Laugier's
    L. hernia
    L. sign
Laumonier's ganglion
Launois-Bensaude syndrome
Launois-Cléret syndrome
laurel fever
Laurence-Moon-Biedl syndrome
Laurer's canal
Lauth's
    L. canal
    L. ligament
    L. violet
lavage
Lavdovsky's nucleoid
Laverania
laveur
law
    all or none l.
    Ambard's l.'s
    Ångström's l.

Arndt's l.
l.'s of association
l. of average localization
Baer's l.
Baruch's l.
Beer's l.
Behring's l.
Bell-Magendie l.
Bell's l.
biogenetic l., l. of biogenesis
Bowditch's l.
Broadbent's l.
Bunsen-Roscoe l.
l. of constant numbers in ovulation
l. of contiguity
l. of contrary innervation
Courvoisier's l.
Dale-Feldberg l.
l. of denervation
Descartes' l.
Donders' l.
Du Bois-Reymond's l
Einthoven's l.
Elliott's l.
l. of excitation
Farr's l.
Fechner-Weber l.
Ferry-Porter l.
Flatau's l.
Galton's l.
Gerhardt-Semon l.
Godélier's l.
Gompertz' l.
Grasset's l.
l. of gravitation
Haeckel's l.
Halsted's l.
Hamburger's l.
Hardy-Weinberg l.
l. of the heart
Heidenhain's l.
Hellin's l.
Hilton's l.
Hooke's l.
l. of independent assortment
l. of initial value
l. of intestine
inverse square l.
l. of isochronism
Jackson's l.
Koch's l.
Landouzy-Grasset l.
Lapicque's l.
Laplace's l.
Le Chatelier's l.
Listing's l.
Louis' l.
Magendie's l.

L

law *(continued)*
>Marey's l.
>Marfan's l.
>Meltzer's l.
>Mendel's first l.
>Mendel's second l.
>l. of the minimum
>Müller's l.
>Nasse's l.
>Newton's l.
>Nysten's l.
>Ochoa's l.
>Pflüger's l.
>Plateau-Talbot l.
>Poiseuille's l.
>l. of polar excitation
>l. of priority
>Profeta's l.
>l. of recapitulation
>reciprocity l.
>l. of referred pain
>l. of refraction
>l. of regression to mean
>Ricco's l.
>Ritter's l.
>Roscoe-Bunsen l.
>Rosenbach's l.
>Rubner's l.'s of growth
>l. of segregation
>Semon's l.
>Sherrington's l.
>l. of similars
>Snell's l.
>Spallanzani's l.
>l. of specific nerve energies
>Starling's l.
>Tait's l.
>Thoma's l.'s
>van der Kolk's l.
>Virchow's l.
>Vogel's l.
>wallerian l.
>Weber-Fechner l.
>Weber's l.
>Weigert's l.
>Wilder's l. of initial value
>Williston's l.
>Wolff's l.

Lawrence-Seip syndrome
laxation
laxator tympani
layer
>ameloblastic l.
>anterior elastic l.
>anterior limiting l. of cornea
>anterior l. of rectus abdominis
> sheath
>bacillary l.

basal l.
basal cell l.
basal l. of choroid
basal l. of ciliary body
l. of Bechterew
blastodermic l.'s
brown l.
cambium l.
l.'s of cerebellar cortex
l.'s of cerebral cortex
cerebral l. of retina
Chievitz' l.
choriocapillary l., choroid
  capillary l.
circular l. of muscular coat
circular l.'s of muscular tunics
circular l. of tympanic membrane
claustral l.
clear l. of epidermis
columnar l.
conjunctival l. of bulb
conjunctival l. of eyelids
corneal l. of epidermis
cornified l. of nail
cutaneous l. of tympanic membrane
deep l.
deep gray l. of superior colliculus
deep l. of levator palpebrae
  superioris muscle
deep l. of temporalis fascia
deep white l. of superior colliculus
elastic l.'s of arteries
elastic l.'s of cornea
enamel l.
ependymal l.
epithelial l.'s
epithelial choroid l.
epitrichial l.
external nuclear l. of retina
fatty l. of superficial fascia
fibrous l.
fillet l.
fusiform l.
ganglionic l. of cerebellar cortex
ganglionic l. of cerebral cortex
ganglionic l. of optic nerve
ganglionic l. of retina
germ l.
germinative l.
germinative l. of nail
glomerular l. of olfactory bulb
granular l. of cerebellar cortex
granular l. of cerebellum
granular l.'s of cerebral cortex
granular l. of epidermis
granular l.'s of retina
granular l. of a vesicular ovarian
  follicle

gray l. of superior colliculus
half-value l.
Henle's l.
Henle's fiber l.
Henle's nervous l.
horny l. of epidermis
horny l. of nail
Huxley's l.
infragranular l.
intermediate l.
internal nuclear l. of retina
investing l. of deep cervical fascia
Kölliker's l.
Langhans' l.
lateral cartilaginous l.
lateral l. of cartilaginous auditory tube
latticed l.
limiting l.'s of cornea
longitudinal l. of muscular coat
longitudinal l.'s of muscular tunics
malpighian l.
mantle l.
marginal l.
medial cartilaginous l.
medial l. of cartilaginous auditory tube
medullary l.'s of thalamus
membranous l.
membranous l. of superficial fascia
meningeal l. of dura mater
Meynert's l.
middle gray l. of superior colliculus
molecular l.
molecular l. of cerebellar cortex
molecular l. of cerebellum
molecular l. of cerebral cortex
molecular l.'s of olfactory bulb
molecular l. of retina
multiform l.
muscular l. of mucosa
neural l. of optic retina
neural l. of retina
neuroepithelial l. of retina
Nitabuch's l.
nuclear l.'s of retina
odontoblastic l.
optic l.
orbital l. of ethmoid bone
osteogenetic l.
palisade l.
papillary l.
parietal l.
parietal l. of leptomeninges
parietal l. of serous pericardium
parietal l. of tunica vaginalis
perforated l. of sclera

periosteal l. of dura mater
pigmented l. of ciliary body
pigmented l. of iris
pigmented l. of retina
piriform neuron l.
l. of piriform neurons
plasma l.
plexiform l.
plexiform l. of cerebral cortex
plexiform l.'s of retina
polymorphous l.
posterior elastic l.
posterior limiting l. of cornea
posterior l. of rectus abdominis sheath
pretracheal l.
prevertebral l.
prickle cell l.
Purkinje's l.
pyramidal cell l.
radiate l. of tympanic membrane
reticular l. of corium
l.'s of retina
l. of rods and cones
rostral l.
Sattler's elastic l.
serous l. of peritoneum
l.'s of skin
sluggish l.
somatic l.
spindle-celled l.
spinous l.
splanchnic l.
still l.
subendocardial l.
subendothelial l.
subpapillary l.
subserous l.
superficial l.
superficial l. of deep cervical fascia
superficial gray l. of superior colliculus
superficial l. of the levator palpebrae superioris muscle
superficial l. of temporalis fascia
suprachoroid l.
Tomes' granular l.
vascular l.
vascular l. of choroid coat of eye
ventricular l.
visceral l.
visceral l. of serous pericardium
visceral l. of tunica vaginalis of testis
Waldeyer's zonal l.
Weil's basal l.
zonular l.

L

layered keratoplasty
lazaret, lazaretto
lazarine leprosy
LCAT deficiency
L-chain
    L.-c. disease
    L.-c. myeloma
LCM virus
l-cone
L-D body
LDH agent
LDL receptor disorder
L^+ dose
L_+ dose
L_r dose
LE
    L. body
    L. cell
    L. cell test
    L. factors
    L. phenomenon
Le
    L. antigens
    L. Chatelier's law
    L. Chatelier's principle
    L. Fort I fracture
    L. Fort II fracture
    L. Fort III craniofacial dysjunction
    L. Fort III fracture
    L. Fort osteotomy
    L. Fort's amputation
    L. Fort sound
lead
    ABC l.'s
    l. anemia
    augmented l.
    bipolar l.
    CB l.
    CF l.
    chest l.'s
    l. chromate
    CL l.
    l. colic
    CR l.
    direct l.
    l. encephalitis
    l. encephalopathy
    esophageal l.
    l. gout
    l. hydroxide stain
    indirect l.
    intracardiac l.
    limb l.
    l. line
    l. neuropathy
    l. palsy
    l. paralysis
    precordial l.'s

    semidirect l.'s
    standard limb l.
    l. stomatitis
    unipolar l.'s
    V l.
leader sequences
leading
    l. ancestor
    l. edge
lead-pipe
    l.-p. colon
    l.-p. rigidity
League of Red Cross Societies
leak point pressure
leapfrog position
Lear complex
learned
    l. drive
    l. helplessness
learning
    l. disability
    incidental l.
    insight l.
    latent l.
    passive l.
    rote l.
    l. set
    state-dependent l.
    l. theory
least
    l. diffusion circle
    l. squares
    l. squares estimator
leather-bottle stomach
Leber's
    L. hereditary optic atrophy
    L. idiopathic stellate neuroretinitis
    L. idiopathic stellate retinopathy
    L. plexus
Le Blood Group (*var. of* Lewis Blood Group)
lecithin
    l.-cholesterol l.
lecithin/sphingomyelin ratio
lecithoblast
LeCompte
    L. maneuver
    L. operation
Lederer's anemia
Ledermann formula
ledge
    dental l.
    enamel l.
leech
leeching
Leede-Rumpel phenomenon
Lee's ganglion
Leeuwenhoek's canals

leeway space
Lee-White method
left
   l. atrioventricular valve
   l. atrium of heart
   l. auricular appendage
   l. axis deviation
   l. branch
   l. colic artery
   l. colic flexure
   l. colic lymph nodes
   l. colic vein
   l. coronary artery
   l. coronary vein
   l. crus of atrioventricular bundle
   l. crus of diaphragm
   l. duct of caudate lobe
   l. fibrous trigone
   l. frontoanterior
   l. frontoposterior
   l. frontotransverse
   l. gastric artery
   l. gastric lymph nodes
   l. gastric vein
   l. gastroepiploic artery
   l. gastroepiploic lymph nodes
   l. gastroepiploic vein
   l. gastro-omental artery
   l. gastro-omental nodes
   l. gastroomental vein
   l. heart
   l. heart bypass
   l. hepatic artery
   l. hepatic duct
   l. hepatic veins
   l. inferior pulmonary vein
   l. lobe
   l. lobe of liver
   l. lumbar lymph nodes
   l. main bronchus
   l. mentoanterior
   l. mentoposterior
   l. mentotransverse
   l. occipitoanterior
   l. occipitoposterior
   l. occipitotransverse
   l. ovarian vein
   l. pulmonary artery
   l. sacroanterior
   l. sacroposterior
   l. sacrotransverse
   l. sagittal fissure
   l. superior intercostal vein
   l. superior pulmonary vein
   l. suprarenal vein
   l. testicular vein
   l. triangular ligament
   l. umbilical vein

   l. ventricle
   l. ventricular ejection time
   l. ventricular failure
   l. ventricular myomectomy
left-footed
left-handed
left-sided
   l.-s. appendicitis
   l.-s. heart failure
left-sidedness
   bilateral l.-s.
left-to-right shunt
left-ventricular assist device
leg
   l. of antihelix
   Barbados l.
   bow-l.
   elephant l.
   milk l.
   l. phenomenon
   restless l.'s
   rider's l.
   tennis l.
   white l.
legal
   l. blindness
   l. dentistry
   l. medicine
   l. psychiatry
Legal's test
Legendre's sign
Legg-Calvé-Perthes disease
Legg-Perthes disease
Legg's disease
Legionella
   L. bozemanii
   L. dumoffii
   L. feeleii
   L. gormanii
   L. longbeachae
   L. micdadei
   L. pneumophila
   L. wadsworthii
legionellosis
Legionnaire's disease
Leichtenstern's
   L. phenomenon
   L. sign
Leigh's disease
Leiner's disease
leiodermia
leiomyofibroma
leiomyoma
   l. cutis
   parasitic l.
   vascular l.
leiomyomatosis
leiomyomectomy

L

leiomyosarcoma
leiotrichous
Leipzig yellow
Leishman-Donovan body
Leishmania
    L. aethiopica
    L. braziliensis
    L. braziliensis braziliensis
    L. braziliensis guyanensis
    L. braziliensis panamensis
    L. donovani archibaldi
    L. donovani chagasi
    L. donovani donovani
    L. donovani infantum
    L. furunculosa
    L. major
    L. mexicana
    L. mexicana amazonensis
    L. mexicana garnhami
    L. mexicana mexicana
    L. mexicana pifanoi
    L. mexicana venezuelensis
    L. peruviana
    L. pifanoi
    L. tropica
    L. tropica major
    L. tropica mexicana
leishmaniasis
    acute cutaneous l.
    American l., l. americana
    anergic l.
    anthroponotic cutaneous l.
    chronic cutaneous l.
    cutaneous l.
    diffuse l.
    diffuse cutaneous l.
    disseminated cutaneous l.
    dry cutaneous l.
    infantile l.
    lupoid l.
    mucocutaneous l.
    nasopharyngeal l.
    New World l.
    Old World l.
    pseudolepromatous l.
    l. recidivans
    rural cutaneous l.
    l. tegumentaria diffusa
    urban cutaneous l.
    visceral l.
    wet cutaneous l.
    zoonotic cutaneous l.
leishmanin test
leishmaniosis
leishmanoid
    dermal l.
    post-kala azar dermal l.

Leishman's
    L. chrome cells
    L. stain
Leiter International Performance Scale
Lejeune syndrome
Lembert suture
lemic
lemmoblast
lemmocyte
lemniscal trigone
lemniscus, pl. **lemnisci**
    acoustic l.
    auditory l.
    gustatory l.
    lateral l.
    l. lateralis
    medial l.
    l. medialis
    spinal l.
    l. spinalis
    trigeminal l.
    l. trigeminalis
lemon yellow
Lendrum's phloxine-tartrazine stain
Lenègre's
    L. disease
    L. syndrome
length
    arch l.
    available arch l.
    crown-heel l.
    crown-rump l.
    greatest l.
    required arch l.
    resting l.
    spinal l.
length-breadth index
lengthening reaction
length-height index
Lenhossék's processes
Lennert
    L. classification
    L. lesion
    L. lymphoma
Lennox-Gastaut syndrome
Lennox syndrome
Lenoir's facet
lens
    achromatic l.
    acoustic l.
    aplanatic l.
    apochromatic l.
    aspheric l.
    astigmatic l.
    biconcave l.
    biconvex l.
    bifocal l.
    l. capsule

cataract l.
l. clock
compound l.
concave l.
concavoconcave l.
concavoconvex l.
contact l.
convex l.
convexoconcave l.
convexoconvex l.
corneal l.
crystalline l.
cylindrical l.
decentered l.
dislocation of l.
double concave l.
double convex l.
eye l.
field l.
Fresnel l.
immersion l.
lighthouse l.
meniscus l.
minus l.
multifocal l.
ocular l.
omnifocal l.
orthoscopic l.
periscopic l.
photochromic l.
l. pits
l. placodes
planoconcave l.
planoconvex l.
plus l.
safety l.
slab-off l.
spherical l.
spherocylindrical l.
l. stars
l. sutures
toric l.
trial l.'s
trifocal l.
l. vesicle
lensectomy
lens-induced uveitis
lensometer
lensopathy
lenticonus
lenticula
lenticular
l. ansa
l. apophysis
l. astigmatism
l. bone
l. capsule
l. colony

l. fasciculus
l. fossa
l. ganglion
l. knife
l. loop
l. nucleus
l. papillae
l. process of incus
l. progressive degeneration
l. syphilid
l. vesicle
lenticuli (*pl. of* lenticulus)
lenticulo-optic
lenticulopapular
lenticulostriate
l. arteries
lenticulothalamic
lenticulus, pl. **lenticuli**
lentiform
l. bone
l. nucleus
lentigines (*pl. of* lentigo)
lentiginosis
centrofacial l.
generalized l.
lentiglobus
lentigo, pl. **lentigines**
l. maligna
senile l.
solar l.
Lentivirinae
lentivirus
lentula, lentulo
leonine facies
leontiasis
l. ossea
leopard
l. fundus
l. retina
LEOPARD syndrome
Leopold's maneuvers
Lepehne-Pickworth stain
leper
lepidic
Lepidoptera
lepidosis
Lepore thalassemia
Leporipoxvirus
lepothrix
lepra
l. cells
leprechaunism
leprid
leprologist
leprology
leproma
lepromatous
l. leprosy

L

lepromin
   l. reaction
   l. test
leprosarium
leprose
leprosery
leprosy
   anesthetic l.
   articular l.
   l. bacillus
   borderline l.
   dimorphous l.
   dry l.
   histoid l.
   indeterminate l.
   lazarine l.
   lepromatous l.
   Lucio's l.
   macular l.
   Malabar l.
   mutilating l.
   nodular l.
   smooth l.
   trophoneurotic l.
   tuberculoid l.
leprotic
leprous
   l. neuropathy
leptocephalous
leptocephaly
leptochroa
leptochromatic
leptocyte
leptocytosis
leptodactylous
leptodermic
leptomeningeal
   l. carcinoma
   l. carcinomatosis
   l. cyst
   l. fibrosis
leptomeninges, leptomeninx,
   sing. **leptomeninx**
leptomeningitis
   basilar l.
leptomere
leptomonad
Leptomonas
leptonema
leptophonia
leptophonic
leptopodia
leptoprosopia
leptoprosopic
leptorrhine
leptoscope
leptosomatic, leptosomic

Leptospira
   L. interrogans
leptospiral jaundice
leptospire
leptospirosis
   anicteric l.
   l. icterohemorrhagica
leptospiruria
leptotene
leptothricosis
Leptothrix
Leptotrichia
   L. buccalis
Leptotrombidium
   L. akamushi
Leriche's
   L. operation
   L. syndrome
Leri's
   L. pleonosteosis
   L. sign
Leri-Weill
   L.-W. disease
   L.-W. syndrome
Lermoyez' syndrome
Lerner homeostasis
lesbian
lesbianism
Lesch-Nyhan syndrome
Leser-Trélat sign
lesion
   Baehr-Lohlein l.
   benign lymphoepithelial l.
   Bracht-Wachter l.
   caviar l.
   coin l. of lungs
   Councilman's l.
   Dreulofoy's l.
   Duret's l.
   Ghon's primary l.
   gross l.
   Hill-Sachs l.
   Janeway l.
   Lennert's l.
   Lohlein-Baehr l.
   lower motor neuron l.
   Mallory-Weiss l.
   precancerous l.
   radial sclerosing l.
   ring-wall l.
   supranuclear l.
   upper motor neuron l.
   wire-loop l.
lesser
   l. alar cartilages
   l. arterial circle of iris
   l. circulation
   l. cul-de-sac

l. curvature of stomach
l. horn of hyoid bone
l. internal cutaneous nerve
l. multangular bone
l. occipital nerve
l. omentum
l. palatine artery
l. palatine foramina
l. palatine nerves
l. pancreas
l. pelvis
l. peritoneal cavity
l. peritoneal sac
l. petrosal nerve
l. rhomboid muscle
l. ring of iris
l. sciatic notch
l. splanchnic nerve
l. superficial petrosal nerve
l. supraclavicular fossa
l. trochanter
l. tubercle of humerus
l. tuberosity of humerus
l. tympanic spine
l. vestibular glands
l. wing of sphenoid bone
l. zygomatic muscle

Lesser's triangle
Lesshaft's triangle
let-down reflex
lethal
clinical l.
l. coefficient
l. dwarfism
l. equivalent
l. factor
l. gene
genetic l.
l. midline granuloma
l. mutation

lethality
l. rate

lethargic hypnosis
lethargy
letter blindness
Letterer-Siwe disease
leucin
leucine hypoglycemia
leucine-induced hypoglycemia
leucinosis
leucinuria
Leucocytozoon
L. marchouxi
L. simondi
L. smithi
leucomethylene blue
Leuconostoc
L. mesenteroides

leuco patent blue
Leudet's tinnitus
leukanemia
leukapheresis
leukasmus
leukemia
acute lymphocytic l.
acute promyelocytic l.
adult T-cell l.
aleukemic l.
basophilic l., basophilocytic l.
l. cutis
embryonal l.
eosinophilic l., eosinophilocytic l.
granulocytic l.
hairy cell l.
leukemic l.
leukopenic l.
lymphatic l.
lymphoblastic l.
lymphocytic l.
lymphoid l.
mast cell l.
mature cell l.
megakaryocytic l.
meningeal l.
micromyeloblastic l.
mixed l., mixed cell l.
monocytic l.
murine l.
myeloblastic l.
myelocytic l., myelogenic l.,
  myelogenous l., myeloid l.
myelomonocytic l.
Naegeli type of monocytic l.
neutrophilic l.
plasma cell l.
polymorphocytic l.
Rieder cell l.
Schilling type of monocytic l.
splenic l.
stem cell l.
subleukemic l.

leukemic
l. hyperplastic gingivitis
l. leukemia
l. myelosis
l. reticuloendotheliosis
l. reticulosis
l. retinitis
l. retinopathy

leukemid
leukemogenesis
leukemogenic
leukemoid
l. reaction

leukemoid reaction
lymphocytic l. r.

L

leukemoid reaction *(continued)*
    monocytic l. r.
    myelocytic l. r.
    plasmocytic l. r.
leukin
leukoagglutinin
leukobilin
leukoblast
    granular l.
leukoblastosis
leukochloroma
leukocidin
leukocoria, leukokoria
leukocytactic
leukocytal
leukocytaxia, leukocytaxis
leukocyte
    acidophilic l.
    l. adherence assay test
    agranular l.
    l. bactericidal assay test
    basophilic l.
    l. common antigen
    l. cream
    cystinotic l.
    endothelial l.
    eosinophilic l.
    filament polymorphonuclear l.
    globular l.
    granular l.
    hyaline l.
    l. inclusions
    l. interferon
    mast l.
    motile l.
    multinuclear l.
    neutrophilic l.
    nonfilament polymorphonuclear l.
    nongranular l.
    nonmotile l.
    oxyphilic l.
    polymorphonuclear l., polynuclear l.
    segmented l.
    transitional l.
    Türk's l.
leukocythemia
leukocytic
    l. pyrogens
    l. sarcoma
leukocytoblast
leukocytoclasis
leukocytoclastic vasculitis
leukocytogenesis
leukocytoid
leukocytolysin
leukocytolysis
leukocytolytic
leukocytoma

leukocytometer
leukocytopenia
leukocytoplania
leukocytopoiesis
leukocytosis
    absolute l.
    agonal l.
    basophilic l.
    digestive l.
    distribution l.
    emotional l.
    eosinophilic l.
    lymphocytic l.
    monocytic l.
    neutrophilic l.
    l. of the newborn
    physiologic l.
    relative l.
    terminal l.
leukocytosis-promoting factor
leukocytotactic
leukocytotaxia
    negative l.
    positive l.
leukocytotoxin
Leukocytozoon
leukocyturia
leukoderma
    acquired l.
    l. acquisitum centrifugum
    l. colli
    syphilitic l.
leukodermatous
leukodontia
leukodystrophia
    l. cerebri progressiva
leukodystrophy
    adrenal l.
    l. with diffuse Rosenthal fiber
      formation
leukoedema
leukoencephalitis
    acute epidemic l.
    acute hemorrhagic l.
    acute necrotizing hemorrhagic l.
    sclerosing l.
    subacute sclerosing l.
leukoencephalopathy
    progressive multifocal l.
leukoerythroblastic anemia
leukoerythroblastosis
leukokeratosis
leukokinetic
leukokinetics
leukokoria *(var. of* leukocoria*)*
leukokoria
leukokraurosis
leukolymphosarcoma

leukolysin
leukolysis
leukolytic
leukoma
    adherent l.
leukomatous
leukomyelitis
    necrotizing hemorrhage l.
leukomyelopathy
leukon
leukonecrosis
leukonychia
    apparent l.
leukopathia, leukopathy
    acquired l.
    l. unguis
leukopedesis
leukopenia
    basophilic l.
    eosinophilic l.
    lymphocytic l.
    monocytic l.
    neutrophilic l.
leukopenic
    l. factor
    l. index
    l. leukemia
    l. myelosis
leukophlegmasia
    l. dolens
leukoplakia
    hairy l.
    l. vulvae
leukoplakic vulvitis
leukopoiesis
leukopoietic
leukorrhagia
leukorrhea
    menstrual l.
leukorrheal
leukosarcoma
leukosarcomatosis
leukosis
leukotactic
leukotaxia
leukotaxine
leukotaxis
leukotic
leukotome
leukotomy
    prefrontal l.
    transorbital l.
leukotoxin
leukotrichia
    l. annularis
leukotrichous
Leukovirus
Levaditi stain

levator
    l. anguli oris muscle
    l. ani muscle
    l. cushion
    l. hernia
    l. labii superioris alaeque nasi muscle
    l. labii superioris muscle
    l. muscle of thyroid gland
    l. palati muscle
    l. palpebrae superioris muscle
    l. prostatae muscle
    l. scapulae muscle
    l. swelling
    l. veli palatini muscle
levatores costarum muscles
Levay antigen
LeVeen shunt
level
    acoustic reference l.
    l. of aspiration
    background l.
    Clark's l.
    hearing l.
    sound pressure l.
    window l.
lever
    dental l.
leverage
Levinea
    L. amalonatica
    L. diversus
    L. malonatica
Levin tube
levitation
Leviviridae
levoatrio-cardinal vein
levocardia
levocardiogram
levoclination
levocycleduction
levocycloduction
levoduction
levogram
levophobia
levotorsion
levoversion
Levret's forceps
Lev's
    L. disease
    L. syndrome
levulosemia
levulosuria
Lewis Blood Group, Le Blood Group
Lewy bodies
Leyden-Möbius muscular dystrophy
Leyden's
    L. ataxia

L

495

Leyden's *(continued)*
    L. crystals
    L. neuritis
Leydig
    L. cell adenoma
    L. cells
leydigarche
Lf, L$_f$
    L. dose
Lhermitte's sign
liberomotor
libidinization
libidinous
libido
    object l.
    l. theory
Libman-Sacks
    L.-S. endocarditis
    L.-S. syndrome
Liborius' method
library
    gene l.
    l. screening
lice (*pl. of* louse)
licensed
    l. practical nurse
    l. vocational nurse
lichen
    l. acuminatus
    l. agrius
    l. albus
    l. amyloidosis
    l. annularis
    l. hemorrhagicus
    l. infantum
    l. iris
    l. myxedematosus
    l. nitidus
    l. nuchae
    l. obtusus
    oral (erosive) l. planus
    l. planopilaris
    l. planus
    l. planus annularis
    l. planus et acuminatus atrophicans
    l. planus follicularis
    l. planus hypertrophicus
    l. planus-like keratosis
    l. planus verrucosus
    l. ruber
    l. ruber moniliformis
    l. ruber planus
    l. ruber verrucosus
    l. sclerosus et atrophicus
    l. scrofulosorum
    l. simplex chronicus
    l. spinulosus
    l. striatus

    l. strophulosus
    l. syphiliticus
    tropical l., l. tropicus
    l. urticatus
    Wilson's l.
lichenification
lichenization
lichenoid
    l. amyloidosis
    l. dermatosis
    l. eczema
    l. keratosis
Lichtheim's sign
lid
    l. crutch spectacles
    granular l.'s
    lower l.
    l. reflex
    upper l.
lid-closure reaction
Liddell-Sherrington reflex
lie
    longitudinal l.
    oblique l.
    transverse l.
lieberkühn
Lieberkühn's
    L. crypts
    L. follicles
    L. glands
Liebermann-Burchard test
Liebermeister's rule
lie detector
lien
    l. accessorius
    l. mobilis
    l. succenturiatus
lienal
    l. artery
lienculus
lienectomy
lienomedullary
lienomyelogenous
lienopancreatic
lienophrenic ligament
lienorenal
    l. ligament
lienteric
    l. diarrhea
lientery
lienunculus
Liesegang rings
Lieutaud's
    L. body
    L. triangle
    L. trigone
    L. uvula

life
  l. cycle
  l. events
  half-l.
  l. instinct
  postnatal l.
  prenatal l.
  sexual l.
  l. stress
  l. table
  vegetative l.
life-belt cataract
lifespan
life-span development
life-style
Li-Fraumeni cancer syndrome
ligament
  accessory l.'s
  accessory plantar l.'s
  accessory volar l.'s
  acromioclavicular l.
  alar l.'s
  alveolodental l.
  annular l.
  annular l. of the radius
  annular l. of the stapes
  annular l.'s of the trachea
  anococcygeal l.
  anterior costotransverse l.
  anterior cruciate l.
  anterior l. of head of fibula
  anterior l. of Helmholtz
  anterior longitudinal l.
  anterior l. of malleus
  anterior meniscofemoral l.
  anterior sacrococcygeal l.
  anterior sacroiliac l.'s
  anterior sacrosciatic l.
  anterior sternoclavicular l.
  anterior talofibular l.
  anterior talotibial l.
  anterior tibiofibular l.
  anterior tibiotalar l.
  apical l. of dens
  Arantius' l.
  arcuate popliteal l.
  arcuate pubic l.
  arterial l.
  l.'s of auditory ossicles
  auricular l.'s
  axis l. of malleus
  Bardinet's l.
  Barkow's l.'s
  Bellini's l.
  Berry's l.'s
  Bertin's l.
  Bichat's l.
  bifurcate l.

bifurcated l.
Bigelow's l.
Botallo's l.
Bourgery's l.
broad l. of the uterus
Brodie's l.
Burns' l.
calcaneocuboid l.
calcaneofibular l.
calcaneonavicular l.
calcaneotibial l.
Caldani's l.
Campbell's l.
Camper's l.
capsular l.
cardinal l.
caroticoclinoid l.
carpometacarpal l.'s
caudal l.
ceratocricoid l.
cervical l. of uterus
check l.'s of eyeball, medial and
  lateral
check l.'s of odontoid
chondroxiphoid l.
ciliary l.
Civinini's l.
Clado's l.
collateral l.
Colles' l.
conoid l.
Cooper's l.'s
coracoacromial l.
coracoclavicular l.
coracohumeral l.
corniculopharyngeal l.
coronary l. of knee
coronary l. of liver
costoclavicular l.
costocolic l.
costotransverse l.
costoxiphoid l.
cotyloid l.
Cowper's l.
cricopharyngeal l.
cricosantorinian l.
cricothyroid l.
cricotracheal l.
crucial l.
cruciate l. of the atlas
cruciate l.'s of knee
cruciate l. of leg
cruciform l. of atlas
Cruveilhier's l.'s
cuboideonavicular l.'s
cuneocuboid l.'s
cuneonavicular l.'s
cystoduodenal l.

ligament *(continued)*

deep dorsal sacrococcygeal l.
deep posterior sacrococcygeal l.
deep transverse metacarpal l.
deep transverse metatarsal l.
deltoid l.
Denonvilliers' l.
dentate l. of spinal cord
denticulate l.
Denucé's l.
diaphragmatic l. of the
  mesonephros
dorsal calcaneocuboid l.
dorsal carpal l.
dorsal carpometacarpal l.'s
dorsal cuboideonavicular l.
dorsal cuneocuboid l.
dorsal cuneonavicular l.'s
dorsal metacarpal l.'s
dorsal metatarsal l.'s
dorsal radiocarpal l.
dorsal sacroiliac l.'s
dorsal talonavicular l.
duodenorenal l.
l. of epididymis
epihyal l.
external collateral l. of wrist
extracapsular l.'s
falciform l.
falciform l. of liver
fallopian l.
Ferrein's l.
fibular collateral l.
fibular collateral l. of ankle
Flood's l.
fundiform l. of foot
fundiform l. of penis
gastrocolic l.
gastrodiaphragmatic l.
gastrolienal l.
gastrophrenic l.
gastrosplenic l.
genital l.
genitoinguinal l.
Gerdy's l.
Gillette's suspensory l.
Gimbernat's l.
gingivodental l.
glenohumeral l.'s
glenoid l.
glossoepiglottic l.
Günz' l.
hammock l.
l. of head of femur
Helmholtz' axis l.
Hensing's l.
hepatocolic l.
hepatoduodenal l.

hepatoesophageal l.
hepatogastric l.
hepatorenal l.
Hesselbach's l.
Hey's l.
Holl's l.
Hueck's l.
Humphry's l.
Hunter's l.
hyalocapsular l.
hyoepiglottic l.
hypsiloid l.
iliofemoral l.
iliolumbar l.
iliopectineal l.
iliotrochanteric l.
inferior calcaneonavicular l.
inferior l. of epididymis
inferior pubic l.
inferior transverse scapular l.
infundibulo-ovarian l.
infundibulopelvic l.
inguinal l.
inguinal l. of the kidney
intercarpal l.'s
interclavicular l.
interclinoid l.
intercornual l.
intercostal l.'s
intercuneiform l.'s
interfoveolar l.
internal collateral l. of the wrist
interosseous cuneocuboid l.
interosseous cuneometatarsal l.'s
interosseous metacarpal l.'s
interosseous metatarsal l.'s
interosseous sacroiliac l.'s
interosseous talocalcaneal l.
interosseous tibiofibular l.
interspinous l.
intertransverse l.
intra-articular l. of costal head
intra-articular sternocostal l.
intracapsular l.'s
ischiocapsular l.
ischiofemoral l.
Jarjavay's l.
jugal l.
Krause's l.
laciniate l.
lacunar l.
Lannelongue's l.'s
lateral arcuate l.
lateral l.'s of the bladder
lateral collateral l. of ankle
lateral costotransverse l.
lateral l. of elbow
lateral l. of knee

lateral malleolar l.
lateral l. of malleus
lateral palpebral l.
lateral puboprostatic l.
lateral sacrococcygeal l.
lateral talocalcaneal l.
lateral temporomandibular l.
lateral l. of temporomandibular joint
lateral thyrohyoid l.
lateral umbilical l.
lateral l. of wrist
Lauth's l.
l. of left superior vena cava
left triangular l.
l. of left vena cava
lienophrenic l.
lienorenal l.
Lisfranc's l.'s
Lockwood's l.
longitudinal l.
long plantar l.
lumbocostal l.
Luschka's l.'s
Mackenrodt's l.
l.'s of malleus
Mauchart's l.'s
Meckel's l.
medial l.
medial arcuate l.
medial collateral l. of elbow
medial l. of knee
medial palpebral l.
medial puboprostatic l.
medial talocalcaneal l.
medial l. of talocrural joint
medial umbilical l.
medial l. of wrist
median arcuate l.
median thyrohyoid l.
median umbilical l.
meniscofemoral l.'s
middle costotransverse l.
middle umbilical l.
nuchal l.
oblique l. of elbow joint
oblique popliteal l.
occipitoaxial l.'s
odontoid l.
orbicular l.
orbicular l. of radius
ovarian l.
palmar l.'s
palmar carpal l.
palmar carpometacarpal l.'s
palmar metacarpal l.'s
palmar radiocarpal l.
palmar ulnocarpal l.

patellar l.
pectinate l.'s of iridocorneal angle
pectinate l.'s of iris
pectineal l.
peridental l.
periodontal l.
Petit's l.
phrenicocolic l.
phrenicolienal l.
phrenicosplenic l.
phrenogastric l.
phrenosplenic l.
pisohamate l.
pisometacarpal l.
pisounciform l.
pisouncinate l.
plantar l.'s
plantar calcaneocuboid l.
plantar calcaneonavicular l.
plantar cuboideonavicular l.
plantar cuneocuboid l.
plantar cuneonavicular l.'s
plantar metatarsal l.'s
posterior costotransverse l.
posterior cricoarytenoid l.
posterior cruciate l.
posterior l. of head of fibula
posterior l. of incus
posterior l. of knee
posterior longitudinal l.
posterior meniscofemoral l.
posterior occipitoaxial l.
posterior sacroiliac l.'s
posterior sacrosciatic l.
posterior sternoclavicular l.
posterior talofibular l.
posterior talotibial l.
posterior tibiofibular l.
posterior tibiotalar l.
Poupart's l.
proper l. of ovary
pterygomandibular l.
pterygospinal l.
pterygospinous l.
pubocapsular l.
pubofemoral l.
puboprostatic l.
pubovesical l.
pulmonary l.
quadrate l.
radial collateral l.
radial collateral l. of elbow
radial collateral l. of wrist
radiate l.
radiate l. of head of rib
radiate sternocostal l.'s
radiate l. of wrist
reflected inguinal l.

L

ligament *(continued)*
  reflex l.
  Retzius' l.
  rhomboid l.
  right triangular l.
  ring l.
  round l. of elbow joint
  round l. of femur
  round l. of liver
  round l. of uterus
  sacrodural l.
  sacrospinous l.
  sacrotuberous l.
  serous l.
  sheath l.'s
  Simonart's l.'s
  Soemmerring's l.
  sphenomandibular l.
  spinoglenoid l.
  spiral l. of cochlea
  splenorenal l.
  spring l.
  Stanley's cervical l.'s
  stellate l.
  sternoclavicular l.
  sternopericardial l.
  stylohyoid l.
  stylomandibular l.
  stylomaxillary l.
  superficial dorsal sacrococcygeal l.
  superficial posterior
    sacrococcygeal l.
  superficial transverse metacarpal l.
  superficial transverse metatarsal l.
  superior costotransverse l.
  superior l. of epididymis
  superior l. of incus
  superior l. of malleus
  superior pubic l.
  superior transverse scapular l.
  suprascapular l.
  supraspinous l.
  suspensory l. of axilla
  suspensory l.'s of breast
  suspensory l. of clitoris
  suspensory l.'s of Cooper
  suspensory l. of esophagus
  suspensory l. of eyeball
  suspensory l. of gonad
  suspensory l. of lens
  suspensory l. of ovary
  suspensory l. of penis
  suspensory l. of testis
  suspensory l. of thyroid gland
  sutural l.
  synovial l.
  talocalcaneal l.
  talonavicular l.

  tarsal l.'s
  tarsometatarsal l.'s
  temporomandibular l.
  Teutleben's l.
  Thompson's l.
  thyroepiglottic l.,
    thyroepiglottidean l.
  tibial collateral l.
  tibiocalcaneal l.
  tibiofibular l.
  tibionavicular l.
  transverse l. of acetabulum
  transverse atlantal l.
  transverse l. of the atlas
  transverse carpal l.
  transverse crural l.
  transverse l. of elbow
  transverse genicular l.
  transverse humeral l.
  transverse l. of knee
  transverse l. of leg
  transverse metacarpal l.
  transverse metatarsal l.
  transverse l. of pelvis
  transverse perineal l.
  transverse l. of perineum
  transverse tibiofibular l.
  trapezoid l.
  Treitz's l.
  triangular l.
  triangular l.'s of liver
  ulnar collateral l.
  ulnar collateral l. of elbow
  ulnar collateral l. of wrist
  urachal l.
  uterosacral l.
  uterovesical l.
  Valsalva's l.'s
  venous l.
  ventral sacrococcygeal l.
  ventral sacroiliac l.'s
  ventricular l.
  vertebropelvic l.'s
  vesicoumbilical l.
  vesicouterine l.
  vestibular l.
  vocal l.
  volar carpal l.
  Weitbrecht's l.
  Winslow's l.
  Wrisberg's l.
  yellow l.
  Y-shaped l.
  Zaglas' l.
  Zinn's l.
ligamenta (*pl. of* ligamentum)
ligamentopexis, ligamentopexy

ligamentous
ligamentum, pl. **ligamenta**
l. acromioclaviculare
ligamenta alaria
l. annulare
l. annulare bulbi
l. annulare digitorum
l. annulare radii
l. annulare stapedis
ligamenta annularia trachealia
l. anococcygeum
l. apicis dentis
l. arcuatum laterale
l. arcuatum mediale
l. arcuatum medianum
l. arcuatum pubis
l. arteriosum
ligamenta auricularia, l. auriculare
  anterius, l. auriculare posterius, l.
  auriculare superius
l. bifurcatum
l. calcaneocuboideum
l. calcaneocuboideum plantare
l. calcaneofibulare
l. calcaneonaviculare
l. calcaneonaviculare plantare
l. calcaneotibiale
l. capitis costae intra-articulare
l. capitis costae radiatum
l. capitis femoris
l. capitis fibulae anterius
l. capitis fibulae posterius
ligamenta capitulorum transversa
l. capsulare
l. carpi dorsale
l. carpi radiatum
l. carpi transversum
l. carpi volare
ligamenta carpometacarpalia
l. carpometacarpalia dorsalia
l. carpometacarpalia palmaria
l. caudale
l. ceratocricoideum
l. collaterale, pl. ligamenta
  collateralia
l. collaterale carpi radiale
l. collaterale carpi ulnare
l. collaterale fibulare
l. collaterale radiale
l. collaterale tibiale
l. collaterale ulnare
ligamenta collateralia (*pl. of* l.
  collaterale)
l. colli costae
l. conoideum
l. coracoacromiale
l. coracoclaviculare
l. coracohumerale

l. corniculopharyngeum
l. coronarium hepatis
l. costoclaviculare
l. costotransversarium
l. costotransversarium anterius
l. costotransversarium laterale
l. costotransversarium posterius
l. costotransversarium superius
l. costoxiphoideum
l. cotyloideum
l. cricoarytenoideum posterius
l. cricopharyngeum
l. cricothyroideum
l. cricotracheale
ligamenta cruciata digitorum
ligamenta cruciata genus
l. cruciatum anterius
l. cruciatum atlantis
l. cruciatum cruris
l. cruciatum posterius
l. cruciatum tertium genus
l. cruciforme atlantis
l. cuboideonavicular
l. cuboideonaviculare dorsale
l. cuboideonaviculare plantare
l. cuneocuboidenum
l. cuneocuboideum dorsale
l. cuneocuboideum interosseum
l. cuneocuboideum plantare
ligamenta cuneometatarsalia
  interossea
l. cuneonaviculare plantare
ligamenta cuneonavicularia dorsalia
l. cuneonavicularia plantaria
l. deltoideum
l. denticulatum
l. ductus venosi
l. duodenorenale
l. epididymidis
l. epididymidis inferius
l. epididymidis superius
ligamenta extracapsularia
l. falciforme
l. falciforme hepatis
l. flavum
l. fundiforme penis
l. gastrocolicum
l. gastrolienale
l. gastrophrenicum
l. gastrosplenicum
l. genitoinguinale
ligamenta glenohumeralia
l. glenoidale
l. hepatocolicum
l. hepatoduodenale
l. hepatoesophageum
l. hepatogastricum
l. hepatorenale

L

ligamentum *(continued)*
l. hyaloideo-capsulario
l. hyoepiglotticum
l. hyothyroideum laterale
l. hyothyroideum medium
l. iliofemorale
l. iliolumbale
l. iliopectineale
l. incudis posterius
l. incudis superius
l. inguinale
ligamenta intercarpalia, l.
   intercarpalia palmaria
l. intercarpalia dorsalia
l. intercarpalia interossea
l. intercarpalia palmaria
l. interclaviculare
ligamenta intercostalia
ligamenta intercuneiformia, l.
   intercuneiformia plantaria
l. intercuneiformia dorsalia
l. intercuneiformia interossea
l. intercuneiformia plantaria
l. interfoveolare
l. interspinale
l. intertransversarium
ligamenta intracapsularia
l. ischiocapsulare
l. ischiofemorale
l. jugale
l. laciniatum
l. lacunare
l. laterale articulationis
   temporomandibularis
l. latum pulmonis
l. latum uteri
l. lienorenale
l. longitudinale
l. longitudinale anterius
l. longitudinale posterius
l. lumbocostale
l. mallei anterius
l. mallei laterale
l. mallei superius
l. malleoli lateralis
l. mediale articulationis talocruralis
l. mediale articulationis
   temporomandibularis
l. medialis
l. menisci lateralis
ligamenta meniscofemorale
l. meniscofemorale anterius
l. meniscofemorale posterius
l. metacarpale transversum
   profundum
l. metacarpale transversum
   superficiale
ligamenta metacarpalia dorsalia

ligamenta metacarpalia interossea
ligamenta metacarpalia palmaria
l. metatarsale transversum
   profundum
l. metatarsale transversum
   superficiale
ligamenta metatarsalia dorsalia
ligamenta metatarsalia interossea
ligamenta metatarsalia plantaria
l. natatorium
ligamenta navicularicuneiformia
l. nuchae
l. orbiculare radii
ligamenta ossiculorum auditus
l. ovarii proprium
ligamenta palmaria
l. palpebrale externum
l. palpebrale laterale
l. palpebrale mediale
l. patellae
l. pectinatum
l. pectinatum anguli iridocornealis
l. pectinatum iridis
l. pectineale
l. phrenicocolicum
l. phrenicolienale
l. phrenicosplenicum
l. pisohamatum
l. pisometacarpeum
l. plantare longum
ligamenta plantaria
l. popliteum arcuatum
l. popliteum obliquum
l. pterygospinale
l. pubicum superius
l. pubocapsulare
l. pubofemorale
l. puboprostaticum
l. puboprostaticum laterale
l. puboprostaticum mediale
l. pubovesicale
l. pulmonale
l. quadratum
l. radiatum
l. radiocarpale dorsale
l. radiocarpale palmare
l. reflexum
l. sacrococcygeum anterius
l. sacrococcygeum laterale
l. sacrococcygeum posterius
   profundum
l. sacrococcygeum posterius
   superficiale
l. sacrodurale
ligamenta sacroiliaca anteriora
ligamenta sacroiliaca interossea
ligamenta sacroiliaca posteriora
l. sacroiliacum posterius

l. sacrospinale
l. sacrospinosum
l. sacrotuberale
l. sacrotuberosum
l. serosum
l. sphenomandibulare
l. spirale cochleae
l. splenorenale
l. sternoclaviculare
l. sternoclaviculare anterius
l. sternoclaviculare posterius
l. sternocostale intra-articulare
ligamenta sternocostalia radiata
ligamenta sternopericardiaca
l. stylohyoideum
l. stylomandibulare
l. supraspinale
ligamenta suspensoria mammae
l. suspensorium clitoridis
l. suspensorium ovarii
l. suspensorium penis
l. talocalcaneare
l. talocalcaneare interosseum
l. talocalcaneare laterale
l. talocalcaneare mediale
l. talofibulare anterius
l. talofibulare posterius
l. talonaviculare
l. talotibiale anterius
l. talotibiale posterius
l. tarsale externum
l. tarsale internum
ligamenta tarsi, l. tarsi dorsalia, l.
    tarsi interossea, l. tarsi plantaria
ligamenta tarsometatarsalia
l. temporomandibulare
l. teres femoris
l. teres hepatis
l. teres uteri
l. testis
l. thyroepiglotticum
l. thyrohyoideum laterale
l. thyrohyoideum medianum
l. tibiofibulare anterius
l. tibiofibulare medium
l. tibiofibulare posterius
l. tibionaviculare
ligamenta trachealia
l. transversale colli
l. transversum acetabuli
l. transversum atlantis
l. transversum cruris
l. transversum genus
l. transversum pelvis
l. transversum perinei
l. transversum scapulae inferius
l. transversum scapulae superius
l. trapezoideum

l. triangulare
l. triangulare dextrum
l. triangulare sinistrum
l. tuberculi costae
l. ulnocarpale palmare
l. umbilicale laterale
l. umbilicale mediale
l. umbilicale medianum
l. venae cavae sinistrae
l. venosum
l. ventriculare
l. vestibulare
l. vocale
ligand
    addressing l.'s
ligand-gated channel
ligate
ligation
    pole l.
    surgical l.
    tooth l.
    tubal l.
ligator
ligature
    elastic l.
    intravascular l.
    nonabsorbable l.
    occluding l.
    provisional l.
    soluble l.
    Stannius l.
    suboccluding l.
    suture l.
    l. wire
light
    l. adaptation
    l. bath
    l. cells of thyroid
    l. chain-related amyloidosis
    l. difference
    l. differential threshold
    l. green SF yellowish
    infrared l.
    invisible l.
    l. micrograph
    l. microscope
    minimum l.
    polarized l.
    reflected l.
    l. reflex
    refracted l.
    l. sense
    l. sleep
    transmitted l.
    l. treatment
    l. wire appliance
    Wood's l.
light-activated resin

L

light-adapted eye
light-cured resin
lightening
lighthouse lens
light-near dissociation
lightning strip
light-touch palpation
Lignac-Fanconi syndrome
ligneous
    l. conjunctivitis
    l. struma
    l. thyroiditis
likelihood
Likert scale
Lillie's
    L. allochrome connective tissue stain
    L. azure-eosin stain
    L. ferrous iron stain
    L. sulfuric acid Nile blue stain
lilliputian hallucination
limb
    ampullary l.'s of semicircular ducts
    anacrotic l.
    anterior l. of internal capsule
    anterior l. of stapes
    l.'s of bony semicircular canals
    l. bud
    common l. of membranous semicircular ducts
    l. of helix
    inferior l.
    lateral l.
    l. lead
    lower l.
    medial l.
    l. myokymia
    pelvic l.
    phantom l.
    posterior l. of internal capsule
    posterior l. of stapes
    retrolenticular l. of internal capsule
    simple membranous l. of semicircular duct
    sublenticular l. of internal capsule
    superior l.
    thoracic l.
    upper l.
limb-girdle muscular dystrophy
limbi (*pl. of* limbus)
limbic
    l. lobe
    l. system
limb-kinetic apraxia
limbus, pl. limbi
    l. acetabuli
    l. alveolaris
    l. of bony spiral lamina

    l. of cornea
    l. corneae
    l. fossae ovalis
    l. laminae spiralis osseae
    l. membranae tympani
    limbi palpebrales
    l. palpebrales anteriores
    l. penicillatus
    l. striatus
    l. of tympanic membrane
    Vieussens' l.
limen, pl. limina
    l. insulae
    l. nasi
limerence
liminal
    l. stimulus
    l. trait
liminometer
limit
    l. dextrinosis
    Hayflick's l.
    permissible exposure l.
    quantum l.
limited range audiometer
limiting
    l. angle
    l. layers of cornea
    l. membrane of retina
    l. sulcus
    l. sulcus of Reil
    l. sulcus of rhomboid fossa
Limnatis nilotica
limnemia
limnemic
limophoitas
limophthisis
limosis
limp
limulus lysate test
Lindau's
    L. disease
    L. tumor
Lindner's bodies
line
    absorption l.'s
    accretion l.'s
    alveolonasal l.
    Amberg's lateral sinus l.
    l. angle
    anocutaneous l.
    anterior axillary l.
    anterior junction l.
    anterior median l.
    arcuate l.
    arcuate l. of ilium
    arcuate l. of rectus sheath
    arterial l.

axillary l.
Baillarger's l.'s
base l.
basinasal l.
Beau's l.'s
l. of Bechterew
bismuth l.
black l.
blue l.
Bolton-nasion l.
Brödel's bloodless l.
Burton's l.
calcification l.'s of Retzius
Camper's l.
cell l.
cement l.
cervical l.
Chamberlain's l.
Chaussier's l.
Clapton's l.
cleavage l.'s
Conradi's l.
contour l.'s of Owen
Correra's l.
costoclavicular l.
costophrenic septal l.'s
Crampton's l.
Daubenton's l.
l. of demarcation
demarcation l. of retina
Dennie's l.
dentate l.
developmental l.'s
Douglas' l.
Eberth's l.'s
Egger's l.
Ehrlich-Türk l.
epiphysial l.
established cell l.
Farre's l.
Feiss l.
l. of fixation
Fleischner l.'s
Fraunhofer's l.'s
fulcrum l.
Futcher's l.
l. of Gennari
germ l.
gluteal l.
Granger's l.
growth arrest l.'s
Gubler's l.
gum l.
Haller's l.
Hampton l.
Harris' l.'s
Head's l.'s
Hensen's l.

highest nuchal l.
high lip l.
Hilton's white l.
His' l.
Holden's l.
Hudson-Stähli l.
Hunter's l.
Hunter-Schreger l.'s
iliopectineal l.
imbrication l.'s of von Ebner
incremental l.'s
incremental l.'s of von Ebner
inferior nuchal l.
inferior temporal l.
infracostal l.
intercondylar l. of femur
intermediate l. of iliac crest
internal oblique l.
interspinal l.
intertrochanteric l.
intertubercular l.
isoelectric l.
l. of Kaes
Kerley A l.'s
Kerley B l.'s
Kerley C l.'s
Kilian's l.
Langer's l.'s
Lanz's l.
lead l.
Looser's l.'s
low lip l.
M l.
Mach l.
mamillary l.
mammary l.
McKee's l.
median l.
Mees' l.'s
mercurial l.
Meyer's l.
midaxillary l.
midclavicular l.
middle axillary l.
milk l.
Monro-Richter l.
Monro's l.
Muehrcke's l.'s
mylohyoid l.
nasobasilar l.
Nélaton's l.
neonatal l.
nipple l.
Obersteiner-Redlich l.
oblique l.
oblique l. of mandible
oblique l. of thyroid cartilage
l. of occlusion

line *(continued)*
    Ogston's l.
    Ohngren's l.
    orbitomeatal l.
    Owen's l.'s
    l. pairs
    paraspinal l.
    parasternal l.
    paravertebral l.
    Paris l.
    Paton's l.'s
    pectinate l.
    pectineal l.
    pectineal l. of pubis
    pleural l.'s
    pleuroesophageal l.
    Poirier's l.
    popliteal l.
    postaxillary l.
    posterior axillary l.
    posterior junction l.
    posterior median l.
    Poupart's l.
    preaxillary l.
    Reid's base l.
    retentive fulcrum l.
    l.'s of Retzius
    Richter-Monro l.
    Roser-Nélaton l.
    rough l.
    sagittal l.
    Salter's incremental l.'s
    S-BP l.
    scapular l.
    Schreger's l.'s
    semicircular l.
    semicircular l. of Douglas
    semilunar l.
    septal l.'s
    Sergent's white l.
    Shenton's l.
    S-N l.
    soleal l.
    l. for soleus muscle
    Spigelius' l.
    spiral l.
    l. spread function
    stabilizing fulcrum l.
    sternal l.
    Stocker's l.
    subcostal l.
    superior nuchal l.
    superior temporal l.
    supracrestal l.
    survey l.
    Sydney l.
    sylvian l.
    temporal l.

    tender l.'s
    terminal l.
    Topinard's l.
    tram l.'s
    transverse l.'s of sacrum
    trapezoid l.
    Ullmann's l.
    Vesling's l.
    vibrating l.
    l. of vision
    Voigt's l.'s
    Wegner's l.
    white l.
    white l. of anal canal
    white l. of Toldt
    Z l.
    l.'s of Zahn
    Zöllner's l.'s
linea, gen. and pl. **lineae**
    l. alba
    lineae albicantes
    l. anocutanea
    l. arcuata
    l. arcuata ossis ilii
    l. arcuata vaginae musculi recti
        abdominis
    l. aspera
    lineae atrophicae
    l. axillaris anterior
    l. axillaris media
    l. axillaris posterior
    l. corneae senilis
    l. epiphysialis
    l. glutea
    l. glutea anterior
    l. glutea inferior
    l. glutea posterior
    l. intercondylaris femoris
    l. intermedia cristae iliacae
    l. interspinalis
    l. intertrochanterica
    l. intertubercularis
    l. mamillaris
    l. mediana anterior
    l. mediana posterior
    l. medio-axillaris
    l. medioclavicularis
    l. musculi solei
    l. mylohyoidea
    l. nigra
    l. nuchae inferior
    l. nuchae mediana
    l. nuchae superior
    l. nuchae suprema
    l. obliqua
    l. obliqua cartilaginis thyroidea
    l. obliqua mandibulae
    l. parasternalis

l. paravertebralis
l. pectinea
l. poplitea
l. postaxillaris
l. preaxillaris
l. scapularis
l. semicircularis
l. semilunaris
l. spiralis
l. splendens
l. sternalis
l. subcostalis
l. supracristalis
l. temporalis inferior
l. temporalis superior
l. terminalis
lineae transversa ossi sacri
l. trapezoidea
lineage
linear
l. absorption coefficient
l. acceleration
l. accelerator
l. amputation
l. atrophy
l. craniectomy
l. energy transfer
l. epidermal nevus
l. fracture
l. IgA bullous disease in children
l. phonocardiograph
l. skull fracture
linebreeding
lined flap
liner
asbestos l.
cavity l.
Lingelsheimia
L. anitrata
lingism
Ling's method
lingua, gen. and pl. **linguae**
l. cerebelli
l. dissecta
l. fissurata
l. frenata
l. geographica
l. nigra
l. plicata
lingual
l. aponeurosis
l. arch
l. artery
l. bar
l. bone
l. branches
l. branch of facial nerve
l. crypt

l. embrasure
l. flange
l. flap
l. follicles
l. frenulum
l. gingiva
l. goiter
l. gyrus
l. hemiatrophy
l. lobe
l. lymph nodes
l. mucosa
l. nerve
l. occlusion
l. papilla
l. plate
l. plexus
l. quinsy
l. rest
l. salivary gland depression
l. septum
l. splint
l. surface of tooth
l. tonsil
l. trophoneurosis
l. vein
lingual-facial-buccal dyskinesia
Linguatula
L. rhinaria
L. serrata
Linguatulidae
linguiform
lingula, pl. **lingulae**
l. cerebelli
l. of cerebellum
l. of left lung
l. of mandible
l. mandibulae
l. pulmonis sinistri
l. sphenoidalis
lingular
l. branch
lingulectomy
linguocervical ridge
linguoclination
linguoclusion
linguodistal
linguofacial trunk
linguogingival
l. fissure
l. groove
l. ridge
linguo-occlusal
linguopapillitis
linguoplate
linguoversion
lining
l. cell

L

linin network
linitis
l. plastica
linkage
l. analysis
l. disequilibrium
genetic l.
l. group
l. marker
medical record l.
record l.
sex l.
linkage map
linked
linker
l. DNA
linker scanning
Linognathus
lint
lion-jaw bone-holding forceps
lip
acetabular l.
anterior l. of uterine os
articular l.
cleft l.
double l.
external l. of iliac crest
glenoidal l.
Hapsburg l.
internal l. of iliac crest
large pudendal l.
lateral l. of linea aspera
lower l.
medial l. of linea aspera
l.'s of mouth
l. pits
posterior l. of uterine os
l. reflex
rhombic l.
small pudendal l.
l. sulcus
tympanic l. of limbus of spiral lamina
upper l.
vestibular l. of limbus of spiral lamina
liparocele
lipase test
lipectomy
lipedema
lipedematous alopecia
lipemia
alimentary l.
diabetic l.
postprandial l.
l. retinalis
lipemic
l. retinopathy

lipid
l. granulomatosis
l. histiocytosis
l. keratopathy
l. pneumonia
lipidemia
lipidolytic
lipidosis, pl. **lipidoses**
cerebral l.
cerebroside l.
ganglioside l.
glycolipid l.
sphingomyelin l.
sulfatide l.
lipoarthritis
lipoatrophia
l. annularis
l. circumscripta
lipoatrophic diabetes
lipoatrophy
insulin l.
partial l.
lipoblast
lipoblastic lipoma
lipoblastoma
lipoblastomatosis
lipocardiac
lipochondrodystrophy
lipochrome
lipocrit
lipocyte
lipodermoid
lipodystrophia
l. intestinalis
l. progessiva superior
lipodystrophy
congenital total l.
familial l.
insulin l.
intestinal l.
membranous l.
partial face-sparing l.
progressive l.
lipoedema
lipofectin
lipofection
lipofibroma
lipofuscin
lipofuscinosis
ceroid l.
neuronal l.
lipogenous diabetes
lipogranuloma
lipogranulomatosis
lipohemia
lipoid
l. dermatoarthritis
l. granuloma

l. granulomatosis
l. nephrosis
l. pneumonia
l. proteinosis
lipoidemia
lipoidosis
cerebroside l.
l. corneae
l. cutis et mucosae
galactosylceramide l.
lipolipoidosis
lipoma
l. annulare colli
l. arborescens
atypical l.
l. capsulare
l. cavernosum
l. fibrosum
infiltrating l.
lipoblastic l.
l. myxomatodes
l. ossificans
l. petrificans
pleomorphic l.
l. sarcomatodes, l. sarcomatosum
spindle cell l.
telangiectatic l.
lipomatoid
lipomatosis
encephalocraniocutaneous l.
mediastinal l.
multiple symmetric l.
l. neurotica
lipomatous
l. hypertrophy
l. infiltration
l. polyp
lipomelanic reticulosis
lipomeningocele
lipomucopolysaccharidosis
Liponyssus
lipopenia
lipophage
lipophagia
l. granulomatosis
lipophagic
l. granuloma
l. intestinal granulomatosis
lipophagy
lipophanerosis
lipoprotein
l. electrophoresis
l. Lp(a)
l. polymorphism
lipoprotein-X
liposarcoma
liposis
liposuction

liposuctioning
lipotrophic
lipotrophy
lipoxenous
lipoxeny
lipping
lippitude, lippitudo
Lipschütz cell
Lipschütz' ulcer
lipuria
lipuric
liquefaction degeneration
liquefactive necrosis
liquid
Cotunnius' l.
l. crystal thermography
l. scatter
liquor, gen. **liquoris**, pl. **liquores**
l. amnii
l. cerebrospinalis
l. cotunnii
l. entericus
l. folliculi
Morgagni's l.
Scarpa's l.
liquorrhea
Lisch nodule
Lisfranc's
L. amputation
L. joints
L. ligaments
L. operation
L. tubercle
Lison-Dunn stain
lisping
lissamine rhodamine B 200
Lissauer's
L. bundle
L. column
L. fasciculus
L. marginal zone
L. tract
lissencephalia
lissencephalic
lissencephaly
lissosphincter
lissotrichic, lissotrichous
Listerella
Listeria
L. *denitrificans*
L. *grayi*
L. *monocytogenes*
listerism
Lister's
L. dressing
L. method
L. tubercle

L

Listing's
  L. law
  L. reduced eye
Liston's
  L. knives
  L. shears
  L. splint
literal agraphia
lithectomy
lithiasis
  l. conjunctivae
  pancreatic l.
lithium
  l. carmine
  l. tungstate
Lithobius
lithoclast
lithogenesis, lithogeny
lithogenic
lithogenous
lithogeny (*var. of* lithogenesis)
lithoid
lithokelyphopedion, lithokelyphopedium
lithokelyphos
litholabe
litholapaxy
litholysis
litholyte
lithomyl
lithonephritis
lithopedion, lithopedium
lithotome
lithotomist
lithotomy
  bilateral l.
  high l.
  lateral l.
  marian l.
  median l.
  perineal l.
  l. position
  prerectal l.
  suprapubic l.
  vaginal l.
  vesical l.
lithotresis
  ultrasonic l.
lithotripsy
  electrohydraulic shock wave l.
  extracorporeal shock wave l.
  shock wave l.
lithotriptor
lithotriptoscopy
lithotrite
lithotrity
lithuresis
lithuria
litigious paranoia

litmus
little
  l. finger
  l. fossa of the cochlear window
  l. fossa of the vestibular round window
  l. fossa of the vestibular window
  l. head of humerus
  L. Leaguer's elbow
Little's
  L. area
  L. disease
littoral cell
Littré's
  L. glands
  L. hernia
littritis
Litzmann obliquity
livebirth, live birth
liveborn infant
livedo
  postmortem l.
  l. racemosa
  l. reticularis
  l. reticularis idiopathica
  l. reticularis symptomatica
  l. telangiectatica
  l. vasculitis
livedoid
  l. dermatitis
liver
  l. acinus
  l. breath
  l. bud
  cardiac l.
  l. cell carcinoma
  fatty l.
  l. flap
  frosted l.
  hobnail l.
  icing l.
  l. kidney syndrome
  lardaceous l.
  nutmeg l.
  l. palm
  pigmented l.
  polycystic l.
  l. spot
  sugar-icing l.
  wandering l.
  waxy l.
liver-shod clamp
livid
lividity
  postmortem l.
living anatomy
livor
LLETZ

L-L factor
Lloyd's reagent
Lo, L$_o$
    L. dose
load
    electronic pacemaker l.
    genetic l.
loading
    l. dose
    salt l.
Loa loa
lobar
    l. bronchi
    l. nephronia
    l. pneumonia
    l. sclerosis
lobate
lobe
    anterior l. of hypophysis
    azygos l. of lung
    caudate l.
    l.'s of cerebrum
    cuneiform l.
    ear l.
    falciform l.
    flocculonodular l.
    frontal l.
    frontal l. of cerebrum
    glandular l. of hypophysis
    Home's l.
    inferior l. of lung
    left l.
    left l. of liver
    limbic l.
    lingual l.
    lower l. of lung
    l.'s of mammary gland
    middle l. of prostate
    middle l. of right lung
    nervous l.
    nervous l. of hypophysis
    occipital l.
    occipital l. of cerebrum
    parietal l.
    parietal l. of cerebrum
    placental l.'s
    polyalveolar l.
    posterior l. of hypophysis
    l. of prostate
    pyramidal l. of thyroid gland
    quadrate l.
    renal l.
    Riedel's l.
    right l.
    right l. of liver
    Spigelius' l.
    superior l. of lung
    supplemental l.

    temporal l.
    l.'s of thyroid gland
    upper l. of lung
lobectomy
lobi (*gen. and pl. of* lobus)
lobitis
Loboa loboi
lobomycosis
lobopodium, pl. **lobopodia**
Lobo's disease
lobose, lobous
lobotomy
    prefrontal l.
    transorbital l.
Lobstein's ganglion
lobster-claw deformity
lobular
    l. carcinoma
    l. carcinoma in situ
    l. glomerulonephritis
    l. neoplasia
lobulate, lobulated
lobule
    ala central l.
    ansiform l.
    anterior lunate l.
    l. of auricle
    biventer l.
    biventral l.
    central l.
    central l. of cerebellum
    cortical l.'s of kidney
    crescentic l.'s of the cerebellum
    l.'s of epididymis
    gracile l.
    hepatic l.
    inferior parietal l.
    inferior semilunar l.
    l.'s of mammary gland
    paracentral l.
    portal l. of liver
    posterior lunate l.
    primary pulmonary l.
    quadrangular l.
    quadrate l.
    renal cortical l.
    respiratory l.
    secondary pulmonary l.
    simple l.
    slender l.
    superior parietal l.
    superior semilunar l.
    l.'s of testis
    l.'s of thymus
    l.'s of thyroid gland
lobulet, lobulette
lobulus, gen. and pl. **lobuli**
    l. auriculae

L

lobulus (*continued*)
  l. biventer
  l. biventralis
  l. centralis cerebelli
  l. clivi
  l. corticalis renalis
  l. culminis
  l. cuneiformis
  lobuli epididymidis
  l. folii
  l. fusiformis
  lobuli glandulae mammariae
  lobuli glandulae thyroideae
  l. gracilis
  l. hepatis
  l. paracentralis
  l. parietalis inferior
  l. parietalis superior
  l. quadrangularis
  l. quadratus
  l. semilunaris inferior
  l. semilunaris superior
  l. simplex
  lobuli testis
  lobuli thymi

lobus, gen. and pl. **lobi**
  l. anterior hypophyseos
  l. appendicularis
  l. azygos
  l. caudatus
  lobi cerebri
  l. clivi
  l. dexter
  l. falciformis
  l. frontalis cerebri
  lobi glandulae mammariae
  lobi glandulae thyroideae
  l. glandularis hypophyseos
  l. hepatis dexter
  l. hepatis sinister
  l. inferior pulmonis
  l. linguiformis
  l. medius prostatae
  l. medius pulmonis dextri
  l. nervosus
  l. occipitalis cerebri
  l. parietalis cerebri
  l. posterior hypophyseos
  l. prostatae
  l. pyramidalis glandulae thyroideae
  l. quadratus
  l. renalis
  l. sinister
  l. superior pulmonis
  l. temporalis

local
  l. anaphylaxis
  l. anemia
  l. anesthesia
  l. anesthetic reaction
  l. asphyxia
  l. bloodletting
  l. death
  l. epilepsy
  l. excitatory state
  l. flap
  l. glomerulonephritis
  l. hormone
  l. immunity
  l. reaction
  l. sign
  l. symptom
  l. syncope
  l. tetanus
  l. tic

localization
  l. agnosia
  auditory l.
  cerebral l.
  germinal l.
  radiotherapy l.
  l. related epilepsy
  spatial l.
  stereotaxic l.

localized
  l. amnesia
  l. mucinosis
  l. nodular tenosynovitis
  l. osteitis fibrosa
  l. pemphigoid of Brunsting-Perry
  l. peritonitis
  l. scleroderma

localizing
  l. electrode
  l. symptom

locator

lochia
  l. alba
  l. cruenta
  l. purulenta
  l. rubra
  l. sanguinolenta
  l. serosa

lochial
lochiometra
lochiometritis
lochioperitonitis
lochiorrhagia
lochiorrhea
loci (*pl. of* locus)
locked
  l. bite
  l. facets
  l. knee
locked-in syndrome
lock finger

lockjaw
Lockwood's ligament
locomotive
locomotor
    l. ataxia
locomotorial
locomotorium
locomotory
locular
loculate
loculated empyema
loculation
    l. syndrome
loculus, pl. loculi
locum
    l. tenant
    l. tenens
locus, pl. loci
    l. ceruleus
    l. cinereus
    complex l.
    l. of control
    l. ferrugineus
    genetic l.
    l. niger
    l. perforatus anticus
    l. perforatus posticus
    sex-linked l.
    X-linked l.
    Y-linked l.
lod method
Loeb's deciduoma
Loeffler's
    L. bacillus
    L. blood culture medium
    L. caustic stain
    L. methylene blue
    L. stain
Loevit's cell
Loewenthal's
    L. bundle
    L. reaction
    L. tract
Löffler's
    L. disease
    L. endocarditis
    L. fibroplastic endocarditis
    L. syndrome
Loffler's parietal fibroplastic
    endocarditis
logagnosia
logagraphia
logamnesia
Logan's bow
logaphasia
logarithm

logarithmic
    l. phase
    l. phonocardiograph
logasthenia
logetronography
logistic
    l. curve
    l. model
logit
    l. transformation
lognormal distribution
logopathy
logopedia
logopedics
logoplegia
logorrhea
logospasm
logotherapy
Lohlein-Baehr lesion
loiasis
loin
Lombard voice-reflex test
long
    l. abductor muscle of thumb
    l. adductor muscle
    l. axis
    l. axis of body
    l. axis view
    l. bone
    l. buccal nerve
    l. central artery
    l. chain
    l. ciliary nerve
    l. cone technique
    l. crus of incus
    l. extensor muscle of great toe
    l. extensor muscle of thumb
    l. extensor muscle of toes
    l. fibular muscle
    l. flexor muscle of great toe
    l. flexor muscle of thumb
    l. flexor muscle of toes
    l. gyrus of insula
    l. head
    l. incubation hepatitis
    l. levatores costarum muscles
    l. muscle of head
    l. muscle of neck
    l. palmar muscle
    l. peroneal muscle
    l. plantar ligament
    l. posterior ciliary artery
    l. process of malleus
    l. pulse
    l. radial extensor muscle of wrist
    l. root of ciliary ganglion
    l. saphenous nerve
    l. saphenous vein

L

long (*continued*)
   l. sight
   l. subscapular nerve
   l. terminal repeat sequences
   l. thoracic artery
   l. thoracic nerve
   l. thoracic vein
   l. vinculum
long-acting thyroid stimulator
longevity
longissimus
   l. capitis muscle
   l. cervicis muscle
   l. muscle
   l. thoracis muscle
longitudinal
   l. aberration
   l. arch of foot
   l. arc of skull
   l. bands of cruciform ligament
   l. canals of modiolus
   l. dissociation
   l. duct of epoöphoron
   l. fissure of cerebrum
   l. fold of duodenum
   l. fracture
   l. layer of muscular coat
   l. layers of muscular tunics
   l. lie
   l. ligament
   l. method
   l. oval pelvis
   l. pontine bundles
   l. pontine fasciculi
   l. relaxation
   l. section
   l. sinus
   l. study
   l. sulcus of heart
   l. vertebral venous sinus
longitudinalis
longitype
long-leg arthropathy
Longmire's operation
Long's
   L. coefficient
   L. formula
long-term memory
longus
   l. capitis muscle
   l. colli muscle
Lon protease
loop
   Biebl l.
   bulboventricular l.
   capillary l.'s
   cervical l.
   cruciform l.'s

[handwritten: Waltman's loop]

   D l.
   displacement l.
   l. electrocautery excision procedure
   l. excision
   gamma l.
   Gerdy's interatrial l.
   Granit's l.
   hairpin l.'s
   Henle's l.
   l. of hypoglossal nerve
   Hyrtl's l.
   lenticular l.
   memory l.
   Meyer-Archambault l.
   nephronic l.
   peduncular l.
   l. resection
   l.'s of spinal nerves
   l. stoma
   subclavian l.
   vector l.
   ventricular l.
   Vieussens' l.
loose
   l. associations
   l. body
   l. cartilage
   l. skin
loosening of association
Looser's
   L. lines
   L. zones
lop-ear, lop ear
lophodont
lophotrichate
lophotrichous
Lorain-Lévi
   L.-L. dwarfism
   L.-L. infantilism
   L.-L. syndrome
Lorain's disease
lordoscoliosis
lordosis
lordotic
   l. albuminuria
   l. pelvis
Lorenz' sign
loss
   hearing l.
Lou Gehrig's disease
Louis'
   L. angle
   L. law
Louis-Bar syndrome
loupe
   binocular l.
louping-ill virus
louse, pl. **lice**

biting l., chewing l., feather l.
l. flies
sucking l.
louse-borne typhus
lousiness
lousy
Lovén reflex
Lovibond's
  L. angle
  L. profile sign
Lovibond's profile sign
low
  l. convex
  l. delirium
  l. flow principle
  l. forceps delivery
  l. frequency transduction
  l. grade astrocytoma
  l. lip line
  l. malignant potential tumor
  l. output failure
  l. purine diet
  l. residue diet
  l. salt diet
  l. salt syndrome
  l. sodium syndrome
  l. spinal anesthesia
  l. tension glaucoma
  l. tone deafness
low-calorie diet
low-density lipoprotein receptors
Löwenberg's
  L. canal
  L. forceps
  L. scala
Lowenstein-Jensen
  L.-J. culture medium
  L.-J. medium
lower
  l. abdominal periosteal reflex
  l. airway
  l. alveolar point
  l. esophageal sphincter
  l. extremity
  l. eyelid
  l. jaw
  l. lateral cutaneous nerve of arm
  l. lid
  l. limb
  l. lip
  l. lobe of lung
  l. motor neuron
  l. motor neuron dysarthria
  l. motor neuron lesion
  l. nephron nephrosis
  l. nodal extrasystole
  l. nodal rhythm
  l. respiratory tract smear

l. ridge slope
l. uterine segment
l. uterine segment cesarean section
Lower's
  L. ring
  L. tubercle
Lowe's syndrome
lowest
  l. lumbar arteries
  l. splanchnic nerve
  l. thyroid artery
Lowe-Terrey-MacLachlan syndrome
low-fat diet
Lown-Ganong-Levine syndrome
low-pass filter
Lowsley tractor
loxia
loxoscelism
Loxotrema ovatum
L-phase variants
Lr dose
Lu antigens
Lubarsch's crystals
Lu Blood Group (*var. of* Lutheran Blood Group)
Lucas' groove
lucent
Lucibacterium
  L. harveyi
lucid
  l. interval
lucidification
lucidity
lucifugal
Lucilia
  L. caesar
  L. illustris
  L. sericata
Lucio's
  L. leprosy
  L. leprosy phenomenon
lucipetal
lückenschädel
Lücke's test
Lucké's virus
lucotherapy
Luc's operation
ludic
Ludloff's sign
Ludwig's
  L. angina
  L. angle
  L. ganglion
  L. labyrinth
  L. nerve
  L. stromuhr
Luer-Lok syringe
Luer syringe

L

lues
l. venerea
luetic
l. mask
Luft's
L. disease
L. potassium permanganate fixative
Lugol's iodine solution
Lukes-Collins classification
lumbago
ischemic l.
lumbar
l. appendicitis
l. artery
l. branch of iliolumbar artery
l. cistern
l. enlargement
l. enlargement of spinal cord
l. flexure
l. ganglia
l. hernia
l. iliocostal muscle
l. interspinales muscles
l. interspinal muscle
l. lymph nodes
l. myelogram
l. nephrectomy
l. nerves
l. part
l. part of diaphragm
l. part of spinal cord
l. plexus
l. puncture
l. puncture needle
l. quadrate muscle
l. region
l. rheumatism
l. rib
l. rotator muscles
l. segments of spinal cord
l. splanchnic nerves
l. triangle
l. trunks
l. veins
l. vertebrae
lumbarization
lumberman's itch
lumbi (*gen. and pl. of* lumbus)
lumboabdominal
lumbocolostomy
lumbocolotomy
lumbocostal
l. ligament
lumbocostoabdominal triangle
lumbodorsal fascia
lumboiliac
lumboinguinal
l. nerve

lumbo-ovarian
lumbosacral
l. angle
l. joint
l. plexus
l. trunk
lumbrical
l. muscle of foot
l. muscle of hand
lumbricalis
lumbricidal
lumbricoid
lumbricosis
lumbricus
lumbus, gen. and pl. **lumbi**
lumen, pl. **lumina, lumens**
residual l.
luminal
luminance
luminous
l. flux
l. retinoscope
lumpectomy
lunacy
Luna-Ishak stain
lunare
lunar periodicity
lunate
l. bone
l. surface of acetabulum
lunatic
lunatomalacia
lung
air-conditioner l.
bird-breeder's l., bird-fancier's l.
black l.
brown l.
l. bud
cardiac l.
cheese worker's l.
collier's l.
coptic l.
endstage l.
farmer's l.
fibroid l.
l. fluke disease
honeycomb l.
hyperlucent l.
iron l.
malt-worker's l.
mason's l.
miner's l.
mushroom-worker's l.
postperfusion l.
pump l.
quiet l.
shock l.
silo-filler's l.

thresher's l.
trench l.
unilateral hyperlucent l.
l. unit
uremic l.
vanishing l.
welder's l.
wet l., white l.
l. window
lungworms
lunula, pl. **lunulae**
    azure l. of nails
    l. of semilunar valve
    l. valvulae semilunaris
Lunyo virus
lupiform
lupoid
    l. hepatitis
    l. leishmaniasis
    l. sycosis
    l. ulcer
lupous
lupus
    l. anticoagulant
    l. band test
    chilblain l.
    chilblain l. erythematosus
    chronic discoid l. erythematosus
    cutaneous l. erythematosus
    discoid l. erythematosus
    disseminated l. erythematosus
    drug-induced l.
    l. erythematodes
    l. erythematosus
    l. erythematosus cell
    l. erythematosus cell test
    l. erythematosus, neonatal
    l. erythematosus panniculitis
    l. erythematosus profundus
    l. livido
    l. lymphaticus
    l. miliaris disseminatus faciei
    l. mutilans
    neonatal l.
    l. nephritis
    l. papillomatosus
    l. pernio
    l. profundus
    l. sebaceus
    l. serpiginosus
    l. superficialis
    systemic l. erythematosus
    l. tuberculosus
    l. verrucosus
    l. vulgaris
lupus-like syndrome
lura
lural

Luschka's
    L. bursa
    L. cartilage
    L. cystic glands
    L. ducts
    L. gland
    L. joints
    L. ligaments
    L. sinus
    L. tonsil
Luse bodies
lute
luteal
    l. cell
    l. phase
    l. phase defect
    l. phase deficiency
lutein cell
luteinization
luteinize
luteinoma
Lutembacher's syndrome
luteogenic
luteolysis
luteolytic
luteoma
    pregnancy l.
luteoplacental shift
luteus
Lutheran Blood Group, Lu Blood Group
luting agent
Lutzomyia
    L. flaviscutellata
    L. intermedius
    L. longipalpis
    L. peruensis
Lutz-Splendore-Almeida disease
luxatio
    l. erecta
    l. perinealis
luxation
    Malgaigne's l.
Luxol fast blue
luxus
Luys' body
lycanthropy
lycopenemia
lycoperdonosis
lycophora
Lyell's
    L. disease
    L. syndrome
lygophilia
Lyme
    L. arthritis
    L. borreliosis
Lymnaea

L

lymph
    aplastic l.
    blood l.
    l. capillary
    l. cell
    l. circulation
    l. cords
    l. corpuscle
    corpuscular l.
    croupous l.
    dental l.
    l. embolism
    euplastic l.
    fibrinous l.
    l. follicle
    l. gland
    inflammatory l.
    intercellular l.
    intravascular l.
    l. node
    l. node permeability factor
    l. nodule
    plastic l.
    l. sacs
    l. scrotum
    l. sinus
    l. space
    tissue l.
    vaccine l., vaccinia l.
    l. varix
    l. vessels
lympha
lymphaden
lymphadenectomy
lymphadenitis
    dermatopathic l.
    paratuberculous l.
    regional l.
    regional granulomatous l.
    tuberculosis l.
    tuberculous l.
lymphadenography
lymphadenoid
    l. goiter
lymphadenoma
lymphadenomatosis
lymphadenopathy
    angioimmunoblastic l. with
      dysproteinemia
    dermatopathic l.
    immunoblastic l.
    persistent generalized l.
lymphadenopathy-associated virus
lymphadenosis
    benign l.
    malignant l.
lymphadenovarix
lymphangeitis

lymphangial
lymphangiectasis, lymphangiectasia
    cavernous l.
    cystic l.
    intestinal l.
    simple l.
lymphangiectatic
lymphangiectodes
lymphangiectomy
lymphangiitis *lymphangitic*
lymphangioendothelioma
lymphangiography
lymphangiology
lymphangioma
    l. capillare varicosum
    l. cavernosum
    l. circumscriptum
    l. cysticum
    l. simplex
    l. superficium simplex
    l. tuberosum multiplex
    l. xanthelasmoideum
lymphangiomatous
lymphangiomyomatosis
lymphangion
lymphangiophlebitis
lymphangioplasty
lymphangiosarcoma
lymphangiotomy
lymphangitis
    l. carcinomatosa
lymphapheresis
lymphatic
    afferent l.
    l. angina
    l. corpuscle
    l. dissemination theory of
      endometriosis
    l. duct
    l. edema
    efferent l.
    l. fistula
    l. follicle
    l. follicles of larynx
    l. follicles of rectum
    l. leukemia
    l. nodule
    l. plexus
    l. ring of cardiac part of stomach
    l. sarcoma
    l. sinus
    l. stroma
    l. system
    l. tissue
    l. valvule
    l. vessels
lymphatic node (*var. of* lymph node)
lymphaticostomy

lymphatics
lymphatitis
lymphatology
lymphatolysis
lymphatolytic
lymphectasia
lymphedema
 congenital l.
 hereditary l.
 l. praecox
 primary l.
lymphedematous keratoderma
lymphemia
lymphization
lymph node, lymphatic node
 l. n.'s of abdominal organs
 accessory nerve l. n.'s
 anorectal l. n.'s
 anterior cervical l. n.'s
 anterior deep cervical l. n.'s
 anterior group of axillary l. n.'s
 anterior jugular l. n.'s
 anterior mediastinal l. n.'s
 anterior superficial cervical l. n.'s
 anterior tibial l. n.
 apical group of axillary l. n.'s
 appendicular l. n.'s
 axillary l. n.'s
 l. n. of azygos arch
 bifurcation l. n.'s
 brachial l. n.'s
 bronchopulmonary l. n.'s
 buccal l. n.
 carinal l. n.'s
 celiac l. n.'s
 central group of axillary l. n.'s
 central mesenteric l. n.'s
 colic l. n.'s
 common iliac l. n.'s
 companion l. n.'s of accessory
  nerve
 cubital l. n.'s
 cystic l. n.
 deep inguinal l. n.'s
 deep parotid l. n.'s
 l. n.'s of elbow
 external iliac l. n.'s
 facial l. n.'s
 fibular l. n.
 foraminal l. n.
 gastroduodenal l. n.'s
 gluteal l. n.'s
 hepatic l. n.'s
 hilar l. n.'s
 ileocolic l. n.'s
 inferior epigastric l. n.'s
 inferior mesenteric l. n.'s
 inferior phrenic l. n.'s

inferior tracheobronchial l. n.'s
infra-auricular deep parotid l. n.'s
infra-auricular subfascial parotid l.
 n.'s
intercostal l. n.'s
interiliac l. n.'s
intermediate lacunar l. n.
intermediate lumbar l. n.'s
internal iliac l. n.'s
interpectoral l. n.'s
intraglandular deep parotid l. n.'s
intraglandular parotid l. n.'s
jugulo-digastric l. n.
jugulo-omohyoid l. n.
juxta-esophageal pulmonary l. n.'s,
 juxta-esophageal l. n.'s
juxta-intestinal l. n.'s
lateral deep cervical l. n.'s
lateral group of axillary l. n.'s
lateral jugular l. n.'s
lateral lacunar l. n.
lateral pericardiac l. n.'s
lateral superficial cervical l. n.'s
left colic l. n.'s
left gastric l. n.'s
left gastroepiploic l. n.'s
left lumbar l. n.'s
l. n. of ligamentum arteriosum
lingual l. n.'s
lumbar l. n.'s
malar l. n.
mandibular l. n.
mastoid l. n.'s
medial lacunar l. n.
mesenteric l. n.'s
mesocolic l. n.'s
middle colic l. n.'s
middle group of mesenteric l. n.'s
middle rectal l. n.
nasolabial l. n.
obturator l. n.'s
occipital l. n.'s
pancreatic l. n.'s
pancreaticoduodenal l. n.'s
pancreaticosplenic l. n.'s
paramammary l. n.'s
pararectal l. n.'s
parasternal l. n.'s
paratracheal l. n.
parauterine l. n.'s
paravaginal l. n.'s
paravesical l. n.'s
parietal l. n.'s
pectoral group of axillary l. n.'s
popliteal l. n.'s
posterior group of axillary l. n.'s
posterior mediastinal l. n.'s
posterior tibial l. n.

L

lymph node (*continued*)
  preauricular deep parotid l. n.'s
  prececal l. n.'s
  prelaryngeal l. n.'s
  prepericardiac l. n.'s
  pretracheal l. n.'s
  prevertebral l. n.'s
  promontory common iliac l. n.'s
  pulmonary l. n.'s
  pyloric l. n.'s
  retroauricular l. n.'s
  retrocecal l. n.'s
  retropharyngeal l. n.'s
  retropyloric l. n.'s
  right colic l. n.'s
  right gastric l. n.'s
  right gastroepiploic l. n.'s
  right gastro-omental l. n.'s
  right lumbar l. n.'s
  sacral l. n.'s
  sigmoid l. n.'s
  splenic l. n.'s
  subaortic l. n.'s
  submandibular l. n.'s
  submental l. n.'s
  subpyloric l. n.'s
  subscapular group of axillary l. n.'s
  superficial inguinal l. n.'s
  superficial parotid l. n.'s
  superior gastric l. n.'s
  superior mesenteric l. n.'s
  superior phrenic l. n.'s
  superior rectal l. n.'s
  superior tracheobronchial l. n.'s
  supraclavicular l. n.'s
  suprapyloric l. n.
  thyroid l. n.'s
  tracheal l. n.'s
  visceral l. n.'s
lymphoadenoma
lymphoblast
lymphoblastic
  l. leukemia
  l. lymphoma
lymphoblastoma
  giant follicular l.
lymphoblastosis
lymphocele
lymphocerastism
lymphocinesis, lymphocinesia
lymphocyst
lymphocytapheresis
lymphocyte
  B l.
  l. function associated antigen
  Rieder's l.
  T l.

  l. transformation
  transformed l.
  tumor-infiltrating l.'s
lymphocyte-mediated cytotoxicity
lymphocythemia
lymphocytic
  l. adenohypophysitis
  l. choriomeningitis
  l. choriomeningitis virus
  l. hypophysitis
  l. interstitial pneumonia
  l. interstitial pneumonitis
  l. leukemia
  l. leukemoid reaction
  l. leukocytosis
  l. leukopenia
  l. series
  l. thyroiditis
lymphocytoblast
lymphocytoma
  benign l. cutis
lymphocytopenia
lymphocytopoiesis
lymphocytosis
lymphocytotoxic antibodies
lymphoderma
lymphoduct
lymphoepithelial cyst
lymphoepithelioma
lymphogenesis
lymphogenic
lymphogenous
  l. embolism
  l. metastasis
lymphoglandula
lymphogranuloma
  l. benignum
  l. inguinale
  l. malignum
  Schaumann's l.
  venereal l., l. venereum
  l. venereum antigen
  l. venereum virus
lymphogranulomatosis
lymphography
lymphohistiocytosis
lymphoid
  l. cell
  l. corpuscle
  l. hemoblast of Pappenheim
  l. hypophysitis
  l. interstitial pneumonia
  l. leukemia
  l. polyp
  l. ring
  l. series
  l. tissue
lymphoidectomy

lymphoidocyte
lymphokines
lymphokinesis
lympholeukocyte
lymphology
lymphoma
 adult T-cell l.
 anaplastic large cell l.
 benign l. of the rectum
 Burkitt's l.
 diffuse small cleaved cell l.
 follicular l.
 follicular predominantly large
 cell l.
 follicular predominantly small
 cleaved cell l.
 histiocytic l.
 Hodgkin's l.
 immunoblastic l.
 Ki-1+ l.
 large cell l.
 Lennert's l.
 lymphoblastic l.
 malignant l.
 Mediterranean l.
 nodular l.
 nodular histiocytic l.
 non-Hodgkin's l.
 poorly differentiated lymphocytic l.
 small lymphocytic l.
 T cell-rich, B cell l.
 well-differentiated lymphocytic l.
lymphomatoid
 l. granulomatosis
 l. papulosis
lymphomatosis
lymphomatous
lymphomyeloma
lymphomyxoma
lymphopathia
 l. venereum
lymphopathy
lymphopenia
lymphopenic thymic dysplasia
lymphoplasmapheresis
lymphoplasty
lymphopoiesis

lymphopoietic
lymphoreticulosis
 benign inoculation l.
lymphorrhagia
lymphorrhea
lymphorrhoid
lymphosarcoma
lymphosarcomatosis
lymphoscintigraphy
lymphosis
lymphostasis
lymphostatic verrucosis
lymphotaxis
lymphotoxicity
lymphotoxin
lymphotrophy
lymphuria
Lyon hypothesis
lyonization
lyra
 l. davidis, lyre of David
 l. uterina
lyre of David
lysemia
lysinemia
lysinogen
lysinogenic
lysinuria
lysis
lysogenic
 l. bacterium
 l. induction
 l. strain
lysogenicity
lysogenization
lysogeny
lysosomal disease
lysosome
 definitive l.'s
 primary l.'s
 secondary l.'s
lysostaphin
lysotype
Lyssavirus
Lyt antigens
lytic

L

M

- M antigen
- M band
- M concentration
- M line
- M protein

Macchiavello's stain
MAC complex
MacConkey agar
Macewen's
- M. sign
- M. symptom
- M. triangle

Mach
- M. band
- M. effect
- M. line
- M. number

Machado-Guerreiro test
Machado-Joseph
machine
- anesthesia m.
- heart-lung m.
- panoramic rotating m.

machinery murmur
Machupo virus
Mackay-Marg tonometer
Mackenrodt's ligament
Mackenzie's
- M. amputation
- M. polygraph

Maclagan's
- M. test
- M. thymol turbidity test

Macleod's
- M. rheumatism
- M. syndrome

maclurin
MacNeal's tetrachrome blood stain
Macracanthorhynchus
- *M. hirudinaceus*

macrencephaly, macrencephalia
macroadenoma
macroamylasemia
macrobacterium
macrobiosis
macrobiote
macrobiotic
- m. diet

macrobiotics
macroblast
macroblepharon
macrobrachia
macrocardia
macrocephalic, macrocephalous

macrocephaly, macrocephalia
macrocheilia, macrochilia
macrocheiria, macrochiria
macrochilia
macrocnemia
macrococcus
macrocolon
macroconidium, pl. **macroconidia**
macrocornea
macrocranium
macrocryoglobulinemia
macrocyst
macrocytase
macrocyte
macrocythemia
- hyperchromatic m.

macrocytic
- m. achylic anemia
- m. anemia
- m. anemia of pregnancy
- m. anemia tropical
- m. hyperchromia

macrocytosis
macrodactylia, macrodactylism, macrodactyly
macrodont
macrodontia, macrodontism
macrodystrophia lipomatosa
macroencephalon
macroerythroblast
macroerythrocyte
macroesthesia
macrofollicular adenoma
macrogamete
macrogametocyte
macrogamont
macrogamy
macrogastria
macrogenitosomia
- m. praecox
- m. praecox suprarenalis

macroglia
- m. cell

macroglobulinemia
- Waldenström's m.

macroglossia
macrognathia
macrography
macrogyria
macrolabia
macroleukoblast
macromastia, macromazia
macromelanosome
macromelia
macromere

M

macromerozoite
macromonocyte
macromyeloblast
macronormoblast
macronormochromoblast
macronucleus
macronychia
macroparasite
macropathology
macropenis
macrophage
  activated m.
  alveolar m.
  armed m.
  associated m.
  m. colony-stimulating factor
  fixed m.
  free m.
  Hansemann m.
  inflammatory m.
  m. inflammatory protein
  m. migration inhibition test
macrophage-activating factor
macrophagocyte
macrophallus
macrophthalmia
macropodia
macropolycyte
macropromyelocyte
macroprosopia
macroprosopous
macropsia
macrorhinia
macroscelia
macroscopic
  m. anatomy
  m. sphincter
macroscopy
macrosigmoid
macrosis
macrosmatic
macrosomia
macrosplanchnic
macrospore
macrostereognosis
macrostomia
macrotia
macrotome
macula, pl. **maculae**
  maculae acusticae
  m. adherens
  m. albida, pl. maculae albidae
  m. atrophica
  m. cerulea
  m. communicans
  m. communis
  m. corneae
  m. cribrosa, m. cribrosa inferior, m.

cribrosa media, m. cribrosa quarta,
m. cribrosa superior, pl. maculae
cribrosae
m. densa
false m.
m. flava
m. germinativa
m. gonorrhoica
honeycomb m.
m. lactea
m. lutea
mongolian m.
m. pellucida
m. retinae
m. of saccule
m. sacculi
Saenger's m.
m. tendinea
m. of utricle
m. utriculi
macular, maculate
m. amyloidosis
m. area
m. arteries
m. atrophy
m. coloboma
m. degeneration
m. drusen
m. dystrophy
m. erythema
m. evasion
m. fasciculus
m. leprosy
m. retinopathy
m. syphilid
maculation
macule
maculocerebral
maculoerythematous
maculopapule
maculopathy
  bull's-eye m.
  cystoid m.
  familial pseudoinflammatory m.
  nicotinic acid m.
  solar m.
mad
  M. Hatter syndrome
madarosis
Maddox's rod
Madelung's
  M. deformity
  M. disease
  M. neck
madescent
madidans
Madlener operation
madness

Madura
    M. boil
    M. foot
Madurella
maduromycosis
maedi virus
Maffucci's syndrome
Magendie-Hertwig
    M.-H. sign
    M.-H. syndrome
Magendie's
    M. foramen
    M. law
    M. spaces
magenstrasse
magenta tongue
maggot
    cheese m.
    surgical m.
magical thinking
magma
    m. reticulare
Magnan's
    M. sign
    M. trombone movement
magnet
    m. reaction
    m. reflex
    superconducting m.
magnetic
    m. field
    m. field gradient
    m. implant
    m. resonance angiography
    m. resonance spectroscopy
magnetism
    animal m.
magnetocardiography
magnetoencephalogram
magnetoencephalography
magnetogyric ratio
magnetometer
magnetotherapy
magnification
    m. angiography
    m. radiography
magnitude
    average pulse m.
    peak m.
magnocellular
magnum
magnus
Magnus' sign
Mahaim fibers
MAI
maidenhead
maidism

Maier's sinus
maim
main
    m. d'accoucheur
    m. en crochet
    m. en griffe
    m. en lorgnette
    m. fourchée
    m. succulente
mainframe
mainstreaming
maintainer
    space m.
maintenance
    m. dose
    m. drug therapy
    m. medication
Maissiat's band
Majocchi
    M. disease
    M. granulomas
major
    m. agglutinin
    m. amblyoscope
    m. amputation
    m. calices
    m. connector
    m. depression
    m. duodenal papilla
    m. epilepsy
    m. fissure
    m. forceps
    m. groove
    m. hippocampus
    m. histocompatibility complex
    m. hypnosis
    m. hysteria
    justo m.
    m. mood disorder
    m. motor seizure
    m. operation
    m. salivary glands
    m. sublingual duct
    m. surgery
Makeham's hypothesis
mal
    m. de Cayenne
    m. de la rosa, m. rosso
    m. de los pintos
    m. de Meleda
    m. de mer
    m. de San Lazaro
    grand m.
    m. perforant
    petit m.
    m. rosso (*var. of* m. de la rosa)
mala

M

Malabar
  M. itch
  M. leprosy
malabsorption
  m. syndrome
Malacarne's
  M. pyramid
  M. space
malacia
malacic
malacoplakia, malakoplakia
malacosis
malacotic
malacotomy
maladie
  m. de Roger
  m. des jambes
maladjustment
  social m.
malady
malaise
malakoplakia (*var. of* malacoplakia)
malalignment
malar
  m. arch
  m. bone
  m. flush
  m. fold
  m. foramen
  m. lymph node
  m. node
  m. point
  m. process
malaria
  acute m.
  algid m.
  autochthonous m.
  benign tertian m.
  bilious remittent m.
  cerebral m.
  chronic m.
  m. comatosa
  double tertian m.
  dysenteric algid m.
  falciparum m.
  gastric algid m.
  induced m.
  intermittent m.
  malariae m.
  malignant tertian m.
  nonan m.
  ovale m., ovale tertian m.
  pernicious m.
  quartan m.
  quotidian m.
  relapsing m.
  remittent m.
  tertian m.

  therapeutic m.
  vivax m.
malariae malaria
malarial
  m. cachexia
  m. crescent
  m. fever
  m. hemoglobinuria
  m. knobs
  m. periodicity
  m. pigment
  m. pigment stain
malariology
malarious
Malassez' epithelial rests
Malassezia
  M. furfur
  M. ovalis
malassimilation
maldigestion
Maldonado-San Jose stain
male
  m. breast
  genetic human m.
  m. gonad
  m. hermaphroditism
  m. homosexuality
  m. hypogonadism
  m. pattern alopecia
  m. pattern baldness
  m. pronucleus
  m. pseudohermaphroditism
  m. sterility
  m. urethra
  XX m.
  XXY m.
  XYY m.
Malecot catheter
malemission
maleruption
malformation
  Arnold-Chiari m.
  cystic adenomatoid m.
malfunction
Malgaigne's
  M. amputation
  M. fossa
  M. hernia
  M. luxation
  M. triangle
Malherbe's calcifying epithelioma
malignancy
malignant
  m. anemia
  m. atrophic papulosis
  m. bubo
  m. carcinoid syndrome
  m. catarrhal fever virus

m. ciliary epithelioma
m. dysentery
m. dyskeratosis
m. endocarditis
m. exophthalmos
m. fibrous histiocytoma
m. glaucoma
m. granuloma
m. hepatoma
m. histiocytosis
m. hyperpyrexia
m. hypertension
m. jaundice
m. lentigo melanoma
m. lymphadenosis
m. lymphoma
m. malnutrition
m. melanoma
m. melanoma in situ
m. meningioma
m. mesenchymoma
m. midline reticulosis
m. mixed müllerian tumor
m. mole syndrome
m. myopia
m. nephrosclerosis
m. pustule
m. scleritis
m. smallpox
m. stupor
m. synovioma
m. tertian fever
m. tertian malaria
m. tertian malarial parasite
m. tumor
malinger
malingerer
malingering
malinterdigitation
mallear
m. fold
m. prominence
m. stripe
malleation
mallei (*gen. and pl. of* malleus)
malleoincudal
malleolar
m. articular surface of fibula
m. articular surface of tibia
m. sulcus
malleolus, pl. **malleoli**
external m.
inner m.
internal m.
lateral m.
m. lateralis
medial m.

m. medialis
outer m.
malleotomy
mallet finger
malleus, gen. and pl. **mallei**
Mallophaga
Mallory bodies
Mallory's
M. aniline blue stain
M. collagen stain
M. iodine stain
M. phloxine stain
M. phosphotungstic acid
hematoxylin stain
M. stain for actinomyces
M. stain for hemofuchsin
M. trichrome stain
M. triple stain
Mallory-Weiss
M.-W. lesion
M.-W. syndrome
M.-W. tear
Mall's
M. formula
M. ridges
malnutrition
malignant m.
protein m.
malocclusion
Maloney
M. bougies
M. leukemia virus
malpighian
m. bodies
m. capsule
m. cell
m. corpuscles
m. glands
m. glomerulus
m. layer
m. nodules
m. pyramid
m. rete
m. stigmas
m. stratum
m. tubules
m. tuft
m. vesicles
malposition
malpractice
malpresentation
malrotation
malt-worker's lung
malum
m. articulorum senilis
m. coxae
m. coxae senile
m. perforans pedis

M

malum *(continued)*
    m. venereum
    m. vertebrale suboccipitale
malunion
mamanpian
mamelon
mamelonated
mamelonation
mamilla, pl. mamillae
mamillare
mamillaria
mamillary
    m. body
    m. ducts
    m. line
    m. process
    m. tubercle
    m. tubercle of hypothalamus
mamillate, mamillated
mamillation
mamilliform
mamillotegmental fasciculus
mamillothalamic
    m. fasciculus
    m. tract
mamma, gen. and pl. mammae
    m. accessoria
    m. erratica
    m. masculina
    supernumerary m.
    m. virilis
mammalgia
mammaplasty
    Arie-Pitanguy m.
    augmentation m.
    reconstructive m.
    reduction m.
mammary
    m. branches
    m. calculus
    m. cancer virus of mice
    m. duct ectasia
    m. ducts
    m. dysplasia
    m. fistula
    m. fold
    m. gland
    m. line
    m. neuralgia
    m. plexus
    m. region
    m. ridge
    m. souffle
    m. tumor virus of mice
mammectomy
mammiform
mammillaplasty
mammillitis

mammitis
mammogram
mammography
mammoplasty
mammose
mammosomatotroph
mammotomy
mammotroph
mammotropic, mammotrophic
managed care
Manchester
    M. operation
    M. ovoid
manchette
Manchurian
    M. fever
    M. hemorrhagic fever
    M. typhus
Mandelin's reagent
mandible
mandibula, pl. mandibulae
mandibular
    m. arch
    m. axis
    m. canal
    m. cartilage
    m. condyle
    m. dentition
    m. disk
    m. foramen
    m. fossa
    m. glide
    m. guide prosthesis
    m. hinge position
    m. joint
    m. lymph node
    m. movement
    m. nerve
    m. nodes
    m. notch
    m. process
    m. protraction
    m. reflex
    m. retraction
    m. tongue
    m. torus
mandibulectomy
mandibuloacral dysostosis
mandibulofacial
    m. dysostosis
    m. dysotosis syndrome
    m. dysplasia
mandibulomaxillary fixation
mandibulo-oculofacial
    m.-o. syndrome
mandibulopharyngeal
mandibulum
mandrel, mandril

mandrin
maneuver
    Adson m.
    Bill's m.
    Bracht m.
    Brandt-Andrews m.
    Buzzard's m.
    Credé's m.'s
    DeLee's m.
    Ejrup m.
    Hampton m.
    Heimlich m.
    Hillis-Müller m.
    Hueter's m.
    Jendrassik's m.
    key-in-lock m.
    LeCompte m.
    Leopold's m.'s
    Mauriceau-Levret m.
    Mauriceau's m.
    McDonald's m.
    McRoberts m.
    Müller's m.
    Pajot's m.
    Pinard's m.
    Prague m.
    Ritgen's m.
    Scanzoni's m.
    Sellick's m.
    Valsalva m.
    Wigand m.
mango dermatitis
mangrove fly
mania
    acute m.
maniac
maniacal
manic
    m. episode
    m. excitement
    m. psychosis
manic-depressive
    m.-d. disorder
    m.-d. illness
    m.-d. psychosis
manicy
manifest
    m. content
    m. hyperopia
    m. strabismus
    m. tetany
    m. vector
manifestation
    behavioral m.
    neurotic m.
    psychophysiologic m.
    psychotic m.

manifesting
    m. carrier
    m. heterozygote
manikin
maniphalanx
Mann-Bollman fistula
mannerism
Mannkopf's sign
mannoproteins
mannose-6-phosphate receptors
mannosidosis
Mann's methyl blue-eosin stain
Mann-Williamson
    M.-W. operation
    M.-W. ulcer
manometer
    aneroid m.
    dial m.
    mercurial m.
manometric
manometry
    esophageal m.
manoscopy
Mansonella
    M. demarquayi
    M. ozzardi
    M. perstans
    M. streptocerca
    M. tucumana
mansonelliasis
mansonellosis
Mansonia
Mansonoides
Manson's
    M. disease
    M. eye worm
    M. pyosis
    M. schistosomiasis
Mantel-Haenszel test
M_1 **antigen**
M_2 **antigen**
M^c **antigen**
M^g **antigen**
mantle
    brain m.
    m. layer
    myoepicardial m.
    m. radiotherapy
    m. sclerosis
    m. zone
Mantoux
    M. pit
    M. test
manual
    Diagnostic and Statistical M.
    m. pelvimetry
    m. ventilation

M

manubriosternal
    m. joint
    m. junction
    m. symphysis
manubrium, pl. manubria
    m. mallei
    m. of malleus
    m. sterni
    m. of sternum
manudynamometer
manus, gen. and pl. manus
    m. cava
    m. extensa
    m. flexa
    m. plana
    m. superextensa
    m. valga
    m. vara
map
    chromosomal m.
    chromosome m.
    m. distance
    fate m.
    genetic m.
map-dot-fingerprint dystrophy
maple
    m. bark disease
    m. syrup urine
maplike skull
mapping
    cardiac m.
    chromosome m.
    m. function
    gene m.
    S1 nuclease m.
Marañón
Marañón's
    M. sign
    M. syndrome
marantic
    m. atrophy
    m. edema
    m. endocarditis
    m. thrombosis
    m. thrombus
marasmic
    m. kwashiorkor
    m. thrombosis
    m. thrombus
marasmoid
marasmus
    nutritional m.
marathon group psychotherapy
marble
    m. bone disease
    m. bones
    m. cutters' phthisis

Marburg
    M. disease
    M. virus
    M. virus disease
Marcacci's muscle
march
    m. fracture
    m. hemoglobinuria
Marchand's
    M. adrenals
    M. rest
    M. wandering cell
Marchant's zone
Marchiafava-Bignami disease
Marchiafava-Micheli
    M.-M. anemia
    M.-M. syndrome
Marchi's
    M. fixative
    M. reaction
    M. stain
    M. tract
marcid
Marcille's triangle
marcor
Marcus
    M. Gunn phenomenon
    M. Gunn pupil
    M. Gunn's sign
    M. Gunn syndrome
Marek's disease virus
Marey's law
marfanoid
Marfan's
    M. disease
    M. law
    M. syndrome
margarine disease
Margaropus
    M. winthemi
margin
    m. of acetabulum
    anterior m.
    articular m.
    cavity m.
    cervical m.
    cervical m. of tooth
    ciliary m. of iris
    corneal m.
    m.'s of eyelids
    falciform m.
    fibular m. of foot
    m. of fossa ovalis
    free m.
    free m. of eyelids
    frontal m.
    gingival m.
    incisal m.

inferior m.
inferolateral m.
inferomedial m.
infraorbital m.
interosseous m.
lacrimal m. of maxilla
lambdoid m. of occipital bone
lateral m.
mastoid m. of occipital bone
medial m.
mesovarian m. of ovary
nasal m. of frontal bone
occipital m.
m. of orbit
orbital m. of eyelids
parietal m.
psoas m.
pupillary m. of iris
right m. of heart
squamous m.
superomedial m.
supraorbital m.
m. of the tongue
ulnar m. of forearm
zygomatic m. of greater wing of
  sphenoid bone

marginal
  m. artery of colon
  m. blepharitis
  m. corneal degeneration
  m. crest
  m. fasciculus
  m. gingivitis
  m. gyrus
  m. integrity of amalgam
  m. keratitis
  m. layer
  M. Line Calculus Index
  m. mandibular branch of facial
    nerve
  m. part of orbicularis oris muscle
  m. rays
  m. ridge
  m. ring ulcer of cornea
  m. sinuses of placenta
  m. sphincter
  m. tentorial branch of internal
    carotid artery
  m. tubercle
  m. tubercle of zygomatic bone
  m. zone

margination
  m. of placenta
marginoplasty
margo, gen. **marginis**, pl. **margines**
  m. acetabularis
  m. anterior fibulae
  m. anterior pancreatis

m. anterior pulmonis
m. anterior radii
m. anterior testis
m. anterior tibiae
m. anterior ulnae
m. ciliaris iridis
m. dexter cordis
m. falciformis
m. fibularis pedis
m. frontalis
m. frontalis ossis parietalis
m. frontalis ossis sphenoidalis
m. incisalis
m. inferior
m. inferior cerebri
m. inferior hepatis
m. inferior pancreatis
m. inferior pulmonis
m. inferior splenis
m. inferolateralis
m. inferomedialis
m. infraorbitalis
m. interosseus
m. interosseus fibulae
m. interosseus radii
m. interosseus tibiae
m. interosseus ulnae
m. lacrimalis maxillae
m. lambdoideus squamae occipitalis
m. lateralis
m. lateralis antebrachii
m. lateralis humerii
m. lateralis pedis
m. lateralis renis
m. lateralis scapulae
m. lateralis unguis
m. liber
m. liber ovarii
m. liber unguis
m. linguae
m. mastoideus squamae occipitalis
m. medialis
m. medialis antebrachii
m. medialis cerebri
m. medialis glandulae suprarenalis
m. medialis humerii
m. medialis pedis
m. medialis renis
m. medialis scapulae
m. medialis tibiae
m. mesovaricus ovarii
m. nasalis ossis frontalis
m. occipitalis
m. occipitalis ossis parietalis
m. occipitalis ossis temporalis
m. occultus unguis
m. palpebrae
m. parietalis

M

margo *(continued)*
    m. parietalis ossis frontalis
    m. parietalis ossis sphenoidalis
    m. parietalis ossis temporalis
    m. posterior fibulae
    m. posterior partis petrosae ossis temporalis
    m. posterior radii
    m. posterior testis
    m. posterior ulnae
    m. pupillaris iridis
    m. radialis antebrachii
    m. sagittalis ossis parietalis
    m. sphenoidalis ossis temporalis
    m. squamosus
    m. squamosus ossis parietalis
    m. squamosus ossis sphenoidalis
    m. superior cerebri
    m. superior glandulae suprarenalis
    m. superior pancreatis
    m. superior partis petrosae ossis temporalis
    m. superior scapulae
    m. superior splenis
    m. superomedialis
    m. supraorbitalis
    m. tibialis pedis
    m. ulnaris antebrachii
    m. uteri
    m. zygomaticus alae majoris
marian lithotomy
Marie-Robinson syndrome
Marie's ataxia
Marie-Strümpell disease
Marinesco-Garland syndrome
Marinesco-Sjögren syndrome
Marinesco's succulent hand
Marion's disease
Mariotte bottle
Mariotte's
    M. blind spot
    M. experiment
mariposia
marital
    m. counseling
    m. therapy
Marjolin's ulcer
mark
    alignment m.
    dhobie m.
    port-wine m.
    strawberry m.
    stretch m.'s
    Unna's m.
    washerman's m.
marked fetal bradycardia
marker
    allotypic m.

    cell m.
    cell surface m.
    m. chromosome
    DNA m.'s
    genetic m.
    linkage m.
    oncofetal m.
    polymorphic genetic m.'s
    time m.
    m. trait
    tumor m.
Markov process
Marme's reagent
marmorated
marmoset virus
Maroteaux-Lamy syndrome
Marquis' reagent
marriage therapy
marrow
    bone m.
    m. canal
    m. cell
    red bone m.
    spinal m.
    yellow bone m.
marrow-lymph gland
Marseilles fever
Marshall
    M. method
    M. oblique vein
    M. syndrome
    M. test
    M. vestigial fold
Marshallagia marshalli
Marshall-Marchetti-Krantz operation
Marshall-Marchetti test
marsh fever
marsupialization
marsupial notch
Martegiani's
    M. area
    M. funnel
Martin-Gruber anastomosis
Martinotti's cell
Martin's
    M. bandage
    M. disease
    M. tube
martius yellow
Martorell's syndrome
Maryland coma scale
maschaladenitis
maschale
maschalephidrosis
maschaloncus
maschalyperidrosis
masculine
    m. pelvis

m. protest
m. uterus
masculinity
masculinity-femininity scale
masculinization
masculinize
masculinovoblastoma
masculinus
Masini's sign
mask
ecchymotic m.
Hutchinson's m.
laryngeal m.
luetic m.
nonrebreathing m.
m. of pregnancy
tropical m.
masked
m. epilepsy
m. gout
m. hyperthyroidism
m. virus
masking
unsharp m.
masklike face
Maslow's hierarchy
masochism
masochist
masochistic personality
Mason operation
Mason-Pfizer virus
mason's lung
masque biliaire
mass
m. action theory
apperceptive m.
filar m.
m. hysteria
m. infection
injection m.
inner cell m.
intermediate m.
lateral m. of atlas
lateral m. of ethmoid bone
m. movement
m. peristalsis
m. reflex
sclerotic cemental m.
m. screening
tubular excretory m.
massa, gen. and pl. **massae**
m. intermedia
m. lateralis atlantis
massage
cardiac m.
closed chest m.
external cardiac m.
gingival m.

heart m.
open chest m.
prostatic m.
vibratory m.
Masselon's spectacles
masseter
m. muscle
m. reflex
masseteric
m. artery
m. fascia
m. nerve
m. tuberosity
m. veins
masseur
masseuse
massive
m. bowel resection syndrome
m. collapse
Masson-Fontana ammoniacal silver stain
Masson's
M. argentaffin stain
M. pseudoangiosarcoma
M. trichrome stain
massotherapy
MASS syndrome
mast
m. cell
m. cell leukemia
m. leukocyte
mastadenitis
mastadenoma
Mastadenovirus
mastalgia
mastatrophy, mastatrophia
mastauxe
mastectomy
extended radical m.
modified radical m.
radical m.
simple m.
subcutaneous m.
total m.
master
m. cast
m. eye
m. gland
M. test
M.'s two-step exercise test
mastery motive
masticate
masticating
m. cycles
m. surface
mastication
masticator nerve
masticatory
m. apparatus

M

masticatory *(continued)*
    m. diplegia
    m. force
    m. nucleus
    m. silent period
    m. spasm
    m. surface
    m. system
Mastigophora
mastigote
mastitis
    chronic cystic m.
    gargantuan m.
    glandular m.
    granulomatous m.
    interstitial m.
    lactational m.
    m. neonatorum
    parenchymatous m.
    phlegmonous m.
    plasma cell m.
    puerperal m.
    retromammary m.
    stagnation m.
    submammary m.
    suppurative m.
mastoccipital
mastocyte
mastocytogenesis
mastocytoma
mastocytosis
    diffuse m.
    diffuse cutaneous m.
    systemic m.
mastodynia
mastoid
    m. abscess
    m. air cells
    m. angle of parietal bone
    m. antrum
    m. artery
    m. bone
    m. border of occipital bone
    m. branches of posterior auricular
      artery
    m. branch of occipital artery
    m. canaliculus
    m. cells
    m. emissary vein
    m. empyema
    m. fontanel
    m. foramen
    m. fossa
    m. groove
    m. lymph nodes
    m. margin of occipital bone
    m. notch
    m. part of the temporal bone

    m. process
    m. sinuses
    m. wall of middle ear
mastoidal
mastoidale
mastoidectomy
    radical m.
mastoiditis
    Bezold's m.
    sclerosing m.
mastoncus
masto-occipital
mastoparietal
mastopathy
mastopexy
mastoplasia
mastoplasty
mastoptosis
mastorrhagia
mastosquamous
mastosyrinx
mastotomy
masturbate
masturbation
    false m.
Masugi's nephritis
mat
    m. burn
    m. gold
Matas' operation
matched groups
mater
materia
    m. alba
material
    base m.
    by-product m.
    contrast m.
    cross-reacting m.
    dental m.
    impression m.
    plastic restoration m.
    restorative dental m.'s
maternal
    m. cotyledon
    m. death
    m. death rate
    m. deprivation syndrome
    m. dystocia
    m. immunity
    m. inheritance
    m. placenta
maternity
    m. hospital
mathematical
    m. chaos
    m. determinant

m. genetics
m. model
mating
assortative m.
cross m.
m. isolate
nonrandom m.
random m.
matrical
matrices (*pl. of* matrix)
matricial
matricide
matrix, pl. **matrices**
amalgam m.
m. band
bone m.
m. calculus
cartilage m.
cell m.
cytoplasmic m.
m. Gla protein
identity m.
mitochondrial m.
nail m.
m. retainer
square m.
territorial m.
m. unguis
matter
gray m., grey m.
pontine gray m.
white m.
mattress suture
maturate
maturation
m. arrest
m. index
m. value
mature
m. bacteriophage
m. cataract
m. cell leukemia
m. neutrophil
m. ovarian follicle
maturity
m. onset diabetes of youth
maturity-onset diabetes
matutinal epilepsy
Mauchart's ligaments
Maurer's
M. clefts
M. dots
Mauriac's syndrome
Mauriceau-Levret maneuver
Mauriceau's maneuver

Mauthner's
M. sheath
M. test
maxilla, gen. and pl. **maxillae**
maxillary
m. angle
m. antrum
m. artery
m. dentition
m. eminence
m. gland
m. hiatus
m. nerve
m. plexus
m. process
m. process of embryo
m. protraction
m. sinus
m. sinus radiograph
m. surface of greater wing of
sphenoid bone
m. surface of palatine bone
m. tuberosity
m. vein
maxillectomy
maxillitis
maxillodental
maxillofacial
m. prosthetics
maxillojugal
maxillomandibular
m. fixation
m. record
m. registration
m. relation
m. traction
maxillopalatine
maxillotomy
maxilloturbinal
maximal
m. dose
m. Histalog test
m. permissible dose
m. stimulus
Maximow's stain for bone marrow
maximum
m. breathing capacity
glucose transport m.
m. likelihood estimator
m. occipital point
m. permissible dose
m. temperature
transport m.
tubular m.
m. urea clearance
m. voluntary ventilation
Mayaro virus

M

**Mayer-Rokitansky-Küster-Hauser
  syndrome**
Mayer's
  M. hemalum stain
  M. mucicarmine stain
  M. mucihematein stain
  M. pessary
  M. reflex
May-Grünwald stain
May-Hegglin anomaly
mayidism
Mayo
  M. bunionectomy
  M. operation
  M. vein
Mayo-Robson's
  M.-R. point
  M.-R. position
May-White syndrome
mazamorra
maze
mazodynia
mazolysis
mazopathy, mazopathia
mazopexy
mazoplasia
Mazzoni corpuscle
Mazzotti
  M. reaction
  M. test
McArdle's
  M. disease
  M. syndrome
McArdle-Schmid-Pearson disease
McBurney's
  M. incision
  M. point
  M. sign
McCarthy's reflexes
McCrea sound
McCune-Albright syndrome
McDonald's maneuver
McGoon's technique
McIndoe operation
McKee's line
McMurray test
McNemar's test
m-cone
McPhail test
McRoberts maneuver
McVay's operation
meadow
  m. dermatitis
  m. grass dermatitis
Meadows' syndrome
meal
  Boyden m.

  test m.
  m. worm
mean
  arithmetic m.
  m. corpuscular hemoglobin
  m. corpuscular hemoglobin
    concentration
  m. corpuscular volume
  m. electrical axis
  m. foundation plane
  geometric m.
  harmonic m.
  m. manifest vector
  regression of the m.
  standard error of the m.
  m. vector
measle
measles
  atypical m.
  black m.
  m. convalescent serum
  German m.
  hemorrhagic m.
  three-day m.
  tropical m.
  m. virus
measure
measured intelligence
measurement
  nasion-pogonion m.
measures of central tendency
meatal
  m. cartilage
  m. spine
meatometer
meatoplasty
meatorrhaphy
meatoscope
meatoscopy
meatotome
meatotomy
meatus, pl. **meatus**
  acoustic m.
  m. acusticus externus, m. acusticus
    externus cartilagineus
  m. acusticus internus
  external acoustic m.
  external auditory m.
  fish-mouth m.
  internal acoustic m.
  internal auditory m.
  nasal m.
  m. nasi, m. nasi inferior, m. nasi
    medius, m. nasi superior
  m. nasopharyngeus
  ureteral m.
  m. urinarius

mechanical
    m. abrasion
    m. alternation of the heart
    m. corepraxy
    m. dysmenorrhea
    m. heart
    m. ileus
    m. intelligence
    m. jaundice
    m. strabismus
    m. vector
    m. ventilation
    m. vertigo
mechanically balanced occlusion
mechanicoreceptor
mechanics
    body m.
mechanism
    association m.
    countercurrent m.
    defense m.
    Douglas m.
    Duncan's m.
    gating m.
    immunological m.
    pressoreceptive m.
    proprioceptive m.
    re-entrant m.
    Schultze's m.
mechanistic school
mechanobullous disease
mechanocardiography
mechanocyte
mechanophobia
mechanoreceptor
mechanoreflex
mechanotherapy
mèche
mecism
Mecistocirrus
Meckel's
    M. band
    M. cartilage *CAVe*
    M. cavity
    M. diverticulum
    M. ganglion
    M. ligament
    M. plane
    M. scan
    M. space
    M. syndrome
Meckel-Gruber syndrome
Mecke's reagent
mecometer
meconial colic
meconiorrhea
meconium
    m. aspiration

    m. blockage syndrome
    m. ileus
    m. peritonitis
media (*pl. of* medium)
mediad
medial
    m. accessory olivary nucleus
    m. angle of eye
    m. antebrachial cutaneous nerve
    m. anterior thoracic nerve
    m. aperture of the fourth ventricle
    m. arcuate ligament
    m. arteriole of retina
    m. arteriosclerosis
    m. atrial vein
    m. basal branch of pulmonary artery
    m. basal segment
    m. bicipital groove
    m. border
    m. border of foot
    m. border of forearm
    m. border of humerus
    m. border of kidney
    m. border of scapula
    m. border of suprarenal gland
    m. border of tibia
    m. brachial cutaneous nerve
    m. branches
    m. calcaneal branches of tibial nerve
    m. canthus
    m. cartilaginous layer
    m. central nucleus of thalamus
    m. cerebral surface
    m. circumflex artery of thigh
    m. circumflex femoral artery
    m. circumflex femoral veins
    m. collateral ligament of elbow
    m. condyle
    m. condyle of femur
    m. condyle of tibia
    m. cord of brachial plexus
    m. crest of fibula
    m. crural cutaneous branches of saphenous nerve
    m. crus
    m. crus of facial canal
    m. crus of greater alar cartilage of nose
    m. crus of the horizontal part of the facial canal
    m. crus of the superficial inguinal ring
    m. cuneiform bone
    m. cutaneous branch
    m. cutaneous nerve of arm
    m. cutaneous nerve of forearm

M

medial *(continued)*
  m. cutaneous nerve of leg
  m. dorsal cutaneous nerve
  m. eminence
  m. epicondylar crest
  m. epicondylar ridge
  m. epicondyle of femur
  m. epicondyle of humerus
  m. femoral circumflex artery
  m. femoral tuberosity
  m. fillet
  m. forebrain bundle
  m. frontobasal artery
  m. geniculate body
  m. great muscle
  m. head
  m. inferior genicular artery
  m. inguinal fossa
  m. lacunar lymph node
  m. lacunar node
  m. lamina of cartilaginous auditory tube
  m. layer of cartilaginous auditory tube
  m. lemniscus
  m. ligament
  m. ligament of knee
  m. ligament of talocrural joint
  m. ligament of wrist
  m. limb
  m. lip of linea aspera
  m. longitudinal arch of foot
  m. longitudinal bundle
  m. longitudinal fasciculus
  m. longitudinal stria
  m. lumbar intertransversarii muscles
  m. lumbar intertransverse muscles
  m. lumbocostal arch
  m. malleolar arteries
  m. malleolar network
  m. malleolar subcutaneous bursa
  m. malleolar surface of talus
  m. malleolus
  m. mammary branches
  m. margin
  m. medullary lamina of corpus striatum
  m. meniscus
  m. midpalmar space
  m. nasal branches of anterior ethmoidal nerve
  m. nasal fold
  m. nasal primordium
  m. nasal process
  m. nasal prominence
  m. nucleus of thalamus
  m. occipital artery
  m. occipitotemporal gyrus

  m. palpebral commissure
  m. palpebral ligament
  m. part of longitudinal arch of foot
  m. part of middle lobar branch of right superior pulmonary vein
  m. part of posterior cervical intertransversarii muscles
  m. patellar retinaculum
  m. pectoral nerve
  m. plantar artery
  m. plantar nerve
  m. plate of pterygoid process
  m. pole of ovary
  m. popliteal nerve
  m. preoptic nucleus
  m. process of calcaneal tuberosity
  m. pterygoid muscle
  m. pterygoid plate
  m. puboprostatic ligament
  m. rectus muscle
  m. root of median nerve
  m. root of optic tract
  m. rotator
  m. segment
  m. striate artery
  m. sulcus of crus cerebri
  m. superior genicular artery
  m. supraclavicular nerve
  m. supracondylar crest
  m. supracondylar ridge
  m. sural cutaneous nerve
  m. surface
  m. surface of arytenoid cartilage
  m. surface of cerebral hemisphere
  m. surface of fibula
  m. surface of lung
  m. surface of ovary
  m. surface of testis
  m. surface of tibia
  m. surface of toes
  m. surface of ulna
  m. talocalcaneal ligament
  m. tarsal artery
  m. tubercle of posterior process of talus
  m. umbilical fold
  m. umbilical ligament
  m. vastus muscle
  m. vein of lateral ventricle
  m. venule of retina
  m. vestibular nucleus
  m. wall of middle ear
  m. wall of orbit
  m. wall of tympanic cavity
medialecithal
medialis

median
m. antebrachial vein
m. anterior maxillary cyst
m. aperture of the fourth ventricle
m. arcuate ligament
m. artery
m. atlantoaxial joint
m. bar of Mercier
m. basilic vein
m. cephalic vein
m. cubital vein
m. eminence
m. frontal sulcus
m. glossoepiglottic fold
m. groove of tongue
m. laryngotomy
m. line
m. lithotomy
m. longitudinal raphe of tongue
m. mandibular point
m. maxillary anterior alveolar cleft
m. nerve
m. palatal cyst
m. palatine suture
m. plane
m. raphe cyst of the penis
m. relation
m. retruded relation
m. rhinoscopy
m. rhomboid glossitis
m. sacral artery
m. sacral crest
m. sacral vein
m. section
m. sternotomy
m. strumectomy
m. sulcus of fourth ventricle
m. thyrohyoid ligament
m. tongue bud
m. umbilical fold
m. umbilical ligament
m. vein of forearm
m. vein of neck
medianus
mediastinal
m. arteries
m. branches
m. branches of internal thoracic artery
m. branches of thoracic aorta
m. emphysema
m. fibrosis
m. lipomatosis
m. part of lung
m. pleura
m. pleurisy
m. space
m. surface of lung

m. veins
m. window
mediastinitis
fibrosing m.
fibrous m.
idiopathic fibrous m.
mediastinography
gaseous m.
mediastinopericarditis
mediastinoscope
mediastinoscopy
mediastinotomy
anterior m.
mediastinum
anterior m.
m. anterius
inferior m.
m. inferius
m. medium
middle m.
posterior m.
m. posterius
superior m.
m. superius
m. testis
mediate
m. auscultation
m. contagion
m. percussion
m. transfusion
medicable
medical
m. anatomy
m. care
m. corps
m. diathermy
m. ethics
m. examiner
m. genetics
m. jurisprudence
m. model
m. mycology
m. pathology
m. psychology
m. record
m. record linkage
m. selection
m. transcriptionist
m. treatment
medication
ionic m.
maintenance m.
medicator
medicephalic
medicinal eruption
medicine
adolescent m.
aerospace m.

M

medicine *(continued)*
   alternative m.
   aviation m.
   behavioral m.
   clinical m.
   community m.
   comparative m.
   defensive m.
   desmoteric m.
   experimental m.
   family m.
   fetal m.
   folk m.
   forensic m.
   geriatric m.
   holistic m.
   hyperbaric m.
   internal m.
   legal m.
   military m.
   neonatal m.
   nuclear m.
   osteopathic m.
   perinatal m.
   physical m.
   podiatric m.
   preventive m.
   psychosomatic m.
   social m.
   socialized m.
   space m.
   sports m.
   tropical m.
medicobiologic, medicobiological
medicochirurgical
medicolegal
medicomechanical
medicophysical
medicopsychology
mediocarpal
medioccipital
mediocolic sphincter
mediodens
mediodorsal
   m. nucleus
mediolateral
medionecrosis
   m. of the aorta
   m. aortae idiopathica cystica
mediopubic reflex
mediotarsal
   m. amputation
mediotrusion
mediotype
medisect

Mediterranean
   M. exanthematous fever
   M. lymphoma
medium, pl. **media**
   m. artery
   clearing m.
   complete m.
   contrast m.
   culture m.
   Czapek-Dox m.
   Dorset's culture egg m.
   Eagle's basal m.
   Eagle's minimum essential m.
   Endo's m.
   high osmolar contrast m.
   Loeffler's blood culture m.
   Lowenstein-Jensen m.
   Lowenstein-Jensen culture m.
   motility test m.
   mounting m.
   Mueller-Hinton m.
   passive m.
   selective m.
   separating m.
   Simmons' citrate m.
   Thayer-Martin m.
   transport m.
   m. vein
medius
medi virus
medulla, pl. **medullae**
   m. of adrenal gland
   m. glandulae suprarenalis
   m. of hair shaft
   m. of kidney
   m. of lymph node
   m. nodi lymphatici
   m. oblongata
   m. ossium
   m. ossium flava
   m. ossium rubra
   renal m.
   m. renalis
   m. spinalis
   suprarenal m.
medullar
medullary
   m. arteries of brain
   m. callus
   m. carcinoma
   m. cavity
   m. center
   m. chemoreceptor
   m. cone
   m. cords
   m. folds
   m. groove
   m. laminae of thalamus

m. layers of thalamus
m. membrane
m. plate
m. pyramid
m. pyramidotomy
m. ray
m. sarcoma
m. sheath
m. space
m. spinal arteries
m. sponge kidney
m. striae of fourth ventricle
m. stria of thalamus
m. substance
m. teniae
m. tube

medullated
m. nerve fiber

medullation
medullectomy
medullization
medulloarthritis
medulloblastoma
desmoplastic m.
melanotic m.

medullocell
medulloepithelioma
adult m.
embryonal m.

medullomyoblastoma
Medusa head
Meeh-Dubois formula
Meeh formula
Mees'
M. lines
M. stripes

Meesman dystrophy
megabacterium
megacalycosis
megacardia
megacaryoblast
megacaryocyte
megacephalia
megacephalic
megacephalous
megacephaly
megacoccus, pl. **megacocci**
megacolon
acquired m.
idiopathic m.
toxic m.

megacystic syndrome
megacystis
megacystitis-megaureter syndrome
megacystitis-microcolon-intestinal
hypoperistalsis syndrome
megadactyly, megadactylia,
megadactylism

megadolichocolon
megadont
megadontism
megaesophagus
megagamete
megagnathia
megakaryoblast
megakaryocyte
megakaryocytic leukemia
megalecithal
megalgia
megaloblast
megaloblastic anemia
megalocardia
megalocephaly, megalocephalia
megalocheiria, megalochiria
megalocornea
megalocystis
megalocyte
megalocythemia
megalocytic anemia
megalocytosis
megalodactylia, megalodactylism,
megalodactyly
megalodont
megalodontia
megaloencephalic
megaloencephalon
megaloencephaly
megaloenteron
megalogastria
megaloglossia
megalographia
megalohepatia
megalokaryocyte
megalomania
megalomaniac
megalomelia
megalonychosis
megalophthalmos
anterior m.
megalopia
megalopodia
megalopsia
megalosplanchnic
megalosplenia
megalospore
megalosyndactyly, megalosyndactylia
megaloureter
megalourethra
megamerozoite
meganucleus
megaprosopia
megaprosopous
megarectum
megaseme
megasigmoid
megasomia

megaspore
megathrombocyte
megaureter
    primary m.
    secondary m.
megophthalmus
megoxycyte
megoxyphil, megoxyphile
megrim
meibomian
    m. blepharitis
    m. conjunctivitis
    m. cyst
    m. glands
    m. sty
meibomitis, meibomianitis
Meige's disease
Meigs' syndrome
Meinicke test
meiosis
meiotic
    m. division
    m. drive
    m. phase
Meissel
Meissner's
    M. corpuscle
    M. plexus
melagra
melalgia
melancholia
    hypochondriacal m.
    involutional m.
melancholic
melancholy
melanedema
melanemia
melanidrosis
melaniferous
melanism
melanoacanthoma
melanoameloblastoma
melanoblast
melanoblastoma
melanocarcinoma
melanocomous
melanocyte
melanocytoma
melanodendrocyte
melanoderma
    m. cachecticorum
    m. chloasma
    parasitic m.
    racial m.
    senile m.
melanodermatitis
melanodermic
melanogenemia

melanoglossia
melanokeratosis
melanoleukoderma
    m. colli
melanoma
    acral lentiginous m.
    amelanotic m.
    benign juvenile m.
    Cloudman m.
    desmoplastic malignant m.
    halo m.
    Harding-Passey m.
    malignant m.
    malignant lentigo m.
    malignant m. in situ
    minimal deviation m.
    nodular m.
    subungual m.
    superficial spreading m.
melanomatosis
melanonychia
melanopathy
melanophage
melanophore
melanoplakia
melanorrhagia
melanorrhea
melanosis
    m. circumscripta precancerosa
    m. coli
    m. corii degenerativa
    neurocutaneous m.
    oculodermal m.
    precancerous m. of Dubreuilh
    Riehl's m.
melanosity
melanosome
    giant m.
melanotic
    m. carcinoma
    m. freckle
    m. medulloblastoma
    m. neuroectodermal tumor of
      infancy
    m. progonoma
    m. whitlow
melanotrichous
melanotroph
melanuria
melanuric
melasma
    m. gravidarum
    m. universale
Melchior
melena
    m. neonatorum
    m. spuria
    m. vera

melenemesis
Meleney's
    M. gangrene
    M. ulcer
melicera, meliceris
melissophobia
melitis
melituria
Melkersson-Rosenthal syndrome
Melnick-Needles syndrome
melocervicoplasty
melodidymus
melomania
melomelia
melonoplasty
melon-seed body
meloplasty
melorheostosis
melosalgia
meloschisis
melotia
Meltzer-Lyon test
Meltzer's law
member
    virile m.
membra (*pl. of* membrum)
membrana, gen. and pl. **membranae**
    m. abdominis
    m. adamantina
    m. adventitia
    m. atlanto-occipitalis anterior
    m. atlanto-occipitalis posterior
    m. basalis ductus semicircularis
    m. basilaris
    m. capsularis
    m. capsulopupillaris
    m. carnosa
    m. cerebri
    m. choriocapillaris
    m. cordis
    m. cricothyroidea
    m. decidua
    m. eboris
    m. fibroelastica laryngis
    m. fibrosa
    m. flaccida
    m. fusca
    m. germinativa
    m. granulosa
    m. hyaloidea
    m. hyothyroidea
    membranae intercostalia
    m. intercostalis externa
    m. intercostalis interna
    m. interossea antebrachii
    m. interossea cruris
    m. limitans
    m. limitans gliae

m. mucosa
m. obturatoria
m. perinei
m. pituitosa
m. preformativa
m. propria ductus semicircularis
m. pupillaris
m. quadrangularis
m. reticularis
m. serosa
m. serotina
m. spiralis
m. stapedis
m. statoconiorum
m. sterni
m. striata
m. succingens
m. suprapleuralis
m. synovialis
m. tectoria
m. tectoria ductus cochlearis
m. tensa
m. thyrohyoidea
m. tympani
m. tympani secundaria
m. versicolor
m. vestibularis
m. vibrans
m. vitellina
m. vitrea
membranaceous
membranate
membrane
    adamantine m.
    alveolocapillary m.
    alveolodental m.
    anal m.
    anterior atlanto-occipital m.
    arachnoid m.
    atlanto-occipital m.
    m. attack complex
    basal m. of semicircular duct
    basement m.
    basilar m.
    Bichat's m.
    Bogros' serous m.
    m. bone
    Bowman's m.
    Bruch's m.
    Brunn's m.
    bucconasal m.
    buccopharyngeal m.
    cell m.
    chorioallantoic m.
    cloacal m.
    closing m.'s
    Corti's m.
    cricothyroid m.

M

membrane *(continued)*
  cricotracheal m.
  cricovocal m.
  croupous m.
  deciduous m.
  Descemet's m.
  diphtheritic m.
  drum m.
  Duddell's m.
  dysmenorrheal m.
  egg m., primary egg m., secondary
    egg m., tertiary egg m.
  elastic m.
  embryonic m.
  enamel m.
  epipapillary m.
  epiretinal m.
  exocelomic m.
  m. expansion theory
  external intercostal m.
  extraembryonic m.
  false m.
  fenestrated m.
  fertilization m.
  fetal m.
  fibroelastic m. of larynx
  fibrous m.
  Fielding's m.
  flaccid m.
  germ m., germinal m.
  glassy m.
  glial limiting m.
  Henle's m.
  Henle's fenestrated elastic m.
  Heuser's m.
  Hunter's m.
  Huxley's m.
  hyaline m.
  hyaloid m.
  hyoglossal m.'s
  intercostal m.'s
  internal intercostal m.
  interosseous m. of forearm
  interosseous m. of leg
  ivory m.
  Jackson's m.
  keratogenous m.
  limiting m. of retina, internal
    limiting m., outer limiting m.
  medullary m.
  mucous m.'s
  mucous m. of tympanic cavity
  Nasmyth's m.
  Nitabuch's m.
  nuclear m.
  obturator m.
  olfactory m.
  oral m.
  oronasal m.
  oropharyngeal m.
  otolithic m.
  outer limiting m. *(var. of*
    limiting m. of retina)
  ovular m.
  Payr's m.
  pericardiopleural m.
  peridental m.
  perineal m.
  periodontal m.
  periorbital m.
  pharyngeal m.'s
  pial-glial m.
  pituitary m.
  placental m.
  plasma m.
  pleuropericardial m.
  pleuroperitoneal m.
  posterior atlanto-occipital m.
  postsynaptic m.
  m. potential
  presynaptic m.
  primary egg m. *(var. of* egg m.)
  primary egg m.
  proligerous m.
  prophylactic m.
  pupillary m.
  pyogenic m.
  quadrangular m.
  Reissner's m.
  reticular m.
  Rivinus' m.
  Ruysch's m.
  Scarpa's m.
  schneiderian m.
  Schultze's m.
  secondary egg m.
  secondary egg m. *(var. of*
    egg m.)
  secondary tympanic m.
  semipermeable m.
  serous m.
  Shrapnell's m.
  spiral m.
  stapedial m.
  statoconial m.
  sternal m.
  striated m.
  suprapleural m.
  synovial m.
  tectorial m.
  tectorial m. of cochlear duct
  tertiary egg m. *(var. of* egg m.)
  tertiary egg m.
  thyrohyoid m.
  Toldt's m.
  Tourtual's m.

tympanic m.
m. of tympanum
undulating m., undulatory m.
unit m.
urogenital m.
urorectal m.
uteroepichorial m.
vaginal synovial m.
vestibular m.
virginal m.
vitelline m.
vitreous m.
Wachendorf's m.
yolk m.
Zinn's m.
membrane-coating granule
membranectomy
membranelle
membraniform
membranocartilaginous
membranoid
membranoproliferative glomerulonephritis
membranous
    m. ampulla
    m. cataract
    m. cochlea
    m. conjunctivitis
    m. dysmenorrhea
    m. glomerulonephritis
    m. labyrinth
    m. lamina of cartilaginous auditory tube
    m. laryngitis
    m. layer
    m. layer of superficial fascia
    m. lipodystrophy
    m. neurocranium
    m. ossification
    m. part of interventricular septum
    m. part of male urethra
    m. part of nasal septum
    m. pharyngitis
    m. septum
    m. urethra
    m. viscerocranium
    m. wall of middle ear
    m. wall of trachea
membrum, pl. **membra**
    m. inferius
    m. muliebre
    m. superius
    m. virile
memory
    affect m.
    anterograde m.
    long-term m.
    m. loop
    remote m.

retrograde m.
screen m.
selective m.
senile m.
short-term m.
m. span
subconscious m.
m. trace
menacme
menarche
menarcheal, menarchial
Mendel-Bechterew reflex
mendelian
    m. character
    m. genetics
    m. inheritance
    m. ratio
    m. trait
Mendelian Inheritance in Man
mendelism
mendelizing
Mendel's
    M. first law
    M. instep reflex
    M. second law
Mendelson's syndrome
Ménétrier's
    M. disease
    M. syndrome
Menge's pessary
Mengo
    M. encephalitis
    M. virus
Ménière's
    M. disease
    M. syndrome
meningeal
    m. branches
    m. branch of internal carotid artery
    m. branch of mandibular nerve
    m. branch of occipital artery
    m. branch of ophthalmic nerve
    m. branch of spinal nerves
    m. branch of vagus nerve
    m. carcinoma
    m. carcinomatosis
    m. hernia
    m. layer of dura mater
    m. leukemia
    m. neurosyphilis
    m. plexus
    m. veins
meningeocortical
meningeorrhaphy
meninges (*pl. of* meninx)
meningioangiomatosis

M

meningioma
 cutaneous m.
 malignant m.
 psammomatous m.
meningiomatosis
meningis (*gen. of* meninx)
meningism
meningitic
 m. streak
meningitis, pl. **meningitides**
 basilar m.
 cerebrospinal m.
 epidemic cerebrospinal m.
 epidural m.
 external m. *BeTA StreP*
 internal m.
 meningococcal m.
 Mollaret's m.
 neoplastic m.
 occlusive m.
 otitic m.
 serous m.
 tuberculous m.
meningocele
 spurious m.
 traumatic m.
meningocerebral cicatrix
meningococcal meningitis
meningococcemia
 acute fulminating m.
meningococcus, pl. **meningococci**
meningocortical
meningocyte
meningoencephalitis
 acute primary hemorrhagic m.
 biundulant m.
 chronic progressive syphilitic m.
 eosinophilic m.
 herpetic m.
 mumps m.
 primary amebic m.
 syphilitic m.
meningoencephalocele
meningoencephalomyelitis
meningoencephalopathy
meningomyelitis
meningomyelocele
meningo-osteophlebitis
meningoradicular
meningoradiculitis
meningorrhachidian
meningorrhagia
meningosis
meningotyphoid fever
meningovascular
 m. neurosyphilis
 m. syphilis

meninguria
meninx, gen. **meningis**, pl. **meninges**
 m. fibrosa
 m. primitiva
 primitive m.
 m. serosa
 m. tenuis
 vascular m.
 m. vasculosa
meniscectomy
menisci (*pl. of* meniscus)
meniscitis
meniscocyte
meniscofemoral ligaments
meniscopexy
meniscorrhaphy
meniscotome
meniscus, pl. **menisci**
 articular m.
 m. articularis
 converging m.
 diverging m.
 lateral m.
 m. lateralis
 m. lens
 medial m.
 m. medialis
 negative m.
 periscopic m.
 positive m.
 tactile m.
 m. tactus
Menkes' syndrome
menocelis
menometrorrhagia
menopausal
 m. syndrome
menopause
menophania
Menopon
menorrhagia
menorrhalgia
menoschesis
menostasis, menostasia
menostaxis
menouria
menoxenia
menses
menstrual
 m. age
 m. colic
 m. cycle
 m. edema
 m. extraction abortion
 m. leukorrhea
 m. molimina
 m. period
 m. sclerosis

menstruant
menstruate
menstruation
    anovular m.
    anovulational m.
    nonovulational m.
    retained m.
    retrograde m.
    supplementary m.
    suppressed m.
    vicarious m.
mensual
mensuration
mentagra
mental
    m. aberration
    m. age
    m. agraphia
    m. apparatus
    m. artery
    m. branches of mental nerve
    m. canal
    m. chronometry
    m. deficiency
    m. disease
    m. disorder
    m. disturbance
    m. foramen
    m. health
    m. hospital
    m. hygiene
    m. illness
    m. image
    m. impairment
    m. impression
    m. nerve
    m. point
    m. process
    m. protuberance
    m. region
    m. retardation
    m. scotoma
    m. spine
    m. symphysis
    m. tubercle
mentalis
    m. muscle
mentality
mentation
menti (*gen. of* mentum)
mentoanterior position
mentolabial
    m. furrow
    m. sulcus
mentolabialis
menton
mentoplasty
mentoposterior position

mentotransverse position
mentum, gen. menti
meralgia
    m. paraesthetica
M:E ratio
mercaptoethanol
Mercier's
    M. bar
    M. sound
    M. valve
mercurial
    m. line
    m. manometer
    m. stomatitis
    m. tremor
mercurialentis
mercury
    m. arc
    m. vapor lamp
Merendino's technique
meridian
    m. of cornea
    m.'s of eye
meridiani
meridianus, pl. meridiani
    meridiani bulbi oculi
meridional
    m. aberration
    m. cleavage
    m. fibers
merispore
meristematic
Merkel
    M. cell tumor
    M. corpuscle
    M. filtrum ventriculi
    M. fossa
    M. muscle
    M. tactile cell
    M. tactile disk
mermaid deformity
meroacrania
meroanencephaly
meroblastic cleavage
merocele
merocrine
    m. gland
merodiastolic
merogastrula
merogenesis
merogenetic, merogenic
merogony
meromelia
meromicrosomia
meront
merorachischisis, merorrhachischisis
merosmia
merosporangium

M

merosystolic
merotomy
merozoite
merozygote
Merrifield knife
Méry's gland
Merzbacher-Pelizaeus disease
mesad
mesal
mesameboid
mesangial
    m. cell
    m. nephritis
    m. proliferative glomerulonephritis
mesangiocapillary glomerulonephritis
mesangium
    extraglomerular m.
mesaortitis
mesareic, mesaraic
mesarteritis
mesaticephalic
mesatipellic, mesatipelvic
    m. pelvis
mesaxon
mesectic
mesectoderm
mesencephalic
    m. flexure
    m. nucleus of trigeminal nerve
    m. tegmentum
    m. tract of trigeminal nerve
    m. veins
mesencephalitis
mesencephalon
mesencephalotomy
mesenchyma
mesenchymal
    m. cells
    m. epithelium
    m. hyloma
    m. tissue
mesenchyme
    interzonal m.
    synovial m.
mesenchymoma
    benign m.
    malignant m.
mesenteric
    m. artery occlusion
    m. glands
    m. hernia
    m. lymph nodes
    m. portion of small intestine
    m. veins
mesentericoparietal
    m. fossa
    m. recess

mesenteriolum
    m. processus vermiformis
mesenteriopexy
mesenteriorrhaphy
mesenteriplication
mesenteritis
mesenterium
    m. dorsale commune
mesenteron
mesentery
    m. of appendix
    m. of cecum
    m. of lung
    m. of sigmoid colon
    m. of transverse colon
    urogenital m.
mesethmoid bone
mesh graft
meshwork
    trabecular m.
mesiad
mesial
    m. angle
    m. caries
    m. displacement
    m. occlusion
    m. surface of tooth
mesiobuccal
mesiobucco-occlusal
mesiobuccopulpal
mesiocervical
mesioclusion
mesiodens
mesiodistal
mesiodistocclusal
mesiogingival
mesiognathic
mesioincisal
mesiolabial
mesiolingual
mesiolinguo-occlusal
mesiolinguopulpal
mesio-occlusal
mesio-occlusion
mesioplacement
mesiopulpal
mesioversion
mesmerism
mesmerize
mesoappendix
mesoarium
mesoblast
mesoblastema
mesoblastemic
mesoblastic
    m. nephroma

m. segment
m. sensibility
mesocardium, pl. **mesocardia**
dorsal m.
ventral m.
mesocarpal
mesocaval shunt
mesocecal
mesocecum
mesocephalic
mesocephalous
mesocolic
m. lymph nodes
m. tenia
mesocolon
mesocolopexy
mesocoloplication
mesocord
mesocuneiform
mesoderm
branchial m.
extraembryonic m.
gastral m.
intermediate m.
intraembryonic m.
lateral m.
lateral plate m.
paraxial m.
primary m.
prostomial m.
secondary m.
somatic m.
somitic m.
splanchnic m.
visceral m.
mesodermic
mesodiastolic
mesodont
mesoduodenal
mesoduodenum
mesoenteriolum
mesoepididymis
mesogaster
mesogastric
mesogastrlum
dorsal m.
ventral m.
mesoglia
mesoglial cells
mesogluteal
mesogluteus
mesognathic
mesognathion
mesognathous
mesoileum
mesojejunum
mesolepidoma
mesolobus

mesolymphocyte
mesomelia
mesomelic
m. dwarfism
mesomere
mesometanephric carcinoma
mesometric pregnancy
mesometritis
mesometrium
mesomorph
mesomorphic
mesonephric
m. adenocarcinoma
m. duct
m. fold
m. rest
m. ridge
m. tissue
m. tubule
mesonephroi (*pl. of* mesonephros)
mesonephroid tumor
mesonephroma
mesonephros, pl. **mesonephroi**
mesoneuritis
nodular m.
meso-ontomorph
mesopexy
mesophil, mesophile
mesophilic
mesophlebitis
mesophragma
mesophryon
mesopic
m. perimetry
mesopneumonium
mesoprosopic
mesopulmonum
mesorchial
mesorchium
mesorectum
mesorrhachischisis
mesorrhaphy
mesorrhine
mesosalpinx
mesoscope
mesoseme
mesosigmoid
mesosigmoiditis
mesosigmoidopexy
mesosomatous
mesosome
mesosomia
mesostenium
mesosternum
mesosyphilis
mesosystolic
mesotarsal
mesotendineum

M

mesotendon
mesothelia (*pl. of* mesothelium)
mesothelial
    m. cell
    m. hyloma
mesothelioma
    benign m.
    benign m. of genital tract
mesothelium, pl. mesothelia
mesothorium
mesotropic
mesouranic
mesovarian
    m. border of ovary
    m. margin of ovary
mesovarium, pl. mesovaria
Mesozoa
mesuranic
meta-analysis
metabasis
metabiosis
metabisulfite test
metabolic
    m. acidosis
    m. alkalosis
    m. calculus
    m. coma
    m. craniopathy
    m. disease
    m. encephalopathy
    m. equivalent
    m. mmucinosis
metabolism
    inborn error of m.
metacarpal
    m. bone
    m. index
    m. veins
metacarpectomy
metacarpi (*pl. of* metacarpus)
metacarpohypothenar reflex
metacarpophalangeal
    m. articulations
    m. joints
metacarpothenar reflex
metacarpus, pl. metacarpi
metacentric
    m. chromosome
metacercaria, pl. metacercariae
metacestode
metachromasia
metachromatic
    m. bodies
    m. granules
    m. stain
metachromatism
metachroming
metachromophil, metachromophile

metachronous
metachrosis
metacone
metaconid
metacontrast
metaconule
metacryptozoite
metacyesis
metadysentery
metafacial angle
Metagonimus
metaherpetic keratitis
metahypophysial diabetes
metaicteric
metainfective
metakinesis, metakinesia
metal
    Babbitt m.
    m. base
    d'Arcet's m.
    m. fume fever
    m. insert teeth
    m. interface
    m. objects
metallic
    m. rale
    m. tremor
metallophilia
metallophobia
metalloscopy
metaluetic
metamere
metameric nervous system
metamorphopsia
metamorphosis
    complete m.
    fatty m.
    heterometabolous m.
    holometabolous m.
    incomplete m.
    retrograde m.
metamorphotic
metamyelocyte
metanephric
    m. blastema
    m. bud
    m. cap
    m. diverticulum
    m. duct
    m. tubule
metanephrogenic, metanephrogenous
    m. tissue
metanephros, pl. metanephroi
metaneutrophil, metaneutrophile
metanil yellow
metaphase
metaphysial, metaphyseal
    m. dysostosis

m. dysplasia
m. fibrous cortical defect
metaphysis, pl. **metaphyses**
metaphysitis
metaplasia
agnogenic myeloid m.
apocrine m.
autoparenchymatous m.
coelomic m.
intestinal m.
myeloid m.
primary myeloid m.
secondary myeloid m.
squamous m.
squamous m. of amnion
symptomatic myeloid m.
metaplasis
metaplasm
metaplastic
m. anemia
m. carcinoma
m. ossification
m. polyp
metaplexus
metapophysis
metapore
metapsychology
metapyretic
metarteriole
metarubricyte
pernicious anemia type m.
metastasis, pl. **metastases**
biochemical m.
calcareous m.
hematogenous m.
lymphogenous m.
pulsating metastases
satellite m.
metastasize
metastasizing septicemia
metastatic
m. abscess
m. calcification
m. carcinoid syndrome
m. carcinoma
m. choroiditis
m. mumps
m. ophthalmia
m. pneumonia
m. retinitis
metasternum
metastrongyle
Metastrongylus
metasyphilis
metasyphilitic
metatarsal
m. artery

m. bone
m. reflex
metatarsalgia
metatarsectomy
metatarsophalangeal
m. articulations
m. joints
metatarsus, pl. **metatarsi**
m. adductovarus
m. adductus
m. atavicus
m. latus
m. varus
metathalamus
metatroph
metatrophic
metatropic
m. dwarfism
metatypical
m. carcinoma
Metchnikoff's theory
metencephalic
metencephalon
Metcnier's sign
meteorism
meteoropathy
meteorotropic
meter
m. angle
rate m.
ventilation m.
Venturi m.
metergasia
metesthesiologist
metesthesiology
Methanobacteriaceae
methanogen
methanol fixative
methemalbumin
methemalbuminemia
methemoglobinemia
acquired m.
congenital m.
enterogenous m.
hereditary m.
primary m.
secondary m.
methemoglobinuria
methenamine-silver
method
Abbott's m.
Abell-Kendall m.
Altmann-Gersh m.
Anel's m.
Antyllus' m.
aristotelian m.
Ashby m.
auxanographic m.

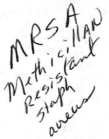
MRSA
Methicillan
Resistant
Staph
aureus

Met

M

method *(continued)*
- Barraquer's m.
- Beck's m.
- Bier's m.
- Born m. of wax plate reconstruction
- Brasdor's m.
- Callahan's m.
- capture-recapture m.
- Carpue's m.
- Charters' m.
- Chayes' m.
- chloropercha m.
- closed circuit m.
- confrontation m.
- cooled-knife m.
- copper sulfate m.
- correlational m.
- Credé's m.'s
- cross-sectional m.
- definitive m.
- Dick m.
- Dieffenbach's m.
- diffusion m.
- direct m. for making inlays
- disk sensitivity m.
- double antibody m.
- Eggleston m.
- Eicken's m.
- encu m.
- ensu m.
- experimental m.
- Fick m.
- flotation m.
- Gärtner's m.
- Gerota's m.
- glucose oxidase m.
- Gräupner's m.
- Gruber's m.
- Hamilton-Stewart m.
- Hammerschlag's m.
- hexokinase m.
- Hilton's m.
- Hirschberg's m.
- Hung's m.
- immunofluorescence m.
- impedance m.
- Indian m.
- indicator dilution m.
- indirect m. for making inlays
- introspective m.
- Italian m.
- ITO m.
- Johnson's m.
- Keating-Hart's m.
- Kety-Schmidt m.
- Klapp's m.
- Krause's m.
- Lamaze m.
- Langendorff's m.
- Lee-White m.
- Liborius' m.
- Ling's m.
- Lister's m.
- Iod m.
- longitudinal m.
- Marshall's m.
- micro-Astrup m.
- microsphere m.
- Moore's m.
- Needles' split cast m.
- Nikiforoff's m.
- Ochsner's m.
- Ollier's m.
- open circuit m.
- Orsi-Grocco m.
- Ouchterlony m.
- Pachon's m.
- paracelsian m.
- parallax m.
- Pavlov m.
- Politzer m.
- Porges m.
- Purmann's m.
- Quick's m.
- reference m.
- Rehfuss m.
- Reverdin's m.
- rhythm m.
- Rideal-Walker m.
- Roux's m.
- Sanger m.
- Scarpa's m.
- Schäfer's m.
- Schede's m.
- Schick m.
- Schweninger's m.
- Somogyi m.
- split cast m.
- Stewart-Hamilton m.
- Stroganoff's m.
- Thane's m.
- Theden's m.
- Thezac-Porsmeur m.
- Thiersch's m.
- twin m.
- ultropaque m.
- u-score m.
- Wardrop's m.
- Westergren m.
- Wheeler m.
- Wilson's m.
- Wolfe's m.
- zinc sulfate flotation centrifugation m.

methodology

3-methoxy-4-hydroxymandelic acid test
methyl
    m. green
    m. green-pyronin stain
    m. violet
    m. yellow
methylase
    dam m.
    deoxyadenosine m.
methylation
    restriction m.
methylene azure
methylene blue
    Kühne's m. b.
    Loeffler's m. b.
    new m. b.
    polychrome m. b.
methylene white
methylenophil, methylenophile
methylenophilic, methylenophilous
N-methylglucamine
methylmalonic acidemia
methylmalonic aciduria
methylrosaniline chloride
methyl-*tert*-butyl ether
metonymy
metopagus
metopic
    m. point
    m. suture
metopion
metopism
metopoplasty
metoposcopy
Metorchis
metoxenous
metoxeny
metra
metratonia
metratrophy, metratrophia
metria
metriocephalic
metritis
metrocyte
metrodynamometer
metrodynia
metrofibroma
metrography
metrolymphangitis
metromalacia
metromania
metronoscope
metroparalysis
metropathia
    m. hemorrhagica
metropathic
metropathy

metroperitoneal fistula
metroperitonitis
metrophlebitis
metroplasty
metrorrhagia
    m. myopathica
metrorrhea
metrorrhexis
metrosalpingitis
metrosalpingography
metroscope
metrostaxis
metrostenosis
metrotomy
metrotrophic test
Meulengracht's diet
Mexican
    M. hat cell
    M. hat corpuscle
    M. spotted fever
    M. typhus
Meycnburg-Altherr-Uehlinger syndrome
Meyenburg's
    M. complex
    M. disease
Meyer-Archambault loop
Meyer-Betz
    M.-B. disease
    M.-B. syndrome
Meyer-Overton rule
Meyer's
    M. cartilages
    M. line
    M. sinus
Meynert's
    M. cells
    M. commissures
    M. decussation
    M. fasciculus
    M. layer
    M. retroflex bundle
MHA-TP test
MHC restriction
mianeh
    m. disease
    m. fever
miasma theory
Mibelli's
    M. angiokeratomas
    M. disease
micatosis
Michaelis-Gutman
Michel's spur
micracoustic
micrencephalia
micrencephalou
micrencephaly

M

microabscess
    Munro's m.
    Pautrier's m.
microadenoma
microaerobion
microaerophil, microaerophile
microaerophilic
microaerophilous
microaerosol
microanastomosis
microanatomist
microanatomy
microaneurysm
microangiography
microangiopathic hemolytic anemia
microangiopathy
    thrombotic m.
microangioscopy
microarteriography
micro-Astrup method
microbe
microbial
    m. associates
    m. genetics
    m. persistence
microbic
microbid
microbiologic
microbiologist
microbiology
microbiotic
microbism
    latent m.
microblast
microblepharia
microblepharism
microblepharon
microbrachia
microbrenner
microcardia
microcentrum
microcephalia
microcephalic
microcephalism
microcephalous
microcephaly
    encephaloclastic m.
    schizencephalic m.
microcheilia, microchilia
microcheiria, microchiria
microcinematography
microcirculation
microccoccaceae
ccus
    candidus
    nglomeratus
    hilus

    M. morrhuae
    M. ureae
    M. varians
micrococcus, pl. micrococci
microcolitis
microcolon
microcolony
microconidium, pl. microconidia
microcoria
microcornea
microcoustic
microcurie
microcyst
microcystic
    m. disease of renal medulla
    m. epithelial dystrophy
microcyte
microcythemia
microcytic anemia
microcytosis
microdactylia
microdactylous
microdactyly
microdissection
microdont
microdontia, microdontism
microdose
microdrepanocytic anemia
microdrepanocytosis
microdysgenesia
microelectrode
microencephaly
microerythrocyte
microetching technique
microevolution
microfibril
microfilament
microfilaremia
microfilaria, pl. microfilariae
microfilarial sheath
microfilm
microflora
microfollicular
    m. adenoma
    m. goiter
microgamete
microgametocyte
microgamont
microgamy
microgastria
microgenia
microgenitalism
microglandular adenosis
microglia
    m. cells
microgliacyte
microglial cells
microglioma

microgliomatosis
microgliosis
microglobulin
    β-m.
microglossia
micrognathia
    m. with peromelia
micrograph
    electron m.
    light m.
micrography
microgyria
microhemagglutination-Treponema
  pallidum test
microhepatia
microincineration
microincision
microinjector
microinvasion
microinvasive carcinoma
microkymatotherapy
microleukoblast
microlith
microlithiasis
    pulmonary alveolar m.
micrology
micromania
micromanipulation
micromanipulator
micromazia
micromelia
micromelic dwarfism
micromere
micromerozoite
micrometastasis
micrometastatic
    m. disease
micrometer
    caliper m.
    filar m.
    ocular m.
    slide m.
micrometry
micromotoscope
micromyelia
micromyeloblast
micromyeloblastic leukemia
microneedle
microneme
micronodular
micronucleus
micronychia
micronystagmus
microorganism
microparasite
micropathology
micropenis
microphage

microphagocyte
microphallus
microphobia
microphone
microphonia, microphony
microphonoscope
microphotograph
microphthalmia
microphthalmos
micropipette, micropipet
microplania
microplasia
microplethysmography
micropodia
micropore
microprecipitation test
micropromyelocyte
microprosopia
micropsia
micropuncture
micropyle
microradiography
microrefractometer
microrespirometer
microsaccades
microscintigraphy
microscope
    binocular m.
    color-contrast m.
    comparator m.
    compound m.
    dark-field m.
    electron m.
    fluorescence m.
    flying spot m.
    infrared m.
    interference m.
    laser m.
    light m.
    opaque m.
    operating m.
    phase m., phase-contrast m.
    polarizing m.
    Rheinberg m.
    scanning electron m.
    simple m., single m.
    stereoscopic m.
    stroboscopic m.
    surgical m.
    television m.
    ultra-m.
    ultrasonic m.
    ultraviolet m.
    x-ray m.
microscopic, microscopical
    m. anatomy
    m. field
    m. hematuria

M

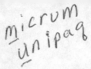

microscopic *(continued)*
   m. section
   m. sphincter
microscopically controlled surgery
microscopy
   electron m.
   fluorescence m.
   immersion m.
   immune electron m.
   immunofluorescence m.
microseme
microsmatic
microsome
microsomia
microspectrophotometry
microspectroscope
microsphere
   m. method
microspherocytosis
microsphygmy
microsphyxia
microsplanchnic
microsplenia
Microspora
Microsporasida
Microsporida
microsporidia
microsporidian keratoconjunctivitis
microsporidiasis
microsporidiosis, microsporidiasis
Microsporum
   M. audouinii
   M. canis
   M. ferrugineum
   M. fulvum
   M. gypseum
microstethophone
microstethoscope
microstomia
microsurgery
microsuture
microsyringe
microthelia
microtia
microtome
microtomy
microtonometer
Microtrombidium
microtropia
microtubule
   subpellicular m.
microvascular anastomosis
microvesicle
microvillus, pl. **microvilli**
Microviridae
microwave therapy
microwelding
microxyphil

microzoon
micrurgical
miction
micturate
micturition
   m. reflex
   m. syncope
midaxillary line
midbody
midbrain
   m. tegmentum
   m. vesicle
midcarpal
   m. joint
midclavicular line
middiastolic murmur
middle
   m. atlantoepistrophic joint
   m. axillary line
   m. cardiac vein
   m. carpal joint
   m. cells
   m. cerebellar peduncle
   m. cerebral artery
   m. cervical cardiac nerve
   m. cervical fascia
   m. cervical ganglion
   m. cluneal nerves
   m. colic artery
   m. colic lymph nodes
   m. colic vein
   m. collateral artery
   m. constrictor muscle of pharynx
   m. costotransverse ligament
   m. cranial fossa
   m. cuneiform bone
   m. ear
   m. ethmoidal air cells
   m. ethmoidal sinuses
   m. finger
   m. frontal convolution
   m. frontal gyrus
   m. frontal sulcus
   m. genicular artery
   m. glossoepiglottic fold
   m. gray layer of superior
     colliculus
   m. group of mesenteric lymph
     nodes
   m. hemorrhoidal artery
   m. hemorrhoidal plexuses
   m. hemorrhoidal veins
   m. hepatic veins
   m. kidney
   m. lobe branch
   m. lobe of prostate
   m. lobe of right lung
   m. lobe syndrome

m. mediastinum
m. meningeal artery
m. meningeal artery groove
m. meningeal branch of maxillary nerve
m. meningeal nerve
m. meningeal veins
m. nasal concha
m. pain
m. palmar space
m. piece
m. radioulnar joint
m. rectal artery
m. rectal lymph node
m. rectal node
m. rectal plexuses
m. rectal veins
m. sacral artery
m. sacral plexus
m. scalene muscle
m. superior alveolar branch of infraorbital nerve
m. supraclavicular nerve
m. suprarenal artery
m. talar articular surface of calcaneus
m. temporal artery
m. temporal convolution
m. temporal gyrus
m. temporal sulcus
m. temporal vein
m. thyroid vein
m. transverse rectal fold
m. trunk of brachial plexus
m. turbinated bone
m. umbilical fold
m. umbilical ligament
midforceps delivery
midgastric transverse sphincter
midget bipolar cells
midgracile
midgut
midlife crisis
midline
m. incision
m. malignant reticulosis granuloma
m. myelotomy
midmenstrual
midnodal extrasystole
midoccipital
midpain
midpalmar space
midplane
midriff
midsagittal
m. plane
m. section
midsection

midsigmoid sphincter
midsternum
midtarsal
m. joint
midwife
midwifery
Miescher's
M. elastoma
M. granuloma
M. tubes
mignon lamp
migraine
abdominal m.
acephalic m.
basilar m.
classic m.
common m.
complicated m.
fulgurating m.
Harris' m.
m. headache
hemiplegic m.
ocular m.
ophthalmoplegic m.
m. without headache
migrating
m. abscess
m. teeth
migration
epithelial m.
m. inhibition test
m. inhibitory factor test
m. of ovum
m. theory
migration-inhibitory factor
migratory
m. cell
m. pneumonia
mika operation
Mikulicz'
M. aphthae
M. cells
M. disease
M. drain
M. operation
M. syndrome
Mikulicz clamp
Mikulicz-Vladimiroff amputation
mild fetal bradycardia
Miles' operation
Miles resection
milia (*pl. of* milium)
Milian's
M. disease
M. erythema
miliaria
m. alba
apocrine m.

M

miliaria *(continued)*
    m. crystallina
    m. profunda
    pustular m.
    m. rubra
miliary
    m. abscess
    m. aneurysm
    m. embolism
    m. fever
    m. papular syphilid
    m. pattern
    m. tuberculosis
milieu
    m. intérieur, m. interne
    m. therapy
military
    m. medicine
    m. neurosis
military antishock trousers
milium, pl. **milia**
    colloid m.
milk
    acidophilus m.
    m. anemia
    m. of calcium
    m. crust
    m. cyst
    m. ducts
    m. factor
    fortified m.
    m. gland
    lactobacillary m.
    m. leg
    m. let-down reflex
    m. line
    m. ridge
    m. scall
    m. spots
    m. tetter
    m. tooth
    uterine m.
    witch's m.
milk-alkali syndrome
milk-ejection reflex
milker's nodule virus
Milkman's syndrome
milkpox
milky
    m. ascites
    m. urine
mill
    m. fever
    m. wheel murmur
Millard-Gubler syndrome
milled-in
    m.-i. curves
    m.-i. paths

Miller-Abbott tube
miller's
    m. asthma
Miller's chemicoparasitic theory
millet seed
milliampere
millibar
millicurie
milligramage
milligram hour
millilambert
milling-in
Millner needle
Millon
    M. clinical multiaxial inventory
    M. Clinical Multiaxial Inventory
       test
milphosis
Milroy's disease
Milton's disease
mimesis
mimetic
    m. chorea
    m. muscles
    m. paralysis
mimic
    m. convulsion
    m. genes
    m. spasm
    m. tic
mimmation
MIM number
Minamata disease
mind
    m. blindness
    m. pain
    prelogical m.
    subconscious m.
mind-reading
mineralization
miner's
    m. asthma
    m. cramps
    m. disease
    m. elbow
    m. lung
    m. nystagmus
Minerva jacket
mini
miniature
    m. scarlet fever
    m. stomach
minicore-multicore myopathy
minilaparotomy
minimal
    m. air
    m. alveolar concentration
    m. amplitude nystagmus

m. anesthetic concentration
m. brain dysfunction
m. deviation melanoma
m. dose
m. infecting dose
m. inhibitory concentration
m. reacting dose

minimal-change
m.-c. disease
m.-c. nephrotic syndrome

minimally invasive surgery

minimum
m. light
m. light threshold
m. temperature

mink enteritis virus

Minnesota
M. Multiphasic Personality Inventory
M. multiphasic personality inventory test

minor
m. agglutinin
m. amputation
m. calices
m. connector
m. duodenal papilla
m. fissure
m. forceps
m. groove
m. hippocampus
m. hypnosis
m. hysteria
justo m.
m. motor seizure
m. operation
m. salivary glands
m. sublingual ducts
m. surgery

Minot-Murphy diet

minus
m. lens
m. strand

minute
m. objects
m. output
m. volume

miodidymus, miodymus
miolecithal
mionectic
miopragia
miopus
miosis
paralytic m.
spastic m.

miosphygmia
miostagmin reaction
miracidium, pl. **miracidia**

Mirchamp's sign
mire
Mirizzi's syndrome
mirror
concave m.
convex m.
m. haploscope
head m.
m. image
m. image dextrocardia
mouth m.
m. speech
van Helmont's m.

mirror-image cell
mirror-writing
miryachit
misandry
misanthropy
miscarriage
miscarry
miscegenation
misdiagnosis
misdirection phenomenon
miserotia
mismatch repair
misogamy
misogyny
misologia
misoneism
misopedia, misopedy
missed
m. abortion
m. labor
m. period

missense
m. suppression

mist bacillus
Mitchell's
M. disease
M. treatment

mite
m. typhus

mite-born typhus
mitella
mitigate
mitis
mitochondrial
m. chromosome
m. gene
m. matrix
m. myopathy
m. sheath

mitochondrion, pl. **mitochondria**
m. of hemoflagellates

mitogen
pokeweed m.

mitogenesis
mitogenetic

M

mitogenic
mitosis, pl. **mitoses**
    heterotype m.
    multipolar m.
    somatic m.
mitotic
    m. division
    m. figure
    m. index
    m. rate
    m. spindle
mitral
    m. area
    m. cells
    m. click
    m. commissurotomy
    m. facies
    m. gradient
    m. incompetence
    m. insufficiency
    m. murmur
    m. orifice
    m. regurgitation
    m. stenosis
    m. tap
    m. valve
    m. valve prolapse
    m. valve prolapse syndrome
    m. valvotomy
mitralization
Mitrofanoff principle
Mitsuda
    M. antigen
    M. reaction
Mitsuo's phenomenon
mittelschmerz
mixed
    m. agglutination
    m. agglutination reaction
    m. agglutination test
    m. aphasia
    m. astigmatism
    m. beat
    m. cell leukemia
    m. chancre
    m. connective-tissue disease
    m. discrete-continuous random
      variable
    m. esotropia
    m. expired gas
    m. gland
    m. glioma
    m. hyperlipemia
    m. hyperlipidemia
    m. hyperlipoproteinemia familial,
      type 5 hyperlipidemia
    m. hypoglycemia
    m. infection

    m. leukemia
    m. lymphocyte culture
    m. lymphocyte culture reaction
    m. lymphocyte culture test
    m. mesodermal tumor
    m. nerve
    m. paralysis
    m. thrombus
    m. tumor
    m. tumor of salivary gland
    m. tumor of skin
mixing
    phenotypic m.
Mixter clamp
Miyagawa bodies
Miyagawanella
MLC test
M-mode
MM virus
M'Naghten rule
mneme
mnemenic, mnemic
mnemism
mnemonic
mnemonics
MNSs antigens
MNSs blood group
mobile
    m. part of nasal septum
    m. spasm
mobilization
    stapes m.
Mobitz
    M. block
    M. types of atrioventricular block
Möbius'
    M. sign
    M. syndrome
modal alteration
modality
mode
model
    additive m.
    animal m.
    Bingham m.
    biomedical m.
    biopsychosocial m.
    computer m.
    m. game
    genetic m.
    logistic m.
    mathematical m.
    medical m.
    multiplicative m.
    multistage m.
    pathological m.
    statistical m.

modeling
    m. composition
    m. compound
    m. plastic
moderate hypothermia
moderator
    m. band
    m. variable
modern genetics
modification
    behavior m.
modified
    m. radical hysterectomy
    m. radical mastectomy
    m. smallpox
    m. zinc oxide-eugenol cement
modifier gene
modiolus, pl. modioli
    m. labii
modulation transfer function
modulus
    bulk m.
    m. of elasticity
    m. of volume elasticity
    Young's m.
Moeller's
    M. glossitis
    M. grass bacillus
Mogen clamp
mogiarthria
mogigraphia
mogilalia
mogiphonia
Mohr
    M. pipette
    M. syndrome
Mohrenheim's
    M. fossa
    M. space
Mohs'
    M. chemosurgery
    M. fresh tissue chemosurgery technique
    M. micrographic surgery
    M. surgery
moist
    m. gangrene
    m. papule
    m. rale
    m. tetter
    m. wart
Mokola virus
molar
    m. behavior
    first m., first permanent m.
    m. glands
    Moon's m.'s
    mulberry m.

    m. pregnancy
    second m.
    sixth-year m.
    third m.
    m. tooth
    twelfth-year m.
molariform
molaris tertius
mold
    m. guide
    pink bread m.
molding
    border m.
    compression m.
    injection m.
    tissue m.
mole
    blood m.
    Breus m.
    carneous m.
    cystic m.
    false m.
    fleshy m.
    grape m.
    hairy m.
    hydatidiform m., hydatid m.
    invasive m.
    spider m.
    vesicular m.
molecular
    m. behavior
    m. disease
    m. dissociation theory
    m. genetics
    m. layer
    m. layer of cerebellar cortex
    m. layer of cerebellum
    m. layer of cerebral cortex
    m. layer of retina
    m. layers of olfactory bulb
    m. pathology
molecule
    accessory m.'s
    adhesion m.'s
    cell adhesion m.
    endothelial-leukocyte adhesion m.
    intercellular adhesion m.-1
molilalia
molimen, pl. molimina
    m. climactericum virile
    menstrual molimina
Mollaret's meningitis
mollities
Moll's glands
molluscous
molluscum
    m. body
    m. conjunctivitis

M

molluscum *(continued)*
- m. contagiosum
- m. contagiosum virus
- m. corpuscle
- m. verrucosum

Moloney
- M. test
- M. virus

molybdenum-99

molybdenum target tube

molysmophobia

momism

Monakow's
- M. bundle
- M. nucleus
- M. syndrome
- M. tract

monaminuria

monangle

monarthric

monarthritis

monarticular

monaster

monathetosis

monaural

monaxonic

Mönckeberg's
- M. arteriosclerosis
- M. calcification
- M. degeneration
- M. medial calcification
- M. sclerosis

Mondini
- M. deafness
- M. dysplasia

Mondonesi's reflex

Mondor's disease

Monera

moneran

monesthetic

Monge's disease

mongolian
- m. fold
- m. macula
- m. spot

monilated

monilethrix

Monilia

Moniliaceae

monilial

moniliasis
- m. pneumonia

moniliform
- m. hair

Moniliformis

moniliid

monism

monistic

monitor
- cardiac m.
- electronic fetal m.
- Holter m.

monitoring

monkey
- m. B virus
- m. hand

monkey-paw

mono-amelia

monoaminergic

monoaminuria

monoamniotic
- m. twins

monoassociated

monoblast

monobrachius

monocardian

monocephalus

monochorea

monochorial
- m. twins

monochorionic
- m. diamniotic placenta
- m. monoamniotic placenta

monochroic

monochromasia

monochromasy
- blue cone m.
- pi cone m.

monochromatic
- m. aberration
- m. rays

monochromatism
- blue cone m.
- pi cone m.
- rod m.

monochromatophil, monochromatophile

monochromic

monochromophil, monochromophile

monocle

monoclonal
- m. antibody
- m. gammopathy
- m. immunoglobulin
- m. peak
- m. protein

monocranius

monocrotic
- m. pulse

monocrotism

monocular
- m. diplopia
- m. heterochromia
- m. strabismus

monoculus

monocyte
- m. chemoattractant protein-1

monocytic
    m. angina
    m. leukemia
    m. leukemoid reaction
    m. leukocytosis
    m. leukopenia
monocytoid cell
monocytopenia
monocytosis
monodactyly, monodactylism
monodermoma
monodisperse
monogametic
monogenesis
monogenetic
monogenic
monogenous
monogerminal
monograph
monoideism
monoinfection
monoiodotyrosine
monokine
monoleptic fever
monolocular
monomania
monomaniac
monomastigote
monomelic
monomicrobic
monomorphic
    m. adenoma
monomphalus
monomyoplegia
monomyositis
mononeural, mononeuric
mononeuralgia
mononeuritis
mononeuropathy
    m. multiplex
mononoea
mononuclear
    m. phagocyte system
mononucleosis
    infectious m.
monoparesis
monoparesthesia
monopathic
monopathy
monopenia
monophagism
monophasia
monophasic
    m. complex
monophobia
monophthalmos
monophthalmus

monophyletic
    m. theory
monophyletism
monophyodont
monoplasmatic
monoplast
monoplastic
monoplegia
    m. masticatoria
monoploid
monopodia
monopolar cautery
monops
monoptychial
monorchia
monorchidic, monorchid
monorchidism
monorchism
monorecidive
    m. chancre
monorhinic
monoscelous
monoscenism
monosomia
monosomic
monosomous
monosomy
monospasm
monospermy
Monosporium apiospermum
Monostoma
monostome
monostotic
    m. fibrous dysplasia
monostratal
monosymptomatic
monosynaptic
monosyphilide
monothermia
monotonic sequence
monotrichate
monotrichous
monovalent antiserum
monovular twins
monoxenous
monozoic
monozygotic, monozygous
    m. twins
Monro-Kellie doctrine
Monro-Richter line
Monro's
    M. doctrine
    M. foramen
    M. line
    M. sulcus
mons, gen. **montis**, pl. **montes**
    m. pubis

M

mons *(continued)*
    m. ureteris
    m. veneris
Monsel solution
Monson curve
monster
Monteggia's fracture
Montenegro test
montes (*pl. of* mons)
Montgomery's
    M. follicles
    M. glands
    M. tubercles
monticulus, pl. **monticuli**
    palmar monticuli
montis (*gen. of* mons)
mood
    m. disorders
    m. swing
mood-congruent hallucination
mood-incongruent hallucination
moon
    m. face
    m. facies
    m. shaped face
Moon's molars
Mooren's ulcer
Moore's
    M. lightning streaks
    M. method
Mooser bodies
moral
    m. ataxia
    m. treatment
Morand's
    M. foot
    M. spur
Morax-Axenfeld diplobacillus
Moraxella
    M. anatipestifer
    M. catarrhalis
    M. conjunctivitis
    M. kingae
    M. lacunata
    M. nonliquefaciens
    M. osloensis
    M. phenylpyruvica
morbid
    m. impulse
    m. obesity
    m. thirst
morbidity
    puerperal m.
    m. rate
morbific
morbigenous
morbility
morbilli

morbilliform
Morbillivirus
morbilous
morbus
morcel
morcellation
    m. operation
morcellement
mordant
Morel's ear
Morerastrongylus costaricensis
mores
Morgagni-Adams-Stokes syndrome
morgagnian cyst
Morgagni's
    M. appendix
    M. cartilage
    M. caruncle
    M. cataract
    M. columns
    M. concha
    M. crypts
    M. disease
    M. foramen
    M. fossa
    M. fovea
    M. frenum
    M. globules
    M. humor
    M. hydatid
    M. lacuna
    M. liquor
    M. nodule
    M. prolapse
    M. retinaculum
    M. sinus
    M. spheres
    M. syndrome
    M. tubercle
    M. valves
    M. ventricle
morgan
Morganella
    M. morganii
Morgan's
    M. bacillus
    M. fold
morgue
moria
moribund
morin
Morison's pouch
Mörner's test
morning
    m. diarrhea
    m. glory anomaly
    m. glory syndrome

m. sickness
m. vomiting
moron
Moro reflex
morphea
m. acroterica
m. alba
m. guttata
m. herpetiformis
m. linearis
m. pigmentosa
morpheme
morphine injector's septicemia
morphogenetic
m. movement
morphologic element
morphometric
morphometry
morphon
morphophysiology
morphosis
morphosynthesis
morphotype
Morquio's
M. disease
M. syndrome
Morquio-Ullrich disease
mors, gen. **mortis**
m. thymica
morsicatio
m. buccarum
mortal
mortality
perinatal m.
m. rate
mortar kidney
Mortierella
mortification
mortified
mortis (*gen. of* mors)
mortise
m. joint
Morton's
M. neuralgia
M. plane
M. syndrome
mortuary
morula
morulation
moruloid
Morvan's
M. chorea
M. disease
mosaic
m. fundus
m. inheritance
m. pattern
m. wart

mosaicism
cellular m.
chromosome m.
gene m.
germinal m., gonadal m.
Moschcowitz' disease
Moschcowitz test
Mosenthal test
Mosler's
M. diabetes
M. sign
mosquito, pl. **mosquitoes**
m. clamp
m. forceps
Mossman fever
Mosso's
M. ergograph
M. sphygmomanometer
Moss tube
mossy
m. cell
m. fibers
m. foot
Motais' operation
mote
blood m.'s
moth-eaten alopecia
mother
m. cell
m. colony
m. cyst
m. star
m. superior complex
surrogate m.
m. surrogate
m. yaw
moth patch
motile
m. leukocyte
motility
m. test
m. test medium
motion
continuous passive m.
m. sickness
motivation
extrinsic m.
intrinsic m.
personal m.
motive
achievement m.
mastery m.
motofacient
motoneuron
motor
m. abreaction
m. agraphia
m. alexia

M

motor *(continued)*
    m. amusia
    m. aphasia
    m. apraxia
    m. area
    m. ataxia
    m. cell
    m. cortex
    m. decussation
    m. endplate
    m. fibers
    m. image
    m. impersistence
    m. nerve
    m. nerve of face
    m. neuron
    m. neuron disease
    m. nuclei
    m. nucleus of facial nerve
    m. nucleus of trigeminal nerve
    m. nucleus of trigeminus
    m. oculi
    m. paralysis
    plastic m.
    m. plate
    m. point
    m. root
    m. root of ciliary ganglion
    m. roots of submandibular ganglion
    m. root of trigeminal nerve
    m. speech center
    m. system disease
    m. unit
    m. urgency
    m. zone
motorial
motormeter
mottle
    quantum m.
mottled
    m. enamel
    m. tooth
mottling
Motulsky dye reduction test
moulage
mould
mounding
Mounier-Kuhn syndrome
mountain
    m. anemia
    m. disease
    m. sickness
mounting
    m. medium
    split cast m.
mourn
mouse
    m. cancer

    m. encephalomyelitis virus
    m. hepatitis virus
    joint m.'s
    m. leukemia viruses
    m. mammary tumor virus
    New Zealand mice
    nude m.
    m. parotid tumor virus
    m. poliomyelitis virus
    m. thymic virus
mousepox virus
mousetail pulse
mouse-tooth forceps
mouth
    m. breathing
    carp m.
    denture sore m.
    m. guard
    m. mirror
    m. rehabilitation
    m. stick
    tapir m.
    trench m.
    m. of the womb
mouth-to-mouth
    m.-t.-m. respiration
    m.-t.-m. resuscitation
movable
    m. heart
    m. joint
    m. kidney
    m. pulse
    m. spleen
    m. testis
movement
    active m.
    adversive m.
    after-m.
    ameboid m.
    assistive m.
    associated m.'s
    Bennett m.
    border m.'s
    border tissue m.'s
    bowel m.
    cardinal ocular m.'s
    choreic m.
    ciliary m.
    circus m.
    cogwheel ocular m.'s
    conjugate m. of eyes
    decomposition of m.
    disconjugate m. of eyes
    drift m.'s
    fetal m.
    fixational ocular m.
    flick m.'s
    free mandibular m.'s

functional mandibular m.'s
fusional m.
hinge m.
intermediary m.'s
lateral m.
Magnan's trombone m.
mandibular m.
mass m.
morphogenetic m.
muscular m.
neurobiotactic m.
non-rapid eye m.
opening m.
paradoxical m. of eyelids
passive m.
pendular m.
protoplasmic m.
rapid eye m.'s
reflex m.
resistive m.
saccadic m.
streaming m.
Swedish m.'s
translatory m.
vermicular m.
Mowry's colloidal iron stain
moyamoya disease
Mozart ear
MP joints
MR angiography
MS-1
M. agent
M. hepatitis
MS-2 agent
MSB trichrome stain
Mu antigen
Mucha-Habermann
M.-H. disease
M.-H. syndrome
Much's bacillus
mucicarmine
mucid
muciferous
muciform
mucigenous
mucihematein
mucilaginous gland
mucin clot test
mucinemia
mucinogen granules
mucinoid degeneration
mucinosis
cutaneous focal m.
follicular m.
localized m.
metabolic m.
oral focal m.
papular m.

reticular erythematous m.
secondary m.
mucinous
m. carcinoma
m. plaque
mucinuria
muciparous
m. gland
mucitis
Muckle-Wells syndrome
mucoalbuminous cells
mucobuccal fold
mucocele
mucoclasis
mucocolitis
mucocolpos
mucocutaneous
m. junction
m. leishmaniasis
m. lymph node syndrome
m. muscle
mucoenteritis
mucoepidermoid
m. carcinoma
m. tumor
mucoepithelial dysplasia
mucoid
m. adenocarcinoma
m. colony
m. degeneration
m. impaction of bronchus
m. medial degeneration
mucolipidosis, pl. mucolipidoses
m. I
m. II
m. III
m. IV
mucolysis
mucolytic
mucomembranous
m. enteritis
mucoperichondrial flap
mucoperiosteal
m. flap
mucoperiosteum
mucopolysaccharide keratin dystrophy
mucopolysaccharidosis, mucopolysaccharidoses
type II m.
type III m.
type IS m.
type IVA, B m.
type V m.
type VI m.
type VII m.
type VIII m.
mucopolysacchariduria

M

mucoprotein
> Tamm-Horsfall m.

mucopurulent
> m. conjunctivitis

mucopus
Mucor
Mucoraceae
mucormycosis
mucosa
> alveolar m.
> m. of auditory tube
> m. of bronchi
> m. of colon
> m. of ductus deferens
> esophageal m.
> m. of female urethra
> m. of gallbladder
> gastric m.
> gingival m.
> laryngeal m.
> lingual m.
> nasal m.
> olfactory m.
> oral m.
> pharyngeal m.
> respiratory m.
> m. of seminal vesicle
> m. of small intestine
> tracheal m.
> m. of tympanic cavity
> m. of ureter
> m. of urinary bladder
> m. of uterine tube
> vaginal m.

mucosal
> m. disease virus
> m. folds of gallbladder
> m. graft
> m. relief radiography
> m. tunics

mucosanguineous, mucosanguinolent
mucosectomy
mucoserous
> m. cells

mucostatic
mucous
> m. cast
> m. cell
> m. colitis
> m. connective tissue
> m. cyst
> m. diarrhea
> m. gland
> m. glands of auditory tube
> m. membranes
> m. membrane of tympanic cavity
> m. neck cell
> m. papule

> m. patch
> m. plaque
> m. plug
> m. polyp
> m. rale
> m. sheath of tendon
> m. tunics

mucoviscidosis
mucro, pl. **mucrones**
> m. cordis
> m. sterni

mucron
mucronate
mucrones (*pl. of* mucro)
mucus
> glairy m.
> m. impaction

mud bed
Muehrcke's lines
Mueller electronic tonometer
Mueller-Hinton
> M.-H. agar
> M.-H. medium

Muellerius capillaris
Muerhrcke's sign
muffle furnace
Muir-Torre syndrome
mulberry
> m. calculus
> m. molar
> m. ovary
> m. spots

Mules' operation
mule-spinner's cancer
mulibrey nanism
muliebria
müllerian
> m. adenosarcoma
> m. duct
> m. duct inhibitory factor
> m. inhibiting factor
> m. inhibiting substance
> m. regression factor

Müller's
> M. capsule
> M. duct
> M. fibers
> M. fixative
> M. law
> M. maneuver
> M. muscle
> M. radial cells
> M. sign
> M. trigone
> M. tubercle

mulling
multangular
> m. bone

multiarticular
multiaxial
    m. classification
    m. joint
multibacillary
multicapsular
multicellular
multicentric reticulohistiocytosis
Multiceps
    M. multiceps
    M. serialis
multicollinearity
multi-colony-stimulating factor
multicore disease
multicuspid
    m. tooth
multicuspidate
multidrug resistance
multifactorial inheritance
multifetation
multifid
multifidus
    m. muscle
multifocal
    m. choroiditis
    m. lens
    m. osteitis fibrosa
multiform
    m. layer
multiformat camera
multiglandular
multigravida
multi-infarct dementia
multi-infection
multilamellar body
multilobar, multilobate, multilobed
multilobular
multilocal
    m. genetics
multilocular
    m. cyst
    m. hydatid cyst
multiloculate hydatid cyst
multimammae
multinodal
multinodular, multinodulate
    m. goiter
multinomial distribution
multinuclear, multinucleate
    m. leukocyte
multinucleosis
multipara
    grand m.
multiparity
multiparous
multipartial
multipennate muscle
multiphasic screening

multiple
    m. amputation
    m. anchorage
    m. chemical sensitivity
    m. ego states
    m. embolism
    m. endocrine adenomatosis
    m. endocrine deficiency syndrome
    m. endocrine neoplasia, type 2
    m. epiphysial dysplasia
    m. exostosis
    m. fission
    m. fracture
    m. glandular deficiency syndrome
    m. hamartoma syndrome
    m. idiopathic hemorrhagic sarcoma
    m. intestinal polyposis
    m. lentigines syndrome
    m. mucosal neuroma syndrome
    m. myeloma
    m. myelomatosis
    m. myositis
    m. neuritis
    m. parasitism
    m. personality
    m. personality disorder
    m. pregnancy
    m. puncture tuberculin test
    m. sclerosis
    m. self-healing squamous
      epithelioma
    m. serositis
    m. sleep latency test
    m. stain
    m. symmetric lipomatosis
    m. vision
multiplicative
    m. division
    m. growth
    m. model
multiplier
    countercurrent m.
multipolar
    m. cell
    m. mitosis
    m. neuron
multirooted
multistage model
multisynaptic
multivariate studies
multivesicular bodies
mummification
    m. necrosis
mummified pulp
mumps
    m. meningoencephalitis
    metastatic m.
    m. sensitivity test

M

mumps *(continued)*
m. skin test antigen
m. virus
mumu fever
Munchausen
M. syndrome
M. syndrome by proxy
Münchhausen syndrome
municipal hospital
Munro's
M. abscess
M. microabscess
M. point
Munson's sign
mural
m. aneurysm
m. cell
m. endocarditis
m. pregnancy
m. thrombosis
m. thrombus
murexide
muriform
murine
m. leukemia
m. sarcoma virus
m. typhus
murmur
accidental m.
anemic m.
aneurysmal m.
aortic m.
arterial m.
atriosystolic m.
Austin Flint m.
bellows m.
brain m.
Cabot-Locke m.
cardiac m.
cardiopulmonary m.
cardiorespiratory m.
Carey Coombs m.
Cole-Cecil m.
continuous m.
cooing m.
Coombs m.
crescendo m.
Cruveilhier-Baumgarten m.
diamond-shaped m.
diastolic m.
Duroziez' m.
dynamic m.
early diastolic m.
ejection m.
endocardial m.
extracardiac m.
Flint's m.
Fräntzel's m.

friction m.
functional m.
Gibson m.
Graham Steell's m.
Hamman's m.
hemic m.
Hodgkin-Key m.
holosystolic m.
hourglass m.
innocent m.
inorganic m.
late apical systolic m.
late diastolic m.
machinery m.
middiastolic m.
mill wheel m.
mitral m.
musical m.
nun's m.
obstructive m.
organic m.
pansystolic m.
pericardial m.
pleuropericardial m.
presystolic m.
pulmonary m., pulmonic m.
regurgitant m.
respiratory m.
Roger's m.
sea gull m.
seesaw m.
Steell's m.
stenosal m.
Still's m.
systolic m.
to-and-fro m.
tricuspid m.
vascular m.
venous m.
vesicular m.
water wheel m.
Murphy
M. button
M. drip
M. percussion
M. sign
Murray
M. Valley encephalitis
M. Valley encephalitis virus
M. Valley rash
Murutucu virus
Musca
muscae volitantes
Muscidae
muscle
m.'s of abdomen
abdominal external oblique m.
abdominal internal oblique m.

abductor digiti minimi m. of foot
abductor digiti minimi m. of hand
abductor m. of great toe
abductor hallucis m.
abductor m. of little finger
abductor m. of little toe
abductor pollicis brevis m.
abductor pollicis longus m.
accessory flexor m. of foot
adductor brevis m.
adductor m. of great toe
adductor hallucis m.
adductor longus m.
adductor magnus m.
adductor minimus m.
adductor pollicis m.
adductor m. of thumb
Aeby's m.
Albinus' m.
anconeus m.
antagonistic m.'s
anterior auricular m.
anterior cervical
  intertransversarii m.'s
anterior cervical intertransverse m.'s
anterior rectus m. of head
anterior scalene m.
anterior serratus m.
anterior tibial m.
antigravity m.'s
antitragicus m.
m. of antitragus
appendicular m.
arrector pili m.'s
articular m.
articular m. of elbow
articularis cubiti m.
articularis genu m.
articular m. of knee
aryepiglottic m.
m.'s of auditory ossicles
axial m.
axillary arch m.
m.'s of the back
Bell's m.
biceps m. of arm
biceps brachii m.
biceps femoris m.
biceps m. of thigh
bipennate m.
Bochdalek's m.
Bovero's m.
Bowman's m.
brachial m.
brachialis m.
brachioradial m.
brachioradialis m.
branchiomeric m.'s

Braune's m.
broadest m. of back
bronchoesophageal m.
Brücke's m.
buccinator m.
bulbocavernosus m.
m. bundle
cardiac m.
Casser's perforated m.
ceratocricoid m.
cervical iliocostal m.
cervical interspinal m.
cervical interspinales m.'s
cervical longissimus m.
cervical rotator m.'s
cheek m.
chin m.
chondroglossus m.
ciliary m.
coccygeal m.
coccygeus m.
m.'s of coccyx
Coiter's m.
compressor m. of lips
coracobrachial m.
coracobrachialis m.
corrugator m.
corrugator cutis m. of anus
corrugator supercilii m.
cowl m.
Crampton's m.
cremaster m.
cricopharyngeus m.
cricothyroid m.
cruciate m.
m. curve
cutaneomucous m.
cutaneous m.
dartos m.
deep m.'s of back
deep flexor m. of fingers
deep transverse perineal m.
deep transverse m. of perineum
deltoid m.
depressor anguli oris m.
depressor m. of epiglottis
depressor m. of eyebrow
depressor labii inferioris m.
depressor m. of lower lip
depressor septi m.
depressor m. of septum
depressor supercilii m.
detrusor m. of urinary bladder
digastric m.
dilator m.
dilator m. of ileocecal sphincter
dilator pupillae m.
dilator m. of pylorus

M

muscle *(continued)*

dorsal m.'s
dorsal interosseous m.'s of foot
dorsal interosseous m.'s of hand
dorsal sacrococcygeal m.
dorsal sacrococcygeus m.
Dupré's m.
Duverney's m.
elevator m. of anus
elevator m. of prostate
elevator m. of rib
elevator m. of scapula
elevator m. of soft palate
elevator m. of thyroid gland
elevator m. of upper eyelid
elevator m. of upper lip
elevator m. of upper lip and wing
  of nose
epicranial m.
epicranius m.
m. epithelium
erector m.'s of hairs
erector spinae m.'s
erector m. of spine
extensor carpi radialis brevis m.
extensor carpi radialis longus m.
extensor carpi ulnaris m.
extensor digiti minimi m.
extensor digitorum m.
extensor digitorum brevis m.
extensor digitorum brevis m. of
  hand
extensor digitorum longus m.
extensor m. of fingers
extensor hallucis brevis m.
extensor hallucis longus m.
extensor indicis m.
extensor m. of little finger
extensor pollicis brevis m.
extensor pollicis longus m.
external intercostal m.'s
external oblique m.
external obturator m.
external pterygoid m.
external sphincter m. of anus
extraocular m.'s
extrinsic m.'s
m.'s of eyeball
facial m.'s
m.'s of facial expression
m. fascicle
femoral m.
fixator m.
flexor carpi radialis m.
flexor carpi ulnaris m.
flexor digiti minimi brevis m. of
  foot

flexor digiti minimi brevis m. of
  hand
flexor digitorum brevis m.
flexor digitorum longus m.
flexor digitorum profundus m.
flexor digitorum superficialis m.
flexor hallucis brevis m.
flexor hallucis longus m.
flexor pollicis brevis m.
flexor pollicis longus m.
frontalis m.
fusiform m.
Gantzer's m.
gastrocnemius m.
Gavard's m.
genioglossal m.
genioglossus m.
geniohyoid m.
gluteus maximus m.
gluteus medius m.
gluteus minimus m.
gracilis m.
great adductor m.
greater pectoral m.
greater posterior rectus m. of head
greater psoas m.
greater rhomboid m.
greater zygomatic m.
Guthrie's m.
hamstring m.'s
m.'s of head
m. of heart
helicis major m.
helicis minor m.
Horner's m.
Houston's m.
hyoglossal m.
hyoglossus m.
iliac m.
iliacus m.
iliacus minor m.
iliococcygeal m.
iliococcygeus m.
iliocostal m.
iliocostalis m.
iliocostalis cervicis m.
iliocostalis lumborum m.
iliocostalis thoracis m.
iliopsoas m.
index extensor m.
inferior constrictor m. of pharynx
inferior gemellus m.
inferior lingual m.
inferior longitudinal m. of tongue
inferior oblique m.
inferior oblique m. of head
inferior posterior serratus m.
inferior rectus m.

inferior tarsal m.
infrahyoid m.'s
infraspinatus m.
innermost intercostal m.
intermediate great m.
intermediate layer of the
  transversospinalis m.'s
intermediate vastus m.
internal intercostal m.
internal oblique m.
internal obturator m.
internal pterygoid m.
internal sphincter m. of anus
interosseous m.'s
interspinal m.'s
interspinales m.'s
intertransversarii m.'s
intertransverse m.'s
intrinsic m.'s
intrinsic m.'s of foot
involuntary m.'s
ischiocavernous m.
Jung's m.
Klein's m.
Kohlrausch's m.
Krause's m.
Landström's m.
Langer's m.
large m. of helix
m.'s of larynx
lateral cricoarytenoid m.
lateral great m.
lateral lumbar intertransversarii m.'s
lateral lumbar intertransverse m.'s
lateral pterygoid m.
lateral rectus m.
lateral rectus m. of the head
lateral vastus m.
latissimus dorsi m.
lesser rhomboid m.
lesser zygomatic m.
levator anguli oris m.
levator ani m.
levatores costarum m.'s
levator labii superioris m.
levator labii superioris alaeque
  nasi m.
levator palati m.
levator palpebrae superioris m.
levator prostatae m.
levator scapulae m.
levator m. of thyroid gland
levator veli palatini m.
long abductor m. of thumb
long adductor m.
long extensor m. of great toe
long extensor m. of thumb
long extensor m. of toes

long fibular m.
long flexor m. of great toe
long flexor m. of thumb
long flexor m. of toes
long m. of head
longissimus m.
longissimus capitis m.
longissimus cervicis m.
longissimus thoracis m.
long levatores costarum m.'s
long m. of neck
long palmar m.
long peroneal m.
long radial extensor m. of wrist
longus capitis m.
longus colli m.
lumbar iliocostal m.
lumbar interspinal m.
lumbar interspinales m.'s
lumbar quadrate m.
lumbar rotator m.'s
lumbrical m. of foot
lumbrical m. of hand
Marcacci's m.
masseter m.
m.'s of mastication
medial great m.
medial lumbar
  intertransversarii m.'s
medial lumbar intertransverse m.'s
medial pterygoid m.
medial rectus m.
medial vastus m.
mentalis m.
Merkel's m.
middle constrictor m. of pharynx
middle scalene m.
mimetic m.'s
mucocutaneous m.
Müller's m.
multifidus m.
multipennate m.
mylohyoid m.
nasal m.
nasalis m.
m.'s of neck
m. of notch of helix
oblique arytenoid m.
oblique m. of auricle
oblique auricular m.
obliquus capitis inferior m.
obliquus capitis superior m.
obturator externus m.
obturator internus m.
occipitalis m.
occipitofrontal m.
occipitofrontalis m.
ocular m.'s

M

muscle *(continued)*
Oehl's m.'s
omohyoid m.
opponens digiti minimi m.
opponens pollicis m.
opposer m. of little finger
opposer m. of thumb
orbicular m.
orbicular m. of eye
orbicularis m.
orbicularis oculi m.
orbicularis oris m.
orbicular m. of mouth
orbital m.
orbitalis m.
palatoglossus m.
palatopharyngeal m.
palatopharyngeus m.
palatouvularis m.
palmar interosseous m.
palmaris brevis m.
palmaris longus m.
papillary m.
pectinate m.'s
pectineal m.
pectineus m.
pectoralis major m.
pectoralis minor m.
pectorodorsal m.
pectorodorsalis m.
pennate m.
perineal m.'s
peroneus brevis m.
peroneus longus m.
peroneus tertius m.
m. phosphorylase deficiency
piriform m.
piriformis m.
plantar m.
plantar interosseous m.
plantaris m.
plantar quadrate m.
m. plate
platysma m.
pleuroesophageal m.
popliteal m.
popliteus m.
posterior auricular m.
posterior cervical
  intertransversarii m.'s
posterior cervical
  intertransverse m.'s
posterior cricoarytenoid m.
posterior scalene m.
posterior tibial m.
Pozzi's m.
procerus m.
pronator quadratus m.

pronator teres m.
psoas major m.
psoas minor m.
pubococcygeal m.
pubococcygeus m.
puboprostatic m.
puborectal m.
puborectalis m.
pubovaginal m.
pubovaginalis m.
pubovesical m.
pubovesicalis m.
pyramidal m.
pyramidal m. of auricle
pyramidal auricular m.
pyramidalis m.
quadrate m.
quadrate m. of loins
quadrate pronator m.
quadrate m. of sole
quadrate m. of thigh
quadrate m. of upper lip
quadratus m.
quadratus femoris m.
quadratus lumborum m.
quadratus plantae m.
quadriceps femoris m.
quadriceps m. of thigh
radial flexor m. of wrist
rectococcygeal m.
rectococcygeus m.
rectourethral m.
rectourethralis m.
rectouterine m.
rectovesical m.
rectovesicalis m.
rectus m. of abdomen
rectus abdominis m.
rectus capitis anterior m.
rectus capitis lateralis m.
rectus capitis posterior major m.
rectus capitis posterior minor m.
rectus femoris m.
rectus m. of thigh
red m.
Reisseisen's m.'s
m. repositioning
m. resection
rhomboideus major m.
rhomboid minor m.
rider's m.'s
Riolan's m.
risorius m.
rotator m.'s
rotatores m.'s
rotatores cervicis m.'s
rotatores lumborum m.'s
rotatores thoracis m.'s

Rouget's m.
round pronator m.
Ruysch's m.
salpingopharyngeal m.
salpingopharyngeus m.
Santorini's m.
sartorius m.
scalenus anterior m.
scalenus medius m.
scalenus minimus m.
scalenus posterior m.
scalp m.
Sebileau's m.
second tibial m.
semimembranosus m.
semispinal m.
semispinal m. of head
semispinalis m.
semispinalis capitis m.
semispinalis cervicis m.
semispinalis thoracis m.
semispinal m. of neck
semispinal m. of thorax
semitendinosus m.
serratus anterior m.
serratus posterior inferior m.
serratus posterior superior m.
m. serum
shawl m.
short abductor m. of thumb
short adductor m.
short extensor m. of great toe
short extensor m. of thumb
short extensor m. of toes
short fibular m.
short flexor m. of great toe
short flexor m. of little finger
short flexor m. of little toe
short flexor m. of thumb
short flexor m. of toes
short levatores costarum m.'s
short palmar m.
short peroneal m.
short radial extensor m. of wrist
Sibson's m.
skeletal m.
smaller m. of helix
smaller pectoral m.
smaller posterior rectus m. of head
smaller psoas m.
smallest scalene m.
smooth m.
Soemmerring's m.
soleus m.
m. sound
m. spasm
sphincter m.
sphincter m. of common bile duct

sphincter m. of pancreatic duct
sphincter m. of pupil
sphincter m. of pylorus
sphincter m. of urethra
sphincter m. of urinary bladder
spinal m.
spinal m. of head
spinalis m.
spinalis capitis m.
spinalis cervicis m.
spinalis thoracis m.
spinal m. of neck
spinal m. of thorax
m. spindle
spindle-shaped m.
splenius capitis m.
splenius cervicis m.
splenius m. of head
splenius m. of neck
stapedius m.
sternal m.
sternalis m.
sternochondroscapular m.
sternoclavicular m.
sternocleidomastoid m.
sternocostalis m.
sternohyoid m.
sternomastoid m.
sternothyroid m.
strap m.'s
striated m.
styloauricular m.
styloglossus m.
stylohyoid m.
stylopharyngeal m.
stylopharyngeus m.
subanconeus m.
subclavian m.
subclavius m.
subcostal m.
subcrural m.
suboccipital m.'s
subquadricipital m.
subscapular m.
subscapularis m.
superficial back m.'s
superficial flexor m. of fingers
superficial lingual m.
superficial transverse perineal m.
superficial transverse m. of
  perineum
superior auricular m.
superior constrictor m. of pharynx
superior gemellus m.
superior longitudinal m. of tongue
superior oblique m.
superior oblique m. of head
superior posterior serratus m.

M

muscle *(continued)*

superior rectus m.
superior tarsal m.
supinator m.
supraclavicular m.
suprahyoid m.'s
supraspinalis m.
supraspinatus m.
supraspinous m.
suspensory m. of duodenum
synergistic m.'s
tailor's m.
temporal m.
temporalis m.
temporoparietal m.
temporoparietalis m.
tensor fasciae latae m.
tensor m. of fascia lata
tensor m. of soft palate
tensor tarsi m.
tensor tympani m.
tensor m. of tympanic membrane
tensor veli palati m.
teres major m.
teres minor m.
Theile's m.
third peroneal m.
thoracic interspinal m.
thoracic interspinales m.'s
thoracic intertransversarii m.'s
thoracic intertransverse m.'s
thoracic longissimus m.
thoracic rotator m.'s
m.'s of thorax
thyroarytenoid m.
thyroepiglottic m.,
  thyroepiglottidean m.
thyrohyoid m.
tibialis anterior m.
tibialis posterior m.
Tod's m.
m.'s of tongue
Toynbee's m.
trachealis m.
tracheloclavicular m.
tragicus m.
m. of tragus
transverse m. of abdomen
transverse arytenoid m.
transverse m. of auricle
transverse auricular m.
transverse m. of chin
transverse m. of nape
transverse m. of thorax
transverse m. of tongue
transversospinal m.
transversospinalis m.
transversus abdominis m.

transversus menti m.
transversus nuchae m.
transversus thoracis m.
trapezius m.
Treitz's m.
triangular m.
triceps m. of arm
triceps brachii m.
triceps m. of calf
triceps coxae m.
triceps m. of hip
triceps surae m.
true m.'s of back
two-bellied m.
ulnar extensor m. of wrist
ulnar flexor m. of wrist
unipennate m.
unstriated m., unstriped m.
m. of uvula
uvulae m.
Valsalva's m.
vastus intermedius m.
vastus lateralis m.
vastus medialis m.
ventral sacrococcygeal m.
ventral sacrococcygeus m.
vertical m. of tongue
vestigial m.
visceral m.
vocal m.
vocalis m.
voluntary m.
white m.
Wilson's m.
wrinkler m. of eyebrow
zygomaticus major m.
zygomaticus minor m.

muscle-bound
muscle-tendon

m.-t. attachment
m.-t. junction

muscle-trimming
muscular

m. artery
m. asthenopia
m. atrophy
m. branches
m. coat
m. coat of bronchi
m. coat of colon
m. coat of ductus deferens
m. coat of esophagus
m. coat of female urethra
m. coat of gallbladder
m. coat of pharynx
m. coat of rectum
m. coat of small intestine
m. coat of stomach

m. coat of trachea
m. coat of ureter
m. coat of urinary bladder
m. coat of uterine tube
m. coat of uterus
m. coat of vagina
m. dystrophy
m. fascia of extraocular muscle
m. fibril
m. hyperesthesia
m. incompetence
m. insufficiency
m. lacuna
m. layer of mucosa
m. movement
m. part of interventricular septum
   of heart
m. process of arytenoid cartilage
m. pulley
m. reflex
m. rheumatism
m. sense
m. subaortic stenosis
m. substance of prostate
m. system
m. tissue
m. triangle
m. trophoneurosis
m. tunic of gallbladder
m. tunics

muscularis
   m. mucosae
muscularity
musculature
musculi (*gen. and pl. of* musculus)
musculoaponeurotic
musculocutaneous
   m. amputation
   m. flap
   m. nerve
   m. nerve of leg
musculomembranous
musculophrenic
   m. artery
   m. veins
musculoskeletal
musculospiral
   m. groove
   m. nerve
   m. paralysis
musculotendinous
   m. cuff
musculotropic
musculotubal canal
musculus, gen. and pl. **musculi**
   musculi abdominis
   m. abductor digiti minimi manus
   m. abductor digiti minimi pedis

m. abductor digiti quinti
m. abductor hallucis
m. abductor pollicis brevis
m. abductor pollicis longus
m. adductor brevis
m. adductor hallucis
m. adductor longus
m. adductor magnus
m. adductor minimus
m. adductor pollicis
m. anconeus
m. antitragicus
musculi arrectores pilorum
m. articularis
m. articularis cubiti
m. articularis genus
m. aryepiglotticus
m. arytenoideus obliquus
m. arytenoideus transversus
m. aryvocalis
m. attollens aurem, m. attollens
   auriculam
m. attrahens aurem, m. attrahens
   auriculam
m. auricularis anterior
m. auricularis posterior
m. auricularis superior
m. azygos uvulae
m. biceps brachii
m. biceps femoris
m. biceps flexor cruris
m. bipennatus
m. biventer mandibulae
m. brachialis
m. brachioradialis
m. bronchoesophageus
m. buccinator
m. buccopharyngeus
musculi bulbi
m. bulbocavernosus
m. bulbospongiosus
m. caninus
musculi capitis
m. cephalopharyngeus
m. ceratocricoideus
m. ceratopharyngeus
m. cervicalis ascendens
m. chondroglossus
m. chondropharyngeus
m. ciliaris
m. cleidoepitrochlearis
m. cleidomastoideus
m. cleido-occipitalis
musculi coccygei
m. coccygeus
musculi colli
m. complexus
m. complexus minor

M

musculus *(continued)*

m. compressor naris
m. compressor urethrae
m. constrictor pharyngis inferior
m. constrictor pharyngis medius
m. constrictor pharyngis superior
m. constrictor urethrae
m. coracobrachialis
m. corrugator cutis ani
m. corrugator supercilii
m. cremaster
m. cricoarytenoideus lateralis
m. cricoarytenoideus posterior
m. cricopharyngeus
m. cricothyroideus
m. cruciatus
m. cutaneomucosus
m. cutaneus
m. deltoideus
m. depressor anguli oris
m. depressor labii inferioris
m. depressor septi
m. depressor supercilii
m. detrusor urinae
m. diaphragma
m. digastricus
m. dilatator
m. dilator
m. dilator iridis
m. dilator naris
m. dilator pupillae
m. dilator pylori gastroduodenalis
m. dilator pylori ilealis
m. dilator tubae
musculi dorsi
m. ejaculator seminis
m. epicranius
m. epitrochleoanconeus
m. erector clitoridis
m. erector penis
m. erector spinae
m. extensor brevis digitorum
m. extensor brevis pollicis
m. extensor carpi radialis brevis
m. extensor carpi radialis longus
m. extensor carpi ulnaris
m. extensor coccygis
m. extensor digiti minimi
m. extensor digiti quinti proprius
m. extensor digitorum
m. extensor digitorum brevis
m. extensor digitorum brevis
  manus
m. extensor digitorum communis
m. extensor digitorum longus
m. extensor hallucis brevis
m. extensor hallucis longus
m. extensor indicis

m. extensor indicis proprius
m. extensor longus digitorum
m. extensor longus pollicis
m. extensor minimi digiti
m. extensor ossis metacarpi pollicis
m. extensor pollicis brevis
m. extensor pollicis longus
musculi faciales
m. fibularis brevis
m. fibularis longus
m. fibularis tertius
m. flexor accessorius
m. flexor brevis digitorum
m. flexor brevis hallucis
m. flexor carpi radialis
m. flexor carpi ulnaris
m. flexor digiti minimi brevis
  manus
m. flexor digiti minimi brevis
  pedis
m. flexor digitorum brevis
m. flexor digitorum longus
m. flexor digitorum profundus
m. flexor digitorum sublimis
m. flexor digitorum superficialis
m. flexor hallucis brevis
m. flexor hallucis longus
m. flexor longus digitorum
m. flexor longus hallucis
m. flexor longus pollicis
m. flexor pollicis brevis
m. flexor pollicis longus
m. flexor profundus
m. flexor sublimis
m. frontalis
m. fusiformis
m. gastrocnemius
m. gemellus inferior
m. gemellus superior
m. genioglossus
m. geniohyoglossus
m. geniohyoideus
m. glossopalatinus
m. glossopharyngeus
m. gluteus maximus
m. gluteus medius
m. gluteus minimus
m. gracilis
m. helicis major
m. helicis minor
m. hyoglossus
m. hypopharyngeus
m. iliacus
m. iliacus minor
m. iliocapsularis
m. iliococcygeus
m. iliocostalis
m. iliocostalis cervicis

m. iliocostalis dorsi
m. iliocostalis lumborum
m. iliocostalis thoracis
m. iliopsoas
m. incisivus labii inferioris
m. incisivus labii superioris
m. incisurae helicis
m. infracostalis, pl. musculi infracostales
musculi infrahyoidei
m. infraspinatus
m. intercostales externi, pl. musculi intercostales externi
m. intercostalis internus, pl. musculi intercostales interni
m. intercostalis intimus, pl. musculi intercostales intimi
musculi interossei
musculi interossei dorsalis manus, pl. musculi interossei dorsales manus
musculi interossei dorsalis pedis, pl. musculi interossei dorsales pedis
m. interosseus palmaris, pl. musculi interossei palmares
m. interosseus plantaris, pl. musculi interossei plantares
m. interosseus volaris
musculi interspinales
m. interspinalis cervicis
m. interspinalis lumborum
m. interspinalis thoracis
m. intertragicus
musculi intertransversarii
musculi intertransversarii anteriores cervicis
musculi intertransversarii laterales lumborum
musculi intertransversarii mediales lumborum
musculi intertransversarii posteriores cervicis
musculi intertransversarii thoracis
m. ischiocavernosus
m. ischiococcygeus
m. keratopharyngeus
musculi laryngis
m. laryngopharyngeus
m. latissimus dorsi
m. levator alae nasi
m. levator anguli oris
m. levator anguli scapulae
m. levator ani
m. levator costae, musculi levatores costarum longi, pl. musculi levatores costarum
musculi levatores costarum
musculi levatores costarum breves
musculi levatores costarum longi

m. levator glandulae thyroideae
m. levator labii inferioris
m. levator labii superioris
m. levator labii superioris alaeque nasi
m. levator palati
m. levator palpebrae superioris
m. levator prostatae
m. levator scapulae
m. levator veli palatini
musculi linguae
m. longissimus
m. longissimus capitis
m. longissimus cervicis
m. longissimus dorsi
m. longissimus thoracis
m. longitudinalis inferior
m. longitudinalis superior
m. longus capitis
m. longus colli
m. lumbricalis manus, pl. musculi lumbricales manus
m. lumbricalis pedis, pl. musculi lumbricales pedis
m. masseter
m. mentalis
m. multifidus
m. multifidus spinae
m. multipennatus
m. mylohyoideus
m. mylopharyngeus
m. nasalis
m. obliquus auriculae
m. obliquus capitis inferior
m. obliquus capitis superior
m. obliquus externus abdominis
m. obliquus inferior
m. obliquus internus abdominis
m. obliquus superior
m. obturator externus
m. obturator internus
m. occipitalis
m. occipitofrontalis
m. omohyoideus
m. opponens digiti minimi
m. opponens digiti quinti
m. opponens minimi digiti
m. opponens pollicis
m. orbicularis
m. orbicularis oculi
m. orbicularis oris
m. orbicularis palpebrarum
m. orbitalis
m. orbitopalpebralis
musculi ossiculorum auditus
m. palatoglossus
m. palatopharyngeus
m. palatosalpingeus

M

musculus *(continued)*
- m. palatostaphylinus
- m. palmaris brevis
- m. palmaris longus
- m. papillaris
- musculi pectinati
- m. pectineus
- m. pectoralis major
- m. pectoralis minor
- musculi perinei
- m. peroneocalcaneus
- m. peroneus brevis
- m. peroneus longus
- m. peroneus tertius
- m. petropharyngeus
- m. petrostaphylinus
- m. pharyngopalatinus
- m. piriformis
- m. plantaris
- m. platysma
- m. platysma myoides
- m. pleuroesophageus
- m. popliteus
- m. procerus
- m. pronator pedis
- m. pronator quadratus
- m. pronator radii teres
- m. pronator teres
- m. prostaticus
- m. psoas major
- m. psoas minor
- m. pterygoideus externus
- m. pterygoideus internus
- m. pterygoideus lateralis
- m. pterygoideus medialis
- m. pterygopharyngeus
- m. pterygospinosus
- m. pubococcygeus
- m. puboprostaticus
- m. puborectalis
- m. pubovaginalis
- m. pubovesicalis
- m. pyramidalis
- m. pyramidalis auriculae
- m. pyramidalis nasi
- m. pyriformis
- m. quadratus
- m. quadratus femoris
- m. quadratus labii inferioris
- m. quadratus labii superioris
- m. quadratus lumborum
- m. quadratus menti
- m. quadratus plantae
- m. quadriceps extensor femoris
- m. quadriceps femoris
- m. rectococcygeus
- m. rectourethralis
- m. rectouterinus
- m. rectovesicalis
- m. rectus abdominis
- m. rectus capitis anterior
- m. rectus capitis anticus major
- m. rectus capitis anticus minor
- m. rectus capitis lateralis
- m. rectus capitis posterior major
- m. rectus capitis posterior minor
- m. rectus capitis posticus major
- m. rectus capitis posticus minor
- m. rectus externus
- m. rectus femoris
- m. rectus inferior
- m. rectus internus
- m. rectus lateralis
- m. rectus medialis
- m. rectus superior
- m. rectus thoracis
- m. retrahens aurem, m. retrahens auriculam
- m. rhomboatloideus
- m. rhomboideus major
- m. rhomboideus minor
- m. risorius
- musculi rotatores
- musculi rotatores cervicis
- musculi rotatores lumborum
- musculi rotatores thoracis
- m. sacrococcygeus anterior
- m. sacrococcygeus dorsalis
- m. sacrococcygeus posterior
- m. sacrococcygeus ventralis
- m. sacrolumbalis
- m. sacrospinalis
- m. salpingopharyngeus
- m. sartorius
- m. scalenus anterior
- m. scalenus anticus
- m. scalenus medius
- m. scalenus minimus
- m. scalenus posterior
- m. scalenus posticus
- m. semimembranosus
- m. semispinalis
- m. semispinalis capitis
- m. semispinalis cervicis
- m. semispinalis colli
- m. semispinalis dorsi
- m. semispinalis thoracis
- m. semitendinosus
- m. serratus anterior
- m. serratus magnus
- m. serratus posterior inferior
- m. serratus posterior superior
- m. skeleti
- m. soleus
- m. sphenosalpingostaphylinus
- m. sphincter

m. sphincter ampullae hepatopancreaticae
m. sphincter ani externus
m. sphincter ani internus
m. sphincter ductus choledochi
m. sphincter ductus pancreatici
m. sphincter oris
m. sphincter pupillae
m. sphincter pylori
m. sphincter urethrae
m. sphincter urethrae membranaceae
m. sphincter vaginae
m. sphincter vesicae
m. spinalis
m. spinalis capitis
m. spinalis cervicis
m. spinalis colli
m. spinalis dorsi
m. spinalis thoracis
m. splenius capitis
m. splenius cervicis
m. splenius colli
m. stapedius
m. sternalis
m. sternochondroscapularis
m. sternoclavicularis
m. sternocleidomastoideus
m. sternofascialis
m. sternohyoideus
m. sternothyroideus
m. styloauricularis
m. styloglossus
m. stylohyoideus
m. stylolaryngeus
m. stylopharyngeus
m. subclavius
m. subcostalis, pl. musculi subcostales
m. subcutaneus colli
musculi suboccipitales
m. subscapularis
m. supinator
m. supinator longus
m. supinator radii brevis
m. supraclavicularis
musculi suprahyoidei
m. supraspinalis
m. supraspinatus
m. suspensorius duodeni
m. tarsalis inferior
m. tarsalis superior
m. temporalis
m. temporoparietalis
m. tensor fasciae femoris
m. tensor fasciae latae
m. tensor palati
m. tensor tarsi
m. tensor tympani

m. tensor veli palatini
m. teres major
m. teres minor
m. tetragonus
musculi thoracis
m. thyroarytenoideus
m. thyroarytenoideus externus
m. thyroarytenoideus internus
m. thyroepiglotticus
m. thyrohyoideus
m. thyropharyngeus
m. tibialis anterior
m. tibialis anticus
m. tibialis gracilis
m. tibialis posterior
m. tibialis posticus
m. tibialis secundus
m. tibiofascialis anterior, m. tibiofascialis anticus
m. trachealis
m. tracheloclavicularis
m. trachelomastoideus
m. tragicus
m. transversalis abdominis
m. transversalis capitis
m. transversalis cervicis, m. transversalis colli
m. transversalis nasi
m. transversospinalis
m. transversus abdominis
m. transversus auriculae
m. transversus linguae
m. transversus menti
m. transversus nuchae
m. transversus perinei profundus
m. transversus perinei superficialis
m. transversus thoracis
m. trapezius
m. triangularis
m. triangularis labii inferioris
m. triangularis labii superioris
m. triangularis sterni
m. triceps brachii
m. triceps coxae
m. triceps surae
m. triticeoglossus
m. unipennatus
m. uvulae
m. vastus externus
m. vastus intermedius
m. vastus internus
m. vastus lateralis
m. vastus medialis
m. ventricularis
m. verticalis linguae
m. vocalis
m. zygomaticus

M

musculus *(continued)*
  m. zygomaticus major
  m. zygomaticus minor
mushbite
mushroom-worker's lung
musical
  m. agraphia
  m. alexia
  m. murmur
music blindness
musician's cramp
musicotherapy
Musset's sign
mussitation
Mustard
  M. operation
  M. procedure
mutacism
mutagenesis
  cassette m.
  insertional m.
mutagenic
mutant
  active m.
  m. gene
  inactive m.
  silent m.
mutation
  back m.
  induced m.
  lethal m.
  natural m.
  neutral m.
  new m.
  m. rate
  reverse m.
  silent m.
  site specific m.
  somatic m.
  spontaneous m.
mute
mutilating
  m. keratoderma
  m. leprosy
mutilation
mutism
  akinetic m.
  elective m.
  voluntary m.
muton
muttering delirium
mutton-fat keratic precipitates
mutualism
mutualist
MVE virus
myalgia
  epidemic m.
  m. thermica

myasthenia
  m. angiosclerotica
  m. gravis
myasthenic
  m. crisis
  m. facies
  m. reaction
  m. syndrome
myatonia, myatony
  m. congenita
myatrophy
mycelia (*pl. of* mycelium)
mycelian
mycelioid
mycelium, pl. **mycelia**
  aerial m.
  nonseptate m.
  septate m.
mycete
mycetism, mycetismus
  m. cerebralis
mycetogenetic, mycetogenic
mycetogenous
mycetoma
  Bouffardi's m.'s
  Bouffardi's black m.
  Bouffardi's white m.
  Brumpt's white m.
  Carter's black m.
  Nicolle's white m.
  Vincent's white m.
mycid
mycobacteria
  atypical m.
  group I m.
  group II m.
  group III m.
  group IV m.
Mycobacteriaceae
mycobacteriosis
Mycobacterium
  M. abscessus
  M. avium
  M. avium-intracellulare complex
  M. bovis
  M. chelonae
  M. chelonae subsp. *abscessus*
  M. fortuitum
  M. intracellulare
  M. kansasii
  M. leprae
  M. marianum
  M. marinum
  M. microti
  M. paratuberculosis
  M. phlei
  M. scrofulaceum
  M. smegmatis

M. *tuberculosis*
M. *ulcerans*
M. *xenopi*
mycobactin
mycodermatitis
mycogastritis
mycologist
mycology
   medical m.
mycomyringitis
mycophage
Mycoplasma
   M. *faucium*
   M. *fermentans*
   M. *genitalium*
   M. *granularum*
   M. *hominis*
   M. *laidlawii*
   M. *pharyngis*
   M. *pneumoniae*
   M. *salivarium*
mycoplasma, pl. **mycoplasmata**
mycoplasmal pneumonia
Mycoplasmatales
mycopus
mycosis, pl. **mycoses**
   m. cutis chronica
   m. framboesioides
   m. fungoides
   Gilchrist's m.
   m. intestinalis
mycotic
   m. aneurysm
   m. endocarditis
   m. keratitis
mycovirus
mydriasis
   alternating m.
   amaurotic m.
   paralytic m.
   spastic m.
myectomy
myectopy, myectopia
myelapoplexy
myelatelia
myelauxe
myelemia
myelencephalon
myelic
myelin
   m. body
   m. figure
   m. sheath
myelinated
   m. nerve
   m. nerve fiber
myelination

myelinic
   m. degeneration
myelinization
myelinoclasis
myelinogenesis
myelinolysis , osmotic
   central pontine m.
myelinopathy
myelitic
myelitis
   acute necrotizing m.
   acute transverse m.
   ascending m.
   bulbar m.
   concussion m.
   demyelinated m.
   Foix-Alajouanine m.
   funicular m.
   postinfectious m.
   postvaccinal m.
   radiation m.
   subacute necrotizing m.
   systemic m.
   transverse m.
myeloarchitectonics
myeloblast
myeloblastemia
myeloblastic
   m. leukemia
   m. protein
myeloblastoma
myeloblastosis
myelocele
myelocyst
myelocystic
myelocystocele
myelocystomeningocele
myelocyte
   m. A
   m. B
   m. C
myelocythemia
myelocytic
   m. crisis
   m. leukemia
   m. leukemoid reaction
myelocytoma
myelocytosis
myelodiastasis
myelodysplasia
myelofibrosis
myelogenesis
myelogenetic, myelogenic
myelogenous
   m. leukemia
myelogone, myelogonium

M

myelogram
  cervical m.
  lumbar m.
myelography
myeloic
myeloid
  m. cell
  m. leukemia
  m. metaplasia
  m. sarcoma
  m. series
  m. tissue
myeloidosis
myeloleukemia
myelolipoma
myelolymphocyte
myelolysis
myeloma
  Bence Jones m.
  endothelial m.
  giant cell m.
  L-chain m.
  multiple m., m. multiplex
  nonsecretory m.
  plasma cell m.
myelomalacia
  angiodysgenetic m.
myelomatosis
  multiple m., m. multiplex
myelomeningocele
myelomere
myelomonocyte
myelomonocytic leukemia
myeloneuritis
myelonic
myeloparalysis
myelopathic
  m. anemia
myelopathy
  carcinomatous m.
  compressive m.
  diabetic m.
  paracarcinomatous m.
  radiation m.
myelopetal
myelophthisic
  m. anemia
myelophthisis
myeloplast
myeloplegia
myelopoiesis
myelopoietic
myeloproliferative
  m. syndromes
myeloradiculitis
myeloradiculodysplasia
myeloradiculopathy
myeloradiculopolyneuronitis

myelorrhagia
myelorrhaphy
myelosarcoma
myelosarcomatosis
myeloschisis
myelosclerosis
myelosis
  aleukemic m.
  chronic nonleukemic m.
  erythremic m.
  funicular m.
  leukemic m.
  leukopenic m., subleukemic m.
myelospongium
myelosyphilis
myelosyringosis
myelotome
myelotomography
myelotomy
  Bischof's m.
  commissural m.
  midline m.
  T m.
myelotoxic
myenteric
  m. plexus
  m. reflex
myenteron
myesthesia
myiasis
  aural m.
  creeping m.
  intestinal m.
  nasal m.
  ocular m.
  m. oestruosa
  subcutaneous m.
  wound m., traumatic m.
myitis
mylohyoid
  m. artery
  m. fossa
  m. groove
  m. line
  m. muscle
  m. nerve
  m. ridge
mylohyoideus
mylopharyngeal part of superior
  pharyngeal constrictor
myoarchitectonic
myoatrophy
myoblast
myoblastic
myoblastoma
  granular cell m.
myobradia
myocardia (*pl. of* myocardium)

myocardial
   m. bridge
   m. depressant factor
   m. infarction
   m. infarction in dumbbell form
   m. insufficiency
   m. ischemia
   m. rigor mortis
myocardiograph
myocardiopathy
   alcoholic m.
   chagasic m.
myocardiorrhaphy
myocarditic
myocarditis
   acute isolated m.
   Fiedler's m.
   fragmentation m.
   giant cell m.
   idiopathic m.
   indurative m.
   toxic m.
myocardium, pl. myocardia
   hibernating m.
   stunned m.
myocardosis
myocele
myocelialgia
myocelitis
myocellulitis
myocerosis
myochronoscope
myocinesimeter
myoclonia
   fibrillary m.
myoclonic
   m. astatic epilepsy
   m. seizure
myoclonus
   m. epilepsy
   m. multiplex
   nocturnal m.
   palatal m.
   stimulus sensitive m.
myocolpitis
myocomma, pl. myocommata
myocrismus
myocutaneous
   m. flap
myocyte
   Anitschkow m.
myocytolysis
   m. of heart
myocytoma
myodegeneration
myodemia
myodermal
   m. flap

myodiastasis
myodynamia
myodynamics
myodynamometer
myodynia
myodystony
myodystrophy, myodystrophia
myoedema
myoelastic
   m. theory
myoelectric
myoendocarditis
myoepicardial mantle
myoepithelial
   m. cell
myoepithelioma
myoepithelium
myoesthesis, myoesthesia
myofacial pain-dysfunction syndrome
myofascial
   m. syndrome
myofascitis
myofibril
myofibrilla, pl. myofibrillae
myofibroblast
myofibroma
myofibromatosis
   infantile m.
myofibrosis
   m. cordis
myofibrositis
myofilaments
myofunctional
   m. therapy
myogenesis
myogenetic, myogenic
myogenous
myoglobinuria
myoglobulinuria
myognathus
myogram
myograph
   palate m.
myographic
myography
myoid cells
myoidema
myoischemia
myokerosis
myokinesimeter
myokymia
   facial m.
   generalized m.
   hereditary m.
   limb m.
myolemma
myolipoma
myologia

M

myologist
myology
    descriptive m.
myolysis
    cardiotoxic m.
myoma
myomalacia
myomatous
    m. polyp
myomectomy
    abdominal m.
    left ventricular m.
    vaginal m.
myomelanosis
myomere
myometer
myometrial
    m. arcuate arteries
    m. radial arteries
myometritis
myometrium
myomitochondrion, pl. myomitochondria
myomotomy
myon
myonecrosis
    clostridial m.
myoneme
myoneural
    m. junction
myoneuralgia
    postural m.
myoneurasthenia
myoneuroma
myonosus
myonymy
myopachynsis
myopalmus
myoparalysis
myoparesis
myopathic
    m. atrophy
    m. facies
    m. scoliosis
myopathy
    carcinomatous m.
    centronuclear m.
    distal m.
    minicore-multicore m.
    mitochondrial m.
    myotubular m.
    nemaline m.
    ocular m.
    rod m.
    thyrotoxic m.
myopericarditis
myoperitonitis
myophone
myophosphorylase deficiency glycogenosis

myopia
    axial m.
    curvature m.
    degenerative m.
    index m.
    malignant m.
    night m.
    pathologic m.
    prematurity m.
    senile lenticular m.
    simple m.
    space m.
    transient m.
myopic
    m. astigmatism
    m. choroidopathy
    m. conus
    m. crescent
    m. degeneration
myoplasm
myoplastic
myoplasty
myopolar
myorhythmia
myorrhaphy
myorrhexis
myosalgia
myosalpingitis
myosalpinx
myosarcoma
myosclerosis
myoseism
myoseptum
myosin filament
myosis
myositic
myositis
    acute disseminated m.
    cervical m.
    epidemic m., m. epidemica acuta
    m. fibrosa
    infectious m.
    interstitial m.
    multiple m.
    m. ossificans
    m. ossificans circumscripta
    m. ossificans progressiva
    proliferative m.
    m. purulenta tropica
    tropical m.
myospasm, myospasmus
    cervical m.
myospherulosis
myosthenometer
myostroma
myotactic
myotasis

myotatic
>m. contraction
>m. irritability
>m. reflex

myotenositis
myotenotomy
myothermic
myotome
myotomy
>cricopharyngeal m.
>Heller m.

myotone
myotonia
>m. acquisita
>m. atrophica
>m. congenita
>m. dystrophica
>m. neonatorum

myotonic
>m. cataract
>m. dystrophy

myotonoid
myotonus
myotony
myotrophy
myotube
myotubular myopathy
myotubule
myovascular sphincter
myovenous sphincter
Myoviridae
myriachit
myringa
myringectomy
myringitis
>m. bulbosa
>bullous m.

myringodermatitis
myringomycosis
myringoplasty
myringostapediopexy
myringotome
myringotomy
myrinx
myrmecia
mysophilia
mysophobia
mytacism
myurous
myxadenitis
>m. labialis

myxadenoma
myxasthenia
myxedema
>circumscribed m.
>congenital m.
>m. heart
>infantile m.
>operative m.
>pituitary m.
>pretibial m.
>m. voice

myxedematoid
myxedematous
>m. infantilism

myxemia
myxochondrofibrosarcoma
myxochondroma
Myxococcidium stegomyiae
myxocyte
myxofibroma
myxofibrosarcoma
myxoid
>m. cyst
>m. degeneration

myxolipoma
myxoma
>atrial m.
>m. enchondromatosum
>m. fibrosum
>m. lipomatosum
>odontogenic m.
>m. sarcomatosum

myxomatosis virus
myxomatous
>m. degeneration

myxomembranous colitis
myxomycete
Myxomycetes
myxoneuroma
myxopapillary ependymoma
myxopapilloma
myxopoiesis
myxorrhea
>m. gastrica

myxosarcoma
Myxospora
myxospore
Myxosporea
myxovirus
Myxozoa

M

nabothian
    n. cyst
    n. follicle
nacreous
    n. ichthyosis
Nadi reaction
Naegeli
    N. syndrome
    N. type of monocytic leukemia
Naegleria
Naffziger
    N. operation
    N. syndrome
Nägele
    N. obliquity
    N. pelvis
    N. rule
Nagel's test
Nageotte cells .
nail
    n. bed
    egg shell n.
    n. extension
    n. fold
    half and half n.
    hippocratic n.'s
    n. horn
    ingrown n.
    Küntscher n.
    n. matrix
    parrot-beak n.
    pincer n.
    n. pits
    n. plate
    n. pulse
    racket n.
    reedy n.
    shell n.
    Smith-Petersen n.
    spoon n.
    Terry's n.'s
    yellow n.
nailing
nail-patella syndrome
Nakanishi's stain
naked virus
NAME syndrome
NANB hepatitis
NANDA
nanism
    mulibrey n.
    renal n.
    symptomatic n.
Nannizzia
nanocephalia

nanocephalous, nanocephalic
nanocephaly
nanocormia
nanoid enamel
nanomelia
nanophthalmia, nanophthalmos
Nanophyetus salmincola
Nanta
nanukayami
    n. fever
nape
    n. nevus
napex
naphthol yellow S
napkin rash
naprapathy
narcissism
    primary n.
    secondary n.
narcissistic
    n. personality
    n. personality disorder
narcohypnia
narcohypnosis
narcolepsy
narcoleptic
    n. tetrad
narcosis
    CO_2 n.
    intravenous n.
    nitrogen n.
narcosynthesis
narcotherapy
narcotic hunger
naris, pl. **nares**
    anterior n.
    external n.
    internal n.
    posterior n.
narrow-angle glaucoma
nasal
    n. arch
    n. atrium
    n. bone
    n. border of frontal bone
    n. calculus
    n. capsule
    n. catarrh
    n. cavity
    n. crest
    n. duct
    n. feeding
    n. foramen
    n. ganglion
    n. glands

N

NASCET
criteria (Arteriogram)

nasal *(continued)*
    n. glioma
    n. height
    n. hemorrhage
    n. index
    n. margin of frontal bone
    n. meatus
    n. mucosa
    n. muscle
    n. myiasis
    n. nerve
    n. notch
    n. part of frontal bone
    n. part of pharynx
    n. pharynx
    n. pits
    n. placodes
    n. point
    n. polyp
    n. process
    n. reflex
    n. region
    n. ridge
    n. sacs
    n. septal cartilage
    n. septum
    n. spine of frontal bone
    n. surface of maxilla
    n. surface of palatine bone
    n. valve
    n. venous arch
    n. venules of retina
nasalis muscle
Nasik vibrio
nasioiniac
nasion
    n. soft tissue
nasion-pogonion measurement
nasion-postcondylar plane
Nasmyth's
    N. cuticle
    N. membrane
nasoalveolar cyst
nasoantral
nasobasilar line
nasobregmatic arc
nasociliary
    n. nerve
    n. root
nasofrontal
    n. vein
nasogastric
    n. tube
nasojugal fold
nasolabial
    n. cyst
    n. groove

    n. lymph node
    n. node
nasolacrimal
    n. canal
    n. duct
nasomandibular fixation
nasomaxillary suture
nasomental reflex
naso-occipital arc
naso-oral
nasopalatine
    n. duct cyst
    n. groove
    n. nerve
nasopharyngeal
    n. groove
    n. leishmaniasis
    n. passage
nasopharyngolaryngoscope
nasopharyngoscope
nasopharyngoscopy
nasopharynx
nasorostral
nasosinusitis
nasotracheal
    n. intubation
    n. tube
Nasse's law
nasus
    n. externus
natal
    n. cleft
    n. tooth
natality
Natal's sore
nates
natiform skull
natimortality
natremia, natriemia
natriuresis
natural
    n. antibody
    n. dentition
    n. dyes
    n. focus of infection
    n. hemolysin
    n. immunity
    n. killer cells
    n. killer cell stimulating factor
    n. mutation
    n. selection
nature-nurture issue
naturopath
naturopathic
naturopathy
Nauheim
    N. bath
    N. treatment

naupathia
nausea
    epidemic n.
    n. gravidarum
nauseate
nauseated
nauseous
Nauta's stain
navel
navicula
navicular
    n. abdomen
    n. articular surface of talus
    n. bone
    n. bone of hand
    n. fossa of urethra
ND virus
near
    n. drowning
    n. point
    n. point of convergence
    n. reaction
    n. reflex
    n. sight
nearsightedness
nearthrosis
near-total thyroidectomy
nebulous urine
Necator
necatoriasis
necessary cause
neck
    anatomical n. of humerus
    buffalo n.
    bull n.
    dental n.
    n. of femur
    n. of fibula
    n. of gallbladder
    n. of glans penis
    n. of hair follicle
    n. of humerus
    Madelung's n.
    n. of malleus
    n. of mandible
    n. of radius
    n. reflexes
    n. of rib
    n. of scapula
    n. sign
    stiff n.
    surgical n. of humerus
    n. of talus
    n. of thigh bone
    n. of tooth
    turkey gobbler n.
    n. of urinary bladder
    n. of uterus

    webbed n.
    n. of womb
    wry n.
necklace
    Casal's n.
    n. of Venus
neck-shaft angle
necrectomy
necrobiosis
    n. lipoidica, n. lipoidica diabeticorum
necrobiotic
    n. xanthogranuloma
necrocytosis
necrogenic
    n. wart
necrogenous
necrogranulomatous
necrologist
necrology
necrolysis
    toxic epidermal n.
necrolytic migratory erythema
necromania
necrometer
necroparasite
necropathy
necrophagous
necrophilia, necrophilism
necrophilous
necrophobia
necropsy
necrosadism
necroscopy
necrose
necrosectomy
necrosis
    aseptic n.
    avascular n.
    n. bacillus
    bridging hepatic n.
    caseous n., caseation n.
    central n.
    coagulation n.
    colliquative n.
    contraction band n.
    cystic medial n.
    epiphysial aseptic n.
    fat n.
    fibrinoid n.
    focal n.
    ischemic n.
    laminar cortical n.
    liquefactive n.
    mummification n.
    progressive emphysematous n.
    renal papillary n.
    simple n.
    subcutaneous fat n. of newborn

N

necrosis *(continued)*
    suppurative n.
    total n.
    Zenker's n.
    zonal n.
necrospermia
necrosteon, necrosteosis
necrotic
    n. angina
    n. cirrhosis
    n. cyst
    n. infectious conjunctivitis
    n. inflammation
    n. pulp
necrotizing
    n. angiitis
    n. arteriolitis
    n. cellulitis
    n. encephalitis
    n. encephalomyelopathy
    n. encephalopathy
    n. enterocolitis　～NEC
    n. fasciitis
    n. hemorrhage leukomyelitis
    n. inflammation
    n. papillitis
    n. scleritis
    n. sialometaplasia
    n. ulcerative gingivitis
necrotomy
    osteoplastic n.
needle
    aneurysm n., artery n.
    aspirating n.
    atraumatic n.
    n. bath
    biopsy n.
    n. biopsy
    cataract n.
    couching n.
    n. culture
    cutting n.
    Deschamps n.
    Emmet's n.
    exploring n.
    n. forceps
    Francke's n.
    Frazier's n.
    Gillmore n.
    Hagedorn n.
    hypodermic n.
    knife n.
    lumbar puncture n.
    Millner n.
    n. point tracing
    Salah's sternal puncture n.
    spatula n.
    stop-n.

    Tuohy n.
    Veress n.
    Vicat n.
needle-holder, needle-carrier, needle-driver
Needles' split cast method
needling
neencephalon
Neethling virus
Neftel's disease
negation
negative
    n. accommodation
    n. afterimage
    n. anergy
    n. base excess
    n. chronotropism
    n. convergence
    n. cytotaxis
    n. electrotaxis
    n. end-expiratory pressure
    false n.
    n. feedback
    n. G
    n. heteropyknosis
    n. image
    n. leukocytotaxia
    n. meniscus
    n. phase
    n. politzerization
    n. pressure
    n. reinforcer
    n. scotoma
    n. stain
    n. stereotropism
    n. strand virus
    n. supporting reaction's
    n. taxis
    n. thermotaxis
    n. transference
    n. tropism
negative hydrotropism *(var. of* hydrotropism)
negatively
    n. bathmotropic
    n. dromotropic
    n. inotropic
negative neutrotaxis *(var. of* neutrotaxis)
negativism
Negishi virus
Negri
    N. bodies
    N. corpuscles
Negro's phenomenon
Neisseria
    N. catarrhalis
    N. caviae
    N. flava

N. *flavescens*
N. *gonorrhoeae*
N. *haemolysans*
N. *meningitidis*
N. *sicca*
N. *subflava*
neisseria, pl. neisseriae
Neisser's
    N. coccus
    N. stain
    N. syringe
Nélaton's
    N. catheter
    N. dislocation
    N. fibers
    N. line
    N. sphincter
Nêlaton's fold
Nelson
    N. syndrome
    N. tumor
nem
nemaline myopathy
nemathelminth
Nemathelminthes
nematicidal, nematocidal
nematization
nematoblast
nematocidal (*var. of* nematicidal)
Nematoda
nematode
Nematodirella longispiculata
nematoid
nematologist
nematology
nematospermia
neoantigens
neoarthrosis
Neoascaris vitulorum
neobiogenesis
neoblastic
neocerebellum
neocortex
neocystostomy
neoencephalon
neofetal
neofetus
neoformation
neogala
neogenesis
neogenetic
neokinetic
neolallism
neologism
neomembrane
neomorph, neomorphism
neonatal
    n. apoplexy

n. calf diarrhea virus
n. conjunctivitis
n. death
n. diagnosis
n. hepatitis
n. herpes
n. hyperbilirubinemia
n. hypoglycemia
n. line
n. lupus
n. medicine
n. mortality rate
n. ring
n. screening
n. tetanus
n. tetany
n. tooth
neonate
neonatologist
neonatology
neopallium
neopathy
neophobia
neophrenia
neoplasia
    cervical intraepithelial n.
    lobular n.
    multiple endocrine n., type 2
    prostatic intraepithelial n.
neoplasm
    histoid n.
neoplastic
    n. arachnoiditis
    n. meningitis
Neospora canium
neostomy
neostriatum
neoteny
Neotestudina rosati
neothalamus
neotype
    n. culture
    n. strain
neovascular glaucoma
neovascularization
nephradenoma
nephralgia
nephralgic
nephratonia, nephratony
nephrectomy
    abdominal n.
    lumbar n.
    posterior n.
nephredema
nephrelcosis

N

nephric
    n. blastema
    n. duct
nephridium, pl. **nephridia**
nephritic
    n. calculus
    n. factor
    n. syndrome
nephritis, pl. **nephritides**
    acute n.
    acute interstitial n.
    analgesic n.
    anti-basement membrane n.
    anti-kidney serum n.
    chronic n.
    Ellis type 1 n.
    focal n.
    glomerular n.
    n. gravidarum
    hemorrhagic n.
    hereditary n.
    immune complex n.
    interstitial n.
    lupus n.
    Masugi's n.
    mesangial n.
    salt-losing n.
    scarlatinal n.
    serum n.
    subacute n.
    suppurative n.
    syphilitic n.
    transfusion n.
    trench n.
    tuberculous n.
    tubulointerstitial n.
    uranium n.
nephritogenic
nephroblastema
nephroblastoma
nephrocalcinosis
nephrocapsectomy
nephrocardiac
nephrocystosis
nephrogenetic, nephrogenic
nephrogenous
nephrogram
nephrography
nephrohydrosis
nephroid
nephrolith
nephrolithiasis
nephrolithotomy
nephrology
nephrolysin
nephrolysis
nephrolytic

nephroma
    mesoblastic n.
nephromalacia
nephromegaly
nephromere
nephron
nephronic loop
nephropathia epidemica
nephropathic
nephropathy
    analgesic n.
    Balkan n.
    Danubian endemic familial n.
    hypokalemic n.
    IgA n.
    IgM n.
    reflux n.
nephropexy
nephrophthisis
    familial juvenile n.
nephroptosis, nephroptosia
nephropyosis
nephrorrhaphy
nephros
nephrosclerosis
    arterial n.
    arteriolar n.
    benign n.
    malignant n.
    senile n.
nephrosclerotic
nephroscope
nephrosis
    acute n.
    acute lobar n.
    amyloid n.
    cholemic n.
    familial n.
    hemoglobinuric n.
    hypoxic n.
    lipoid n.
    lower nephron n.
    osmotic n.
    toxic n.
    vacuolar n.
nephrospasia, nephrospasis
nephrostogram
nephrostoma, nephrostome
nephrostomy
    percutaneous n.
    n. tube
nephrotic
    n. edema
    n. syndrome
nephrotome
nephrotomic
nephrotomogram
nephrotomography

nephrotomy
  anatrophic n.
nephrotoxic
nephrotoxicity
nephrotoxin
nephrotrophic
nephrotropic
nephrotuberculosis
nephroureterectomy
nephroureterocystectomy
nepiology
Neptune's girdle
Néri's sign
Nernst's equation
nerve
  abdominopelvic splanchnic n.'s
  abducent n.
  accelerator n.'s
  accessory n.
  accessory phrenic n.'s
  acoustic n.
  afferent n.
  Andersch's n.
  anococcygeal n.'s
  anterior ampullar n.
  anterior antebrachial n.
  anterior auricular n.'s
  anterior crural n.
  anterior cutaneous n.'s of abdomen
  anterior ethmoidal n.
  anterior femoral cutaneous n.'s
  anterior interosseous n.
  anterior labial n.'s
  anterior scrotal n.'s
  anterior supraclavicular n.
  anterior tibial n.
  aortic n.
  Arnold's n.
  articular n.
  auditory n.
  augmentor n.'s
  auriculotemporal n.
  autonomic n.
  n. avulsion
  axillary n.
  baroreceptor n.
  Bell's respiratory n.
  n. block
  n. block anesthesia
  Bock's n.
  buccal n.
  buccinator n.
  cardiopulmonary splanchnic n.'s
  caroticotympanic n.
  n. to carotid sinus
  carotid sinus n.
  cavernous n.'s of clitoris
  cavernous n.'s of penis

  n. cell
  n. cell body
  centrifugal n.
  centripetal n.
  cervical n.'s
  cervical splanchnic n.'s
  circumflex n.
  coccygeal n.
  cochlear n.
  common fibular n.
  common palmar digital n.'s
  common peroneal n.
  common plantar digital n.'s
  n. conduction
  n. conduction velocity
  cranial n.'s
  crural interosseous n.
  cubital n.
  cutaneous n.
  cutaneous cervical n.
  Cyon's n.
  dead n.
  n. deafness
  n. decompression
  deep fibular n.
  deep peroneal n.
  deep petrosal n.
  deep temporal n.'s
  dental n.
  depressor n. of Ludwig
  dorsal n. of clitoris
  dorsal digital n.'s
  dorsal digital n.'s of foot
  dorsal digital n.'s of hand
  dorsal interosseous n.
  dorsal lateral cutaneous n.
  dorsal medial cutaneous n.
  dorsal n. of penis
  dorsal n. of scapula
  dorsal scapular n.
  dorsal n.'s of toes
  efferent n.
  eighth n.
  eighth cranial n.
  eleventh cranial n.
  n. ending
  esodic n.
  excitor n.
  excitoreflex n.
  exodic n.
  n. of external acoustic meatus
  external carotid n.'s
  external respiratory n. of Bell
  external saphenous n.
  external spermatic n.
  facial n.
  n. fascicle
  femoral n.

nerve *(continued)*
    n. fiber
    n. field
    fifth cranial n.
    first cranial n.
    n. force
    fourth cranial n.
    fourth lumbar n.
    frontal n.
    furcal n.
    Galen's n.
    gangliated n.
    n. ganglion
    genitocrural n.
    genitofemoral n.
    glossopharyngeal n.
    n. graft
    great auricular n.
    greater occipital n.
    greater palatine n.
    greater petrosal n.
    greater splanchnic n.
    greater superficial petrosal n.
    great sciatic n.
    n. growth factor antiserum
    hemorrhoidal n.'s
    Hering's sinus n.
    hypogastric n.
    hypoglossal n.
    iliohypogastric n.
    ilioinguinal n.
    n. implantation
    inferior alveolar n.
    inferior cervical cardiac n.
    inferior cluneal n.'s
    inferior dental n.
    inferior gluteal n.
    inferior hemorrhoidal n.'s
    inferior laryngeal n.
    inferior lateral brachial
      cutaneous n.
    inferior maxillary n.
    inferior rectal n.'s
    inferior vesical n.'s
    infraorbital n.
    infratrochlear n.
    inhibitory n.
    intercarotid n.
    intercostal n.'s
    intercostobrachial n.'s
    intercostohumeral n.'s
    intermediary n.
    intermediate n.
    intermediate dorsal cutaneous n.
    intermediate supraclavicular n.
    internal carotid n.
    internal saphenous n.
    interosseous n. of leg

Jacobson's n.
jugular n.
lacrimal n.
Latarget's n.
lateral ampullar n.
lateral antebrachial cutaneous n.
lateral anterior thoracic n.
lateral cutaneous n. of calf
lateral cutaneous n. of forearm
lateral cutaneous n. of thigh
lateral dorsal cutaneous n.
lateral femoral cutaneous n.
lateral pectoral n.
lateral plantar n.
lateral popliteal n.
lateral supraclavicular n.
lateral sural cutaneous n.
lesser internal cutaneous n.
lesser occipital n.
lesser palatine n.'s
lesser petrosal n.
lesser splanchnic n.
lesser superficial petrosal n.
lingual n.
long buccal n.
long ciliary n.
long saphenous n.
long subscapular n.
long thoracic n.
lower lateral cutaneous n. of arm
lowest splanchnic n.
Ludwig's n.
lumbar n.'s
lumbar splanchnic n.'s
lumboinguinal n.
mandibular n.
masseteric n.
masticator n.
maxillary n.
medial antebrachial cutaneous n.
medial anterior thoracic n.
medial brachial cutaneous n.
medial cutaneous n. of arm
medial cutaneous n. of forearm
medial cutaneous n. of leg
medial dorsal cutaneous n.
medial pectoral n.
medial plantar n.
medial popliteal n.
medial supraclavicular n.
medial sural cutaneous n.
median n.
mental n.
middle cervical cardiac n.
middle cluneal n.'s
middle meningeal n.
middle supraclavicular n.
mixed n.

motor n.
motor n. of face
musculocutaneous n.
musculocutaneous n. of leg
musculospiral n.
myelinated n.
mylohyoid n.
n. to mylohyoid
nasal n.
nasociliary n.
nasopalatine n.
ninth cranial n.
obturator n.
oculomotor n.
olfactory n.'s
ophthalmic n.
optic n.
orbital n.
n. pain
n. papilla
parasympathetic n.
pathetic n.
pelvic splanchnic n.'s
perineal n.'s
peroneal communicating n.
phrenic n.
n. plexus
pneumogastric n.
popliteal communicating n.
posterior ampullar n.
posterior antebrachial n.
posterior antebrachial cutaneous n.
posterior auricular n.
posterior brachial cutaneous n.
posterior cutaneous n. of arm
posterior cutaneous n. of forearm
posterior cutaneous n. of thigh
posterior ethmoidal n.
posterior femoral cutaneous n.
posterior interosseous n.
posterior labial n.'s
posterior scapular n.
posterior scrotal n.'s
posterior supraclavicular n.
posterior thoracic n.
presacral n.
pressor n.
pressoreceptor n.
proper palmar digital n.'s
proper plantar digital n.'s
pterygoid n.
n. of pterygoid canal
pterygopalatine n.'s
pudendal n.
pudic n.
radial n.
recurrent n.
recurrent laryngeal n.

recurrent meningeal n.
n. to rhomboid
n. root
n. root sleeve
saccular n.
sacral n.'s
sacral splanchnic n.'s
saphenous n.
sciatic n.
second cranial n.
secretomotor n.
secretory n.
sensory n.
seventh cranial n.
short ciliary n.
short saphenous n.
sinus n. of Hering
sinuvertebral n.'s
sixth cranial n.
small deep petrosal n.
smallest splanchnic n.
small sciatic n.
n. of smell
somatic n.
space n.
spinal n.'s
spinal accessory n.
splanchnic n.
n. to stapedius muscle
statoacoustic n.
n. stroma
subclavian n.
subcostal n.
sublingual n.
suboccipital n.
subscapular n.'s
sudomotor n.'s
superficial cervical n.
superficial fibular n.
superficial peroneal n.
superior alveolar n.'s
superior cervical cardiac n.
superior cluneal n.'s
superior dental n.'s
superior gluteal n.
superior laryngeal n.
superior lateral brachial
  cutaneous n.
superior maxillary n.
supraorbital n.
suprascapular n.
supratrochlear n.
sural n.
n. suture
sympathetic n.
temporomandibular n.
n. of tensor tympani muscle
n. of tensor veli palatini muscle

N

nerve *(continued)*
    tenth cranial n.
    tentorial n.
    terminal n.'s
    third cranial n.
    third occipital n.
    thoracic cardiac n.'s
    thoracic spinal n.'s
    thoracic splanchnic n.'s
    thoracoabdominal n.'s
    thoracodorsal n.
    n. to thyrohyoid muscle
    tibial n.
    tibial communicating n.
    Tiedemann's n.
    n. tract
    transverse cervical n.
    transverse n. of neck
    trifacial n.
    trigeminal n.
    trochlear n.
    n. trunk
    twelfth cranial n.
    tympanic n.
    n. of tympanic membrane
    ulnar n.
    unmyelinated n.
    upper lateral cutaneous n. of arm
    upper subscapular n.
    upper thoracic splanchnic n.'s
    utricular n.
    utriculoampullar n.
    vaginal n.'s
    vagus n.
    Valentin's n.
    vascular n.
    vasomotor n.
    vertebral n.
    vestibular n.
    vestibulocochlear n.
    vidian n.
    visceral n.
    volar interosseous n.
    Wrisberg's n.
    zygomatic n.
nervi (*gen. and pl. of* nervus)
nervimotility
nervimotion
nervimotor
nervosism
nervous
    n. asthenopia
    n. asthma
    n. breakdown
    n. dyspepsia
    n. dysphagia
    n. force
    n. indigestion

n. lobe
n. lobe of hypophysis
n. part of retina
n. system
n. tissue
n. tunic of eyeball
nervousness
nervus, gen. and pl. **nervi**
    n. abducens
    n. accessorius
    n. acusticus
    nervi alveolares superiores
    n. alveolaris inferior
    n. ampullaris anterior
    n. ampullaris lateralis
    n. ampullaris posterior
    nervi anococcygei
    n. antebrachii anterior
    n. antebrachii posterior
    n. articularis
    nervi auriculares anteriores
    n. auricularis magnus
    n. auricularis posterior
    n. auriculotemporalis
    n. axillaris
    n. buccalis
    n. canalis pterygoidei
    nervi cardiaci thoracici
    n. cardiacus cervicalis inferior
    n. cardiacus cervicalis medius
    n. cardiacus cervicalis superior
    nervi carotici externi
    n. caroticotympanicus, pl. nervi
      caroticotympanici
    n. caroticus internus
    nervi cavernosi clitoridis
    nervi cavernosi penis
    nervi cervicales
    n. cervicalis superficialis
    n. ciliaris brevis, pl. nervi ciliares
      breves
    n. ciliaris longus, pl. nervi ciliares
      longi
    nervi clunium inferiores
    nervi clunium medii
    nervi clunium superiores
    n. coccygeus
    n. cochlearis
    n. communicans fibularis
    n. communicans peroneus
    nervi craniales
    n. cutaneus
    n. cutaneus antebrachii lateralis
    n. cutaneus antebrachii medialis
    n. cutaneus antebrachii posterior
    n. cutaneus brachii lateralis inferior
    n. cutaneus brachii lateralis
      superior

n. cutaneus brachii medialis
n. cutaneus brachii posterior
n. cutaneus dorsalis intermedius
n. cutaneus dorsalis lateralis
n. cutaneus dorsalis medialis
n. cutaneus femoris lateralis
n. cutaneus femoris posterior
n. cutaneus surae lateralis
n. cutaneus surae medialis
nervi digitales dorsales
nervi digitales dorsales pedis
nervi digitales palmares communes
nervi digitales palmares proprii
nervi digitales plantares communes
nervi digitales plantares proprii
n. dorsalis clitoridis
n. dorsalis penis
n. dorsalis scapulae
nervi erigentes
n. ethmoidalis anterior
n. ethmoidalis posterior
n. facialis
n. femoralis
n. fibularis communis
n. fibularis profundus
n. fibularis superficialis
n. frontalis
n. furcalis
n. genitofemoralis
n. glossopharyngeus
n. gluteus inferior
n. gluteus superior
n. hemorrhoidalis
n. hypogastricus
n. hypoglossus
n. iliohypogastricus
n. ilioinguinalis
n. impar
n. infraorbitalis
n. infratrochlearis
nervi intercostales
nervi intercostobrachiales
n. intermedius
n. interosseus anterior
n. interosseus cruris
n. interosseus dorsalis
n. interosseus posterior
n. ischiadicus
n. jugularis
nervi labiales anteriores
nervi labiales posteriores
n. lacrimalis
n. laryngeus inferior
n. laryngeus recurrens
n. laryngeus superior
n. lingualis
nervi lumbales
n. mandibularis

n. massetericus
n. maxillaris
n. meatus acustici externi
n. medianus
n. mentalis
n. musculocutaneus
n. mylohyoideus
n. nasociliaris
n. nasopalatinus
nervi nervorum
n. obturatorius
n. occipitalis major
n. occipitalis minor
n. occipitalis tertius
n. octavus
n. oculomotorius
nervi olfactorii
n. ophthalmicus
n. opticus
nervi palatini minores
n. palatinus major
n. pectoralis lateralis
n. pectoralis medialis
nervi pelvici splanchnici
nervi perineales
n. peroneus communis
n. peroneus profundus
n. peroneus superficialis
n. petrosus major
n. petrosus minor
n. petrosus profundus
nervi phrenici accessorii
n. phrenicus
n. plantaris lateralis
n. plantaris medialis
n. presacralis
n. pterygoideus
nervi pterygopalatini
n. pudendus
n. radialis
nervi rectales inferiores
n. saccularis
nervi sacrales
n. saphenus
n. sciaticus
nervi scrotales anteriores
nervi scrotales posteriores
n. spermaticus externus
nervi sphenopalatini
nervi spinales
n. spinosus
nervi splanchnici lumbales
nervi splanchnici sacrales
n. splanchnicus imus
n. splanchnicus major
n. splanchnicus minor
n. stapedius
n. statoacusticus

N

nervus *(continued)*
    n. subclavius
    n. subcostalis
    n. sublingualis
    n. suboccipitalis
    nervi subscapulares
    n. supraclavicularis intermedius
    n. supraclavicularis lateralis
    n. supraclavicularis medialis
    n. supraorbitalis
    n. suprascapularis
    n. supratrochlearis
    n. suralis
    nervi temporales profundi
    n. tensoris tympani
    n. tensoris veli palatini
    n. tentorii
    nervi terminales
    nervi thoracici
    n. thoracicus longus
    n. thoracodorsalis
    n. tibialis
    n. transversus colli
    n. trigeminus
    n. trochlearis
    n. tympanicus
    n. ulnaris
    n. utricularis
    n. utriculoampullaris
    nervi vaginales
    n. vagus
    n. vascularis
    n. vertebralis
    n. vestibularis
    n. vestibulocochlearis
    n. zygomaticus
nesidiectomy
nesidioblast
nesidioblastoma
nesidioblastosis
nesslerize
nest
    Brunn's n.'s
    cell n.'s
    epithelial n.
    isogenous n.
net
    Chiari's n.
    chromidial n.
    n. flux
    n. knot
Netherton's syndrome
nettle rash
nettling hairs
network
    acromial arterial n.
    arteriolar n.
    articular n.

    articular vascular n.
    articular vascular n. of elbow
    articular vascular n. of knee
    calcaneal arterial n.
    chromatin n.
    dorsal carpal n.
    dorsal venous n. of foot
    dorsal venous n. of hand
    lateral malleolar n.
    linin n.
    medial malleolar n.
    neurofibrillar n.
    patellar n.
    peritarsal n.
    plantar venous n.
    Purkinje's n.
    subpapillary n.
    trabecular n.
Neubauer's artery
Neufeld
    N. capsular swelling
    N. reaction
Neumann's
    N. cells
    N. disease
    N. sheath
neuragmia
neural
    n. arch
    n. axis
    n. canal
    n. crest
    n. crest syndrome
    n. cyst
    n. deafness
    n. folds
    n. ganglion
    n. groove
    n. layer of optic retina
    n. layer of retina
    n. part of hypophysis
    n. plate
    n. segment
    n. spine
    n. tube
neuralgia
    atypical facial n.
    atypical trigeminal n.
    epileptiform n.
    facial n.
    n. facialis vera
    Fothergill's n.
    geniculate n.
    glossopharyngeal n.
    hallucinatory n.
    Hunt's n.
    idiopathic n.
    intercostal n.

mammary n.
Morton's n.
occipital n.
periodic migrainous n.
red n.
sciatic n.
Sluder's n.
sphenopalatine n.
stump n.
suboccipital n.
supraorbital n.
symptomatic n.
trifacial n.
trigeminal n.
neuralgic
n. amyotrophy
neuralgiform
neuramebimeter
α₂-neuraminoglycoprotein
neuranagenesis
neurapophysis
neurapraxia
neurarchy
neurasthenia
angiopathic n., angioparalytic n.
gastric n.
n. gravis
n. praecox
primary n.
pulsating n.
sexual n.
traumatic n.
neurasthenic
n. helmet
n. personality
neuraxis
neuraxon, neuraxone
neurectasis, neurectasia, neurectasy
neurectomy
occipital n.
presacral n.
retrogasserian n.
neurectopia, neurectopy
neurenteric
n. canal
n. cysts
neurepithelium
neurergic
neurexeresis
neurilemma
n. cells
neurilemoma
acoustic n.
Antoni type A n.
Antoni type B n.
neurility
neurimotility

neurimotor
neurinoma
acoustic n.
neurit, neurite
neuritic
n. atrophy
n. plaque
neuritis, pl. **neuritides**
adventitial n.
ascending n.
axial n.
brachial n.
central n.
descending n.
Eichhorst's n.
endemic n.
fallopian n.
interstitial n.
intraocular n.
Leyden's n.
multiple n.
occipital n.
optic n.
parenchymatous n.
retrobulbar n.
sciatic n.
segmental n.
suboccipital n.
toxic n.
traumatic n.
neuroallergy
neuroanastomosis
neuroanatomy
neuroarthropathy
neuroaugmentation
neuroaugmentive
neuroaxonal dystrophy
neurobiology
neurobiotactic movement
neurobiotaxis
neuroblast
neuroblastoma
olfactory n.
neuroborreliosis
neurocardiac
neurocele
neurocentral
n. joint
n. suture
n. synchondrosis
neurochitin
neurochorioretinitis
neurochoroiditis
neurochronaxic theory
neurocirculatory asthenia
neurocladism
neurocranial granulomatous arteritis

N

neurocranium
    cartilaginous n.
    membranous n.
neurocristopathy
neurocutaneous
    n. melanosis
    n. syndrome
neurocyte
neurocytolysis
neurocytoma
neurodendrite
neurodendron
neurodermatitis
neurodermatosis
neurodynamic
neurodynia
neuroectoderm
neuroectodermal
    n. junction
neuroectomy
neuroencephalomyelopathy
neuroendocrine
    n. cell
    n. transducer cell
neuroendocrinology
neuroepithelial
    n. body
    n. cells
    n. layer of retina
neuroepithelium
    n. of ampullary crest
    n. cristae ampullaris
    n. of macula
    n. maculae
neurofibril
neurofibrillar
    n. nerve
neurofibrillary
    n. degeneration
    n. tangle
neurofibroma
    plexiform n.
    storiform n.
neurofibromatosis
    abortive n.
    central type n.
    incomplete n.
neurofilament
neuroganglion
neurogastric
neurogenesis
neurogenic, neurogenetic
    n. atrophy
    n. bladder
    n. fracture
    n. tonus
neurogenous

neuroglia
    n. cells
neurogliacyte
neuroglial, neurogliar
neurogliomatosis
neurogram
neurography
neurohemal
    n. organs
neurohistology
neurohumoral transmission
neurohypophysial
neurohypophysis
neuroid
neurokeratin
neurolemma
    n. cells
neuroleptanalgesia
neuroleptanesthesia
neuroleptic malignant syndrome
neurolinguistics
neurologist
neurology
neurolymph
neurolymphomatosis
neurolysin
neurolysis
neurolytic
neuroma
    acoustic n.
    amputation n.
    n. cutis
    false n.
    fibrillary n.
    plexiform n.
    n. telangiectodes
    traumatic n.
    Verneuil's n.
neuromalacia
neuromatosis
neuromelanin
neuromeningeal
neuromere
neuromimesis
neuromuscular
    n. junction
    n. spindle
    n. system
neuromyasthenia
    epidemic n.
neuromyelitis
    n. optica
neuromyopathy
    carcinomatous n.
neuromyositis
neuron
    autonomic motor n.

autonomic motor n.'s (*var. of* motor n.)
bipolar n.
gamma motor n.'s
ganglionic motor n.
Golgi type I n.
Golgi type II n.
intercalary n.
internuncial n.
lower motor n.
motor n., autonomic motor n.'s, somatic motor n.'s, visceral motor n.'s
multipolar n.
non-adrenergic, non-cholinergic n.
polymorphic n.
postganglionic motor n.
preganglionic motor n.
pseudounipolar n.
sensory n.
somatic motor n.'s (*var. of* motor n.)
somatic motor n.
unipolar n.
upper motor n.
visceral motor n.'s (*var. of* motor n.)
visceral motor n.

neuronal
n. ceroid lipofuscinosis
n. hyperplasia
n. intestinal dysplasia

neurone
neuronephric
neuronevus
neuronitis
vestibular n.

neuronopathy
sensory n.

neuronophage
neuronophagia, neuronophagy
neuronyxis
neuro-oncology
neuro-ophthalmology
neuro-otology
neuroparalysis
neuroparalytic
n. keratitis
n. keratopathy

neuropath
neuropathic
n. albuminuria
n. arthritis
n. arthropathy
n. bladder
n. joint

neuropathogenesis
neuropathology

neuropathy
asymmetric motor n.
brachial plexus n.
chronic interstitial hypertrophic n.
compression n.
dapsone n.
diabetic n.
diphtheritic n.
entrapment n.
familial amyloid n.
giant axonal n.
Graves' optic n.
heavy metal n.
hereditary hypertrophic n.
hereditary sensory radicular n.
hypertrophic interstitial n.
ischemic n.
ischemic optic n.
isoniazid n.
lead n.
leprous n.
onion bulb n.
symmetric distal n.
vitamin B_{12} n.

neuropeptide
n. Y

neurophilic
neurophonia
neurophysiology
neuropil, neuropile
neuroplasm
neuroplasty
neuroplegic
neuroplexus
neuropodia
neuropore
anterior n.
caudal n.
cranial n.
posterior n.
rostral n.

neuropraxia
neuropsychiatry
neuropsychologic, neuropsychological
n. disorder

neuropsychology
neuropsychopathic
neuropsychopathy
neuroradiology
neurorelapse
neuroretinitis
Leber's idiopathic stellate n.
stellate n.

neurorrhaphy
neurosarcocleisis
neurosarcoidosis
neurosarcoma
neuroschwannoma

N

neurosciences
neurosecretion
neurosecretory
    n. cells
    n. substance
neurosis, pl. **neuroses**
    accident n.
    anxiety n.
    association n.
    battle n.
    cardiac n.
    character n.
    combat n.
    compensation n.
    compulsive n.
    conversion n.
    conversion hysteria n.
    depressive n.
    expectation n.
    experimental n.
    hypochondriacal n.
    hysterical n.
    military n.
    noogenic n.
    obsessional n.
    obsessive-compulsive n.
    occupational n., professional n.
    oedipal n.
    pension n.
    postconcussion n.
    posttraumatic n.
    n. tarda
    torsion n.
    transference n.
    traumatic n.
    vasomotor n.
    war n.
neurosomatic junction
neurosplanchnic
neurospongium
Neurospora
neurostimulator
neurosurgeon
neurosurgery
    functional n.
neurosuture
neurosyphilis
    asymptomatic n.
    meningeal n.
    meningovascular n.
    paretic n.
    tabetic n.
neurotaxis
neurotendinous
    n. organ
    n. spindle
neurotension
neurothekeoma

neurothele
neurotherapeutics, neurotherapy
neurothlipsis, neurothlipsia
neurotic
    n. excoriation
    n. manifestation
neuroticism
neurotization
neurotize
neurotmesis
neurotology
neurotome
neurotomy
    retrogasserian n.
neurotonic reaction
neurotransmission
neurotrauma
neurotripsy
neurotrophic
    n. atrophy
    n. keratitis
neurotrophy
neurotropic
    n. attraction
    n. virus
neurotropy, neurotropism
neurotrosis
neurotubule
neurovaccine
neurovaricosis, neurovaricosity
neurovascular
    n. flap
    n. sheath
neurovegetative
neurovirus
neurovisceral
neurula, pl. **neurulae**
neurulation
Neusser's granules
neutral
    n. axis of straight beam
    n. buffered formalin fixative
    n. lipid storage disease
    n. mutation
    n. occlusion
    n. stain
    n. zone
neutralization
    n. plate
    n. test
    viral n.
neutralizing antibody
neutral red
neutroclusion
neutron radiation
neutropenia
    cyclic n.
    periodic n.

neutropenic angina
neutrophil, neutrophile
    n. activating factor
    n. activating protein
    band n.
    n. chemotactant factor
    n. granule
    hypersegmented n.
    immature n.
    juvenile n.
    mature n.
    segmented n.
    stab n.
neutrophilia
neutrophilic
    n. leukemia
    n. leukocyte
    n. leukocytosis
    n. leukopenia
neutrophilopenia
neutrophilous
neutrotaxis, indifferent neutrotaxis,
    negative neutrotaxis, positive
    neutrotaxis
nevi (*pl. of* nevus)
nevocyte
nevoid
    n. amentia
    n. elephantiasis
    n. hypertrichosis
nevolipoma
nevose, nevous
nevoxanthoendothelioma
nevus, pl. **nevi**
    acquired n.
    n. anemicus
    n. angiectodes
    n. arachnoideus
    n. araneus
    balloon cell n.
    basal cell n.
    bathing trunk n.
    Becker's n.
    blue n.
    blue rubber-bleb nevi
    capillary n.
    n. cavernosus
    n. cell
    n. cell, A-type
    n. cell, B-type
    n. cell, C-type
    cellular blue n.
    n. comedonicus, comedo n.
    compound n.
    congenital n.
    dysplastic n.
    n. elasticus of Lewandowski

    epidermic-dermic n.
    epithelioid cell n.
    faun tail n.
    n. flammeus, flame n.
    n. follicularis keratosis
    giant pigmented n.
    halo n.
    intradermal n.
    Ito's n.
    Jadassohn's n.
    Jadassohn-Tièche n.
    junction n.
    linear epidermal n.
    n. lipomatodes, n. lipomatosus
    n. lymphaticus
    nape n.
    oral epithelial n.
    organoid n.
    Ota's n.
    n. papillomatosus
    pigmented hair epidermal n.
    n. pigmentosus
    n. pilosus
    n. sanguineus
    n. sebaceus
    spider n.
    n. spilus
    spindle cell n.
    Spitz n.
    strawberry n.
    Sutton's n.
    systematized n.
    n. unius lateris
    n. vascularis, n. vasculosus
    n. venosus
    verrucous n.
    white sponge n.
    woolly-hair n.
new
    n. combination
    n. growth
    N. Hampshire rule
    n. methylene blue
    n. mutation
    N. World leishmaniasis
    N. York Heart Association
      classification
    N. Zealand mice
newborn
Newcastle disease virus
Newcomer's fixative
newtonian
    n. aberration
    n. flow
    n. fluid
    n. viscosity

N

Newton's
  N. disk
  N. law
nexus, pl. nexus
Neyman-Pearson statistical hypothesis
Nezelof
  N. syndrome
  N. type of thymic alymphoplasia
NGF antiserum
niacin test
nib
niche
  enamel n.
  Haudek's n.
nickel dermatitis
Nickerson-Kveim test
nicking
  arteriovenous n.
Nick's procedure
Nicolas-Favre disease
Nicolle's
  N. stain for capsules
  N. white mycetoma
Nicol prism
nicotine stomatitis
nicotinic
  n. acid maculopathy
  n. receptors
nictation
nictitate
nictitating spasm
nictitation
nidal
nidation
nidus, pl. nidi
  n. avis
  n. hirundinis
Nieden's syndrome
Niemann
  N. disease
  N. splenomegaly
Niemann-Pick
  N.-P. cell
  N.-P. disease
Niewenglowski rays
night
  n. blindness
  n. hospital
  n. myopia
  n. pain
  n. sight
  n. sweats
  n. vision
nightguard
nightmare
night-terrors
nigra
nigricans

nigrities
  n. linguae
nigrosin, nigrosine
Nigrospora
nigrostriatal
nihilism
  therapeutic n.
nihilistic delusion
Nikiforoff's method
Nikolsky's sign
nil disease
Nile blue A
ninhydrin reaction
ninhydrin-Schiff stain for proteins
ninth cranial nerve
ninth-day erythema
nipple
  aortic n.
  n. line
  n. shield
nirvana principle
Nissen's operation *fundoplication*
Nissl
  N. bodies
  N. degeneration
  N. granules
  N. stain
  N. substance
nit
Nitabuch's
  N. layer
  N. membrane
  N. stria
niter paper
nitinol filter
nitric oxide
  n. o. synthase
nitritoid reaction
nitrituria
nitroblue
  n. tetrazolium
  n. tetrazolium test
nitro dyes
nitrofurantoin
  n. polyneuropathy
nitrogen
  blood urea n.
  n. distribution
  n. equivalent
  n. narcosis
  n.ous equilibrium
  n. partition
  undetermined n.
  urea n.
  urinary n.
nitrogen lag
nitroprusside test
njovera

NK cells
NLN
NMR imaging
Noack's syndrome
Noble-Collip procedure
Noble's
    N. position
    N. stain
Nocardia
    N. asteroides
    N. brasiliensis
    N. caviae
    N. gibsonii
    N. leishmanii
    N. lurida
    N. lutea
    N. madurae
    N. mediterranei
    N. orientalis
nocardia, pl. **nocardiae**
Nocardiaceae
Nocardia dacryoliths
nocardiae (*pl. of* nocardia)
nocardiasis
nocardioform
nocardiosis
    granulomatous n.
nociceptive
    n. reflex
nociceptor
nocifensor
    n. reflex
noci-influence
nociperception
noctalbuminuria
noctambulation
noctambulism
noctiphobia
noctograph
nocturia
nocturnal
    n. amblyopia
    n. diarrhea
    n. dyspnea
    n. emission
    n. enuresis
    n. epilepsy
    n. myoclonus
    n. periodicity
    n. vertigo
nodal
    n. bigeminy
    n. bradycardia
    n. fever
    n. plane
    n. point
    n. rhythm

    n. tachycardia
    n. tissue
nodding spasm
node
    anterior tibial n.
    n. of Aschoff and Tawara
    atrioventricular n.
    Babès' n.'s
    buccinator n., buccal n.
    n. of Cloquet
    coronary n.
    cystic n.
    delphian n.
    diaphragmatic n.'s
    ductus n.'s
    Dürck's n.'s
    epitrochlear n.'s
    fibular n.
    Flack's n.
    foraminal n.
    Haygarth's n.'s
    Heberden's n.'s
    hemolymph n.
    Hensen's n.
    intermediate lacunar n.
    jugulodigastric n.
    jugulo-omohyoid n.
    Keith and Flack n.
    Keith's n.
    Koch's n.
    lateral lacunar n.
    left gastro-omental n.'s
    n. of ligamentum arteriosum
    lymph n.
    malar n.
    mandibular n.'s
    medial lacunar n.
    middle rectal n.
    nasolabial n.
    Osler n.
    parietal n.'s
    peroneal n.
    posterior tibial n.
    primitive n.
    Ranvier's n.
    retropyloric n.'s
    Rosenmüller's n.
    n. of Rouviere
    signal n.
    singer's n.'s
    sinoatrial n.
    sinuatrial n.
    sinus n.
    subdigastric n.
    subpyloric n.
    suprapyloric n.
    Tawara's n.
    teachers' n.'s

sentinal node

N

node *(continued)*
    Troisier's n.
    Virchow's n.
    visceral n.'s
    vital n.
nodi (*pl. of* nodus)
nodi lymphatici (*pl. of* nodus lymphaticus)
nodose
    n. ganglion
    n. rheumatism
nodositas
    n. crinium
nodosity
    Haygarth's n.'s
    Heberden's n.'s
nodous, nodular, nodulate, nodulated
nodoventricular fibers
nodulation
nodule
    aggregated lymphatic n.'s
    Albini's n.'s
    apple jelly n.'s
    Arantius' n.
    Aschoff n.'s
    Bianchi's n.
    Bohn's n.'s
    Caplan's n.'s
    cold n.
    Dalen-Fuchs n.'s
    enamel n.
    Gamna-Gandy n.'s
    Hoboken's n.'s
    hot n.
    Jeanselme's n.'s
    juxta-articular n.'s
    Lisch n.
    lymph n.
    lymphatic n.
    malpighian n.'s
    Morgagni's n.
    picker's n.'s
    primary n.
    pulp n.
    rheumatoid n.'s
    Sakurai-Lisch n.
    Schmorl's n.
    secondary n.
    n. of semilunar valve
    siderotic n.'s
    singer's n.'s
    Sister Joseph's n.
    solitary n.'s of intestine
    splenic lymph n.'s
    vocal cord n.'s
nodulous
nodulus, pl. **noduli**
    n. caroticus

    n. lymphaticus
    n. valvulae semilunaris, pl. noduli valvularum semilunarium
nodus, pl. **nodi**
    n. atrioventricularis
    n. buccinatorius
    n. cysticus
    n. fibularis
    n. foraminalis
    nodi lymphatici iliaci communes promontorii
    nodi lymphatici iliaci externi laterales
    n. jugulodigastricus
    n. jugulo-omohyoideus
    n. lacunaris intermedius
    n. lacunaris lateralis
    n. lacunaris medialis
    n. ligamenti arteriosi
    n. malaris
    n. mandibularis
    n. nasolabialis
    n. rectalis medius
    nodi retropylorici
    n. sinuatrialis
    n. sinuatrialis echo
    nodi subpylorici
    n. suprapyloricus
    n. tibialis anterior
    n. tibialis posterior
    nodi viscerales
nodus lymphaticus, pl. **nodi lymphatici**
    l. arcus venae azygos
    nodi lymphatici axillares
    nodi lymphatici axillares apicales
    nodi lymphatici axillares subscapulares
    nodi lymphatici axillaris pectorales
    nodi lymphatici brachiales
    nodi lymphatici bronchopulmonales
    nodi lymphatici cavales laterales (*var. of* nodi lymphatici lumbales dextri)
    nodi lymphatici cervicales anteriores
    nodi lymphatici cervicales anteriores profundi
    nodi lymphatici cervicales anteriores superficiales
    nodi lymphatici cervicales laterales profundi
    nodi lymphatici cervicales laterales superficiales
    nodi lymphatici coeliaci
    nodi lymphatici colici
    nodi lymphatici colici dextri
    nodi lymphatici colici medii
    nodi lymphatici colici sinistri

nodi lymphatici comitantes nervi
accessorii
nodi lymphatici cubitales
nodi lymphatici epigastrici
inferiores
nodi lymphatici faciales
nodi lymphatici gastrici dextri
nodi lymphatici gastrici sinistri
nodi lymphatici gastro-omentales
dextri
nodi lymphatici gastro-omentales
sinistri
nodi lymphatici gluteales
nodi lymphatici hepatici
nodi lymphatici ileocolici
nodi lymphatici iliaci communes,
nodi lymphatici iliaci communes
laterales, nodi lymphatici iliaci
communes subaortici
nodi lymphatici iliaci externi
nodi lymphatici iliaci externi
mediales
nodi lymphatici iliaci interni
nodi lymphatici inguinales profundi
nodi lymphatici inguinales
superficiales
nodi lymphatici intercostales
nodi lymphatici interiliaci
nodi lymphatici interpectorales
nodi lymphatici jugulares anteriores
nodi lymphatici jugulares laterales
nodi lymphatici juxta-esophageales
pulmonales
nodi lymphatici juxta-intestinales
nodi lymphatici lienales
nodi lymphatici linguales
nodi lymphatici lumbales dextri,
nodi lymphatici cavales laterales,
nodi lymphatici precavales
nodi lymphatici lumbales intermedii
nodi lymphatici lumbales sinistri,
nodi lymphatici ortici laterales, nodi
lymphatici preaortici, nodi
lymphatici prececales
nodi lymphatici abdominis
viscerales
nodi lymphatici anorectales
nodi lymphatici appendiculares
nodi lymphatici centrales
nodi lymphatici mesenterici
inferiores
nodi lymphatici mesenterici
superiores
nodi lymphatici mastoidei
nodi lymphatici mediastinales
anteriores
nodi lymphatici mediastinales
posteriores

nodi lymphatici mesenterici
nodi lymphatici mesocolici
nodi lymphatici obturatorii
nodi lymphatici occipitales
nodi lymphatici ortici laterales
(*var. of* nodi lymphatici lumbales
sinistri)
nodi lymphatici pancreatici, nodi
lymphatici pancreatici inferiores
nodi lymphatici pancreatici
inferiores
nodi lymphatici pancreatici
superiores
nodi lymphatici
pancreaticoduodenales
nodi lymphatici pancreticolienales
nodi lymphatici paracolici
nodi lymphatici paramammarii
nodi lymphatici pararectales
nodi lymphatici parasternales
nodi lymphatici paratracheales
nodi lymphatici parauterini
nodi lymphatici paravaginales
nodi lymphatici paravesiculares
nodi lymphatici parietales
nodi lymphatici parotidei
intraglandulares
nodi lymphatici parotidei profundi
nodi lymphatici parotidei profundi
infra-auriculares
nodi lymphatici parotidei profundi
preauriculares
nodi lymphatici parotidei
superficiales
nodi lymphatici pericardiales
laterales
nodi lymphatici phrenici inferiores
nodi lymphatici phrenici superiores
nodi lymphatici popliteales
nodi lymphatici postcavales
nodi lymphatici postvesiculares
nodi lymphatici preaortici (*var. of*
nodi lymphatici lumbales sinistri)
nodi lymphatici precavales (*var. of*
nodi lymphatici lumbales dextri)
nodi lymphatici prececales (*var. of*
nodi lymphatici lumbales sinistri)
nodi lymphatici prececales
nodi lymphatici prelaryngeales
nodi lymphatici prepericardiales
nodi lymphatici pretracheales
nodi lymphatici prevertebrales
nodi lymphatici prevesiculares
nodi lymphatici promontorii
nodi lymphatici pulmonales
nodi lymphatici pylorici
nodi lymphatici rectales superiores
nodi lymphatici retrocecales

N

nodus lymphaticus (*continued*)
    nodi lymphatici retropharyngeales
    nodi lymphatici sacrales
    nodi lymphatici sigmoidei
    nodi lymphatici splenici
    nodi lymphatici subaortici
    nodi lymphatici submandibulares
    nodi lymphatici submentales
    nodi lymphatici superiores centrales
    nodi lymphatici supraclaviculares
    nodi lymphatici thyroidei
    nodi lymphatici tracheobronchiales inferiores
    nodi lymphatici tracheobronchiales superiores
    nodi lymphatici vesicales laterales
noematic
noesis
noetic
    n. anxiety
noeud vital
Noguchia
noise
    n. pollution
    structured n.
noise–induced deafness
noma
Nomarski optics
nomatophobia
nomenclatural type
Nomenklatur Kommission
Nomina Anatomica
nominal aphasia
nomogram
    blood volume n.
    d'Ocagne n.
    Radford n.
    Siggaard-Andersen n.
nomograph
nomothetic
    n. approach
nomotopic
non-A
    n.-A, non-B hepatitis
    n.-A, non-B hepatitis virus
    n.-A, non-B, non-C hepatitis
nonabsorbable ligature
nonaccommodative esotropia
non-adrenergic, non-cholinergic neuron
nonallele
nonan
    n. malaria
nonanatomic teeth
non-arcon articulator
nonbacterial
    n. thrombotic endocarditis
    n. verrucous endocarditis

nonbullous congenital ichthyosiform erythroderma
nonbursate
noncariogenic
noncellular
nonchromaffin paraganglioma
nonchromogens
nonclonogenic cell
noncohesive gold
noncommunicating
    n. hydrocele
    n. hydrocephalus
noncomplementary role
non compos mentis
nonconjugative plasmid
nonconvulsive seizure
nondeciduous placenta
nondepolarizing block
nondiabetic glycosuria
nondirective psychotherapy
nondisease
nondisjunction
    primary n.
    secondary n.
nonepileptic seizure
nonfenestrated forceps
nonfilament polymorphonuclear leukocyte
nonfluent aphasia
nongonococcal urethritis
nongranular leukocyte
non-Hodgkin's lymphoma
nonhomologous chromosomes
nonhyperglycemic glycosuria
nonimmune
    n. agglutination
    n. fetal hydrops
    n. serum
nonimmunity
noninfectious
noninfiltrating lobular carcinoma
noninflammatory edema
non-insulin-dependent diabetes mellitus
noninvasive
nonionic
nonisolated proteinuria
nonketotic
    n. hyperglycemia
    n. hyperglycinemia
nonlamellar bone
nonlipid histiocytosis
nonmaleficence
nonmedullated
    n. fibers
nonmotile leukocyte
nonmyelinated
nonneoplastic
nonneurogenic neurogenic bladder

non-newtonian fluid
non-nucleated
nonobstructive jaundice
nonoccluded virus
nonocclusion
nonorganic aphonia
nonossifying fibroma
nonosteogenic fibroma
nonovulational menstruation
nonoxynol 9
nonparous
nonparticipant observer
nonpedunculated hydatid
nonpenetrance
nonpenetrant trait
nonpenetrating
    n. keratoplasty
    n. wound
nonphasic sinus arrhythmia
nonpitting edema
nonprecipitable antibody
nonprecipitating antibody
nonrandom mating
non-rapid eye movement
nonreactive depression
nonrebreathing
    n. anesthesia
    n. mask
    n. valve
nonrefractive accommodative esotropia
nonrenal azotemia
nonreset nodus sinuatrialis
nonresponder tolerance
nonrotation
    n. of intestine
    n. of kidney
nonsecretor
nonsecretory myeloma
nonsense
    n. suppression
    n. syndrome
nonseptate mycelium
nonsexual generation
nonspecific
    n. anergy
    n. immunity
    n. protein
    n. system
    n. therapy
    n. urethritis
    n. vaginitis
nonstress test
nonsuppressible insulin-like activity
nonthrombocytopenic purpura
nontoxic goiter
nontransmural myocardial infarction
nontropical sprue
nonunion

nonvascular
nonvenereal syphilis
nonverbal
nonviable
nonvital
    n. pulp
    n. tooth
noogenic neurosis
Noonan's syndrome
no reflow phenomenon
norm
norma, pl. normae
    n. anterior
    n. basilaris
    n. facialis
    n. frontalis
    n. inferior
    n. lateralis
    n. occipitalis
    n. posterior
    n. sagittalis
    n. superior
    n. temporalis
    n. ventralis
    n. verticalis
normal
    n. animal
    n. antibody
    n. antithrombin
    n. bite
    n. cholesteremic xanthomatosis
    n. distribution
    n. electrical axis
    n. hearing
    n. horse serum
    n. human plasma
    n. occlusion
    n. opsonin
    n. ovariotomy
    n. pressure hydrocephalus
    n. serum
    n. values
normally posed tooth
normative
normobaric
normoblast
normoblastosis
normocapnia
normocephalic
normochromia
normochromic
    n. anemia
normocyte
normocytic anemia
normocytosis
normoerythrocyte
normoglycemia

N

normoglycemic
  n. glycosuria
normokalemia, normokaliemia
normokalemic periodic paralysis
normoplasia
normospermatogenic sterility
normosthenuria
normotensive
normothermia
normotonic
normotopia
normotopic
normovolemia
normoxia
Norrie's disease
Norris' corpuscles
North
  N. American blastomycosis
  N. Queensland tick fever
  N. Queensland tick typhus
Northern blot analysis
Norton's operation
Norwalk
  N. agent
  N. virus
Norway itch
Norwegian scabies
Norwood
  N. operation
  N. procedure
nose
  brandy n.
  cleft n.
  copper n.
  dog n.
  external n.
  hammer n.
  potato n.
  rum n.
  saddle n.
  toper's n.
nosebleed
nose-bridge-lid reflex
nose-eye reflex
Nosema
  N. corneum
Nosematidae
nosepiece
nosetiology
nosochthonography
nosocomial
  n. gangrene
nosogenesis, nosogeny
nosogenic
nosogeography
nosographic
nosography
nosologic

nosology
  psychiatric n.
nosomania
nosometry
nosomycosis
nosonomy
nosophilia
nosophobia
nosophyte
nosopoietic
Nosopsyllus
nosotaxy
nosotoxicosis
nosotrophy
nosotropic
nostalgia
nostomania
nostophobia
nostril
  internal n.
notal
notalgia
  n. paresthetica
notancephalia
notanencephalia
notch
  acetabular n.
  angular n.
  antegonial n.
  anterior cerebellar n.
  anterior n. of cerebellum
  anterior n. of ear
  aortic n.
  n. of apex of heart
  auricular n.
  cardiac n.
  cardiac n. of left lung
  n.'s in cartilage of external
    acoustic meatus
  clavicular n. of sternum
  costal n.
  cotyloid n.
  craniofacial n.
  dicrotic n.
  digastric n.
  ethmoidal n.
  fibular n.
  frontal n.
  greater sciatic n.
  hamular n.
  Hutchinson's crescentic n.
  iliosciatic n.
  inferior thyroid n.
  interarytenoid n.
  interclavicular n.
  intercondyloid n.
  intertragic n.
  intervertebral n.

ischiatic n.
jugular n. of occipital bone
jugular n. of temporal bone
Kernohan's n.
lacrimal n.
lesser sciatic n.
mandibular n.
marsupial n.
mastoid n.
nasal n.
pancreatic n.
parietal n.
parotid n.
popliteal n.
posterior cerebellar n.
posterior n. of cerebellum
preoccipital n.
presternal n.
pterygoid n.
pterygomaxillary n.
radial n.
Rivinus' n.
n. for round ligament of liver
sacrosciatic n.
scapular n.
semilunar n.
sigmoid n.
sphenopalatine n.
sternal n.
superior thyroid n.
supraorbital n.
suprascapular n.
suprasternal n.
tentorial n.
n. of tentorium
terminal n. of auricle
trochlear n.
tympanic n.
ulnar n.
umbilical n.
vertebral n.
notched
    n. teeth
note blindness
notencephalocele
Nothnagel's syndrome
no-threshold concept
notochord
notochordal
    n. canal
    n. plate
    n. process
    n. sheath
Notoedres cati
noumenal
Novy and MacNeal's blood agar
noxa
noxious

NS echo
nubecula
nucha
nuchal
    n. fascia
    n. ligament
    n. plane
    n. region
    n. tubercle
Nuck's
    N. diverticulum
    N. hydrocele
nuclear
    n. bag
    n. bag fiber
    n. cataract
    n. chain fiber
    n. envelope
    n. family
    n. hyaloplasm
    n. inclusion bodies
    n. jaundice
    n. layers of retina
    n. magnetic resonance imaging
    n. magnetic resonance tomography
    n. medicine
    n. membrane
    n. ophthalmoplegia
    n. pacemaker
    n. pore
    n. sap
    n. sclerosis
    n. spindle
    n. stain
nuclear-cytoplasmic ratio
nucleated
nuclei (*pl. of* nucleus)
nucleic acid probe
nucleiform
nucleocapsid
nucleochylema
nucleochyme
nucleocortical fibers
nucleofugal
nucleoid
    Lavdovsky's n.
nucleolar
    n. chromosome
    n. organizer
    n. zone
nucleolar-nuclear ratio
nucleoli (*pl. of* nucleolus)
nucleoliform
nucleoloid
nucleolonema
nucleolus, pl. **nucleoli**
    chromatin n.

nucleolus *(continued)*
    false n.
    n. organizer region
nucleomicrosome
nucleopetal
Nucleophaga
nucleoplasm
nucleoplasmic index
nucleoplasmin
nucleoreticulum
nucleorrhexis
nucleosome
nucleospindle
nucleotide deletion
nucleotoxin
nucleus, pl. nuclei
    abducens n., n. abducentis, n. of
      abducent nerve
    accessory cuneate n.
    accessory olivary nuclei
    n. accumbens septi
    n. acusticus
    n. alae cinereae
    almond n.
    ambiguous n.
    n. ambiguus
    n. amygdalae
    amygdaloid n.
    nuclei anteriores thalami
    anterior nuclei of thalamus
    n. anterodorsalis
    anterodorsal thalamic n.
    n. anteromedialis
    anteromedial thalamic n.
    n. anteroventralis
    anteroventral thalamic n.
    arcuate nuclei
    arcuate n.
    arcuate n. of thalamus
    nuclei arcuati
    n. arcuatus
    n. arcuatus thalami
    auditory n.
    autonomic nuclei
    basal nuclei
    nuclei basales
    basal n. of Ganser
    n. basalis of Ganser
    Bechterew's n.
    Blumenau's n.
    branchiomotor nuclei
    Burdach's n.
    caudate n.
    n. caudatus
    n. centralis lateralis thalami
    n. centralis tegmenti superior
    central lateral n. of thalamus
    centromedian n.

n. centromedianus
cerebellar nuclei
ceruleus n.
Clarke's n.
cochlear nuclei
nuclei cochleares
n. colliculi inferioris
convergence n. of Perlia
n. corporis geniculati medialis
nuclei corporis mamillaris
nuclei of cranial nerves
cuneate n.
n. of cuneate fasciculus
n. cuneatus
n. cuneatus accessorius
n. of Darkschewitsch
Deiters' n.
dentate n. of cerebellum
n. dentatus cerebelli
descending n. of the trigeminus
diploid n.
dorsal n.
dorsal accessory olivary n.
n. dorsalis
n. dorsalis corporis trapezoidei
n. dorsalis nervi vagi
dorsal motor n. of vagus
dorsal n. of trapezoid body
dorsal vagal n.
dorsal n. of vagus
dorsal n. of vagus nerve
dorsomedial n.
dorsomedial hypothalamic n.
dorsomedial n. of hypothalamus
n. dorsomedialis hypothalami
droplet nuclei
Edinger-Westphal n.
emboliform n.
n. emboliformis
external cuneate n.
facial n.
n. facialis
facial motor n.
n. fasciculi gracilis
fastigial n.
n. fastigii
n. fibrosus linguae
filiform n.
n. filiformis
n. funiculi cuneati
n. funiculi gracilis
gametic n.
n. gelatinosus
gelatinous n.
geniculatus lateralis n.
germ n.
n. gigantocellularis medullae
  oblongatae

gigantocellular n. of medulla
  oblongata
n. globosus
globosus n.
n. of Goll
gonad n.
gracile n.
n. gracilis
Gudden's tegmental nuclei
gustatory n.
n. habenulae
habenular n.
hypoglossal n.
n. of hypoglossal nerve
n. of inferior colliculus
inferior olivary n.
inferior salivary n.
inferior salivatory n.
inferior vestibular n.
intercalated n.
n. intercalatus
intermediolateral n.
n. intermediolateralis
intermediomedial n.
n. intermediomedialis
interpeduncular ñ.
n. interpeduncularis
interpositus n.
n. interpositus
interstitial n.
interstitial n. of Cajal
n. interstitialis
nuclei intralaminares thalami
intralaminar nuclei of thalamus
Klein-Gumprecht shadow nuclei
lateral cervical nuclei
lateral cuneate n.
n. of lateral geniculate body
n. lateralis medullae oblongatae
n. lateralis thalami
n. of lateral lemniscus
lateral n. of medulla oblongata
lateral preoptic n.
lateral reticular n.
lateral n. of thalamus
lateral tuberal nuclei
lateral vestibular n.
n. lemnisci lateralis
n. of lens
lenticular n., lentiform n.
n. lentiformis
n. lentis
n. of Luys
n. of the mamillary body
nuclei of mamillary body
n. masticatorius
masticatory n.
medial accessory olivary n.

medial central n. of thalamus
n. of medial geniculate body
n. medialis centralis thalami
n. medialis thalami
medial preoptic n.
medial n. of thalamus
medial vestibular n.
mediodorsal n.
mesencephalic n. of trigeminal
  nerve
Monakow's n.
motor nuclei
motor n. of facial nerve
n. motorius nervi trigemini
motor n. of trigeminal nerve
motor n. of trigeminus
n. nervi abducentis
nuclei nervi cochlearis
n. nervi facialis
n. nervi hypoglossi
n. nervi oculomotorii
n. nervi trochlearis
nuclei nervi vestibulocochlearis
nuclei nervorum cranialium
n. niger
oculomotor n.
n. of oculomotor nerve
n. olivaris
n. olivaris accessorius dorsalis
n. olivaris accessorius medialis
Onuf's n.
nuclei of origin
nuclei originis
parabrachial nuclei
nuclei parabrachiales
n. paracentralis thalami
paracentral n. of thalamus
paraventricular n.
n. paraventricularis
perihypoglossal nuclei
Perlia's n.
phrenic n.
pontine nuclei
nuclei pontis
pontis nervi trigeminalis n.
n. posterior hypothalami
posterior hypothalamic n.
posterior medial n. of thalamus
  (*var. of* ventral posteromedial n.
  of thalamus)
posterior periventricular n.
n. preopticus lateralis
n. preopticus medialis
prerubral n.
pretectal n.
principal sensory n. of trigeminal
  nerve

N

nucleus *(continued)*
    principal sensory n. of the
      trigeminus
    n. pulposus
    pulvinar n.
    n. pyramidalis
    raphe nuclei
    nuclei raphes
    red n.
    reduction n.
    reproductive n.
    reticular nuclei of the brainstem
    n. reticularis thalami
    reticular n. of thalamus
    rhombencephalic gustatory n.
    Roller's n.
    roof n.
    n. ruber
    n. salivatorius inferior
    n. salivatorius superior
    Schwalbe's n.
    secondary sensory nuclei
    segmentation n.
    semilunar n. of Flechsig
    n. sensorius principalis nervi
      trigemini
    n. sensorius superior nervi
      trigemini
    sensory nuclei
    shadow n.
    sole nuclei
    n. of solitary tract
    somatic n.
    somatic motor nuclei
    special visceral efferent nuclei
    special visceral motor nuclei
    sperm n.
    spherical n.
    spinal n. of accessory nerve
    n. spinalis nervi accessorii
    spinal trigeminal n.
    spinal n. of the trigeminus
    Spitzka's n.
    Staderini's n.
    Stilling's n.
    subceruleus n.
    subthalamic n.
    n. subthalamicus
    superior central tegmental n.
    superior olivary n.
    superior salivary n.
    superior salivatory n.
    superior vestibular n.
    n. suprachiasmatica
    supraoptic n.
    supraoptic n. of hypothalamus
    n. supraopticus hypothalami
    tectal n.

    n. tecti
    tegmental nuclei
    nuclei tegmenti, n. tegmenti pontis
      caudalis, n. tegmenti pontis oralis
    terminal nuclei, nuclei terminales
    nuclei terminationis
    thalamic gustatory n.
    thoracic n.
    n. thoracicus
    n. tractus mesencephali nervi
      trigemini
    n. tractus solitarii
    n. tractus spinalis nervi trigemini
    triangular n.
    trochlear n.
    n. of trochlear nerve
    trophic n.
    tuberal nuclei
    nuclei tuberales
    ventral anterior n. of thalamus
    ventral intermediate n. of thalamus
    n. ventralis anterior thalami
    n. ventralis corporis trapezoidei
    n. ventralis intermedius thalami
    n. ventralis lateralis
    n. ventralis posterior intermedius
      thalami
    n. ventralis posterior thalami
    n. ventralis posterolateralis thalami
    n. ventralis posteromedialis thalami
    n. ventralis thalami
    ventral lateral n. of thalamus
    ventral posterior intermediate n. of
      thalamus
    ventral posterior n. of thalamus
    ventral posterolateral n. of
      thalamus, ventral posterior
      lateral n. of thalamus
    ventral posteromedial n. of
      thalamus, posterior medial n. of
      thalamus
    ventral n. of thalamus
    ventral tier thalamic nuclei
    ventral n. of trapezoid body
    ventrobasal n.
    ventromedial n. of hypothalamus
    n. ventromedialis hypothalami
    vestibular n.
    n. vestibularis
    vestibulocochlear nuclei
nude mouse
Nuel's space
Nuhn's gland
null
    n. cells
    n. hypothesis
null-cell adenoma
nulligravida

nullipara
nulliparity
nulliparous
number
    Brinell hardness n.
    CT n.
    Hogben n.
    Hounsfield n.
    Kestenbaum's n.
    Knoop hardness n.
    Mach n.
    MIM n.
    Reynolds n.
    wave n.
numbness
numerical
    n. aperture
    n. hypertrophy
nummiform
nummular
    n. dermatitis
    n. eczema
    n. sputum
    n. syphilid
nummulation
nunnation
nun's murmur
nurse
    n. cells
    certified registered n. anesthetist
    charge n.
    clinical n. specialist
    community n.
    community health n.
    dry n.
    n. epidemiologist
    flight n.
    general duty n.
    graduate n.
    head n.
    home health n.
    hospital n.
    infection control n.
    licensed practical n.
    licensed vocational n.
    practical n.
    n. practitioner
    private n.
    private duty n.
    public health n.
    registered n.
    school n.
    scrub n.
    special n.
    student n.
    visiting n.
    wet n.
nursemaid's elbow

nursing
    n. assignment
    n. audit
    n. bottle caries
    n. home
    n. model
    n. plan of care
    n. process
Nussbaum's
    N. bracelet
    N. experiment
nutation
nutmeg liver
nutrient
    n. agar
    n. arteries of humerus
    n. artery
    n. artery of femur
    n. artery of fibula
    n. artery of the tibia
    n. canal
    n. enema
    essential n.'s
    n. foramen
    n. vessel
nutrition
    total parenteral n.
nutritional
    n. amblyopia
    n. anemia
    n. dropsy
    n. edema
    n. hemosiderosis
    n. macrocytic anemia
    n. marasmus
    n. polyneuropathy
    n. type cerebellar atrophy
nutritive equilibrium
nutriture
Nuttallia
nyctalgia
nyctalopia
    n. with congenital myopia
nyctanopia
nycterine
nycterohemeral
nyctohemeral
nyctophilia
nyctophobia
Nyctotherus
nycturia
nymph
nympha, pl. **nymphae**
nymphal
nymphectomy
nymphitis
nymphocaruncular sulcus
nymphohymenal sulcus

N

nympholabial
nympholepsy
nymphomania
nymphomaniac
nymphomaniacal
nymphoncus
nymphotomy
nystagmic
nystagmiform
nystagmogram
nystagmograph
nystagmography
nystagmoid
nystagmus
    after-n.
    amaurotic n.
    n. blockage syndrome
    Bruns' n.
    caloric n.
    cervical n.
    compressive n.
    congenital n.
    conjugate n.
    convergence-retraction n.
    deviational n.
    dissociated n.
    downbeat n.
    dysjunctive n.

    end-point n.
    fixation n.
    galvanic n.
    gaze paretic n.
    incongruent n.
    irregular n.
    jerky n.
    labyrinthine n.
    latent n.
    miner's n.
    minimal amplitude n.
    ocular n.
    opticokinetic n.
    optokinetic n.
    palatal n.
    pendular n.
    positional n.
    railroad n.
    rotational n.
    rotatory n.
    seesaw n.
    n. test
    upbeat n.
    vertical n.
    vestibular n.
    voluntary n.
Nysten's law
nyxis

O
O agglutinin
O antigen
O colony
oasthouse urine disease
oat
o. cell
o. cell carcinoma
oatmeal-tomato paste agar
OAV
O. dysplasia
O. syndrome
obdormition
O'Beirne's
O. sphincter
O. valve
obeliac
obeliad
obelion
Obermayer's test
Obermeier's spirillum
Obersteiner-Redlich
O.-R. line
O.-R. zone
obese
obesity
hypothalamic o.
hypothalamic o. with hypogonadism
o. index
morbid o.
simple o.
obex
obfuscation
object
o. blindness
o. choice
o. constancy
o. glass
good o.
o. libido
o. relationship
sex o.
test o.
objective
achromatic o.
apochromatic o.
o. assessment data
immersion o.
o. optometer
o. perimetry
o. probability
o. psychology
o. sensation
o. sign
o. symptom

o. synonyms
o. vertigo
obligate
o. aerobe
o. anaerobe
o. parasite
oblique
o. amputation
o. arytenoid muscle
o. auricular muscle
o. bandage
o. bundle of pons
o. cord
o. diameter
o. facial cleft
o. fibers of stomach
o. fissure
o. fissure of lung
o. fracture
o. head
o. illumination
o. lie
o. ligament of elbow joint
o. line
o. line of mandible
o. line of thyroid cartilage
o. muscle of auricle
o. part of cricothyroid muscle
o. pericardial sinus
o. pontine fasciculus
o. popliteal ligament
o. projection
o. ridge
o. ridge of trapezium
o. section
o. sinus of pericardium
o. vein of left atrium
obliquity
Litzmann o.
Nägele o.
obliquus
o. capitis inferior muscle
o. capitis superior muscle
obliterating
o. arteritis
o. endarteritis
o. pericarditis
obliteration
obliterative
o. arachnoiditis
o. bronchitis
oblong
o. fovea of arytenoid cartilage
o. pit of arytenoid cartilage
oblongata

O

obnubilation
OBS
observer
    nonparticipant o.
    participant o.
obsession
    impulsive o.
    inhibitory o.
obsessional neurosis
obsessive
    o. behavior
    o. personality
obsessive-compulsive
    o.-c. disorder
    o.-c. neurosis
    o.-c. personality
    o.-c. personality disorder
obsolescence
obstacle sense
obstetric, obstetrical
    o. conjugate
    o. conjugate diameter
    o. conjugate of pelvic outlet
    o. position
    o. ultrasound
obstetrician
obstetrics
obstinate
obstipation
obstruction
    closed-loop o.
    ureteropelvic o.
    ureteropelvic junction o.
    ureterovesical o.
obstructive
    o. apnea
    o. appendicitis
    o. dysmenorrhea
    o. hydrocephalus
    o. jaundice
    o. murmur
    o. pneumonia
    o. pulmonary overinflation
    o. thrombus
    o. uropathy
obtund
obturating embolism
obturation
    intermittent self-o.
obturator
    o. appliance
    o. artery
    o. canal
    o. crest
    o. externus muscle
    o. fascia
    o. foramen
    o. groove

    o. hernia
    o. internus muscle
    o. lymph nodes
    o. membrane
    o. nerve
    o. tubercle
    o. vein
obtuse
obtusion
Occam's razor
occipital
    o. anchorage
    o. angle of parietal bone
    o. artery
    o. belly of occipitofrontalis muscle
    o. bone
    o. border
    o. border of parietal bone
    o. border of temporal bone
    o. branch
    o. cerebral veins
    o. condyle
    o. emissary vein
    o. fontanel
    o. groove
    o. gyri
    o. horn
    o. lobe
    o. lobe of cerebrum
    o. lobe epilepsy
    o. lymph nodes
    o. margin
    o. neuralgia
    o. neurectomy
    o. neuritis
    o. operculum
    o. part of corpus callosum
    o. plane
    o. plexus
    o. point
    o. pole
    o. pole of cerebrum
    o. region of head
    o. sinus
    o. somite
    o. squama
    o. triangle
    o. vein
occipitalis
    o. muscle
occipitalization
occipitis (*gen. of* occiput)
occipitoanterior position
occipitoatloid
occipitoaxial, occipitoaxoid
    o. ligaments
occipitobregmatic
occipitocollicular tract

occipitofacial
occipitofrontal
    o. diameter
    o. fasciculus
    o. muscle
occipitofrontalis
    o. muscle
occipitomastoid
    o. suture
occipitomental
    o. diameter
    o. projection
occipitoparietal
occipitopontine tract
occipitoposterior position
occipitotectal tract
occipitotemporal
    o. sulcus
occipitothalamic
    o. radiation
occipitotransverse position
occiput, gen. **occipitis**
occlude
occluded virus
occluder
occluding
    o. centric relation record
    o. frame
    o. ligature
    o. paper
    o. relation
occlusal
    o. adjustment
    o. analysis
    o. balance
    o. caries
    o. clearance
    o. correction
    o. curvature
    o. disharmony
    o. embrasure
    o. force
    o. form
    o. harmony
    o. imbalance
    o. path
    o. pattern
    o. pivot
    o. plane
    o. position
    o. pressure
    o. radiograph
    o. rest
    o. rest bar
    o. rim
    o. scheme
    o. surface
    o. system

    o. table
    o. trauma
    o. vertical dimension
    o. wear
occlusion
    abnormal o.
    afunctional o.
    anterior o.
    balanced o.
    bimaxillary protrusive o.
    buccal o.
    centric o.
    coronary o.
    distal o.
    eccentric o.
    edge-to-edge o.
    end-to-end o.
    functional o.
    gliding o.
    hyperfunctional o.
    labial o.
    lateral o.
    lingual o.
    mechanically balanced o.
    mesenteric artery o.
    mesial o.
    neutral o.
    normal o.
    pathogenic o.
    physiologic o.
    physiologically balanced o.
    posterior o.
    postnormal o.
    protrusive o.
    o. of pupil
    retrusive o.
    o. rim
    spherical form of o.
    torsive o.
    traumatic o.
    traumatogenic o.
    working o.
occlusive
    o. dressing
    o. ileus
    o. meningitis
occlusometer
occult
    o. bleeding
    o. blood
    o. border of nail
    o. carcinoma
    o. fracture
    o. hydrocephalus
occupational
    o. deafness
    o. disease
    o. neurosis

O

occupational *(continued)*
    o. spasm
    o. therapy
Oceanospirillum
ocellus, pl. ocelli
ochlophobia
Ochoa's law
ochrodermia
ochrometer
ochronosis
    exogenous o.
ochronotic
    o. arthritis
Ochsner clamp
Ochsner's method
octan
octaploidy
octavus
Octomitidae
Octomitus hominis
ocular
    o. albinism
    o. bobbing
    compensating o.
    o. cone
    o. crisis
    o. cup
    o. dysmetria
    o. flutter
    o. humor
    Huygens' o.
    o. hypertelorism
    o. larva migrans
    o. lens
    o. micrometer
    o. migraine
    o. motor
    o. motor apraxia
    o. muscles
    o. myiasis
    o. myopathy
    o. nystagmus
    o. onchocerciasis
    o. paralysis
    o. pemphigoid
    o. prosthesis
    Ramsden's o.
    o. rigidity
    o. scoliosis
    o. sparganosis
    o. tension
    o. torticollis
    o. vertigo
    o. vesicle
    wide field o.
ocularist
ocular-mucous membrane syndrome
oculi (*gen. and pl. of* oculus)

oculist
oculoauriculovertebral
    o. dysplasia
oculobuccogenital syndrome
oculocardiac
    o. reflex
oculocephalic reflex
oculocephalogyric reflex
oculocerebrorenal
    o. syndrome
oculocutaneous
    o. albinism
    o. syndrome
oculodentodigital
    o. dysplasia
oculodermal
    o. melanosis
oculodynia
oculoencephalic angiomatosis
oculofacial
oculography
    photosensor o.
oculogravic illusion
oculogyral illusion
oculogyria
oculogyric
    o. crises
oculomandibulodyscephaly
oculomandibulofacial syndrome
oculomotor
    o. nerve
    o. nucleus
    o. response
    o. root of ciliary ganglion
    o. system
oculomotorius
oculonasal
oculopathy
oculopharyngeal
    o. dystrophy
    o. syndrome
oculoplethysmography
oculopneumoplethysmography
oculopupillary
oculosympathetic
oculovagal reflex
oculovertebral
    o. dysplasia
    o. syndrome
oculovestibulo-auditory syndrome
oculozygomatic
oculus, gen. and pl. oculi
od
odaxesmus
odd chromosome
Oddi's sphincter
odditis
odds

Odland body
odogenesis
odontagra
odontalgia
    o. dentalis
odontalgic
odontectomy
odonterism
odontiasis
odontinoid
odontitis
odontoameloblastoma
odontoblast
odontoblastic
    o. layer
    o. process
odontoblastoma
odontoclast
odontodynia
odontodysplasia
odontogenesis
    o. imperfecta
odontogenic
    o. cyst
    o. dysplasia
    o. fibroma
    o. keratocyst
    o. myxoma
odontogeny
odontoid
    o. ligament
    o. process
    o. process of epistropheus
    o. vertebra
odontology
    forensic o.
odontoloxia, odontoloxy
odontolysis
odontoma
    ameloblastic o.
    complex o.
    compound o.
odontoneuralgia
odontonomy
odontonosology
odontoparallaxis
odontopathy
odontophobia
odontoplasty
odontoprisis
odontoptosis
odontorrhagia
odontoschism
odontoscope
odontoscopy
odontosis
odontotherapy

odontotomy
    prophylactic o.
odor
odorant
    o. binding protein
odoratism
odoriferous
odorimeter
odorimetry
odorivection
odorography
odorous
O'Dwyer's tube
odynacusis
odynometer
odynophagia
odynophonia
oedipal
    o. neurosis
    o. period
    o. phase
oedipism
Oedipus complex
Oehler's symptom
Oehl's muscles
Oesophagostomum
    O. apiostomum
    O. brevicaudum
    O. brumpti
    O. columbianum
    O. dentatum
    O. georgianum
    O. quadrispinulatum
    O. radiatum
    O. stephanostomum
    O. venulosum
oestrids
Oestrus
OFD syndrome
officer
    house o.
Ofuji's disease
Ogilvie's syndrome
Ogino-Knaus rule
Ogston-Luc operation
Ogston's line
Oguchi's disease
Ogura operation
O'Hara forceps
17-OH-corticoids test
ohne Hauch
Ohngren's line
oidiomycin
oidium, pl. oidia
oil
    o. cyst
    o. embolism
    o. immersion

O

oil *(continued)*
    joint o.
    o. pneumonia
    o. red O
    o. retention enema
    o. tumor
oily granuloma
OKT cells
Old World leishmaniasis
olecranon
    o. bursitis
    o. fossa
    o. process
    o. reflex
oleogranuloma
oleoma
oleosus
oleotherapy
olfactie, olfacty
olfaction
olfactology
olfactometer
olfactometry
olfactophobia
olfactory
    o. angle
    o. area
    o. bulb
    o. bundle
    o. cells
    o. cortex
    o. epithelium
    o. esthesioneuroblastoma
    o. fila
    o. foramen
    o. glands
    o. glomerulus
    o. groove
    o. hallucination
    o. hyperesthesia
    o. hypesthesia
    o. membrane
    o. mucosa
    o. nerves
    o. neuroblastoma
    o. organ
    o. peduncle
    o. pits
    o. placodes
    o. pyramid
    o. receptor cells
    o. region of tunica mucosa of
      nose
    o. roots
    o. striae
    o. sulcus
    o. sulcus of nasal cavity

    o. tract
    o. trigone
    o. tubercle
olfacty *(var. of* olfactie)
olfacty
oligamnios
oligemia
oligemic
    o. shock
olighemia
olighidria, oligidria
oligoamnios
oligocholia
oligochylia
oligochymia
oligoclonal band
oligocystic
oligodactyly, oligodactylia
oligodendria
oligodendroblast
oligodendroblastoma
oligodendrocyte
oligodendroglia
    o. cells
oligodendroglioma
    anaplastic o.
    pleomorphic o.
oligodipsia
oligodontia
oligodynamic
oligogalactia
oligohydramnios
oligohydruria
oligolecithal
oligomenorrhea
oligomorphic
oligonephronic
oligopepsia
oligopeptide
oligoplastic
oligopnea
oligoptyalism
oligoria
oligosialia
oligospermia, oligospermatism
oligosymptomatic
oligosynaptic
oligothymia
oligotrichia
oligotrichosis
oligotrophia, oligotrophy
oligozoospermatism, oligozoospermia
oliguresia, oliguresis
oliguria
oliva, pl. **olivae**
    o. inferior
    o. superior

olivary
- o. body
- o. eminence

olive
- inferior o.
- superior o.

olive-tipped catheter
olivifugal
olivipetal
olivocerebellar tract
olivocochlear
- o. bundle
- o. fibers
- o. tract

olivopontocerebellar
- o. atrophy
- o. degeneration

olivospinal tract
Ollier
- O. disease
- O. graft
- O. method
- O. theory

Ollier-Thiersch graft
olophonia
olympian forehead
Ombrédanne operation
ombrophobia
Omenn's syndrome
omenta (*pl. of* omentum)
omental
- o. branches
- o. bursa
- o. enterocleisis
- o. graft
- o. sac
- o. tenia
- o. tuber

omentectomy
omentitis
omentofixation
omentopexy
omentoplasty
omentorrhaphy
omentovolvulus
omentulum
omentum, pl. **omenta**
- gastrocolic o.
- gastrohepatic o.
- gastrosplenic o.
- greater o.
- lesser o.
- o. majus
- o. minus

omentumectomy
omission of duty
Ommaya reservoir
omnifocal lens

omnipotence of thought
omnivorous
omoclavicular
- o. triangle

omohyoid
- o. muscle

omophagia
omothyroid
omotracheal triangle
omphalectomy
omphalelcosis
omphalic
omphalitis
omphaloangiopagous twins
omphaloangiopagus
omphalocele
omphaloenteric
omphalomesenteric
- o. artery
- o. cord
- o. cyst
- o. duct
- o. duct cyst

omphalopagus
omphalophlebitis
omphalorrhagia
omphalorrhea
omphalorrhexis
omphalos
omphalosite
omphalospinous
omphalotomy
omphalotripsy
omphalovesical
omphalus
Omsk
- O. hemorrhagic fever
- O. hemorrhagic fever virus

onanism
Onchocerca
- *O. volvulus*

onchocerciasis
- ocular o.

onchocercid
Onchocercidae
onchocercosis
Oncocerca
oncocyte
oncocytic hepatocellular tumor
oncocytoma
oncofetal
- o. antigens
- o. marker

oncogene
oncogenesis
oncogenic
- o. virus

oncogenous

O

oncograph
oncography
oncoides
oncologist
    radiation o.
oncology
    radiation o.
oncolysis
oncolytic
Oncomelania
oncometer
oncometric
oncometry
oncoplastic carcinoma
oncornaviruses
oncosis
oncosphere
    o. embryo
oncotherapy
oncotic
oncotomy
Oncovirinae
oncovirus
Ondine's curse
one-horned uterus
oneiric
oneirism
oneirocritical
oneirodynia
    o. activa
    o. gravis
oneirogmus
oneirology
oneirophrenia
oneiroscopy
oniomania
onion
    o. bodies
    o. bulb neuropathy
oniric
onlay
    o. graft
Onodi cell
on-off phenomenon
onomatomania
onomatophobia
onomatopoiesis
ontogenesis
ontogenetic, ontogenic
ontogeny
ontology
Onuf's nucleus
onyalai
onychalgia
onychatrophia, onychatrophy
onychauxis
onychectomy

onychia
    o. lateralis
    o. maligna
    o. periungualis
    o. sicca
onychitis
onychoclasis
onychocryptosis
onychodystrophy
onychograph
onychogryphosis
onychogryposis
onychoheterotopia
onychoid
onychology
onycholysis
onychoma
onychomadesis
onychomalacia
onychomycosis
onychonosus
onycho-osteodysplasia
onychopathic
onychopathology
onychopathy
onychophagy, onychophagia
onychophosis
onychophyma
onychoplasty
onychoptosis
onychorrhexis
onychoschizia
onychosis
onychostroma
onychotillomania
onychotomy
onychotrophy
o'nyong-nyong
    o.-n. fever
    o.-n. virus
onyx
onyxis
onyxitis
oocyesis
oocyst
oocyte
    primary o.
    secondary o.
oogenesis
oogenetic
oogenic, oogenous
oogonium, pl. oogonia
ookinesis, ookinesia
ookinete
oolemma
oophagia, oophagy
oophoralgia
oophorectomy

oophoritic cyst
oophoritis
oophorocystectomy
oophorocystosis
oophorohysterectomy
oophoroma
oophoron
oophoropathy
oophoropeliopexy
oophoropexy
oophoroplasty
oophororrhaphy
oophorosalpingectomy
oophorosalpingitis
oophorostomy
oophorotomy
oophorrhagia
ooplasm
oosome
oosporangium
oospore
ootheca
ootid
ootype
opacification
opacifying gallstones
opacity
    nodular o.
    snowball o.
opalescent
    o. dentin
opaline patch
Opalski cell
opaque
    o. microscope
opeidoscope
open
    o. angiography
    o. biopsy
    o. bite
    o. chest massage
    o. circuit method
    o. comedo
    o. cordotomy
    o. dislocation
    o. drainage
    o. drop anesthesia
    o. flap
    o. fracture
    o. head injury
    o. heart surgery
    o. hospital
    o. laparoscopy
    o. pneumothorax
    o. reduction of fractures
    o. skull fracture
    o. spaces

    o. tuberculosis
    o. wound
open-angle glaucoma
opening
    access o.
    aortic o.
    o. axis
    cardiac o.
    o. to cerebral aqueduct
    o. contraction
    esophageal o.
    o. of external acoustic meatus
    external o. of urethra
    femoral o.
    ileocecal o.
    o. of inferior vena cava
    o. of internal acoustic meatus
    internal urethral o.
    lacrimal o.
    o. movement
    orbital o.
    pharyngeal o. of auditory tube
    pharyngeal o. of eustachian tube
    piriform o.
    o. of pulmonary trunk
    o.'s of pulmonary veins
    saphenous o.
    o. snap
    o. of the sphenoidal sinus
    o. of superior vena cava
    tendinous o.
    tympanic o. of auditory tube
    tympanic o. of canaliculi for
      chorda tympani
    tympanic o. of eustachian tube
    ureteral o.
    urethral o.'s
    uterine o. of uterine tubes
    o. of uterus
    vaginal o.
    vertical o.
operable
opera-glass hand
operant
    o. behavior
    o. conditioning
operating
    o. microscope
    o. table
operation
    Abbe o.
    Arie-Pitanguy o.
    Arlt's o.
    arterial switch o.
    Baldy's o.
    Ball's o.
    Barkan's o.
    Bassini's o.

O

operation (*continued*)

Baudelocque's o.
Belsey Mark IV o.
Billroth's o. I
Billroth's o. II
Blalock-Hanlon o.
Blalock-Taussig o.
bloodless o.
Bozeman's o.
Bricker o.
Brock o.
Brunschwig's o.
Burow's o.
Caldwell-Luc o.
capital o.
Carmody-Batson o.
cesarean o.
commando o.
concrete o.'s
Cotte's o.
Dana's o.
Dandy o.
Daviel's o.
debulking o.
decompression o.'s
Doyle's o.
Dupuy-Dutemps o.
Elliot's o.
Emmet's o.
Esser o.
Estes o.
Estlander o.
fenestration o.
Filatov's o.
filtering o.
Finney's o.
flap o.
Foley o.
Fontan o.
formal o.'s
Fothergill's o.
Frazier-Spiller o.
Fredet-Ramstedt o.
Freund's o.
Gigli's o.
Gilliam's o.
Gillies' o.
Gil-Vernet o.
Glenn's o.
Graefe's o.
Gritti's o.
Halsted's o.
Hartmann's o.
Heaney's o.
Heller o.
Hill o.
Hoffa's o.
Hofmeister's o.

Huggins' o.
Hummelsheim's o.
Hunter's o.
Indian o.
interval o.
Italian o.
Jacobaeus o.
Jansen's o.
Kasai o.
Kazanjian's o.
Keen's o.
Keller-Madlener o.
Kelly's o.
Killian's o.
Koerte-Ballance o.
Kondoleon o.
Kraske's o.
Krönlein o.
Ladd's o.
Lambrinudi o.
Laroyenne's o.
Lash's o.
LeCompte o.
Leriche's o.
Lisfranc's o.
Longmire's o.
Luc's o.
Madlener o.
major o.
Manchester o.
Mann-Williamson o.
Marshall-Marchetti-Krantz o.
Mason o.
Matas' o.
Mayo's o.
McIndoe o.
McVay's o.
mika o.
Mikulicz' o.
Miles' o.
minor o.
morcellation o.
Motais' o.
Mules' o.
Mustard o.
Naffziger o.
Nissen's o.
Norton's o.
Norwood's o.
Ogston-Luc o.
Ogura o.
Ombrédanne o.
Payne o.
plastic o.
Pólya's o.
Pomeroy's o.
Porro o.
Potts' o.

pubovaginal o.
Putti-Platt o.
radical o. for hernia
Ramstedt o.
Rastelli's o.
Récamier's o.
Ridell's o.
Roux-en-Y o.
Saenger's o.
Schauta vaginal o.
Schönbein's o.
Schroeder's o.
Schuchardt's o.
scleral buckling o.
Scott o.
second-look o.
Senning o.
seton o.
Shirodkar o.
Sistrunk o.
Smith-Boyce o.
Smith-Indian o.
Smith-Robinson o.
Smith's o.
Soave o.
Spinelli o.
stapes mobilization o.
Stoffel's o.
Stookey-Scarff o.
Sturmdorf's o.
subcutaneous o.
Syme's o.
tagliacotian o.
talc o.
TeLinde o.
Thiersch's o.
Thiersch's graft o.
Torek o.
Trendelenburg's o.
Urban's o.
Waters' o.
Waterston o.
Webster's o.
Weir's o.
Wertheim's o.
Wheelhouse's o.
Whipple's o.
Whitehead's o.
operative
  o. dentistry
  o. myxedema
operator
opercula (*pl. of* operculum)
opercular
  o. fold
  o. part
operculated

operculitis
operculum, gen. **operculi**, pl. **opercula**
  o. ilei
  occipital o.
  trophoblastic o.
operon
  Lac o.
ophiasis
ophidiophobia
ophritis
ophryitis
ophryogenes
ophryon
Ophryoscolecidae
ophryosis
ophryospinal angle
ophthalmalgia
ophthalmia
  catarrhal o.
  caterpillar-hair o.
  o. eczematosa
  Egyptian o.
  gonorrheal o.
  granular o.
  metastatic o.
  o. neonatorum
  o. nivalis
  o. nodosa
  phlyctenular o.
  purulent o.
  spring o.
  sympathetic o.
  transferred o.
ophthalmic
  o. artery
  o. hyperthyroidism
  o. nerve
  o. plexus
  o. scoliosis
  o. veins
  o. vesicle
ophthalmodynamometer
  Bailliart's o.
  suction o.
ophthalmodynamometry
ophthalmolith
ophthalmologist
ophthalmology
ophthalmomalacia
ophthalmomandibulomelic dysplasia
ophthalmomelanosis
ophthalmometer
ophthalmomycosis
ophthalmomyiasis
ophthalmopathy
  endocrine o.
  external o.

O

ophthalmopathy *(continued)*
    Graves' o.
    internal o.
ophthalmoplegia
    chronic progressive external o.
    exophthalmic o.
    o. externa
    external o.
    fascicular o.
    fibrotic o.
    o. interna
    internal o.
    o. internuclearis
    nuclear o.
    orbital o.
    Parinaud's o.
    o. partialis
    o. progressiva
    o. totalis
ophthalmoplegic
    o. migraine
ophthalmoscope
    binocular o.
    demonstration o.
    direct o.
    indirect o.
ophthalmoscopic
ophthalmoscopy
    direct o.
    indirect o.
    o. with reflected light
ophthalmotrope
ophthalmovascular
opiate receptors
opisthenar
opisthiobasial
opisthion
opisthionasial
opisthocheilia, opisthochilia
opisthomastigote
opisthoporeia
opisthorchid
Opisthorchiidae
Opisthorchis
    O. felineus
    O. sinensis
    O. viverrini
opisthotic
opisthotonic
opisthotonoid
opisthotonos, opisthotonus
opodidymus
Oppenheim's
    O. disease
    O. reflex
    O. syndrome
oppilation
oppilative

opponens
    o. digiti minimi muscle
    o. pollicis muscle
opponent color
opportunistic
    o. pathogen
opposer
    o. muscle of little finger
    o. muscle of thumb
oppositional disorder
opposure
opsinogen
opsiuria
opsoclonus
opsogen
opsomania
opsonic
    o. index
opsonin
    common o.
    immune o.
    normal o.
    specific o.
    thermolabile o.
    thermostable o.
opsonization
opsonocytophagic
opsonometry
opsonophilia
opsonophilic
optic, optical
    o. agnosia
    o. ataxia
    o. axis
    o. canal
    o. capsule
    o. chiasm
    o. cup
    o. decussation
    o. disk
    o. fissure
    o. foramen
    o. groove
    o. layer
    o. nerve
    o. nerve drusen
    o. nerve glioma
    o. nerve head
    o. nerve hypoplasia
    o. nerve sheath decompression
    o. nerve sheath fenestration
    o. neuritis
    o. papilla
    o. part of retina
    o. pit
    o. placodes
    o. radiation
    o. recess

o. stalk
o. tract
o. vesicle
optician
opticianry
opticociliary
opticokinetic nystagmus
opticopupillary
optics
Nomarski o.
optimism
therapeutic o.
optimum
o. dose
o. temperature
optokinetic
o. nystagmus
optomeninx
optometer
objective o.
optometrist
optometry
optomyometer
optotypes
ora (*pl. of* os)
ora, pl. **orae**
o. serrata
orad
oral
o. biology
o. cavity
o. cavity proper
o. epithelial ncvus
o. (erosive) lichen planus
o. fissure
o. focal mucinosis
o. hygiene
O. Hygiene Index
o. lactose tolerance test
o. membrane
o. mucosa
o. part of pharynx
o. pathology
o. pharynx
o. phase
o. physiotherapy
o. plate
o. primacy
o. region
o. shields
o. smear
o. stereotypy
o. submucous fibrosis
o. surgeon
o. surgery
o. teeth
o. vestibule
orale

orality
orange
o. G
o. wood
Orbeli effect
orbicular
o. bone
o. ligament
o. ligament of radius
o. muscle
o. muscle of eye
o. muscle of mouth
o. process
o. zone
orbiculare
orbicularis
o. muscle
o. oculi muscle
o. oculi reflex
o. oris muscle
o. phenomenon
o. pupillary reflex
orbiculus cillaris
orbit
orbita, gen. **orbitae**
orbital
o. abscess
o. artery
o. axis
o. branch of middle meningeal
artery
o. branch of pterygopalatine
ganglion
o. cavity
o. decompression
o. eminence of zygomatic bone
o. exenteration
o. fasciae
o. fat-pad
o. gyri
o. height
o. hernia
o. implant
o. index
o. lamina of ethmoid bone
o. layer of ethmoid bone
o. margin of eyelids
o. muscle
o. nerve
o. opening
o. ophthalmoplegia
o. part of frontal bone
o. part of lacrimal gland
o. part of optic nerve
o. part of orbicularis oculi muscle
o. plane
o. plate
o. plate of ethmoid bone

O

orbital *(continued)*
    o. process
    o. region
    o. rim
    o. septum
    o. sulci
    o. surface
    o. syndrome
    o. tubercle of zygomatic bone
    o. width
orbitale
orbitalis muscle
orbitofrontal
    o. artery
    o. cortex
orbitography
    positive contrast o.
orbitomeatal
    o. line
    o. plane
orbitonasal
    o. index
orbitonometer
orbitonometry
orbitopagus
orbitopathy
    Graves' o.
orbitosphenoid
orbitotomy
Orbivirus
orcein
orchectomy
orchella
orchialgia
orchichorea
orchidectomy
orchidic
orchiditis
orchidometer
orchidoptosis
orchidorraphy
orchiectomy
orchiepididymitis
orchil
orchiocele
orchiococcus
orchiodynia
orchioncus
orchioneuralgia
orchiopathy
orchiopexy
    transseptal o.
orchioplasty
orchiorrhaphy
orchiotherapy
orchiotomy
orchis, pl. **orchises**
orchitic

orchitis
    o. parotidea
    traumatic o.
    o. variolosa
orchotomy
order
    pecking o.
orderly
ordinal scale
ordinate
orectic
orexia
orexigenic
orf virus
organ
    accessory o.'s
    accessory o.'s of the eye
    annulospiral o.
    auditory o.
    Chievitz' o.
    circumventricular o.'s
    Corti's o.
    critical o.
    o. culture
    enamel o.
    end o.
    external female genital o.'s
    external male genital o.'s
    floating o.
    flower-spray o. of Ruffini
    genital o.'s
    Golgi tendon o.
    gustatory o.
    o. of hearing
    internal female genital o.'s
    internal male genital o.'s
    intromittent o.
    Jacobson's o.
    neurohemal o.'s
    neurotendinous o.
    olfactory o.
    ptotic o.
    o. of Rosenmüller
    sense o.'s
    o. of smell
    spiral o.
    subcommissural o.
    subfornical o.
    supernumerary o.'s
    tactile o.
    target o.
    o. of taste
    o. of touch
    urinary o.'s
    vestibular o.
    vestibulocochlear o.
    vestigial o.
    o. of vision

visual o.
vomeronasal o.
wandering o.
Weber's o.
o.'s of Zuckerkandl
organa (*pl. of* organon) (*pl. of* organum)
organelle
cell o.
paired o.'s
organic
o. brain syndrome
o. contracture
o. deafness
o. delusions
o. dental cement
o. disease
o. evolution
o. hallucinosis
o. headache
o. mental disorder
o. mental syndrome
o. mood syndrome
o. murmur
o. pain
o. stricture
o. vertigo
organicism
organicist
organification defect
organism
calculated mean o.
fastidious o.
hypothetical mean o.
pleuropneumonia-like o.'s
organization
health maintenance o.
preferred provider o.
pregenital o.
organize
organized pneumonia
organizer
nucleolar o.
primary o.
procentriole o.
organoaxial
organogenesis
organogenetic, organogenic
organogeny
organography
organoid
o. nevus
o. tumor
organoleptic
organology
organoma
organomegaly
organon, pl. **organa**

organonomy
organonymy
organopathy
organopexy, organopexia
organotaxis
organotherapy
organotropic
organotropism
organotropy
organ-specific antigen
organum, pl. **organa**
o. auditus
organa genitalia
organa genitalia feminina externa
organa genitalia feminina interna
organa genitalia masculina externa
organa genitalia masculina interna
o. gustus
organa oculi accessoria
o. olfactus
organa sensuum
o. spirale
o. tactus
organa urinaria
o. vestibulocochleare
o. visus
o. vomeronasale
orgasm
orgasmic, orgastic
Oriboca virus
Oriental
O. boil
O. button
O. ringworm
O. schistosomiasis
O. sore
O. ulcer
orienting
o. reflex
o. response
orifice
anal o.
aortic o.
cardiac o.
esophagogastric o.
o. of external acoustic meatus
external urethral o.
gastroduodenal o.
golf-hole ureteral o.
ileocecal o.
o. of inferior vena cava
o. of internal acoustic meatus
internal urethral o.
mitral o.
pulmonary o.
pyloric o.
root canal o.
o. of superior vena cava

O

orifice *(continued)*
    tricuspid o.
    ureteric o.
    vaginal o.
orificial
orificium, pl. orificia
    o. externum uteri
    o. internum uteri
    o. ureteris
    o. urethrae externum
    o. vaginae
origin
    apparent o.
    deep o.
    ectal o.
    ental o.
    real o.
    o. of replication
    superficial o.
oris *(gen. of* os)
Ormond's disease
ornate
Ornish
    O. prevention diets
    O. reversal diet
ornithinemia
ornithinuria
Ornithodoros
    O. coriaceus
    O. erraticus
    O. hermsi
    O. lahorensis
    O. moubata complex
    O. pappilipes
    O. parkeri
    O. rudis
    O. savigni
    O. talajé
    O. tholozani
    O. turicata
    O. venezuelensis
    O. verrucosus
Ornithonyssus
ornithosis virus
oroantral fistula
orodigitofacial
    o. dysostosis
orofacial
    o. fistula
orofaciodigital syndrome
orolingual
oronasal
    o. fistula
    o. membrane
oropharyngeal
    o. membrane
    o. passage
oropharynx

orotic aciduria
orotracheal
    o. intubation
    o. tube
Oroya fever
orphan
    o. disease
    o. drugs
    o. viruses
orseillin BB
Orsi-Grocco method
orthergasia
orthesis
orthetics
orthoarteriotony
orthobiosis
orthocephalic
orthocephalous
orthochorea
orthochromatic
orthochromophil, orthochromophile
orthocytosis
orthodeoxia
orthodigita
orthodontia
orthodontic
    o. appliance
    o. band
    o. therapy
orthodontics
    surgical o.
orthodontist
orthodromic
orthogenesis
orthogenic
orthogenics
orthoglycemic glycosuria
orthognathia
orthognathic, orthognathous
    o. surgery
orthograde
    o. conduction
    o. degeneration
orthokeratology
orthokeratosis
orthokinetics
orthomechanical
orthomechanotherapy
orthomelic
orthometer
orthomolecular
    o. psychiatry
    o. therapy
Orthomyxoviridae
orthopaedic, orthopedic
    o. surgery
orthopaedics, orthopedics
orthopaedist, orthopedist

orthopedic (*var. of* orthopaedic)
orthopedics
    dental o.
    functional jaw o.
orthopercussion
orthophoria
orthophoric
orthophrenia
orthopnea
    o. position
orthopneic
    o. position
Orthopoxvirus
orthoprosthesis
orthopsychiatry
Orthoptera
orthoptic
orthoptics
orthoptist
orthoscope
orthoscopic
    o. lens
    o. spectacles
orthosis, pl. **orthoses**
orthostatic
    o. albuminuria
    o. hypopiesis
    o. hypotension
    o. proteinuria
    o. tachycardia
orthostereoscope
orthosympathetic
orthothanasia
orthotics
orthotist
orthotonos, orthotonus
orthotopic
    o. graft
orthotropic
orthovoltage
Orth's
    O. fixative
    O. stain
os, gen. **ossis, oris**, pl. **ossa, ora**
    o. acromiale
    o. basilare
    o. breve
    o. calcis
    o. capitatum
    ossa carpi
    o. centrale
    o. centrale tarsi
    o. clitoridis
    o. coccygis
    o. costale
    o. coxae
    ossa cranii
    o. cuboideum

o. cuneiforme intermedium
o. cuneiforme laterale
o. cuneiforme mediale
ossa digitorum
o. ethmoidale
external o. of uterus
ossa faciei
o. femoris
o. frontale
o. hamatum
o. iliacum
o. ilium
o. incae
o. incisivum
incompetent cervical o.
o. innominatum
o. intermaxillare
o. intermedium
o. intermetatarseum
o. interparietale
o. irregulare
o. ischii
o. japonicum
o. lacrimale
o. longum
o. lunatum
o. magnum
o. malare
ossa membri inferioris
ossa membri superioris
o. metacarpale, pl. ossa metacarpalia
o. metatarsale, pl. ossa metatarsalia
o. multangulum majus
o. multangulum minus
o. nasale
o. naviculare
o. naviculare manus
o. occipitale
o. odontoideum
o. orbiculare
o. palatinum
o. parietale
o. pisiforme
o. planum
o. pneumaticum
o. premaxillare
o. pterygoideum
o. pubis
o. pyramidale
o. sacrum
Scanzoni's second o.
o. scaphoideum
o. sesamoideum, pl. ossa sesamoidea
o. sphenoidale
o. subtibiale
o. suprasternale, pl. ossa
  suprasternalia
ossa suturarum

O

os *(continued)*
  o. sylvii
  ossa tarsi
  o. temporale
  o. tibiale posterius, o. tibiale posticum
  o. trapezium
  o. trapezoideum
  o. triangulare
  o. tribasilare
  o. trigonum
  o. triquetrum
  o. unguis
  o. uteri externum
  o. uteri internum
  o. vesalianum
  o. zygomaticum
oscheal
oscheitis
oschelephantiasis
oscheohydrocele
oscheoplasty
oscillating vision
oscillation
oscillatory potential
oscillograph
oscillography
oscillometer
oscillometric
oscillometry
oscillopsia
oscilloscope
  cathode ray o.
  storage o.
oscitate
oscitation
osculum, pl. **oscula**
Osgood-Schlatter disease
Osler
  O. disease
  O. node
  O. sign
Osler-Vaquez disease
osmatic
osmesis
osmic acid
osmic acid fixative
osmicate
osmication, osmification
osmics
osmidrosis
osmification (*var. of* osmication)
osmiophilic
osmiophobic
osmium
  o. tetroxide
osmoceptor
osmodysphoria

osmogram
osmolal clearance
osmolality
  calculated serum o.
osmophil, osmophilic
osmophobia
osmoreceptor
osmotherapy
osmotic
  o. diuresis
  o. fragility
  o. nephrosis
  o. shock
osphresiolagnia
osphresiologic
osphresiology
osphresiophilia
osphresiophobia
osphresis
osphretic
ossa (*pl. of* os)
osseocartilaginous
osseomucin
osseous
  o. ampulla
  o. cell
  o. hydatid cyst
  o. labyrinth
  o. lacuna
  o. part of skeletal system
  o. polyp
  o. spiral lamina
  o. tissue
ossicle
  Andernach's o.'s
  auditory o.'s
  Bertin's o.'s
  epactal o.'s
  Kerckring's o.
ossicula (*pl. of* ossiculum)
ossicular
  o. chain
ossiculectomy
ossiculotomy
ossiculum, pl. **ossicula**
  ossicula auditus
  ossicula mentalia
ossiferous
ossific
  o. center
ossification
  endochondral o.
  intramembranous o.
  membranous o.
  metaplastic o.
ossiform
ossify
ossifying cartilage

ossis (*gen. of* os)
osteal
ostealgia
ostealgic
osteanagenesis
osteanaphysis
ostectomy
osteitic
osteitis
 alveolar o.
 caseous o.
 central o.
 o. condensans ilii
 condensing o.
 cortical o.
 o. deformans
 o. fibrosa circumscripta
 o. fibrosa cystica
 o. fibrosa disseminata
 focal condensing o.
 hematogenous o.
 localized o. fibrosa
 multifocal o. fibrosa
 o. pubis
 renal o. fibrosa
 sclerosing o.
 o. tuberculosa multiplex cystica
ostembryon
ostemia
ostempyesis
osteoanagenesis
osteoarthritis
osteoarthropathy
 idiopathic hypertrophic o.
 pneumogenic o.
 pulmonary o.
osteoarthrosis
osteoblast
osteoblastic
osteoblastoma
osteocalcin
osteocarcinoma
osteocartilaginous
osteochondritis
 o. deformans juvenilis
 o. deformans juvenilis dorsi
 o. dissecans
 syphilitic o.
osteochondrodysplasia
osteochondrodystrophia deformans
osteochondrodystrophy
osteochondrogenic cell
osteochondroma
osteochondromatosis
 synovial o.
osteochondrosarcoma
osteochondrosis
osteochondrous

osteoclasis, osteoclasia
osteoclast
 o. activating factor
osteoclastic
osteoclastoma
osteocollagenous fibers
osteocranium
osteocystoma
osteocyte
osteodentin
osteodermatopoikilosis
osteodermatous
osteodermia
osteodesmosis
osteodiastasis
osteodynia
osteodysplasty
osteodystrophy
 Albright's hereditary o.
 renal o.
osteoectasia
osteoectomy
osteoepiphysis
osteofibroma
osteofibrosis
 periapical o.
osteogen
osteogenesis
 o. imperfecta, o. imperfecta
  congenita, o. imperfecta tarda
osteogenic, osteogenetic
 o. cell
 o. sarcoma
 o. tissue
osteogenous
osteogeny
osteography
osteohalisteresis
osteohypertrophy
osteoid
 o. osteoma
 o. tissue
osteolipochondroma
osteologia
osteologist
osteology
osteolysis
osteolytic
osteoma
 o. cutis
 dental o.
 giant osteoid o.
 o. medullare
 osteoid o.
 o. spongiosum
osteomalacia
 infantile o., juvenile o.
 senile o.

O

osteomalacic
    o. pelvis
osteomatoid
osteomere
osteometry
osteomyelitis
    chronic diffuse sclerosing o.
    chronic focal sclerosing o.
    Garré's o.
osteomyelodysplasia
osteomyelofibrotic syndrome
osteon, osteone
osteoncus
osteonecrosis
osteopath
osteopathia
    o. condensans
    o. hemorrhagica infantum
    o. striata
osteopathic
    o. medicine
    o. physician
    o. scoliosis
osteopathology
osteopathy
    alimentary o.
osteopedion
osteopenia
osteoperiosteal graft
osteoperiostitis
osteopetrosis
    o. acro-osteolytica
osteopetrotic
osteophage
osteophlebitis
osteophony
osteophyma
osteophyte
osteoplaque
osteoplast
osteoplastic
    o. amputation
    o. craniotomy
    o. necrotomy
osteoplasty
osteopoikilosis
osteoponin
osteoporosis
    o. circumscripta cranii
    juvenile o.
    posttraumatic o.
osteoporotic
    o. marrow defect
osteoprogenitor cell
osteoradiologist
osteoradiology
osteoradionecrosis
osteorrhaphy

osteosarcoma
    parosteal o.
    periosteal o.
osteosclerosis
osteosclerotic
    o. anemia
osteosis
    o. cutis
    o. eburnisans monomelica
    parathyroid o.
    renal fibrocystic o.
osteospongioma
osteosteatoma
osteosuture
osteosynthesis
osteothrombosis
osteotome
osteotomy
    "C" sliding o.
    horizontal o.
    Le Fort o.
    sagittal split mandibular o.
    segmental alveolar o.
    sliding oblique o.
    vertical o.
osteotribe
osteotrite
osteotrophy
osteotympanic
ostia (*pl. of* ostium)
ostial
    o. sphincter
ostiomeatal
    o. complex
    o. unit
ostitic
ostitis
ostium, pl. ostia
    o. abdominale tubae uterinae
    abdominal o. of uterine tube
    o. aortae
    aortic o.
    o. appendicis vermiformis
    o. arteriosum
    o. atrioventriculare dextrum
    o. atrioventriculare sinistrum
    o. cardiacum
    o. ileocecale
    o. internum
    o. pharyngeum tubae auditivae
    o. primum
    o. pyloricum
    o. secundum
    o. trunci pulmonalis
    o. tympanicum tubae auditivae
    o. ureteris
    o. urethrae externum
    o. urethrae internum

o. uteri
o. uteri externum
o. uteri internum
uterine o. of uterine tubes
o. uterinum tubae
o. vaginae
o. venae cavae inferioris
o. venae cavae superioris
ostia venarum pulmonalium
o. venosum cordis
o. of vermiform appendix

ostomate
ostomy
ostosis
ostraceous
Ostrum-Furst syndrome
otalgia

geniculate o.
reflex o.

otalgic
Ot antigen
Ota's nevus
Othello syndrome
other-directed
otic

o. abscess
o. barotrauma
o. capsule
o. ganglion
o. pits
o. placodes
o. vesicle

otitic

o. hydrocephalus
o. meningitis

otitis

adhesive o.
aviation o.
o. desquamativa
o. externa
o. interna
o. media
reflux o. media
secretory o. media
serous o.

Otobius
otocephaly
otocerebritis
otoconia, sing. **otoconium**
otocranial
otocranium
otocyst
Otodectes
otodectic
otodynia
otoencephalitis
otoganglion
otogenic, otogenous

otolaryngologist
otolaryngology
otolithic membrane
otoliths, otolites
otologic
otologist
otology
otomandibular

o. dysostosis
o. syndrome

otomucormycosis
otomycosis
otoneuralgia
otopalatodigital

o. syndrome

otopathy
otopharyngeal

o. tube

otoplasty
otorhinolaryngology
otorrhea

cerebrospinal fluid o.

otosalpinx
otosclerosis
otoscope

Siegle's o.

otoscopy

pneumatic o.

otosteal
ototoxic
ototoxicity
Otto

O. disease
O. pelvis

Ottoson potential
Ouchterlony

O. method
O. test

outbreak epidemic
outer

o. cone fiber
o. limiting membrane
o. malleolus
o. table of skull

outlet

o. forceps delivery
pelvic o.

outlier
outline form
outpatient

o. anesthesia

out of phase
output

cardiac o.
minute o.
pacemaker o.
stroke o.

ova (*pl. of* ovum)

O

oval
    o. amputation
    o. area of Flechsig
    o. corpuscle
    o. fasciculus
    o. foramen
    o. fossa
    o. window
ovale
    o. malaria
    o. tertian malaria
ovalocytic anemia
ovalocytosis
ovaria (*pl. of* ovarium)
ovarialgia
ovarian
    o. amenorrhea
    o. artery
    o. branch of uterine artery
    o. bursa
    o. colic
    o. cycle
    o. cyst
    o. dysmenorrhea
    o. fimbria
    o. follicle
    o. fossa
    o. ligament
    o. plexus
    o. pregnancy
    o. tubular adenoma
    o. varicocele
    o. veins
    o. vein syndrome
ovariectomy
ovarioabdominal pregnancy
ovariocele
ovariocentesis
ovariocyesis
ovariodysneuria
ovariogenic
ovariohysterectomy
ovariolytic
ovarioncus
ovariopathy
ovariorrhexis
ovariosalpingectomy
ovariosalpingitis
ovariosteresis
ovariostomy
ovariotomy
    normal o.
ovaritis
ovarium, pl. **ovaria**
    o. bipartitum
    o. disjunctum
    o. gyratum

    o. lobatum
    o. masculinum
ovary
    mulberry o.
    polycystic o.
    third o.
overanxious disorder
overbite
overclosure
overcompensation
overcorrection
overdenture
overdetermination
overdominance
overdominant
overdrive
overeruption
overextension
overflow
    o. incontinence
    o. wave
overgrafting
overhang
overhanging restoration
overhead projector
overhydration
overinflation
    obstructive pulmonary o.
overjet, overjut
overlap
    horizontal o.
    o. hybridization
    vertical o.
overlay
    o. denture
    emotional o.
overlearning
overproduction theory
overresponse
overriding
    o. aorta
overripe cataract
oversensing
overshoot
overt homosexuality
overtone
    psychic o.
overvalued idea
overventilation
overwintering
ovi (*gen. of* ovum)
ovicidal
oviducal
oviduct
oviductal
oviferous
oviform
ovigenesis

ovigenetic, ovigenic
ovigenous
ovigerus
oviposit
oviposition
ovipositor
ovocyte
ovogenesis
ovogonium
ovoid
    fetal o.
    Manchester o.
ovolarviparous
ovoplasm
ovotestis
ovula (*pl. of* ovulum)
ovular
    o. membrane
    o. transmigration
ovulation
    paracyclic o.
ovulational sclerosis
ovulatory
ovule
ovulocyclic
    o. porphyria
ovulum, pl. ovula
ovum, gen. ovi, pl. ova
    alecithal o.
    blighted o.
    centrolecithal o.
    fertilized o.
    isolecithal o.
    Peters' o.
    telolecithal o.
Owen's lines
own controls
Owren's disease
ox
    o. bots
    o. heart
oxalate calculus
oxalemia
oxalosis
oxaluria
oxazin
    o. dyes
oxidase
    o. reaction
    o. test
oximeter
    cuvette o.
oximetry
oxyacoia, oxyakoia, oxyecoia

oxyaphia
oxycephalia
oxycephalic, oxycephalous
oxycephaly
oxychromatic
oxychromatin
oxyecoia (*var. of* oxyacoia)
oxyesthesia
oxygen
    o. affinity anoxia
    o. affinity hypoxia
    o. capacity
    o. consumption
    o. debt
    o. deficit
    o. derived free radicals
    o. effect
    hyperbaric o., high pressure o.
    o. poisoning
    o. tent
    o. therapy
    o. toxicity
    o. utilization coefficient
oxygenation
    apneic o.
    hyperbaric o.
oxygeusia
oxyntic
    o. cell
    o. gland
oxyosmia
oxyosphresia
oxyphil, oxyphile
    o. adenoma
    o. cells
    o. chromatin
    o. granule
oxyphilic
    o. leukocyte
oxyphonia
oxyrhine
oxyrygmia
Oxyspirura mansoni
oxytalan
oxytocia
oxyurid
Oxyuridae
Oxyuris
ozena
ozenous
ozochrotia
ozonator
ozostomia

O

P

P antigens
P cell
P elements
P factor
P and P test
P wave

P-A

P.-A. conduction time
P.-A. interval

Paas' disease
pabular
pabulum
pacchionian

p. bodies
p. corpuscles
p. depressions
p. glands
p. granulations

pacefollower
pacemaker

artificial p.
demand p.
diaphragmatic p.
ectopic p.
electric cardiac p.
electronic p.
external p.
p. failure
fixed-rate p.
nuclear p.
p. output
pervenous p.
p. potential
runaway p.
p. sensitivity
shifting p.
subsidiary atrial p.
p. syndrome
transthoracic p.
wandering p.

Pacheco's parrot disease virus
pachometer
Pachon's

P. method
P. test

pachyblepharon
pachycephalia
pachycephalic, pachycephalous
pachycephaly
pachycheilia, pachychilia
pachycholia
pachychromatic
pachychymia
pachydactylia

pachydactylous
pachydactyly
pachyderma

p. laryngis
p. lymphangiectatica
p. verrucosa
p. vesicae

pachydermatocele
pachydermatosis
pachydermatous
pachydermia
pachydermic
pachydermoperiostosis

p. syndrome

pachyglossia
pachygnathous
pachygyria
pachyhymenia
pachyhymenic
pachyleptomeningitis
pachylosis
pachymenia
pachymenic
pachymeningitis   *pAchy menges*

p. externa   *pAchymeningeAl*
hemorrhagic p.
hypertrophic cervical p.
p. interna
pyogenic p.

pachymeningopathy
pachymeninx
pachymeter

optical p.

pachynema
pachynsis
pachyntic
pachyonychia

p. congenita

pachyotia
pachyperiostitis
pachyperitonitis
pachypleuritis
pachypodous
pachysalpingitis
pachysalpingo-ovaritis
pachysomia
pachytene
pachyvaginalitis
pachyvaginitis

p. cystica

pacing catheter
pacinian corpuscles
pacinitis
pack

cold p.

P

643

pack *(continued)*
    dry p.
    hot p.
    wet p.
packed cell volume
packer
packing
    denture p.
    p. process
paclitaxel
pad
    abdominal p.
    dinner p.
    fat p.
    knuckle p.'s
    laparotomy p.
    Passavant's p.
    periarterial p.
    pharyngoesophageal p.'s
    retromolar p.
    sucking p., suctorial p.
Padykula-Herman stain for myosin ATPase
Paecilomyces
Pagenstecher's circle
Paget-Eccleston stain
pagetic
pagetoid
    p. cells
    p. reticulosis
Paget's
    P. cells
    P. disease
Paget-von Schrötter syndrome
pagophagia
Pahvant
    P. Valley fever
    P. Valley plague
paidology
pain
    after-p.'s
    bearing-down p.
    dream p.
    expulsive p.'s
    false p.'s
    girdle p.
    growing p.'s
    hunger p.
    intermenstrual p.
    intractable p.
    labor p.'s
    middle p.
    mind p.
    nerve p.
    night p.
    organic p.
    phantom limb p.
    postprandial p.

    psychogenic p.
    p. reaction
    referred p.
    rest p.
    somatoform p.
    soul p.
    p. threshold
    p. tolerance
painful
    p. anesthesia
    p. heel
    p. hematuria
    p. paraplegia
    p. point
    p. toe
painful-bruising syndrome
painless
    p. hematuria
    p. jaundice
pain-pleasure principle
painter's colic
pair
    chromosome p.
    line p.'s
    p. production
paired
    p. allosome
    p. associates
    p. beats
    p. organelles
pairing
    chromosome p.
pajaroello
Pajot's maneuver
palatal
    p. abscess
    p. bar
    p. index
    p. myoclonus
    p. nystagmus
    p. papillomatosis
    p. plate
    p. reflex
    p. seal
    p. shelf
    p. triangle
palate
    bony p.
    Byzantine arch p.
    cleft p.
    falling p.
    Gothic p.
    hard p.
    p. hook
    p. myograph
    pendulous p.
    primary p.
    primitive p.

secondary p.
soft p.
palati (*pl. of* palatum)
palatiform
palatine
    p. aponeurosis
    p. bone
    p. crest
    p. glands
    p. groove
    p. index
    p. papilla
    p. process
    p. raphe
    p. reflex
    p. ridge
    p. spines
    p. surface of horizontal plate of
      palatine bone
    p. tonsil
    p. torus
    p. uvula
    p. vein
palatitis
palatoethmoidal suture
palatoglossal
    p. arch
palatoglossus
    p. muscle
palatognathous
palatogram
palatograph
palatomaxillary
    p. index
    p. suture
palatomyograph
palatonasal
palatopharyngeal
    p. arch
    p. muscle
    p. sphincter
palatopharyngeus
    p. muscle
palatopharyngoplasty
palatopharyngorrhaphy
palatoplasty
palatoplegia
palatorrhaphy
palatosalpingeus
palatoschisis
palatouvularis muscle
palatovaginal
    p. canal
    p. groove
palatum, pl. **palati**
    p. durum
    p. fissum

p. molle
p. osseum
pale
    p. globe
    p. hypertension
    p. infarct
    p. thrombus
paleencephalon
paleocerebellum
paleocortex
paleokinetic
paleopathology
paleostriatal
    p. syndrome
paleostriatum
paleothalamus
Palfyn's sinus
palikinesia, palicinesia
palilalia
palinal
palindromia
palindromic
    p. encephalopathy
palinopsia
paliphrasia
palisade
    p. layer
pallanesthesia
pallescense
pallesthesia
pallesthetic
    p. sensibility
pallial
palliate
palliative
    p. treatment
pallidal
    p. syndrome
pallidectomy
pallidoamygdalotomy
pallidoansotomy
pallidotomy
pallidum
pallium
pallor
    cachectic p.
palm
    p. grasp
    liver p.
palma, pl. **palmae**
    p. manus
palmar
    p. aponeurosis
    p. branch of median nerve
    p. branch of ulnar nerve
    p. carpal branch of radial artery
    p. carpal branch of ulnar artery
    p. carpal ligament

P

palmar *(continued)*
    p. carpometacarpal ligaments
    p. crease
    p. digital veins
    p. fascia
    p. fibromatosis
    p. flexion
    p. interosseous artery
    p. interosseous muscle
    p. ligaments
    p. metacarpal artery
    p. metacarpal ligaments
    p. metacarpal veins
    p. monticuli
    p. radiocarpal ligament
    p. reflex
    p. surface of fingers
    p. syphilid
    p. ulnocarpal ligament
palmaris
    p. brevis muscle
    p. longus muscle
palmate folds
palm-chin reflex
palmellin
Palmer acid test for peptic ulcer
palmi *(pl. of* palmus)
palmic
palmin test
palmitin test
palmodic
palmomental reflex
palmoplantar keratoderma
palmoscopy
palmus, pl. **palmi**
palpable
    p. rale
palpate
palpation
    bimanual p.
    light-touch p.
palpatopercussion
palpatory percussion
palpebra, pl. **palpebrae**
    p. inferior
    p. superior
palpebral
    p. arteries
    p. branches of infratrochlear nerve
    p. conjunctiva
    p. fissure
    p. glands
    p. part of lacrimal gland
    p. part of orbicularis oculi muscle
    p. raphe
    p. veins
palpebralis
palpebrate

palpebration
palpebronasal fold
palpitatio cordis
palpitation
palsy
    Bell's p.
    birth p.
    brachial birth p.
    bulbar p.
    cerebral p.
    craft p.
    creeping p.
    crutch p.
    Dejerine-Klumpke p.
    diver's p.
    Erb p.
    extrapyramidal cerebral p.
    facial p.
    Klumpke p.
    lead p.
    obstetrical p.
    posticus p.
    pressure p.
    progressive bulbar p.
    progressive supranuclear p.
    scrivener's p.
    shaking p., trembling p.
    wasting p.
paludal
    p. fever
pampiniform
    p. body
    p. plexus
pampinocele
panacea
panacinar emphysema
panagglutinable
panagglutinins
panangiitis
panarteritis
panarthritis
panatrophy
panblastic
panbronchiolitis
    diffuse p.
pancake kidney
pancarditis
pancervical smear
Pancoast
    P. suture
    P. syndrome
    P. tumor
pancolectomy
pancreas, pl. **pancreata**
    p. accessorium
    accessory p.
    annular p.
    Aselli's p.

p. divisum
dorsal p.
lesser p.
p. minus
small p.
uncinate p., unciform p.
ventral p.
Willis' p.
Winslow's p.
pancreatalgia
pancreatectomy
pancreatemphraxis
pancreatic
p. abscess
p. branches
p. calculus
p. cholera
p. colic
p. cystoduodenostomy
p. diarrhea
p. diverticula
p. duct
p. encephalopathy
p. infantilism
p. islands
p. islets
p. lithiasis
p. lymph nodes
p. notch
p. plexus
p. polypeptide
p. sphincter
p. steatorrhea
p. veins
pancreaticoduodenal
p. arterial arcades
p. lymph nodes
p. transplantation
p. veins
pancreaticoenteric recess
pancreaticosplenic lymph nodes
pancreatitis
acute hemorrhagic p.
calcareous p.
calcific p.
chronic p.
chronic fibrosing p.
chronic relapsing p.
pancreatocholecystostomy
pancreatoduodenectomy
pancreatoduodenostomy
pancreatogastrostomy
pancreatogenic, pancreatogenous
pancreatography
pancreatojejunostomy
pancreatolith
pancreatolithectomy
pancreatolithiasis

pancreatolithotomy
pancreatolysis
pancreatolytic
pancreatomegaly
pancreatomy
pancreatopathy
pancreatotomy
pancreatropic
pancreectomy
pancreolith
pancreopathy
pancreoprivic
pancreozymin-secretin test
pancytopenia
congenital p.
Fanconi's p.
pandemic
pandemicity
pandiculation
Pandy's
P. reaction
P. test
panencephalitis
nodular p.
subacute sclerosing p.
panendoscope
panesthesia
Paneth's granular cells
pang
breast p.
panglossia
panhidrosis
panhyperemia
panhypopituitarism
panic
p. attack
p. disorder
homosexual p.
panidrosis
panimmunity
panleukopenia virus of cats
panlobular emphysema
panmixis
panmyelophthisis
panmyelosis
Panner's disease
panneuritis
p. endemica
panni (*pl. of* pannus)
pannicular hernia
panniculectomy
panniculitis
α-1 antitrypsin deficiency p.
cytophagic histiocytic p.
lupus erythematosus p.
nodular nonsuppurative p.
poststeroid p.

P

panniculitis *(continued)*
    relapsing febrile nodular
      nonsuppurative p.
    subacute migratory p.
panniculus, pl. **panniculi**
    p. adiposus
    p. carnosus
pannus, pl. **panni**
    corneal p., p. crassus, p. siccus, p.
      tenuis
    phlyctenular p.
    trachomatous p.
panodic
panophthalmitis
panoptic
    p. stain
panoramic
    p. radiograph
    p. rotating machine
    p. x-ray film
panotitis
panphobia
panplegia
Pansch's fissure
pansclerosis
pansinuitis
pansinusitis
panspermia, panspermatism
pansporoblast
pansporoblastic
pansystolic
    p. murmur
pant
pantachromatic
pantalgia
pantaloon
    p. embolism
    p. hernia
pantamorphia
pantamorphic
pantanencephaly, pantanencephalia
pantankyloblepharon
pantaphobia
pantatrophia, pantatrophy
panthodic
pantograph
pantomogram
pantomograph
pantomography
pantomorphia
pantomorphic
pantoscopic
    p. spectacles
pantropic virus
Panum's area
panzerherz
PAP
    P. technique

Pap
    P. smear
    P. test
Papanicolaou
    P. examination
    P. smear
    P. smear test
    P. stain
paper
    articulating p.
    Congo red p.
    p. mill worker's disease
    niter p.
    occluding p.
    p. plate
    potassium nitrate p.
    saltpeter p.
Papez circuit
papilla, pl. **papillae**
    acoustic p.
    Bergmeister's p.
    bile p.
    p. of breast
    circumvallate p.
    clavate papillae
    conic papillae
    papillae conicae
    conical papillae
    papillae corii
    papillae of corium
    dental p.
    dentinal p.
    p. dentis
    dermal papillae
    papillae dermis
    p. duodeni major
    p. duodeni minor
    filiform papillae
    papillae filiformes
    papillae foliatae
    foliate papillae
    fungiform papillae
    papillae fungiformes
    hair p.
    p. incisiva
    incisive p.
    interdental p.
    interproximal p.
    lacrimal p.
    p. lacrimalis
    lenticular papillae
    lingual p.
    p. lingualis, pl. papillae linguales
    major duodenal p.
    p. mammae
    minor duodenal p.
    nerve p.
    p. nervi optici

optic p.
palatine p.
parotid p.
p. parotidea
p. pili
renal p.
p. renalis, pl. papillae renales
retrocuspid p.
tactile p.
urethral p., p. urethralis
p. vallata, pl. papillae vallatae
vallate p.
vascular papillae
p. of Vater
papillary, papillate
p. adenocarcinoma
p. adenoma of large intestine
p. carcinoma
p. cystadenoma lymphomatosum
p. cystic adenoma
p. ducts
p. ectasia
p. foramina of kidney
p. hidradenoma
p. layer
p. muscle
p. muscle dysfunction
p. muscle syndrome
p. process
p. stasis
p. tumor
papillectomy
papilledema
papilliferous
papilliform
papillitis
foliate p.
necrotizing p.
papilloadenocystoma
papillocarcinoma
papilloma
p. acuminatum
basal cell p.
p. canaliculum
p. diffusum
duct p.
p. durum
hard p.
Hopmann's p.
p. inguinale tropicum
intracystic p.
intraductal p.
inverted p.
p. molle
Shope p.
soft p.
transitional cell p.
p. venereum

villous p.
p. virus
zymotic p.
papillomatosis
confluent and reticulate p.
florid oral p.
juvenile p.
laryngeal p.
palatal p.
subareolar duct p.
papillomatous
Papillomavirus
Papillon-Léage and Psaume syndrome
Papillon-Lefèvre syndrome
papilloretinitis
papillotomy
papillula, pl. **papillulae**
Papovaviridae
papovavirus
pappataci
p. fever
p. fever viruses
Pappenheimer
P. bodies
Pappenheim's stain
pappose, pappous
pappus
PA projection
papula, pl. **papulae**
papular
p. acrodermatitis of childhood
p. dermatitis of pregnancy
p. fever
p. mucinosis
p. scrofuloderma
p. stomatitis virus of cattle
p. syphilid
p. tuberculid
p. urticaria
papulation
papule
Celsus' p.'s
follicular p.
moist p., mucous p.
piezogenic pedal p.
pruritic urticarial p.'s and plaques
of pregnancy
split p.'s
papuliferous
papuloerythematous
papulonecrotic tuberculid
papulopustular
papulopustule
papulosis
bowenoid p.
lymphomatoid p.
malignant atrophic p.

P

649

papulosquamous
    p. syphilid
papulovesicle
papulovesicular
papyraceous
    p. plate
    p. scars
par
para, para I, para II
para-actinomycosis
para-aortic bodies
para-appendicitis
paraballism
parabasal
    p. body
    p. filament
parabiosis
parabiotic
    p. flap
paraboloid condenser
parabrachial nuclei
parabulia
paracanthoma
paracanthosis
paracarcinomatous
    p. encephalomyelopathy
    p. myelopathy
paracarmine
    p. stain
paracelsian method
paracenesthesia
paracentesis
paracentetic
paracentral
    p. artery
    p. fissure
    p. lobule
    p. nucleus of thalamus
    p. scotoma
paracentric inversion
paracervical
    p. block anesthesia
paracervix
paracholera
parachordal
    p. cartilage
    p. plate
parachroma
parachromatosis
parachute
    p. deformity
    p. mitral valve
    p. reflex
paracinesia, paracinesis
paracmasis
paracmastic
paracme
paracoccidioidal granuloma

Paracoccidioides brasiliensis
paracoccidioidin
paracoccidioidomycosis
paracolic
    p. gutters
    p. recesses
paracolitis
paracolon bacillus
paracolpitis
paracolpium
paracone
paraconid
paracortex
paracousis
paracrine
paracusis, paracusia
    false p.
    p. loci
    Willis' p.
paracyclic ovulation
paracyesis
paracystic
    p. pouch
paracystitis
paracystium
paracytic
paradenitis
paradental
paradentium
paradidymal
paradidymis, pl. **paradidymides**
paradipsia
paradox
    Weber's p.
paradoxical
    p. contraction
    p. diaphragm phenomenon
    p. embolism
    p. extensor reflex
    p. flexor reflex
    p. incontinence
    p. movement of eyelids
    p. patellar reflex
    p. pulse
    p. pupil
    p. pupillary phenomenon
    p. pupillary reflex
    p. reflex
    p. respiration
    p. sleep
    p. triceps reflex
paraduodenal
    p. fold
    p. fossa
    p. hernia
    p. recess
paradysentery bacillus
paraesophageal hernia

paraesthesia
paraffin
    p. cancer
    p. tumor
paraffinoma
Parafilaria multipapillosa
paraflagellate
paraflagellum, pl. **paraflagella**
parafollicular
    p. cells
parafrenal abscess
parafuchsin
paragammacism
paraganglioma
    nonchromaffin p.
paraganglion, pl. **paraganglia**
paraganglionic cells
paragene
paragenital
    p. tubules
parageusia
parageusic
paraglenoid
    p. groove
    p. sulcus
paragnathus
paragnomen
paragonimiasis
Paragonimus
    P. kellicotti
    P. ringeri
    P. westermani
paragonorrheal
paragrammatism
paragraphia
parahemophilia
parahepatic
parahiatal hernia
parahidrosis
parahippocampal gyrus
parahypnosis
parahypophysis
para I (*var. of* para)
para II (*var. of* para)
parainfluenza viruses
parajejunal fossa
parakappacism
parakeratosis
    p. ostracea
    p. psoriasiformis
    p. pustulosa
    p. scutularis
    p. variegata
parakinesia, parakinesis
paralalia
    p. literalis
paralambdacism
paraleprosis

paralepsy
paralexia
paralgesia
paralgia
paralipophobia
parallactic
parallax
    binocular p.
    heteronymous p.
    homonymous p.
    p. method
    stereoscopic p.
    p. test
    vertical p.
parallel
    p. attachment
    p. rays
parallelism
parallelometer
parallergic
paralogia, paralogism, paralogy
    thematic p.
paraluteal cell
paralutein cell
paralysis, pl. **paralyses**
    acute ascending p.
    acute atrophic p.
    p. agitans
    ascending p.
    Brown-Séquard's p.
    bulbar p.
    central p.
    compression p.
    crossed p.
    crutch p.
    diphtheritic p.
    diver's p.
    Duchenne-Erb p.
    Erb p.
    Erb spinal p.
    facial p.
    familial periodic p.
    faucial p.
    flaccid p.
    generalized p.
    ginger p.
    global p.
    glossolabiolaryngeal p., glossolabiopharyngeal p.
    glossopalatolabial p.
    glossopharyngeolabial p.
    Gubler's p.
    hyperkalemic periodic p.
    hypokalemic periodic p.
    hysterical p.
    immune p.
    immunological p.
    jake p.

P

paralysis *(continued)*
    Klumpke's p.
    Landry's p.
    lead p.
    mimetic p.
    mixed p.
    motor p.
    musculospiral p.
    myogenic p.
    normokalemic periodic p.
    obstetrical p.
    ocular p.
    periodic p.
    peripheral facial p.
    postdiphtheritic p.
    posticus p.
    Pott's p.
    pressure p.
    progressive bulbar p.
    pseudobulbar p.
    sensory p.
    sleep p.
    sodium-responsive periodic p.
    spastic spinal p.
    spinal p.
    supranuclear p.
    Todd's p.
    Todd's postepileptic p.
    vasomotor p.
    wasting p.
    Zenker's p.
paralytic
    p. dementia
    p. ectropion
    p. ileus
    p. miosis
    p. mydriasis
    p. scoliosis
    p. strabismus
paralyze
paralyzing vertigo
paramammary lymph nodes
paramastigote
paramastoid
    p. process
Paramecium
paramedian
    p. incision
paramedic
paramedical
paramenia
paramesial
paramesonephric
    p. duct
parametria (*pl. of* parametrium)
parametrial

parametric
    p. abscess
    p. test
parametrismus
parametritic
    p. abscess
parametritis
parametrium, pl. **parametria**
paramimia
paramnesia
Paramoeba
paramolar
Paramphistomatidae
Paramphistomum
paramusia
paramyloidosis
paramyoclonus multiplex
paramyotonia
    ataxic p.
    congenital p., p. congenita
paramyotonus
Paramyxoviridae
Paramyxovirus
paranalgesia
paranasal
    p. sinuses
paraneoplasia
paraneoplastic
    p. acrokeratosis
    p. encephalomyelopathy
    p. syndrome
paranephric
    p. abscess
    p. body
paranephros, pl. **paranephroi**
paranesthesia
paraneural
    p. infiltration
paraneurone
parangi
paranoia
    acute hallucinatory p.
    litigious p.
    p. originaria
    p. querulans
paranoiac
paranoid
    p. disorder
    p. personality
    p. personality disorder
    p. schizophrenia
paranomia
paranuclear
    p. body
paranucleate
paranucleolus
paranucleus
paraomphalic

paraoperative
paraoral
paraovarian
parapancreatic
paraparesis
paraparetic
parapedesis
paraperitoneal
    p. hernia
parapestis
parapharyngeal space
paraphasia
    thematic p.
paraphasic
paraphia
paraphilia
paraphimosis
    p. palpebrae
paraphonia
paraphora
paraphrasia
paraphysial, paraphyseal
    p. body
    p. cysts
paraphysis, pl. paraphyses
parapineal
paraplasm
paraplastic
paraplectic
paraplegia
    ataxic p.
    congenital spastic p.
    p. dolorosa
    p. in extension
    p. in flexion
    infantile spastic p.
    painful p.
    Pott's p.
    spastic p.
    superior p.
paraplegic
Parapoxvirus
parapraxia
paraproctitis
paraproctium, pl. paraproctia
paraprostatitis
paraprotein
paraproteinemia
parapsia
parapsoriasis
    p. en plaque
    p. guttata
    p. lichenoides
    p. lichenoides et varioliformis acuta
    small plaque p.
    p. varioliformis
parapsychology
pararama

pararectal
    p. fossa
    p. lymph nodes
    p. pouch
parareflexia
pararenal
pararhotacism
pararosanilin
pararrhythmia
parasaccular hernia
parasacral
parasagittal
    p. plane
    p. section
parasalpingitis
Parascaris equorum
parascarlatina
parasecretion
paraseptal
    p. cartilage
    p. emphysema
parasexuality
parasigmatism
parasinoidal
    p. sinuses
parasite
    autistic p.
    autochthonous p.
    commensal p.
    euroxenous p.
    facultative p.
    heterogenetic p.
    heteroxenous p.
    incidental p.
    inquiline p.
    malignant tertian malarial p.
    obligate p.
    quartan p.
    specific p.
    stenoxous p.
    temporary p.
    tertian p.
parasite-host ecosystem
parasitemia
parasitic
    p. chylocele
    p. cyst
    p. disease
    p. granuloma
    p. hemoptysis
    p. leiomyoma
    p. melanoderma
    p. thyroiditis
    p. twin
parasiticidal
parasitism
    multiple p.
parasitize

P

parasitocenose
parasitogenesis
parasitogenic
parasitoid
parasitologist
parasitology
parasitome
parasitophobia
parasitophorous vacuole
parasitosis
parasol insertion
parasomnia
paraspinal line
parastasis
parasternal
    p. hernia
    p. line
    p. lymph nodes
parastriate
    p. area
    p. cortex
Parastrongylus
parastruma
parasympathetic
    p. ganglia
    p. nerve
    p. nervous system
    p. part
    p. root of ciliary ganglion
parasympathotonia
parasynapsis
parasynovitis
parasyphilis
parasyphilitic
parasyphilosis
parasystole
parasystolic beat
parataxia
parataxic
    p. distortion
parataxis
paratenesis
paratenic host
paratenon
paraterminal
    p. body
    p. gyrus
parathymia
parathyroid
    p. gland
    p. hormonelike protein
    p. insufficiency
    p. osteosis
    p. tetany
parathyroidectomy
parathyroprival tetany
parathyrotropic, parathyrotrophic
paratope

paratracheal lymph node
paratrichosis
paratripsis
paratriptic
paratrophic
paratuberculous lymphadenitis
paratyphlitis
paratyphoid
    p. bacillus
    p. fever
paraumbilical
    p. veins
paraurethral
    p. ducts
    p. glands
parauterine lymph nodes
paravaccinia virus
paravaginal
    p. hysterectomy
    p. lymph nodes
paravaginitis
paravalvular
paravenous
paraventricular nucleus
paravertebral
    p. anesthesia
    p. ganglia
    p. gutter
    p. line
    p. triangle
paravesical
    p. fossa
    p. lymph nodes
    p. pouch
paraxial
    p. mesoderm
    p. rays
paraxon
Parazoa
parazoon
parchment
    p. crackling
    p. heart
    p. skin
parectasis, parectasia
parectropia
parencephalia
parencephalitis
parencephalocele
parencephalous
parenchyma
    p. testis
parenchymal
    p. atelectasis
    p. cell
parenchymatitis
parenchymatous
    p. cartilage

p. cell of corpus pineale
p. degeneration
p. goiter
p. hemorrhage
p. mastitis
p. neuritis
parent
p. artery
p. cell
p. cyst
parental
p. generation
p. rejection
parenteral
p. absorption
p. alimentation
p. hyperalimentation
p. therapy
parenteric fever
parepicele
parepididymis
parepithymia
parerethisis
parergasia
paresis
general p.
Paré's suture
paresthesia
paresthetic
paretic
p. impotence
p. neurosyphilis
pareunia
paridrosis
paries, gen. **parietis**, pl. **parietes**
p. anterior gastris
p. anterior vaginae
p. caroticus cavi tympani
p. externus ductus cochlearis
p. inferior orbitae
p. jugularis cavi tympani
p. labyrinthicus cavi tympani
p. lateralis orbitae
p. mastoideus cavi tympani
p. medialis orbitae
p. membranaceus cavi tympani
p. membranaceus tracheae
p. posterior gastris
p. posterior vaginae
p. superior orbitae
p. tegmentalis cavi tympani
p. tympanicus ductus cochlearis
p. vestibularis ductus cochlearis
parietal
p. angle
p. arteries
p. bone

p. border
p. border of frontal bone
p. border of sphenoid bone
p. border of temporal bone
p. branch
p. branch of medial occipital artery
p. branch of middle meningeal artery
p. branch of superficial temporal artery
p. cell
p. eminence
p. emissary vein
p. eye
p. fistula
p. foramen
p. hernia
p. layer
p. layer of leptomeninges
p. layer of serous pericardium
p. layer of tunica vaginalis
p. lobe
p. lobe of cerebrum
p. lobe epilepsy
p. lymph nodes
p. margin
p. nodes
p. notch
p. pelvic fascia
p. peritoneum
p. plate
p. pleura
p. region
p. thrombus
p. tuber
p. veins
p. wall
parietofrontal
parietography
parietomastoid
p. suture
parieto-occipital
p.-o. artery
p.-o. fissure
p.-o. sulcus
parietopontine tract
parietosphenoid
parietosplanchnic
parietosquamosal
parietotemporal
parietovisceral
Parinaud's
P. conjunctivitis
P. oculoglandular syndrome
P. ophthalmoplegia
P. syndrome

P

Paris
    P. line
    P. yellow
parity
Parker-Kerr suture
parkinsonian
parkinsonism
Parkinson's
    P. disease
    P. facies
Park's aneurysm
Park-Williams
    P.-W. bacillus
    P.-W. fixative
paroccipital
    p. process
parodontitis
parodontium
parodynia
parole
parolfactory
    p. area
parolivary
paromphalocele
Parona's space
paroneiria, paroniria
    p. salax
paronychia
paronychial
paroophoritic cyst
paroophoritis
paroöphoron
parorchidium
parorchis
parorexia
parosmia
parosphresia
parosteal
    p. fasciitis
    p. osteosarcoma
parosteitis
parosteosis, parostosis
parostitis
parotic
parotid
    p. abscess
    p. bed
    p. branches
    p. bubo
    p. duct
    p. fascia
    p. gland
    p. notch
    p. papilla
    p. recess
    p. sheath
    p. space
    p. veins

parotidectomy
parotideomasseteric fascia
parotiditis
    epidemic p.
    postoperative p.
    punctate p.
parotidoauricularis
parotitis
parous
parovarian
parovariotomy
parovaritis
parovarium
paroxysm
paroxysmal
    p. cerebral dysrhythmia
    p. cold hemoglobinuria
    p. nocturnal dyspnea
    p. nocturnal hemoglobinuria
    p. sleep
    p. tachycardia
parricide
parrot
    p. jaw
    p. virus
parrot-beak nail
Parrot's disease
parry fracture
Parry's disease
pars, pl. partes
    p. abdominalis aortae
    p. abdominalis ductus thoracici
    p. abdominalis esophagi
    p. abdominalis ureteris
    p. alaris musculi nasalis
    p. alveolaris mandibulae
    p. amorpha
    p. annularis vaginae fibrosae
    p. anterior
    p. anterior commissurae anterioris cerebri
    p. anterior commissurae rostralis
    p. anterior faciei diaphragmatis hepatis
    p. anterior fornicis vaginae
    p. ascendens aortae
    p. ascendens duodeni
    p. atlantica
    p. autonomica
    p. basalis arteriae pulmonalis
    p. basilaris ossis occipitalis
    p. basilaris pontis
    p. buccopharyngea musculi constrictoris pharyngei superioris
    p. cardiaca gastris
    p. cardiaca ventriculi
    p. cartilaginea septi nasi
    p. cartilaginea tubae auditivae

p. cartilaginosa systematis skeletalis
p. cavernosa
p. cavernosa arteriae carotidis internae
p. ceca retinae
p. centralis
p. centralis ventriculi lateralis
p. ceratopharyngea musculi constrictoris pharyngis medii
p. cerebralis arteriae carotidis internae
p. cervicalis arteriae carotidis internae
p. cervicalis ductus thoracici
p. cervicalis esophagi
p. cervicalis medullae spinalis
p. chondropharyngea musculi constrictoris pharyngea medii
p. ciliaris retinae
p. clavicularis musculi pectoralis majoris
p. coccygea medullae spinalis
p. cochlearis nervi vestibulocochlearis
p. convoluta lobuli corticalis renis
p. corneoscleralis reticuli trabecularis
partes corporis humani
p. corticalis
p. corticalis arteriae cerebralis mediae
p. costalis diaphragmatis
p. cricopharyngea musculi constrictoris pharyngis inferioris
p. cruciformis vaginae fibrosae
p. cupularis recessus epitympanici
p. cystica
p. descendens aortae
p. descendens duodeni
p. dextra faciei diaphragmaticae hepatis
p. distalis
p. dorsalis pontis
p. endocrina pancreatis
p. exocrina pancreatis
p. fetalis placentae
p. flaccida membranae tympani
p. frontalis corporis callosi
partes genitales femininae externae
partes genitales masculinae externae
p. glossopharyngea musculi constrictoris pharyngis superioris
p. granulosa
p. hepatica
p. horizontalis duodeni
p. inferior
p. inferior duodeni
p. inferior ganglii vestibularis

p. inferior rami lingularis
p. infraclavicularis plexus brachialis
p. infralobaris rami posterioris venae pulmonalis dextrae
p. infrasegmentalis
p. infundibularis
p. insularis
p. insularis arteriae cerebralis mediae
p. interarticularis
p. intercartilaginea rimae glottidis
p. intermedia
p. intermedia adenohypophyseos
p. intermedia bulborum
p. intermedia commissura bulborum
p. intermembranacea rimae glottidis
p. intersegmentalis
p. intracanaliculus nervi optici
p. intracranialis arteriae vertebralis
p. intracranialis nervi optici
p. intralaminaris nervi optici
p. intralobaris venae pulmonalis dextrae superioris
p. intraocularis nervi optici
p. intrasegmentalis
p. iridica retinae
p. labialis musculi orbicularis oris
p. lacrimalis musculi orbicularis oculi
p. laryngea pharyngis
p. lateralis arcus pedis longitudinalis
p. lateralis fornicis vaginae
p. lateralis musculorum intertransversariorum posteriorum cervicis
p. lateralis ossis occipitalis
p. lateralis ossis sacri
p. lateralis rami lobi medii venae pulmonalis dexter superior
p. lumbalis diaphragmatis
p. lumbalis medullae spinalis
p. marginalis musculi orbicularis oris
p. mastoidea ossis temporalis
p. medialis arcus pedis longitudinalis
p. medialis musculorum intertransversariorum posteriorum cervicis
p. medialis rami lobii medii venae pulmonis dextrae superioris
p. mediastinalis pulmonis
p. membranacea septi atriorum
p. membranacea septi interventricularis
p. membranacea septi nasi

P

657

pars *(continued)*

p. membranacea urethrae masculinae
p. mobilis septi nasi
p. muscularis septi interventricularis cordis
p. mylopharyngeus musculi constrictoris pharyngis superioris
p. nasalis ossis frontalis
p. nasalis pharyngis
p. nervosa hypophyseos
p. nervosa retinae
p. obliqua musculi cricothyroidei
p. occipitalis corporis callosi
p. opercularis
p. optica retinae
p. oralis pharyngis
p. orbitalis glandulae lacrimalis
p. orbitalis musculi orbicularis oculi
p. orbitalis nervi optici
p. orbitalis ossis frontalis
p. ossea septi nasi
p. ossea systematis skeletalis
p. ossea tubae auditivae
p. palpebralis glandulae lacrimalis
p. palpebralis musculi orbicularis oculi
p. parasympathica
p. pelvina
p. pelvina ureteris
p. peripherica
p. perpendicularis
p. petrosa arteriae carotidis internae
p. petrosa ossis temporalis
p. phallica
p. pharyngea hypophyseos
p. pigmentosa
p. plana
p. postcommunicalis arteria cerebri anterior
p. posterior commissurae anterioris
p. posterior faciei diaphragmatis hepatis
p. posterior fornicis vaginae
p. postlaminaris nervi optici
p. postsulcalis
p. precommunicalis arteriae cerebri anterior
p. prelaminaris nervi optici
p. presulcalis
p. profunda glandulae parotideae
p. profunda musculi masseteri
p. profunda musculi sphincteri ani externi
p. prostatica urethrae
p. pterygopharyngea musculi constrictoris pharyngis superioris

p. pylorica gastris
p. pylorica ventriculi
p. quadrata hepatis
p. radiata lobuli corticalis renis
p. recta musculi cricothyroidei
p. retrolentiformis capsulae internae
p. sacralis medullae spinalis
p. sellaris
p. sphenoidalis arteriae cerebralis mediae
p. spinalis nervi accessorii
p. spongiosa urethrae masculinae
p. squamosa ossis temporalis
p. sternalis diaphragmatis
p. sternocostalis musculi pectoralis majoris
p. subcutanea musculi sphincteri ani externi
p. sublentiformis capsulae internae
p. superficialis glandulae parotideae
p. superficialis musculi masseteri
p. superficialis musculi sphincteri ani externi
p. superior duodeni
p. superior faciei diaphragmaticae hepatis
p. superior ganglii vestibularis
p. superior rami lingularis venae pulmonis sinistri
p. supraclavicularis plexus brachialis
p. sympathica
p. tecta, p. tecta duodeni, p. tecta pancreatis, p. tecta renalis, p. tecta ureteralis
p. tensa membranae tympani
p. terminalis
p. thoracica aortae
p. thoracica ductus thoracici
p. thoracica esophagi
p. thoracica medullae spinalis
p. thyropharyngea musculi constrictoris pharyngis inferioris
p. tibiocalcanea ligamenti medialis
p. tibionavicularis ligamenti medialis
p. tibiotalaris anterior ligamenti medialis
p. tibiotalaris posterior ligamenti medialis
p. transversa musculi nasalis
p. transversa rami sinistri venae portae hepatis
p. transversaria arteriae vertebralis
p. triangularis
p. tuberalis
p. tympanica ossis temporalis
p. umbilicalis rami sinistri venae portae hepatis

p. uterina placentae
p. uterina tubae uterinae
p. uvealis reticuli trabecularis
p. vagalis nervi accessorii
p. ventralis pontis
p. vertebralis faciei costalis
  pulmonis
p. vestibularis nervi
  vestibulocochlearis
Parsonage-Turner syndrome
pars-planitis
part
abdominal p. of aorta
abdominal p. of esophagus
abdominal p. of thoracic duct
abdominal p. of ureter
alar p. of nasalis muscle
alveolar p. of mandible
annular p. of fibrous digital sheath
anterior p.
anterior p. of anterior commissure
  of brain
anterior p. of diaphragmatic surface
  of liver
anterior p. of fornix of vagina
anterior p. of pons
anterior tibiotalar p. of deltoid
  ligament
ascending p. of aorta
ascending p. of duodenum
atlantic p. of vertebral artery
autonomic p.
basal p. of occipital bone
basal p. of pulmonary artery
basilar p. of the occipital bone
basilar p. of pons
bony p. of auditory tube
bony p. of external acoustic
  meatus
bony p. of nasal septum
buccopharyngeal p. of superior
  pharyngeal constrictor
cardiac p. of stomach
cartilaginous p. of auditory tube
cartilaginous p. of external acoustic
  meatus
cartilaginous p. of skeletal system
cavernous p. of internal carotid
  artery
ceratopharyngeal p. of middle
  pharyngeal constrictor
cerebral p. of arachnoid
cerebral p. of dura mater
cerebral p. of internal carotid
  artery
cervical p. of esophagus
cervical p. of internal carotid
  artery

cervical p. of spinal cord
cervical p. of thoracic duct
chondropharyngeal p. of middle
  pharyngeal constrictor
ciliary p. of retina
clavicular p. of pectoralis major
  muscle
coccygeal p. of spinal cord
cochlear p. of vestibulocochlear
  nerve
convoluted p. of kidney lobule
corneoscleral p. of trabecular
  reticulum
cortical p.
cortical p. of middle cerebral
  artery
costal p. of diaphragm
cricopharyngeal p. of inferior
  pharyngeal constrictor
cruciform p. of fibrous digital
  sheath
cruciform p. of fibrous sheath
cupular p. of epitympanic recess
deep p. of external anal sphincter
deep p. of flexor retinaculum
deep p. of masseter muscle
deep p. of parotid gland
descending p. of aorta
descending p. of duodenum
descending p. of facial canal
distal p. of anterior lobe of
  hypophysis
dorsal p. of pons
endocrine p. of pancreas
exocrine p. of pancreas
flaccid p. of tympanic membrane
frontal p. of corpus callosum
glossopharyngeal p. of superior
  pharyngeal constrictor
hidden p.
horizontal p. of duodenum
horizontal p. of facial canal
p.'s of human body
inferior p.
inferior p. of duodenum
inferior p. of lingular branch of
  left pulmonary vein
inferior p. of vestibular ganglion
inferior p. of vestibulocochlear
  nerve
infraclavicular p. of brachial plexus
infralobar p. of posterior branch of
  right pulmonary vein
infrasegmental p.
infundibular p.
insular p.
insular p. of middle cerebral artery

P

part *(continued)*

intercartilaginous p. of glottic opening
intercartilaginous p. of rima glottidis
intermediate p.
intermediate p. of adenohypophysis
intermediate p. of vestibular bulb
intermembranous p. of glottic opening
intermembranous p. of rima glottidis
intersegmental p. of pulmonary vein
intracanicular p. of optic nerve
intracranial p. of optic nerve
intracranial p. of vertebral artery
intralaminar p. of optic nerve
intralobar p. of the right superior pulmonary vein
intraocular p. of optic nerve
intrasegmental p.
iridial p. of retina
labial p. of orbicularis oris muscle
lacrimal p. of orbicularis oculi muscle
laryngeal p. of pharynx
lateral p. of longitudinal arch of foot
lateral p. of middle lobar branch of right superior pulmonary vein
lateral p. of occipital bone
lateral p. of posterior cervical intertransversarii muscles
lateral p. of sacrum
lateral p. of vaginal fornix
lumbar p.
lumbar p. of diaphragm
lumbar p. of spinal cord
marginal p. of orbicularis oris muscle
mastoid p. of the temporal bone
medial p. of longitudinal arch of foot
medial p. of middle lobar branch of right superior pulmonary vein
medial p. of posterior cervical intertransversarii muscles
mediastinal p. of lung
membranous p. of interventricular septum
membranous p. of male urethra
membranous p. of nasal septum
mobile p. of nasal septum
muscular p. of interventricular septum of heart
mylopharyngeal p. of superior pharyngeal constrictor

nasal p. of frontal bone
nasal p. of pharynx
nervous p. of retina
neural p. of hypophysis
oblique p. of cricothyroid muscle
occipital p. of corpus callosum
opercular p.
optic p. of retina
oral p. of pharynx
orbital p. of frontal bone
orbital p. of lacrimal gland
orbital p. of optic nerve
orbital p. of orbicularis oculi muscle
osseous p. of skeletal system
palpebral p. of lacrimal gland
palpebral p. of orbicularis oculi muscle
parasympathetic p.
pelvic p.
pelvic p. of ureter
peripheral p.
petrous p. of internal carotid artery
petrous p. of temporal bone
pigmented p. of retina
postcommunical p. of anterior cerebral artery
posterior p.
posterior p. of the diaphragmatic surface of the liver
posterior tibiotalar p. of deltoid ligament
postlaminar p. of optic nerve
postsulcal p. of tongue
precommunical p. of anterior cerebral artery
prelaminar p. of optic nerve
presulcal p. of tongue
prevertebral p. of vertebral artery
pterygopharyngeal p. of superior constrictor muscle of pharynx
pyloric p. of stomach
quadrate p. of liver
retrolenticular p. of internal capsule
right p. of diaphragmatic surface of liver
sacral p. of spinal cord
soft p.'s
sphenoidal p. of middle cerebral artery
spinal p. of accessory nerve
spinal p. of arachnoid
spongy p. of the male urethra
squamous p. of frontal bone
squamous p. of occipital bone
squamous p. of temporal bone
sternal p. of diaphragm

sternocostal p. of pectoralis major muscle
straight p. of cricothyroid muscle
subcutaneous p. of external anal sphincter
sublenticular p. of internal capsule
suboccipital p. of vertebral artery
superficial p. of duodenum
superficial p. of external anal sphincter
superficial p. of masseter muscle
superficial p. of parotid gland
superior p. of diaphragmatic surface of liver
superior p. of duodenum
superior p. of lingular branch of left pulmonary vein
superior p. of vestibular ganglion
superior p. of vestibulocochlear nerve
supraclavicular p. of brachial plexus
sympathetic p.
tense p. of the tympanic membrane
terminal p.
thoracic p. of aorta
thoracic p. of esophagus
thoracic p. of spinal cord
thoracic p. of thoracic duct
thyropharyngeal p. of inferior pharyngeal constrictor muscle
tibiocalcaneal p. of deltoid ligament
tibionavicular p. of deltoid ligament
transversarial p. of vertebral artery
transverse p. of left branch of portal vein
transverse p. of nasalis muscle
triangular p.
tympanic p. of temporal bone
umbilical p. of left branch of portal vein
uterine p. of uterine tube
uveal p. of trabecular reticulum
vagal p.
vagal p. of accessory nerve
ventral p. of pons
vertebral p. of the costal surface of the lungs
vertebral p. of diaphragm
vestibular p. of vestibulocochlear nerve

partes (*pl. of* pars)
parthenogenesis
parthenophobia

partial
  p. adrenocortical insufficiency
  p. agglutinin
  p. anencephaly
  p. aneuploidy
  p. anodontia
  p. antigen
  p. breech extraction
  p. cystectomy
  p. denture
  p. denture, distal extension
  p. denture impression
  p. denture retention
  p. enterocele
  p. epilepsy
  p. face-sparing lipodystrophy
  p. heart block
  p. ileal bypass
  p. lipoatrophy
  p. sclerectasia
  p. seizure
  p. thromboplastin time
partial-thickness
  p.-t. burn
  p.-t. flap
  p.-t. graft
participant observer
particle
  chromatin p.'s
  Dane p.'s
  defective interfering p.
  D.I. p.
  elementary p.
  kappa p.'s
  signal recognition p.
  Zimmermann's elementary p.
particulate
particulates
parturient
  p. canal
parturiometer
parturition
parulis, pl. **parulides**
parumbilical
paruresis
parvilocular cyst
Parvobacteriaceae
parvocellular
Parvoviridae
Parvovirus
Parvovirus B 19 *tARgus wAve forms*
parvus
Pascheff's conjunctivitis
Paschen bodies
passage
  blind p.
  nasopharyngeal p.

P

passage (*continued*)
    oropharyngeal p.
    serial p.
Passalurus ambiguus
Passavant's
    P. bar
    P. cushion
    P. pad
    P. ridge
passion
passional attitudes
passive
    p. agglutination
    p. anaphylaxis
    p. atelectasis
    p. clot
    p. congestion
    p. cutaneous anaphylactic reaction
    p. cutaneous anaphylaxis
    p. cutaneous anaphylaxis test
    p. duction
    p. eruption
    p. hemagglutination
    p. hyperemia
    p. immunity
    p. immunization
    p. incontinence
    p. learning
    p. length-tension curve
    p. medium
    p. movement
    p. prophylaxis
    p. transference
    p. tremor
    p. vasoconstriction
    p. vasodilation
passive-aggressive
    p.-a. behavior
    p.-a. personality
passivism
PAS stain
paster
Pasteurella
pasteurella, pl. **pasteurellae**
Pasteur pipette
Pastia's sign
pastil, pastille
    Sabouraud's p.'s
pastoral counseling
past-pointing
patagium, pl. **patagia**
    cervical p.
Patau's syndrome
patch
    butterfly p.
    cotton-wool p.'s
    herald p.

    Hutchinson's p.
    moth p.
    mucous p.
    opaline p.
    Peyer's p.'s
    salmon p.
    shagreen p.
    smoker's p.'s
    soldier's p.'s
    p. test
patchy atelectasis
patefaction
patella, gen. and pl. **patellae**
    floating p.
    slipping p.
patellalgia
patellar
    p. fossa of vitreous
    p. ligament
    p. network
    p. reflex
    p. retinaculum
    p. surface of femur
    p. tendon reflex
patellectomy
patelliform
patello-adductor reflex
patellometer
patency
    probe p.
patent
    p. blue V
    p. ductus arteriosus
Paterson-Brown-Kelly syndrome
Paterson-Kelly syndrome
path
    p. analysis
    condyle p.
    generated occlusal p.
    incisal p.
    p. of insertion
    milled-in p.'s
    occlusal p.
pathema
pathematic aphasia
pathergasia
pathergy
pathetic
    p. nerve
pathfinder
pathic
pathobiology
pathoclisis
pathocrinia
pathodixia
pathodontia
pathoformic

pathogen
    behavioral p.
    opportunistic p.
pathogenesis
pathogenic, pathogenetic
    p. occlusion
pathogenicity
pathogeny
pathognomonic
    p. symptom
pathognomy
pathognostic
pathography
patholesia
pathologic, pathological
    p. absorption
    p. amenorrhea
    p. amputation
    p. calcification
    p. diagnosis
    p. fracture
    p. glycosuria
    p. histology
    p. myopia
    p. physiology
    p. retraction ring
    p. rigidity
    p. sphincter
    p. startle syndromes
pathologist
pathology
    anatomical p.
    cellular p.
    clinical p.
    dental p.
    functional p.
    humoral p.
    medical p.
    molecular p.
    oral p.
    speech p.
    surgical p.
pathometric
pathometry
pathomimesis
pathomimicry
pathomiosis
pathomorphism
pathonomia, pathonomy
pathophobia
pathophysiology
pathopoiesis
pathosis
pathway, biochemical pathway
    auditory p.
    visual p.
patient
    p. controlled analgesia

    target p.
    P. Zero
Patois virus
Paton's lines
patricide
Patrick's test
patrilineal
patten
pattern
    airspace-filling p.
    airway p.
    alveolar p.
    ballerina-foot p.
    butterfly p.
    ground-glass p.
    honeycomb p.
    hourglass p.
    interstitial p.
    juvenile p.
    miliary p.
    mosaic p.
    occlusal p.
    reticulonodular p.
    p. sensitive epilepsy
    wax p.
patterned alopecia
patulous
paucibacillary
paucisynaptic
Paul-Bunnell test
Paul's
    P. reaction
    P. test
pause
    apneic p.
    compensatory p.
    postextrasystolic p.
    preautomatic p.
    respiratory p.
    sinus p.
Pautrier's
    P. abscess
    P. microabscess
Pauzat's disease
pavement epithelium
pavex
Pavlov
    P. method
    P. pouch
    P. reflex
    P. stomach
pavlovian conditioning
pavor nocturnus
Pavy's disease
Paxton's disease
Payne operation
Payr's
    P. clamp

P

Payr's *(continued)*
    P. membrane
    P. sign
PBI test
P-congenitale
P-dextrocardiale
PDL
peak
    biclonal p.
    p. expiratory flow
    p. flow rate
    juxtaphrenic p.
    p. magnitude
    monoclonal p.
pearl
    p. cyst
    Elschnig p.'s
    enamel p.
    epithelial p.
    Epstein's p.'s
    gouty p.
    keratin p.
    Laënnec's p.'s
    squamous p.
pearl-worker's disease
pear-shaped area
peau d'orange
peccant
    p. humors
peccatiphobia
pecking order
Pecquet's
    P. cistern
    P. duct
    P. reservoir
pecten
    anal p.
    p. analis
    p. band
    p. ossis pubis
    p. pubis
pectenitis
pectenosis
pectinate
    p. fibers
    p. ligaments of iridocorneal angle
    p. ligaments of iris
    p. line
    p. muscles
    p. zone
pectineal
    p. ligament
    p. line
    p. line of pubis
    p. muscle
pectineus
    p. muscle

pectiniform
    p. septum
pectora (*pl. of* pectus)
pectoral
    p. and abdominal anterior
        cutaneous branch of intercostal
        nerves
    p. branch of thoracoacromial artery
    p. fascia
    p. girdle
    p. glands
    p. group of axillary lymph nodes
    p. reflex
    p. region
    p. regions
    p. ridge
    p. veins
pectoralgia
pectoralis
    p. major muscle
    p. minor muscle
pectoriloquy
    aphonic p.
    whispered p., whispering p.
pectoris (*gen. of* pectus)
pectorodorsalis muscle
pectorodorsal muscle
pectorophony
pectus, gen. **pectoris**, pl. **pectora**
    p. carinatum
    p. excavatum
    p. recurvatum
pedal
    p. system
pedatrophia, pedatrophy
pederast
pederasty
Pedersen's speculum
pedes (*pl. of* pes)
pediatric
    p. dentistry
    p. radiology
pediatrician
pediatrics
pediatrist
pediatry
pedicel
pedicellate
pedicellation
pedicle
    p. of arch of vertebra
    Filatov-Gillies tubed p.
    p. flap
    p. graft
    vascular p.
pedicular
pediculate
pediculation

pediculi (*pl. of* pediculus)
Pediculoides ventricosus
pediculophobia
pediculosis
    p. capitis
    p. corporis
    p. palpebrarum
    p. pubis
    p. vestimenti, p. vestimentorum
pediculous
    p. blepharitis
Pediculus
pediculus, pl. **pediculi**
    p. arcus vertebrae
pedicure
pedigree
    p. analysis
pediluvium
pedionalgia
pedioneuralgia
pediophobia
pediphalanx
pedis (*gen. of* pes)
pedodontia
pedodontics
pedodontist
pedodynamometer
pedogenesis
pedogram
pedograph
pedography
pedologist
pedology
pedometer
pedomorphism
pedophilia
pedophilic
peduncle
    cerebral p.
    p. of corpus callosum
    p. of flocculus
    inferior cerebellar p.
    inferior thalamic p.
    lateral thalamic p.
    p. of mamillary body
    middle cerebellar p.
    olfactory p.
    superior cerebellar p.
    ventral thalamic p.
peduncular
    p. ansa
    p. loop
    p. veins
pedunculate
pedunculated
    p. hydatid
    p. polyp
pedunculi (*pl. of* pedunculus)

pedunculomamillary fasciculus
pedunculotomy
pedunculus, pl. **pedunculi**
    p. cerebellaris inferior
    p. cerebellaris medius
    p. cerebellaris superior
    p. cerebri
    p. corporis callosi
    p. corporis mamillaris
    p. flocculi
    p. of pineal body
    p. thalami inferior
    p. thalami lateralis
    p. thalami ventralis
    p. vitellinus
peel
    face p.
peeling
    chemical p.
peenash
peer review
peg
    rete p.'s
peg-and-socket
    p.-a.-s. articulation
    p.-a.-s. joint
pegged tooth
pejorism
PEL
pelade
Pel-Ebstein
    P.-E. disease
    P.-E. fever
Pelger-Huët nuclear anomaly
pelidnoma
pelioma
peliosis
    bacterial p.
    p. hepatis
    p. hepatitis
Pelizaeus-Merzbacher disease
pellagra
    infantile p.
    secondary p.
    p. sine p.
pellagroid
pellagrous
Pellegrini's disease
Pellegrini-Stieda disease
pellicle
    acquired p.
    brown p.
pellicular, pelliculous
Pellizzi's syndrome
pellucid
    p. zone
pelma
pelmatic

P

pelmatogram
pelopathy
pelotherapy
pelta
peltation
pelves (*pl. of* pelvis)
pelvic
    p. abscess
    p. axis
    p. brim
    p. canal
    p. cavity
    p. cellulitis
    p. diaphragm
    p. direction
    p. exenteration
    p. fascia
    p. ganglia
    p. girdle
    p. hematocele
    p. index
    p. inflammatory disease
    p. inlet
    p. kidney
    p. limb
    p. outlet
    p. part
    p. part of ureter
    p. peritonitis
    p. plane of greatest dimensions
    p. plane of inlet
    p. plane of least dimensions
    p. plane of outlet
    p. plexus
    p. pole
    p. presentation
    p. promontory
    p. splanchnic nerves
    p. surface of sacrum
    p. version
pelvicephalography
pelvicephalometry
pelvifixation
pelvigraph
pelvilithotomy
pelvimeter
pelvimetry
    manual p.
    radiographic p.
pelviolithotomy
pelvioperitonitis
pelvioplasty
pelvioscopy
pelviotomy, pelvitomy
pelviperitonitis
pelvirectal sphincter
pelvis, pl. pelves
    android p.

anthropoid p.
assimilation p.
beaked p.
brachypellic p.
caoutchouc p.
contracted p.
cordate p., cordiform p.
Deventer's p.
dolichopellic p.
dwarf p.
false p.
flat p.
frozen p.
funnel-shaped p.
p. of gallbladder
greater p.
gynecoid p.
hardened p.
heart-shaped p.
inverted p.
p. justo major
p. justo minor
juvenile p.
kyphoscoliotic p.
kyphotic p.
large p.
lesser p.
longitudinal oval p.
lordotic p.
p. major
masculine p.
mesatipellic p.
p. minor
Nägele's p.
p. nana
p. obtecta
osteomalacic p.
Otto p.
p. plana
platypellic p.
platypelloid p.
Prague p.
pseudo-osteomalacic p.
rachitic p.
renal p.
p. renalis
reniform p.
Robert's p.
Rokitansky's p.
rostrate p.
round p.
rubber p.
scoliotic p.
small p.
spider p.
split p.
spondylolisthetic p.
p. spuria

transverse oval p.
true p.
ureteric p.
p. vera
pelvisacral
pelviscope
pelvitherm
pelvitomy (*var. of* pelviotomy)
pelviureterography
pelvivertebral angle
pelvocephalography
pelvofemoral muscular dystrophy
pelvoscopy
pelvospondylitis ossificans
pemphigoid
benign mucosal p.
bullous p.
cicatricial p.
localized p. of Brunsting-Perry
ocular p.
p. syphilid
pemphigus
p. acutus
benign familial chronic p.
Brazilian p.
p. contagiosus
p. erythematosus
p. foliaceus
p. gangrenosus
p. leprosus
p. vegetans
p. vulgaris
pencil tenderness
pendelluft
Pendred's syndrome
pendular
p. movement
p. nystagmus
pendulous
p. abdomen
p. heart
p. palate
pendulum rhythm
penectomy
penes (*pl. of* penis)
penetrance
genetic p.
penetrant trait
penetrate
penetrating
p. keratoplasty
p. ulcer
p. wound
penetration
penetrometer
pen grasp
penial
peniaphobia

penicillary
penicillate
penicillus, pl. **penicilli**
penile
p. epispadias
p. fibromatosis
p. hypospadias
p. implant
p. raphe
p. urethra
penis, pl. **penes**
bifid p.
buried p.
clubbed p.
concealed p.
p. envy
p. femineus
gryposis p.
p. lunatus
p. muliebris
p. palmatus
webbed p.
penischisis
penitis
pennate
p. muscle
penniform
penopubic epispadias
penoscrotal
p. hypospadias
p. transposition
penotomy
Penrose drain
pension neurosis
pentad
Reynolds p.
pentadactyl, pentadactyle
pentagastrin test
pentalogy
p. of Cantrell
p. of Fallot
pentamer
Pentastoma
Pentastomida
Pentatrichomonas
penton
p. antigen
pentosuria
alimentary p.
primary p.
penumbra
peotillomania
peplomer
peplos
pepper
p. and salt fundus
Pepper syndrome
pepsinuria

P

peptic
>p. cell
>p. esophagitis
>p. gland
>p. ulcer

peptide
>atrial natriuretic p.
>calcitonin gene related p.
>corticotropin-like intermediate-
>lobe p.

peptidergic
Peptococcaceae
Peptococcus
>*P. aerogenes*
>*P. asaccharolyticus*
>*P. constellatus*
>*P. niger*

Peptostreptococcus
>*P. anaerobius*
>*P. asaccharolyticus*
>*P. evolutus*
>*P. foetidus*
>*P. intermedius*
>*P. magnus*
>*P. micros*
>*P. morbillorum*
>*P. paleopneumoniae*
>*P. parvulus*
>*P. plagarumbelli*
>*P. productus*
>*P. putridus*

per
>p. anum
>p. contiguum
>p. continuum
>p. os
>p. primam
>p. rectum
>p. saltum
>p. tubam
>p. vias naturales

peracephalus
peracute
perambulating ulcer
perarticulation
peratodynia
peraxillary
percentile
percept
>p. analysis

perception
>depth p.
>extrasensory p.
>simultaneous p.

perceptive
>p. deafness

perceptivity
perceptorium

perceptual expansion
percuss
percussion
>auscultatory p.
>bimanual p.
>clavicular p.
>deep p.
>direct p.
>finger p.
>immediate p.
>mediate p.
>Murphy's p.
>palpatory p.
>piano p.
>p. sound
>threshold p.
>p. wave

percussor
percutaneous
>p. absorption
>p. cholangiography
>p. endoscopic gastrostomy
>p. nephrostomy
>p. radiofrequency gangliolysis
>p. stimulation
>p. transhepatic cholangiography
>p. transluminal angioplasty
>p. transluminal coronary angioplasty

perencephaly
Perez reflex
Perez' sign
perfect
>p. fungus
>p. stage
>p. state

perfectionism
perflation
perflubron
perfluorooctyl bromide
perforans
perforated
>p. layer of sclera
>p. space
>p. ulcer

perforating
>p. abscess
>p. appendicitis
>p. arteries
>p. arteries of foot
>p. arteries of hand
>p. arteries of internal mammary
>p. branches
>p. branches of internal thoracic
>artery
>p. branches of palmar metacarpal
>arteries
>p. branches of plantar metatarsal
>arteries

p. branch of peroneal artery
p. fibers
p. folliculitis
p. keratoplasty
p. peroneal artery
p. ulcer of foot
p. veins
p. wound
perforation
perforator
perforin
performance test
performic acid reaction
perfrigeration
perfusate
perfuse
perfusion
p. cannula
regional p.
periaccretio pericardii
periacinal, periacinous
periadenitis
p. mucosa necrotica recurrens
perialveolar wiring
perianal
periangiocholitis
periangitis
periaortic
periaortitis
periapex
periapical
p. abscess
p. cemental dysplasia
p. curettage
p. cyst
p. granuloma
p. osteofibrosis
p. radiograph
p. tissue
periappendiceal abscess
periappendicitis
p. decidualis
periappendicular
periarterial
p. pad
p. plexus
p. plexus of maxillary artery
p. plexus of vertebral artery
p. sympathectomy
periarteritis
p. nodosa
periarthric
periarthritis
periarticular
p. abscess
periatrial
periauricular
periaxial

periaxillary
periaxonal
periblast
peribronchial
peribronchiolar ~ chun
peribronchiolitis
peribronchitis
peribuccal
peribulbar
peribursal
pericallosal artery
pericanalicular
p. fibroadenoma
pericapillary cell
pericardectomy
pericardia (*pl. of* pericardium)
pericardiac, pericardial
pericardiacophrenic
p. artery
p. veins
pericardicentesis
pericardiectomy
radical p.
pericardii
pericardiocentesis
pericardioperitoneal
p. canal
pericardiophrenic
pericardiopleural
p. membrane
pericardiorrhaphy
pericardiostomy
pericardiotomy
pericarditic
pericarditis
acute fibrinous p.
adhesive p.
bacterial p.
p. calculosa
carcinomatous p.
chronic constrictive p.
constrictive p.
dry p.
p. epistenocardica
fibrinous p.
fibrous p.
hemorrhagic p.
internal adhesive p.
p. obliterans
obliterating p.
postmyocardial infarction p.
postpericardiotomy p.
posttraumatic p.
purulent p.
rheumatic p.
p. sicca
tuberculous p.
uremic p.

P

pericarditis *(continued)*
   p. villosa
   viral p.
   p. with effusion
pericardium, pl. pericardia
   adherent p.
   bread-and-butter p.
   p. fibrosum
   fibrous p.
   hydrops pericardii
   periaccretio pericardii
   p. serosum
   serous p.
   shaggy p.
   visceral p.
pericardotomy
pericecal
pericellular
pericemental
   p. abscess
   p. attachment
pericementitis
pericentral
   p. fibrosis
   p. scotoma
pericentric inversion
perichareia
pericholangitis
perichondral, perichondrial
   p. bone
perichondritis
   peristernal p.
   relapsing p.
perichondrium
perichord
perichordal
perichoroidal
   p. space
perichoroid space
perichrome
periclaustral lamina
pericolic
   p. membrane syndrome
pericolitis
   p. dextra
   p. sinistra
pericolonitis
pericolpitis
periconchal
   p. sulcus
pericorneal
pericoronal
   p. abscess
   p. flap
pericoronitis
pericorpuscular synapse
pericranial
pericranitis

pericranium
pericystic
pericystitis
pericystium
pericyte
pericytial
pericytic venules
peridens
peridental
   p. ligament
   p. membrane
peridentitis
peridentium
periderm, periderma
peridermal, peridermic
peridesmic
peridesmitis
peridesmium
perididymis
perididymitis
peridium
peridiverticulitis
periduodenitis
peridural
   p. anesthesia
periencephalitis
perienteric
perienteritis
periependymal
periesophageal
periesophagitis
perifocal
perifollicular
perifolliculitis
   p. abscedens et suffodiens
   superficial pustular p.
perifuse
perifusion
periganglionic
perigastric
perigastritis
perigemmal
periglandulitis
periglottic
periglottis
perihepatic
perihepatitis
perihernial
perihypoglossal nuclei
peri-implantoclasia
peri-infarction block
perijejunitis
perikaryon, pl. perikarya
perikeratic
perikymata, sing. perikyma
perilabyrinthitis
perilaryngeal
perilenticular

pericollicular

periligamentous
perilimbal suction cup
perilunar dislocation
perilymph
perilympha
perilymphangial
perilymphangitis
perilymphatic
    p. duct
    p. space
perimeningitis
perimenopause
perimeter
    arc p.
    Goldmann p.
    projection p.
    Tübinger p.
perimetria (*pl. of* perimetrium)
perimetric
perimetritic
perimetritis
perimetrium, pl. **perimetria**
perimetry
    computed p.
    flicker p.
    kinetic p.
    mesopic p.
    objective p.
    quantitative p.
    scotopic p.
    static p.
perimolysis
perimortem delivery
perimuscular fibrosis
perimyelis
perimyelitis
perimyocarditis
perimyositis
perimysia (*pl. of* perimysium)
perimysial
perimysiitis, **perimysitis**
perimysium, pl. **perimysia**
    p. externum
    p. internum
perinatal
    p. death
    p. medicine
    p. mortality
    p. mortality rate
    p. torsion
perinate
perinatologist
perinatology
perinea (*pl. of* perineum)
perineal
    p. artery
    p. body

    p. branches of posterior femoral
      cutaneous nerve
    p. flexure of rectum
    p. hernia
    p. hypospadias
    p. lithotomy
    p. membrane
    p. muscles
    p. nerves
    p. raphe
    p. region
    p. section
    p. spaces
    p. urethrostomy
    p. urethrotomy
perineocele
perineometer
perineoplasty
perineorrhaphy
perineoscrotal
perineostomy
perineosynthesis
perineotomy
perineovaginal
    p. fistula
perinephria (*pl. of* perinephrium)
perinephrial
perinephric
    p. abscess
perinephritis
perinephrium, pl. **perinephria**
perineum, pl. **perinea**
    watering-can p.
perineural
    p. anesthesia
    p. infiltration
perineuria (*pl. of* perineurium)
perineurial
perineuritis
perineurium, pl. **perineuria**
perineuronal satellite
perinuclear
    p. cataract
    p. space
periocular
period
    absolute refractory p.
    critical p.
    eclipse p.
    effective refractory p.
    ejection p.
    extrinsic incubation p.
    fertile p.
    functional refractory p.
    incubation p.
    induction p.
    intrapartum p.
    isoelectric p.

P

period *(continued)*
    isometric p. of cardiac cycle
    isometric contraction p.
    isometric relaxation p.
    latency p.
    latent p.
    masticatory silent p.
    menstrual p.
    missed p.
    oedipal p.
    preejection p.
    prepatent p.
    prodromal p.
    puerperal p.
    pulse p.
    quarantine p.
    refractory p.
    refractory p. of electronic
      pacemaker
    relative refractory p.
    silent p.
    total refractory p.
    vulnerable p., vulnerable p. of heart
    Wenckebach p.
periodic
    p. acid-Schiff stain
    p. arthralgia
    p. catatonia
    p. disease
    p. edema
    p. fever
    p. filariasis
    p. migrainous neuralgia
    p. neutropenia
    p. paralysis
    p. peritonitis
    p. polyserositis
periodicity
    diurnal p.
    filarial p.
    lunar p.
    malarial p.
    nocturnal p.
    subperiodic p.
periodontal
    p. abscess
    p. anesthesia
    p. atrophy
    P. Disease Index
    p. file
    P. Index
    p. ligament
    p. ligament fibers
    p. membrane
    p. pocket
    p. probe
periodontia
periodontia (*pl. of* periodontium)

periodontics
periodontist
periodontitis
    apical p.
    p. complex
    juvenile p.
    p. simplex
    suppurative p.
periodontium, pl. **periodontia**
periodontoclasia
periodontolysis
periodontosis
periomphalic
perionychium, pl. **perionychia**
perionyx
perionyxis
perioophoritis
perioophorosalpingitis
perioperative
periophthalmic
periophthalmitis
perioral
periorbit
periorbita
periorbital
    p. membrane
periorchitis
    p. hemorrhagica
periost
periostea (*pl. of* periosteum)
periosteal
    p. bone
    p. bud
    p. chondroma
    p. elevator
    p. ganglion
    p. graft
    p. implantation
    p. layer of dura mater
    p. osteosarcoma
    p. reaction
    p. reflex
    p. sarcoma
periosteitis
periosteoma
periosteomedullitis
periosteomyelitis
periosteopathy
periosteophyte
periosteoplastic amputation
periosteosis
periosteotome
periosteotomy
periosteous
periosteum, pl. **periostea**
    alveolar p., p. alveolare
    p. cranii
periostitis

periostoma
periostosis, pl. periostoses
periostosteitis
periostotome
periostotomy
periotic
    p. bone
    p. cartilage
periovaritis
periovular
peripachymeningitis
peripancreatitis
peripapillary
peripartum cardiomyopathy
peripatetic
peripenial
peripharyngeal
    p. space
peripherad
peripheral
    p. aneurysm
    p. anterior synechia
    p. apnea
    p. arteriosclerosis
    p. cataract
    p. chemoreceptor
    p. dysostosis
    p. facial paralysis
    p. glare
    p. iridectomy
    p. nervous system
    p. ossifying fibroma
    p. part
    p. resistance
    p. scotoma
    p. seal
    p. tabes
    p. vision
peripheralis
peripherocentral
periphery
periphlebitic
periphlebitis
Periplaneta
peripolar cell
peripolesis
periporitis
periportal
    p. cirrhosis
    p. space of Mall
periproctic
periproctitis
periprostatic
periprostatitis
peripylephlebitis
peripylic
peripyloric

perirectal
    p. abscess
perirectitis
perirenal
    p. fascia
    p. insufflation
perirhinal
perirhizoclasia
perisalpingitis
perisalpingo-ovaritis
perisalpinx
periscopic
    p. lens
    p. meniscus
perisigmoiditis
perisinuous
perisinusoidal space
perispermatitis
    p. serosa
perisplanchnic
perisplanchnitis
perisplenic
perisplenitis
perispondylic
perispondylitis
peristalsis
    mass p.
    reversed p.
peristaltic
peristasis
peristatic hyperemia
peristernal perichondritis
peristole
peristolic
peristoma
peristomal, peristomatous
peristome
peristriate
    p. area
    p. cortex
peristrumous
perisynovial
perisystolic
peritarsal network
peritectomy
peritendineum, pl. peritendinea
peritendinitis
    p. calcarea
    p. serosa
peritenon
peritenontitis
perithecium, pl. perithecia
perithelia (*pl. of* perithelium)
perithelial cell
perithelioma
perithelium, pl. perithelia
    Eberth's p.
perithoracic

P

perithyroiditis
peritomist
peritomy
peritonea (*pl. of* peritoneum)
peritoneal
    p. button
    p. cavity
    p. dialysis
    p. fossae
    p. transfusion
    p. villi
peritonealgia
peritoneocentesis
peritoneoclysis
peritoneopathy
peritoneopericardial
peritoneopexy
peritoneoplasty
peritoneoscope
peritoneoscopy
peritoneotomy
peritoneovenous shunt
peritoneum, pl. **peritonea**
    parietal p.
    p. parietale
    visceral p.
    p. viscerale
peritonism
peritonitis
    adhesive p.
    benign paroxysmal p.
    bile p.
    chemical p.
    chyle p.
    circumscribed p.
    p. deformans
    diaphragmatic p.
    diffuse p.
    p. encapsulans
    fibrocaseous p.
    gas p.
    general p.
    localized p.
    meconium p.
    pelvic p.
    periodic p.
    productive p.
    tuberculous p.
peritonsillar
    p. abscess
peritonsillitis
peritracheal
    p. glands
peritrichal, peritrichate, peritrichic
Peritrichida
peritrichous
peritrochanteric

peritubular
    p. contractile cells
    p. dentin
    p. zone
perityphlic
perityphlitis
    perityphlitis p.
periumbilical
periungual
    p. fibroma
periureteral, periureteric
    p. abscess
periureteritis
    p. plastica
periurethral
    p. abscess
periurethritis
periuterine
periuvular
perivaginitis
perivascular
    p. cuffs
    p. fibrous capsule
perivasculitis
perivenous
periventricular fibers
perivertebral
perivesical
perivisceral
    p. cavity
perivisceritis
perivitelline
    p. space
perkinism
perlèche
Perlia's nucleus
perlingual
Perls'
    P. Prussian blue stain
    P. test
permanent
    p. callus
    p. cartilage
    p. dominant idea
    p. pedicle flap
    p. restoration
    p. stricture
    p. tooth
permeation
permissible exposure limit
perna disease
perniciosiform
pernicious
    p. anemia
    p. anemia type metarubricyte
    p. anemia type prorubricyte
    p. anemia type rubriblast

p. malaria
p. vomiting
perniosis
perobrachius
perocephalus
perochirus
perodactyly, perodactylia
peromelia, peromely
perone
peroneal
    p. anastomotic ramus
    p. artery
    p. bone
    p. communicating branch
    p. communicating nerve
    p. muscular atrophy
    p. node
    p. phenomenon
    p. pulley
    p. retinaculum
    p. trochlea of calcaneus
    p. veins
peroneotibial
peroneus
    p. brevis muscle
    p. longus muscle
    p. tertius muscle
peropus
peroral
    p. endoscopy
perosplanchnia
perosseous
peroxidase
    p. reaction
    p. stain
perpendicular
    p. fasciculus
    p. plate
    p. plate of ethmoid bone
    p. plate of palatine bone
perpetual arrhythmia
perpetually growing tooth
persecution complex
persecutory
    p. delusion
    p. type of paranoid disorder
perseveration
Persian
    P. Gulf syndrome
    P. relapsing fever
persistence
    microbial p.
persistent
    p. anterior hyperplastic primary
      vitreous
    p. atrioventricular canal
    p. chronic hepatitis
    p. cloaca

p. ectopic pregnancy
p. generalized lymphadenopathy
p. müllerian duct syndrome
p. posterior hyperplastic primary
  vitreous
p. tremor
p. truncus arteriosus
persistently growing tooth
persister
persona
personal
    p. equation
    p. growth laboratory
    p. motivation
    p. probability
    p. space
personality
    allotropic p.
    anancastic p.
    antisocial p.
    asthenic p.
    authoritarian p.
    avoidant p.
    basic p.
    borderline p.
    compulsive p.
    cyclothymic p.
    dependent p.
    p. disorder
    dual p.
    p. formation
    histrionic p., hysterical p.
    inadequate p.
    p. integration
    p. inventory
    masochistic p.
    multiple p.
    narcissistic p.
    neurasthenic p.
    obsessive p.
    obsessive-compulsive p.
    paranoid p.
    passive-aggressive p.
    p. profile
    psychopathic p.
    schizoid p.
    schizotypical p.
    shut-in p.
    syntonic p.
    p. test
    type A p., type B p.
person-years
perspiration
    insensible p.
    sensible p.
perspiratory glands
persuasion
pertechnetate

P

Perthes disease
Perthes' test
Pertik's diverticulum
pertrochanteric fracture
pertussis
    p. syndrome
pertussis-like syndrome
Peruvian
    P. tarantula
    P. wart
pervasive developmental disorder
pervenous pacemaker
perversion
    polymorphous p.
    sexual p.
pervert
perverted
pervigilium
pes, gen. **pedis**, pl. **pedes**
    p. abductus
    p. adductus
    p. anserinus
    p. cavus
    p. equinovalgus
    p. equinovarus
    p. febricitans
    p. gigas
    p. hippocampi
    p. planus
    p. pronatus
    p. valgus
    p. varus
pessary
    p. cell
    p. corpuscle
    cube p.
    diaphragm p.
    Dumontpallier's p.
    Gariel's p.
    Hodge's p.
    Mayer's p.
    Menge's p.
    ring p.
pessimism
    therapeutic p.
pesticemia
pestis
    p. ambulans
    p. bubonica
    p. fulminans
    p. major
    p. minor
    p. siderans
Pestivirus
petechiae, sing. **petechia**
    calcaneal p.
    Tardieu's petechiae

petechial
    p. angiomas
    p. hemorrhage
petechiasis
Peters'
    P. anomaly
    P. ovum
Petersen's bag
petiolate, petiolated
petiole
petioled
petiolus
    p. epiglottidis
petit
    p. mal
    p. mal epilepsy
    p. mal seizure
Petit's
    P. aponeurosis
    P. canals
    P. hernia
    P. herniotomy
    P. ligament
    P. lumbar triangle
    P. sinus
Petri dish
petrifaction
pétrissage
petroccipital
petromastoid
petro-occipital
    p.-o. fissure
    p.-o. joint
petropharyngeus
petrosa, pl. **petrosae**
petrosal
    p. bone
    p. branch of middle meningeal
      artery
    p. foramen
    p. fossa
    p. fossula
    p. ganglion
    p. impression of the pallium
    p. sinus
    p. vein
petrosalpingostaphylinus
petrositis
petrosomastoid
petrosphenoid
petrosphenoidal syndrome
petrosquamosal, petrosquamous
petrostaphylinus
petrotympanic fissure
petrous
    p. bone
    p. ganglion
    p. part of internal carotid artery

p. part of temporal bone
p. pyramid
petrousitis
Pette-Döring disease
Peutz-Jeghers syndrome
Peutz's syndrome
pexis
Peyer's
P. glands
P. patches
Peyronie's disease
Peyrot's thorax
Pezzer catheter
Pfannenstiel's incision
Pfaundler-Hurler syndrome
Pfeifferella
Pfeiffer's
P. bacillus
P. blood agar
P. phenomenon
P. syndrome
Pflüger's law
Pfuhl's sign
pH
blood pH
phacoanaphylactic uveitis
phacoanaphylaxis
phacocele
phacocyst
phacocystectomy
phacodonesis
phacoemulsification
phacoerysis
phacofragmentation
phacogenic
p. glaucoma
p. uveitis
phacoid
phacolysis
phacolytic
p. glaucoma
phacoma
phacomalacia
phacomatosis
phacomorphic glaucoma
phacoscope
Phaenicia sericata
phaeomycotic cyst
phage
β p.
defective p.
Lambda p.
phagedena
p. gangrenosa
p. nosocomialis
sloughing p.
p. tropica

phagedenic
p. ulcer
phagocyte
p. dysfunction
phagocytic
p. dysfunction disorders
immunodeficiency
p. dysfunction immunodeficiency
p. index
p. pneumonocyte
phagocytin
phagocytize
phagocytoblast
phagocytolysis
phagocytolytic
phagocytose
phagocytosis
induced p.
spontaneous p.
phagodynamometer
phagolysis
phagolysosome
phagolytic
phagomania
phagophobia
phagosome
phagotype
phakic eye
phakoma
phakomatosis
phalangeal
p. cell
p. joints
phalangectomy
phalanges
phalanx, gen. **phalangis**, pl. **phalanges**
tufted p.
ungual p.
phallalgia
phallectomy
phalli (*pl. of* phallus)
phallic
p. phase
p. tubercle
phallicism
phalliform
phallism
phallitis
phallocampsis
phallocrypsis
phallodynia
phalloid
phalloncus
phalloplasty
phallotomy
phallus, pl. **phalli**
phanerogenic
phaneromania

P

phaneroscope
phanerosis
  fatty p.
phanerozoite
phantasia
phantasm
phantasmagoria
phantasmatomoria
phantasmology
phantasmoscopia, phantasmoscopy
phantom
  p. aneurysm
  p. corpuscle
  p. limb
  p. limb pain
  p. pregnancy
  Schultze's p.
  p. tumor
phantomize
pharmacoepidemiology
pharmacologic stress imaging
pharmacomania
pharmacophilia
pharmacophobia
pharmacopsychosis
pharmacoresistent epilepsy
pharyngeal
  p. arches
  p. branch of the artery of
    pterygoid canal
  p. branch of the ascending
    pharyngeal artery
  p. branch of descending palatine
    artery
  p. branches
  p. branch of glossopharyngeal
    nerve
  p. branch of inferior thyroid artery
  p. branch of pterygopalatine
    ganglion
  p. branch of vagus nerve
  p. bursa
  p. calculus
  p. canal
  p. cartilages
  p. fistula
  p. flap
  p. fornix
  p. glands
  p. grooves
  p. hypophysis
  p. isthmus
  p. membranes
  p. mucosa
  p. opening of auditory tube
  p. opening of eustachian tube
  p. pituitary
  p. plexus

  p. pouches
  p. pouch syndrome
  p. raphe
  p. recess
  p. reflex
  p. ridge
  p. space
  p. tonsil
  p. tubercle
  p. veins
pharyngectomy
pharyngei
pharynges (*pl. of* pharynx)
pharyngeus
pharyngis (*gen. of* pharynx)
pharyngismus
pharyngitic
pharyngitis
  atrophic p.
  gangrenous p.
  membranous p.
  p. sicca
  ulcerative p.
  ulceromembranous p.
pharyngobasilar fascia
pharyngobranchial ducts
pharyngocele
pharyngoconjunctival
  p. fever
  p. fever virus
pharyngoepiglottic, pharyngoepiglottidean
  p. fold
pharyngoesophageal
  p. cushions
  p. diverticulum
  p. pads
pharyngoesophagoplasty
pharyngoglossal
pharyngoglossus
pharyngolaryngeal
pharyngolaryngitis
pharyngolith
pharyngomaxillary
  p. space
pharyngomycosis
pharyngonasal
  p. cavity
pharyngo-oral
pharyngopalatine
  p. arch
pharyngopalatinus
pharyngoplasty
  Hynes p.
pharyngoplegia
pharyngorhinoscopy
pharyngoscope
pharyngoscopy
pharyngospasm

pharyngostaphylinus
pharyngostenosis
pharyngotomy
pharyngotonsillitis
pharyngotympanic
    p. groove
    p. tube
pharynx, gen. **pharyngis**, pl. **pharynges**
    laryngeal p.
    nasal p.
    oral p.
phase
    anal p.
    cis p.
    coupling p.
    eclipse p.
    p. encoding
    eruptive p.
    genital p.
    growth p.
    horizontal growth p.
    p. I block
    p. II block
    p. image
    in p.
    lag p.
    latency p.
    logarithmic p.
    luteal p., short luteal p.
    meiotic p.
    p. microscope
    negative p.
    oedipal p.
    oral p.
    phallic p.
    positive p.
    postmeiotic p.
    postreduction p.
    pregenital p.
    premeiotic p.
    pre-oedipal p.
    prereduction p.
    radial growth p.
    reduction p.
    p. shift
    short luteal p. (*var. of* luteal p.)
    supernormal recovery p.
    synaptic p.
    trans p.
    vertical growth p.
    vulnerable p.
phase-contrast microscope
phasic
    p. reflex
    p. sinus arrhythmia
phasmid
Phasmidia
phasmophobia

phatnorrhagia
P-H conduction time
Phemister graft
phenacetolin
phengophobia
phenocopy
phenol coefficient
phenolemia
phenology
phenolsulfonphthalein test
phenoluria
phenomenology
phenomenon, pl. **phenomena**
    adhesion p.
    AFORMED p.
    Anrep p.
    aqueous influx p.
    Arias-Stella p.
    arm p.
    Arthus p.
    Ascher's aqueous influx p.
    Aschner's p.
    Ashman's p.
    Aubert's p.
    Austin Flint p.
    autoscopic p.
    Babinski's p.
    Bell's p.
    Bombay p.
    Bordet-Gengou p.
    breakoff p., breakaway p.
    Brücke-Bartley p.
    Capgras' p.
    cervicolumbar p.
    cogwheel p.
    constancy p.
    crossed phrenic p.
    Cushing p.
    Danysz p.
    dawn p.
    Debré p.
    declamping p.
    déjà vu p.
    Dejerine-Lichtheim p.
    Dejerine's hand p.
    Denys-Leclef p.
    d'Herelle p.
    dip p.
    Donath-Landsteiner p.
    Doppler p.
    Duckworth's p.
    Ehret's p.
    Ehrlich's p.
    erythrocyte adherence p.
    escape p.
    facialis p.
    finger p.
    Flynn p.

P

phenomenon *(continued)*
    Friedreich's p.
    Galassi's pupillary p.
    Gallavardin's p.
    gap p.
    Gärtner's vein p.
    generalized Shwartzman p.
    Gengou p.
    gestalt p.
    Glover p.
    Goldblatt p.
    Grasset-Gaussel p.
    Grasset's p.
    Gunn p.
    Hill's p.
    hip p.
    hip-flexion p.
    Hoffmann's p.
    hunting p.
    Hunt's paradoxical p.
    immune adherence p.
    jaw-winking p.
    Jod-Basedow p.
    knee p.
    Köbner's p.
    Koch's p.
    Kohnstamm's p.
    Kühne's p.
    LE p.
    Leede-Rumpel p.
    leg p.
    Leichtenstern's p.
    Lucio's leprosy p.
    Marcus Gunn p.
    misdirection p.
    Mitsuo's p.
    Negro's p.
    no reflow p.
    on-off p.
    orbicularis p.
    paradoxical diaphragm p.
    paradoxical pupillary p.
    peroneal p.
    Pfeiffer's p.
    phi p.
    Pool's p.
    pseudo-Graefe's p.
    psi p.
    Purkinje's p.
    quellung p.
    radial p.
    Raynaud's p.
    rebound p.
    red cell adherence p.
    reentry p.
    release p.
    Ritter-Rollet p.
    R-on-T p.

    Rumpel-Leede p.
    Rust's p.
    Sanarelli p.
    Sanarelli-Shwartzman p.
    Schellong-Strisower p.
    Schiff-Sherrington p.
    Schüller's p.
    Schultz-Charlton p.
    Sherrington p.
    shot-silk p.
    Shwartzman p.
    Somogyi p.
    Splendore-Hoeppli p.
    staircase p.
    Staub-Traugott p.
    steal p.
    Strassman's p.
    Strümpell's p.
    Theobald Smith's p.
    tibial p.
    toe p.
    tongue p.
    Tournay's p.
    Tullio's p.
    Twort p.
    Twort-d'Herelle p.
    Tyndall p.
    vacuum disk p.
    Wenckebach p.
    Westphal-Piltz p.
    Westphal's p.
    Wever-Bray p.

phenotype
phenotypic
    p. mixing
    p. threshold
    p. value
phenozygous
phentolamine test
phenylamine
phenylhydrazine hemolysis
phenylpyruvic amentia
pheochrome
    p. cell
pheochromoblast
pheochromoblastoma
pheochromocyte
pheochromocytoma
pheomelanogenesis
pheomelanosome
pheresis
phialide
phialoconidium, pl. **phialoconidia**
Phialophora
Phialophore-type conidiophore
Philadelphia chromosome
philanthropic hospital
philiater

Philippe's triangle
Philippine hemorrhagic fever
Philip's glands
Phillips' catheter
Phillipson's reflex
philomimesia
Philopia casei
philoprogenitive
phimosis, pl. **phimoses**
    p. clitoridis
    p. vaginalis
phimotic
phi phenomenon
phlebalgia
phlebectasia
phlebectomy
phlebeurysm
phlebitic
phlebitis
    adhesive p.
    p. nodularis necrotisans
    puerperal p.
    septic p.
    sinus p.
phleboclysis
    drip p.
phlebodynamics
phlebogram
phlebograph
phlebography
phleboid
phlebolite
phlebolith
phlebolithiasis
phlebology
phlebomanometer
phlebometritis
phlebomyomatosis
phlebophlebostomy
phleboplasty
phleborrhagia
phleborrhaphy
phleborrhexis
phlebosclerosis
phlebostasis
phlebostenosis
phlebostrepsis
phlebothrombosis
phlebotomine
phlebotomist
Phlebotomus
    P. argentipes
    P. chinensis
    P. flaviscutellatus
    P. longipalpis
    P. major
    P. noguchi
    P. orientalis

    P. papatasii
    P. perniciosus
    P. sergenti
    P. verrucarum
phlebotomus
    p. fever
    p. fever viruses
phlebotomy
    bloodless p.
Phlebovirus
phlegm
phlegmasia
    p. alba dolens
    cellulitic p.
    p. cerulea dolens
    p. dolens
    p. malabarica
    thrombotic p.
phlegmatic
phlegmon
    diffuse p.
    emphysematous p.
    gas p.
phlegmonous
    p. abscess
    p. cellulitis
    p. enteritis
    p. erysipelas
    p. gastritis
    p. mastitis
    p. ulcer
phlogocyte
phlogocytosis
phlogogenic, phlogogenous
phlogosin
phlogotherapy
phloridzin glycosuria
phlorizin
    p. diabetes
    p. glycosuria
phloxine
phlyctena, pl. **phlyctenae**
phlyctenar
phlyctenoid
phlyctenosis
phlyctenous
phlyctenula, pl. **phlyctenulae**
phlyctenular
    p. conjunctivitis
    p. keratitis
    p. ophthalmia
    p. pannus
phlyctenule
phlyctenulosis
phobanthropy
phobia
    school p.
phobic

P

phobophobia
phocomelia, phocomely
phocomelic dwarfism
Phoma
phonacoscope
phonacoscopy
phonal
phonarteriogram
phonarteriography
phonasthenia
phonation
phonatory
phoneme
phonemic
    p. regression
phonendoscope
phonetic
phonetics
phoniatrics
phonic
    p. spasm
phonoangiography
phonocardiogram
phonocardiograph
    linear p.
    logarithmic p.
    spectral p.
    stethoscopic p.
phonocardiography
phonocatheter
phonogram
phonology
phonomania
phonometer
phonomyoclonus
phonomyography
phonopathy
phonophobia
phonophore
phonophotography
phonopsia
phonoreceptor
phonoscope
phonoscopy
phonosurgery
phoresy
phoria
Phoroptor
phorozoon
phosphastat
phosphate
    p. diabetes
    p. tetany
phosphatemia
phosphaturia
phosphene
    accommodation p.
phosphohexose isomerase deficiency

phospholipid syndrome
phosphopenia
phosphor
    photostimulable p.
    p. plate
phosphorhidrosis
phosphoridrosis
phosphorpenia
phosphoruria
phosphotungstic
    p. acid hematoxylin
    p. acid stain
phosphotungstic acid
phosphuresis
phosphuria
phot
photalgia
photaugiaphobia
photechic effect
photesthesia
photic
    p. driving
    p. stimulation
photism
photoablation
photoactinic
photoallergic sensitivity
photoallergy
photoautotrophic
Photobacterium
    P. harveyi
    P. phosphoreum
photobacterium, pl. photobacteria
photobiology
photobiotic
photo cell
photoceptor
photochemotherapy
photochromic
    p. lens
    p. spectacles
photochromogens
photocoagulation
photocoagulator
    laser p.
    xenon-arc p.
photodermatitis
photodistribution
photodynamic sensitization
photodynia
photodysphoria
photoelectric absorption
photoerythema
photoesthetic
photofluorography
photogastroscope
photogen
photogenic epilepsy

photohemotachometer
photoheterotrophic
photoinactivation
photokeratoscope
photokinesis
photokinetic
photokinetics
photokymograph
photomacrography
photomania
photometer
    flame p.
    flicker p.
photometry
photomicrograph
photomicrography
photomultiplier tube
photomyoclonus
    hereditary p.
photon
    p. density
photoncia
photonosus
photo-patch test
photopathy
photopeak
photoperceptive
photoperiodism
photophobia
photophobic
photophore
photophoresis
    extracorporeal p.
photophthalmia
photopia
photopic
    p. adaptation
    p. eye
    p. vision
photopsia
photopsy
photoptarmosis
photoradiation
    p. therapy
photoreceptive
photoreceptor
    p. cells
photorefractive keratectomy
photoretinitis
photoretinopathy
photoscan
photosensitive
photosensitivity
photosensitization
photosensor
    p. oculography
photostethoscope
photostimulable phosphor

photostress
    p. test
phototherapy
photothermal
phototimer
phototoxic
    p. sensitivity
phototoxis
photuria
phragmoplast
phren
phrenalgia
phrenectomy
phrenemphraxis
phrenetic
phrenic
    p. ampulla
    p. ganglia
    p. nerve
    p. nucleus
    p. pleura
    p. plexus
    p. pressure test
    p. veins
phrenicectomy
phreniclasia
phrenicoabdominal branch of phrenic
  nerve
phrenicocolic
    p. ligament
phrenicocostal sinus
phrenicoexeresis
phrenicogastric
phrenicoglottic, phrenoglottic
phrenicohepatic
phrenicolienal ligament
phrenicomediastinal recess
phreniconeurectomy
phrenicopleural fascia
phrenicosplenic, phrenosplenic
    p. ligament
phrenicotomy
phrenicotripsy
phrenocardia
phrenocolic
phrenocolopexy
phrenogastric
    p. ligament
phrenoglottic (*var. of* phrenicoglottic)
phrenograph
phrenohepatic
phrenologist
phrenology
phrenopericardial angle
phrenoplegia
phrenoptosia
phrenospasm

P

phrenosplenic (*var. of* phrenicosplenic)
    p. ligament
phrenotropic
phrictopathic
phrygian cap
phrynoderma
phthalein test
phthinoid
    p. chest
phthiriophobia
Phthirus
phthisic, phthisical
phthisiologist
phthisis
    aneurysmal p.
    p. bulbi
    essential p. bulbi
    marble cutters' p.
Phycomycetes
phycomycetosis
phycomycosis
    subcutaneous p.
phylacagogic
phylaxis
phyletic
phyllode
phyllodes tumor
phyloanalysis
phylogenesis
phylogenetic, phylogenic
phylogeny
phyma
phymatoid
phymatorrhysin
phymatosis
Physa
physaliferous
physaliform
physaliphore
physaliphorous
    p. cell
physalis
Physaloptera
physeal
physiatrician
physiatrics
physiatrist
physiatry
physical
    p. age
    p. allergy
    p. anthropology
    p. diagnosis
    p. elasticity of muscle
    p. examination
    p. fitness
    p. half-life
    p. medicine

    p. sign
    p. therapy
physician
    p. assistant
    attending p.
    family p.
    osteopathic p.
    resident p.
Physick's pouches
physics
    radiation p.
physiogenic
physiognomy
physiognosis
physiologic
    p. age
    p. albuminuria
    p. amenorrhea
    p. anemia
    p. anisocoria
    p. congestion
    p. cup
    p. dead space
    p. dwarfism
    p. elasticity of muscle
    p. equilibrium
    p. excavation
    p. hypertrophy
    p. icterus
    p. jaundice
    p. leukocytosis
    p. occlusion
    p. rest position
    p. retraction ring
    p. sclerosis
    p. scotoma
    p. tremor
    p. unit
    p. vertigo
physiological
    p. anatomy
    p. drives
    p. sphincter
physiologically balanced occlusion
physiologicoanatomical
physiologist
physiology
    comparative p.
    general p.
    hominal p.
    pathologic p.
physiomedical
physiopathologic
physiopathology
physiopsychic
physiopyrexia
physiotherapeutic
physiotherapist

physiotherapy
    oral p.
physique
physocele
Physocephalus sexalatus
physocephaly
physometra
Physopsis
physopyosalpinx
phytoagglutinin
phytodermatitis
Phytoflagellata
phytoid
Phytomastigina
Phytomastigophorasida
Phytomastigophorea
phytomitogen
phytophagous
phytophlyctodermatitis
phytophotodermatitis
phytopneumoconiosis
phytosis
pi
    p. cone monochromatism
pia
pia-arachnitis
pia-arachnoid
pial
    p. funnel
pial-glial membrane
pia mater
    p. m. cranialis [encephali]
    p. m. spinalis
pian
    p. bois
    hemorrhagic p.
pianist's cramp
piano percussion
piano-player's cramp
piarachnoid
piblokto, pibloktog
pica
Picchini
Picchini's syndrome
Pick cell
picker's nodules
pickling
Pick's
    P. atrophy
    P. bodies
    P. bundle
    P. disease
    P. syndrome
    P. tubular adenoma
pickwickian syndrome
Picornaviridae
picornavirus

picrocarmine
    p. stain
picroformol
    p. fixative
picro-Mallory trichrome stain
picronigrosin
    p. stain
pictograph
picture
    p. element
    p. frame vertebra
piebald
    p. eyelash
    p. skin
piebaldism
piebaldness
piece
    end p.
    Fab p.
    Fc p.
    middle p.
    principal p.
piedra
    black p.
    p. nostras
    white p.
Piedraia
pieds terminaux
Pierre Robin syndrome
piesesthesia
piesimeter, piesometer
    Hales' p.
piesis
piezoelectric
    p. effect
    p. transducer
piezogenic
    p. pedal papule
PIG
pigbel
pigeon
    p. breast
    p. chest
pigment
    p. cell
    p. cells of iris
    p. cell of skin
    p. cells of retina
    p. cirrhosis
    p. epitheliopathy
    p. epithelium
    p. epithelium of optic retina
    formalin p.
    hematogenous p.
    hepatogenous p.
    p. induration of the lung
    malarial p.

P

pigmentary
    p. cirrhosis
    p. glaucoma
    p. retinopathy
    p. syphilid
pigmentation
    arsenic p.
    exogenous p.
pigmented
    p. ameloblastoma
    p. dermatofibrosarcoma protuberans
    p. epulis
    p. hair epidermal nevus
    p. keratic precipitates
    p. layer of ciliary body
    p. layer of iris
    p. layer of retina
    p. liver
    p. part of retina
    p. purpuric lichenoid dermatosis
    p. villonodular synovitis
pigmentolysin
pigmentum nigrum
pigmy
Pignet's formula
pig skin
pigtail catheter
pilar, pilary
    p. cyst
    p. tumor of scalp
pile
    sentinel p.
pileous
    p. gland
piles
pileus
pili (*pl. of* pilus)
piliferous cyst
pilimiction
pilin
pillar
    anterior p. of fauces
    anterior p. of fornix
    p. cells
    p. cells of Corti
    Corti's p.'s
    p.'s of fauces
    p.'s of fornix
    p. of iris
    posterior p. of fauces
    posterior p. of fornix
pill-rolling
    p.-r. tremor
pilocystic
piloerection
piloid
    p. astrocytoma
    p. gliosis

pilojection
pilomatrixoma
pilomotor
    p. fibers
    p. reflex
pilon fracture
pilonidal
    p. cyst
    p. fistula
    p. sinus
pilose
pilosebaceous
pilosis
Piltz sign
pilus, pl. **pili**
    pili annulati
    F p.
    F pili
    I pili
    pili multigemini
    R pili
    pili torti
pimelorrhea
pimelorthopnea
pimple
pin
    p. amalgam
    p. implant
    Steinmann p.
pinacyanol
Pinard's maneuver
pincement
pincer nail
pinch graft
Pindborg tumor
pineal
    p. body
    p. cells
    p. cyst
    p. eye
    p. gland
    p. habenula
    p. recess
    p. stalk
pinealectomy
pinealocyte
pinealoma
    ectopic p.
    extrapineal p.
pinealopathy
Pinel's system
pineoblastoma
pineocytoma
ping-pong
    p.-p. bone
    p.-p. fracture
pinguecula, pinguicula
pinhole pupil

piniform
pink
    p. bread mold
    p. disease
Pinkus tumor
pinledge
pinna, pl. pinnae
    p. nasi
pinnal
pinocyte
pinocytosis
pinocytotic vesicle
pinosome
Pins'
    P. sign
    P. syndrome
pinta
    p. fever
pintids
pintoid
pinus
pinworm
    p. vaginitis
piorthopnea
pipe
    p. bone
    p. stem cirrhosis
pipecuronium
Piper's forceps
pipe-smoker's cancer
pipestem
    p. arteries
    p. fibrosis
pipette, pipet
    blowout p.
    graduated p.
    Mohr p.
    Pasteur p.
    serologic p.
PIP joints
Pirenella
Pirie's bone
piriform
    p. area
    p. cortex
    p. fossa
    p. muscle
    p. neuron layer
    p. opening
    p. recess
    p. sinus
piriformis muscle
Pirogoff's
    P. amputation
    P. angle
    P. triangle
Piroplasmida

Pirquet's
    P. index
    P. reaction
    P. test
pisciform cataract
pisiform
    p. bone
pisohamate ligament
pisometacarpal ligament
pisotriquetral joint
pisounciform ligament
pisouncinate ligament
pistol-shot
    p.-s. femoral sound
    p.-s. sound
piston pulse
pit
    anal p.
    articular p. of head of radius
    p. of atlas for dens
    auditory p.'s
    buccal p.
    p. carics
    central p.
    commisural p.'s
    costal p. of transverse process
    p. and fissure caries
    gastric p.
    granular p.'s
    p. of head of femur
    inferior articular p. of atlas
    inferior costal p.
    iris p.'s
    lens p.'s
    lip p.'s
    Mantoux p.
    nail p.'s
    nasal p.'s
    oblong p. of arytenoid cartilage
    olfactory p.'s
    optic p.
    otic p.'s
    postnatal p. of the newborn
    primitive p.
    pterygoid p.
    p. of stomach
    sublingual p.
    superior articular p. of atlas
    superior costal p.
    suprameatal p.
    triangular p. of arytenoid cartilage
    trochlear p.
pitch wart
pitch-worker's cancer
pithecoid
pithode
Pitot tube

P

Pitres'
> P. area
> P. sign

pitted keratolysis

pitting
> p. edema

Pittsburgh
> P. pneumonia
> P. pneumonia agent

pituicyte

pituicytoma

pituita

pituitarism

pituitarium

pituitary
> p. adamantinoma
> p. adenoma
> p. ameloblastoma
> p. apoplexy
> p. cachexia
> p. diverticulum
> p. dwarf
> p. dwarfism
> p. fossa
> p. gigantism
> p. gland
> p. infantilism
> p. membrane
> p. myxedema
> pharyngeal p.
> p. stalk
> p. stalk section

pituitous

pityriasic

pityriasis
> p. alba
> p. alba atrophicans
> p. amiantacea
> p. capitis
> p. circinata
> p. lichenoides
> p. lichenoides chronica
> p. lichenoides et varioliformis acuta
> p. linguae
> p. maculata
> p. nigra
> p. rosea
> p. rubra
> p. rubra pilaris
> p. sicca
> p. versicolor

pityroid

Pityrosporum
> P. orbiculare
> P. ovale

pivot
> adjustable occlusal p.
> p. joint

> occlusal p.
> p. shift test

pixel

P-J interval

P-K
> P.-K. antibodies
> P.-K. test

pkv

placebo
> active p.

placenta
> accessory p.
> p. accreta
> p. accreta vera
> adherent p.
> annular p.
> battledore p.
> bidiscoidal p.
> p. biloba
> p. bipartita
> central p. previa
> chorioallantoic p.
> chorioamnionic p.
> p. circumvallata
> cotyledonary p.
> deciduate p.
> dichorionic diamniotic p.
> dichorionic diamniotic p. (*var. of* twin p.)
> p. diffusa
> p. dimidiata
> disperse p.
> p. duplex
> endotheliochorial p.
> endothelio-endothelial p.
> epitheliochorial p.
> p. extrachorales
> p. fenestrata
> fetal p., p. fetalis
> hemochorial p.
> hemoendothelial p.
> horseshoe p.
> incarcerated p.
> p. increta
> labyrinthine p.
> p. marginata
> maternal p.
> p. membranacea
> monochorionic diamniotic p. (*var. of* twin p.)
> monochorionic diamniotic p.
> monochorionic monoamniotic p. (*var. of* twin p.)
> monochorionic monoamniotic p.
> p. multiloba
> nondeciduous p.
> p. panduraformis
> p. percreta

placenta sercreta (strickler) [handwritten]

p. previa
p. previa centralis
p. previa marginalis
p. previa partialis
p. reflexa
p. reniformis
retained p.
Schultze's p.
p. spuria
succenturiate p.
supernumerary p.
total p. previa
p. triloba
p. tripartita
p. triplex
twin p., dichorionic diamniotic p., monochorionic diamniotic p., monochorionic monoamniotic p.
p. uterina
p. velamentosa
villous p.
zonary p.

placental
p. barrier
p. circulation
p. dysfunction
p. dysfunction syndrome
p. dysmature
p. dystocia
p. lobes
p. membrane
p. multipartita
p. parasitic twin
p. plasmodium
p. polyp
p. presentation
p. septa
p. site trophoblastic tumor
p. souffle
p. sulfatase deficiency
p. thrombosis
p. transfusion

placentascan
placentation
placentitis
placentography
indirect p.
placentoma
placentotherapy
place theory
Placido da Costa's disk
placode
auditory p.'s
epibranchial p.'s
lens p.'s
nasal p.'s
olfactory p.'s

optic p.'s
otic p.'s
pladaroma, pladarosis
plafond
plagiocephalic
plagiocephalism
plagiocephalous
plagiocephaly
plague
ambulant p., ambulatory p.
p. bacillus
black p.
bubonic p.
glandular p.
hemorrhagic p.
larval p.
Pahvant Valley p.
p. pneumonia
pneumonic p.
pulmonic p.
p. septicemia
septicemic p.
plain film
plakins
plana (*pl. of* planum)
plane
Addison's clinical p.'s
Aeby's p.
auriculo-infraorbital p.
axial p.
axiolabiolingual p.
axiomesiodistal p.
bite p.
Bolton p.
Bolton-Broadbent p.
Bolton-nasion p.
Broca's visual p.
Camper's p.
canthomeatal p.
coronal p.
cove p.
datum p.
Daubenton's p.
equatorial p.
eye-ear p.
facial p.
first parallel pelvic p.
fourth parallel pelvic p.
Frankfort p.
Frankfort horizontal p.
frontal p.
guide p.
horizontal p.
p. of incidence
infraorbitomeatal p.
p. of inlet
interspinal p.
intertubercular p.

P

plane *(continued)*
    p. joint
    labiolingual p.
    p. of least pelvic dimensions
    mean foundation p.
    Meckel's p.
    median p.
    p. of midpelvis
    midsagittal p.
    Morton's p.
    nasion-postcondylar p.
    nodal p.
    nuchal p.
    occipital p.
    occlusal p., p. of occlusion
    orbital p.
    orbitomeatal p.
    p. of outlet
    parasagittal p.
    p. of pelvic canal
    pelvic p. of greatest dimensions
    pelvic p. of inlet
    pelvic p. of least dimensions
    pelvic p. of outlet
    popliteal p. of femur
    principal p.
    p.'s of reference
    p. of regard
    sagittal p.
    second parallel pelvic p.
    spectacle p.
    sternal p.
    subcostal p.
    supracrestal p.
    supracristal p.
    supraorbitomeatal p.
    suprasternal p.
    p. suture
    temporal p.
    third parallel pelvic p.
    tooth p.
    transaxial p.
    transpyloric p.
    transverse p.
    p. wart
    wide p.
planigraphy
planimeter
planimetry
planing
planithorax
plankter
plankton
planktonic
planocellular
planoconcave
    p. lens

planoconvex
    p. lens
planography
planomania
Planorbis
planotopokinesia
planovalgus
plant
    p. agglutinin
    p. dermatitis
    p. viruses
planta, gen. and pl. **plantae**
    p. pedis
plantalgia
plantar
    p. aponeurosis
    p. arch
    p. arterial arch
    p. calcaneocuboid ligament
    p. calcaneonavicular ligament
    p. cuboideonavicular ligament
    p. cuneocuboid ligament
    p. cuneonavicular ligaments
    p. digital veins
    p. fascia
    p. fibromatosis
    p. flexion
    p. interosseous muscle
    p. ligaments
    p. metatarsal artery
    p. metatarsal ligaments
    p. metatarsal veins
    p. muscle
    p. muscle reflex
    p. quadrate muscle
    p. reflex
    p. space
    p. surface of toe
    p. syphilid
    p. tendon sheath of peroneus
      longus muscle
    p. venous arch
    p. venous network
    p. wart
plantaris
    p. muscle
planula, pl. **planulae**
    invaginate p.
planum, pl. **plana**
    p. interspinale
    p. intertuberculare
    p. occipitale
    p. orbitale
    p. popliteum
    p. semilunatum
    p. sphenoidale
    p. sternale
    p. subcostale

p. supracristale
p. temporale
p. transpyloricum

planuria

plaque
atheromatous p.
bacterial p.
bacteriophage p.
dental p.
Hollenhorst p.'s
P. Index
mucous p., mucinous p.
neuritic p.
pleural p.
Randall's p.'s
senile p.

plasma
p. accelerator globulin
p. cell
p. cell balanitis
p. cell dyscrasia
p. cell gingivitis
p. cell hepatitis
p. cell leukemia
p. cell mastitis
p. cell myeloma
p. factor X
p. fibronectin
p. iodoprotein disorder
p. labile factor
p. layer
p. marinum
p. membrane
normal human p.
p. renin activity
salted p.
p. scalpel
p. stain
p. therapy
p. thromboplastin antecedent
p. thromboplastin component
p. thromboplastin factor
p. thromboplastin factor B

plasmablast

plasmacrit
p. test

plasmacyte

plasmacytoblast

plasmacytoma

plasmacytosis

plasmagene

plasmalemma

plasmal reaction

plasmapheresis

plasmapheretic

plasmatic
p. stain

plasmatogamy

plasmic
p. stain

plasmid
bacteriocinogenic p.'s
conjugative p.
F p.
infectious p.
nonconjugative p.
R p.'s
resistance p.'s
transmissible p.

plasmin prothrombins conversion factor

plasmocytic leukemoid reaction

plasmodia (*pl. of* plasmodium)

plasmodial
p. trophoblast

plasmodiotrophoblast

Plasmodium
P. aethiopicum
P. berghei
P. falciparum
P. knowlesi
P. kochi
P. malariae
P. ovale
P. vivax

plasmodium, pl. plasmodia
placental p.

Plasmodromata

plasmogamy

plasmogen

plasmokinin

plasmolemma

plasmolysis

plasmolytic

plasmolyze

plasmorrhexis

plasmoschisis

plasmotomy

plasmotropic

plasmotropism

plasmotype

plasmozyme

plaster
p. bandage
p. of Paris disease
p. splint

plastic
p. anatomy
Bingham p.
p. bronchitis
p. corpuscle
p. cyclitis
p. induration
p. iritis
p. lymph
modeling p.
p. motor

P

691

plastic *(continued)*
    p. operation
    p. pleurisy
    p. restoration material
    p. section stain
    p. surgery
    p. teeth
plasticity
plastid
    blood p.
plastogamy
plastron
plasty
plate
    alar p. of neural tube
    anal p.
    axial p.
    basal p. of neural tube
    base p.
    blood p.
    bone p.
    buttress p.
    cardiogenic p.
    chorionic p.
    cloacal p.
    cribriform p. of ethmoid bone
    cutis p.
    dorsal p. of neural tube
    dorsolateral p. of neural tube
    end p.
    epiphysial p.
    equatorial p.
    ethmovomerine p.
    flat p.
    floor p.
    foot p.
    frontal p.
    horizontal p. of palatine bone
    Kühne's p.
    Lane's p.'s
    lateral p.
    lateral pterygoid p.
    lateral p. of pterygoid process
    lingual p.
    medial pterygoid p.
    medial p. of pterygoid process
    medullary p.
    p. of modiolus
    motor p.
    muscle p.
    nail p.
    neural p.
    neutralization p.
    notochordal p.
    oral p.
    orbital p.
    orbital p. of ethmoid bone
    palatal p.

    paper p., papyraceous p.
    parachordal p.
    parietal p.
    perpendicular p.
    perpendicular p. of ethmoid bone
    perpendicular p. of palatine bone
    phosphor p.
    polar p.'s
    prechordal p.
    prochordal p.
    pterygoid p.'s
    quadrigeminal p.
    roof p.
    secondary spiral p.
    segmental p.
    sieve p.
    spiral p.
    suction p.
    tarsal p.'s
    terminal p.
    p. thrombosis
    tympanic p. of temporal bone
    urethral p.
    ventral p.
    ventral p. of neural tube
    vertical p.
    visceral p.
    wing p.
plateau
    p. iris
    p. pulse
    ventricular p.
Plateau-Talbot law
platelet
    p. actomyosin
    p. aggregation test
    p. cofactor I
    p. cofactor II
    p. factor 3
    p. thrombosis
    p. tissue factor
platelet-activating factor
platelet-aggregating factor
plateletpheresis
platelike atelectasis
plating
    compression p.
    replica p.
platinum foil
platybasia
platycephaly
platycnemia
platycnemic
platycnemism
platycrania
platycyte
platyglossal
platyhelminth

Platyhelminthes
platyhieric
platymeric
platymorphia
platyopia
platyopic
platypellic
    p. pelvis
platypelloid
    p. pelvis
platypnea
platyrrhine
platyrrhiny
platysma, pl. **platysmas, platysmata**
    p. muscle
platyspondylia, platyspondylisis
platystencephaly
Plaut's bacillus
play therapy
Pleasure
    P. curve
pleasure principle
plectridium
pledgetted suture
pleiotropic
    p. gene
pleiotropy, pleiotropia
    functional p.
    structural p.
Pleistophora
pleochroic
pleochroism
pleochromatic
pleochromatism
pleocytosis
pleomastia, pleomazia
pleomorphic
    p. adenoma
    p. lipoma
    p. oligodendroglioma
    p. xanthoastrocytoma
pleomorphism
pleomorphous
pleonasm
pleonectic
pleonexia
pleonosteosis
    Leri's p.
pleoptics
pleoptophor
plerocercoid
Piesiomonas
    P. shigelloides
plesiomorphic
plesiomorphism
plesiomorphous
plessesthesia
plessimeter

plessimetric
plessor
plethora
plethoric
plethysmograph
    body p.
    digital p.
    pressure p.
    volume-displacement p.
plethysmographic goggle
plethysmography
    impedance p.
    venous occlusion p.
plethysmometry
pleura, gen. and pl. **pleurae**
    cervical p.
    costal p.
    p. costalis
    diaphragmatic p.
    p. diaphragmatica
    mediastinal p.
    p. mediastinalis
    parietal p.
    p. parietalis
    p. pericardiaca, pericardial p.
    phrenic p.
    p. phrenica
    p. pulmonalis
    pulmonary p.
    visceral p.
    p. visceralis
pleuracentesis
pleural
    p. calculus
    p. canal
    p. cavity
    p. crackles
    p. cupula
    p. effusion
    p. fluid
    p. fremitus
    p. friction rub
    p. lines
    p. plaque
    p. poudrage
    p. pressure
    p. rale
    p. reaction
    p. recesses
    p. rub
    p. sinuses
    p. space
    p. stripe
    p. villi
pleuralgia
pleurapophysis
pleurectomy

P

pleurisy
    adhesive p.
    benign dry p.
    bilateral p.
    chronic p.
    costal p.
    diaphragmatic p.
    double p.
    dry p.
    encysted p.
    epidemic benign dry p.
    epidemic diaphragmatic p.
    fibrinous p.
    hemorrhagic p.
    interlobular p.
    mediastinal p.
    plastic p.
    productive p.
    proliferating p.
    pulmonary p.
    purulent p.
    sacculated p.
    serofibrinous p.
    serous p.
    suppurative p.
    typhoid p.
    visceral p.
    wet p.
    p. with effusion
pleuritic
    p. pneumonia
    p. rub
pleuritis
pleuritogenous
pleurocele
pleurocentesis
pleurocentrum
pleuroclysis
pleurodesis
pleurodynia
    epidemic p.
pleuroesophageal
    p. line
    p. muscle
pleurogenic
pleurogenous
pleurography
pleurohepatitis
pleurolith
pleurolysis
pleuropericardial
    p. canals
    p. fold
    p. hiatus
    p. membrane
    p. murmur
pleuropericarditis

pleuroperitoneal
    p. canal
    p. cavity
    p. fold
    p. foramen
    p. hiatus
    p. membrane
pleuropneumonia-like organisms
pleuropulmonary
pleuroscopy
pleurothotonos, pleurothotonus
pleurotomy
pleurotyphoid
pleurovisceral
plexal
plexectomy
plexiform
    p. layer
    p. layer of cerebral cortex
    p. layers of retina
    p. neurofibroma
    p. neuroma
pleximeter
plexitis
    brachial p.
plexogenic
    p. pulmonary arteriopathy
plexometer
plexor
plexus, pl. **plexus, plexuses**
    abdominal aortic p.
    acromial p.
    annular p.
    p. annularis
    p. of anterior cerebral artery
    anterior coronary p.
    aortic lymphatic p.
    p. aorticus
    p. aorticus abdominalis
    p. aorticus thoracicus
    areolar venous p.
    p. arteriae cerebri anterioris
    p. arteriae cerebri mediae
    p. arteriae choroideae
    ascending pharyngeal p.
    Auerbach's p.
    p. auricularis posterior
    autonomic plexuses
    p. autonomici
    p. axillaris
    axillary p.
    basilar p.
    p. basilaris
    Batson's p.
    brachial p.
    p. brachialis
    cardiac p.
    p. cardiacus

p. cardiacus profundus
p. cardiacus superficialis
p. caroticus communis
p. caroticus externus
p. caroticus internus
p. cavernosi concharum
p. cavernosus
cavernous p. of clitoris
cavernous p. of conchae
cavernous p. of penis
celiac p.
celiac (lymphatic) p.
celiac (nervous) p.
p. celiacus
cervical p.
p. cervicalis
choroid p.
p. of choroid artery
p. choroideus
p. choroideus ventriculi lateralis
p. choroideus ventriculi quarti
p. choroideus ventriculi tertii
choroid p. of fourth ventricle
choroid p. of lateral ventricle
choroid p. of third ventricle
ciliary ganglionic p.
coccygeal p.
p. coccygeus
common carotid p.
p. coronarius cordis
coronary p.
Cruveilhier's p.
deep cardiac p.
deferential p.
p. deferentialis
p. dentalis inferior
p. dentalis superior
enteric p.
p. entericus
esophageal p.
p. esophageus
Exner's p.
external carotid p.
external iliac p.
external maxillary p.
facial p.
femoral p.
p. femoralis
p. gangliosus ciliaris
gastric plexuses of autonomic
  system
p. gastrici systematis autonomici
p. gulae
Haller's p.
Heller's p.
hemorrhoidal p.
hepatic p.
p. hepaticus

p. hypogastricus inferior
p. hypogastricus superior
iliac p.
p. iliaci
p. iliacus externus
inferior dental p.
inferior hemorrhoidal plexuses
inferior hypogastric p.
inferior mesenteric p.
inferior rectal plexuses
inferior thyroid p.
inferior vesical p.
inguinal p.
p. inguinalis
intermesenteric p.
p. intermesentericus
internal carotid (nervous) p.
internal carotid venous p.
internal mammary p.
internal maxillary p.
internal thoracic p.
internal thoracic lymphatic p.
intracavernous p.
p. intraparotideus
intraparotid p. of facial nerve
ischiadic p.
Jacobson's p.
Jacques' p.
jugular p.
p. jugularis
Leber's p.
p. lienalis
lingual p.
p. lingualis
p. lumbalis
lumbar p.
lumbosacral p.
p. lumbosacralis
lymphatic p.
p. lymphaticus
p. mammarius
p. mammarius internus
mammary p.
p. maxillaris externus
p. maxillaris internus
maxillary p.
Meissner's p.
meningeal p.
p. meningeus
p. mesentericus inferior
p. mesentericus superior
p. of middle cerebral artery
middle hemorrhoidal plexuses
middle rectal plexuses
middle sacral p.
myenteric p.
p. myentericus
nerve p.

P

plexus *(continued)*
p. nervorum spinalium
p. nervosus
occipital p.
p. occipitalis
ophthalmic p.
p. ophthalmicus
ovarian p.
p. ovaricus
pampiniform p.
p. pampiniformis
pancreatic p.
p. pancreaticus
pelvic p.
p. pelvinus
periarterial p.
p. periarterialis
periarterial p. of maxillary artery
periarterial p. of vertebral artery
pharyngeal p.
p. pharyngeus
p. pharyngeus ascendens
phrenic p., p. phrenicus
popliteal p., p. popliteus
posterior auricular p.
posterior coronary p.
prostatic p.
prostaticovesical p.
p. prostaticovesicalis
p. prostaticus
prostatic venous p.
pterygoid p.
p. pterygoideus
p. pudendalis
p. pudendus nervosus
p. pulmonalis
pulmonary p.
Quénu's hemorrhoidal p.
Ranvier's p.
rectal plexuses
p. rectales inferiores
p. rectales medii
p. rectalis superior
rectal venous p.
Remak's p.
renal p.
p. renalis
sacral p.
p. sacralis
p. sacralis medius
sacral venous p.
Santorini's p.
Sappey's p.
sciatic p.
solar p.
spermatic p.
p. of spinal nerves
splenic p.

p. splenicus
Stensen's p.
stroma p.
subclavian p.
subclavian periarterial p.
p. subclavius
submucosal p.
p. submucosus
suboccipital venous p.
p. subserosus
subserous p.
superficial cardiac p.
superficial temporal p.
superior dental p.
superior hemorrhoidal p.
superior hypogastric p.
superior mesenteric p.
superior rectal p.
superior thyroid p.
suprarenal p.
p. suprarenalis
sympathetic plexuses
p. temporalis superficialis
testicular p.
p. testicularis
thoracic aortic p.
p. thyroideus impar
p. thyroideus inferior
p. thyroideus superior
tympanic p.
p. tympanicus
ureteric p.
p. uretericus
uterine venous p.
uterovaginal p.
p. uterovaginalis
vaginal venous p.
vascular p.
p. vasculosus
p. venosus
p. venosus areolaris
p. venosus canalis hypoglossi
p. venosus caroticus internus
p. venosus foraminis ovalis
p. venosus prostaticus
p. venosus rectalis
p. venosus sacralis
p. venosus suboccipitalis
p. venosus uterinus
p. venosus vaginalis
p. venosus vertebralis, p. venosus
    vertebralis externus anterior, p.
    venosus vertebralis externus
    posterior, p. venosus vertebralis
    internus anterior, p. venosus
    vertebralis internus posterior
p. venosus vesicalis
venous p.

venous p. of bladder
venous p. of foramen ovale
venous p. of hypoglossal canal
vertebral p.
p. vertebralis
vertebral venous p.
vesical p.
p. vesicalis
p. vesicalis inferior
vesicular venous p.
Walther's p.

plica, gen. and pl. **plicae**
plicae adiposae
plicae alares
plicae ampullares tubae uterinae
p. aryepiglottica
p. axillaris
plicae cecales
p. cecalis vascularis
p. chordae tympani
p. choroidea
plicae ciliares
plicae circulares
p. duodenalis inferior
p. duodenalis superior
p. duodenojejunalis
p. duodenomesocolica
p. epigastrica
plicae epiglottica
p. fimbriata
plicae gastricae
plicae gastropancreaticae
p. glossoepiglottica lateralis
p. glossoepiglottica mediana
p. gubernatrix
p. hypogastrica
p. ileocecalis
p. incudis
p. inguinalis
p. interdigitalis
p. interureterica
plicae iridis
p. lacrimalis
p. longitudinalis duodeni
p. lunata
p. mallearis
p. membranae tympani
p. nervi laryngei
p. palatina transversa
plicae palmatae
p. palpebronasalis
p. paraduodenalis
plicae recti
p. rectouterina
p. rectovaginalis
p. salpingopalatina
p. salpingopharyngea
p. semilunaris

p. semilunaris of colon
p. semilunaris of eye
p. sigmoidea
p. spiralis ductus cystici
p. stapedis
p. sublingualis
p. synovialis
p. synovialis infrapatellaris
p. synovialis patellaris
plicae transversales recti
p. triangularis
plicae tubariae tubae uterinae
p. tubopalatina
plicae tunicae mucosae vesicae
    felleae
p. umbilicalis lateralis
p. umbilicalis media
p. umbilicalis medialis
p. umbilicalis mediana
p. urachi
p. ureterica
p. uterovesicalis
p. venae cavae sinistrae
p. ventricularis
p. vesicalis transversa
p. vesicouterina
p. vestibularis
p. vestibuli
p. villosa
p. vocalis

plicate
plication
plicotomy
Plimmer's bodies
plocytic astrocytoma
ploidy
plombage
plosive
Plotz bacillus
plug
    Dittrich's p.'s
    epithelial p.
    laminated epithelial p.
    mucous p.
    Traube's p.'s
plugger
    automatic p.
    back-action p.
    foot p.
    root canal p.
plugging instrument
Plummer's
    P. dilator
    P. disease
Plummer-Vinson syndrome
plumose
plural pregnancy
pluricausal

P

pluriglandular
plurilocular
plurinuclear
pluripotent, pluripotential
    p. cells
pluriresistant
plus
    p. lens
    p. strand
plutomania
plutonism
PMA index
P-mitrale
pneocardiac reflex
pneodynamics
pneometer
pneometry
pneopneic reflex
pneoscope
pneumarthrogram
pneumarthrography
pneumarthrosis
pneumatic
    p. antishock garment
    p. bone
    p. otoscopy
    p. retinopexy
    p. space
    p. tire injury
    p. tonometer
pneumatinuria
pneumatization
pneumatized
pneumatocardia
pneumatocele
    extracranial p.
    intracranial p.
pneumatoenteric
    p. recess
pneumatohemia
pneumatometer
pneumatorrhachis
pneumatoscope
pneumatosis
    p. coli
    p. cystoides intestinalis
pneumaturia
pneumatype
pneumoangiography
pneumoarthrography
pneumobacillus
pneumobulbar
pneumocardial
pneumocele
    extracranial p.
    intracranial p.
pneumocentesis
pneumocephalus

pneumocholecystitis
pneumococcal
    p. empyema
    p. pneumonia
pneumococcal/suppurative keratitis
pneumococcemia
pneumococci (*pl. of* pneumococcus)
pneumococcidal
pneumococcolysis
pneumococcosis
pneumococcosuria
pneumococcus, pl. pneumococci
    Fraenkel's p.
    Fraenkel-Weichselbaum p.
pneumocolon
pneumoconiosis, pneumokoniosis,
    pl. pneumoconioses
        bauxite p.
        p. of coal workers
        collagenous p.
        p. siderotica
pneumocranium
Pneumocystis carinii
pneumocystography
pneumocystosis
pneumocyte
pneumoderma
pneumodynamics
pneumoempyema
pneumoencephalogram
pneumoencephalography
pneumoenteric recess
pneumogastric
    p. nerve
pneumogastrography
pneumogenic osteoarthropathy
pneumogram
pneumograph
pneumography
pneumohemia
pneumohemopericardium
pneumohemothorax
pneumohydrometra
pneumohydropericardium
pneumohydroperitoneum
pneumohydrothorax
pneumohypoderma
pneumokoniosis (*var. of* pneumoconiosis)
pneumokoniosis
pneumolith
pneumolithiasis
pneumology
pneumolysis
pneumomalacia
pneumomassage
pneumomediastinum
pneumomelanosis
pneumometer

pneumometry
pneumomycosis
pneumomyelography
pneumonectomy
pneumonia
  acute interstitial p.
  alcoholic p.
  anthrax p.
  apex p., apical p.
  aspiration p.
  atypical p.
  bacterial p.
  bilious p.
  bronchial p.
  caseous p.
  central p.
  chemical p.
  chronic p.
  chronic eosinophilic p.
  congenital p.
  contusion p.
  core p.
  deglutition p.
  desquamative p.
  desquamative interstitial p.
  p. dissecans
  double p.
  Eaton agent p.
  embolic p.
  eosinophilic p.
  fibrous p.
  Friedländer's p.
  Friedländer's bacillus p.
  gangrenous p.
  giant cell p.
  Hecht's p.
  hypostatic p.
  influenzal p.
  influenzal virus p.
  p. interlobularis purulenta
  interstitial giant cell p.
  interstitial plasma cell p.
  intrauterine p.
  lipid p., lipoid p.
  lobar p.
  lymphocytic interstitial p.
  lymphoid interstitial p.
  p. malleosa
  metastatic p.
  migratory p.
  moniliasis p.
  mycoplasmal p.
  obstructive p.
  oil p.
  organized p.
  Pittsburgh p.
  plague p.
  pleuritic p.

  pneumococcal p.
  postoperative p.
  primary atypical p.
  purulent p.
  rheumatic p.
  septic p.
  staphylococcal p.
  streptococcal p.
  suppurative p.
  terminal p.
  traumatic p.
  tularemic p.
  typhoid p.
  unresolved p.
  uremic p.
  usual interstitial p. of Liebow
  p. virus of mice
  wandering p.
  woolsorter's p.
pneumonic
  p. plague
pneumonitis
  acute interstitial p.
  hypersensitivity p.
  lymphocytic interstitial p.
  radiation p.
  uremic p.
pneumonocele
pneumonocentesis
pneumonococcal
pneumonococcus
pneumonoconiosis, pneumonokoniosis
pneumonocyte
  granular p.'s
  phagocytic p.
pneumonokoniosis
pneumonomelanosis
pneumonomoniliasis
pneumonomycosis
pneumonopathy
  eosinophilic p.
pneumonopexy
pneumonopleuritis
pneumonorrhaphy
pneumonotomy
pneumo-orbitography
pneumopericardium
pneumoperitoneum
pneumoperitonitis
pneumopexy
pneumophagia
pneumopleuritis
pneumopyelography
pneumopyothorax
pneumoradiography
pneumoresection
pneumoretroperitoneum
pneumoroentgenography

P

pneumorrhachis
pneumoscope
pneumoserothorax
pneumosilicosis
pneumotachogram
pneumotachograph
    Fleisch p.
    Silverman-Lilly p.
pneumotachometer
pneumothermomassage
pneumothorax
    artificial p.
    extrapleural p.
    open p.
    pressure p.
    p. simplex
    spontaneous p.
    tension p.
    therapeutic p.
    valvular p.
pneumotomy
pneumoventricle
Pneumovirus
pneusis
pnigophobia
PNP syndrome
pock
pocket
    gingival p.
    infrabony p., intrabony p.
    periodontal p.
    Rathke's p.
    Seessel's p.
    subcrestal p.
    Tröltsch's p.'s
pocketed calculus
pockmark
poculum
    p. diogenis
podagra
podagral, podagric, podagrous
podalgia
podalic
    p. extraction
    p. version
podarthritis
podedema
podiatric
    p. medicine
podiatrist
podiatry
podismus
poditis
podobromidrosis
podocyte
pododynamometer
pododynia
podogram

podograph
podologist
podology
podomechanotherapy
podometer
podospasm, podospasmus
Podoviridae
POEMS syndrome
pogoniasis
pogonion
poietin
poikiloblast
poikilocyte
poikilocythemia
poikilocytosis
poikilodentosis
poikiloderma
    p. atrophicans and cataract
    p. atrophicans vasculare
    p. of Civatte
    p. congenitale
poikilothrombocyte
poikilothymia
point
    p. A
    absorbent p.'s
    alveolar p.
    p. angle
    anterior focal p.
    apophysary p., apophysial p.
    auricular p.
    axial p.
    p. B
    Cannon's p.
    Capuron's p.'s
    cardinal p.'s
    central-bearing p.
    Clado's p.
    cold-rigor p.
    congruent p.'s
    conjugate p.
    contact p.
    p.'s of convergence
    craniometric p.'s
    p. deletion
    p. of elbow
    far p.
    p. of fixation
    focal p.
    Guéneau de Mussy's p.
    gutta-percha p.'s
    Hallé's p.
    heat-rigor p.
    incident p.
    incisal p.
    J p.
    jugal p.
    lower alveolar p.

malar p.
p. of maximal impulse
maximum occipital p.
Mayo-Robson's p.
McBurney's p.
median mandibular p.
mental p.
metopic p.
motor p.
Munro's p.
nasal p.
near p.
nodal p.
occipital p.
p. of ossification
painful p.
posterior focal p.
power p.
preauricular p.
pressure p.
primary p. of ossification
principal p.
p. of proximal contact
p. of regard
retention p.
secondary p. of ossification
silver p.
p. source
spinal p.
subnasal p.
Sudeck's critical p.
supra-auricular p.
supranasal p.
supraorbital p.
sylvian p.
p. system test types
tender p.'s
trigger p.
Trousseau's p.
Valleix's p.'s
Weber's p.
zygomaxillary p.
pointed
p. condyloma
p. objects
p. wart
pointillage
pointing
Poirier's
P. gland
P. line
Poiseuille's
P. law
P. space
poisoning
bacterial food p.
carbon monoxide p.
oxygen p.

radiation p.
Staphylococcus food p.
Poisson distribution
Poisson-Pearson formula
Poitou colic
poker
p. back
p. spine
pokeweed mitogen
Poland's syndrome
polar
p. anemia
p. body
p. cataract
p. cell
p. globule
p. hypogenesis
p. plates
p. presentation
p. ring
p. star
p. zone
polarimeter
polarimetry
polariscope
polariscopic
polariscopy
polarized light
polarizer
polarizing microscope
pole
abapical p.
animal p.
anterior p. of eyeball
anterior p. of lens
cephalic p.
frontal p.
frontal p. of cerebrum
germinal p.
inferior p.
inferior p. of kidney
inferior p. of testis
lateral p.
p. ligation
medial p. of ovary
occipital p.
occipital p. of cerebrum
pelvic p.
posterior p. of eyeball
posterior p. of lens
superior p.
superior p. of kidney
superior p. of testis
temporal p.
temporal p. of cerebrum
vegetal p., vegetative p.
vitelline p.
poli (*pl. of* polus)

P

polio
  French p.
polioclastic
poliodystrophia
  p. cerebri progressiva infantilis
poliodystrophy
  progressive cerebral p.
polioencephalitis
  p. infectiva
  inferior p.
  superior p.
  superior hemorrhagic p.
polioencephalomeningomyelitis
polioencephalomyelitis
polioencephalopathy
poliomyelencephalitis
poliomyelitis
  acute anterior p.
  acute bulbar p.
  chronic anterior p.
  p. vaccines
  p. virus
poliomyeloencephalitis
poliomyelopathy
poliosis
  ciliary p.
poliovirus
  p. hominis
polishing
  p. brush
Politzer
  P. bag
  P. luminous cone
  P. method
politzerization
  negative p.
polka fever
polkissen of Zimmermann
pollakidipsia
pollakiuria
pollen
  p. antigen
pollenosis
pollex, gen. **pollicis**, pl. **pollices**
  p. pedis
pollicization
pollinosis
pollodic
pollution
  noise p.
polocyte
polster
polus, pl. **poli**
  p. anterior bulbi oculi
  p. anterior lentis
  p. frontalis cerebri
  poli lienalis inferior et superior
  p. occipitalis cerebri

  p. posterior bulbi oculi
  p. posterior lentis
  poli renalis inferior et superior
  p. temporalis cerebri
poly
Pólya
  P. gastrectomy
  P. operation
polyadenitis
  p. maligna
polyadenopathy
polyadenosis
polyadenous
polyallelism
polyalveolar lobe
polyangiitis
polyarteritis
  p. nodosa
polyarthric
polyarthritis
  p. chronica
  p. chronica villosa
  epidemic p.
  p. rheumatica acuta
  vertebral p.
polyarticular
polyavitaminosis
polyaxial joint
polyblast
polyblennia
polycarboxylate cement
polycardia
polycentric
polycheiria, polychiria
polychondritis
  chronic atrophic p.
  relapsing p.
polychromasia
polychromatic
  p. cell
polychromatocyte
polychromatophil, polychromatophile
  p. cell
polychromatophilia
polychromatophilic
polychromatosis
polychrome methylene blue
polychromemia
polychromia
polychromophil
polychromophilia
polychylia
polycinematosomnography
polyclinic
polyclonal
  p. activator
  p. antibody
  p. gammopathy

polyclonia
polycoria
polycrotic
polycrotism
polycyesis
polycystic
    p. disease of kidneys
    p. kidney
    p. liver
    p. liver disease
    p. ovary
    p. ovary syndrome
polycythemia
    compensatory p.
    p. hypertonica
    relative p.
    p. rubra
    p. rubra vera
    p. vera
polydactylism
polydactylous
polydactyly
polydentia
polydipsia
    hysterical p.
    psychogenic p.
    psychogenic nocturnal p.
polydysplasia
polydystrophic
    p. dwarfism
polydystrophy
polyembryony
polyendocrine deficiency syndrome
polyendocrinopathy
polyergic
polyester resin
polyesthesia
polygalactia
polyganglionic
polygene
polygenic
    p. inheritance
polyglandular
    p. deficiency syndrome
polygnathus
polygraph
    Mackenzie's p.
polygyria
polyhedral
    p. body
polyhidrosis
polyhybrid
polyhydramnios
polyhypermenorrhea
polyhypomenorrhea
polyidrosis
polykaryocyte

polyleptic
    p. fever
polylogia
polymastia
polymastigote
polymazia
polymegethism
polymelia
polymenorrhea
polymeria
polymetacarpalia, polymetacarpalism
polymetatarsalia, polymetatarsalism
polymicrolipomatosis
polymitus
polymorph
polymorphic
    p. genetic markers
    p. neuron
    p. reticulosis
    p. superficial keratitis
polymorphism
    balanced p.
    corneal endothelial p.
    genetic p.
    lipoprotein p.
    restriction fragment length p.
polymorphocellular
polymorphocytic leukemia
polymorphonuclear
    p. leukocyte
polymorphous
    p. layer
    p. light eruption
    p. perversion
polymyalgia
    p. arteritica
    p. rheumatica
polymyoclonus
polymyositis
polynesic
polyneural
polyneuralgia
polyneuritic psychosis
polyneuritis
    acute idiopathic p.
    chronic familial p.
    infectious p.
    postinfectious p.
polyneuronitis
polyneuropathy
    acute inflammatory p.
    alcoholic p.
    arsenical p.
    axonal p.
    axon loss p.
    buckthorn p.
    chronic inflammatory
      demyelinating p.

P

polyneuropathy *(continued)*
    critical illness p.
    demyelinating p.
    diabetic p.
    isoniazid p.
    nitrofurantoin p.
    nutritional p.
    progressive hypertrophic p.
    segmental demyelinating p.
    uremic p.
polynuclear, polynucleate
    p. leukocyte
polynucleosis
polyodontia
Polyomavirus
polyoma virus
polyoncosis, polyonchosis
polyonychia
polyopia, polyopsia
polyorchism, polyorchidism
polyostotic
    p. fibrous dysplasia
polyotia
polyovular
    p. ovarian follicle
polyovulatory
polyp
    adenomatous p.
    bleeding p.
    bronchial p.
    cardiac p.
    cellular p.
    choanal p.
    cystic p.
    dental p.
    fibrinous p.
    fibroepithelial p.
    fibrous p.
    fleshy p.
    gelatinous p.
    Hopmann's p.
    hydatid p.
    hyperplastic p.
    inflammatory p.
    juvenile p.
    laryngeal p.
    lipomatous p.
    lymphoid p.
    metaplastic p.
    mucous p.
    myomatous p.
    nasal p.
    osseous p.
    pedunculated p.
    placental p.
    pulp p.
    regenerative p.
    retention p.

    sessile p.
    tooth p.
    vascular p.
polypapilloma
polypathia
polypectomy
    p. snare
polypeptide
    pancreatic p.
    trefoil p.
polyphagia
polyphalangism
polyphallic
polyphenic
    p. gene
polyphobia
polyphrasia
polyphyletic
    p. theory
polyphyletism
polyphyodont
polypi (*pl. of* polypus)
polypiform
polyplasmia
polyplastic
Polyplax
polyploid
polyploidy
polypnea
polypodia
polypoid
    p. adenoma
polyporous
polyposia
polyposis
    p. coli
    familial intestinal p.
    multiple intestinal p.
polypotome
polypotrite
polypous
    p. endocarditis
    p. gastritis
polypragmasy
polyptychial
polypus, pl. **polypi**
polyradiculitis
polyradiculomyopathy
polyradiculoneuropathy
polyradiculopathy
    diabetic p.
polyrrhea
polyscelia
polyscope
polyserositis
    familial paroxysmal p.
    familial recurrent p.

periodic p.
recurrent p.
polysinusitis
polysomia
polysomic
polysomnogram
polysomnography
polysomy
polyspermia, polyspermism
polyspermy
polysplenia
p. syndrome
polysteraxic
polystichia
polysulfide rubber
polysymbrachydactyly
polysynaptic
polysyndactyly
polytendinitis
polytene
p. chromosome
polythelia
polytomography
polytrichia
polytrichosis
polytrophic
polyunguia
polyuria
p. test
polyvalent
p. allergy
p. antiserum
p. serum
polyzoic
polyzygotic
p. twins
pomade acne
Pomeroy's operation
Pompe's disease
pompholyx
pomphus
ponceau D xylidine
ponderal index
pond fracture
Ponfick's shadow
ponograph
ponopalmosis
ponophobia
ponos
pons, pl. **pontes**
p. cerebelli
p. hepatis
p. varolii
pontic
ponticulus
p. hepatis
p. nasi
p. promontorii

pontile, pontine
pontis nervi trigeminalis nucleus
pontobulbar body
pontocerebellar recess
ponto-geniculo-occipital spike
pontomedullary groove
pool
abdominal p.
gene p.
vaginal p.
Pool-Schlesinger sign
Pool's phenomenon
poorly
p. compliant bladder
p. differentiated lymphocytic
   lymphoma
poples
popliteal
p. arch
p. artery
p. communicating nerve
p. entrapment syndrome
p. fascia
p. fossa
p. groove
p. line
p. lymph nodes
p. muscle
p. notch
p. plane of femur
p. plexus
p. region
p. space
p. surface of femur
p. vein
popliteus
p. muscle
population
p. genetics
p. pyramid
porcelain
p. gallbladder
p. inlay
porcine
p. adenoviruses
p. graft
p. hemagglutinating
   encephalomyelitis virus
p. valve
porcupine skin
pore
dilated p.
external acoustic p., external
   auditory p.
gustatory p.
interalveolar p.'s
internal acoustic p., auditory p.
Kohn's p.'s

P

705

pore *(continued)*
    nuclear p.
    skin p.
    slit p.'s
    sweat p.
    taste p.
porencephalia
porencephalic
porencephalitis
porencephalous
porencephaly
Porges-Meier test
Porges method
pori *(pl. of* porus)
poria *(pl. of* porion)
Porifera
poriomania
porion, pl. **poria**
pornolagnia
porocele
Porocephalus
    P. armillatus
poroconidium
porokeratosis
    actinic p.
poroma
    eccrine p.
porosis, pl. **poroses**
    cerebral p.
porosity
porospore
porotic
porous
porphyria
    acute intermittent p., acute p.
    p. cutanea tarda
    p. cutanea tarda hereditaria
    p. cutanea tarda symptomatica
    erythropoietic p.
    hepatic p.
    p. hepatica
    intermittent acute p.
    ovulocyclic p.
    South African type p.
    symptomatic p.
    variegate p.
porphyrinopathy
porphyrinuria
porphyrism
porphyruria
porrigo
    p. decalvans
    p. favosa
    p. furfurans
    p. larvalis
    p. lupinosa
    p. scutulata

Porro
    P. hysterectomy
    P. operation
porta, pl. **portae**
    p. hepatis
    p. lienis
    p. pulmonis
    p. renis
portable radiography
portacaval
    p. anastomoses
    p. shunt
portae (*pl. of* porta)
portal
    anterior intestinal p.
    p. canals
    p. circulation
    p. cirrhosis
    p. fissure
    p. hypertension
    p. hypophysial circulation
    p. lobule of liver
    posterior intestinal p.
    p. pyemia
    p. system
    p. triad
    p. vein
portal-systemic
    p.-s. anastomoses
    p.-s. encephalopathy
portasystemic shunt
Porter's fascia
Porter-Silber
    P.-S. chromogens
    P.-S. chromogens test
    P.-S. reaction
portio, pl. **portiones**
    p. intermedia
    p. major nervi trigemini
    p. minor nervi trigemini
    p. supravaginalis
    p. vaginalis
portion
    accessory p. of spinal accessory
      nerve
    mesenteric p. of small intestine
    subcutaneous p. of external anal
      sphincter
    supravaginal p. of cervix
    vaginal p. of cervix
portiplexus
portobilioarterial
portoenterostomy
portogram
portography
portosystemic
portovenography
Portuguese-Azorean disease

port-wine
    p.-w. mark
    p.-w. stain
porus, pl. **pori**
    p. acusticus externus
    p. acusticus internus
    p. crotaphytico-buccinatorius
    p. gustatorius
    p. opticus
    p. sudoriferus
Posadas disease
position
    p. agnosia
    anatomical p. _AbeR position_
    Bozeman's p.
    Casselberry p.
    centric p.
    condylar hinge p.
    dorsal p.
    dorsosacral p.
    eccentric p.
    p. effect
    electrical heart p.
    Elliot's p.
    English p.
    flank p.
    Fowler's p.
    frontoanterior p., left frontoanterior, right frontoanterior
    frontoposterior p., left frontoposterior, right frontoposterior
    frontotransverse p., left frontotransverse, right frontotransverse
    genucubital p.
    genupectoral p.
    heart p.
    hinge p.
    intercuspal p.
    knee-chest p.
    knee-elbow p.
    lateral recumbent p.
    leapfrog p.
    left frontoanterior (*var. of* frontoanterior p.)
    left frontoposterior (*var. of* frontoposterior p.)
    left frontotransverse (*var. of* frontotransverse p.)
    left occipitoanterior (*var. of* occipitoanterior p.)
    left occipitoposterior (*var. of* occipitoposterior p.)
    left occipitotransverse (*var. of* occipitotransverse p.)
    left sacroanterior (*var. of* sacroanterior p.)
    left sacroposterior (*var. of* sacroposterior p.)
    left sacrotransverse (*var. of* sacrotransverse p.)
    lithotomy p.
    mandibular hinge p.
    Mayo-Robson's p.
    mentoanterior p., left mentoanterior, right mentoanterior
    mentoposterior p., left mentoposterior, right mentoposterior
    mentotransverse p., left mentotransverse, right mentotransverse
    Noble's p.
    obstetric p.
    occipitoanterior p., left occipitoanterior, right occipitoanterior
    occipitoposterior p., left occipitoposterior, right occipitoposterior
    occipitotransverse p., left occipitotransverse, right occipitotransverse
    occlusal p.
    orthopnea p.
    orthopneic p.
    physiologic rest p.
    postural p., postural resting p.
    prone p.
    protrusive p.
    rest p.
    reverse Trendelenburg p.
    right frontoanterior (*var. of* frontoanterior p.)
    right frontoposterior (*var. of* frontoposterior p.)
    right frontotransverse (*var. of* frontotransverse p.)
    right mentoanterior (*var. of* mentoanterior p.)
    right mentoposterior (*var. of* mentoposterior p.)
    right mentotransverse (*var. of* mentotransverse p.)
    right occipitoanterior (*var. of* occipitoanterior p.)
    right occipitoposterior (*var. of* occipitoposterior p.)
    right occipitotransverse (*var. of* occipitotransverse p.)
    Rose's p.
    sacroanterior p., left sacroanterior, right sacroanterior
    sacroposterior p., left sacroposterior, right sacroposterior
    sacrotransverse p., left

P

position *(continued)*
    sacrotransverse, right
    sacrotransverse
    Scultetus' p.
    semiprone p.
    p. sense
    Simon's p.
    Sims' p.
    supine p.
    terminal hinge p.
    Trendelenburg's p.
    Valentine's p.
    Walcher p.
positional
    p. nystagmus
    p. vertigo of Bárány
positioner
positive
    p. accommodation
    p. afterimage
    p. afterpotential
    p. anergy
    p. chronotropism
    p. contrast orbitography
    p. convergence
    p. cytotaxis
    p. electrotaxis
    p. end-expiratory pressure
    false p.
    p. feedback
    p. G
    p. heteropyknosis
    p. leukocytotaxia
    p. meniscus
    p. phase
    p. rays
    p. reinforcer
    p. scotoma
    p. stain
    p. stereotropism
    p. supporting reactions
    p. taxis
    p. thermotaxis
    p. transference
    p. tropism
positive hydrotropism *(var. of* hydrotropism)
positively
    p. bathmotropic
    p. dromotropic
    p. inotropic
positive-negative pressure breathing
positive neutrotaxis *(var. of* neutrotaxis)
positron emission tomography
post
    p. dam
    p. dam area
    p. implant

postacetabular
postadolescence
postadrenalectomy syndrome
postage stamp grafts
postanal
    p. gut
postanesthetic
postapoplectic
postarsphenamine jaundice
postaxial
postaxillary line
postbasic stare
postbrachial
postcapillary venules
postcardinal
postcardiotomy syndrome
postcava
postcaval
    p. ureter
postcentral
    p. area
    p. artery
    p. fissure
    p. gyrus
    p. sulcal artery
    p. sulcus
postcholecystectomy syndrome
postchroming
postcibal
postclavicular
postcloacal gut
postcoital
postcoitus
postcommissurotomy syndrome
postcommunical part of anterior cerebral artery
postconcussion
    p. neurosis
    p. syndrome
postcordial
postcostal
    p. anastomosis
postcrown
postcubital
postdam
postdiastolic
postdicrotic
postdiphtheritic
    p. paralysis
postdormital
postdormitum
postdrive depression
postductal
postencephalitic
postepileptic
posterior
    p. alveolar artery
    p. ampullar nerve

p. antebrachial cutaneous nerve
p. antebrachial nerve
p. antebrachial region
p. anterior jugular vein
p. aphasia
p. arch of atlas
p. articular surface of dens
p. asynclitism
p. atlanto-occipital membrane
p. auricular artery
p. auricular groove
p. auricular muscle
p. auricular nerve
p. auricular plexus
p. auricular vein
p. axillary fold
p. axillary line
p. basal branch
p. basal segment
p. belly of digastric muscle
p. border of eyelids
p. border of fibula
p. border of petrous part of temporal bone
p. border of radius
p. border of testis
p. border of ulna
p. brachial cutaneous nerve
p. brachial region
p. branches
p. branch of great auricular nerve
p. branch of inferior pancreaticoduodenal artery
p. branch of lateral cerebral sulcus
p. branch of obturator artery
p. branch of obturator nerve
p. branch of recurrent ulnar artery
p. branch of renal artery
p. branch of right branch of portal vein
p. branch of right hepatic duct
p. branch of right superior pulmonary vein
p. branch of spinal nerves
p. branch of superior thyroid artery
p. canaliculus of chorda tympani
p. cardinal veins
p. carpal region
p. cecal artery
p. cells
p. central convolution
p. central gyrus
p. centriole
p. cerebellar notch
p. cerebral artery
p. cerebral commissure
p. cervical intertransversarii muscles

p. cervical intertransverse muscles
p. chamber of eye
p. choroidal artery
p. choroiditis
p. circumflex humeral artery
p. column
p. column cordotomy
p. column of spinal cord
p. communicating artery
p. condyloid foramen
p. conjunctival artery
p. cord of brachial plexus
p. coronary plexus
p. costotransverse ligament
p. cranial fossa
p. cricoarytenoid ligament
p. cricoarytenoid muscle
p. cruciate ligament
p. crural region
p. crus of stapes
p. cubital region
p. cusp of atrioventricular valve
p. cutaneous nerve of arm
p. cutaneous nerve of forearm
p. cutaneous nerve of thigh
p. dental artery
p. descending artery
p. elastic layer
p. embryotoxon
p. ethmoidal air cells
p. ethmoidal artery
p. ethmoidal nerve
p. extremity
p. facial vein
p. femoral cutaneous nerve
p. focal point
p. fontanel
p. funiculus
p. group of axillary lymph nodes
p. horn
p. humeral circumflex artery
p. hypothalamic area
p. hypothalamic nucleus
p. hypothalamic region
p. inferior cerebellar artery
p. inferior cerebellar artery syndrome
p. inferior iliac spine
p. inferior nasal branches of greater palatine nerve
p. intercondylar area of tibia
p. intercostal arteries 1–2
p. intercostal arteries 3-11
p. intercostal veins
p. intermediate groove
p. intermediate sulcus
p. interosseous artery
p. interosseous nerve

P

posterior *(continued)*

p. interventricular artery
p. interventricular groove
p. intestinal portal
p. intraoccipital joint
p. intraoccipital synchondrosis
p. junction line
p. knee region
p. labial arteries
p. labial commissure
p. labial nerves
p. labial veins
p. lacrimal crest
p. lateral nasal arteries
p. layer of rectus abdominis sheath
p. ligament of head of fibula
p. ligament of incus
p. ligament of knee
p. limb of internal capsule
p. limb of stapes
p. limiting layer of cornea
p. lip of uterine os
p. lobe of hypophysis
p. longitudinal bundle
p. longitudinal ligament
p. lunate lobule
p. marginal vein
p. medial nucleus of thalamus
p. median fissure of the medulla oblongata
p. median fissure of spinal cord
p. median line
p. median sulcus of medulla oblongata
p. median sulcus of spinal cord
p. mediastinal arteries
p. mediastinal lymph nodes
p. mediastinum
p. medullary velum
p. meningeal artery
p. meniscofemoral ligament
p. myocardial infarction
p. naris
p. nasal spine
p. neck region
p. nephrectomy
p. neuropore
p. notch of cerebellum
p. occipitoaxial ligament
p. occlusion
p. palatal seal
p. palatal seal area
p. palatine arch
p. palatine foramina
p. palatine spine
p. pancreaticoduodenal artery
p. parietal artery
p. parolfactory sulcus

p. parotid veins
p. part
p. part of the diaphragmatic surface of the liver
p. pelvic exenteration
p. perforated substance
p. pericallosal vein
p. periventricular nucleus
p. peroneal arteries
p. pillar of fauces
p. pillar of fornix
p. pole of eyeball
p. pole of lens
p. primary division
p. probability
p. process of septal cartilage
p. process of talus
p. pyramid of the medulla
p. quadrigeminal body
p. recess
p. recess of tympanic membrane
p. region of arm
p. region of elbow
p. region of forearm
p. region of leg
p. region of neck
p. region of thigh
p. rhinoscopy
p. rhizotomy
p. root
p. sacroiliac ligaments
p. sacrosciatic ligament
p. sagittal diameter
p. scalene muscle
p. scapular nerve
p. scleritis
p. sclerosis
p. sclerotomy
p. scrotal branch of internal pudendal artery
p. scrotal nerves
p. scrotal veins
p. segment
p. segmental artery of kidney
p. segment of eyeball
p. semicircular canals
p. septal artery of nose
p. spinal artery
p. spinal sclerosis
p. spinocerebellar tract
p. staphyloma
p. sternoclavicular ligament
p. subcapsular cataract
p. superior alveolar artery
p. superior alveolar branches of maxillary nerve
p. superior iliac spine

p. superior lateral nasal branches of pterygopalatine ganglion
p. superior medial nasal branches of pterygopalatine ganglion
p. supraclavicular nerve
p. surface
p. surface of arm
p. surface of arytenoid cartilage
p. surface of cornea
p. surface of elbow
p. surface of eyelids
p. surface of fibula
p. surface of forearm
p. surface of iris
p. surface of kidney
p. surface of leg
p. surface of lens
p. surface of lower limb
p. surface of pancreas
p. surface of petrous part of temporal bone
p. surface of prostate
p. surface of radius
p. surface of shaft of humerus
p. surface of suprarenal gland
p. surface of thigh
p. surface of tibia
p. surface of ulna
p. symblepharon
p. synechia
p. talar articular surface of calcaneus
p. talofibular ligament
p. talotibial ligament
p. teeth
p. temporal artery
p. thalamic radiations
p. thoracic nerve
p. tibial artery
p. tibial lymph node
p. tibial muscle
p. tibial node
p. tibial recurrent artery
p. tibial veins
p. tibiofibular ligament
p. tibiotalar ligament
p. tibiotalar part of deltoid ligament
p. tooth form
p. triangle of neck
p. tubercle of atlas
p. tubercle of cervical vertebrae
p. tympanic artery
p. urethra
p. urethral valves
p. urethritis
p. uveitis

p. vaginal hernia
p. vaginismus
p. vein of left ventricle
p. vein of septum pellucidum
p. vitrectomy
p. wall of middle ear
p. wall of stomach
p. wall of tympanic cavity
p. wall of vagina
posterius
posteroanterior
p. projection
posteroclusion
posteroexternal
posterointernal
posterolateral
p. central arteries
p. fissure
p. fontanel
p. groove
p. sulcus
posteromedial
p. central arteries
posteromedian
posteroparietal
posterosuperior
posterotemporal
posteruption cuticle
postesophageal
postextrasystolic
p. pause
p. T wave
postfebrile
postganglionic
p. fibers
p. motor neuron
postgastrectomy syndrome
postglenoid foramen
posthemiplegic
p. athetosis
p. chorea
posthemorrhagic
p. anemia
posthepatic
posthepatitic cirrhosis
posthetomy
posthioplasty
posthippocampal fissure
posthitis
postholith
posthyoid
posthypnotic
p. amnesia
p. psychosis
p. suggestion
posthypoglycemic hyperglycemia
postictal

posticus
- p. palsy
- p. paralysis

postinfarction ventricular septal defect
postinfectious
- p. bradycardia
- p. myelitis
- p. polyneuritis
- p. psychosis

postinfluenzal
postischial
post-kala azar dermal leishmanoid
postlaminar part of optic nerve
postlingual
- p. deafness
- p. fissure

postlunate fissure
postmalarial
post-marketing surveillance
postmastoid
postmature
- p. infant

postmaturity syndrome
postmedian
postmediastinal
postmediastinum
postmeiotic phase
postmeningitic hydrocephalus
postmenopausal
- p. atrophy

postminimus
postmortem
- p. clot
- p. delivery
- p. examination
- p. hypostasis
- p. livedo
- p. lividity
- p. pustule
- p. rigidity
- p. suggillation
- p. thrombus
- p. tubercle
- p. wart

postmyocardial
- p. infarction pericarditis
- p. infarction syndrome

postnarial
postnaris
postnasal
- p. drip

postnatal
- p. life
- p. pit of the newborn

postnecrotic
- p. cirrhosis

post-necrotic cirrhosis
postneuritic

postnormal occlusion
postocular
postoperative
- p. bronchopneumonia
- p. parotiditis
- p. pneumonia
- p. pressure alopecia
- p. tetany

postoral
- p. arches

postorbital
postpalatal
- p. seal
- p. seal area

postpalatine
postparalytic
postpartum
- p. alopecia
- p. amenorrhea
- p. cardiomyopathy
- p. hemorrhage
- p. hypertension
- p. pituitary necrosis syndrome
- p. psychosis
- p. tetanus

postperfusion lung
postpericardiotomy
- p. pericarditis
- p. syndrome

postpharyngeal
- p. space

postphlebitic syndrome
postpneumonic
postprandial
- p. lipemia
- p. pain

postprimary tuberculosis
postpuberal, postpubertal
postpuberty
postpubescent
postpyknotic
postpyloric sphincter
postpyramidal fissure
postreduction phase
postrenal albuminuria
postrhinal fissure
postrolandic
postrubella syndrome
postsacral
postscapular
postscarlatinal
postsphenoid bone
postsphygmic
postsplenic
post-stenotic dilation
poststeroid panniculitis
postsulcal part of tongue

postsynaptic
 p. membrane
posttarsal
posttecta
post-term infant
postthrombotic syndrome
posttibial
posttransverse
posttraumatic
 p. arterial thrombosis
 p. delirium
 p. dementia
 p. epilepsy
 p. hydrocephalus
 p. leptomeningeal cyst
 p. neck syndrome
 p. neurosis
 p. osteoporosis
 p. pericarditis
 p. psychosis
 p. stress disorder
 p. stress syndrome
 p. syndrome
 p. venous thrombosis
posttrematic
posttussis
 p. suction sound
posttussive suction
posttyphoid
postulate
 Koch's p.'s
postural
 p. albuminuria
 p. contraction
 p. drainage
 p. hypotension
 p. ischemia
 p. myoneuralgia
 p. position
 p. proteinuria
 p. reflex
 p. resting position
 p. set
 p. syncope
 p. tremor
 p. version
 p. vertigo
posture
 p. sense
 Stern's p.
posturography
 dynamic platform p.
postuterine
postvaccinal
 p. encephalitis
 p. encephalomyelitis
 p. myelitis
postvalvar, postvalvular

Potain's sign
potamophobia
potassium
 p. inhibition
 p. nitrate paper
potato
 p. dextrose agar
 p. nose
 p. tumor of neck
potency
 sexual p.
potential
 action p.
 after-p.
 bioelectric p.
 biotic p.
 brain p.
 demarcation p.
 early receptor p.
 p. energy
 evoked p.
 excitatory junction p.
 excitatory postsynaptic p.
 generator p.
 inhibitory junction p.
 inhibitory postsynaptic p.
 injury p.
 membrane p.
 myogenic p.
 oscillatory p.
 Ottoson p.
 pacemaker p.
 S p.
 somatosensory evoked p.
 spike p.
 transmembrane p.
 visual evoked p.
 zeta p.
Potter-Bucky diaphragm
Potter's
 P. disease
 P. facies
 P. syndrome
 P. version
Potts'
 P. anastomosis
 P. clamp
 P. operation
Pott's
 P. abscess
 P. aneurysm
 P. curvature
 P. disease
 P. fracture
 P. gangrene
 P. paralysis
 P. paraplegia
 P. puffy tumor

P

pouch
    antral p.
    branchial p.'s
    Broca's p.
    deep perineal p.
    Denis Browne's p.
    p. of Douglas
    Douglas' p.
    endodermal p.'s
    Hartmann's p.
    Heidenhain p.
    hepatorenal p.
    hypophyseal p.
    ileoanal p.
    Kock p.
    laryngeal p.
    Morison's p.
    paracystic p.
    pararectal p.
    paravesical p.
    Pavlov p.
    pharyngeal p.'s
    Physick's p.'s
    Prussak's p.
    Rathke's p.
    rectouterine p.
    rectovaginouterine p.
    rectovesical p.
    Seessel's p.
    superficial inguinal p.
    superficial perineal p.
    ultimobranchial p.
    uterovesical p.
    vesicouterine p.
    Willis' p.

J-pouch (handwritten annotation)

pouchitis
poudrage
    pleural p.
poultry handler's disease
poultryman's itch
Poupart's
    P. ligament
    P. line
Powassan
    P. encephalitis
    P. virus
powdered gold
power
    back vertex p.
    carbon dioxide combining p.
    equivalent p.
    p. failure
    p. injector
    p. point
    resolving p.
    statistical p.
pox
    Kaffir p.

Poxviridae
poxvirus
    p. officinalis
Pozzi's muscle
P-P interval
P-pulmonale
P-Q interval
P-R
    P.-R. interval
    P.-R. segment
practical
    p. anatomy
    p. nurse
practice
    extramural p.
    family p.
    general p.
    group p.
    intramural p.
practitioner
    nurse p.
Prader-Willi syndrome
pragmatagnosia
pragmatamnesia
pragmatics
pragmatism
Prague
    P. maneuver
    P. pelvis
prairie
    p. conjunctivitis
    p. itch
prandial
Pratt
    P. dilators
    P. symptom
Prausnitz-Küstner
    P.-K. antibody
    P.-K. reaction
praxiology
praxis
preagonal
preanal
preanesthetic
preantiseptic
preaortic
preaseptic
preataxic
preauricular
    p. deep parotid lymph nodes
    p. groove
    p. point
    p. sulcus
preautomatic pause
preaxial
preaxillary line
precancer

precancerous
    p. lesion
    p. melanosis of Dubreuilh
precapillary
    p. anastomosis
precardiac
precardinal
precartilage
precava
prececal lymph nodes
precentral
    p. area
    p. artery
    p. cerebellar vein
    p. gyrus
    p. sulcal artery
    p. sulcus
precervical sinus
prechiasmatic sulcus
prechordal
    p. plate
prechroming
precipitate
    keratic p.'s
    p. labor
    mutton-fat keratic p.'s
    pigmented keratic p.'s
precipitating
    p. antibody
    p. cause
precipitation
    double antibody p.
    immune p.
    p. test
precipitin
    p. reaction
    p. test
precipitinogen
precipitinogenoid
precipitogen
precipitoid
precipitophore
precision
    p. attachment
    p. rest
preclinical
precocious
    p. pseudopuberty
    p. puberty
precocity
precognition
precollagenous fibers
precommissural
    p. bundle
    p. septal area
    p. septum
precommunical part of anterior cerebral artery

preconceptual stage
preconscious
preconvulsive
precordia
precordial
    p. catch syndrome
    p. electrocardiography
    p. leads
precordialgia
precordium
precorneal film
precostal
    p. anastomosis
precritical
precuneal
    p. artery
precuneate
precuneus
precursory cartilage
predecidual
predentin
prediabetes
prediastole
prediastolic
predicrotic
predictive
    p. validity
    p. value
predigestion
predispose
predisposing
    p. cause
    p. factors
predisposition
predormital
predormitum
predorsal bundle
preductal
preeclampsia
    superimposed p.
preejection period
preepiglottic
preeruptive
preexcitation
    p. syndrome
preextraction record
preferred provider organization
prefrontal
    p. area
    p. cortex
    p. leukotomy
    p. lobotomy
    p. veins
preganglionic
    p. fibers
    p. motor neuron

P

pregenital
    p. organization
    p. phase
pregnancy
    abdominal p.
    aborted ectopic p.
    ampullar p.
    bigeminal p.
    p. cells
    cervical p.
    combined p.
    compound p.
    cornual p.
    p. diabetes
    ectopic p.
    extraamniotic p.
    extrachorial p.
    extramembranous p.
    extrauterine p.
    fallopian p.
    false p.
    heterotopic p.
    hydatid p.
    hysterical p.
    interstitial p.
    intraligamentary p.
    intramural p.
    intraperitoneal p.
    p. luteoma
    mesometric p.
    molar p.
    multiple p.
    mural p.
    ovarian p.
    ovarioabdominal p.
    persistent ectopic p.
    phantom p.
    plural p.
    secondary abdominal p.
    spurious p.
    tubal p.
    tuboabdominal p.
    tubo-ovarian p.
    tubouterine p.
    p. tumor
    twin p.
    uterine p.
    uteroabdominal p.
pregnant
pregranulosa cells
prehallux
prehelicine
prehemiplegic
prehensile
prehension
prehyoid
    p. gland
preictal

preinduction
preinfarction
    p. angina
    p. syndrome
preinterparietal bone
Preisz-Nocard bacillus
prelacrimal
prelaminar part of optic nerve
prelaryngeal
    p. lymph nodes
preleptotene
preleukemia
prelimbic
preliminary impression
prelingual deafness
preload
    ventricular p.
prelogical
    p. mind
    p. thinking
premalignant
premammary abscess
premaniacal
premature
    p. alopecia
    p. beat
    p. birth
    p. contact
    p. contraction
    p. delivery
    p. ejaculation
    p. labor
    p. senility syndrome
    p. systole
prematurity
    p. myopia
premaxilla
premaxillary
    p. bone
    p. suture
premedication
premeiotic phase
premelanosome
premenstrual
    p. edema
    p. salivary syndrome
    p. syndrome
    p. tension
    p. tension syndrome
premenstruum
premolar
    p. tooth
premonocyte
premorbid
premotor
    p. area
    p. cortex
    p. syndrome

premunition
premunitive
premyeloblast
premyelocyte
prenaris, pl. prenares
prenatal
    p. diagnosis
    p. life
    p. screening
preneoplastic
prenodular fissure
Prentice's rule
preoccipital notch
pre-oedipal phase
preoperative
    p. record
preoptic
    p. area
    p. region
preoral
    p. gut
preosteoblast
preoxygenation
prepalatal
prepapillary sphincter
preparalytic
preparation
    cavity p.
    corrosion p.
    cytologic filter p.
    heart-lung p.
prepatellar
    p. bursa
    p. bursitis
prepatent period
prepericardiac lymph nodes
preperitoneal
prepiriform gyrus
preplacental
prepotential
preprostate urethral sphincter
prepsychotic
prepuberal, prepubertal
prepubescent
prepuce
    p. of clitoris
    hooded p.
preputia (pl. of preputium)
preputial
    p. calculus
    p. glands
    p. sac
preputiotomy
preputium, pl. preputia
    p. clitoridis
prepyloric
    p. sphincter
    p. vein

prepyramidal tract
prerectal
    p. lithotomy
prereduced
prereduction phase
prerenal
    p. albuminuria
    p. azotemia
preretinal
pre-Rolandic artery
prerubral
    p. field
    p. nucleus
presacral
    p. anesthesia
    p. nerve
    p. neurectomy
    p. sympathectomy
presbyacousia
presbyacusis, presbyacusia
presbyatrics
presbycusis
presbyopia
presbyopic
prescribe
presenile
    p. dementia
    p. spontaneous gangrene
presenility
presenium
present
presentation
    acromion p.
    breech p., full breech p.,
      incomplete foot p., incomplete
      knee p.
    brow p.
    cephalic p.
    face p.
    footling p., foot p.
    frank breech p.
    head p.
    incomplete foot p.
    incomplete foot p. (var. of
      breech p.)
    incomplete knee p. (var. of
      breech p.)
    knee p.
    pelvic p.
    placental p.
    polar p.
    shoulder p.
    sincipital p.
    transverse p.
    vertex p.
presenting symptom
presomite
    p. embryo

P

presphenoid
>   p. bone

presphygmic

prespinal

presplenic fold

prespondylolisthesis

pressor
>   p. fibers
>   p. nerve

pressoreceptive
>   p. mechanism

pressoreceptor
>   p. nerve
>   p. reflex
>   p. system

pressosensitive

pressosensitivity
>   reflexogenic p.

pressure
>   abdominal p.
>   acoustic p.
>   p. alopecia
>   p. amaurosis
>   p. anesthesia
>   p. atrophy
>   back p.
>   biting p.
>   blood p.
>   central venous p.
>   cerebrospinal p.
>   p. collapse
>   continuous positive airway p.
>   coronary perfusion p.
>   detrusor p.
>   diastolic p.
>   differential blood p.
>   Donders' p.
>   p. dressing
>   p. epiphysis
>   p. gangrene
>   intracranial p.
>   intraocular p.
>   leak point p.
>   negative p.
>   negative end-expiratory p.
>   occlusal p.
>   p. palsy
>   p. paralysis
>   p. plethysmograph
>   pleural p.
>   p. pneumothorax
>   p. point
>   positive end-expiratory p.
>   pulmonary p.
>   pulmonary capillary wedge p.
>   pulp p.
>   pulse p.
>   p. reversal

>   selection p.
>   p. sense
>   p. sore
>   p. stasis
>   systolic p.
>   transmural p.
>   transpulmonary p.
>   transthoracic p.
>   p. urticaria
>   ventricular filling p.
>   wedge p.
>   zero end-expiratory p.

pressure-controlled respirator

pressure-volume index

presternal
>   p. notch
>   p. region

presternum

prestriate area

presulcal part of tongue

presumed ocular histoplasmosis

presumptive region

presuppurative

presynaptic
>   p. membrane

presystole

presystolic
>   p. gallop
>   p. murmur
>   p. thrill

pretarsal

pretecta

pretectal
>   p. area
>   p. nucleus
>   p. region

pretectum

preterm infant

prethyroid, prethyroideal, prethyroidean

pretibial
>   p. fever
>   p. myxedema

pretracheal
>   p. fascia
>   p. layer
>   p. lymph nodes

pretrematic

pretympanic

prevalence

preventive
>   p. dentistry
>   p. dose
>   p. medicine
>   p. treatment

prevertebral
>   p. fascia
>   p. ganglia
>   p. layer

p. lymph nodes
p. part of vertebral artery
prevesical
previllous chorion
previus
Prevotella
    P. disiens
    P. melaninogenica
    P. oralis
    P. oris
prezone
priapism
priapus
Price-Jones curve
prickle
    p. cell
    p. cell layer
prickly heat
primacy
    genital p.
    oral p.
primal
    p. repression
    p. scene
primaquine sensitivity
primary
    p. adhesion
    p. adrenocortical insufficiency
    p. aerodontalgia
    p. aldosteronism
    p. amebic meningoencephalitis
    p. amenorrhea
    p. amputation
    p. amyloidosis
    p. anesthetic
    p. atelectasis
    p. atypical pneumonia
    p. biliary cirrhosis
    p. brain vesicle
    p. bronchus
    p. bubo
    p. carcinoma
    p. cardiomyopathy
    p. caries
    p. cementum
    p. center of ossification
    p. choana
    p. coccidioidomycosis
    p. color
    p. complex
    p. constriction
    p. dementia
    p. dental lamina
    p. dentin
    p. dentition
    p. deviation
    p. disease
    p. drives

p. dysmenorrhea
p. egg membrane
p. embryonic cell
p. erythroblastic anemia
p. extrapulmonary coccidioidomycosis
p. fissure of cerebellum
p. gain
p. generalized epilepsy
p. gout
p. hemochromatosis
p. hemorrhage
p. herpetic stomatitis
p. hydrocephalus
p. hyperoxaluria and oxalosis
p. hyperparathyroidism
p. hypertension
p. hyperthyroidism
p. hypogammaglobulinemia
p. hypogonadism
p. idiopathic macular atrophy
p. immune response
p. impression
p. interatrial foramen
p. irritant
p. irritant dermatitis
p. labial groove
p. lateral sclerosis
p. lymphedema
p. lysosomes
p. macular atrophy of skin
p. medical care
p. megaureter
p. mesoderm
p. methemoglobinemia
p. myeloid metaplasia
p. narcissism
p. neurasthenia
p. neuroendocrine carcinoma of the skin
p. neuronal degeneration
p. nodule
p. nondisjunction
p. oocyte
p. organizer
p. ovarian follicle
p. palate
p. pentosuria
p. pigmentary degeneration of retina
p. point of ossification
p. process
p. progressive cerebellar degeneration
p. pulmonary lobule
p. pyoderma
p. radiation
p. reaction

P

primary *(continued)*
   p. refractory anemia
   p. reinforcement
   p. rejection
   p. renal calculus
   p. renal tubular acidosis
   p. reninism
   p. sclerosing cholangitis
   p. screw-worm
   p. senile dementia
   p. sensation
   p. sequestrum
   p. sex characters
   p. shock
   p. skin graft
   p. spermatocyte
   p. syphilis
   p. telangiectasia
   p. tooth
   p. tuberculosis
   p. union
   p. uterine inertia
   p. villus
   p. visual area
   p. visual cortex
   p. vitreous
primer extension
primerite
primigravida
primipara
primiparity
primiparous
primite
primitive
   p. aorta
   p. choana
   p. chorion
   p. costal arches
   p. furrow
   p. groove
   p. gut
   p. knot
   p. meninx
   p. neuroectodermal tumor
   p. node
   p. palate
   p. perivisceral cavity
   p. pit
   p. reticular cell
   p. ridge
   p. streak
primordial
   p. cartilage
   p. cell
   p. cyst
   p. dwarfism

   p. germ cell
   p. gigantism
   p. ovarian follicle
primordium, pl. **primordia**
   frontonasal p.
   lateral nasal p.
   medial nasal p.
primulin
primus
princeps, pl. **principes**
   p. cervicis
   p. cervicis artery
   p. pollicis
   p. pollicis artery
Princeteau's tubercle
principal
   p. artery of thumb
   p. focus
   p. optic axis
   p. piece
   p. plane
   p. point
   p. sensory nucleus of trigeminal nerve
   p. sensory nucleus of the trigeminus
principes (*pl. of* princeps)
principle
   azygos vein p.
   closure p.
   consistency p.
   Fick p.
   founder p.
   Huygens' p.
   p. of inertia
   Le Chatelier's p.
   low flow p.
   Mitrofanoff p.
   nirvana p.
   pain-pleasure p.
   pleasure p.
   reality p.
   repetition-compulsion p.
   Stewart-Hamilton p.
Pringle's disease
Prinzmetal's angina
prion
   p. protein
prior probability
prism
   p. bar
   p. cover test
   p. diopter
   enamel p.'s
   Fresnel p.
   Nicol p.

Risley's rotary p.
p. vergence test
prisma, pl. **prismata**
prismata adamantina
prismatic
prison fever typhus
privacy
private
p. antigens
p. blood group
p. duty nurse
p. hospital
p. nurse
privet cough
privileged site
proaccelerin
proacrosomal
p. granules
proactivator
C3 p.
C3 p. convertase
proactive inhibition
proal
proamnion
probability
conditional p.
p. curve
joint p.
objective p.
personal p.
posterior p.
prior p.
p. sample
subjective p.
probacteriophage
defective p.
proband
probe
Bowman's p.
p. gorget
nucleic acid p.
p. patency
periodontal p.
radioactive p.
p. syringe
vertebrated p.
viral p.
probiosis
probiotic
problem
problem-oriented record
proboscis, pl. **proboscides, proboscises**
Probstymayria vivipara
procapsid
Procaryotae
procaryote
procaryotic
procatarctic

procatarxis
procedure
Belsey Mark IV p.
Belsey Mark V p.
Chamberlain p.
Clagett p. for empyema
Collis-Belsey p.
commando p.
Damus-Kaye-Stancel p.
dideoxy p.
Dor p.
Eloesser p.
endorectal pull-through p.
Ewart's p.
Fontan p.
Girdlestone p.
Jatene p.
Konno p.
Konno-Rastan p.
loop electrocautery excision p.
Mustard p.
Nick's p.
Noble-Collip p.
Norwood p.
Puestow p.
push-back p.
Putti-Platt p.
Rittenhouse-Manogian p.
shelf p.
Snow p.
Stanley Way p.
Sugiura p.
Thal p.
Vineberg p.
V-Y p.
W p.
Z p.
procelia
procelous
procentriole
p. organizer
procephalic
procercoid
procerus
p. muscle
process
accessory p.
acromial p.
alar p.
alveolar p.
anterior p. of malleus
apical p.
articular p.
ascending p.
auditory p.
axonal p.
basilar p.
basilar p. of occipital bone

[handwritten annotations: "DicoPAC - for Schillings Test", "TIPS"]

process *(continued)*
    binary p.
    Burns' falciform p.
    calcaneal p. of cuboid bone
    caudate p.
    ciliary p.
    Civinini's p.
    clinoid p.
    cochleariform p.
    complex learning p.'s
    condylar p.
    condyloid p.
    conoid p.
    coracoid p.
    coronoid p.
    costal p.
    dendritic p.
    dental p.
    ensiform p.
    ethmoidal p.
    falciform p.
    follian p.
    Folli's p.
    foot p.
    frontal p. of maxilla
    frontal p. of zygomatic bone
    frontonasal p.
    frontosphenoidal p.
    funicular p.
    globular p.
    hamular p. of lacrimal bone
    hamular p. of sphenoid bone
    head p.
    intrajugular p.
    jugular p.
    lacrimal p.
    lateral p. of calcaneal tuberosity
    lateral p. of malleus
    lateral nasal p.
    lateral p. of talus
    Lenhossék's p.'s
    lenticular p. of incus
    long p. of malleus
    malar p.
    mamillary p.
    mandibular p.
    Markov p.
    mastoid p.
    maxillary p.
    maxillary p. of embryo
    medial p. of calcaneal tuberosity
    medial nasal p.
    mental p.
    muscular p. of arytenoid cartilage
    nasal p.
    notochordal p.
    odontoblastic p.
    odontoid p.

    odontoid p. of epistropheus
    olecranon p.
    orbicular p.
    orbital p.
    packing p.
    palatine p.
    papillary p.
    paramastoid p.
    paroccipital p.
    posterior p. of septal cartilage
    posterior p. of talus
    primary p.
    progressive p.'s
    pterygoid p.
    pterygospinous p.
    pyramidal p.
    Rau's p.
    Ravius' p.
    retromandibular p. of parotid gland
    p. schizophrenia
    secondary p.
    sheath p. of sphenoid bone
    short p. of malleus
    slender p. of malleus
    sphenoid p.
    sphenoid p. of palatine bone
    sphenoid p. of septal cartilage
    spinous p.
    spinous p. of tibia
    Stieda's p.
    stochastic p.
    styloid p. of fibula
    styloid p. of radius
    styloid p. of temporal bone
    styloid p. of third metacarpal bone
    styloid p. of ulna
    superior articular p. of sacrum
    supracondylar p.
    supraepicondylar p.
    temporal p.
    Tomes' p.'s
    transverse p.
    trochlear p.
    uncinate p. of ethmoid bone
    uncinate p. of pancreas
    vaginal p.
    vaginal p. of peritoneum
    vaginal p. of sphenoid bone
    vaginal p. of testis
    vermiform p.
    vocal p.
    vocal p. of arytenoid cartilage
    xiphoid p.
    zygomatic p. of frontal bone
    zygomatic p. of maxilla
    zygomatic p. of temporal bone
processus, pl. **processus**
    p. accessorius

p. alveolaris
p. anterior mallei
p. articularis
p. articularis superior ossis sacri
p. ascendens
p. brevis
p. calcaneus ossis cuboidei
p. caudatus
p. ciliaris
p. clinoideus
p. cochleariformis
p. condylaris
p. coracoideus
p. coronoideus
p. costalis
p. ethmoidalis
p. falciformis
p. ferreini
p. frontalis maxillae
p. frontalis ossis zygomatici
p. gracilis
p. intrajugularis
p. jugularis
p. lacrimalis
p. lateralis mallei
p. lateralis tali
p. lateralis tuberis calcanei
p. lenticularis incudis
p. mamillaris
p. mastoideus
p. maxillaris
p. medialis tuberis calcanei
p. muscularis cartilaginis arytenoidei
p. orbitalis
p. palatinus
p. papillaris
p. paramastoideus
p. posterior cartilaginis septi nasi
p. posterior tali
p. pterygoideus
p. pterygospinosus
p. pyramidalis
p. ravii
p. retromandibularis
p. retromandibularis glandulae
  parotidis
p. sphenoidalis
p. sphenoidalis cartilaginis septi
  nasi
p. spinosus
p. styloideus ossis metacarpalis III
p. styloideus ossis temporalis
p. styloideus radii
p. styloideus ulnae
p. supraepicondylaris humeri
p. temporalis
p. transversus
p. trochleariformis

p. trochlearis
p. uncinatus ossis ethmoidalis
p. uncinatus pancreatis
p. vaginalis ossis sphenoidalis
p. vaginalis peritonei
p. vaginalis of peritoneum
p. vermiformis
p. vocalis cartilaginis arytenoidei
p. xiphoideus
p. zygomaticus maxillae
p. zygomaticus ossis frontalis
p. zygomaticus ossis temporalis
procheilia, prochilia
procheilon, prochilon
prochondral
prochordal
   p. plate
procidentia
   p. uteri
proconvertin
procreate
procreation
procreative
proctagra
proctalgia
   p. fugax
proctatresia
proctectasia
proctectomy
proctencleisis, proctenclisis
procteurynter
proctitis
   chronic ulcerative p.
   epidemic gangrenous p.
   idiopathic p.
proctocele
proctoclysis
proctococcypexy
proctocolectomy
proctocolitis
proctocolonoscopy
proctocolpoplasty
proctocystocele
proctocystoplasty
proctocystotomy
proctodeal
proctodeum, pl. **proctodea**
proctodynia
proctoelytroplasty
proctologic
proctologist
proctology
proctoparalysis
proctoperineoplasty
proctoperineorrhaphy
proctopexy
proctophobia
proctoplasty

P

proctoplegia
proctopolypus
proctoptosia, proctoptosis
proctorrhagia
proctorrhaphy
proctorrhea
proctoscope
    Tuttle's p.
proctoscopy
proctosigmoid
proctosigmoidectomy
proctosigmoiditis
proctosigmoidoscope
proctosigmoidoscopy
proctospasm
proctostasis
proctostat
proctostenosis
proctostomy
proctotome
proctotomy
proctotresia
proctovalvotomy
procumbent
procursive
    p. chorea
    p. epilepsy
procurvation
prodromal
    p. period
    p. stage
prodromic, prodromous
    p. sign
prodromus, pl. **prodromi**
product
    double p.
    fibrin/fibrinogen degradation p.'s
productive
    p. inflammation
    p. peritonitis
    p. pleurisy
product-moment correlation
proemial
proencephalon
proerythroblast
proerythrocyte
professional
    p. neurosis
    p. spasm
Profeta's law
profile
    biochemical p.
    biophysical p.
    facial p.
    personality p.
    p. record
    test p.
    urethral pressure p.

profiling
    DNA p.
profilometer
profound hypothermia
profunda
    p. brachii artery
    p. femoris artery
profundus
profusion
progenia
progenitalis
progenitor
progeny
progeria
    p. with cataract, p. with
        microphthalmia
proglossis
proglottid
proglottis, pl. **proglottides**
prognathic
prognathism
    basilar p.
prognathous
prognose
prognosis
    denture p.
prognostic
prognosticate
prognostician
progonoma
    p. of jaw
    melanotic p.
prograde
program
progranulocyte
progress
progressive
    p. bacterial synergistic gangrene
    p. bulbar palsy
    p. bulbar paralysis
    p. cataract
    p. cerebellar tremor
    p. cerebral poliodystrophy
    p. choroidal atrophy
    p. circumscribed cerebral atrophy
    p. cleavage
    p. emphysematous necrosis
    p. familial scleroderma
    p. hypertrophic polyneuropathy
    p. infantile spinal muscular atrophy
    p. lipodystrophy
    p. multifocal leukoencephalopathy
    p. muscular atrophy
    p. muscular dystrophy
    p. pigmentary dermatosis
    p. pneumonia virus
    p. processes
    p. spinal amyotrophy

p. spinal muscular atrophy
p. staining
p. subcortical encephalopathy
p. supranuclear palsy
p. tapetochoroidal dystrophy
p. torsion spasm
p. vaccinia
proiosystolia
projectile vomiting
projection
anteroposterior p.
AP p.
apical lordotic p.
axial p.
base p.
Caldwell p.
cross-table lateral p.
enamel p.
erroneous p.
false p.
p. fibers
frog-leg lateral p.
Granger p.
half-axial p.
lateral p.
oblique p.
occipitomental p.
PA p.
p. perimeter
posteroanterior p.
Rhese p.
Stenvers p.
submental vertex p.
submentovertical p.
p. system
Towne p.
visual p.
Waters' p.
projective test
Prokaryotae
prokaryote
prokaryotic
prolabial
prolabium
prolactin cell
prolactinoma
prolactin-producing adenoma
prolapse
p. of the corpus luteum
mitral valve p.
Morgagni's p.
p. of umbilical cord
p. of the uterus, first degree p.,
  second degree p., third degree p.
valvular p.
prolective
prolepsis
proleptic

proleukocyte
proliferate
proliferating
p. endarteritis
p. pleurisy
p. systematized
  angioendotheliomatosis
p. tricholemmal cyst
proliferation
p. cyst
diffuse mesangial p.
gingival p.
p. therapy
proliferative, proliferous
p. arthritis
p. bronchiolitis
p. choroiditis
p. cyst
p. fasciitis
p. gingivitis
p. glomerulonephritis
p. inflammation
p. intimitis
p. myositis
p. retinopathy
prolific
proligerous
p. disk
p. membrane
promastigote
promegaloblast
prometaphase
p. banding
prominence
Ammon's p.
canine p.
cardiac p.
p. of facial canal
forebrain p.
frontonasal p.
hepatic p.
hypothenar p.
laryngeal p.
lateral nasal p.
p. of lateral semicircular canal
mallear p.
medial nasal p.
spiral p.
styloid p.
thenar p.
tubal p.
p. of venous valvular sinus
prominens
prominent heel
prominentia, pl. prominentiae
p. canalis facialis
p. canalis semicircularis lateralis
p. laryngea

P

prominentia (*continued*)
    p. mallearis
    p. spiralis
    p. styloidea
promonocyte
promontorium, pl. **promontoria**
    p. cavi tympani
    p. ossis sacri
promontory
    p. common iliac lymph nodes
    pelvic p.
    sacral p.
    p. of the sacrum
    tympanic p.
    p. of tympanic cavity
promoting agent
promotion
    health p.
promyelocyte
pronasion
pronate
pronation
    p. of foot
    p. of forearm
pronator
    p. quadratus muscle
    p. reflex
    p. ridge
    p. teres muscle
pronatus
prone
    p. position
pronephric
    p. duct
    p. tubule
pronometer
pronormoblast
pronucleus, pl. **pronuclei**
    female p.
    male p.
pro-opiomelanocortin
prootic
propagate
propagated thrombus
propagation
propagative
propalinal
proper
    p. fasciculi
    p. hepatic artery
    p. ligament of ovary
    p. palmar digital artery
    p. palmar digital nerves
    p. plantar digital artery
    p. plantar digital nerves
    p. substance
properdin
    p. factor A

    p. factor B
    p. factor D
    p. factor E
    p. system
properitoneal
    p. inguinal hernia
property emergence
prophage
    defective p.
prophase
prophlogistic
prophylactic
    p. membrane
    p. odontotomy
    p. treatment
prophylaxis, pl. **prophylaxes**
    active p.
    chemical p.
    dental p.
    passive p.
Propionibacterium
    P. acnes
    P. freudenreichii
    P. jensenii
    P. propionicus
proplasia
proplasmacyte
proplexus
proportional counter
proportionate infantilism
propositus, pl. **propositi**
proprietary hospital
proprioception
proprioceptive
    p. mechanism
    p. reflexes
    p. sensibility
proprioceptive-oculocephalic reflex
proprioceptor
propriospinal
proptometer
proptosis
proptotic
propulsion
prorsad
prorubricyte
    pernicious anemia type p.
proscolex
prosecretion granules
prosect
prosector
prosectorium
prosector's
    p. tubercle
    p. wart
prosencephalon
proserum prothrombin conversion
    accelerator

prosodemic
prosopagnosia
prosopagus
prosopalgia
prosopalgic
prosopectasia
prosoplasia
prosopoanoschisis
prosopodiplegia
prosoponeuralgia
prosopopagus
prosopoplegia
prosopoplegic
prosoposchisis
prosopospasm
prosopothoracopagus
prospective fate
prospermia
prostata
prostatalgia
prostate
    female p.
    p. gland
prostatectomy
prostate-specific antigen
prostatic
    p. adenoma
    p. calculus
    p. catheter
    p. ducts
    p. ductules
    p. fluid
    p. intraepithelial neoplasia
    p. massage
    p. plexus
    p. sheath
    p. sinus
    p. urethra
    p. utricle
    p. venous plexus
prostaticovesical
    p. plexus
prostatism
prostatitis
prostatocystitis
prostatodynia
prostatolith
prostatolithotomy
prostatomegaly
prostatomy
prostatorrhea
prostatoseminalvesiculectomy
prostatotomy
prostatovesiculectomy
prostatovesiculitis
prosternation
prostheon
prosthesis, pl. prostheses

    cardiac valve p.
    cochlear p.
    definitive p.
    dental p.
    heart valve p.
    hybrid p.
    mandibular guide p.
    ocular p.
    provisional p.
    surgical p.
    testicular p.
    tilting disc valve p.
prosthetic
    p. dentistry
    p. valves
prosthetics
    dental p.
    maxillofacial p.
prosthetist
prosthetophacos
prosthion
prosthodontia
prosthodontics
prosthodontist
Prosthogonimus macrorchis
prosthokeratoplasty
prostomial mesoderm
prostration
    heat p.
protanomaly
protanopia
protean
protease
    Lon p.
protection
    p. test
protective
    p. block
    p. laryngeal reflex
    p. protein
    p. spectacles
    p. zone
Proteeae
protein
    acute phase p.
    androgen binding p.
    antiviral p.
    C-reactive p.
    docking p.
    p. fever
    G-p.
    heat shock p.'s
    immune p.
    M p.
    macrophage inflammatory p.
    p. malnutrition
    matrix Gla p.
    monoclonal p.

P

protein *(continued)*
    monocyte chemoattractant p.-1
    myeloblastic p.
    neutrophil activating p.
    nonspecific p.
    odorant binding p.
    parathyroid hormonelike p.
    prion p.
    protective p.
    p. quotient
    p. S
    p. shock
    p. shock therapy
    Tamm-Horsfall p.
    unwinding p.'s
    vitamin D-binding p.
protein-bound iodine test
protein-losing enteropathy
proteinosis
    lipoid p.
    pulmonary alveolar p.
proteinuria
    Bence Jones p.
    gestational p.
    isolated p.
    nonisolated p.
    orthostatic p., postural p.
protensity
Proteomyxidia
Proteus
    P. inconstans
    P. mirabilis
    P. morganii
    P. rettgeri
    P. vulgaris
prothoracic glands
prothrombase
prothrombin
    p. accelerator
    p. and proconvertin test
    p. test
    p. time
prothrombinase
prothrombinogen
prothrombinopenia
prothrombokinase
prothymia
protist
Protista
protistologist
protistology
protobe
protobiology
protochordal knot
protocol
protocone
protoconid

protocoproporphyria
    p. hereditaria
Protoctista
protoderm
protodiastolic
    p. gallop
protoduodenum
protoerythrocyte
protofilament
protogonoplasm
protoleukocyte
protomerite
protometrocyte
protoneuron
proton pump
proto-oncogene
protopathic
    p. sensibility
protopianoma
protoplasm
    totipotential p.
protoplasmatic, protoplasmic
protoplasmolysis
protoplast
protoporphyria
    erythropoietic p.
protospore
protostoma
protostome
prototaxic
Prototheca
protothecosis
prototroph
prototrophic
    p. strains
prototype
protovertebra
protovertebral
Protozoa
protozoa (*pl. of* protozoon)
protozoal
protozoan
    p. cyst
protozoiasis
protozoologist
protozoology
protozoon, pl. **protozoa**
protozoophage
protraction
    mandibular p.
    maxillary p.
protractor
protrude
protruded disk
protruding teeth
protrusio acetabuli
protrusion
    bimaxillary p.

bimaxillary dentoalveolar p.
double p.

protrusive
p. excursion
p. interocclusal record
p. jaw relation
p. occlusion
p. position
p. record
p. relation

protuberance
Bichat's p.
external occipital p.
internal occipital p.
mental p.

protuberant abdomen
protuberantia
p. laryngea
p. mentalis
p. occipitalis externa
p. occipitalis interna

proud flesh
Proust's space
provertebra
Providencia
P. alcalifaciens
P. rettgeri
P. stuartii

provirus
provisional
p. callus
p. cortex
p. denture
p. ligature
p. prosthesis

provocation typhoid
provocative
p. test
p. Wassermann test

Prowazek bodies
Prowazek-Greeff bodies
Prowazekia
proxemics
proximad
proximal
p. border of nail
p. caries
p. centriole
p. contact
p. femoral focal deficiency
p. interphalangeal joints
p. radioulnar articulation
p. radioulnar joint
p. spiral septum
p. tibiofibular joint
p. urethral sphincter

proximalis

proximate
p. cause
p. contact

proximoataxia
proximobuccal
proximolabial
proximolingual
prozone
p. reaction

prozygosis
prune
p. belly
p. belly syndrome

prune-juice
p.-j. expectoration
p.-j. sputum

pruriginous
prurigo
actinic p.
p. aestivalis
p. agria
Besnier's p.
p. ferox
p. gestationis
Hebra's p.
p. infantilis
p. mitis
p. nodularis
p. simplex
summer p.

pruritic
p. urticarial papules and plaques
of pregnancy

pruritus
p. aestivalis
p. ani
aquagenic p.
p. balnea
bath p.
essential p.
p. hiemalis
p. senilis, senile p.
symptomatic p.
p. vulvae

Prussak's
P. fibers
P. pouch
P. space

Prussian
P. blue
P. blue stain

prussiate
psalterial cord
psammocarcinoma
psammoma
p. bodies
Virchow's p.

P

psammomatous
    p. meningioma
psammous
pselaphesis, pselaphesia
psellism
pseudacromegaly
pseudagraphia
pseudalbuminuria
Pseudallescheria boydii
pseudallescheriasis
Pseudamphistomum
pseudangina
pseudankylosis
pseudaphia
pseudarthrosis
pseudelminth
pseudesthesia
pseudinoma
pseudoacanthosis nigricans
pseudoacephalus
pseudoachondroplasia
pseudoachondroplastic spondyloepiphysial
   dysplasia
pseudoactinomycosis
pseudoagglutination
pseudoagrammatism
pseudoagraphia
pseudoainhum
pseudoalbuminuria
pseudoallelic
pseudoallelism
pseudoalopecia areata
pseudoanaphylactic
    p. shock
pseudoanaphylaxis
pseudoanemia
pseudoaneurysm
pseudoangina
pseudoangiosarcoma
    Masson's p.
pseudoanodontia
pseudoapoplexy
pseudoappendicitis
pseudoapraxia
pseudoarthrosis
pseudoataxia
pseudoauthenticity
pseudobacillus
pseudobacterium
pseudobulbar
    p. paralysis
pseudocarcinomatous hyperplasia
pseudocartilage
pseudocartilaginous
pseudocast
pseudocele
pseudocelom

pseudocephalocele
pseudochancre
pseudocholinesterase deficiency
pseudochorea
pseudochromesthesia
pseudochromidrosis, pseudochromhidrosis
pseudochylous ascites
pseudocirrhosis
pseudoclonus
pseudocoarctation
    p. of the aorta
pseudocolloid
    p. of lips
pseudocollusion
pseudocoma
pseudocowpox virus
pseudocoxalgia
pseudocrisis
pseudocroup
pseudocryptorchism
pseudocyesis
pseudocylindroid
pseudocyst
pseudodeciduosis
pseudodementia
pseudodextrocardia
pseudodiabetes
pseudodiastolic
pseudodiphtheria
pseudodipsia
pseudodiverticulum
pseudodysentery
pseudoedema
pseudoepitheliomatous hyperplasia
pseudoerysipelas
pseudoesthesia
pseudoexfoliation
    p. of lens capsule
pseudoexfoliative capsular glaucoma
pseudofluctuation
pseudofolliculitis
pseudofracture
pseudofusion beat
pseudoganglion
pseudo-Gaucher cell
pseudogeusesthesia
pseudogeusia
pseudoglioma
pseudoglomerulus
pseudoglucosazone
pseudogout
pseudo-Graefe sign
pseudo-Graefe's phenomenon
pseudogynecomastia
pseudohematuria
pseudohemoptysis
pseudohermaphrodite

pseudohermaphroditism
female p.
male p.
pseudohernia
pseudoheterotopia
pseudo-Hurler disease
pseudohydrocephaly
pseudohydronephrosis
pseudohyperkalemia
pseudohyperparathyroidism
pseudohypertelorism
pseudohypertrophic
p. muscular dystrophy
pseudohypertrophy
pseudohypha
pseudohyponatremia
pseudoicterus
pseudoileus
pseudoinfarction
pseudoinfluenza
pseudointraligamentous
pseudoisochromatic
pseudojaundice
pseudolepromatous leishmaniasis
pseudolipoma
pseudolithiasis
pseudologia
p. phantastica
pseudolymphocyte
pseudolymphocytic choriomeningitis virus
pseudolymphoma
Spiegler-Fendt p.
pseudolysogenic
p. strain
pseudolysogeny
pseudomalignancy
pseudomamma
pseudomania
pseudomasturbation
pseudomegacolon
pseudomelanosis
pseudomembrane
pseudomembranous
p. bronchitis
p. colitis
p. conjunctivitis
p. enteritis
p. enterocolitis
p. gastritis
p. inflammation
pseudomeningitis
pseudomenstruation
pseudometaplasia
pseudomnesia
pseudomonad
Pseudomonas
P. acidovorans
P. aeruginosa

P. cepacia
P. diminuta
P. fluorescens
P. maltophilia
P. piscicida
P. pseudoalcaligenes
P. pseudomallei
P. putrefaciens
P. stutzeri
P. vesicularis
pseudomucinous cyst
pseudomycelium
pseudomyopia
pseudomyxoma
p. peritonei
pseudoneoplasm
pseudoneurogenic bladder
pseudoneuroma
pseudoneurotic schizophrenia
pseudonit
pseudo-osteomalacia
pseudo-osteomalacic
p.-o. pelvis
pseudopapilledema
pseudoparalysis
arthritic general p.
congenital atonic p.
pseudoparaplegia
Basedow's p.
pseudoparasite
pseudoparenchyma
pseudoparesis
pseudopelade
p. of Brocq
pseudopericarditis
pseudoperitonitis
pseudophacos
pseudophakia
pseudophakodonesis
pseudophlegmon
Hamilton's p.
pseudophotesthesia
pseudophyllid
Pseudophyllidea
pseudoplastic fluid
pseudoplatelet
pseudoplegia
pseudopocket
pseudopod
pseudopodium, pl. **pseudopodia**
pseudopolydystrophy
pseudopolyp
pseudoporphyria
pseudoprognathism
pseudo psychosis
pseudopterygium
pseudoptosis

P

pseudopuberty
  precocious p.
pseudorabies virus
pseudoreaction
pseudoreplica
pseudoretinitis pigmentosa
pseudorheumatism
pseudorickets
pseudorosette
pseudorubella
pseudosarcoma
pseudosarcomatous fasciitis
pseudoscarlatina
pseudosclerosis
  Westphal's p.
  Westphal-Strümpell p.
pseudoseizure
pseudosmallpox
pseudosmia
Pseudostertagia bullosa
pseudostoma
pseudostrabismus
pseudostratified epithelium
pseudotabes
  pupillotonic p.
pseudotrichinosis, pseudotrichiniasis
pseudotruncus arteriosus
pseudotubercle
pseudotubular degeneration
pseudotumor
  p. cerebri
  inflammatory p.
pseudounipolar
  p. cell
  p. neuron
pseudovacuole
pseudovariola
pseudoventricle
pseudovomiting
pseudoxanthoma cell
pseudoxanthoma elasticum
psilosis
psilothin
psilotic
P-sinistrocardiale
psi phenomenon
psittacosis
  p. inclusion bodies
  p. virus
psoas
  p. abscess
  p. major muscle
  p. margin
  p. minor muscle
psomophagia, psomophagy
psora
psorelcosis
psorenteritis

Psorergates
psoriasic
psoriasiform
psoriasis
  p. annularis, p. annulata
  p. arthropica
  p. circinata
  p. diffusa, diffused p.
  p. discoidea
  generalized pustular p. of
    Zambusch
  p. geographica
  p. guttata
  p. gyrata
  p. inveterata
  p. nummularis
  p. orbicularis
  p. ostreacea
  p. punctata
  pustular p.
  p. rupioides
  p. spondylitica
  p. universalis
psoriatic
  p. arthritis
psoric
psoroid
Psoroptes
psoroptic acariasis
psorous
psychagogy
psychalgalia
psychalgia
psychalia
psychanopsia
psychataxia
psyche
psychedelic therapy
psychentonia
psychiatric
  p. nosology
psychiatrics
psychiatric trend
psychiatrist
psychiatry
  analytic p.
  biological p.
  community p.
  contractual p.
  cross-cultural p.
  descriptive p.
  dynamic p.
  existential p.
  forensic p., legal p.
  industrial p.
  orthomolecular p.
  psychoanalytic p.
  social p.

psychic
  p. blindness
  p. contagion
  p. determinism
  p. energy
  p. force
  p. impotence
  p. inertia
  p. overtone
  p. seizure
  p. tic
  p. trauma
psychical
psychism
psychoacoustics
psychoallergy
psychoanalysis
  active p.
  adlerian p.
  freudian p.
  jungian p.
psychoanalyst
psychoanalytic
  p. psychiatry
  p. psychotherapy
  p. situation
  p. therapy
psychoauditory
psychobiology
psychocardiac reflex
psychocatharsis
psychochrome
psychochromesthesia
psychodiagnosis
Psychodidae
psychodometry
psychodrama
psychodynamics
psychoendocrinology
psychoexploration
psychogalvanic
  p. reaction
  p. reflex
  p. response
  p. skin reaction
  p. skin reflex
  p. skin response
psychogalvanometer
psychogender
psychogenesis
psychogenic, psychogenetic
  p. deafness
  p. nocturnal polydipsia
  p. nocturnal polydipsia syndrome
  p. pain
  p. pain disorder
  p. polydipsia
  p. purpura

  p. seizure
  p. torticollis
  p. tremor
  p. vomiting
psychogeny
psychogeusic
psychogogic
psychographic
psychography
psychohistory
psychokinesis, psychokinesia
psychokym
psycholagny
psycholepsy
psycholinguistics
psychologic, psychological
psychologist
psychology
  adlerian p.
  analytical p.
  animal p.
  atomistic p.
  behavioral p.
  behavioristic p.
  child p.
  clinical p.
  cognitive p.
  community p.
  constitutional p.
  counseling p.
  criminal p.
  depth p.
  developmental p.
  dynamic p.
  educational p.
  environmental p.
  existential p.
  experimental p.
  forensic p.
  genetic p.
  gestalt p.
  health p.
  holistic p.
  humanistic p.
  individual p.
  industrial p.
  medical p.
  objective p.
  subjective p.
psychometrics
psychometry
psychomotor
  p. epilepsy
  p. retardation
  p. seizure
  p. tests
psychoneuroimmunology

P

psychoneurosis
    p. maidica
psychoneurotic
psychonomic
psychonomy
psychonosology
psychonoxious
psycho-oncology
psychopath
psychopathic
    p. personality
psychopathist
psychopathologist
psychopathology
psychopathy
psychophysical
psychophysics
psychophysiologic
    p. disorder
    p. manifestation
psychophysiology
psychoprophylaxis
psychorelaxation
psychorrhea
psychorrhythmia, psychorhythmia
psychosensory, psychosensorial
    p. aphasia
psychosexual
    p. development
    p. dysfunction
psychosis, pl. **psychoses**
    affective p.
    alcoholic psychoses
    amnestic p.
    arteriosclerotic p.
    bipolar p.
    Cheyne-Stokes p.
    climacteric p.
    depressive p.
    drug p.
    dysmnesic p.
    exhaustion p.
    febrile p.
    functional p.
    gestational p.
    hysterical p.
    ICU p.
    infection-exhaustion p.
    involutional p.
    Korsakoff's p.
    manic p.
    manic-depressive p.
    polyneuritic p.
    posthypnotic p.
    postinfectious p.
    postpartum p.
    posttraumatic p.
    pseudo p.

    puerperal p.
    schizo-affective p.
    senile p.
    situational p.
    toxic p.
    traumatic p.
    Windigo p., Wittigo p.
psychosocial
psychosomatic
    p. disorder
    p. medicine
psychosurgery
psychosynthesis
psychotechnics
psychotherapeutic
psychotherapeutics
psychotherapist
psychotherapy
    anaclitic p.
    autonomous p.
    brief p.
    contractual p.
    directive p.
    dyadic p.
    dynamic p.
    existential p.
    group p.
    heteronomous p.
    hypnotic p.
    intensive p.
    marathon group p.
    nondirective p.
    psychoanalytic p.
    reconstructive p.
    suggestive p.
    supportive p.
    transactional p.
psychotic
    p. manifestation
psychroalgia
psychroesthesia
psychrophile, psychrophil
psychrophilic
psychrophobia
psychrophore
ptarmus
PTA stain
pterion   *OR pterionA) (BRAIN)*
pterygium
    p. colli
    p. syndrome
    p. unguis
pterygoid
    p. branch of maxillary artery
    p. canal
    p. chest
    p. depression
    p. fissure

p. fossa
p. fovea
p. hamulus
p. laminae
p. nerve
p. notch
p. pit
p. plates
p. plexus
p. process
p. ridge of sphenoid bone
p. tubercle
p. tuberosity
pterygomandibular
p. ligament
p. raphe
p. space
pterygomaxillare
pterygomaxillary
p. fissure
p. fossa
p. notch
pterygopalatine
p. canal
p. fossa
p. ganglion
p. groove
p. nerves
pterygopharyngeal part of superior constrictor muscle of pharynx
pterygospinal ligament
pterygospinous
p. ligament
p. process
pthiriasis
p. capitis
p. corporis
p. pubis
Pthirus
ptomainemia
ptosed
ptosis, pl. **ptoses**
p. adiposa
p. sympathetica
ptotic
p. organ
ptyalectasis
ptyalism
ptyalocele
ptyalography
ptyalolith
ptyalolithiasis
ptyalolithotomy
ptyocrinous
pubarche
puberal, pubertal
pubertas praecox

puberty
precocious p.
pubes
pubescence
pubescent
pubic
p. angle
p. arch
p. arteries
p. baldness
p. body
p. bone
p. branch of inferior epigastric artery
p. branch of obturator artery
p. crest
p. rami
p. region
p. spine
p. symphysis
p. tubercle
pubiotomy
pubic
p. antigens
p. health
p health dentistry
p. health nurse
P. Health Service
p. hospital
pubocapsular
p. ligament
pubococcygeal
p. muscle
pubococcygeus muscle
pubofemoral
p. ligament
pubomadesis
puboprostatic
p. ligament
p. muscle
puborectal
p. muscle
puborectalis muscle
pubourethral triangle
pubovaginal
p. muscle
p. operation
pubovaginalis muscle
pubovesical
p. ligament
p. muscle
pubovesicalis muscle
Puchtler-Sweat
P.-S. stain for basement membranes
P.-S. stain for hemoglobin and hemosiderin
P.-S. stains

P

puddle sign
pudendal
- p. anesthesia
- p. canal
- p. cleavage
- p. cleft
- p. hematocele
- p. hernia
- p. nerve
- p. sac
- p. slit
- p. ulcer
- p. veins

pudendum, pl. **pudenda**
- p. femininum
- p. muliebre

pudic
- p. nerve

puerile respiration
puerpera, pl. **puerperae**
puerperal
- p. convulsions
- p. eclampsia
- p. fever
- p. mastitis
- p. morbidity
- p. period
- p. phlebitis
- p. psychosis
- p. sepsis
- p. septicemia
- p. tetanus

puerperant
puerperium, pl. **puerperia**
Puestow procedure
puff
- veiled p.

Pulex
- *P. cheopis*
- *P. fasciatus*
- *P. irritans*
- *P. penetrans*
- *P. serraticeps*

pulley
- annular p.
- cruciform p.
- p. of humerus
- muscular p.
- peroneal p.
- p. of talus

pullulate
pullulation
pulmo, gen. **pulmonis**, pl. **pulmones**
- p. dexter
- p. sinister

pulmoaortic
pulmolith
pulmometer

pulmometry
pulmonary
- p. acinus
- p. adenomatosis
- p. alveolar microlithiasis
- p. alveolar proteinosis
- p. alveolus
- p. amebiasis
- p. anthrax
- p. arc
- p. area
- p. artery
- p. artery aneurysm
- p. artery banding
- p. aspergillosis
- p. atresia
- p. branch of autonomic nervous system
- p. bulla
- p. capillary wedge pressure
- p. cavity
- p. circulation
- p. cirrhosis
- p. collapse
- p. cone
- p. conus
- p. distomiasis
- p. dysmaturity syndrome
- p. edema
- p. embolism
- p. emphysema
- p. encephalopathy
- p. fistula
- p. glomangiosis
- p. glomus
- p. hamartoma
- p. heart
- p. hemosiderosis
- p. hypertension
- p. hypostasis
- p. incompetence
- p. insufficiency
- p. ligament
- p. lymph nodes
- p. murmur
- p. orifice
- p. osteoarthropathy
- p. pleura
- p. pleurisy
- p. plexus
- p. pressure
- p. ridges
- p. salient
- p. schistosomiasis
- p. siderosis
- p. sinuses
- p. stenosis
- p. sulcus

p. surface of heart
p. talcosis
p. toilet
p. transpiration
p. trunk
p. tuberculosis
p. tularemia
p. valve
p. veins
p. ventilation
pulmonectomy
pulmones (*pl. of* pulmo)
pulmonic
p. incompetence
p. murmur
p. plague
p. regurgitation
p. tularemia
p. valve
pulmonis (*gen. of* pulmo)
pulmonitis
pulmonocoronary reflex
pulmotor
pulp
p. abscess
p. amputation
p. atrophy
p. calcification
p. calculus
p. canal
p. cavity
p. chamber
coronal p.
dead p.
dental p., dentinal p.
digital p.
enamel p.
exposed p.
p. of finger
p. horn
mummified p.
necrotic p.
p. nodule
nonvital p.
p. polyp
p. pressure
putrescent p.
radicular p.
red p.
splenic p.
p. stone
p. test
tooth p.
vertebral p.
vital p.
white p.
pulpa
p. coronalis

p. dentis
p. lienis
p. radicularis
p. splenica
pulpal
p. wall
pulpalgia
pulpar cell
pulpation
pulpectomy
pulpifaction
pulpiform
pulpify
pulpitis
hyperplastic p.
hypertrophic p.
irreversible p.
reversible p.
suppurative p.
pulpit spectacles
pulpless
p. tooth
pulpodontia
pulposus
pulpotomy
pulpy
pulsate
pulsatile
p. hematoma
pulsatility index
pulsating
p. empyema
p. metastases
p. neurasthenia
pulsation
balloon counter p.
suprasternal p.
pulsator
pulse
abdominal p.
alternating p.
anacrotic p., anadicrotic p.
bigeminal p.
bisferious p.
bulbar p.
cannonball p.
capillary p.
carotid p.
catacrotic p.
catadicrotic p.
collapsing p.
cordy p.
Corrigan's p.
coupled p.
p. curve
p. deficit
dicrotic p.
p. duration

pulse *(continued)*
    entoptic p.
    filiform p.
    gaseous p.
    p. generator
    p. granuloma
    guttural p.
    hard p.
    p. height analyzer
    intermittent p.
    irregular p.
    jugular p.
    Kussmaul's p.
    Kussmaul's paradoxical p.
    labile p.
    long p.
    monocrotic p.
    mousetail p.
    movable p.
    nail p.
    paradoxical p.
    p. period
    piston p.
    plateau p.
    p. pressure
    quadrigeminal p.
    Quincke's p.
    radial p.
    radiofrequency p.
    p. rate
    respiratory p.
    reversed paradoxical p.
    Riegel's p.
    sequence p.
    soft p.
    tense p.
    thready p.
    trigeminal p.
    triphammer p.
    undulating p.
    unequal p.
    vagus p.
    venous p.
    vermicular p.
    water-hammer p.
    p. wave
    wiry p.
pulsed dye laser
pulsed-field gel electrophoresis
pulseless disease
pulsellum
pulsimeter, pulsometer
pulsion
    p. diverticulum
pulsus
    p. abdominalis
    p. alternans
    p. anadicrotus

    p. bigeminus
    p. bisferiens
    p. caprisans
    p. catacrotus
    p. catadicrotus
    p. celer
    p. celerrimus
    p. cordis
    p. debilis
    p. differens
    p. duplex
    p. durus
    p. filiformis
    p. fluens
    p. formicans
    p. fortis
    p. frequens
    p. heterochronicus
    p. inaequalis
    p. incongruens
    p. infrequens
    p. intercidens
    p. intercurrens
    p. irregularis perpetuus
    p. magnus
    p. mollis
    p. monocrotus
    p. myurus
    p. paradoxus
    p. parvus
    p. parvus et tardus
    p. quadrigeminus
    p. rarus
    p. respiratione intermittens
    p. tardus
    p. tremulus
    p. trigeminus
    p. vacuus
    p. venosus
pultaceous
pulvinar
    p. nucleus
pulvinate
pump
    breast p.
    calf p.
    Carrel-Lindbergh p.
    constant infusion p.
    dental p.
    p. failure
    hydrogen p.
    intra-aortic balloon p.
    jet ejector p.
    p. lung
    proton p.
    saliva p.
    stomach p.
pump-oxygenator

puna
punch
p. biopsy
p. card
p. grafts
punchdrunk
p. syndrome
puncta (*pl. of* punctum)
punctate
p. basophilia
p. cataract
p. hemorrhage
p. hyalosis
p. keratitis
p. keratoderma
p. parotiditis
p. retinitis
punctiform
punctum, gen. **puncti**, pl. **puncta**
p. cecum
p. coxale
p. dolorosum
lacrimal p.
p. lacrimale
p. luteum
p. ossificationis
p. ossificationis primarium
p. ossificationis secundarium
p. proximum
p. remotum
p. vasculosum
puncture
Bernard's p.
cisternal p.
diabetic p.
lumbar p.
Quincke's p.
spinal p.
sternal p.
p. wound
pungent
pupa, pl. **pupae**
pupil
Adie's p.
amaurotic p.
Argyll Robertson p.
artificial p.
Bumke's p.
catatonic p.
cat's-eye p.
fixed p.
Gunn p.
Holmes-Adie p.
Horner's p.
Hutchinson's p.
keyhole p.
Marcus Gunn p.
paradoxical p.

pinhole p.
Robertson p.
seclusion of p.
tadpole-shaped p.
tonic p.
pupilla, pl. **pupillae**
pupillary
p. axis
p. block glaucoma
p. border of iris
p. distance
p. light-near dissociation
p. margin of iris
p. membrane
p. reflex
relative afferent p. defect
p. zone
pupillary ruff
pupillary-skin reflex
pupillography
pupillometer
pupillometry
pupillomotor
pupillostatometer
pupillotonic pseudotabes
pupiparous
pure
p. absence
p. aphasias
p. color
p. culture
p. flutter
p. random drift
p. red cell anemia
p. red cell aplasia
p. tone audiogram
pure-tone
p.-t. audiometer
p.-t. audiometry
puriform
purine-free diet
purinemia
purine-restricted diet
purity
radiochemical p.
radioisotopic p.
radionuclidic p.
radiopharmaceutical p.
Purkinje
P. cells
P. conduction
P. corpuscles
P. fibers
P. figures
P. images
P. layer
P. network
P. phenomenon

P

Purkinje *(continued)*
  P. shift
  P. system
Purkinje
Purkinje-Sanson images
Purmann's method
puromucous
purple
purpura
  acute vascular p.
  allergic p.
  anaphylactoid p.
  p. angioneurotica
  p. annularis telangiectodes
  factitious p.
  fibrinolytic p.
  p. fulminans
  Henoch's p.
  Henoch-Schönlein p.
  hyperglobulinemic p.
  idiopathic thrombocytopenic p.
  immune thrombocytopenic p.
  p. iodica, iodic p.
  p. nervosa
  nonthrombocytopenic p.
  psychogenic p.
  p. pulicans, p. pulicosa
  p. rheumatica
  Schönlein's p.
  p. senilis
  p. simplex
  p. symptomatica
  thrombocytopenic p.
  thrombopenic p.
  thrombotic thrombocytopenic p.
  p. urticans
  Waldenström's p.
purpuric
purpurinuria
purr
pursed lips breathing
purse-string
  p.-s. corepexy
  p.-s. instrument
  p.-s. suture
Purtscher's
  P. disease
  P. retinopathy
purulence, purulency
purulent
  p. conjunctivitis
  p. cyclitis
  p. encephalitis
  p. inflammation
  p. ophthalmia
  p. pericarditis
  p. pleurisy
  p. pneumonia

  p. retinitis
  p. synovitis
puruloid
pus
  p. basin
  blue p.
  p. cell
  cheesy p.
  p. corpuscle
  curdy p.
  green p.
  ichorous p.
  laudable p.
  sanious p.
  p. tube
push-back procedure
pustular
  p. blepharitis
  p. miliaria
  p. psoriasis
  p. syphilid
pustulation
pustule
  malignant p.
  postmortem p.
  spongiform p. of Kogoj
pustuliform
pustulocrustaceous
pustulosis
  p. palmaris et plantaris
  p. vacciniformis acuta
putamen
Putnam-Dana syndrome
putrescent pulp
putrid bronchitis
Putti-Platt
  P.-P. operation
  P.-P. procedure
putty kidney
puzzle
  blood p.'s
PVM virus
pyarthrosis
pyelectasis, pyelectasia
pyelitic
pyelitis
pyelocaliceal
pyelocaliectasis
pyelocalyceal
pyelocystitis
pyelofluoroscopy
pyelogram
pyelography
  antegrade p.
  intravenous p.
  retrograde p.
pyelolithotomy
pyelolymphatic

pyelonephritic kidney
pyelonephritis
    acute p.
    ascending p.
    chronic p.
    xanthogranulomatous p.
pyelonephrosis
pyeloplasty
    Anderson-Hynes p.
    capsular flap p.
    Culp p.
    disjoined p., dismembered p.
    Foley Y-plasty p.
    Scardino vertical flap p.
pyeloplication
pyeloscopy
pyelostomy
pyelotomy
    extended p.
pyelotubular reflux
pyeloureterectasis
pyeloureterography
pyelovenous
    p. backflow
pyemesis
pyemia
    cryptogenic p.
    portal p.
pyemic
    p. abscess
    p. embolism
Pyemotes tritici
pyencephalus
pyesis
pygal
pygalgia
pygmalionism
pygmy
pygoamorphus
pygodidymus
pygomelus
pygopagus
pyknic
pyknodysostosis
pyknoepilepsy, pyknolepsy
pyknolepsy
pyknomorphous
pyknophrasia
pyknosis
pyknotic
pyla
pylar
pylemphraxis
pylephlebectasis, pylephlebectasia
pylephlebitis
pylethrombophlebitis
pylethrombosis
pylic

pylon
pyloralgia
pylorectomy
pylori (*pl. of* pylorus)
pyloric
    p. antrum
    p. artery
    p. canal
    p. cap
    p. constriction
    p. glands
    p. incompetence
    p. insufficiency
    p. lymph nodes
    p. orifice
    p. part of stomach
    p. sphincter
    p. stenosis
    p. valve
    p. vein
pyloristenosis
pyloritis
pylorodiosis
pyloroduodenitis
pylorogastrectomy
pyloromyotomy
pyloroplasty
    Finney p.
    Heineke-Mikulicz p.
    Jaboulay p.
pyloroptosis, pyloroptosia
pylorospasm
pylorostenosis
pylorostomy
pylorotomy
pylorus, pl. pylori
Pym's fever
pyocele
pyocelia
pyocephalus
    circumscribed p.
    external p.
    internal p.
pyochezia
pyocin
pyococcus
pyocolpocele
pyocolpos
pyocyanic
pyocyanogenic
pyocyanolysin
pyocyst
pyocystis
pyocyte
pyoderma
    chancriform p.
    p. gangrenosum
    primary p.

P

pyoderma *(continued)*
    secondary p.
    p. vegetans
pyodermatitis
pyodermatosis
pyogen
pyogenesis
pyogenic, pyogenetic
    p. arthritis
    p. bacterium
    p. fever
    p. granuloma
    p. infection
    p. membrane
    p. pachymeningitis
    p. salpingitis
pyogenous
pyohemia
pyohemothorax
pyoid
pyometra
pyometritis
pyomyositis
    tropical p.
pyonephritis
pyonephrolithiasis
pyonephrosis
pyo-ovarium
pyopericarditis
pyopericardium
pyoperitoneum
pyoperitonitis
pyophysometra
pyopneumocholecystitis
pyopneumohepatitis
pyopneumopericardium
pyopneumoperitoneum
pyopneumoperitonitis
pyopneumothorax
    subdiaphragmatic p., subphrenic p.
pyopoiesis
pyopoietic
pyoptysis
pyopyelectasis
pyorrhea
pyosalpingitis
pyosalpingo-oophoritis
pyosalpingo-oothecitis
pyosalpinx
pyosemia
pyosepticemia
pyosis
    Manson's p.
    p. palmaris
    p. tropica
pyospermia
pyostomatitis
    p. vegetans

pyothorax
pyourachus
pyoureter
pyoxanthin
pyoxanthose
pyramid
    anterior p.
    cerebellar p.
    Ferrein's p.
    Lallouette's p.
    p. of light
    Malacarne's p.
    malpighian p.
    p. of medulla oblongata
    medullary p.
    olfactory p.
    petrous p.
    population p.
    posterior p. of the medulla
    renal p.
    p. sign
    p. of thyroid
    p. of tympanum
    p. of vermis
    p. of vestibule
pyramidal
    p. auricular muscle
    p. bone
    p. cataract
    p. cell layer
    p. cells
    p. decussation
    p. eminence
    p. fibers
    p. fracture
    p. lobe of thyroid gland
    p. muscle
    p. muscle of auricle
    p. process
    p. radiation
    p. tract
    p. tractotomy
pyramidale
pyramidalis
    p. muscle
pyramidotomy
    medullary p.
    spinal p.
pyramis, pl. **pyramides**
    p. medullae oblongatae
    p. renalis, pl. pyramides renales
    p. tympani
    p. vermis
    p. vestibuli
pyrectic
pyrenemia
Pyrenochaeta romeroi
pyrenoid

pyretic
pyretogenesis
pyretotherapy
pyrexia
pyrexial
pyrexiophobia
pyriform
       p. aperture wiring
       p. apparatus
pyrogen
       endogenous p.
       exogenous p.'s
       leukocytic p.'s
pyroglobulins
pyrolagnia
pyromania
pyromaniac
pyronin
       p. B

p. G
p. Y
pyroninophilia
pyrophobia
pyrophosphate
       ^{99m}Tc p.
pyroptothymia
pyrosis
pyrotherapy
pyrotoxin
pyrrhol cell
pyrrol
       p. blue
       p. cell
pyruvate kinase deficiency
Pythium insidiosum
pythogenesis
pythogenic, pythogenous
pyuria

P

Q
- Q angle
- Q disks
- Q tip test
- Q wave

Q$_0$, Q$_{O2}$
Q-banding
- Q.-b. stain

Q-RB interval
Q-R interval
QRS
- Q. complex
- Q. interval

Q-S$_2$ interval
Q-T interval
quack
quackery
quadrangular
- q. cartilage
- q. lobule
- q. membrane
- q. space
- q. therapy

quadrant
quadrantanopia
quadrantic
- q. hemianopia
- q. scotoma

quadrate
- q. ligament
- q. lobe
- q. lobule
- q. muscle
- q. muscle of loins
- q. muscle of sole
- q. muscle of thigh
- q. muscle of upper lip
- q. part of liver
- q. pronator muscle

quadratus
- q. femoris muscle
- q. lumborum muscle
- q. muscle
- q. plantae muscle

quadriceps
- q. femoris muscle
- q. muscle of thigh
- q. reflex

quadricepsplasty
quadricuspid
quadridigitate
quadrigeminal
- q. bodies
- q. lamina
- q. plate
- q. pulse
- q. rhythm

quadrigeminum
quadrigeminus
quadrigeminy
quadrilateral space
quadriparesis
quadripedal extensor reflex
quadriplegia
quadriplegic
quadripolar
quadrisect
quadrisection
quadritubercular
quadruple
- q. amputation
- q. rhythm

quadruplet
quail bronchitis virus
qualimeter
qualitative
- q. alteration
- q. trait

quality
- q. assurance
- q. control
- q. control chart
- q. factor

quanta (*pl. of* quantum)
quantile
quantitative
- q. alteration
- q. genetics
- q. hypertrophy
- q. perimetry

Quant's sign
quantum, pl. **quanta**
- q. limit
- q. mottle
- q. sink

Quaranfil virus
quarantine
- q. period

quark
quartan
- double q.
- q. fever
- q. malaria
- q. parasite
- triple q.

quartisect
quartz glass
quasidominance
quasidominant
quaternary syphilis

Quatrefages' angle
Queckenstedt-Stookey test
Queensland tick typhus
quellung
    q. phenomenon
    q. reaction
    q. test
quenching
    fluorescence q.
Quénu-Muret sign
Quénu's hemorrhoidal plexus
querulent
questionnaire
    Holmes-Rahe q.
Quetelet
quick
quickening
Quick's
    Q. method
    Q. test
quiescent
quiet
    q. hip disease
    q. iritis
    q. lung
quilted suture
quin-2
quinacrine chromosome banding stain

Quincke's
    Q. disease
    Q. edema
    Q. pulse
    Q. puncture
    Q. sign
quinine
    q. carbacrylic resin
    q. carbacrylic resin test
Quinlan's test
quinquedigitate
quinquetubercular
quinsy
    lingual q.
quintan
    q. fever
quintuplet
quotidian
    q. fever
    q. malaria
quotient
    achievement q.
    Ayala's q.
    cognitive laterality q.
    intelligence q.
    protein q.
    respiratory q.
    spinal q.

R

R antigen
R factors
R pili
R plasmids
R wave

r

rabbeting

rabbit

r. fever
r. fibroma
r. fibroma virus
r. myxoma virus

rabbitpox virus

rabies

r. virus, Flury strain
r. virus, Kelev strain

raccoon eyes

racemose

r. aneurysm
r. gland
r. hemangioma

rachial

rachicentesis

rachides (*pl. of* rachis)

rachidial

rachidian

rachigraph

rachilysis

rachiocampsis

rachiocentesis

rachiochysis

rachiometer

rachiopagus

rachiopathy

rachioplegia

rachioscoliosis

rachiotome

rachiotomy

rachipagus

rachis, pl. **rachides, rachises**

rachischisis

r. partialis
r. totalis

rachitic

r. diet
r. pelvis
r. rosary
r. scoliosis

rachitis

r. fetalis
r. fetalis annularis
r. fetalis micromelica
r. intrauterina, r. uterina
r. tarda

rachitism

rachitogenic

rachitome

rachitomy

racial melanoderma

racket

r. amputation
r. nail

racquet hypha

radarkymography

radectomy

Radford nomogram

radiability

radiable

radiad

radial

r. acceleration
r. aplasia-thrombocytopenia syndrome
r. artery
r. border of forearm
r. bursa
r. clubhand
r. collateral artery
r. collateral ligament
r. collateral ligament of elbow
r. collateral ligament of wrist
r. eminence of wrist
r. flexor muscle of wrist
r. fossa of humerus
r. growth phase
r. head
r. immunodiffusion
r. index artery
r. keratotomy
r. nerve
r. notch
r. phenomenon
r. pulse
r. recurrent artery
r. reflex
r. scar
r. sclerosing lesion
r. styloid tendovaginitis
r. tuberosity
r. veins

radialis

r. indicis artery

radiant

radiate

r. crown
r. layer of tympanic membrane
r. ligament
r. ligament of head of rib

radiate *(continued)*
  r. ligament of wrist
  r. sternocostal ligaments
radiatio, pl. **radiationes**
  r. acustica
  r. corporis callosi
  r. optica
  r. pyramidalis
radiation
  acoustic r.
  alpha r.
  r. anemia
  annihilation r.
  anterior thalamic r.'s
  background r.
  beta r.
  r. biology
  r. burn
  r. caries
  r. cataract
  central thalamic r.'s
  Cerenkov r.
  characteristic r.
  r. chimera
  r. of corpus callosum
  corpuscular r.
  r. dermatosis
  electromagnetic r.
  gamma r.
  geniculocalcarine r.
  Gratiolet's r.
  heterogeneous r.
  homogeneous r.
  ionizing r.
  K-r.
  L-r.
  r. myelitis
  r. myelopathy
  neutron r.
  occipitothalamic r.
  r. oncologist
  r. oncology
  optic r.
  r. physics
  r. pneumonitis
  r. poisoning
  posterior thalamic r.'s
  primary r.
  pyramidal r.
  r. risks
  scattered r.
  secondary r.
  r. sickness
  r. therapy
  r. weighting factor
  Wernicke's r.
radical
  r. cystectomy

  r. hysterectomy
  r. mastectomy
  r. mastoidectomy
  r. operation for hernia
  oxygen derived free r.'s
  r. pericardiectomy
radices (*pl. of* radix)
radicis (*gen. of* radix)
radicle
radicotomy
radicula
radiculalgia
radicular
  r. abscess
  r. arteries
  r. cyst
  r. fila
  r. pulp
  r. syndrome
radiculectomy
radiculitis
  acute brachial r.
radiculoganglionitis
radiculomeningomyelitis
radiculomyelopathy
radiculoneuropathy
radiculopathy
  diabetic thoracic r.
radiectomy
radii (*gen. and pl. of* radius)
radioactive
  r. cow
  r. iodide uptake test
  r. probe
radioactivity
  artificial r.
  induced r.
radioallergosorbent test
radioautogram
radioautography
radiobicipital
  r. reflex
radiobiology
radiocalcium
radiocardiogram
radiocardiography
radiocarpal
  r. articulation
  r. joint
radiocephalpelvimetry
radiochemical purity
radiocholangiography
radiocholecystography
radiocineangiocardiography
radiocineangiography
radiocinematography
radiocurable
radiodense

radiodensity
radiodermatitis
radiodiagnosis
radiodigital
radioelectrophysiologram
radioelectrophysiolograph
radioelectrophysiolography
radioepidermitis
radioepithelitis
radiofrequency
    r. pulse
radiogallium
radiogenesis
radiogenic
radiogenics
radiogram
radiograph
    bitewing r.
    cephalometric r.
    decubitus r.
    lateral decubitus r.
    lateral oblique r.
    lateral ramus r.
    lateral skull r.
    maxillary sinus r.
    occlusal r.
    panoramic r.
    periapical r.
    scout r.
    submental vertex r.
    submentovertex r.
    Towne projection r.
    transcranial r.
    Trendelenburg r.
    Waters' view r.
radiographer
radiographic
    r. parallel line shadows
    r. pelvimetry
radiography
    advanced multiple-beam
      equalization r.
    air-gap r.
    bedside r.
    computed r.
    digital r.
    electron r.
    magnification r.
    mucosal relief r.
    portable r.
    scanning equalization r.
    sectional r.
    serial r.
    spot-film r.
radiohumeral
radioimmunity
radioimmunoassay
radioimmunodiffusion

R

radioimmunoelectrophoresis
radioimmunoprecipitation
radioimmunosorbent test
radioisotopic purity
radiolesion
radioligand
radiologic, radiological
radiologist
radiology
    cardiovascular r.
    chest r.
    interventional r.
    pediatric r.
radiolucency
radiolucent
radiolus
radiometer
radiomicrometer
radiomimetic
radiomuscular
radionecrosis
radioneuritis
radionuclide
    r. angiocardiography
    r. angiography
    r. cisternography
    r. generator
    r. ventriculography
radionuclidic purity
radiopacity
radiopalmar
radiopaque
radiopathology
radiopelvimetry
radioperiosteal reflex
radiopharmaceutical
    r. chemistry
    r. purity
radiophobia
radiopill
radioreaction
radioreceptor
    r. assay
radioresistant
radioscopy
radiosensitive
radiosensitivity
radiosensitization
radiosensitizer
radiostereoscopy
radiosurgery
radiotelemetering capsule
radiotherapeutic
radiotherapeutics
radiotherapist
radiotherapy
    r. localization
    mantle r.

radiothermy
radiothyroidectomy
radiotoxemia
radiotracer
radiotransparent
radiotropic
radioulnar
    r. articular disk
    r. disk
    r. syndesmosis
radisectomy
radium
    r. beam therapy
    r. emanation
radius, gen. and pl. **radii**
    r. fixus
    radii lentis
radix, gen. **radicis**, pl. **radices**
    r. anterior
    r. arcus vertebrae
    r. brevis ganglii ciliaris
    r. clinica
    r. cochlearis
    radices craniales
    r. dentis
    r. dorsalis
    r. facialis
    r. inferior ansae cervicalis
    r. inferior nervi vestibulocochlearis
    r. lateralis nervi mediani
    r. lateralis tractus optici
    r. linguae
    r. longa ganglii ciliaris
    r. medialis nervi mediani
    r. medialis tractus optici
    r. mesenterii
    r. motoria
    r. motoria nervi trigemini
    r. nasi
    r. nasociliaris
    r. nervi facialis
    radices nervi trigemini
    r. oculomotoria ganglii ciliaris
    r. parasympathica ganglii ciliaris
    r. penis
    r. pili
    r. posterior
    r. pulmonis
    r. sensoria
    r. sensoria ganglii ciliaris
    r. sensoria ganglii pterygopalatini
    r. sensoria nervi trigemini
    radices spinales nervi accessorii
    r. superior ansae cervicalis
    r. superior nervi vestibulocochlearis
    r. sympathica ganglii ciliaris
    r. unguis

    r. ventralis
    r. vestibularis
Raeder's paratrigeminal syndrome
rage
    sham r.
ragpicker's disease
ragsorter's, rag-sorter's
    r.'s disease
Rahe-Holmes social readjustment rating scale
Rahn-Otis sample
Raillietina
railroad
    r. disease
    r. nystagmus
    r. sickness
rainbow symptom
Rainey's corpuscles
RAI test
Raji
    R. cell
    R. cell radioimmune assay
rale
    amphoric r.
    atelectatic r.
    bubbling r.
    cavernous r.
    clicking r.
    consonating r.
    crackling r.
    crepitant r.
    dry r.
    gurgling r.
    guttural r.
    metallic r.
    moist r.
    mucous r.
    palpable r.
    pleural r.
    sibilant r.
    Skoda's r.
    sonorous r.
    subcrepitant r.
    vesicular r.
    whistling r.
ramal
Rambourg's
    R. chromic acid-phosphotungstic acid stain
    R. periodic acid-chromic methenamine-silver stain
    R. stains
ramex
rami (*pl. of* ramus)
ramicotomy
ramification
ramify
ramisection

ramitis
ramose, ramous
ramp
Ramsay Hunt's syndrome
Ramsden's ocular
Ramstedt operation
ramulus, pl. **ramuli**
ramus, pl. **rami**
    r. acetabularis
    r. acromialis arteriae suprascapularis
    r. acromialis arteriae
      thoracoacromialis
    rami ad pontem
    rami alveolares superiores anteriores
      nervi infraorbitalis
    rami alveolares superiores
      posteriores nervi maxillaris
    r. alveolaris superior medius nervi
      infraorbitalis
    r. anastomoticus
    r. anastomoticus arteriae meningeae
      mediae cum lacrimali
    r. anterior
    r. anterior ascendens
    r. anterior descendens
    r. anterior lateralis
    r. apicalis
    r. apicalis lobi inferioris arteriae
      pulmonalis dextrae
    r. apicoposterior venae pulmonalis
      sinistrae superioris
    rami articulares
    rami articulares arteriae
      descendentis genicularis
    r. ascendens
    rami atriales
    rami auriculares anteriores arteriae
      temporalis superficialis
    r. auricularis arteriae occipitalis
    r. auricularis nervi vagi
    r. basalis anterior
    r. basalis lateralis
    r. basalis medialis
    r. basalis posterior
    r. basalis tentorii arteriae carotidis
      internae
    rami bronchiales
    rami bronchiales segmentorum
    rami buccales nervi facialis
    rami calcanei
    rami calcanei laterales nervi suralis
    rami calcanei mediales nervi
      tibialis
    r. calcarinus arteriae occipitalis
      medialis
    rami capsulae internae
    rami capsulares arteriae renalis

    rami cardiaci cervicales inferiores
      nervi vagi
    rami cardiaci cervicales superiores
      nervi vagi
    rami cardiaci thoracici nervi vagi
    r. cardiacus
    rami caroticotympanici
    r. carpalis dorsalis arteriae radialis
    r. carpalis dorsalis arteriae ulnaris
    r. carpalis palmaris arteriae radialis
    r. carpalis palmaris arteriae ulnaris
    r. carpeus dorsalis arteriae radialis
    r. carpeus dorsalis arteriae ulnaris
    r. carpeus palmaris arteriae radialis
    r. carpeus palmaris arteriae ulnaris
    rami caudae nuclei caudati
    rami caudati
    rami celiaci nervi vagi
    rami centrales anteromediales
    cephalic arterial rami
    r. cervicalis nervi facialis
    r. chiasmaticus
    rami choroidei
    r. choroidei posteriores laterales
    r. choroidei posteriores mediales
    r. choroidei ventriculi lateralis
    r. choroidei ventriculi quarti
    r. choroidei ventriculi tertii
    r. cingularis
    r. circumflexus arteriae coronariae
      sinistrae
    r. circumflexus fibularis arteriae
      tibialis posterioris
    r. clavicularis arteriae
      thoracoacromialis
    r. clivi
    r. cochlearis arteriae labyrinthi
    r. collateralis arteriarum
      intercostalium posteriorum III–XI
    r. colli nervi facialis
    r. communicans, pl. rami
      communicantes
    r. communicans arteriae fibularis
    r. communicans arteriae peroneae
    r. communicans cum chorda
      tympani
    r. communicans cum nervo
      glossopharyngeo
    r. communicans fibularis nervi
      fibularis communis
    r. communicans ganglii otici cum
      nervo auriculotemporali
    r. communicans ganglii otici cum
      nervo pterygoideo mediali
    r. communicans ganglii otici cum
      ramo meningeo nervi mandibularis
    r. communicans nervi facialis cum
      plexu tympanico

R

ramus *(continued)*

r. communicans nervi glossopharyngei cum ramo auriculari nervi vagalis

r. communicans nervi lacrimalis cum nervo zygomatico

r. communicans nervi laryngei recurrentis cum ramo laryngeo interno

r. communicans nervi laryngei superioris cum nervo laryngeo recurrenti

r. communicans nervi mediani cum nervo ulnari

r. communicans nervi nasociliaris cum ganglio ciliari

r. communicans peroneus nervi peronei communis

r. communicans ulnaris nervi radialis

rami communicantes (*pl. of* r. communicans)

communicating rami of spinal nerves

communicating rami of sympathetic trunk

rami corporis amygdaloidei

r. corporis callosi dorsalis

rami corporis geniculati lateralis

r. costalis lateralis arteriae thoracicae internae

r. cricothyroideus

rami cutanei anteriores nervi femoralis

rami cutanei anteriores pectoralis et abdominalis nervorum intercostalium

rami cutanei cruris mediales nervi sapheni

r. cutaneus anterior nervi iliohypogastrici

r. cutaneus anterior (pectoralis et abdominalis) nervorum thoracicorum

r. cutaneus lateralis

r. cutaneus lateralis nervi iliohypogastrici

r. cutaneus lateralis ramorum posteriorum arteriae intercostalium

r. cutaneus medialis

r. cutaneus medialis rami dorsalis arteriarum intercostalium posteriorum III–XI

r. cutaneus medialis ramorum dorsalium nervorum thoracicorum

r. cutaneus rami anterioris nervi obturatorii

r. deltoideus

dental rami

rami dentales

rami dentales arteriae alveolaris inferioris

rami dentales arteriae alveolaris superioris posterioris

rami dentales inferiores

rami dentales inferiores plexus dentalis inferioris

rami dentales superiores

rami dentales superiores plexus dentalis superioris

r. descendens

r. descendens arteriae circumflexae femoris lateralis

r. descendens arteriae occipitalis

r. dexter

r. dexter arteriae hepaticae propriae

r. dexter venae portae hepatis

r. digastricus nervi facialis

rami dorsales arteriae intercostalis supremae

rami dorsales arteriae subcostalis

rami dorsales linguae arteriae lingualis

rami dorsales nervi ulnaris

r. dorsalis, rami dorsales

r. dorsalis arteriae lumbalium

r. dorsalis arteriarum intercostalium posteriorum III–XI

r. dorsalis nervorum spinalium

r. dorsalis venarum intercostalium posteriorum IV–XI

dorsal primary r. of spinal nerve

rami duodenales arteriae pancreaticoduodenalis superioris

rami epiploicae

rami esophageales

rami esophageales aortae thoracicae

rami esophageales arteriae gastricae sinistrae

rami esophageales arteriae thyroideae inferioris

rami esophagei

rami esophagei nervi laryngei recurrentis

rami esophagei nervi vagi

r. externus nervi accessorii

r. externus nervi laryngei superioris

rami fauciales nervi lingualis

r. femoralis nervi genitofemoralis

r. frontalis anteromedialis

r. frontalis arteriae temporalis superficialis

r. frontalis interomedialis

r. frontalis posteromedialis

rami ganglii submandibularis

rami communicantes ganglii

submandibularis cum nervo linguali

r. ganglii trigeminalis

rami ganglionares

rami ganglionici nervi maxillaris

rami gastrici anteriores nervi vagi

rami gastrici posteriores nervi vagi

r. genitalis nervi genitofemoralis

rami gingivales inferiores plexus dentalis inferioris

rami gingivales superiores plexus dentalis superioris

rami glandulares

r. glandulares anterior/lateralis/posterior arteriae thyroideae superioris

rami glandulares arteriae facialis

rami glandulares arteriae thyroideae inferioris

rami glandulares ganglii submandibularis

rami globi pallidi

gray rami communicantes

rami hepatici nervi vagi

r. hypothalamicus

r. iliacus arteriae iliolumbalis

r. inferior

r. inferior arteriae gluteae superioris

inferior dental rami

rami inferiores nervi transversi cervicalis [colli]

r. inferior nervi oculomotorii

r. inferior ossis pubis

r. infrahyoideus arteriae thyroidea superioris

r. infrapatellaris nervi sapheni

rami inguinales arteriae pudendae externae

rami intercostales anteriores

rami intercostalis anteriores arteria thoracica interna

rami interganglionares

interganglionic rami

internal r. of accessory nerve

r. internus nervi accessorii

r. internus nervi laryngei superioris

rami interventriculares septales

r. interventricularis anterior arteriae coronariae sinistrae

r. interventricularis posterior arteriae coronariae dextrae

ischial r.

ischiopubic r.

rami isthmi faucium nervi lingualis

rami labiales anteriores arteriae pudendae externae

rami labiales inferiores nervi mentalis

rami labiales posteriores arteriae pudendae internae

rami labiales superiores nervi infraorbitalis

rami laryngopharyngei ganglii cervicalis superioris

rami laterales

rami laterales arteriarum centralium anterolateralium

rami laterales rami sinistri venae portae hepatis

rami laterales ramorum dorsalium nervorum cervicalium/thoracalium/lumbalium-/sac

r. lateralis ductus hepatici sinistri

r. lateralis interventricularis anterioris arteriae coronariae sinistrae

r. lateralis nervi supraorbitalis

r. lateralis ramorum dorsalium nervorum thoracicorum

r. lateralis ramorum lobaris medium arteriorum pulmonalium dextrorum

rami lienales arteriae lienalis

rami linguales

rami linguales nervi glossopharyngei

rami linguales nervi hypoglossi

rami linguales nervi lingualis

r. lingualis

r. lingularis inferior

r. lingularis nervi facialis

r. lingularis superior

r. lobi medii

r. lobi medii arteriae pulmonalis dextrae

r. lobi medii venae pulmonalis dextrae superioris

r. lumbalis arteriae iliolumbalis

rami malleolares laterales

rami malleolares mediales

rami mammarii

rami mammarii laterales

rami mammarii laterales arteriae thoracicae lateralis

rami mammarii laterales nervorum intercostalium

rami mammarii laterales rami cutanei lateralis nervorum intercostalium

rami mammarii laterales rami cutanei lateralis nervorum thoracicorum

rami mammarii mediales

ramus *(continued)*

rami mammarii mediales rami cutanei anterioris nervorum intercostalium

rami mammarii mediales rami cutanei anterioris ramorum ventralium nervorum thoracicorum

rami mammarii mediales rami perforantis arteriae thoracicae internae

r. of mandible

r. mandibulae

r. marginalis mandibulae nervi facialis

r. marginalis tentorii arteriae carotidis internae

rami mastoidei arteriae auricularis posterioris

r. mastoideus arteriae occipitalis

r. meatus acustici interni

rami mediales

rami mediales arteriarum centralium anterolateralium

rami mediales rami sinistri venae portae hepatis

r. medialis ductus hepatici sinistri

r. medialis nervi supraorbitalis

r. medialis rami lobaris medii arteriorum pulmonalium dextrorum

r. medialis ramorum dorsalium nervorum cervicalium/thoracicorum/lumbalium-/sacralium

rami mediastinales

rami mediastinales aortae thoracicae

rami mediastinales arteriae thoracicae internae

rami medullares laterales

rami medullares mediales

r. membranae tympani nervi auriculotemporalis

rami meningei

r. meningeus accessorius arteriae meningeae mediae

r. meningeus anterior arteriae vertebralis

r. meningeus arteriae carotidis internae

r. meningeus arteriae occipitalis

r. meningeus medius nervi maxillaris

r. meningeus nervi mandibularis

r. meningeus nervi vagi

r. meningeus nervorum spinalium

r. meningeus posterior

rami mentales nervi mentalis

rami musculares

r. musculi stylopharyngei nervi glossopharyngei

r. mylohyoideus arteriae alveolaris inferioris

rami nasales externi

rami nasales externi nervi ethmoidalis anterioris

rami nasales externi nervi infraorbitalis

rami nasales interni

rami nasales interni nervi ethmoidalis anterioris

rami nasales interni nervi infraorbitalis

rami nasales laterales nervi ethmoidalis anterioris

rami nasales mediales nervi ethmoidalis anterioris

rami nasales posteriores inferiores nervi palatini majoris

rami nasales posteriores superiores laterales ganglii pterygopalatini

rami nasales posteriores superiores mediales ganglii pterygopalatini

rami communicantes nervi auriculotemporalis cum nervo faciali

rami communicantes nervi lingualis cum nervo hypoglosso

r. nervi oculomotorii arteriae communicantis posterioris

rami communicantes nervorum spinalium

r. nodi atrioventricularis

r. nodi sinuatrialis arteriae coronaria dextra

rami nucleorum hypothalamicorum

r. obturatorius arteriae epigastricae inferioris

rami occipitales arteriae auricularis posterioris

rami occipitales arteriae occipitis

rami occipitales nervi auricularis posterioris

r. occipitalis

r. occipitotemporalis

rami omentales

r. orbitalis arteriae meningeae mediae

r. orbitalis ganglii pterygopalatini

r. orbitofrontalis lateralis

r. orbitofrontalis medialis

r. ossis ischii

r. ovaricus arteriae uterinae

r. palmaris nervi mediani

r. palmaris nervi ulnaris

r. palmaris profundus arteriae ulnaris

r. palmaris superficialis arteriae
  radialis
rami palpebrales nervi
  infratrochlearis
rami pancreatici
rami pancreatici arteriae
  pancreaticoduodenalis superioris
rami pancreatici arteriae splenicae
rami parietales
r. parietalis arteriae meningeae
  mediae
r. parietalis arteriae occipitalis
  medialis
r. parietalis arteriae temporalis
  superficialis
r. parieto-occipitalis
rami parotidei
r. parotidei arteriae temporalis
  superficialis
rami parotidei nervi
  auriculotemporalis
rami parotidei venae facialis
rami pectorales arteriae
  thoracoacromialis
rami pedunculares
r. perforans
r. perforans arteriae fibularis
r. perforantes arteriae thoracicae
  internae
r. perforantes arteriarum
  metacarpalium palmarium
r. perforantes arteriarum
  metatarsearum plantarium
rami pericardiaci aortae thoracicae
r. pericardiacus nervi phrenici
rami perineales nervi cutanei
  femoris posterioris
peroneal anastomotic r.
r. petrosus arteriae meningeae
  mediae
rami pharyngeales
rami pharyngeales arteriae
  pharyngeae ascendentis
rami pharyngeales arteriae
  thyroideae inferioris
rami pharyngei nervi
  glossopharyngei
rami pharyngei nervi vagi
r. pharyngeus arteriae canalis
  pterygoidei
r. pharyngeus arteriae palatini
  descendens
r. pharyngeus ganglii pterygopalatini
rami phrenicoabdominales nervi
  phrenici
r. plantaris profundus arteriae
  dorsalis pedis
r. posterior arteriae obturatoriae

r. posterior arteriae
  pancreaticoduodenalis inferioris
r. posterior arteriae recurrentis
  ulnaris
r. posterior arteriae renalis
r. posterior arteriae thyroideae
  superioris
r. posterior ascendens
r. posterior descendens
r. posterior ductus hepatici dextri
rami posteriores
rami posteriores nervorum
  spinalium
r. posterior nervi auricularis magni
r. posterior nervi obturatorii
r. posterior rami dextri venae
  portae hepatis
r. posterior sulci lateralis cerebri
r. posterior venae pulmonalis
  dextrae superioris
rami profundi arteriae circumflexae
  femoris medialis
rami profundi arteriae transversae
  cervicis
r. profundus
r. profundus arteriae circumflexae
  femoris medialis
r. profundus arteriae transversae
  colli
r. profundus arteria scapularis
  descendens
r. profundus nervi plantaris lateralis
r. profundus nervi radialis
r. profundus nervi ulnaris
rami pterygoidei arteriae maxillaris
pubic rami
r. pubicus arteriae epigastricae
  inferioris
r. pubicus arteriae obturatoriae
rami pulmonales systematis
  autonomici
rami radiculares
rami renales nervi vagi
r. renalis nervi splanchnici minoris
r. saphenus arteriae descendentis
  genicularis
rami scrotales anteriores arteriae
  pudendae externae
rami scrotales posteriores arteriae
  pudendae internae
rami septales
r. sinister
r. sinister arteriae hepaticae
  propriae
r. sinister venae portae hepatis
r. sinus carotici
r. sinus cavernosi

R

ramus *(continued)*
 r. sinus cavernosi arteriae carotidis
  arteriae
 rami spinales
 rami splenici arteriae splenicae
 r. stapedius arteriae stylomastoideae
 rami sternales arteriae thoracicae
  internae
 rami sternocleidomastoidei arteriae
  occipitalis
 r. sternocleidomastoideus arteriae
  thyroideae superioris
 r. stylohyoideus nervi facialis
 rami subscapulares arteriae axillaris
 rami substantiae nigrae
 r. superficialis
 r. superficialis arteriae gluteae
  superioris
 r. superficialis arteriae plantaris
  medialis
 r. superficialis nervi plantaris
  lateralis
 r. superficialis nervi radialis
 r. superficialis nervi ulnaris
 r. superior, rami superiores
 r. superior arteriae gluteae
  superioris
 superior dental rami
 r. superior nervi oculomotorii
 r. superior nervi transversalis
  cervicalis (colli)
 r. superior ossis pubis
 superior pubic r.
 r. superior venae pulmonalis
  dextrae/sinistrae inferioris
 r. suprahyoideus arteriae lingualis
 r. sympathicus [sympatheticus] ad
  ganglion submandibulare
 rami temporales anteriores
 rami temporales intermedii mediales
 rami temporales nervi facialis
 rami temporales posteriores
 rami temporales superficiales nervi
  auriculotemporalis
 r. tentorii
 rami thalamici
 r. thalamicus
 rami thymici
 r. thyrohyoideus ansae cervicalis
 r. tonsillae cerebellae
 rami tonsillares nervi
  glossopharyngei
 r. tonsillaris arteriae facialis
 rami tracheales
 rami tracheales arteriae thyroideae
  inferioris
 rami tracheales nervi laryngei
  recurrentis

 rami tractus optici
 r. transversus
 r. transversus arteriae circumflexae
  femoris lateralis
 r. transversus arteriae circumflexae
  femoris medialis
 r. tubarius
 r. tubarius arteriae uterinae
 r. tubarius plexus tympanici
 rami tuberis cinerei
 r. ulnaris nervi cutanei antebrachii
  medialis
 rami ureterici
 rami ureterici arteriae ovaricae
 rami ureterici arteriae renalis
 rami ureterici arteriae testicularis
 rami ureterici partis patentis
  arteriae umbilicale
 rami ventrales nervorum
  cervicalium
 rami ventrales nervorum lumbalium
 rami ventrales nervorum sacralium
 rami ventralis
 r. ventralis nervi spinalis
 ventral primary rami of cervical
  spinal nerves
 ventral primary rami of lumbar
  spinal nerves
 ventral primary rami of sacral
  spinal nerves
 ventral primary r. of spinal nerve
 rami vestibulares arteriae labyrinthi
 white rami communicantes
 rami zygomatici nervi facialis
 r. zygomaticofacialis nervi
  zygomatici
 r. zygomaticotemporalis nervi
  zygomatici
Randall
 R. plaques
 R. stone forceps
random
 r. mating
 r. mating equilibrium
 r. pattern flap
 r. sample
 r. sampling
 r. variable
 r. waves
randomization
randomized controlled trial
range
 r. of accommodation
 r. of convergence
ranine
 r. artery
 r. tumor
rank

rank-difference correlation
Ranke's
    R. angle
    R. formula
Rankin's clamp
Ransohoff's sign
RANTES
ranula
    r. pancreatica
ranular
Ranvier's
    R. crosses
    R. disks
    R. node
    R. plexus
    R. segment
rape
raphe
    r. anococcygea
    anogenital r.
    r. corporis callosi
    lateral palpebral r.
    r. linguae
    median longitudinal r. of tongue
    r. medullae oblongatae
    r. nuclei
    r. palati
    palatine r.
    palpebral r.
    r. palpebralis lateralis
    penile r.
    r. penis
    perineal r.
    r. perinei
    pharyngeal r.
    r. pharyngis
    r. pontis
    pterygomandibular r.
    r. pterygomandibularis
    r. retinae
    scrotal r.
    r. scroti
    Stilling's r.
raphespinal fibers
rapid
    r. canities
    r. decompression
    r. eye movements
    r. eye movement sleep
    r. film changer
    r. plasma reagin test
rapidly progressive glomerulonephritis
Rapoport test
Rappaport
    R. R.
    R. acinus
rapport
rapture of the deep

rare-earth screen
rarefaction
rarefy
rasceta
rash
    ammonia r.
    antitoxin r.
    astacoid r.
    black currant r.
    butterfly r.
    caterpillar r.
    crystal r.
    diaper r.
    drug r.
    heat r.
    hydatid r.
    Murray Valley r.
    napkin r.
    nettle r.
    serum r.
    summer r.
    wildfire r.
Rasmussen
    R. a. aneurysm
    bundle of R. a.
raspatory
raspberry tongue
Rastelli's operation
rat-bite
    r.-b. disease
    r.-b. fever
rate
    abortion r.
    age-specific r.
    average flow r.
    baseline fetal heart r.
    birth r.
    concordance r.
    critical r.
    death r.
    erythrocyte sedimentation r.
    fatality r.
    fetal death r.
    fetal heart r.
    five year survival r.
    general fertility r.
    glomerular filtration r.
    gross reproduction r.
    growth r.
    growth r. of population
    hazard r.
    heart r.
    inception r.
    incidence r.
    infant mortality r.
    lethality r.
    maternal death r.
    r. meter

R

rate *(continued)*
   mitotic r.
   morbidity r.
   mortality r.
   mutation r.
   neonatal mortality r.
   peak flow r.
   perinatal mortality r.
   pulse r.
   recurrence r.
   repetition r.
   respiration r.
   sedimentation r.
   shear r.
   slew r.
   steroid metabolic clearance r.
   steroid production r.
   steroid secretory r.
   stillbirth r.
   voiding flow r.

Rathke's
   R. bundles
   R. cleft cyst
   R. diverticulum
   R. pocket
   R. pouch
   R. pouch tumor

ratio
   absolute terminal innervation r.
   accommodative convergence-
     accommodation r.
   albumin-globulin r.
   ALT:AST r.
   amylase-creatinine clearance r.
   body-weight r.
   cardiothoracic r.
   case fatality r.
   r. of decayed and filled surfaces
   r. of decayed and filled teeth
   extraction r.
   fertility r.
   flux r.
   functional terminal innervation r.
   grid r.
   gyromagnetic r.
   hand r.
   IRI/G r.
   lecithin/sphingomyelin r.
   magnetogyric r.
   M:E r.
   mendelian r.
   nuclear-cytoplasmic r.
   nucleolar-nuclear r.
   respiratory exchange r.
   r. scale
   segregation r.
   sex r.
   signal-to-noise r.

   standardized mortality r.
   systolic/diastolic r.
   variance r.
   ventilation/perfusion r.
   zeta sedimentation r.

rational
   r. therapy
rationalization
rat mite dermatitis
Rauscher
   R. leukemia virus
   R. virus
Rau's process
Raussly disease
Ravius' process
raw score
ray
   actinic r.
   anode r.'s
   Becquerel r.'s
   cathode r.'s
   chemical r.
   direct r.'s
   Dorno r.'s
   r. fungus
   gamma r.'s
   glass r.'s
   grenz r.
   H r.'s
   hard r.'s
   incident r.
   indirect r.'s
   infrared r.
   intermediate r.'s
   marginal r.'s
   medullary r.
   monochromatic r.'s
   Niewenglowski r.'s
   parallel r.'s
   paraxial r.'s
   positive r.'s
   reflected r.
   roentgen r.
   secondary r.'s
   soft r.'s
   supersonic r.'s
   r. therapeutics
   ultrasonic r.'s
   ultraviolet r.'s
   W r.'s
   x-r.
Rayer's disease
rayl
Rayleigh
   R. equation
   R. test
Raynaud's
   R. disease

R. phenomenon
R. sign
R. syndrome
R-banding
R.-b. stain
R.C.P.C.
R.C.S.C.
RCT
reactant
acute phase r.'s
reaction
accelerated r.
acute phase r.
acute situational r.
acute stress r.
alarm r.
allergic r.
amphoteric r.
anamnestic r.
anaphylactic r.
anxiety r.
Arias-Stella r.
arousal r.
Arthus r.
Ascoli r.
Berthelot r.
Bittorf's r.
Bordet and Gengou r.
Brunn r.
capsular precipitation r.
Carr-Price r.
catastrophic r.
cell-mediated r.
r. center
Chantemesse r.
cholera-red r.
chromaffin r.
circular r.
cocarde r., cockade r.
colloidal gold r.
complement-fixation r.
consensual r.
constitutional r.
conversion r.
cross r.
cutaneous r.
cutaneous graft versus host r.
cytotoxic r.
Dale r.
decidual r.
r. of degeneration
delayed r.
depot r.
depressive r.
dermotuberculin r.
diazo r.
dissociative r.
dystonic r.

early r.
echo r.
Ehrlich's benzaldehyde r.
Ehrlich's diazo r.
eye-closure pupil r.
false-negative r.
false-positive r.
Fernandez r.
Feulgen r.
fight or flight r.
fixation r.
flocculation r.
focal r.
r. formation
Forssman r.
Forssman antigen-antibody r.
Frei-Hoffmann r.
fright r.
fuchsinophil r.
furfurol r.
galvanic skin r.
gel diffusion r.'s
Gell and Coombs r.'s
gemistocytic r.
general adaptation r.
Gerhardt's r.
graft versus host r.
group r.
Gruber's r.
Gruber-Widal r.
harlequin r.
heel-tap r.
hemoclastic r.
Henle's r.
Herxheimer's r.
homograft r.
hunting r.
hypersensitivity r.
id r.
r. of identity
immediate r.
immediate hypersensitivity r.
immune r.
incompatible blood transfusion r.
indirect pupillary r.
intracutaneous r., intradermal r.
iodate r. of epinephrine
iodine r. of epinephrine
irreversible r.
Jaffe r.
Jarisch-Herxheimer r.
Jolly's r.
late r.
lengthening r.
lepromin r.
leukemoid r.
lid-closure r.
local r.

flare reaction to chemotherapy

R

reaction *(continued)*
  local anesthetic r.
  Loewenthal's r.
  magnet r.
  Marchi's r.
  Mazzotti r.
  miostagmin r.
  Mitsuda r.
  mixed agglutination r.
  mixed lymphocyte culture r.
  myasthenic r.
  Nadi r.
  near r.
  negative supporting r.'s (*var. of*
    supporting r.'s)
  Neufeld r.
  neurotonic r.
  ninhydrin r.
  nitritoid r.
  r. of nonidentity
  oxidase r.
  pain r.
  Pandy's r.
  r. of partial identity
  passive cutaneous anaphylactic r.
  Paul's r.
  performic acid r.
  periosteal r.
  peroxidase r.
  Pirquet's r.
  plasmal r.
  pleural r.
  Porter-Silber r.
  positive supporting r.'s (*var. of*
    supporting r.'s)
  Prausnitz-Küstner r.
  precipitin r.
  primary r.
  prozone r.
  psychogalvanic r., psychogalvanic
    skin r.
  quellung r.
  reversed Prausnitz-Küstner r.
  Sakaguchi r.
  Schultz r.
  Schultz-Charlton r.
  Schultz-Dale r.
  serum r.
  shortening r.
  Shwartzman r.
  skin r.
  specific r.
  startle r.
  stress r.
  supporting r.'s, negative
    supporting r.'s, positive
    supporting r.'s

  symptomatic r.
  thermoprecipitin r.
  r. time
  Treponema pallidum
    immobilization r.
  type III hypersensitivity r.
  vaccinoid r.
  Voges-Proskauer r.
  Wassermann r.
  Weidel's r.
  Weil-Felix r.
  Weinberg's r.
  Wernicke's r.
  wheal-and-erythema r.
  wheal-and-flare r.
  whitegraft r.
  Widal's r.
  Yorke's autolytic r.
reactive
  r. astrocyte
  r. attachment disorder
  r. cell
  r. depression
  r. hyperemia
  r. perforating collagenosis
  r. schizophrenia
reagent
  Drabkin's r.
  Esbach's r.
  Frohn's r.
  Girard's r.
  Hahn's oxine r.
  Ilosvay r.
  Kasten's fluorescent Schiff r.'s
  Lloyd's r.
  Mandelin's r.
  Marme's r.
  Marquis' r.
  Mecke's r.
  Rosenthaler-Turk r.
  Schaer's r.
  Scheibler's r.
  Schiff's r.
reagin
  atopic r.
reaginic
  r. antibody
real
  r. focus
  r. image
  r. origin
reality
  r. adaptation
  r. awareness
  r. principle
  r. testing
real-time ultrasonography

reamer
    engine r.
    intramedullary r.
reattachment
rebase
rebound
    r. phenomenon
    r. tenderness
rebreathing
    r. anesthesia
    r. technique
Rebuck skin window technique
RecA
recalcification
recall
Récamier's operation
recanalization
recapitulation
    r. theory
receiver
    r. operating characteristic
    r. operating characteristic curve
receptaculum, pl. **receptacula**
    r. chyli
    r. ganglii petrosi
    r. pecqueti
receptive
    r. aphasia
    r. field
receptoma
receptor
    ANP r.'s
    ANP clearance r.'s
    B cell antigen r.'s
    Fc r.
    low-density lipoprotein r.'s
    mannose-6-phosphate r.'s
    nicotinic r.'s
    opiate r.'s
    sensory r.'s
    stretch r.'s
    T cell antigen r.'s
recess
    anterior r.
    anterior r. of tympanic membrane
    azygoesophageal r.
    cecal r.
    cerebellopontine r.
    cochlear r.
    costodiaphragmatic r.
    costomediastinal r.
    duodenojejunal r.
    elliptical r.
    epitympanic r.
    hepatoenteric r.
    hepatorenal r.
    Hyrtl's epitympanic r.
    inferior duodenal r.

    inferior ileocecal r.
    inferior omental r.
    infundibular r.
    intersigmoid r.
    Jacquemet's r.
    lateral r. of fourth ventricle
    mesentericoparietal r.
    optic r.
    pancreaticoenteric r.
    paracolic r.'s
    paraduodenal r.
    parotid r.
    pharyngeal r.
    phrenicomediastinal r.
    pineal r.
    piriform r.
    pleural r.'s
    pneumatoenteric r., pneumoenteric r.
    pontocerebellar r.
    posterior r.
    posterior r. of tympanic membrane
    Reichert's cochlear r.
    retrocecal r.
    retroduodenal r.
    Rosenmüller's r.
    sacciform r.
    sphenoethmoidal r.
    spherical r.
    splenic r.
    subhepatic r.
    subphrenic r.'s
    subpopliteal r.
    superior azygoesophageal r.
    superior duodenal r.
    superior ileocecal r.
    superior r. of lesser peritoneal sac
    superior omental r.
    superior r. of tympanic membrane
    suprapineal r.
    supratonsillar r.
    triangular r.
    Tröltsch's r.'s
    tubotympanic r.
recession
    clitoral r.
    gingival r.
    tendon r.
recessitivity
recessive
    r. character
    r. inheritance
    r. trait
recessus, pl. **recessus**
    r. anterior
    r. cochlearis
    r. costodiaphragmaticus
    r. costomediastinalis
    r. duodenalis inferior

recessus *(continued)*
   r. duodenalis superior
   r. ellipticus
   r. epitympanicus
   r. hepatorenalis
   r. ileocecalis inferior
   r. ileocecalis superior
   r. inferior omentalis
   r. infundibuli
   r. infundibuliformis
   r. intersigmoideus
   r. lateralis ventriculi quarti
   r. lienalis
   r. membranae tympani anterior
   r. membranae tympani posterior
   r. membranae tympani superior
   r. opticus
   r. paraduodenalis
   r. parotideus
   r. pharyngeus
   r. phrenicomediastinalis
   r. pinealis
   r. piriformis
   r. pleurales
   r. posterior
   r. retrocecalis
   r. retroduodenalis
   r. sacciformis
   r. sphenoethmoidalis
   r. sphericus
   r. splenicus
   r. subhepaticus
   r. subphrenici
   r. subpopliteus
   r. superior omentalis
   r. suprapinealis
   r. triangularis
recidivation
recidivism
recidivist
recipient
recipiomotor
reciprocal
   r. anchorage
   r. arm
   r. beat
   r. bigeminy
   r. forces
   r. inhibition
   r. innervation
   r. rhythm
   r. transfusion
   r. translocation
reciprocating rhythm
reciprocation
reciprocity law
Recklinghausen's
   R. disease of bone

   R. disease type I
   R. tumor
reclination
recognition
   r. factors
   r. time
recoil wave
recollection
recombinant
   r. strain
   r. vector
recombination
   r. fraction
   genetic r.
   site specific r.
recombinatorial repair
recon
reconstruction
reconstructive
   r. mammaplasty
   r. psychotherapy
   r. surgery
record
   anesthesia r.
   r. base
   face-bow r.
   functional chew-in r.
   hospital r.
   interocclusal r., centric
     interocclusal r., eccentric
     interocclusal r., lateral
     interocclusal r., protrusive
     interocclusal r.
   r. linkage
   maxillomandibular r.
   medical r.
   occluding centric relation r.
   preextraction r.
   preoperative r.
   problem-oriented r.
   profile r.
   protrusive r.
   protrusive interocclusal r. *(var. of*
     interocclusal r.)
   r. rim
   terminal jaw relation r.
   three-dimensional r.
recording
   clinical r.
   depth r.
recovery
   creep r.
   inversion r.
   r. room
   r. score
   short TI inversion r.
   spontaneous r.
   ultrasonic egg r.

R

recrudescence
recrudescent
   r. typhus
   r. typhus fever
recruiting response
recruitment
recta (*pl. of* rectum)
rectal
   r. alimentation
   r. ampulla
   r. anesthesia
   r. columns
   r. disease
   r. folds
   r. plexuses
   r. reflex
   r. shelf
   r. sinuses
   r. valves
   r. valvotomy
   r. venous plexus
rectalgia
rectangular amputation
rectectomy
rectifier
   r. tube
rectitis
rectoabdominal
rectocardiac reflex
rectocele
rectoclysis
rectococcygeal
   r. muscle
rectococcygeus muscle
rectococcypexy
rectocolitis
rectolabial fistula
rectolaryngeal reflex
rectoperineal
rectoperineorrhaphy
rectopexy
rectophobia
rectoplasty
rectorrhaphy
rectoscope
rectoscopy
rectosigmoid
   r. junction
   r. sphincter
rectostenosis
rectostomy
rectotome
rectotomy
rectourethral
   r. fistula
   r. muscle
rectourethralis muscle

rectouterine
   r. fold
   r. muscle
   r. pouch
rectovaginal
   r. fistula
   r. septum
rectovaginouterine pouch
rectovesical
   r. fascia
   r. fistula
   r. fold
   r. muscle
   r. pouch
   r. septum
rectovesicalis muscle
rectovestibular
   r. fistula
rectovulvar fistula
rectum, pl. **rectums, recta**
rectus
   r. abdominis muscle
   r. capitis anterior muscle
   r. capitis lateralis muscle
   r. capitis posterior major muscle
   r. capitis posterior minor muscle
   r. femoris muscle
   r. muscle of abdomen
   r. muscle of thigh
   r. sheath
recumbent
recuperate
recuperation
recurrence
   r. rate
   r. risk
recurrent
   r. albuminuria
   r. aphthous stomatitis
   r. aphthous ulcers
   r. appendicitis
   r. artery
   r. artery of Heubner
   r. caries
   r. central retinitis
   r. corneal erosion
   r. encephalopathy
   r. fever
   r. herpetic stomatitis
   r. hypopyon
   r. interosseous artery
   r. laryngeal nerve
   r. meningeal branch of spinal
     nerves
   r. meningeal nerve
   r. nerve
   r. polyserositis
   r. pyogenic cholangitis

recurrent *(continued)*
    r. radial artery
    r. scarring aphthae
    r. stricture
    r. ulcerative stomatitis
    r. ulnar artery
recurring digital fibromas of childhood
recurvation
red
    r. atrophy
    r. blood cell
    r. blood cell cast
    r. bone marrow
    r. cell adherence phenomenon
    r. cell adherence test
    r. cell cast
    r. corpuscle
    R. Cross
    r. degeneration
    r. fever
    r. fever of the Congo
    r. fibers
    r. half-moon
    r. hepatization
    r. induration
    r. infarct
    r. muscle
    r. neuralgia
    r. nucleus
    r. pulp
    r. pulp cords
    r. reflex
    r. strawberry tongue
    r. sweat
    r. test
    r. thrombus
    r. vision
redifferentiation
redintegration
redressement forcé
redressment
reduced
    r. enamel epithelium
    r. eye
    r. interarch distance
reducible hernia
reducing
    r. diet
    r. valve
reduction
    r. of chromosomes
    closed r. of fractures
    r. deformity
    r. division
    r. en masse
    r. mammaplasty
    r. nucleus
    open r. of fractures

    r. phase
    selective r.
    tuberosity r.
reduplicated cataract
reduplication
reduvid, reduviid
Reduviidae
Reed
    R. cells
Reed-Frost theory of epidemics
reed instrument theory
Reed-Sternberg cells
reedy nail
reefing
    stomach r.
reel foot
reenactment
re-entrant mechanism
reentry
    r. phenomenon
    r. theory
Rees-Ecker fluid
refect
refection
refeeding gynecomastia
reference
    r. method
    r. values
referred
    r. pain
    r. sensation
Refetoff syndrome
reflect
reflected
    r. colors
    r. inguinal ligament
    r. light
    r. ray
reflecting retinoscope
reflection
    r. coefficient
reflex
    abdominal r.'s
    abdominocardiac r.
    Abrams' heart r.
    accommodation r.
    Achilles r., Achilles tendon r.
    acousticopalpebral r.
    acquired r.
    acromial r.
    adductor r.
    allied r.'s
    anal r.
    r. angina
    ankle r.
    antagonistic r.'s
    aortic r.
    aponeurotic r.

r. arc
Aschner-Dagnini r.
Aschner's r.
r. asthma
attitudinal r.'s
auditory r.
auditory oculogyric r.
auricular r.
auriculopalpebral r.
auriculopressor r.
auropalpebral r.
axon r.
Babinski r.
back of foot r., dorsum of foot r.
Bainbridge r.
Barkman's r.
basal joint r.
Bechterew-Mendel r.
behavior r.
Benedek's r.
Bezold-Jarisch r.
biceps r.
biceps femoris r.
Bing's r.
bladder r.
body righting r.'s
bone r.
brachioradial r.
Brain's r.
bregmocardiac r.
Brissaud's r.
bulbocavernosus r.
bulbomimic r.
Capps' r.
cardiac depressor r.
carotid sinus r.
celiac plexus r.
cephalic r.'s
cephalopalpebral r.
Chaddock r.
chain r.
chin r.
Chodzko's r.
ciliospinal r.
clasping r.
cochleo-orbicular r.
cochleopalpebral r.
cochleopupillary r.
cochleostapedial r.
conditioned r.
conjunctival r.
consensual light r.
contralateral r.
r. control
convulsive r.
coordinated r.
corneal r.
costal arch r.

costopectoral r.
cough r.
r. cough
craniocardiac r.
cremasteric r.
crossed r.
crossed adductor r.
crossed extension r.
crossed knee r.
crossed r. of pelvis
crossed spino-adductor r.
cry r.
cuboidodigital r.
cutaneous r.
cutaneous pupil r., cutaneous-
  pupillary r.
darwinian r.
deep r.
deep abdominal r.'s
defense r.
deglutition r.
Dejerine's r.
delayed r.
depressor r.
r. detrusor contraction
diffused r.
digital r.
diving r.
dorsal r.
dorsum of foot r. (*var. of* back of
  foot r.)
dorsum pedis r.
r. dyspepsia
elbow r.
enterogastric r.
epigastric r.
r. epilepsy
erector-spinal r.
esophagosalivary r.
external oblique r.
eye r.
eyeball compression r.
eyeball-heart r.
eye-closure r.
facial r.
faucial r.
femoral r.
femoroabdominal r.
finger-thumb r.
flexor r.
forced grasping r.
front-tap r.
fundus r.
gag r.
Galant's r.
galvanic skin r.
gastrocolic r.
gastroileac r.

R

reflex *(continued)*
  Geigel's r.
  Gifford's r.
  gluteal r.
  Gordon r.
  grasp r.
  grasping r.
  great-toe r.
  Guillain-Barré r.
  gustatory-sudorific r.
  H r.
  r. headache
  hepatojugular r.
  Hering-Breuer r.
  Hoffmann's r.
  hypochondrial r.
  hypogastric r.
  inborn r.
  r. incontinence
  r. inhibition
  innate r.
  interscapular r.
  intrinsic r.
  inverted r.
  inverted radial r.
  investigatory r.
  ipsilateral r.
  r. iridoplegia
  Jacobson's r.
  jaw r.
  jaw-working r.
  Joffroy's r.
  Kisch's r.
  knee r.
  knee-jerk r.
  labyrinthine r.'s
  labyrinthine righting r.'s
  lacrimal r.
  lacrimo-gustatory r.
  laryngeal r.
  laryngospastic r.
  latent r.
  laughter r.
  let-down r.
  lid r.
  Liddell-Sherrington r.
  r. ligament
  light r.
  lip r.
  Lovén r.
  lower abdominal periosteal r.
  magnet r.
  mandibular r.
  mass r.
  masseter r.
  Mayer's r.
  McCarthy's r.'s
  mediopubic r.

  Mendel-Bechterew r.
  Mendel's instep r.
  metacarpohypothenar r.
  metacarpothenar r.
  metatarsal r.
  micturition r.
  milk-ejection r.
  milk let-down r.
  Mondonesi's r.
  Moro r.
  r. movement
  muscular r.
  myenteric r.
  myotatic r.
  nasal r.
  nasomental r.
  near r.
  neck r.'s
  r. neurogenic bladder
  nociceptive r.
  nocifensor r.
  nose-bridge-lid r.
  nose-eye r.
  oculocardiac r.
  oculocephalic r.
  oculocephalogyric r.
  oculovagal r.
  olecranon r.
  Oppenheim's r.
  optical righting r.'s
  orbicularis oculi r.
  orbicularis pupillary r.
  orienting r.
  r. otalgia
  palatal r., palatine r.
  palmar r.
  palm-chin r.
  palmomental r.
  parachute r.
  paradoxical r.
  paradoxical extensor r.
  paradoxical flexor r.
  paradoxical patellar r.
  paradoxical pupillary r.
  paradoxical triceps r.
  patellar r.
  patellar tendon r.
  patello-adductor r.
  Pavlov's r.
  pectoral r.
  Perez r.
  pericardial r.
  periosteal r.
  pharyngeal r.
  phasic r.
  Phillipson's r.
  pilomotor r.
  plantar r.

plantar muscle r.
pneocardiac r.
pneopneic r.
postural r.
pressoreceptor r.
pronator r.
proprioceptive r.'s
proprioceptive-oculocephalic r.
protective laryngeal r.
psychocardiac r.
psychogalvanic r., psychogalvanic
  skin r.
pulmonocoronary r.
pupillary r.
pupillary-skin r.
quadriceps r.
quadripedal extensor r.
radial r.
radiobicipital r.
radioperiosteal r.
rectal r.
rectocardiac r.
rectolaryngeal r.
red r.
Remak's r.
renal r.
righting r.'s
Roger's r.
rooting r.
Rossolimo's r.
scapular r.
scapulohumeral r.
scapuloperiosteal r.
Schäffer's r.
semimembranosus r.,
  semitendinosus r.
r. sensation
shot-silk r.
sinus r.
skin r.'s
skin-muscle r.'s
skin-pupillary r.
snapping r.
snout r.
sole r.
sole tap r.
spinal r.
spino-adductor r.
Starling's r.
startle r.
static r.
statokinetic r.
statotonic r.'s
sternobrachial r.
stretch r.
Strümpell's r.
styloradial r.
superficial r.

supination r.
supinator r., supinator longus r.
supporting r.'s
supraorbital r.
suprapatellar r.
supraumbilical r.
swallowing r.
r. sympathetic dystrophy
r. symptom
synchronous r.
r. tachycardia
tarsophalangeal r.
tendo Achillis r.
tendon r.
r. therapy
thumb r.
tonic r.
trace conditioned r.
trained r.
triceps r.
triceps surae r.
trigeminofacial r.
trochanter r.
Trömner's r.
ulnar r.
unconditioned r.
upper abdominal periosteal r.
urinary r.
utricular r.'s
vagovagal r.
vasopressor r.
venorespiratory r.
vesical r.
vestibular ocular r.
vestibulospinal r.
visceral traction r.
viscerogenic r.
visceromotor r.
viscerosensory r.
viscerotrophic r.
visual orbicularis r.
vomiting r.
Weingrow's r.
Westphal's pupillary r.
white pupillary r.
wink r.
withdrawal r.
wrist clonus r.
reflexogenic
  r. pressosensitivity
  r. zone
reflexogenous
reflexograph
reflexology
reflexometer
reflexophil, reflexophile
reflexotherapy

reflux
    abdominojugular r.
    r. conjunctivitis
    esophageal r., gastroesophageal r.
    r. esophagitis
    hepatojugular r.
    intrarenal r.
    r. nephropathy
    r. otitis media
    pyelotubular r.
    ureterorenal r.
    vesicoureteral r.
reformat
refract
refractable
refracted light
refracting angle of a prism
refraction
    double r.
    dynamic r.
    static r.
refractionist
refractionometer
refractive
    r. accommodative esotropia
    r. amblyopia
    r. index
    r. keratoplasty
    r. keratotomy
refractivity
refractometer
refractometry
refractory
    r. anemia
    r. cast
    r. flask
    r. investment
    r. period
    r. period of electronic pacemaker
    r. rickets
    r. state
refracture
refrangible
refresh
refrigeration
    r. anesthesia
refringence
refringency
refringent
Refsum's
    R. disease
    R. syndrome
refusion
regainer
Regaud's fixative
regenerate
regeneration
    aberrant r.

regenerative polyp
regimen
regio, gen. **regionis**, pl. **regiones**
    regiones abdominis
    r. analis
    r. antebrachialis anterior
    r. antebrachialis posterior
    r. axillaris
    r. brachialis anterior
    r. brachialis posterior
    r. buccalis
    r. calcanea
    regiones capitis
    r. carpalis anterior
    r. carpalis posterior
    regiones cervicales
    r. cervicalis anterior
    r. cervicalis lateralis
    r. cervicalis posterior
    regiones corporis
    r. cruralis anterior
    r. cruralis posterior
    r. cubitalis anterior
    r. cubitalis posterior
    r. deltoidea
    regiones dorsales
    r. epigastrica
    regiones faciales
    r. femoralis
    r. femoralis anterior
    r. femoralis posterior
    r. frontalis capitis
    r. genus anterior
    r. genus posterior
    r. glutealis
    r. hypochondriaca
    r. infraclavicularis
    r. inframammaria
    r. infraorbitalis
    r. infrascapularis
    r. inguinalis
    r. lateralis
    r. lumbalis
    r. mammaria
    regiones membri inferioris
    regiones membri superioris
    r. mentalis
    r. nasalis
    r. nuchalis
    r. occipitalis capitis
    r. olfactoria tunicae mucosae nasi
    r. oralis
    r. orbitalis
    r. parietalis capitis
    regiones pectorales
    r. pectoralis
    r. perinealis
    r. plantaris

R

r. presternalis
r. pubica
r. respiratoria tunicae mucosae nasi
r. sacralis
r. scapularis
r. sternocleidomastoidea
r. suralis
r. talocruralis
r. temporalis capitis
r. umbilicalis
r. urogenitalis
r. vertebralis
r. zygomatica

region
abdominal r.'s
anal r.
ankle r.
anterior antebrachial r.
anterior r. of arm
anterior brachial r.
anterior carpal r.
anterior crural r.
anterior cubital r.
anterior r. of elbow
anterior r. of forearm
anterior hypothalamic r.
anterior knee r.
anterior r. of leg
anterior r. of neck
anterior r. of thigh
axillary r.
r.'s of back
r.'s of body
buccal r.
calcaneal r.
r.'s of chest, r. of chest
chromosomal r.
complementarity determining r.'s
deltoid r.
dorsal hypothalamic r.
epigastric r.
r.'s of face
femoral r.
frontal r. of head
gluteal r.
r.'s of head
hypervariable r.'s
hypochondriac r.
I r.
iliac r.
r.'s of inferior limb
inframammary r.
infraorbital r.
infrascapular r.
inguinal r.
r. of interest
intermediate hypothalamic r.
lateral r.

lateral hypothalamic r.
lateral r. of neck
r.'s of lower limb
lumbar r.
mammary r.
mental r.
nasal r.
r.'s of neck
nuchal r.
nucleolus organizer r.
occipital r. of head
r. of olfactory mucosa
olfactory r. of tunica mucosa of
  nose
oral r.
orbital r.
parietal r.
pectoral r., pectoral r.'s
perineal r.
popliteal r.
posterior antebrachial r.
posterior r. of arm
posterior brachial r.
posterior carpal r.
posterior crural r.
posterior cubital r.
posterior r. of elbow
posterior r. of forearm
posterior hypothalamic r.
posterior knee r.
posterior r. of leg
posterior r. of neck
posterior neck r.
posterior r. of thigh
preoptic r.
presternal r.
presumptive r.
pretectal r.
pubic r.
r. of respiratory mucosa
respiratory r. of tunica mucosa of
  nose
sacral r.
scapular r.
sternocleidomastoid r.
suboccipital r.
r.'s of superior limb
sural r.
temporal r. of head
umbilical r.
r.'s of upper limb
urogenital r.
vertebral r.
Wernicke's r.
zygomatic r.
regional
r. anatomy
r. anesthesia

regional *(continued)*
    r. enteritis
    r. enterocolitis
    r. granulomatous lymphadenitis
    r. hypothermia
    r. ileitis
    r. lymphadenitis
    r. perfusion
regiones (*pl. of* regio)
regionis (*gen. of* regio)
register
registered nurse
registration
    maxillomandibular r.
    tissue r.
registry
regnancy
regressing atypical histiocytosis
regression
    r. analysis
    r. of the mean
    phonemic r.
regressive
    r. staining
regressive-reconstructive approach
regular astigmatism
regulation
regulatory albuminuria
regurgitant
    r. fraction
    r. murmur
regurgitate
regurgitation
    aortic r.
    ischemic mitral r.
    r. jaundice
    mitral r.
    pulmonic r.
    valvular r.
rehabilitation
    mouth r.
rehearsal
Rehfuss
    R. method
    R. stomach tube
Reichel-Pólya stomach resection
Reichert's
    R. cartilage
    R. cochlear recess
Reid's base line
Reifenstein's syndrome
Reil's
    R. ansa
    R. band
    R. ribbon
    R. triangle
reimplantation

reinfection
    r. tuberculosis
reinforced anchorage
reinforcement
    primary r.
    secondary r.
reinforcer
    negative r.
    positive r.
Reinke
    R. crystalloids
    R. space
reinnervation
reinoculation
Reinsch's test
reintegration
reinversion
Reisseisen's muscles
Reissner's
    R. fiber
    R. membrane
Reiter
    R. disease
    R. syndrome
    R. test
rejection
    accelerated r.
    acute r.
    acute cellular r.
    allograft r.
    chronic r.
    chronic allograft r.
    first-set r.
    hyperacute r.
    parental r.
    primary r.
    second set r.
rejuvenescence
relapse
relapsing
    r. appendicitis
    r. febrile nodular nonsuppurative
      panniculitis
    r. fever
    r. malaria
    r. perichondritis
    r. polychondritis
relation
    acquired centric r.
    acquired eccentric r.
    buccolingual r.
    centric jaw r., centric r.
    dynamic r.'s
    eccentric r.
    intermaxillary r.
    maxillomandibular r.
    median retruded r., median r.
    occluding r.

protrusive r.
protrusive jaw r.
rest r.
rest jaw r.
ridge r.
static r.'s
unstrained jaw r.
relational threshold
relationship
blood r.
dose-response r.
dual r.'s
hypnotic r.
object r.
sadomasochistic r.
relative
r. accommodation
r. afferent pupillary defect
r. biological effectiveness
blood r.
r. humidity
r. immunity
r. incompetence
r. leukocytosis
r. polycythemia
r. refractory period
r. risk
r. scotoma
r. sensitivity
r. specificity
r. viscosity
relax
relaxation
cardioesophageal r.
isometric r.
isovolumetric r.
isovolumic r.
longitudinal r.
r. response
spin-lattice r.
spin-spin r.
r. suture
transverse r.
relearning
release phenomenon
reliability
r. coefficient
equivalent form r.
interjudge r.
interrater r.
test-retest r.
relief
r. area
r. chamber
relieve
religious objects
reline

REM
R. behavior disorder
R. sleep
R. syndrome
Remak's
R. fibers
R. ganglia
R. nuclear division
R. plexus
R. reflex
R. sign
remediable
remedial
remineralization
reminiscence
reminiscent aura
remission
spontaneous r.
remit
remittence
remittent
r. fever
r. malaria
r. malarial fever
remnant
remodeling
remote memory
removable
r. bridge
r. partial denture
ren, gen. **renis**, pl. **renes**
renal
r. adenocarcinoma
r. agenesis
r. amyloidosis
r. artery
r. ballottement
r. branch of lesser splanchnic nerve
r. branch of vagus nerve
r. calculus
r. capsulotomy
r. carbuncle
r. carcinosarcoma
r. cast
r. cell carcinoma
r. colic
r. collar
r. columns
r. corpuscle
r. cortex
r. cortical adenoma
r. cortical lobule
r. diabetes
r. epistaxis
r. failure
r. fascia
r. fibrocystic osteosis

renal (*continued*)
    r. ganglia
    r. glycosuria
    r. hematuria
    r. hemorrhage
    r. hypertension
    r. hypoplasia
    r. impression
    r. infantilism
    r. insufficiency
    r. labyrinth
    r. lobe
    r. medulla
    r. nanism
    r. osteitis fibrosa
    r. osteodystrophy
    r. papilla
    r. papillary necrosis
    r. pelvis
    r. plexus
    r. portal system
    r. pyramid
    r. reflex
    r. retinopathy
    r. rickets
    r. segments
    r. sinus
    r. surface of spleen
    r. surface of suprarenal gland
    r. surface of the suprarenal gland
    r. threshold
    r. transplantation
    r. tubular acidosis
    r. veins
renal-splanchnic steal
renal-splenic venous shunt
Renaut body
renculus
Rendu-Osler-Weber syndrome
renes (*pl. of* ren)
renicapsule
renicardiac
reniculus, pl. **reniculi**
renifleur
reniform
    r. pelvis
renin-angiotensin-aldosterone system
reniportal
renis (*gen. of* ren)
renocutaneous
renogastric
renogenic
renogram
renography
renointestinal
renomegaly
renopathy
renoprival

renopulmonary
renotrophic
renotrophin
renotropic
renotropin
renovascular
    r. hypertension
Renpenning's syndrome
Renshaw cells
renunculus
Reoviridae
REO virus
Reovirus
reovirus-like agent
repair
    error-prone r.
    mismatch r.
    recombinatorial r.
    SOS r.
repand
reparative
    r. dentin
    r. giant cell granuloma
reperfusion injury
repetition
    r. rate
    r. time
repetition-compulsion
    r.-c. principle
replacement
    r. bone
    r. fibrosis
    r. therapy
replant
replantation
    intentional r.
repletion
replica
    r. plating
replicate
replicative intermediate
replicator
repolarization
repositioning
    gingival r.
    jaw r.
    muscle r.
repositor
repressed
repression
    primal r.
repressor gene
reproduction
    asexual r.
    cytogenic r.
    sexual r.
    somatic r.
    vegetative r.

R

reproductive
r. assimilation
r. cycle
r. nucleus
r. system
reptilase
repullulation
required arch length
resect
resectable
resection
gum r.
loop r.
Miles r.
muscle r.
Reichel-Pólya stomach r.
root r.
scleral r.
transurethral r.
wedge r.
resectoscope
r. sheath
reserve
r. air
breathing r.
cardiac r.
r. force
r. tooth germ
reservoir
r. bag
r. host
r. of infection
Ommaya r.
Pecquet's r.
r. of spermatozoa
vitelline r.
reset nodus sinuatrialis
resident
r. physician
residual
r. abscess
r. air
r. body
r. body of Regaud
r. capacity
r. cleft
r. cyst
r. error
r. inhibition
r. inhibitor
r. lumen
r. ovary syndrome
r. ridge
r. schizophrenia
r. urine
r. volume
residue
day r.

resilience
resin
acrylic r.
r. cement
chemically cured r.
composite r.
direct filling r.
dual-cure r.
epoxy r.
light-activated r.
light-cured r.
polyester r.
quinine carbacrylic r.
resistance
airway r.
bacteriophage r.
dicumarol r.
expiratory r.
r. factors
r. form
impact r.
insulin r.
multidrug r.
peripheral r.
r. plasmids
synaptic r.
systemic vascular r.
total peripheral r.
resistance-inducing factor
resistance-transfer factor
resistance-transferring episomes
resistant ovary syndrome
resistive movement
resistivity
resistor
resolution
r. acuity
resolvase
resolve
resolving power
resonance
amphoric r.
bandbox r.
bellmetal r.
cavernous r.
cracked-pot r.
hydatid r.
skodaic r.
r. theory of hearing
tympanitic r.
vesicular r.
vesiculotympanitic r.
vocal r.
wooden r.
resonant frequency
resorb

resorcinol
  r. phthalic anhydride
  r. test
resorcinolphthalein
  r. sodium
resorption
  r. atelectasis
  bone r.
  gingival r.
  horizontal r.
  internal r.
  r. lacunae
  ridge r.
  root r.
respirable
respiration
  abdominal r.
  amphoric r.
  artificial r.
  assisted r.
  Biot's r.
  bronchial r.
  bronchovesicular r.
  cavernous r.
  Cheyne-Stokes r.
  cogwheel r.
  controlled r.
  costal r.
  diffusion r.
  electrophrenic r.
  external r.
  forced r.
  internal r.
  interrupted r.
  jerky r.
  Kussmaul r.
  Kussmaul-Kien r.
  labored r.
  mouth-to-mouth r.
  paradoxical r.
  puerile r.
  r. rate
  stertorous r.
  thoracic r.
  tissue r.
  tubular r.
  vesicular r.
  vesiculocavernous r.
respirator
  r. brain
  cuirass r.
  Drinker r.
  pressure-controlled r.
  tank r.
  volume-controlled r.
respiratory
  r. acidosis
  r. airway

  r. alkalosis
  r. apparatus
  r. arrhythmia
  r. ataxia
  r. bronchioles
  r. burst
  r. capacity
  r. center
  r. coefficient
  r. dead space
  r. distress syndrome of the
    newborn
  r. enteric orphan virus
  r. epithelium
  r. exchange ratio
  r. frequency
  r. hippus
  r. insufficiency
  r. lobule
  r. minute volume
  r. mucosa
  r. murmur
  r. pause
  r. pulse
  r. quotient
  r. region of tunica mucosa of
    nose
  r. scleroma
  r. sound
  r. syncytial virus
  r. system
  r. tract
respire
respirometer
  Dräger r.
  Wright r.
respondent
  r. behavior
  r. conditioning
response
  anamnestic r.
  biphasic r.
  booster r.
  conditioned r.
  Cushing r.
  depletion r.
  early-phase r.
  evoked r.
  flight or fight r.
  galvanic skin r.
  Henry-Gauer r.
  r. hierarchy
  immune r.
  isomorphic r.
  late-phase r.
  oculomotor r.
  orienting r.
  primary immune r.

psychogalvanic r., psychogalvanic
   skin r.
recruiting r.
relaxation r.
secondary immune r.
sonomotor r.
target r.
triple r.
unconditioned r.
response-produced cues
rest
adrenal r.
r. area
bed r.
r. bite
r. body
cingulum r.
incisal r.
r. jaw relation
lingual r.
Malassez' epithelial r.'s
Marchand's r.
mesonephric r.
occlusal r.
r. pain
r. position
precision r.
r. relation
r. seat
r.'s of Serres
r. vertical dimension
Walthard's cell r.
wolffian r.
restenosis
restiform
r. body
r. eminence
resting
r. cell
r. length
r. saliva
r. stage
r. tidal volume
r. tremor
r. wandering cell
restitope
restitution
restless
r. legs
r. legs syndrome
restoration
acid-etched r.
combination r.
compound r.
direct acrylic r.
direct composite resin r.
direct resin r.
overhanging r.

permanent r.
root canal r.
silicate r.'s
temporary r.
restorative
r. dental materials
r. dentistry
restored cycle
restrained beam
restraint
restriction
r. fragment length polymorphism
r. methylation
MHC r.
restrictive cardiomyopathy
restructured cell
resuscitate
resuscitation
cardiopulmonary r.
mouth-to-mouth r.
resuscitator
retained
r. menstruation
r. placenta
retainer
continuous bar r.
direct r.
extracoronal r.
Hawley r.
indirect r.
intracoronal r.
matrix r.
space r.
retardate
retardation
mental r.
psychomotor r.
retarded dentition
retarder
retch
retching
rete, pl. **retia**
r. acromiale
r. arteriosum
r. articulare cubiti
r. articulare genus
r. calcaneum
r. canalis hypoglossi
r. carpi dorsale
r. carpi posterius
r. cords
r. cutaneum corii
r. cyst of ovary
r. foraminis ovalis
Haller's r., r. halleri
r. malleolare laterale
r. malleolare mediale
malpighian r.

rete (continued)
r. mirabile
r. ovarii
r. patellae
r. pegs
r. ridges
r. subpapillare
r. testis
r. vasculosum articulare
r. venosum dorsale manus
r. venosum dorsale pedis
r. venosum plantare
retention
r. area
r. arm
r. cyst
denture r.
direct r.
r. form
r. groove
indirect r.
r. jaundice
partial denture r.
r. point
r. polyp
r. suture
r. vomiting
retentive
r. arm
r. circumferential clasp arm
r. fulcrum line
retia (pl. of rete)
retial
reticula (pl. of reticulum)
reticular, reticulated
r. activating system
r. cartilage
r. cell
r. degeneration
r. dystrophy of cornea
r. erythematous mucinosis
r. fibers
r. formation
r. lamina
r. layer of corium
r. membrane
r. nuclei of the brainstem
r. nucleus of thalamus
r. substance
r. tissue
reticularis cell
reticulation
reticulocyte
reticulocytopenia
reticulocytosis
reticuloendothelial
r. cell
r. system

reticuloendothelioma
reticuloendotheliosis
leukemic r.
reticuloendothelium
reticulohistiocytic granuloma
reticulohistiocytoma
reticulohistiocytosis
multicentric r.
reticuloid
actinic r.
reticulonodular pattern
reticulopenia
reticulosis
benign inoculation r.
histiocytic medullary r.
leukemic r.
lipomelanic r.
malignant midline r.
midline malignant reticulosis r.
pagetoid r.
polymorphic r.
reticulospinal
r. tract
reticulotomy
reticulum, pl. reticula
agranular endoplasmic r.
r. cell sarcoma
Ebner's r.
Golgi internal r.
granular endoplasmic r.
Kölliker's r.
rough-surfaced endoplasmic r.
sarcoplasmic r.
smooth-surfaced endoplasmic r.
stellate r.
trabecular r.
r. trabeculare sclerae
retiform
r. cartilage
r. tissue
retina
albedo r.'s
coarctate r.
detached r.
flecked r.
fleck r. of Kandori
leopard r.
shot-silk r.
tigroid r.
retinaculum, gen. retinaculi, pl. retinacula
antebrachial flexor r.
r. of articular capsule of hip
r. capsulae articularis coxae
caudal r.
r. caudale
r. cutis
extensor r.
retinacula of extensor muscles

r. extensorum
flexor r.
flexor r. of forearm
flexor r. of lower limb
r. of flexor muscles
r. flexorum
inferior extensor r.
inferior r. of extensor muscles
lateral patellar r.
medial patellar r.
Morgagni's r.
r. musculorum extensorum inferius
r. musculorum extensorum superius
retinacula musculorum fibularium
r. musculorum flexorum
retinacula musculorum peroneorum
retinacula of nail
r. patellae laterale
r. patellae mediale
patellar r.
peroneal r.
retinacula of peroneal muscles
r. of skin
superior extensor r.
superior r. of extensor muscles
r. tendinum
retinacula unguis

retinal
r. adaptation
r. anlage tumor
r. blood vessels
r. camera
r. cones
r. detachment
r. disparity
r. dysplasia
r. embolism
r. fold
r. image

retinectomy
retinitis
albuminuric r.
apoplectic r.
azotemic r.
central angiospastic r.
circinate r.
diabetic r.
exudative r., r. exudativa
gravidic r.
leukemic r.
metastatic r.
r. pigmentosa
r. proliferans
punctate r.
purulent r.
recurrent central r.
r. sclopetaria

secondary r.
septic r.
serous r.
simple r.
r. syphilitica, syphilitic r.
retinoblastoma
retinochoroid
retinochoroiditis
bird shot r.
r. juxtapapillaris
retinodialysis
retinoic acid
13-*cis*-r. a.
retinopapillitis
r. of premature infants
retinopathy
arteriosclerotic r.
central angiospastic r.
central serous r.
circinate r.
compression r.
diabetic r.
dysproteinemic r.
eclamptic r.
electric r.
external exudative r.
gravidic r.
hypertensive r.
Leber's idiopathic stellate r.
leukemic r.
lipemic r.
macular r.
pigmentary r.
r. of prematurity
proliferative r.
r. punctata albescens
Purtscher's r.
renal r.
rubella r.
sickle cell r.
solar r.
toxemic r. of pregnancy
toxic r.
transient r.
traumatic r.
venous-stasis r.
retinopexy
fluid r.
gas r.
pneumatic r.
retinopiesis
retinoschisis
juvenile r.
senile r.
retinoscope
luminous r.
reflecting r.

retinoscopy
    cylinder r.
    fogging r.
retinotomy
retoperithelium
Retortamonas
retothelioma
retract
retractile
    r. testis
retraction
    gingival r.
    mandibular r.
    r. syndrome
retractor
retrad
retrahens aurem, retrahens auriculam
retreat from reality
retrenchment
retrieval
retroactive inhibition
retroadductor space
retroauricular
    r. lymph nodes
retrobuccal
retrobulbar
    r. abscess
    r. anesthesia
    r. neuritis
retrocalcaneobursitis
retrocaval ureter
retrocecal
    r. abscess
    r. lymph nodes
    r. recess
retrocedent gout
retrocervical
retrocession
retroclusion
retrocochlear deafness
retrocolic
retrocollic
    r. spasm
retrocollis
retroconduction
retrocursive
retrocuspid papilla
retrodeviation
retrodisplacement
retroduodenal
    r. artery
    r. fossa
    r. recess
retroesophageal
retrofilling
retroflected
retroflection
retroflexed

retroflex fasciculus
retroflexion
    r. of iris
retrogasserian
    r. neurectomy
    r. neurotomy
retrognathic
retrognathism
retrograde
    r. amnesia
    r. aortography
    r. beat
    r. block
    r. cardioplegia
    r. chromatolysis
    r. conduction
    r. degeneration
    r. embolism
    r. hernia
    r. intussusception
    r. memory
    r. menstruation
    r. metamorphosis
    r. P wave
    r. pyelography
    r. urography
retrography
retrogression
retrohyoid bursa
retroiliac ureter
retroinguinal space
retroiridian
retrojection
retrojector
retrolental
    r. fibroplasia
retrolenticular
    r. limb of internal capsule
    r. part of internal capsule
retrolingual
retromammary
    r. mastitis
retromandibular
    r. fossa
    r. process of parotid gland
    r. vein
retromastoid
retromolar
    r. fossa
    r. pad
retromorphosis
retromylohyoid space
retronasal
retro-ocular
retroperitoneal
    r. fibrosis
    r. hernia
    r. space

retroperitoneum
retroperitonitis
    idiopathic fibrous r.
retropharyngeal
    r. abscess
    r. lymph nodes
    r. space
retropharynx
retroplacental
retroplasia
retroposed
retroposition
retropubic
    r. hernia
    r. space
retropulsion
retropyloric
    r. lymph nodes
    r. nodes
retrospection
retrospective
    r. falsification
retrospondylolisthesis
retrosternal
    r. hernia
    r. space
retrotarsal
    r. fold
retrouterine
retroversioflexion
retroversion
retroverted
Retroviridae
retrovirus
retrusion
retrusive
    r. excursion
    r. occlusion
Rett's syndrome
return extrasystole
returning cycle
Retzius'
    R. cavity
    R. fibers
    R. foramen
    R. gyrus
    R. ligament
    R. space
    R. striae
    R. veins
reunient
Reuss'
    R. color tables
    R. formula
    R. test
revaccination
revascularization
reverberating circuit

reverberation
Reverdin
    R. graft
    R. method
reversal
    pressure r.
    sex r.
reverse
    r. banding
    r. bevel
    r. curve
    r. Eck fistula
    r. genetics
    r. Kingsley splint
    r. mutation
    r. passive hemagglutination
    r. Trendelenburg position
reversed
    r. anaphylaxis
    r. coarctation
    r. paradoxical pulse
    r. passive anaphylaxis
    r. peristalsis
    r. Prausnitz-Küstner reaction
    r. reciprocal rhythm
    r. shunt
reversed-three sign
reversible
    r. calcinosis
    r. decortication
    r. pulpitis
    r. shock
reversion
revertant
Revilliod's sign
revivescence
revivification
revulsion
reward
rewarming
Rexed
Reye's syndrome
Reynolds
    R. number
    R. pentad
Rh
    R. antigens
    R. blocking test
    R. null syndrome
rhabditiform
    r. larva
Rhabditis
    R.-like
rhabdocyte
rhabdoid
rhabdomyoblast
rhabdomyolysis
    acute recurrent r.

rhabdomyolysis *(continued)*
    exertional r.
    familial paroxysmal r.
    idiopathic paroxysmal r.
rhabdomyoma
rhabdomyosarcoma
    embryonal r.'s
rhabdophobia
rhabdosarcoma
rhabdosphincter
Rhabdoviridae
rhabdovirus
rhagades
rhagadiform
rhagiocrine cell
rhaphe
rhathymia
rhegma
rhegmatogenous
    r. retinal detachment
Rheinberg microscope
rheobase
rheobasic
rheocardiography
rheoencephalogram
rheoencephalography
rheometry
rheostosis
rheotaxis
rheotropism
Rhese projection
rhestocythemia
rhesus disease
rheum
rheumatalgia
rheumatic
    r. arteritis
    r. carditis
    r. chorea
    r. disease
    r. endocarditis
    r. fever
    r. heart disease
    r. pericarditis
    r. pneumonia
    r. tetany
    r. torticollis
    r. valvulitis
rheumatid
rheumatism
    articular r.
    cerebral r.
    chronic r.
    gonorrheal r.
    r. of the heart
    inflammatory r.
    lumbar r.
    Macleod's r.

    muscular r.
    nodose r.
    subacute r.
    tuberculous r.
rheumatismal
rheumatocelis
rheumatoid
    r. arteritis
    r. arthritis
    r. disease
    r. factors
    r. nodules
    r. spondylitis
rheumatologist
rheumatology
rhexis
rhigosis
rhigotic
rhinal
    r. fissure
    r. sulcus
rhinalgia
rhinedema
rhinencephalic
rhinencephalon
rhinenchysis
rhinion
rhinism
rhinitis
    acute r.
    allergic r.
    atrophic r.
    r. caseosa, caseous r.
    chronic r.
    gangrenous r.
    hypertrophic r.
    r. medicamentosa
    r. nervosa
    scrofulous r.
    r. sicca
    vasomotor r.
rhinoanemometer
rhinocanthectomy
rhinocele
rhinocephaly, rhinocephalia
rhinocheiloplasty, rhinochiloplasty
Rhinocladiella
rhinocleisis
rhinodacryolith
rhinodymia
rhinodynia
Rhinoestrus purpureus
rhinogenous
rhinokyphectomy
rhinokyphosis
rhinolalia
    r. aperta
    r. clausa

rhinolite
rhinolith
rhinolithiasis
rhinologic
rhinologist
rhinology
rhinomanometer
rhinomanometry
rhinomucormycosis
rhinomycosis
rhinonecrosis
rhinopathy
rhinopharyngeal
rhinopharyngolith
rhinopharynx
rhinophonia
rhinophycomycosis
rhinophyma
rhinoplasty
    English r.
    Indian r.
    Italian r.
    Joseph r.
rhinorrhea
    cerebrospinal fluid r.
    gustatory r.
rhinosalpingitis
rhinoscleroma
rhinoscope
rhinoscopic
rhinoscopy
    anterior r.
    median r.
    posterior r.
rhinosporidiosis
Rhinosporidium seeberi
rhinostenosis
rhinotomy
Rhinovirus
rhinovirus
    bovine r.'s
    equine r.'s
Rhipicephalus
rhizoid
rhizomelia
rhizomeningomyelitis
rhizoplast
Rhizopoda
Rhizopodasida
Rhizopodea
Rhizopus
rhizotomy
    anterior r.
    facet r.
    posterior r.
    trigeminal r.
rhodamine B
rhodanile blue

Rhodesian trypanosomiasis
Rhodococcus
Rhodotorula
rhombencephalic
    r. gustatory nucleus
    r. isthmus
    r. tegmentum
rhombencephalon
rhombic
    r. grooves
    r. lip
rhomboatloideus
rhombocele
rhomboid, rhomboidal
    r. fossa
    r. impression
    r. ligament
    r. minor muscle
rhomboideus
    r. major muscle
rhombomere
rhonchal, rhonchial
    r. fremitus
rhonchus, pl. rhonchi
    cavernous r.
    sibilant r.
    sonorous r.
rhopheocytosis
rhoptry, pl. rhoptries
rhotacism
Rhus
    R. toxicodendron antigen
    R. venenata antigen
rhus
    r. dermatitis
rhyparia
rhypophagy
rhypophobia
rhythm
    agonal r.
    alpha r.
    atrioventricular junctional r., lower
     nodal r., upper nodal r.
    A-V junctional r.
    basic electrical r.
    Berger r.
    beta r.
    bigeminal r.
    cantering r.
    circadian r.
    circus r.
    coronary nodal r.
    coronary sinus r.
    coupled r.
    delta r.
    diurnal r.
    ectopic r.
    escape r.

R

rhythm *(continued)*
    gallop r.
    idiojunctional r.
    idionodal r.
    idioventricular r.
    junctional r.
    lower nodal r. *(var. of*
      atrioventricular junctional r.)
    r. method
    nodal r.
    pendulum r.
    quadrigeminal r.
    quadruple r.
    reciprocal r.
    reciprocating r.
    reversed reciprocal r.
    sinus r.
    systolic gallop r.
    theta r.
    tic-tac r.
    trainwheel r.
    trigeminal r.
    triple r.
    ultradian r.
    upper nodal r. *(var. of*
      atrioventricular junctional r.)
    ventricular r.
rhythmic chorea
rhytidectomy
rhytidoplasty
rhytidosis
    r. retinae
rib
    bicipital r.
    bifid r.
    cervical r.
    false r.'s
    floating r.'s
    lumbar r.
    r. notching
    slipping r.
    r. spreader
    true r.'s
    vertebral r.'s
    vertebrochondral r.'s
    vertebrosternal r.'s
Ribas-Torres disease
Ribbert's theory
ribbon
    r. arch
    r. arch appliance
    Reil's r.
Ribes' ganglion
riboflavin deficiency
ribonuclease
    r. D
    r. P
ribophorins

ribosome-lamella complex
ribosuria
ribovirus
ribozyme
Ricco's law
rice
    r. body
    r. diet
    r. disease
    r. itch
rice-field fever
rice-Tween agar
rice-water stool
Richard's fringes
Richards-Rundle syndrome
Richter-Monro line
Richter's
    R. hernia
    R. syndrome
rickets
    acute r.
    adult r.
    celiac r.
    hemorrhagic r.
    late r.
    refractory r.
    renal r.
    scurvy r.
    vitamin D-resistant r.
Rickettsia
    R. akari
    R. australis
    R. burnetii
    R. canis
    R. conorii
    R. prowazekii
    R. psittaci
    R. rickettsii
    R. sennetsu
    R. sibirica
    R. tsutsugamushi
    R. typhi
rickettsial
rickettsialpox
rickettsiosis
    vesicular r.
rickety
Rickles test
Rida virus
Rideal-Walker
    R.-W. coefficient
    R.-W. method
Ridell's operation
rider's
    r. bone
    r. bursa
    r. leg
    r. muscles

ridge
- alveolar r.
- apical ectodermal r.
- basal r.
- bicipital r.'s
- buccocervical r.
- buccogingival r.
- bulbar r.
- bulboventricular r.
- dental r.
- epidermal r.'s
- epipericardial r.
- r. extension
- external oblique r.
- ganglion r.
- genital r.
- gluteal r.
- gonadal r.
- interpapillary r.'s
- key r.
- lateral epicondylar r.
- lateral supracondylar r.
- linguocervical r.
- linguogingival r.
- Mall's r.'s
- mammary r.
- marginal r.
- medial epicondylar r.
- medial supracondylar r.
- mesonephric r.
- milk r.
- mylohyoid r.
- nasal r.
- oblique r.
- oblique r. of trapezium
- palatine r.
- Passavant's r.
- pectoral r.
- pharyngeal r.
- primitive r.
- pronator r.
- pterygoid r. of sphenoid bone
- pulmonary r.'s
- r. relation
- residual r.
- r. resorption
- rete r.'s
- skin r.'s
- sphenoidal r.'s
- superciliary r.
- supplemental r.
- supraorbital r.
- taste r.
- temporal r.
- transverse r.
- transverse palatine r.
- trapezoid r.
- triangular r.

- urogenital r.
- wolffian r.

riding embolism

Ridley's
- R. circle
- R. sinus

Riedel's
- R. disease
- R. lobe
- R. struma
- R. thyroiditis

Rieder
- R. cell leukemia
- R. cells
- R. lymphocyte

Riegel's pulse

Rieger's
- R. anomaly
- R. syndrome

Riehl's melanosis

Rift Valley fever virus

Riga-Fede disease

right
- r. angle clamp
- r. atrioventricular valve
- r. atrium of heart
- r. auricular appendage
- r. axis deviation
- r. border of heart
- r. branch
- r. branch of portal vein
- r. branch of proper hepatic artery
- r. colic artery
- r. colic flexure
- r. colic lymph nodes
- r. colic vein
- r. coronary artery
- r. crus of atrioventricular bundle
- r. crus of diaphragm
- r. duct of caudate lobe
- r. fibrous trigone
- r. frontoanterior
- r. frontoposterior
- r. frontotransverse
- r. gastric artery
- r. gastric lymph nodes
- r. gastric vein
- r. gastroepiploic artery
- r. gastroepiploic lymph nodes
- r. gastroepiploic vein
- r. gastro-omental artery
- r. gastro-omental lymph nodes
- r. gastroomental vein
- r. heart
- r. heart bypass
- r. hepatic artery
- r. hepatic duct
- r. hepatic veins

R

right *(continued)*
  r. inferior pulmonary vein
  r. or left lateral decubitus film
  r. lobe
  r. lobe of liver
  r. lumbar lymph nodes
  r. lymphatic duct
  r. main bronchus
  r. margin of heart
  r. mentoanterior
  r. mentoposterior
  r. mentotransverse
  r. occipitoanterior
  r. occipitoposterior
  r. occipitotransverse
  r. ovarian vein
  r. ovarian vein syndrome
  r. parasternal impulses
  r. part of diaphragmatic surface of liver
  r. pulmonary artery
  r. sacroanterior
  r. sacroposterior
  r. sacrotransverse
  r. sagittal fissure
  r. superior intercostal vein
  r. superior pulmonary vein
  r. suprarenal vein
  r. testicular vein
  r. triangular ligament
  r. ventricle
  r. ventricular failure
  r. ventricular hypoplasia
right-eyed
right-footed
right-handed
righting reflexes
right-to-left shunt
rigid dysarthria
rigidity
  anatomic r.
  cadaveric r.
  catatonic r.
  cerebellar r.
  clasp-knife r.
  cogwheel r.
  decerebrate r.
  decorticate r.
  lead-pipe r.
  ocular r.
  pathologic r.
  postmortem r.
  scleral r.
rigor
  calcium r.
  r. mortis
  myocardial r. mortis
Riley-Day syndrome

rim
  bite r.
  occlusal r.
  occlusion r.
  orbital r.
  record r.
rima, gen. and pl. **rimae**
  r. glottidis
  r. oris
  r. palpebrarum
  r. pudendi
  r. respiratoria
  r. vestibuli
  r. vocalis
  r. vulvae
Rimini's test
rimose
rimula
rinderpest virus
Rindfleisch's
  R. cells
  R. folds
ring
  abdominal r.
  r. abscess
  amnion r.
  annuloplasty r.
  anterior limiting r.
  Bandl's r.
  Bickel's r.
  Cannon's r.
  cardiac lymphatic r.
  casting r.
  choroidal r.
  r. chromosome
  ciliary r.
  common tendinous r.
  conjunctival r.
  constriction r.
  crural r.
  deep inguinal r.
  Donders' r.'s
  r. enhancement
  external inguinal r.
  femoral r.
  fibrocartilaginous r. of tympanic membrane
  fibrous r.
  fibrous r. of heart
  fibrous r. of intervertebral disc
  r. finger
  Fleischer's r.
  Fleischer-Strumpell r.
  Flieringa's r.
  glaucomatous r.
  Graefenberg r.
  greater r. of iris
  Imlach's r.

R

internal inguinal r.
r. of iris
Kayser-Fleischer r.
lesser r. of iris
Liesegang r.'s
r. ligament
Lower's r.
lymphatic r. of cardiac part of stomach
lymphoid r.
neonatal r.
pathologic retraction r.
r. pessary
physiologic retraction r.
polar r.
r. precipitin test
Schatzki's r.
Schwalbe's r.
scleral r.
r. scotoma
signet r.
r. of Soemmerring
subcutaneous r.
superficial inguinal r.
r. syringe
r. test
tonsillar r.
tracheal r.
tympanic r.
r. ulcer of cornea
umbilical r.
vascular r.
Vieussens' r.
Vossius' lenticular r.
Waldeyer's throat r.
Zinn's r.
ringed hair
ring-knife
ring-like corneal dystrophy
ring-wall lesion
ringworm
r. of beard
black-dot r.
r. of body
crusted r.
r. of foot
r. of genitocrural region
honeycomb r.
r. of nails
Oriental r.
r. of scalp
scaly r.
Tokelau r.
r. yaws
Rinne's test
Riolan's
R. anastomosis
R. arc

R. arcades
R. bones
R. bouquet
R. muscle
riparian
Ripault's sign
ripe cataract
ripening
rise time
risk
attributable r.
competing r.
empiric r.
r. factor
radiation r.'s
recurrence r.
relative r.
Risley's rotary prism
risorius
r. muscle
risus
r. caninus
r. sardonicus
Ritgen's maneuver
Rittenhouse-Manogian procedure
Ritter-Rollet phenomenon
Ritter's
R. law
R. opening tetanus
ritual
ritualistic behavior
rivalry
binocular r.
r. of retina
sibling r.
Riva-Rocci sphygmomanometer
river blindness
Rivero-Carvallo effect
Rivinus'
R. canals
R. ducts
R. gland
R. incisure
R. membrane
R. notch
rivus lacrimalis
riziform
RNA
R. tumor viruses
R. virus
Roach clasp
Roaf's syndrome
Robertshaw tube
robertsonian translocation
Robertson pupil
Robert's pelvis
Roberts syndrome

Robinow
  R. dwarfism
  R. syndrome
Robinson
  R. catheter
  R. disease
  R. index
Robin's syndrome
robotic
robustness
roccellin
ROC curve
Rochalimaea
  R. henselae
  R. quintana
Rocher's sign
rocket immunoelectrophoresis
Rocky Mountain spotted fever
rod
  analyzing r.
  Auer r.'s
  basal r.
  r. cell of retina
  Corti's r.'s
  r. disks
  enamel r.'s
  r. fiber
  germinal r.
  r. granule
  Maddox's r.
  r. monochromatism
  r. myopathy
  r. nuclear cell
  r. vision
rodent ulcer
rodonalgia
roentgen
  r.-equivalent-man
  r.-equivalent-physical
  r. ray
  r. unit
roentgenkymogram
roentgenkymograph
roentgenkymography
roentgenogram
roentgenograph
roentgenography
roentgenologist
roentgenology
roentgenometer
roentgenometry
roentgenoscope
roentgenoscopy
roentgenotherapy
Roesler-Bressler infarct
roetheln (*var. of* röteln)
roetheln
Roger-Anderson pin fixation appliance

Roger's
  R. bruit
  R. disease
  R. murmur
  R. reflex
Rogers' sphygmomanometer
Röhrer's index
Rohr's stria
Rokitansky-Aschoff sinuses
Rokitansky-Küster-Hauser syndrome
Rokitansky's
  R. disease
  R. hernia
  R. pelvis
Rolandic
  R. artery
rolandic epilepsy
Rolando's
  R. angle
  R. area
  R. cells
  R. column
  R. gelatinous substance
  R. substance
  R. tubercle
role
  complementary r.
  r. conflict
  gender r.
  noncomplementary r.
  sex r.
  sick r.
role-playing
roll
  iliac r.
  scleral r.
  r. tube
roller
  r. bandage
Roller's nucleus
Rolleston's rule
Rollet's stroma
rolling circle
roll-tube culture
Romaña's sign
Roman fever
Romano-Ward syndrome
Romanowsky's blood stain
Romberg
  R. disease
  R. sign
  R. symptom
  R. syndrome
  R. test
  R. trophoneurosis
Romberg-Howship symptom
rombergism
Römer's test

R

rongeur
Rónne's nasal step
R-on-T phenomenon
roof
    r. of fourth ventricle
    r. of mouth
    r. nucleus
    r. of orbit
    r. plate
    r. of skull
    r. of tympanic cavity
    r. of tympanum
roofplate
room
    recovery r.
    r. temperature
root
    r. abscess
    r. amputation
    anatomical r.
    anterior r.
    r. apex
    r. avulsion
    r. canal file
    r. canal orifice
    r. canal plugger
    r. canal restoration
    r. canal spreader
    r. canal therapy
    r. canal of tooth
    r. canal treatment
    r. caries
    r. caries index
    clinical r.
    cochlear r. of vestibulocochlear
      nerve
    cochlear r. of VIII nerve
    conjoined nerve r. (*var. of*
      nerve r.)
    cranial r.'s
    cranial r. of accessory nerve
    r. dehiscence
    dorsal r.
    r. end cyst
    r. end granuloma
    facial r.
    r. of facial nerve
    r. filaments
    r. of foot
    r. foramen
    hair r.
    inferior r. of ansa cervicalis
    inferior r. of vestibulocochlear
      nerve
    lateral r. of median nerve
    lateral r. of optic tract
    long r. of ciliary ganglion
    r. of lung

    medial r. of median nerve
    medial r. of optic tract
    r. of mesentry
    motor r.
    motor r. of ciliary ganglion
    motor r.'s of submandibular
      ganglion
    motor r. of trigeminal nerve
    r. of nail
    nasociliary r.
    nerve r., conjoined nerve r.
    r. of nose
    oculomotor r. of ciliary ganglion
    olfactory r.'s
    r.'s of olfactory tract, lateral and
      medial
    parasympathetic r. of ciliary
      ganglion
    r. of penis
    r. planing
    posterior r.
    r. resection
    r. resorption
    sensory r. of ciliary ganglion
    sensory r. of pterygopalatine
      ganglion
    sensory r. of trigeminal nerve
    r. sheath
    short r. of ciliary ganglion
    spinal r. of accessory nerve
    superior r. of ansa cervicalis
    superior r. of vestibulocochlear
      nerve
    sympathetic r. of ciliary ganglion
    r. tip
    r. of tongue
    r. of tooth
    r.'s of trigeminal nerve
    ventral r.
    vestibular r.
    vestibular r. of vestibulocochlear
      nerve
rooting reflex
rootlets
ropalocytosis
rope
    r. burn
    r. flap
Ropes test
Rorschach test
rosacea
    granulomatous r.
    hypertrophic r.
    tuberculoid r.
rosacea-like tuberculid
Rosai-Dorman disease
rosanilin dyes

rosary
  rachitic r.
Roscoe-Bunsen law
rose
  r. bengal
  r. bengal radioactive (^{131}I) test
  r. cephalic tetanus
  r. cold
  r. spots
Rose-Bradford kidney
Rosenbach-Gmelin test
Rosenbach's
  R. disease
  R. law
  R. sign
  R. test
Rosenmüller's
  R. fossa
  R. gland
  R. node
  R. recess
  R. valve
Rosenthal
  R. canal
  R. fiber
  R. vein
Rosenthaler-Turk reagent
roseola
  epidemic r.
  idiopathic r.
  r. infantilis, r. infantum
  syphilitic r.
roseolous
Roser-Nélaton line
Rose's
  R. cephalic tetanus
  R. position
rosette
  E r.
  EAC r.
  Homer-Wright r.'s
  r. test
  Wintersteiner r.'s
rosette-forming cells
Rose-Waaler test
Ross
  R. River fever
  R. River virus
Ross-Jones test
Rossolimo's
  R. reflex
  R. sign
rostellum
  armed r.
  unarmed r.
rostra (*pl. of* rostrum)
rostrad

rostral
  r. lamina
  r. layer
  r. neuropore
  r. transtentorial herniation
rostralis
rostrate
  r. pelvis
rostriform
rostrum, pl. **rostra, rostrums**
  r. corporis callosi
  r. of corpus callosum
  r. sphenoidale
  r. of the sphenoid bone
rot
  Barcoo r.
rotameter
rotary joint
rotating
  r. anode
  r. anode tube
rotation
  r. flap
  intestinal r.
  r. therapy
rotational
  r. axis
  r. nystagmus
rotator
  r. cuff of shoulder
  medial r.
  r. muscles
rotatores
  r. cervicis muscles
  r. lumborum muscles
  r. muscles
  r. thoracis muscles
rotatory
  r. joint
  r. nystagmus
  r. spasm
  r. tic
rotavirus
Rotch's sign
rote learning
röteln, roetheln
Roth-Bernhardt disease
Rothera's nitroprusside test
Rothia
  R. dentocariosa
Rothmund's syndrome
Rothmund-Thomson syndrome
Roth's
  R. disease
  R. spots
Rotor's syndrome
rotoscoliosis
rototome

Rouget-Neumann sheath
Rouget's
    R. bulb
    R. muscle
rough
    r. colony
    r. line
rough-surfaced endoplasmic reticulum
Roughton-Scholander
    R.-S. apparatus
    R.-S. syringe
Rougnon-Heberden disease
rouleau, pl. **rouleaux**
round
    r. atelectasis
    r. bur
    r. cell sarcoma
    r. eminence
    r. fasciculus
    r. foramen
    r. heart
    r. ligament of elbow joint
    r. ligament of femur
    r. ligament of liver
    r. ligament of uterus
    r. pelvis
    r. pronator muscle
    r. window
roundworm
Rous
    R. sarcoma
    R. sarcoma virus
    R. tumor
Rous-associated virus
Roussy-Lévy
    R.-L. disease
    R.-L. syndrome
Roux
    R. method
    R. spatula
    R. stain
Roux-en-Y
    R.-e.-Y. anastomosis
    R.-e.-Y. operation
Rovsing's sign
Rowntree and Geraghty test
royal touch
RPR test
R-R interval
RST segment
Rs virus
RU-486
rub
    friction r.
    pericardial r., pericardial friction r.
    pleural r.
    pleural friction r.
    pleuritic r.

Rubarth's disease virus
rubber
    r. dam
    r. dam clamp
    r. dam clamp forceps
    r. pelvis
    r. shod clamp
    r. tissue
rubber-bulb syringe
rubber-shod clamp
rubeanic acid
rubedo
rubefacient
rubefaction
rubella
    r. cataract
    r. HI test
    r. retinopathy
    r. virus
rubeola
    r. virus
rubeosis
    r. iridis diabetica
rubescent
rubin S, rubine
Rubinstein-Taybi syndrome
Rubin test
Rubivirus
Rubner's
    R. laws of growth
    R. test
rubor
rubriblast
    pernicious anemia type r.
rubric
rubricyte
rubrobulbar tract
rubroreticular
    r. fasciculi
    r. tract
rubrospinal
    r. decussation
    r. tract
ruby spots
ructus
rudiment
rudimentary
rudimentum, pl. **rudimenta**
    r. hippocampi
Rud's syndrome
Ruffini's corpuscles
rufous
    r. albinism
ruga, pl. **rugae**
    r. gastrica
    r. palatina
    rugae of stomach

R

ruga *(continued)*
    rugae of vagina
    rugae vaginales
rugal columns of vagina
rugger jersey vertebra
rugine
rugitus
rugose
rugosity
rugous
rule
    American Law Institute r.
    r. of bigeminy
    Clark's weight r.
    Cowling's r.
    Durham r.
    Goriaew's r.
    Haase's r.
    His' r.
    Jackson's r.
    Liebermeister's r.
    Meyer-Overton r.
    M'Naghten r.
    Nägele's r.
    New Hampshire r.
    r. of nines
    Ogino-Knaus r.
    r. of outlet
    Prentice's r.
    Rolleston's r.
    Trusler's r. for pulmonary artery
      banding
    Young's r.
rum-blossom
rumination disorder
ruminative
Rummel tourniquet
rum nose
Rumpel-Leede
    R.-L. phenomenon
    R.-L. sign
    R.-L. test
runaround, runround
runaway pacemaker
Runeberg's formula
runoff
runround *(var. of* runaround)

runt disease
runting syndrome
rupia
    r. escharotica
rupial
    r. syphilid
rupioid
rupture
ruptured
    r. aneurysm
    r. disk
rural cutaneous leishmaniasis
Rushton bodies
Russell
    R. bodies
    R. effect
    R. Periodontal Index
    R. sign
    R. syndrome
    R. traction
    R. viper venom clotting time
Russian
    R. autumn encephalitis
    R. autumn encephalitis virus
    R. influenza
    R. spring-summer encephalitis
      (Eastern subtype)
    R. spring-summer encephalitis virus
    R. spring-summer encephalitis
      (Western subtype)
    R. tick-borne encephalitis
Rust's
    R. disease
    R. phenomenon
rusts
rusty sputum
ruthenium red
rutherford
rutidosis
Ruysch's
    R. membrane
    R. muscle
    R. tube
    R. veins
Rye classification
Ryle's tube

S

S antigen
S factor
S potential
S sign of Golden
S wave
S1 nuclease mapping
saber
s. shin
s. tibia
saber-sheath trachea
Sabin-Feldman dye test
S-A block
sabot heart
Sabouraud-Noiré instrument
Sabouraud's
S. agar
S. dextrose agar
S. pastils
sabulous
saburra
saburral
sac
abdominal s.
allantoic s.
alveolar s.
amniotic s.
aneurysmal s.
aortic s.
chorionic s.
conjunctival s.
cupular blind s.
dental s.
endolymphatic s.
heart s.
hernial s.
Hilton's s.
lacrimal s.
lesser peritoneal s.
lymph s.'s
nasal s.'s
omental s.
preputial s.
pudendal s.
tear s.
tooth s.
vestibular blind s.
vitelline s.
yolk s.
saccade
saccadic
s. movement
saccate
saccharephidrosis
Saccharomyces

Saccharomycetaceae
Saccharomycetales
saccharorrhea
saccharosuria
sacci (*pl. of* saccus)
sacciform
s. recess
saccular
s. aneurysm
s. bronchiectasis
s. gland
s. nerve
s. spot
sacculated
s. aneurysm
s. pleurisy
sacculation
s.'s of colon
saccule
s. of larynx
sacculocochlear
sacculus, pl. **sacculi**
s. communis
s. endolymphaticus
s. lacrimalis
s. laryngis
s. proprius
s. vestibuli
saccus, pl. **sacci**
s. conjunctivae
s. endolymphaticus
s. lacrimalis
s. reuniens
s. vaginalis
Sachs' bacillus
Sachs-Georgi test
sacra (*pl. of* sacrum)
sacrad
sacral
s. anesthesia
s. canal
s. cornua
s. crest
s. flexure
s. flexure of rectum
s. foramen
s. ganglia
s. hiatus
s. horns
s. index
s. lymph nodes
s. nerves
s. part of spinal cord
s. plexus
s. promontory

S

sacral *(continued)*
- s. region
- s. splanchnic nerves
- s. triangle
- s. tuberosity
- s. veins
- s. venous plexus
- s. vertebrae

sacralgia
sacralization
sacrectomy
sacred
- s. bone
- s. objects

sacroanterior position
sacrococcygeal
- s. disc
- s. joint
- s. junction
- s. teratoma

sacrococcygeus
sacrodural ligament
sacrodynia
sacrogenital folds
sacroiliac
- s. articulation
- s. joint

sacroiliitis
sacrolisthesis
sacrolumbalis
sacrolumbar
sacropelvic surface of ilium
sacroposterior position
sacrosciatic
- s. notch

sacrospinal
sacrospinous ligament
sacrotomy
sacrotransverse position
sacrotuberous ligament
sacrouterine fold
sacrovaginal fold
sacrovertebral
sacrovesical fold
sacrum, pl. sacra
- assimilation s.

saddle
- s. anesthesia
- s. back
- s. block anesthesia
- s. embolism
- s. head
- s. joint
- s. nose
- Turkish s.

sadism
sadist
sadistic

sadomasochism
sadomasochistic relationship
Saemisch's
- S. section
- S. ulcer

Saenger's
- S. macula
- S. operation
- S. sign

Saethre-Chotzen syndrome
safe sex
safety
- s. lens
- s. spectacles

safranin O
safranophil, safranophile
sagitta
sagittal
- s. axis
- s. border of parietal bone
- s. fontanel
- s. groove
- s. line
- s. plane
- s. section
- s. split mandibular osteotomy
- s. sulcus
- s. suture
- s. synostosis

sagittalis
sago spleen
sailor's skin
sail sound
Saint
- S. Anthony's dance
- S. Ignatius' itch
- S. John's dance
- S. triad
- S. Vitus dance

Sakaguchi reaction
Sakati-Nyhan syndrome
Sakurai
Sakurai-Lisch nodule
sakushu fever
salaam
- s. attack
- s. convulsions
- s. spasm

Salah's sternal puncture needle
salient
- pulmonary s.

saline agglutinin
Salinem
- S. fever
- S. infection

Salisbury common cold viruses
saliva
- chorda s.

s. ejector
ganglionic s.
s. pump
resting s.
sympathetic s.
salivant
salivary
s. calculus
s. colic
s. corpuscle
s. duct
s. fistula
s. gland
s. gland disease
s. gland virus
s. gland virus disease
s. virus
salivate
salivation
salivator
salivolithiasis
Salmonella
S. paratyphi A
S. schottmülleri
S. typhi
S. typhosa
salmon patch
salpingectomy
abdominal s.
salpingemphraxis
salpinges (*pl. of* salpinx)
salpingian
salpingioma
salpingitic
salpingitis
chronic interstitial s.
foreign body s.
gonorrheal s.
s. isthmica nodosa
pyogenic s.
salpingocele
salpingocyesis
salpingography
salpingolysis
salpingo-oophorectomy
abdominal s.-o.
salpingo-oophoritis
salpingo-oophorocele
salpingo-ovariectomy
salpingopalatine fold
salpingoperitonitis
salpingopexy
salpingopharyngeal
s. fold
s. muscle
salpingopharyngeus
s. muscle
salpingoplasty

salpingorrhagia
salpingorrhaphy
salpingoscopy
salpingostomatomy
salpingostomy
salpingotomy
abdominal s.
salpinx, pl. **salpinges**
s. uterina
salt
s. depletion
s. depletion syndrome
diazonium s.'s
s. dye
s. edema
s. fever
hexazonium s.'s
s. loading
s. sensitivity
tetrazonium s.'s
s. wasting
s. water boils
saltation
saltatory
s. chorea
s. conduction
s. evolution
s. spasm
salt-depletion crisis
salted
s. plasma
s. serum
Salter-Harris classification of epiphysial plate injuries
Salter's incremental lines
salt-losing
s.-l. defect
s.-l. nephritis
s.-l. syndrome
saltpeter paper
salubrious
saluresis
saluretic
salutarium
salutary
salvage
s. chemotherapy
s. cystectomy
s. therapy
Salzmann's nodular corneal degeneration
sample
cluster s.
end-tidal s.
Haldane-Priestley s.
probability s.
Rahn-Otis s.

S

sample (*continued*)
    random s.
    stratified s.
sampling
    biological s.
    chemical s.
    haphazard s.
    random s.
    snowball s.
Samter's syndrome
San
    S. Joaquin fever
    S. Joaquin Valley disease
    S. Joaquin Valley fever
    S. Miguel sea lion virus
Sanarelli phenomenon
Sanarelli-Shwartzman phenomenon
sanative
sanatorium
sanatory
Sanchez Salorio syndrome
sand
    s. bodies
    brain s.
    hydatid s.
    intestinal s.
    s. tumor
    urinary s.
sandal
    s. foot
    s. strap dermatitis
sandfly
    s. fever
    s. fever viruses
Sandhoff's disease
sandpaper
    s. disks
    s. gallbladder
Sandström's bodies
sandworm
    s. disease
sane
Sanfilippo's syndrome
Sanger method
sanguifacient
sanguiferous
sanguification
sanguine
sanguineous
    s. cyst
sanguinolent
sanguinopurulent
Sanguisuga
sanguivorous
sanies
saniopurulent
sanioserous

sanious
    s. pus
sanitarian
sanitarium
sanitary
sanitation
sanitization
sanity
Sansom's sign
Sanson's images
Santini's booming sound
Santorini's
    S. canal
    S. cartilage
    S. concha
    S. duct
    S. fissures
    S. incisures
    S. labyrinth
    S. major caruncle
    S. minor caruncle
    S. muscle
    S. plexus
    S. tubercle
    S. vein
São Paulo
    S. P. fever
    S. P. typhus
sap
    nuclear s.
saphena
saphenectomy
saphenous
    s. branch of descending genicular
      artery
    s. hiatus
    s. nerve
    s. opening
    s. veins
Sappey's
    S. fibers
    S. plexus
    S. veins
sapphism
sapremia
saprobe
saprobic
saprodontia
saprogen
saprogenic, saprogenous
saprophilous
saprophyte
    facultative s.
saprophytic
saprozoic
Sarcina
    S. maxima
    S. ventriculi

sarcoblast
sarcocele
Sarcocystis
    S. *bovihominis*
    S. *fusiformis*
    S. *hominis*
    S. *lindemanni*
    S. *miescheriana*
    S. *suihominis*
    S. *tenella*
sarcode
Sarcodina
sarcogenic cell
sarcoglia
sarcoid
    Boeck's s.
    Spiegler-Fendt s.
sarcoidal granuloma
sarcoidosis
    hypercalcemic s.
sarcolemma
sarcolemmal, sarcolemmic, sarcolemmous
sarcology
sarcoma
    alveolar soft part s.
    ameloblastic s.
    angiolithic s.
    avian s.
    botryoid s.
    endometrial stromal s.
    Ewing's s.
    fascicular s.
    giant cell s.
    giant cell monstrocellular s. of
      Zülch
    granulocytic s.
    immunoblastic s.
    Jensen's s.
    juxtacortical osteogenic s.
    Kaposi's s.
    leukocytic s.
    lymphatic s.
    medullary s.
    multiple idiopathic hemorrhagic s.
    myelogenic s.
    myeloid s.
    osteogenic s.
    periosteal s.
    reticulum cell s.
    round cell s.
    Rous s.
    spindle cell s.
    synovial s.
    telangiectatic osteogenic s.
Sarcomastigophora
sarcomatoid
    s. carcinoma
sarcomatosis

sarcomatous
sarcomere
sarconeme
sarcoplasm
sarcoplasmic
    s. reticulum
sarcoplast
sarcopoietic
Sarcopsylla penetrans
Sarcopsyllidae
sarcoptic
    s. acariasis
sarcoptid
sarcosinemia
sarcosis
sarcosome
sarcostosis
sarcotic
sarcotripsy
sarcotubules
sarcous
sardonic grin
sarmassation
sartorius
    s. bursae
    s. muscle
satellite
    s. abscess
    s. cells
    s. cell of skeletal muscle
    chromosome s.
    s. metastasis
    perineuronal s.
satellite-rich heterochromatin
satellitosis
satiation
satiety center
Sattler's
    S. elastic layer
    S. veil
saturated color
saturation
    s. analysis
    s. index
    secondary s.
saturnine
    s. colic
    s. encephalopathy
    s. gout
    s. tremor
satyriasis
satyrism
saucerization
saucer-shaped cataract
Saundby's test
sauriasis
sauriderma
sauriosis

S

sauroderma
sausage fingers
Savage
>S. perineal body
>S. syndrome

Savary bougies
saw
>Gigli's s.
>Stryker s.

saxitoxin
Sayre's
>S. jacket
>S. suspension apparatus
>S. suspension traction

S-BP line
scab
scabbard trachea
scabies
>Norwegian s.

scabious
scabrities
>s. unguium

scala, pl. **scalae**
>Löwenberg's s.
>s. media
>s. tympani
>s. vestibuli

scalar electrocardiogram
scald
scalded skin syndrome
scalding
scale
>activities of daily living s.
>adaptive behavior s.'s
>Bayley s.'s of Infant Development
>Binet s.
>Binet-Simon s.
>Brazelton's Neonatal Behavioral
> Assessment s.'s
>Cattell Infant Intelligence S.
>Charrière s.
>Columbia Mental Maturity S.
>coma s.
>digital gray s.
>French s.
>Gaffky s.
>Glasgow coma s.
>gray s.
>interval s.
>Karnofsky s.
>Leiter International Performance S.
>Likert s.
>masculinity-femininity s.
>ordinal s.
>Rahe-Holmes social readjustment
> rating s.
>ratio s.
>Shipley-Hartford s.

>Stanford-Binet intelligence s.
>Wechsler-Bellevue s.
>Wechsler intelligence s.'s
>Zubrod s.

scalene
>s. hiatus
>s. tubercle
>s. tubercle of Lisfranc

scalenectomy
scalenotomy
scalenus
>s. anterior muscle
>s. anterior syndrome
>s. medius muscle
>s. minimus muscle
>s. posterior muscle

scaler
>hoe s.
>ultrasonic s.

scaling
scall
>milk s.

scalloping
scalp
>s. contusion
>s. hair
>s. infection
>s. laceration
>s. muscle

scalpel
>plasma s.

scalpriform
scalprum
scaly
>s. ringworm
>s. tetter

scamping speech
scan
>duplex Doppler s.
>EMI s.
>Meckel s.
>sector s.
>ventilation-perfusion s.

scanner
scanning
>s. electron microscope
>s. equalization radiography
>s. speech

scanogram
Scanzoni's
>S. maneuver
>S. second os

scapha
scaphocephalic
scaphocephalism
scaphocephalous
scaphocephaly
scaphohydrocephalus, scaphohydrocephaly

scaphoid
- s. abdomen
- s. bone
- s. fossa
- s. fossa of sphenoid bone
- s. scapula
- s. tuberosity
- s. type of scapula

scapi (*pl. of* scapus)

scapula, gen. and pl. **scapulae**
- s. alata
- s. elevata
- scaphoid s., scaphoid type of s.
- winged s.

scapulalgia

scapular
- s. line
- s. notch
- s. reflex
- s. region

scapulary

scapulectomy

scapuloclavicular

scapulocostal syndrome

scapulodynia

scapulohumeral
- s. atrophy
- s. muscular dystrophy
- s. reflex

scapuloperiosteal reflex

scapulopexy

scapus, pl. **scapi**
- s. penis
- s. pili

scar
- s. cancer
- s. cancer of the lungs
- s. carcinoma
- cigarette-paper s.'s
- hypertrophic s.
- papyraceous s.'s
- radial s.
- shilling s.'s

Scardino vertical flap pyeloplasty

scarf bandage

scarification
- s. test

scarificator

scarify

scarlatina
- anginose s., s. anginosa
- s. hemorrhagica
- s. latens, latent s.
- s. maligna
- s. rheumatica
- s. simplex

scarlatinal
- s. nephritis

scarlatinella

scarlatiniform
- s. erythema

scarlatinoid

scarlet
- s. fever

Scarpa's
- S. fascia
- S. fluid
- S. foramina
- S. ganglion
- S. habenula
- S. hiatus
- S. liquor
- S. membrane
- S. method
- S. sheath
- S. staphyloma
- S. triangle

scarring alopecia

scatemia

scatologic

scatology

scatoma

scatophagy

scatoscopy

scatter
- Compton s.
- liquid s.

scattered radiation

scattergram

scattering
- Compton s.

scavenger cell

Scedosporium apiospermum

scelalgia

scent

Schacher's ganglion

Schaeffer-Fulton stain

Schaer's reagent

Schäfer's method

Schäffer's reflex

Schaffer's test

Schamberg's dermatitis

Schanz syndrome

Schapiro's sign

Schatzki's ring

Schaudinn's fixative

Schaumann
- S. bodies
- S. lymphogranuloma
- S. syndrome

Schauta vaginal operation

Schede's
- S. clot
- S. method

schedule
- s.'s of reinforcement, continuous

schedule (*continued*)
    reinforcement s., fixed-interval
    reinforcement s., fixed-ratio
    reinforcement s., intermittent
    reinforcement s., variable-interval
    reinforcement s.
Scheibe's deafness
Scheibler's reagent
Scheie's syndrome
Scheiner's experiment
Schellong-Strisower phenomenon
Schellong test
schema, pl. **schemata**
    body s.
schematic
    s. eye
schematograph
scheme
    occlusal s.
Schenck's disease
Scheuermann's disease
Schick
    S. method
    S. test
Schiff-Sherrington phenomenon
Schiff's reagent
Schilder's disease
Schiller's test
Schilling
    S. band cell
    S. blood count
    S. index
    S. test
    S. type of monocytic leukemia
schindylesis
schindyletic joint
Schiötz tonometer
Schirmer test
schistocelia
schistocormia
schistocystis
schistocyte
schistocytosis
schistoglossia
schistomelia
schistorrhachis
Schistosoma
    S. haematobium
    S. intercalatum
    S. japonicum
    S. malayensis
    S. mansoni
schistosomal dermatitis
schistosome
    s. granuloma
schistosomia
schistosomiasis
    Asiatic s.

    bladder s.
    cutaneous s. japonica
    ectopic s.
    s. haematobium
    s. intercalatum
    intestinal s.
    s. japonica, Japanese s.
    s. mansoni
    Manson's s.
    s. mekongi
    Oriental s.
    pulmonary s.
    urinary s.
schistosomulum, pl. **schistosomula**
schistosternia
schistothorax
schizamnion
schizaxon
schizencephalic microcephaly
schizencephaly
schizo-affective
    s.-a. psychosis
schizocyte
schizocytosis
schizogenesis
schizogony
schizogyria
schizoid
    s. personality
schizoidism
schizomycete
Schizomycetes
schizomycetic
schizomycosis
schizont
schizonychia
schizophasia
schizophrenia
    acute s.
    ambulatory s.
    catatonic s.
    childhood s.
    disorganized s.
    hebephrenic s.
    latent s.
    paranoid s.
    process s.
    pseudoneurotic s.
    reactive s.
    residual s.
    simple s.
schizophrenic
schizophreniform disorder
schizothemia
schizotonia
schizotrichia
Schizotrypanum cruzi
schizotypical personality

schizozoite
schlammfieber
Schlatter-Osgood disease
Schlatter's disease
Schlemm's canal
Schlesinger's sign
Schmidel's anastomoses
Schmid-Fraccaro syndrome
Schmidt
    S. diet
    S. syndrome
Schmidt-Lanterman
    S.-L. clefts
    S.-L. incisures
Schmidt-Strassburger diet
Schmorl's
    S. bacillus
    S. ferric-ferricyanide reduction stain
    S. jaundice
    S. nodule
    S. picrothionin stain
schneiderian
    s. first rank symptoms
    s. membrane
Schneider's
    S. carmine
    S. first rank symptoms
Schneidersitz
Scholander apparatus
Scholz' disease
Schönbein's
    S. operation
    S. test
Schönlein-Henoch syndrome
Schönlein's
    S. disease
    S. purpura
school
    biometrical s.
    iatromathematical s.
    mechanistic s.
    s. nurse
    s. phobia
Schottmueller's
    S. bacillus
    S. disease
Schott treatment
Schreger's lines
Schridde's cancer hairs
Schroeder's operation
Schuchardt's operation
Schüffner's
    S. dots
    S. granules
Schüller's
    S. disease
    S. ducts

    S. phenomenon
    S. syndrome
Schultz
    S. reaction
    S. stain
Schultz-Charlton
    S.-C. phenomenon
    S.-C. reaction
Schultz-Dale reaction
Schultze's
    S. cells
    S. mechanism
    S. membrane
    S. phantom
    S. placenta
    S. sign
Schütz' bundle
Schwabach test
Schwalbe's
    S. corpuscle
    S. nucleus
    S. ring
    S. spaces
Schwann
    S. cells
    S. cell unit
    S. white substance
schwannoma
    acoustic s.
schwannosis
Schwartz
    S. syndrome
    S. tractotomy
Schweninger-Buzzi anetoderma
Schweninger's method
sciage
sciatic
    s. foramen
    s. hernia
    s. nerve
    s. neuralgia
    s. neuritis
    s. plexus
    s. scoliosis
    s. spine
sciatica
science
scimitar sign
scinticisternography
scintigram
scintigraphic
    s. angiography
scintigraphy
scintillating scotoma
scintillation
    s. camera
    s. counter
scintiphotograph

scintiphotography
scintiscan
scintiscanner
scion
sciosophy
scirrhencanthis
scirrhosity
scirrhous
    s. carcinoma
scirrhus
scissiparity
scissor gait
scissors
    de Wecker's s.
    Smellie's s.
scissors-shadow
scissura, pl. scissurae
    s. pilorum
scissure
sclera, pl. scleras, sclerae
    blue s.
scleradenitis
scleral
    s. buckling operation
    s. ectasia
    s. resection
    s. rigidity
    s. ring
    s. roll
    s. spur
    s. staphyloma
    s. sulcus
    s. veins
scleras (pl. of sclera)
scleratogenous
sclerectasia
    partial s.
    total s.
sclerectomy
scleredema
    s. adultorum
sclerema
    s. adiposum
    s. neonatorum
sclerencephaly, sclerencephalia
scleriasis
scleritis
    annular s.
    anterior s.
    brawny s.
    deep s.
    gelatinous s.
    malignant s.
    necrotizing s.
    nodular s.
    posterior s.
scleroatrophy
scleroblastema

sclerochoroidal
sclerochoroiditis
    s. anterior
    s. posterior
scleroconjunctival
sclerocornea
sclerocorneal junction
sclerocystic disease of the ovary
sclerodactyly, sclerodactylia
scleroderma
    localized s.
    progressive familial s.
sclerodermatitis
sclerodermatous
sclerogenous, sclerogenic
scleroid
scleroiritis
sclerokeratitis
sclerokeratoiritis
scleroma
    respiratory s.
scleromalacia
scleromere
scleromyxedema
scleronychia
sclero-oophoritis
sclerophthalmia
scleroplasty
sclerosal
sclerosant
sclerose
sclerosing
    s. adenosis
    s. hemangioma
    s. inflammation
    s. keratitis
    s. leukoencephalitis
    s. mastoiditis
    s. osteitis
    s. therapy
sclerosis, pl. scleroses
    Alzheimer's s.
    arterial s.
    arteriocapillary s.
    arteriolar s.
    bone s.
    Canavan's s.
    central areolar choroidal s.
    combined s.
    s. corii
    s. cutanea
    diffuse infantile familial s.
    disseminated s.
    endocardial s.
    focal s.
    glomerular s.
    hippocampal s.

idiopathic hypercalcemic s. of
  infants
insular s.
laminar cortical s.
lateral spinal s.
lobar s.
mantle s.
menstrual s.
Mönckeberg's s.
multiple s.
nodular s.
nuclear s.
ovulational s.
physiologic s.
posterior s.
posterior spinal s.
primary lateral s.
systemic s.
tuberous s.
unicellular s.
valvular s.
vascular s.
s. of white matter
sclerostenosis
Sclerostoma
sclerostomy
sclerotherapy
sclerothrix
sclerotia (*pl. of* sclerotium)
sclerotic
  s. bodies
  s. cemental mass
  s. coat
  s. dentin
  s. gastritis
  s. kidney
  s. stomach
  s. teeth
sclerotica
sclerotium, pl. **sclerotia**
sclerotome
sclerotomy
  anterior s.
  posterior s.
sclerotrichia
sclerotylosis
sclerous
scoleces (*pl. of* scolex)
scoleciasis
scoleciform
scolecoid
scolecology
scolex, pl. **scoleces, scolices**
scoliokyphosis
scoliometer
scoliosis
  coxitic s.
  empyemic s.

habit s.
myopathic s.
ocular s., ophthalmic s.
osteopathic s.
paralytic s.
rachitic s.
sciatic s.
static s.
scoliotic
  s. pelvis
scoliotone
Scolopendra
s-cone
scoop
scopophilia
scopophobia
Scopulariopsis
scorbutic
  s. anemia
scorbutigenic
scorbutus
scordinema
score
  APACHE s.
  Apgar s.
  Dubowitz s.
  Gleason's s.
  raw s.
  recovery s.
  standard s.
  symptom s.
scorpion
Scorpionida
scotochromogens
scotograph
scotoma, pl. **scotomata**
  absolute s.
  annular s.
  arcuate s.
  Bjerrum's s.
  cecocentral s.
  central s.
  color s.
  flittering s.
  glaucomatous nerve-fiber bundle s.
  hemianopic s.
  mental s.
  negative s.
  paracentral s.
  pericentral s.
  peripheral s.
  physiologic s.
  positive s.
  quadrantic s.
  relative s.
  ring s.
  scintillating s.
  Seidel's s.

S

scotoma *(continued)*
    sickle s.
    zonular s.
scotomatous
scotometer
scotometry
scotophilia
scotophobia
scotopia
scotopic
    s. adaptation
    s. eye
    s. perimetry
    s. vision
scotoscopy
Scott operation
scotty dog
scout
    s. film
    s. radiograph
scrape
scratch test
screen
    Bjerrum s.
    s. defense
    s.-film contact
    fluorescent s.
    Hess s.
    intensifying s.
    s. memory
    rare-earth s.
    tangent s.
    vestibular s.
screening
    s. audiometry
    carrier s.
    cytologic s.
    familial s.
    mass s.
    multiphasic s.
    neonatal s.
    prenatal s.
    s. test
screw
    afterloading s.
    s. arteries
    s. elevator
    s. joint
screwdriver teeth
screw-worm
    primary s.-w.
    secondary s.-w.
scribe
Scribner shunt
scrivener's palsy
scrobiculate
scrobiculus cordis
scrofula

scrofuloderma
    s. gummosa
    papular s.
    verrucous s.
scrofulous
    s. keratitis
    s. rhinitis
scroll
    s. bones
    s. ear
scrota (*pl. of* scrotum)
scrotal
    s. arteries
    s. hernia
    s. raphe
    s. septum
    s. swelling
    s. tongue
    s. veins
scrotectomy
scrotiform
scrotitis
scrotocele
scrotoplasty
scrotum, pl. **scrota, scrotums**
    lymph s.
    watering-can s.
scrub
    s. nurse
    s. typhus
Scultetus'
    S. bandage
    S. position
scurf
scurvy
    Alpine s.
    hemorrhagic s.
    infantile s.
    land s.
    s. rickets
    sea s.
scuta (*pl. of* scutum)
scutate
scute
    tympanic s.
scutiform
Scutigera
scutular
scutulum, pl. **scutula**
scutum, pl. **scuta**
scybala
scybalous
scybalum, pl. **scybala**
scyphiform
scyphoid
sea
    s. gull murmur
    s. scurvy

s. sickness
s. urchin granuloma
sea-blue
s.-b. histiocyte
s.-b. histiocyte disease
seal
border s.
s. fingers
palatal s.
peripheral s.
posterior palatal s.
postpalatal s.
velopharyngeal s.
sealant
dental s.
fissure s.
sealed jar technique
seal-fin deformity
seamstress's cramp
searcher
Seashore test
seasickness
season
seat
basal s.
rest s.
seatworm
sebaceous
s. adenoma
s. cyst
s. epithelioma
s. follicles
s. glands
s. horn
s. tubercle
sebaceus
sebiagogic
sebiferous
Sebileau's
S. hollow
S. muscle
sebiparous
sebolith
seborrhea
s. adiposa
s. capitis
s. cerea
concrete s.
s. corporis
eczematoid s.
s. faciei, s. of face
s. furfuracea
s. nigra
s. oleosa
s. sicca
s. squamosa neonatorum
seborrheic
s. blepharitis

s. blepharoconjunctivitis
s. dermatitis
s. dermatosis
s. eczema
s. keratosis
s. verruca
s. wart
sebum
s. cutaneum
s. preputiale
Secernentasida
Secernentia
Seckel
S. dwarfism
S. syndrome
seclusion of pupil
second
s. cranial nerve
s. cuneiform bone
s. degree A-V block
s. degree burn
s. degree prolapse
s. finger
s. gas effect
s. heart sound
s. incisor
s. molar
s. parallel pelvic plane
s. set rejection
s. sight
s. signaling system
s. sound
s. temporal convolution
s. tibial muscle
s. tooth
secondaries
secondarily generalized tonic-clonic
seizure
secondary
s. abdominal pregnancy
s. adhesion
s. adrenocortical insufficiency
s. aerodontalgia
s. agammaglobulinemia
s. aldosteronism
s. amenorrhea
s. amputation
s. amyloidosis
s. anesthetic
s. antibody deficiency
s. aortic area
s. atelectasis
s. axis
s. buffer
s. carcinoma
s. cardiomyopathy
s. caries
s. cataract

S

secondary (*continued*)
s. cementum
s. center of ossification
s. choana
s. coccidioidomycosis
s. constriction
s. degeneration
s. dementia
s. dentin
s. dentition
s. deviation
s. dextrocardia
s. disease
s. drives
s. drowning
s. dysmenorrhea
s. egg membrane
s. elaboration
s. encephalitis
s. fissure of cerebellum
s. follicle
s. gain
s. generalized epilepsy
s. glaucoma
s. gout
s. hemochromatosis
s. hemorrhage
s. host
s. hydrocephalus
s. hyperparathyroidism
s. hypertension
s. hyperthyroidism
s. hypogammaglobulinemia
s. hypogonadism
s. hypothyroidism
s. immune response
s. immunodeficiency
s. infection
s. interatrial foramen
s. lysosomes
s. medical care
s. megaureter
s. mesoderm
s. methemoglobinemia
s. mucinosis
s. myeloid metaplasia
s. narcissism
s. nodule
s. nondisjunction
s. oocyte
s. palate
s. pellagra
s. point of ossification
s. process
s. pulmonary lobule
s. pyoderma
s. radiation
s. rays

s. refractory anemia
s. reinforcement
s. renal calculus
s. renal tubular acidosis
s. retinitis
s. saturation
s. screw-worm
s. sensory cortex
s. sensory nuclei
s. sex characters
s. spermatocyte
s. spiral lamina
s. spiral plate
s. suture
s. syphilid
s. syphilis
s. telangiectasia
s. thrombus
s. tuberculosis
s. tympanic membrane
s. union
s. uterine inertia
s. villus
s. visual area
s. visual cortex
s. vitreous
s. X zone
second-look operation
second-order conditioning
secreta
Secrétan's syndrome
secrete
secretin test
secretion
cytocrine s.
external s.
secretomotor, secretomotory
s. nerve
secretor
s. factor
secretory
s. canaliculus
s. carcinoma
s. component
s. cyst
s. duct
s. granule
s. immunoglobulin
s. immunoglobulin A
s. nerve
s. otitis media
sectile
sectio, pl. **sectiones**
section
abdominal s.
attached cranial s.
axial s.
cesarean s.

classical cesarean s.
coronal s.
cross s.
detached cranial s.
diagonal s.
frontal s.
frozen s.
Latzko's cesarean s.
longitudinal s.
lower uterine segment cesarean s.
median s.
microscopic s.
midsagittal s.
oblique s.
parasagittal s.
perineal s.
pituitary stalk s.
Saemisch's s.
sagittal s.
serial s.
thin s., ultrathin s.
transverse s.

sectional
s. impression
s. radiography
sectiones (*pl. of* sectio)
sector
s. iridectomy
s. scan
sectoranopia
secular equilibrium
secundigravida
secundina, pl. **secundinae**
secundines
secundipara
sedate
sedigitate
sedimentary cataract
sedimentation rate
sedimentator
sedimentometer
sedimentum
s. lateritium
seed corn
Seeligmüller's sign
seesaw
s. murmur
s. nystagmus
Seessel's
S. pocket
S. pouch
segment
anterior s.
anterior basal s.
anterior inferior s.
anterior ocular s.
anterior superior s.

apical s.
apicoposterior s.
arterial s.'s of kidney
bronchopulmonary s.
cardiac s.
cervical s.'s of spinal cord
coccygeal s.'s of spinal cord
hepatic s.'s
hepatic venous s.'s
inferior s.
inferior lingular s.
interannular s.
intermaxillary s.
internodal s.
Lanterman's s.'s
lateral s.
lateral basal s.
s.'s of liver
lower uterine s.
lumbar s.'s of spinal cord
medial s.
medial basal s.
mesoblastic s.
neural s.
posterior s.
posterior basal s.
posterior s. of eyeball
P-R s.
Ranvier's s.
renal s.'s
RST s.
s.'s of spinal cord
s.'s of spleen
S-T s.
subapical s.
subsuperior s.
superior s.
superior lingular s.
sympathetic s.
upper uterine s.
venous s.'s of the kidney
venous s.'s of liver
segmenta (*pl. of* segmentum)
segmental
s. alveolar osteotomy
s. anesthesia
s. arteries of kidney
s. atelectasis
s. bronchus
s. demyelinating polyneuropathy
s. fracture
s. glomerulonephritis
s. neuritis
s. plate
s. sphincter
s. tubule
s. zone

S

805

segmentation
- s. cavity
- s. nucleus

segmentectomy

segmented
- s. cell
- s. leukocyte
- s. neutrophil

segmenter

Segmentina

segmenting body

segmentum, pl. **segmenta**
- s. anterius
- s. anterius inferius
- s. anterius superius
- s. apicale
- s. apicoposterius
- s. basale anterius
- s. basale laterale
- s. basale mediale
- s. basale posterius
- s. bronchopulmonale
- s. cardiacum
- segmenta hepatis
- s. inferius
- s. internodale
- s. laterale
- segmenta lienis
- s. lingulare inferius
- s. lingulare superius
- s. mediale
- segmenta medullae spinalis
- segmenta medullae spinalis cervicalia
- segmenta medullae spinalis coccygea
- segmenta medullae spinalis lumbaria
- segmenta medullae spinalis sacralia
- segmenta medullae spinalis thoracica
- s. posterius
- segmenta renalia
- s. subapicale
- s. subsuperius
- s. superius

segregation
- s. analysis
- s. ratio

segregator

Seidel's
- S. scotoma
- S. sign

Seiler's cartilage

seismocardiogram

seismotherapy

seizure
- absence s.
- akinetic s.
- anosognosic s.'s
- atonic s.
- atypical absence s.
- audiogenic s.
- clonic s.
- complex partial s.
- convulsive s.
- early s.
- electrographic s.
- epileptic s.
- febrile s.
- focal motor s.
- gelastic s.
- generalized s.
- generalized tonic-clonic s.
- grand mal s.
- jacksonian s.
- late s.
- major motor s.
- minor motor s.
- myoclonic s.
- nonconvulsive s.
- nonepileptic s.
- partial s.
- petit mal s.
- psychic s.
- psychogenic s.
- psychomotor s.
- secondarily generalized tonic-clonic s.
- simple partial s.
- subclinical s.
- tonic s.
- tonic-clonic s.
- versive s.

sejunction

selaphobia

Seldinger technique

selectins

selection
- s. coefficient
- medical s.
- natural s.
- s. pressure
- sexual s.

selective
- s. angiography
- s. grinding
- s. hypoaldosteronism
- s. inattention
- s. injection
- s. medium
- s. memory
- s. reduction
- s. stain

selene unguium

Selenomonas

self
- s. concept
- subliminal s.

self-accusation
self-analysis
self-awareness
self-centeredness
self-commitment
self-control
self-differentiation
self-discovery
self-efficacy
self-fertilization
self-infection
self-knowledge
self-limited
- s.-l. disease

self-love
self-poisoning
self-regulation
self-retaining catheter
self-stimulation
Selivanoff's test
sella
- empty s.
- s. turcica

sellar
Sellick's maneuver
semantic aphasia
semantics
semeiography (*var. of* semiography)
semeiologic (*var. of* semiologic)
semeiology (*var. of* semiology)
semeiopathic (*var. of* semiopathic)
semeiotic (*var. of* semiotic)
semeiotics (*var. of* semiotics)
semelincident
semen, pl. **semina, semens**
semenuria
semicanal
- s. of auditory tube
- s. for tensor tympani muscle

semicanalis, pl. **semicanales**
- s. musculi tensoris tympani
- s. tubae auditivae

semicartilaginous
semicircular
- s. canals
- s. ducts
- s. line
- s. line of Douglas

semi-closed
- s.-c. anesthesia
- s.-c. circle

semicoma
semicomatose
semiconscious
semiconservative

semicrista
- s. incisiva

semidecussation
semidirect leads
semiflexion
semihorizontal heart
semilunar
- s. bone
- s. cartilage
- s. cusp
- s. fascia
- s. fasciculus
- s. fibrocartilage
- s. fold
- s. fold of colon
- s. ganglion
- s. hiatus
- s. line
- s. notch
- s. nucleus of Flechsig
- s. valve

semilunare
semiluxation
semimembranosus
- s. muscle
- s. reflex

semimembranous
semina (*pl. of* semen)
seminal
- s. capsule
- s. colliculus
- s. duct
- s. fluid
- s. gland
- s. granule
- s. hillock
- s. lake
- s. vesical cyst
- s. vesicle

semination
seminiferous
- s. epithelium
- s. tubule
- s. tubule dysgenesis

seminoma
- spermacytic s.

seminomatous
seminuria
semiography, semeiography
semiologic, semeiologic
semiology, semeiology
semiopathic, semeiopathic
semi-open anesthesia
semiorbicular
semiotic, semeiotic
semiotics, semeiotics
semioval center
semipenniform

semipermeable membrane
semipronation
semiprone
    s. position
semispinal
    s. muscle
    s. muscle of head
    s. muscle of neck
    s. muscle of thorax
semispinalis
    s. capitis muscle
    s. cervicis muscle
    s. muscle
    s. thoracis muscle
Semisulcospina
semisulcus
semisupination
semisupine
semitendinosus
    s. muscle
    s. reflex
semitendinous
semitertian
semivertical heart
Semon-Hering theory
Semon's law
Sendai virus
Senear-Usher
    S.-U. disease
    S.-U. syndrome
seneciosis
senescence
    dental s.
senescent
Sengstaken-Blakemore tube
senile
    s. amyloidosis
    s. arteriosclerosis
    s. atrophoderma
    s. atrophy
    s. cataract
    s. chorea
    s. degeneration
    s. delirium
    s. dementia
    s. dental caries
    s. deterioration
    s. dwarfism
    s. ectasia
    s. emphysema
    s. fibroma
    s. gangrene
    s. halo
    s. hemangioma
    s. hip disease
    s. involution
    s. keratoderma
    s. keratoma

    s. keratosis
    s. lenticular myopia
    s. lentigo
    s. melanoderma
    s. memory
    s. nephrosclerosis
    s. osteomalacia
    s. plaque
    s. pruritus
    s. psychosis
    s. retinoschisis
    s. sebaceous hyperplasia
    s. tremor
    s. vaginitis
    s. wart
senility
senior synonym
senium
Senning operation
sensate
sensation
    cincture s.
    delayed s.
    general s.
    girdle s.
    objective s.
    primary s.
    referred s.
    reflex s.
    special s.
    subjective s.
    s. time
    transferred s.
sense
    color s.
    s. of equilibrium
    geometrical s.
    s. of identity
    joint s.
    kinesthetic s.
    light s.
    muscular s.
    obstacle s.
    s. organs
    position s.
    posture s.
    pressure s.
    seventh s.
    sixth s.
    space s.
    special s.
    static s.
    tactile s.
    temperature s.
    thermal s., thermic s.
    time s.
    visceral s.
    weight s.

sensibility
    articular s.
    bone s.
    cortical s.
    deep s.
    dissociation s.
    electromuscular s.
    epicritic s.
    mesoblastic s.
    pallesthetic s.
    proprioceptive s.
    protopathic s.
    splanchnesthetic s.
    vibratory s.

sensible
    s. perspiration

sensiferous
sensigenous
sensimeter
sensitivity
    acquired s.
    analytical s.
    antibiotic s.
    clinical s.
    contrast s.
    diagnostic s.
    idiosyncratic s.
    induced s.
    multiple chemical s.
    pacemaker s.
    photoallergic s.
    phototoxic s.
    primaquine s.
    relative s.
    salt s.
    spectral s.
    s. training group

sensitization
    autoerythrocyte s.
    covert s.
    photodynamic s.

sensitize
sensitized
    s. antigen
    s. cell
    s. culture

sensitizer
sensitizing
    s. dose
    s. substance

sensitometry
sensomobile
sensomobility
sensomotor
sensor
sensoria (*pl. of* sensorium)
sensorial
    s. areas

sensoriglandular
sensorimotor
    s. area
    s. theory

sensorimuscular
sensorineural deafness
sensorium, pl. **sensoria, sensoriums**
sensorivascular
sensorivasomotor
sensory
    s. alexia
    s. amblyopia
    s. amusia
    s. aphasia
    s. areas
    s. ataxia
    s. cell
    s. cortex
    s. crossway
    s. decussation of medulla oblongata
    s. deprivation
    s. epilepsy
    s. ganglion
    s. image
    s. inattention
    s. nerve
    s. neuron
    s. neuronopathy
    s. nuclei
    s. paralysis
    s. precipitated epilepsy
    s. receptors
    s. root of ciliary ganglion
    s. root of pterygopalatine ganglion
    s. root of trigeminal nerve
    s. speech center
    s. tract
    s. urgency

sensual
sensualism
sensuality
sentient
sentiment
sentinel
    s. animal
    s. gland
    s. loop sign
    s. pile
    s. spinous process fracture
    s. tag

separating
    s. medium
    s. wire

separation
    s. anxiety
    s. anxiety disorder
    jaw s.
    s. of retina

separation *(continued)*
   sternochondral s.
   s. of teeth
sepsis, pl. **sepses**
   intestinal s.
   s. lenta
   puerperal s.
septa *(pl. of* septum)
septal
   s. area
   s. artery
   s. bone
   s. branches
   s. cartilage
   s. cell
   s. cusp of tricuspid valve
   s. gingiva
   s. lines
septan
Septata
septate
   s. hymen
   s. mycelium
   s. uterus
   s. vagina
septectomy
septemia
septi *(gen. of* septum)
septic
   s. abortion
   s. endocarditis
   s. fever
   s. infarct
   s. intoxication
   s. phlebitis
   s. pneumonia
   s. retinitis
   s. shock
   s. wound
septicemia
   acute fulminating meningococcal s.
   anthrax s.
   cryptogenic s.
   metastasizing s.
   morphine injector's s.
   plague s.
   puerperal s.
   typhoid s.
septicemic
   s. abscess
   s. plague
septicopyemia
septicopyemic
septimetritis
septodermoplasty
septomarginal
   s. fasciculus

   s. trabecula
   s. tract
septonasal
septo-optic dysplasia
septoplasty
septorhinoplasty
septostomy
septulum, pl. **septula**
   s. testis
   septula of testis
septum, gen. **septi**, pl. **septa**
   s. accessorium
   alveolar s.
   aortopulmonary s.
   atrioventricular s.
   s. atrioventriculare
   s. of auditory tube
   Bigelow's s.
   bony nasal s.
   bulbar s.
   s. bulbi urethrae
   s. canalis musculotubarii
   cartilaginous s.
   s. cervicale intermedium
   s. clitoridis
   Cloquet's s.
   comblike s.
   s. corporum cavernosorum clitoridis
   crural s.
   distal spiral s.
   endovenous s., s. endovenosum
   femoral s.
   s. femorale
   s. of frontal sinuses
   gingival s.
   s. glandis
   s. of glans penis
   hanging s.
   interalveolar s.
   s. interalveolare, pl. septa
     interalveolaria
   interatrial s.
   s. interatriale
   interdental s.
   interlobular s.
   intermediate cervical s.
   s. intermedium
   intermuscular s.
   s. intermusculare
   interpulmonary s.
   interradicular septa
   septa interradicularia
   interventricular s.
   s. interventriculare
   intra-alveolar septa
   s. linguae
   lingual s.
   s. lucidum

s. mediastinale
s. membranaceum ventriculorum
membranous s.
s. mobile nasi
s. musculare ventriculorum
s. of musculotubal canal
nasal s.
s. nasi
s. nasi osseum
orbital s.
s. orbitale
pectiniform s., s. pectiniforme
s. pellucidum
s. penis
placental septa
precommissural s.
s. primum
proximal spiral s.
rectovaginal s.
s. rectovaginale
rectovesical s.
s. rectovesicale
scrotal s.
s. scroti
s. secundum
sinus s.
s. sinuum frontalium
s. sinuum sphenoidalium
s. of sphenoidal sinuses
spiral s.
spiral bulbar s.
s. spurium
s. of testis
s. of tongue
transparent s.
transverse s.
s. tubae
urogenital s.
urorectal s.
ventricular s.
sequela, pl. **sequelae**
sequence
Alu s.'s
chi-s.'s
leader s.'s
long terminal repeat s.'s
monotonic s.
s. pulse
sequential
s. analysis
sequester
sequestra (*pl. of* sequestrum)
sequestral
sequestration
bronchopulmonary s.
s. cyst
s. dermoid
sequestrectomy

sequestrotomy
sequestrum, pl. **sequestra**
primary s.
sequoiosis
sera (*pl. of* serum)
serendipity
Sergent's white line
serial
s. extraction
s. film changer
s. passage
s. radiography
s. section
series, pl. **series**
erythrocytic s.
granulocytic s.
lymphocytic s., lymphoid s.
myeloid s.
small bowel s.
thrombocytic s.
upper GI s.
seriograph
seriography
serioscopy
seriscission
serocolitis
seroconversion
serocystic
serodiagnosis
seroenteritis
seroepidemiology
serofast
serofibrinous
s. inflammation
s. pleurisy
serofibrous
serologic
s. pipette
serology
seroma
seromembranous
seromucous
s. cells
s. gland
seromyotomy
seronegative
seropositive
seropurulent
seropus
seroreversion
serosa
s. of colon
s. of gallbladder
s. of liver
s. of small intestine
s. of stomach
s. of urinary bladder

811

serosa *(continued)*
    s. of uterine tube
    s. of uterus
serosamucin
serosanguineous
seroserous
serositis
    multiple s.
serosity
serosynovial
serosynovitis
serotaxis
serotherapy
serotina
serotype
    heterologous s.
    homologous s.
serous
    s. atrophy
    s. cell
    s. coat
    s. cyst
    s. demilunes
    s. diarrhea
    s. gland
    s. hemorrhage
    s. inflammation
    s. iritis
    s. layer of peritoneum
    s. ligament
    s. membrane
    s. meningitis
    s. otitis
    s. pericardium
    s. pleurisy
    s. retinitis
    s. synovitis
    s. tunic
serovaccination
serovar
serozyme
serpentine aneurysm
serpent ulcer of cornea
serpiginous
    s. choroidopathy
    s. corneal ulcer
    s. keratitis
    s. ulcer
serpigo
serrate, serrated
    s. suture
Serratia
    S. marcescens
serration
serratus
    s. anterior muscle
    s. posterior inferior muscle
    s. posterior superior muscle

serrefine
serrenoeud
Serres'
    S. angle
    S. glands
serrulate, serrulated
Sertoli
    S. cells
    S. cell tumor
    S. columns
Sertoli-cell-only syndrome
serum, pl. **serums, sera**
    s. accelerator
    s. accident
    s. agar
    s. agglutinin
    anticomplementary s.
    antiepithelial s.
    antilymphocyte s.
    antireticular cytotoxic s.
    bacteriolytic s.
    blood s.
    convalescent s.
    Coombs' s.
    s. disease
    s. eruption
    foreign s.
    s. hepatitis
    s. hepatitis virus
    human measles immune s.
    human pertussis immune s.
    human scarlet fever immune s.
    hyperimmune s.
    immune s.
    inactivated s.
    measles convalescent s.
    muscle s.
    s. nephritis
    nonimmune s.
    normal s.
    normal horse s.
    polyvalent s.
    s. prothrombin conversion
      accelerator
    s. rash
    s. reaction
    salted s.
    s. shock
    s. sickness
    specific s.
    s. therapy
    thyrotoxic s.
serumal
    s. calculus
serum-fast
serums (*pl. of* serum)
servation
Servetus' circulation

service
    denture s.
    Public Health S.
servomechanism
sesamoid
    s. bone
    s. cartilage of larynx
    s. cartilages of nose
sessile
    s. hydatid
    s. polyp
set
    haploid s.
    s. of idiotopes
    learning s.
    postural s.
seta, pl. **setae**
setaceous
Setaria
    S. cervi
    S. equina
setback
setiferous
setigerous
seton
    s. operation
    s. wound
setting
    s. expansion
    s. sun sign
set-up
seven-day fever
seventh
    s. cranial nerve
    s. sense
severe
    s. combined immunodeficiency
    s. combined immunodeficient mice
    s. postanoxic encephalopathy
sewing spasm
sex
    s. cell
    s. chromatin
    s. chromosome imbalance
    s. chromosomes
    s. cords
    s. determination
    s. factor
    s. linkage
    s. object
    s. ratio
    s. reversal
    s. role
    safe s.
sexdigitate
sexduction
sex-influenced
    s.-i. inheritance

sex-limited
    s.-l. inheritance
sex-linked
    s.-l. character
    s.-l. inheritance
    s.-l. locus
sexology
sextan
sexual
    s. abuse
    s. deviation
    s. dimorphism
    s. dwarfism
    s. dysfunction
    s. generation
    s. gland
    s. infantilism
    s. instinct
    s. life
    s. neurasthenia
    s. perversion
    s. potency
    s. preference
    s. reproduction
    s. selection
sexuality
    infantile s.
sexualization
sexually transmitted disease
Sézary
    S. cell
    S. erythroderma
    S. syndrome
S_7 gallop
shadow
    acoustic s.
    s. cells
    s. corpuscle
    Gumprecht's s.'s
    hilar s.
    s. nucleus
    Ponfick's s.
    radiographic parallel line s.'s
    s. test
shadow-casting
shaft
    s. of femur
    s. of fibula
    hair s.
    s. of humerus
    s. of radius
    s. of tibia
    s. of ulna
shaggy
    s. aorta
    s. chorion
    s. pericardium

S

shagreen
    s. patch
    s. skin
shake
    s. culture
    smelter's s.'s
    s. test
shaking palsy
shallow breathing
sham
    s. feeding
    s. rage
sham-movement vertigo
shank
shaping
shared psychotic disorder
sharp
    s. spoon
Sharpey's fibers
shave biopsy
Shaver's disease
shaving cramp
shawl muscle
shear
    s. flow
    Liston's s.'s
    s. rate
    s. stress
shearing edge
sheath
    axillary s.
    carotid s.
    caudal s.
    common flexor s.
    common peroneal tendon s.
    crural s.
    dentinal s.
    dural s.
    dural s. of optic nerve
    enamel rod s.
    external s. of optic nerve
    external root s.
    s. of eyeball
    fascial s.'s of extraocular muscles
    fascial s. of eyeball
    femoral s.
    fenestrated s.
    fibrous s.'s
    fibrous digital s.'s of foot
    fibrous digital s.'s of hand
    fibrous tendon s.
    Henle's s.
    Hertwig's s.
    Huxley's s.
    infundibuliform s.
    internal s. of optic nerve
    internal root s.
    intertubercular s.

    s. of Key and Retzius
    s. ligaments
    Mauthner's s.
    medullary s.
    microfilarial s.
    mitochondrial s.
    mucous s. of tendon
    myelin s.
    Neumann's s.
    neurovascular s.
    notochordal s.
    parotid s.
    plantar tendon s. of peroneus longus muscle
    s. process of sphenoid bone
    prostatic s.
    rectus s.
    resectoscope s.
    root s.
    Rouget-Neumann s.
    Scarpa's s.
    s. of Schwann
    s. of Schweigger-Seidel
    s. of styloid process
    synovial s.
    synovial s.'s of digits of foot
    synovial s.'s of digits of hand
    synovial tendon s.
    tail s.
    tendon s. of abductor pollicis longus and extensor pollicis brevis muscles
    tendon s. of extensor carpi radialis muscles
    tendon s. of extensor carpi ulnaris muscle
    tendon s. of extensor digiti minimi muscle
    tendon s. of extensor digitorum and extensor indicis muscles
    tendon s. of extensor digitorum longus muscle of foot
    tendon s. of extensor hallucis longus muscle
    tendon s. of extensor pollicis longus muscle
    tendon s. of flexor carpi radialis muscle
    tendon s. of flexor digitorum longus muscle of foot
    tendon s. of flexor hallucis longus muscle
    tendon s. of flexor pollicis longus muscle
    tendon s. of superior oblique muscle
    tendon s. of tibialis anterior muscle

tendon s. of tibialis posterior muscle
s. of thyroid gland
vascular s.'s
s.'s of vessels
Waldeyer's s.
sheathed artery
Sheehan's syndrome
sheep bots
sheep-pox virus
sheet
beta s.'s
shelf
Blumer's s.
dental s.
palatal s.
s. procedure
rectal s.
vocal s.
shell
cytotrophoblastic s.
diffusion s.
K s.
s. nail
s. shock
shellac base
Shenton's line
Shepherd's fracture
Sherrington
S. law
S. phenomenon
Shibley's sign
shield
embryonic s.
nipple s.
oral s.'s
shift
antigenic s.
axis s.
chemical s.
Doppler s.
s. to the left
luteoplacental s.
phase s.
Purkinje s.
s. to the right
threshold s.
shifting
s. dullness
s. pacemaker
Shiga bacillus
Shiga-Kruse bacillus
Shigella
S. boydii
S. dysenteriae
S. flexneri
S. sonnei
shigellosis

shilling scars
shim
shimamushi disease
shin
s. bone
s. bone fever
saber s.
toasted s.'s
shingles
shin-splints
ship
s. beriberi
Fabricius' s.
s. fever
Shipley-Hartford scale
shipping fever virus
Shirodkar operation
shirt-stud abscess
shiver
shock
anaphylactic s.
anaphylactoid s.
anesthetic s.
s. antigen
break s.
cardiac s.
cardiogenic s.
chronic s.
counter-s.
cultural s.
declamping s.
deferred s., delayed s.
delirious s.
diastolic s.
electric s.
endotoxin s.
erethistic s.
hemorrhagic s.
hypovolemic s.
s. index
insulin s.
irreversible s.
s. lung
oligemic s.
osmotic s.
primary s.
protein s.
pseudoanaphylactic s.
reversible s.
septic s.
serum s.
shell s.
spinal s.
systolic s.
s. therapy
toxic s.
s. treatment
vasogenic s.

S

shock *(continued)*
    s. wave lithotripsy
    wet s.
shocking dose
shoddy fever
Shone's
    S. anomaly
    S. complex
    S. syndrome
shook jong
Shope
    S. fibroma
    S. fibroma virus
    S. papilloma
    S. papilloma virus
shop typhus
short
    s. abductor muscle of thumb
    s. adductor muscle
    s. bone
    s. central artery
    s. chain
    s. ciliary nerve
    s. crus of incus
    s. extensor muscle of great toe
    s. extensor muscle of thumb
    s. extensor muscle of toes
    s. fibular muscle
    s. flexor muscle of great toe
    s. flexor muscle of little finger
    s. flexor muscle of little toe
    s. flexor muscle of thumb
    s. flexor muscle of toes
    s. gastric arteries
    s. gastric veins
    s. gyri of insula
    s. head
    s. head of biceps brachii muscle
    s. head of biceps femoris muscle
    s. incubation hepatitis
    s. levatores costarum muscles
    s. luteal phase
    s. palmar muscle
    s. peroneal muscle
    s. posterior ciliary artery
    s. process of malleus
    s. radial extensor muscle of wrist
    s. root of ciliary ganglion
    s. saphenous nerve
    s. saphenous vein
    s. sight
    s. TI inversion recovery
    s. vinculum
    s. wave diathermy
short-bowel syndrome
shortening reaction
shortsightedness
short-term memory

shot-feel
shot-silk
    s.-s. phenomenon
    s.-s. reflex
    s.-s. retina
shotted suture
shoulder
    s. blade
    frozen s.
    s. girdle
    s. joint
    s. presentation
shoulder-girdle syndrome
shoulder-hand syndrome
show
Shrapnell's membrane
shudder
    carotid s.
Shulman's syndrome
shunt
    arteriovenous s.
    Blalock s.
    Blalock-Taussig s.
    cavopulmonary s.
    s. cyanosis
    Denver s.
    dialysis s.
    distal splenorenal s.
    Glenn s.
    H s.
    jejunoileal s.
    left-to-right s.
    LeVeen s.
    mesocaval s.
    peritoneovenous s.
    portacaval s.
    portasystemic s.
    renal-splenic venous s.
    reversed s.
    right-to-left s.
    Scribner s.
    splenorenal s.
    Torkildsen s.
    transjugular intrahepatic portosystemic s.
    Warren s.
    Waterston s.
shut-in personality
Shwachman syndrome
Shwartzman
    S. phenomenon
    S. reaction
Shy-Drager syndrome
sialaden
sialadenitis
sialadenoncus
sialadenotropic
sialectasis

sialemesis, sialemesia
sialic
sialidosis
sialine
sialism, sialismus
sialoadenectomy
sialoadenitis
sialoadenotomy
sialoaerophagy
sialoangiectasis
sialoangiitis
sialocele
sialodochitis
sialodochoplasty
sialogenous
sialogram
sialography
sialolith
sialolithiasis
sialolithotomy
sialometaplasia
    necrotizing s.
sialometry
sialorrhea
sialoschesis
sialosemiology, sialosemeiology
sialosis
sialostenosis
Siamese twins
sib
Siberian tick typhus
sibilant
    s. rale
    s. rhonchus
sibilus
sibling
    s. rivalry
sibship
Sibson's
    S. aortic vestibule
    S. aponeurosis
    S. fascia
    S. groove
    S. muscle
sicca
    s. complex
    s. syndrome
sicchasia
sick
    s. building syndrome
    s. euthyroid syndrome
    s. headache
    s. role
    s. sinus syndrome
sickle
    s. cell
    s. cell anemia
    s. cell C disease

    s. cell crisis
    s. cell dactylitis
    s. cell disease
    s. cell retinopathy
    s. cell test
    s. cell-thalassemia disease
    s. cell trait
    s. flap
    s. form
    s. scotoma
sicklemia
sickling
sickness
    acute African sleeping s.
    aerial s.
    African sleeping s.
    air s.
    balloon s.
    black s.
    caisson s.
    car s.
    cave s.
    chronic African sleeping s.
    chronic mountain s.
    decompression s.
    East African sleeping s.
    falling s.
    green s.
    green tobacco s.
    Indian s.
    Jamaican vomiting s.
    laughing s.
    morning s.
    motion s.
    mountain s.
    radiation s.
    railroad s.
    sea s.
    serum s.
    sleeping s.
    space s.
    spotted s.
    West African sleeping s.
side
    balancing s.
    working s.
sideration
sideroachrestic anemia
sideroblast
sideroblastic anemia
siderocyte
sideroderma
siderofibrosis
siderogenous
sideropenia
sideropenic
    s. dysphagia
siderophage

S

siderophil, siderophile
siderophilous
siderophone
siderophore
siderosilicosis
siderosis
    pulmonary s.
siderotic
    s. cataract
    s. nodules
Siegert's sign
Siegle's otoscope
sieve
    s. bone
    s. graft
    s. plate
Siggaard-Andersen nomogram
sigh
sight
    s. blindness
    day s.
    far s.
    long s.
    near s.
    night s.
    second s.
    short s.
sigma
    s. effect
sigmatism
sigmoid
    s. arteries
    s. colon
    s. flexure
    s. fossa
    s. groove
    s. kidney
    s. lymph nodes
    s. notch
    s. sinus
    s. sulcus
    s. veins
    s. volvulus
sigmoidectomy
sigmoiditis
sigmoidopexy
sigmoidoproctostomy
sigmoidorectostomy
sigmoidoscope
sigmoidoscopy
sigmoidostomy
sigmoidotomy
sigmoidovesical fistula
sigmoscope
sign
    Aaron's s.
    Abadie's s. of tabes dorsalis
    Abrahams' s.

accessory s.
Allis' s.
Amoss' s.
Anghelescu's s.
antecedent s.
assident s.
Auenbrugger's s.
Aufrecht's s.
Babinski's s.
Baccelli's s.
Ballance's s.
Bamberger's s.
bandage s.
Bárány's s.
Barré's s.
Bassler's s.
Bastedo's s.
Battle's s.
B6 bronchus s.
beak s.
Bechterew's s.
Beevor's s.
Bezold's s.
Biederman's s.
Bielschowsky's s.
Biermer's s.
Biernacki's s.
Biot's s.
Biot's breathing s.
Bird's s.
Bjerrum's s.
s. blindness
blue dot s.
Blumberg's s.
Bonhoeffer's s.
Bozzolo's s.
Branham's s.
Braxton Hicks s.
Broadbent's s.
Brockenbrough s.
Brudzinski's s.
Bryant's s.
burning drops s.
calcium s.
Calkins' s.
Cantelli's s.
Carman's s.
Carnett's s.
Carvallo's s.
Castellani-Low s.
Chaddock s.
Chadwick's s.
chandelier s.
Chaussier's s.
Chvostek's s.
Claybrook's s.
Cleemann's s.
clenched fist s.

Codman's s.
Collier's s.
Collier's tucked lid s.
colon cutoff s.
Comby's s.
comet s.
comet tail s.
commemorative s.
Comolli's s.
contralateral s.
conventional s.'s
Coopernail's s.
Corrigan's s.
Courvoisier's s.
Crichton-Browne's s.
Cruveilhier-Baumgarten s.
Cullen's s.
Dalrymple's s.
Dance's s.
Danforth's s.
Darier's s.
Dawbarn's s.
Dejerine's s.
Delbet's s.
de Musset's s.
D'Éspine's s.
dimple s.
doll's eye s.
Dorendorf's s.
double bubble s.
double track s.
drawer s.
drooping lily s.
Drummond's s.
Duchenne's s.
Dupuytren's s.
Duroziez' s.
Ebstein's s.
s. of edema of lower eyelid
Epstein's s.
Erb s.
Erb-Westphal s.
Erichsen's s.
Escherich's s.
Ewart's s.
Ewing's s.
external malleolar s.
eyelash s.
Faget's s.
fan s.
Fischer's s.
fissure s.
flag s.
Forchheimer's s.
Fothergill's s.
Friedreich's s.
Froment's s.
Gaenslen's s.

Gauss' s.
Gerhardt's s.
Glasgow's s.
gloved-finger s.
Goggia's s.
Goldstein's toe s.
Goldthwait's s.
Goodell's s.
Gordon's s.
Gorlin's s.
Graefe's s.
Grasset's s.
Grey Turner's s.
Griesinger's s.
Grisolle's s.
Grocco's s.
groove s.
Gunn's s.
Gunn's crossing s.
Guyon's s.
halo s.
halo s. of hydrops
Hamman's s.
Hegar's s.
Heim-Kreysig s.
Helbings' s.
Hennebert's s.
Higoumenakia s.
Hill's s.
Hoagland's s.
Hoffmann's s.
Homans' s.
Hoover's s.'s
Hueter's s.
iconic s.'s
indexical s.'s
inferior triangle s.
Jackson's s.
Joffroy's s.
Keen's s.
Kehr's s.
Kernig's s.
Kestenbaum's s.
Kocher's s.
Kreysig's s.
Kussmaul's s.
Lancisi's s.
Landolfi's s.
Lasègue's s.
Laugier's s.
Legendre's s.
Leichtenstern's s.
Leri's s.
Leser-Trélat s.
Lhermitte's s.
Lichtheim's s.
local s.
Lorenz' s.

S

sign *(continued)*

Lovibond's profile s.
Ludloff's s.
Macewen's s.
Magendie-Hertwig s.
Magnan's s.
Magnus' s.
Mannkopf's s.
Marañón's s.
Marcus Gunn's s.
Masini's s.
McBurney's s.
Metenier's s.
Mirchamp's s.
Möbius' s.
Mosler's s.
Muerhrcke's s.
Müller's s.
Munson's s.
Murphy's s.
Musset's s.
neck s.
Néri's s.
Nikolsky's s.
objective s.
s. of the orbicularis
Osler's s.
Pastia's s.
Payr's s.
Perez' s.
Pfuhl's s.
physical s.
Piltz s.
Pins' s.
Pitres' s.
Pool-Schlesinger s.
Potain's s.
prodromic s.
pseudo-Graefe s.
puddle s.
pyramid s.
Quant's s.
Quénu-Muret s.
Quincke's s.
Ransohoff's s.
Raynaud's s.
Remak's s.
reversed-three s.
Revilliod's s.
Ripault's s.
Rocher's s.
Romaña's s.
Romberg's s.
Rosenbach's s.
Rossolimo's s.
Rotch's s.
Rovsing's s.
Rumpel-Leede s.

Russell's s.
Saenger's s.
Sansom's s.
Schapiro's s.
Schlesinger's s.
Schultze's s.
scimitar s.
Seeligmüller's s.
Seidel's s.
sentinel loop s.
setting sun s.
S s. of Golden
Shibley's s.
Siegert's s.
Signorelli's s.
silhouette s. of Felson
Simon's s.
Skoda's s.
Snellen's s.
spinal s.
spine s.
Steinberg thumb s.
Stellwag's s.
Sternberg's s.
Stewart-Holmes s.
Stierlin's s.
Straus' s.
string s.
subjective s.
Sumner's s.
superior triangle s.
ten Horn's s.
Thomson's s.
Tinel's s.
Toma's s.
Topolanski's s.
Tournay s.
Traube's s.
Trélat's s.
Trendelenburg's s.
Tresilian's s.
Trousseau's s.
Trunecek's s.
Uhthoff's s.
Vierra's s.
Vipond's s.
vital s.'s
von Graefe's s.
Weber's s.
Weiss' s.
Wernicke's s.
Westermark's s.
Westphal-Erb s.
Westphal's s.
Wilder's s.
Winterbottom's s.
wrist s.

signal
    s. node
    s. recognition particle
    s. void
signal-to-noise ratio
signet
    s. ring
    s. ring cells
signet-ring cell carcinoma
significance
    statistical s.
significant
Signorelli's sign
siguatera
silastic band
silent
    s. allele
    s. area
    s. electrode
    s. gallstones
    s. gap
    s. ischemia
    s. mutant
    s. mutation
    s. myocardial infarction
    s. period
silhouette sign of Felson
silica granuloma
silicate
    s. cement
    s. restorations
silicatosis
silicoanthracosis
silicone
    s. implant
    s.-related disease problems
silicoproteinosis
silicosiderosis
silicosis
silicotic granuloma
silicotuberculosis
siliqua olivae
silk
    floss s.
    virgin s.
silo-filler's
    s.-f. disease
    s.-f. lung
silver
    s. cell
    s. cone
    s. impregnation
    s. point
    s. protein stain
    s. stain
silver-ammoniacal silver stain

silver-fork
    s.-f. deformity
    s.-f. fracture
Silverman-Lilly pneumotachograph
Silver-Russell
    S.-R. dwarfism
    S.-R. syndrome
Silverskiöld's syndrome
silver-tin alloy
Simbu virus
simian
    s. crease
    s. hand
    s. vacuolating virus No. 40
    s. virus
    s. virus 40
similia similibus curantur
similimum, simillimum
Simmonds' disease
Simmons' citrate medium
Simonart's
    S. bands
    S. ligaments
    S. threads
Simonea folliculorum
Simon's
    S. position
    S. sign
Simons' disease
Simonsiella
simple
    s. absence
    s. acne
    s. anchorage
    s. anisocoria
    s. beam
    s. bone cyst
    s. color
    s. conjunctivitis
    s. crus of semicircular duct
    s. diplopia
    s. dislocation
    s. epithelium
    s. fission
    s. fracture
    s. glaucoma
    s. goiter
    s. heterochromia
    s. hyperopic astigmatism
    s. hypertrophy
    s. joint
    s. lobule
    s. lymphangiectasis
    s. mastectomy
    s. membranous limb of semicircular duct
    s. microscope
    s. myopia

S

simple *(continued)*
- s. myopic astigmatism
- s. necrosis
- s. obesity
- s. partial seizure
- s. pulmonary eosinophilia
- s. retinitis
- s. schizophrenia
- s. skull fracture
- s. squamous epithelium
- s. ulcer
- s. urethritis

simple-central anisocoria
Simplified Oral Hygiene Index
Simpson
- S. forceps
- S. uterine sound

Sims' position
Sims uterine sound
simulated hypertrophy
simulation
- computer s.

simulator
Simulium
- *S. rugglesi*

simultagnosia
simultanagnosia
simultaneous
- s. contrast
- s. perception

sincipital
- s. presentation

sinciput, pl. **sincipita, sinciputs**
Sindbis
- S. fever
- S. virus

sinew
singer's
- s. nodes
- s. nodules

single
- s. ascertainment
- s. (gel) diffusion precipitin test in one dimension
- s. (gel) diffusion precipitin test in two dimensions
- s. immunodiffusion
- s. microscope
- s. photon emission computed tomography
- s. ventricle

singultation
singultous
singultus
sinister
sinistrad
sinistral
sinistrality

sinistrocardia
sinistrocerebral
sinistrocular
sinistrogyration
sinistromanual
sinistropedal
sinistrorotation
sinistrorse
sinistrotorsion
sinistrous
sinoatrial
- s. block
- s. conduction time
- s. nodal artery
- s. node
- s. recovery time

sinoauricular block
sinography
sinopulmonary
sinovaginal
sinoventricular conduction
sinuatrial
- s. chamber
- s. nodal branch of right coronary artery
- s. node
- s. node artery

sinus, pl. **sinus, sinuses**
- s. alae parvae
- anterior sinuses
- s. aortae
- aortic s.
- Arlt's s.
- barber's pilonidal s.
- basilar s.
- Breschet's s.
- s. caroticus
- carotid s.
- s. cavernosus
- cavernous s.
- cerebral sinuses
- cervical s.
- circular s.
- s. circularis
- coccygeal s.
- s. coronarius
- coronary s.
- costomediastinal s.
- cranial sinuses
- dermal s.
- s. durae matris
- dural venous sinuses
- sinuses of dura mater
- Englisch's s.
- s. epididymidis
- s. of epididymis
- ethmoidal sinuses
- s. ethmoidales

s. ethmoidales anteriores
s. ethmoidales mediae
s. ethmoidales posteriores
frontal s.
s. frontalis
Guérin's s.
Huguier's s.
inferior longitudinal s.
inferior petrosal s.
inferior sagittal s.
s. intercavernosi
intercavernous sinuses
jugular s., s. jugularis
s. lactiferi
lactiferous s.
laryngeal s.
s. laryngeus
lateral s.
s. lienis
longitudinal s.
longitudinal vertebral venous s.
Luschka's s.
lymph s.
lymphatic s.
Maier's s.
marginal sinuses of placenta
mastoid sinuses
s. maxillaris
maxillary s.
Meyer's s.
middle ethmoidal sinuses
Morgagni's s.
s. of nail
oblique pericardial s.
oblique s. of pericardium
s. obliquus pericardii
occipital s.
s. occipitalis
Palfyn's s.
paranasal sinuses
s. paranasales
parasinoidal sinuses
Petit's s.
petrosal s.
s. petrosus inferior
s. petrosus superior
phrenicocostal s.
pilonidal s.
piriform s.
pleural sinuses
s. pocularis
s. posterior
precervical s.
prostatic s.
s. prostaticus
pulmonary sinuses
rectal sinuses
s. rectus

renal s.
s. renalis
s. reuniens
rhomboidal s., s. rhomboidalis
Ridley's s.
Rokitansky-Aschoff sinuses
s. sagittalis inferior
s. sagittalis superior
sigmoid s.
s. sigmoideus
sphenoidal s.
s. sphenoidalis
sphenoparietal s.
s. sphenoparietalis
splenic s.
straight s.
superior longitudinal s.
superior petrosal s.
superior sagittal s.
tarsal s.
s. tarsi
tentorial s.
terminal s., s. terminalis
s. tonsillaris
Tourtual's s.
transverse s.
transverse pericardial s.
transverse s. of pericardium
s. transversus
s. transversus pericardii
s. trunci pulmonalis
s. tympani
tympanic s.
s. unguis
urogenital s.
s. urogenitalis
uterine s.
uteroplacental sinuses
Valsalva's s.
s. of the vena cava
s. venarum cavarum
s. venosus
s. venosus sclerae
venous sinuses
venous s. of sclera
s. vertebrales longitudinales
sinusitis
frontal s.
sinusoid
uterine s.
sinusoidal
s. capillary
sinusotomy
sinuvertebral nerves
siphon
siphonage
Siphona irritans
Siphonaptera

S

Siphoviridae
Sipple's syndrome
sippy diet
sireniform
sirenomelia
siriasis
SISI test
sismotherapy
sister
    s. chromatid exchange
Sister Joseph's nodule
Sistrunk operation
site
    antibody combining s.
    antigen-binding s.
    antigen-combining s.
    combining s.
    fragile s.
    immunologically privileged s.'s
    privileged s.
    s. specific mutation
    s. specific recombination
sitotaxis
sitotropism
situation
    s. anxiety
    psychoanalytic s.
situational
    s. psychosis
    s. test
situs
    s. inversus
    s. inversus viscerum
    s. perversus
    s. solitus
    s. transversus
sitz bath
sixth
    s. cranial nerve
    s. disease
    s. sense
    s. venereal disease
    s. ventricle
sixth-year molar
size
    burst s.
    focal spot s.
sizer
Sjögren-Larsson syndrome
Sjögren's
    S. disease
    S. syndrome
Sjöqvist tractotomy
skein
    s. cell
    choroid s.
skeletal
    s. extension

    s. muscle
    s. muscle fibers
    s. muscle tissue
    s. survey
    s. system
    s. traction
skeletology
skeleton
    appendicular s.
    s. appendiculare
    articulated s.
    axial s.
    s. axiale
    cardiac s.
    cardiac fibrous s.
    fibrous s. of heart
    s. of free inferior limb
    s. of free superior limb
    gill arch s.
    s. hand
    s. of heart
    jaw s.
    s. thoracicus
    visceral s.
skeneitis, skenitis
skeneoscope
Skene's
    S. glands
    S. tubules
skenitis (var. of skeneitis)
skew
    s. deviation
    s. distribution
skiascopy
Skillern's fracture
skin
    alligator s.
    bronzed s.
    deciduous s.
    diamond s.
    s. dose
    elastic s.
    farmer's s.
    fish s.
    s. flap
    s. furrows
    glabrous s.
    glossy s.
    golfer's s.
    s. graft
    s. grooves
    hidden nail s.
    loose s.
    parchment s.
    piebald s.
    pig s.
    porcupine s.
    s. pore

s. reaction
s. reflexes
s. ridges
sailor's s.
shagreen s.
s. stones
s. tag
s. of teeth
s. test
toad s.
s. traction
s. writing
yellow s.
skinbound disease
skin-muscle reflexes
Skinner box
skinnerian conditioning
skin-puncture test
skin-pupillary reflex
skip areas
skipped generation
Sklowsky symptom
skodaic resonance
Skoda's
S. rale
S. sign
S. tympany
skull
cloverleaf s.
s. fracture
maplike s.
natiform s.
steeple s., tower s.
skullcap
sky blue
slab-off
s.-o. lens
slant culture
slaty anemia
sleep
s. apnea
s. apnea syndrome
crescendo s.
s. dissociation
s. drunkenness
electric s.
electrotherapeutic s.
s. epilepsy
hypnotic s.
light s.
paradoxical s.
s. paralysis
paroxysmal s.
s. phase delay syndrome
rapid eye movement s., REM s.
s. spindle
s. terror

s. terror disorder
twilight s.
sleep-induced apnea
sleepiness
sleeping sickness
sleeplessness
sleeptalking
sleepwalker
sleepwalking
sleeve
nerve root s.
sleeve graft
SLE-like syndrome
slender
s. fasciculus
s. lobule
s. process of malleus
slew rate
slide
s. micrometer
sliding
s. esophageal hiatal hernia
s. filament hypothesis
s. flap
s. hernia
s. hiatal hernia
s. hook
s. oblique osteotomy
slime fever
sling
slipped hernia
slipping
s. patella
s. rib
s. rib cartilage
slit
Cheatle s.
filtration s.'s
s. lamp
s. pores
pudendal s.
s. ventricle syndrome
vulvar s.
slitlamp
slope
s. culture
lower ridge s.
slotted attachment
slough
sloughing
s. phagedena
s. ulcer
slow
s. fever
s. virus
slow-reacting
s.-r. factor of anaphylaxis

slow-reacting *(continued)*
    s.-r. substance
    s.-r. substance of anaphylaxis
Sluder's neuralgia
sludge
sludged blood
sluggish layer
sluice
sluiceway
slurring speech
small
    s. arteries
    s. bowel
    s. bowel enema
    s. bowel series
    s. canal of chorda tympani
    s. cardiac vein
    s. cell carcinoma
    s. cleaved cell
    s. deep petrosal nerve
    s. increment sensitivity index
    s. increment sensitivity index test
    s. interarch distance
    s. intestine
    s. lymphocytic lymphoma
    s. pancreas
    s. pelvis
    s. plaque parapsoriasis
    s. pudendal lip
    s. saphenous vein
    s. sciatic nerve
    s. trochanter
    s. vein
smaller
    s. muscle of helix
    s. pectoral muscle
    s. posterior rectus muscle of head
    s. psoas muscle
smallest
    s. cardiac veins
    s. scalene muscle
    s. splanchnic nerve
smallpox
    confluent s.
    discrete s.
    fulminating s.
    hemorrhagic s.
    malignant s.
    modified s., varicelloid s.
    s. virus
    West Indian s.
Sm antigen
smear
    alimentary tract s.
    bronchoscopic s.
    buccal s.
    cervical s.
    colonic s.

    cul-de-sac s.
    s. culture
    cytologic s.
    duodenal s.
    ectocervical s.
    endocervical s.
    endometrial s.
    esophageal s.
    fast s.
    FGT cytologic s., female genital tract cytologic s.
    gastric s.
    lateral vaginal wall s.
    lower respiratory tract s.
    oral s.
    pancervical s.
    Pap s.
    Papanicolaou s.
    sputum s.
    urinary s.
    VCE s.
smegma
    s. clitoridis
    s. preputii
smegmalith
smell
smell-brain
Smellie's scissors
smelter's
    s. chills
    s. fever
    s. shakes
Smith-Boyce operation
Smith-Indian operation
Smith-Lemli-Opitz syndrome
Smith-Petersen nail
Smith-Riley syndrome
Smith-Robinson operation
Smith's
    S. fracture
    S. operation
smoker's
    s. patches
    s. tongue
smooth
    s. broach
    s. chorion
    s. colony
    s. diet
    s. leprosy
    s. muscle
    s. muscle tissue
    s. muscular sphincter
    s. surface caries
smooth-surfaced endoplasmic reticulum
smudge cells
smut
S-N-A angle

snail
    s. fever
snap
    closing s.
    s. finger
    opening s.
snapping
    s. hip
    s. reflex
snare
    cold s.
    galvanocaustic s., hot s.
S-N-B angle
Sneddon's syndrome
Sneddon-Wilkinson disease
sneeze
Snellen's
    S. sign
    S. test types
Snell's law
sniff test
S-N line
snore
snout reflex
snow
    s. blindness
    s. conjunctivitis
snowball
    s. opacity
    s. sampling
snowman abnormality
Snow procedure
snowshoe hare virus
snub-nose dwarfism
snuffbox
    anatomical s.
snuff-box
snuffles
Snyder's test
soapsuds enema
Soave operation
socia
    s. parotidis
social
    s. adaptation
    s. control
    s. diseases
    s. instinct
    s. intelligence
    s. maladjustment
    s. medicine
    s. network therapy
    s. psychiatry
    s. therapy
socialization
socialized medicine
sociocentric
sociocentrism

sociocosm
sociogenesis
sociogram
sociomedical
sociometric distance
sociometry
sociopath
sociopathy
socket
    dry s.
    eye s.
    s. joint
    tooth s.
sodium
    s. tungstoborate
sodium-responsive periodic paralysis
sodoku
sodomist, sodomite
sodomy
Soemmerring's
    S. ganglion
    S. ligament
    S. muscle
    S. spot
soft
    s. cataract
    s. chancre
    s. corn
    s. diet
    s. palate
    s. papilloma
    s. parts
    s. pulse
    s. rays
    s. sore
    s. tissue window
    s. tubercle
    s. ulcer
    s. wart
software
Sohval-Soffer syndrome
sokosho
solar
    s. blindness
    s. cheilitis
    s. dermatitis
    s. elastosis
    s. fever
    s. ganglia
    s. keratosis
    s. lentigo
    s. maculopathy
    s. plexus
    s. retinopathy
    s. therapy
    s. treatment
    s. urticaria
solder

S

soldier's
    s. heart
    s. patches
sole
    s. of foot
    s. nuclei
    s. reflex
    s. tap reflex
soleal line
Solenopotes capillatus
sole-plate ending
soleus
    s. muscle
solid
    color s.
    s. edema
    s. phase immunoassay
solid-state detector
solipsism
solitary
    s. bone cyst
    s. bundle
    s. fasciculus
    s. fibrous tumor
    s. follicles
    s. foramen
    s. glands
    s. lymphatic follicles
    s. nodules of intestine
    s. osteocartilaginous exostosis
    s. tract
solubility test
soluble
    s. antigen
    s. ligature
solum
solution
    Benedict's s.
    s. of contiguity
    s. of continuity
    disclosing s.
    Earle's s.
    Fonio's s.
    Gallego's differentiating s.
    Hartman's s.
    Hayem's s.
    Lange's s.
    Lugol's iodine s.
    Monsel s.
    Weigert's iodine s.
solvent drag
soma
somasthenia
somatagnosia
somatalgia
somatasthenia
somatesthesia
somatesthetic

somatic
    s. agglutinin
    s. antigen
    s. arteries
    s. cell genetics
    s. cell hybridization
    s. cells
    s. crossing-over
    s. death
    s. delusion
    s. layer
    s. mesoderm
    s. mitosis
    s. motor neuron
    s. motor neurons
    s. motor nuclei
    s. mutation
    s. mutation theory of cancer
    s. nerve
    s. nucleus
    s. reproduction
    s. sensory cortex
    s. swallow
    s. teniasis
somaticosplanchnic
somaticovisceral
somatist
somatization
    s. disorder
somatochrome
somatocrinin
somatoform
    s. disorder
    s. pain
somatogenic
somatology
somatomedins
somatometry
somatopagus
somatopathic
somatopathy
somatophrenia
somatoplasm
somatopleure
somatoprosthetics
somatopsychic
somatopsychosis
somatoscopy
somatosensory
    s. cortex
    s. evoked potential
somatosexual
somatostatinoma
somatotherapy
somatotopagnosis
somatotopic
somatotopy
somatotroph

somatotrophic
somatotropic
somatotype
somatotypology
somesthesia
somesthetic
    s. area
    s. system
somite
    s. cavity
    occipital s.
somitic mesoderm
somnambulance
somnambulic epilepsy
somnambulism
somnambulist
somnambulistic trance
somnifacient
somniferous
somnific
somnifugous
somniloquence, somniloquism
somniloquist
somniloquy
somnipathist
somnipathy
somnocinematograph
somnocinematography
somnolence, somnolency
somnolent
somnolentia
somnolescent
somnolism
Somogyi
    S. effect
    S. method
    S. phenomenon
    S. unit
Sondermann's canal
sone
Songo fever
sonic
    s. waves
sonicate
sonication
sonification
sonifier
sonify
Sonne
    S. bacillus
    S. dysentery
sonogram
sonograph
sonographer
sonography
sonolucent
sonomicrometer

sonomotor
    s. response
sonorous
    s. rhonchus
sonorous rale
soot wart
sopor
soporiferous
soporose, soporous
sordes
sore
    bay s.
    bed s.
    canker s.'s
    cold s.
    Delhi s.
    desert s.
    fungating s.
    hard s.
    Lahore s.
    Natal's s.
    Oriental s.
    pressure s.
    soft s.
    s. throat
    tropical s.
    veldt s.
    venereal s.
    water s.
soremouth virus
Soret band
soroche
    chronic s.
Sorsby's
    S. macular degeneration
    S. syndrome
SOS
    S. genes
    S. repair
Sotos' syndrome
souffle
    cardiac s.
    fetal s.
    funic s., funicular s.
    mammary s.
    placental s.
    umbilical s.
    uterine s.
soul pain
sound
    after-s.
    amphoric voice s.
    anvil s.
    atrial s.
    auscultatory s.
    bell s.
    bowel s.'s
    Campbell s.

S

sound *(continued)*
cannon s.
cardiac s.
cavernous voice s.
coconut s.
cracked-pot s.
Davis interlocking s.
double-shock s.
eddy s.'s
ejection s.'s
first heart s.
fourth heart s.
friction s.
gallop s.
heart s.'s
hippocratic succussion s.
Jewett s.
Korotkoff s.'s
Le Fort s.
McCrea s.
Mercier's s.
muscle s.
percussion s.
pericardial friction s.
pistol-shot s.
pistol-shot femoral s.
posttussis suction s.
s. pressure level
respiratory s.
sail s.
Santini's booming s.
second s.
second heart s.
Simpson uterine s.
Sims uterine s.
splitting of heart s.'s
succussion s.
tambour s.
third s.
third heart s.
tic-tac s.'s
to-and-fro s.
van Buren s.
waterwheel s.
water-whistle s.
Winternitz' s.
xiphisternal crunching s.

soundex code

South
S. African tick-bite fever
S. African type porphyria
S. American blastomycosis
S. American trypanosomiasis

Southern blot analysis

Southey's tubes

spa

space
s. adaptation syndrome

alveolar dead s.
anatomical dead s.
antecubital s.
anterior clear s.
apical s.
axillary s.
Berger's s.
Bogros' s.
Böttcher's s.
Bowman's s.
Burns' s.
capsular s.
cartilage s.
central palmar s.
Chassaignac's s.
Cloquet's s.
Colles' s.
corneal s.
Cotunnius' s.
cranial epidural s.
dead s.
deep perineal s.
denture s.
disk s.
Disse's s.
s. of Donders
epidural s.
episcleral s.
epitympanic s.
filtration s.
Fontana's s.'s
freeway s.
gingival s.
haversian s.'s
Henke's s.
His' perivascular s.
infraglottic s.
interalveolar s.
intercostal s.
interfascial s.
interglobular s.
interglobular s. of Owen
interocclusal rest s.
interosseous metacarpal s.'s
interosseous metatarsal s.'s
interpleural s.
interproximal s.
interradicular s.
interseptovalvular s.
intersheath s.'s of optic nerve
intervaginal s. of optic nerve
intervillous s.'s
intraretinal s.
s.'s of iridocorneal angle
Kiernan's s.
Kretschmann's s.
Kuhnt's s.'s
lateral central palmar s.

lateral midpalmar s.
lateral pharyngeal s.
leeway s.
lymph s.
Magendie's s.'s
s. maintainer
Malacarne's s.
Meckel's s.
medial midpalmar s.
mediastinal s.
s. medicine
medullary s.
middle palmar s.
midpalmar s.
Mohrenheim's s.
s. myopia
s. nerve
Nuel's s.
parapharyngeal s.
Parona's s.
parotid s.
perforated s.
perichoroid s.
perichoroidal s.
perilymphatic s.
perineal s.'s
perinuclear s.
peripharyngeal s.
periportal s. of Mall
perisinusoidal s.
perivitelline s.
personal s.
pharyngeal s.
pharyngomaxillary s.
physiologic dead s.
plantar s.
pleural s.
pneumatic s.
Poiseuille's s.
popliteal s.
postpharyngeal s.
Proust's s.
Prussak's s.
pterygomandibular s.
quadrangular s.
quadrilateral s.
Reinke's s.
respiratory dead s.
s. retainer
retroadductor s.
retroinguinal s.
retromylohyoid s.
retroperitoneal s.
retropharyngeal s.
retropubic s.
retrosternal s.
Retzius' s.
Schwalbe's s.'s

s. sense
s. sickness
subarachnoid s.
subchorial s.
subdural s.
subgingival s.
superficial perineal s.
suprahepatic s.'s
suprasternal s.
Tarin's s.
Tenon's s.
thenar s.
Traube's semilunar s.
Trautmann's triangular s.
vertebral epidural s.
Virchow-Robin s.
Waldeyer's s.
Westberg's s.
zonular s.'s

spaced teeth
spade
s. fingers
s. hand

spall
Spallanzani's law
spallation
span
memory s.
Spanish influenza
spannungs-P
sparganoma
sparganosis
ocular s.
sparganum
spasm
s. of accommodation
affect s.'s
anorectal s.
Bell's s.
cadaveric s.
canine s.
carpopedal s.
clonic s.
cynic s.
dancing s.
diffuse esophageal s.
epidemic transient diaphragmatic s.
esophageal s.
facial s.
functional s.
habit s.
histrionic s.
infantile s.
intention s.
masticatory s.
mimic s.
mobile s.
muscle s.

S

spasm *(continued)*
    nictitating s.
    nodding s.
    occupational s., professional s.
    phonic s.
    progressive torsion s.
    retrocollic s.
    rotatory s.
    salaam s.
    saltatory s.
    sewing s.
    synclonic s.
    tailor's s.
    tonic s.
    tonoclonic s.
    tooth s.'s
    torsion s.
    vasomotor s.
    winking s.

spasmodic
    s. asthma
    s. dysmenorrhea
    s. laryngitis
    s. stricture
    s. tic
    s. torticollis

spasmogen
spasmogenic
spasmology
spasmolygmus
spasmolysis
spasmophilia
spasmophilic
    s. diathesis

spasmus
    s. caninus
    s. coordinatus
    s. glottidis
    s. nictitans
    s. nutans

spastic
    s. abasia
    s. anemia
    s. aphonia
    s. colon
    s. diplegia
    s. dysarthria
    s. dysphonia
    s. ectropion
    s. entropion
    s. flat foot
    s. gait
    s. hemiplegia
    s. ileus
    s. miosis
    s. mydriasis
    s. paraplegia

    s. speech
    s. spinal paralysis

spasticity
    clasp-knife s.

spatial
    s. acuity
    s. contiguity
    s. localization
    s. vector
    s. vectorcardiography

spatium, pl. **spatia**
    spatia anguli iridocornealis
    s. episclerale
    s. intercostale
    s. interfasciale
    s. interglobulare, pl. spatia
      interglobularia
    spatia interossea metacarpi
    spatia interossea metatarsi
    s. intervaginale bulbi oculi
    spatia intervaginalia nervi optici
    s. lateropharyngeum
    s. perichoroideale
    s. perilymphaticum
    s. perinei profundum
    s. perinei superficiale
    s. peripharyngeum
    s. retroinguinale
    s. retroperitoneale
    s. retropharyngeum
    s. retropubicum
    s. subdurale
    spatia zonularia

spatula
    s. needle
    Roux s.

spatulate
spatulated
spatulation
special
    s. anatomy
    s. hospital
    s. nurse
    s. sensation
    s. sense
    s. somatic afferent column
    s. visceral efferent column
    s. visceral efferent nuclei
    s. visceral motor nuclei

specialist
specialization
specialize
specialized transduction
specialty
speciation
species, pl. **species**
    type s.

species-specific
    s.-s. antigen
specific
    s. active immunity
    s. anergy
    s. antigens
    s. antiserum
    s. bactericide
    s. cause
    s. compliance
    s. disease
    s. epithet
    s. hemolysin
    s. immunity
    s. indication
    s. opsonin
    s. parasite
    s. passive immunity
    s. reaction
    s. serum
    s. therapy
    s. transduction
    s. urethritis
specificity
    analytical s.
    diagnostic s.
    relative s.
specillum, pl. **specilla**
specimen
    cytologic s.
speck finger
spectacle plane
spectacles
    bifocal s.
    clerical s.
    divers' s.
    divided s.
    Franklin s.
    half-glass s.
    hemianopic s.
    lid crutch s.
    Masselon's s.
    orthoscopic s.
    pantoscopic s.
    photochromic s.
    protective s.
    pulpit s.
    safety s.
    stenopeic s., stenopaic s.
    telescopic s.
spectra (*pl. of* spectrum)
spectral
    s. phonocardiograph
    s. sensitivity
spectrophobia
spectroscopy
    magnetic resonance s.
spectrum, pl. **spectra, spectrums**

    antimicrobial s.
    fortification s.
    frequency s.
    infrared s.
    invisible s.
    thermal s.
    toxin s.
    ultraviolet s.
    wide s.
specular
    s. glare
    s. image
speculum, pl. **specula**
    bivalve s.
    Cooke's s.
    duckbill s.
    eye s.
    s. forceps
    Kelly's rectal s.
    Pedersen's s.
    stop-s.
speech
    alaryngeal s.
    s. audiogram
    s. audiometer
    s. audiometry
    s. bulb
    s. centers
    cerebellar s.
    clipped s.
    echo s.
    esophageal s.
    explosive s.
    helium s.
    mirror s.
    s. pathology
    scamping s.
    scanning s.
    slurring s.
    spastic s.
    staccato s.
    subvocal s.
    syllabic s.
    tracheoesophageal s.
spelencephaly
Spens' syndrome
sperm
    s. aster
    s. cell
    s. crystal
    s. nucleus
spermacytic seminoma
spermagglutination
sperm-aster
spermatic
    s. cord
    s. duct
    s. filament

spermatic *(continued)*
    s. fistula
    s. plexus
    s. vein
spermatid
spermatoblast
spermatocele
spermatocyst
spermatocytal
spermatocyte
    primary s.
    secondary s.
spermatocytogenesis
spermatogenesis
spermatogenetic
spermatogenic
spermatogenous
spermatogeny
spermatogone
spermatogonium
spermatoid
spermatology
spermatolysin
spermatolysis
spermatolytic
spermatophobia
spermatophore
spermatopoietic
spermatorrhea
spermatoxin
spermatozoal, spermatozoan
spermatozoon, pl. **spermatozoa**
spermaturia
spermia (*pl. of* spermium)
spermiduct
spermin crystal
spermiogenesis
spermium, pl. **spermia**
spermolith
spermolysis
spermotoxin
sphacelate
sphacelation
sphacelism
sphaceloderma
sphacelous
sphacelus
sphenethmoid
sphenion
sphenobasilar
sphenoccipital
sphenocephaly
sphenoethmoid
sphenoethmoidal
    s. recess
    s. suture
    s. synchondrosis

sphenofrontal
    s. suture
sphenoid
    s. angle
    s. bone
    s. crest
    s. process
    s. process of palatine bone
    s. process of septal cartilage
sphenoidal
    s. angle
    s. angle of parietal bone
    s. border of temporal bone
    s. conchae
    s. fissure
    s. fontanel
    s. herniation
    s. part of middle cerebral artery
    s. ridges
    s. sinus
    s. sinus aperture
    s. spine
    s. turbinated bones
sphenoidale
sphenoiditis
sphenoidostomy
sphenoidotomy
sphenomalar
sphenomandibular ligament
sphenomaxillary
    s. fissure
    s. fossa
    s. suture
spheno-occipital
    s.-o. joint
    s.-o. suture
    s.-o. synchondrosis
spheno-orbital suture
sphenopalatine
    s. artery
    s. foramen
    s. ganglion
    s. neuralgia
    s. notch
sphenoparietal
    s. sinus
    s. suture
sphenopetrosal
    s. fissure
    s. synchondrosis
sphenopetrous synchondrosis
sphenorbital
sphenosalpingostaphylinus
sphenosquamosal
sphenosquamous suture
sphenotemporal

sphenotic
  s. center
  s. foramen
sphenoturbinal
sphenovomerine
  s. suture
sphenozygomatic
  s. suture
sphere
  attraction s.
  Morgagni's s.'s
spheresthesia
spherical
  s. aberration
  s. amalgam
  s. form of occlusion
  s. lens
  s. nucleus
  s. recess
spherocylinder
spherocylindrical lens
spherocyte
spherocytic
  s. anemia
  s. jaundice
spherocytosis
  hereditary s.
spheroid, spheroidal
  s. articulation
  s. colony
  s. joint
spherometer
spherophakia
spheroplast
spheroprism
spherospermia
spherule
sphincter
  anatomical s.
  s. angularis, angular s.
  s. ani, anal s.
  s. ani tertius
  annular s.
  antral s.
  s. antri
  s. of antrum
  artificial s.
  basal s.
  bicanalicular s.
  Boyden's s.
  canalicular s.
  choledochal s.
  colic s.
  s. of common bile duct
  s. constrictor cardiae
  duodenal s.
  duodenojejunal s.
  external anal s.

external urethral s.
extrinsic s.
first duodenal s.
functional s.
s. of gastric antrum
Glisson's s.
s. of hepatic flexure of colon
hepatopancreatic s.
s. of hepatopancreatic ampulla
Hyrtl's s.
ileal s.
ileocecocolic s.
iliopelvic s.
inferior esophageal s.
s. intermedius
internal anal s.
internal urethral s.
intrinsic s.
lower esophageal s.
macroscopic s.
marginal s.
mediocolic s.
microscopic s.
midgastric transverse s.
midsigmoid s.
s. muscle
s. muscle of common bile duct
s. muscle of pancreatic duct
s. muscle of pupil
s. muscle of pylorus
s. muscle of urethra
s. muscle of urinary bladder
myovascular s.
myovenous s.
Nélaton's s.
O'Beirne's s.
s. oculi
s. of Oddi dysfunction
Oddi's s.
s. oris
ostial s.
palatopharyngeal s.
pancreatic s.
s. of pancreatic duct
pathologic s.
pelvirectal s.
s. of the pharyngeal isthmus
physiological s.
postpyloric s.
prepapillary s.
preprostate urethral s.
prepyloric s.
proximal urethral s.
s. pupillae
pyloric s.
radiological s.
rectosigmoid s.
segmental s.

S

sphincter *(continued)*
    smooth muscular s.
    striated muscular s.
    superior esophageal s.
    s. of third portion of duodenum
    unicanalicular s.
    s. urethrae
    s. vaginae
    Varolius' s.
    velopharyngeal s.
    s. vesicae
    s. vesicae biliaris
sphincteral
sphincteralgia
sphincterectomy
sphincterial, sphincteric
sphincterismus
sphincteritis
sphincteroid
    s. tract of ileum
sphincterolysis
sphincteroplasty
sphincteroscope
sphincteroscopy
sphincterotome
sphincterotomy
    external s.
    transduodenal s.
sphingolipidosis
    cerebral s., adult type, early juvenile
      type, infantile type, late juvenile
      type
sphingolipodystrophy
sphingomyelin lipidosis
sphygmic
    s. interval
sphygmocardiograph
sphygmocardioscope
sphygmochronograph
sphygmogram
sphygmograph
sphygmographic
sphygmography
sphygmoid
sphygmomanometer
    Mosso's s.
    Riva-Rocci s.
    Rogers' s.
sphygmomanometry
sphygmometer
sphygmometroscope
sphygmo-oscillometer
sphygmopalpation
sphygmophone
sphygmoscope
    Bishop's s.
sphygmoscopy
sphygmosystole

sphygmotonograph
sphygmotonometer
sphygmoviscosimetry
spica, pl. **spicae**
    s. bandage
spicula (*pl. of* spiculum)
spicular
spicule
spiculum, pl. **spicula**
spider
    s. angioma
    arterial s.
    s. cancer
    s. finger
    s. hemangioma
    s. mole
    s. nevus
    s. pelvis
    s. telangiectasia
    vascular s.
spider-burst
Spiegelberg's criteria
Spiegler-Fendt
    S.-F. pseudolymphoma
    S.-F. sarcoid
Spielmeyer's acute swelling
Spielmeyer-Sjögren disease
Spielmeyer-Stock disease
Spielmeyer-Vogt disease
spigelian hernia
Spigelius'
    S. line
    S. lobe
spike
    ponto-geniculo-occipital s.
    s. potential
    s. and wave complex
spill
    cellular s.
spillway
spiloma
spiloplaxia
spilus
spin
    s. density
    s. echo
spina, gen. and pl. **spinae**
    s. angularis
    s. bifida
    s. bifida aperta
    s. bifida cystica
    s. bifida manifesta
    s. bifida occulta
    s. dorsalis
    s. frontalis
    s. helicis
    s. iliaca anterior inferior
    s. iliaca anterior superior

s. iliaca posterior inferior
s. iliaca posterior superior
s. ischiadica
s. meatus
s. mentalis
s. nasalis anterior
s. nasalis ossis frontalis
s. nasalis posterior
s. ossis sphenoidalis
spinae palatinae
s. pedis
s. peronealis
s. pubis
s. scapulae
s. suprameatica
s. trochlearis
s. tympanica major
s. tympanica minor
s. ventosa

spinach stools
spinal

s. accessory nerve
s. analgesia
s. anesthesia
s. anesthetic
s. apoplexy
s. arteries
s. ataxia
s. block
s. canal
s. column
s. concussion
s. cord
s. cord concussion
s. curvature
s. decompression
s. fusion
s. ganglion
s. headache
s. induction
s. instability
s. lemniscus
s. length
s. marrow
s. muscle
s. muscle of head
s. muscle of neck
s. muscle of thorax
s. nerves
s. nucleus of accessory nerve
s. nucleus of the trigeminus
s. paralysis
s. part of accessory nerve
s. part of arachnoid
s. point
s. puncture
s. pyramidotomy
s. quotient

s. reflex
s. root of accessory nerve
s. shock
s. sign
s. stroke
s. tap
s. tract
s. tractotomy
s. tract of trigeminal nerve
s. trigeminal nucleus
s. veins

spinalis

s. capitis muscle
s. cervicis muscle
s. muscle
s. thoracis muscle

spinate
spindle

aortic s.
s. cataract
s. cell
s. cell carcinoma
s. cell lipoma
s. cell nevus
s. cell sarcoma
central s.
cleavage s.
s. fiber
His' s.
Krukenberg's s.
Kühne's s.
mitotic s.
muscle s.
neuromuscular s.
neurotendinous s.
nuclear s.
sleep s.

spindle-celled layer
spindle-shaped muscle
spine

alar s.
angular s.
anterior inferior iliac s.
anterior nasal s.
anterior superior iliac s.
bamboo s.
s. cell
cleft s.
dendritic s.'s
dorsal s.
s. fusion
greater tympanic s.
s. of helix
Henle's s.
iliac s.
ischiadic s.
ischial s.
lesser tympanic s.

spine *(continued)*
    meatal s.
    mental s.
    nasal s. of frontal bone
    neural s.
    palatine s.'s
    poker s.
    posterior inferior iliac s.
    posterior nasal s.
    posterior palatine s.
    posterior superior iliac s.
    pubic s.
    s. of scapula
    sciatic s.
    s. sign
    sphenoidal s.
    Spix's s.
    suprameatal s.
    thoracic s.
    trochlear s.
Spinelli operation
spinifugal
spinipetal
spin-lattice relaxation
spinnbarkeit
spino-adductor reflex
spinobulbar
spinocerebellar
    s. ataxia
    s. tracts
spinocerebellum
spinocervicothalamic tract
spinocollicular
spinocostalis
spinogalvanization
spinoglenoid
    s. ligament
spinomuscular
spinoneural
spino-olivary tract
spinoreticular
    s. fibers
    s. tract
spinose
spinotectal
    s. tract
spinothalamic
    s. cordotomy
    s. tract
    s. tractotomy
spinotransversarius
spinous
    s. layer
    s. process
    s. process of tibia
spin-spin relaxation
spintharicon
spiracle

spiradenitis
spiradenoma
    eccrine s.
spiral
    s. artery
    s. bandage
    s. bulbar septum
    s. canal of cochlea
    s. canal of modiolus
    s. cochlear ganglion
    s. computed tomography
    s. crest
    s. CT
    Curschmann's s.'s
    s. fold of cystic duct
    s. foraminous tract
    s. fracture
    s. ganglion of cochlea
    s. groove
    s. hyphae
    s. joint
    s. ligament of cochlea
    s. line
    s. membrane
    s. organ
    s. plate
    s. prominence
    s. septum
    s. suture
    s. of Tillaux
    s. tip catheter
    s. tubule
    s. valve of cystic duct
    s. vein of modiolus
spirem, spireme
spirilla (*pl. of* spirillum)
Spirillaceae
spirillar
    s. dysentery
spirillosis
Spirillum
    S. minus
    S. volutans
spirillum, pl. **spirilla**
    s. fever
    Obermeier's s.
    Vincent's s.
spirit lamp
Spirocerca lupi
Spirochaeta
    S. obermeieri
    S. plicatilis
Spirochaetaceae
Spirochaetales
spirochetal
    s. jaundice
spirochete
spirochetemia

spirochetolysis
spirochetosis
    bronchopulmonary s.
spirochetotic
spirogram
spirograph
spiro-index
spirometer
    chain-compensated s.
    Krogh s.
    Tissot s.
    wedge s.
Spirometra
    S. mansoni
    S. mansonoides
spirometry
spironolactone test
spiroscope
spiruroid
    s. larva migrans
Spiruroidea
spitting
spittle
Spitzer's theory
Spitzka's
    S. marginal tract
    S. marginal zone
    S. nucleus
Spitz nevus
Spix's spine
splanchnapophysial, splanchnapophyseal
splanchnapophysis
splanchnectopia
splanchnemphraxis
splanchnesthesia
splanchnesthetic sensibility
splanchnic
    s. afferent column
    s. anesthesia
    s. cavity
    s. efferent column
    s. ganglion
    s. layer
    s. mesoderm
    s. nerve
    s. wall
splanchnicectomy
splanchnicotomy
splanchnocele
splanchnocranium
splanchnodiastasis
splanchnography
splanchnolith
splanchnologia
splanchnology
splanchnomegaly
splanchnomicria
splanchnopathy

splanchnopleural
splanchnopleure
splanchnopleuric
splanchnoptosis, splanchnoptosia
splanchnosclerosis
splanchnoskeletal
splanchnoskeleton
splanchnosomatic
splanchnotomy
splanchnotribe
splay
spleen
    accessory s.
    diffuse waxy s.
    floating s.
    lardaceous s.
    movable s.
    sago s.
    sugar-coated s.
    waxy s.
splen
    s. accessorius
splenalgia
splenauxe
Splendore-Hoeppli phenomenon
splenectomy
splenectopia, splenectopy
splenelcosis
splenemphraxis
spleneolus
splenetic
splenia (*pl. of* splenium)
splenial
    s. gyrus
splenic
    s. anemia
    s. artery
    s. branches of splenic artery
    s. cells
    s. cords
    s. corpuscles
    s. flexure
    s. flexure syndrome
    s. index
    s. leukemia
    s. lymph follicles
    s. lymph nodes
    s. lymph nodules
    s. plexus
    s. portal venography
    s. pulp
    s. recess
    s. sinus
    s. vein
spleniculus
spleniform
spleniserrate

S

splenitis
splenium, pl. **splenia**
    s. corporis callosi
    s. of corpus callosum
splenius
    s. capitis muscle
    s. cervicis muscle
    s. muscle of head
    s. muscle of neck
splenocele
splenocleisis
splenocolic
splenodynia
splenogonadal fusion
splenohepatomegaly, splenohepatomegalia
splenoid
splenolymphatic
splenoma
splenomalacia
splenomedullary
splenomegaly, splenomegalia
    congestive s.
    Egyptian s.
    hemolytic s.
    hyperreactive malarious s.
    Niemann's s.
    tropical s.
splenomyelogenous
splenomyelomalacia
splenoncus
splenonephric
splenopancreatic
splenopathy
splenopexy, splenopexia
splenophrenic
splenoportogram
splenoportography
splenoptosis, splenoptosia
splenorenal
    s. ligament
    s. shunt
splenorrhagia
splenorrhaphy
splenosis
splenotomy
splenotoxin
splenule
splenulus, pl. **splenuli**
splenunculus, pl. **splenunculi**
splint
    acid etch cemented s.
    active s.
    air s.
    airplane s.
    anchor s.
    Anderson s.
    backboard s.
    Balkan s.

    cap s.
    coaptation s.
    contact s.
    Cramer wire s.
    Denis Browne s.
    dynamic s.
    Essig s.
    Frejka pillow s.
    functional s.
    Gunning s.
    Hodgen s.
    inflatable s.
    interdental s.
    Kingsley s.
    labial s.
    ladder s.
    lingual s.
    Liston's s.
    plaster s.
    reverse Kingsley s.
    surgical s.
    Taylor's s.
    Thomas s.
    Tobruk s.
    wire s.
splinted abutment
splintered fracture
splinter hemorrhages
splinting
split
    s. brain
    s. cast method
    s. cast mounting
    s. genes
    s. hand
    s. papules
    s. pelvis
    s. renal function test
    s. tolerance
split-skin graft
split-thickness
    s.-t. flap
    s.-t. graft
splitting of heart sounds
split-virus vaccine
spodogenous
spodogram
spodography
spodophorous
spoke-shave
spondaic
spondee
Spondweni virus
spondylalgia
spondylarthritis
spondylarthrocace
spondylitic

spondylitis
    ankylosing s.
    s. deformans
    Kümmell's s.
    rheumatoid s.
    tuberculous s.
spondylocace
spondyloepiphysial dysplasia
spondylolisthesis
spondylolisthetic
    s. pelvis
spondylolysis
spondylomalacia
spondylopathy
spondyloptosis
spondylopyosis
spondyloschisis
spondylosis
    cervical s.
    hyperostotic s.
spondylosyndesis
spondylothoracic
spondylotomy
spondylous
sponge
    Bernays' s.
    s. biopsy
    bronchoscopic s.
    compressed s.
    contraceptive s.
    s. tent
spongiform
    s. encephalopathy
    s. pustule of Kogoj
spongioblast
spongioblastoma
spongiocyte
spongioid
spongiose
spongiosis
spongiositis
spongy
    s. body of penis
    s. bone
    s. degeneration of infancy
    s. part of the male urethra
    s. spot
    s. substance
    s. urethra
spontaneous
    s. abortion
    s. agglutination
    s. amputation
    s. breech extraction
    s. cephalic delivery
    s. correction of placenta previa
    s. evolution
    s. fracture

    s. gangrene of newborn
    s. intermittent mandatory ventilation
    s. mutation
    s. phagocytosis
    s. pneumothorax
    s. recovery
    s. remission
    s. version
spoon
    cataract s.
    Daviel's s.
    s. nail
    sharp s.
    Volkmann's s.
sporadin
sporangiophore
sporangium
spore
    black s.
sporicidal
sporicide
sporidium, pl. **sporidia**
sporoagglutination
sporoblast
sporocyst
Sporocystinea
sporodochium
sporogenesis
sporogenous
sporogeny
sporogony
sporont
sporophore
sporoplasm
sporotheca
Sporothrix
sporotrichosis
sporotrichositic chancre
Sporotrichum
sporozoan
Sporozoasida
Sporozoea
sporozoite
sporozooid
sporozoon
sport
sports medicine
sporular
sporulation
sporule
spot
    acoustic s.'s
    Bitot's s.'s
    blind s.
    blood s.'s
    blue s.
    Brushfield's s.'s
    café au lait s.'s

S

spot *(continued)*
    cherry-red s.
    corneal s.
    cotton-wool s.'s
    De Morgan's s.'s
    Elschnig's s.'s
    Filatov's s.'s
    s. film
    flame s.'s
    focal s.
    Fordyce's s.'s
    Fuchs' black s.
    Graefe's s.'s
    hot s.
    hypnogenic s.
    Koplik's s.'s
    liver s.
    Mariotte's blind s.
    milk s.'s
    mongolian s.
    mulberry s.'s
    rose s.'s
    Roth's s.'s
    ruby s.'s
    saccular s.
    Soemmerring's s.
    spongy s.
    Tardieu's s.'s
    Tay's cherry-red s.
    temperature s.
    tendinous s.
    s. test for infectious mononucleosis
    Trousseau's s.
    utricular s.
    white s.
    yellow s.
spot-film radiography
spotted
    s. fever
    s. sickness
spouse, spousal
    s. abuse
sprain
    s. fracture
spread
    common vehicle s.
spreader
    gutta-percha s.
    rib s.
    root canal s.
spreading depression
Sprengel's deformity
spring
    s. conjunctivitis
    s. finger
    s. lancet
    s. ligament
    s. ophthalmia

sprout
    syncytial s.
sprue
    celiac s.
    nontropical s.
    tropical s.
sprue-former
spud
Spumavirinae
Spumavirus
spur
    Fuchs' s.
    Grunert's s.
    Michel's s.
    Morand's s.
    scleral s.
    vascular s.
spurious
    s. ankylosis
    s. cast
    s. meningocele
    s. pregnancy
    s. torticollis
sputum, pl. **sputa**
    s. aerogenosum
    globular s.
    green s.
    nummular s.
    prune-juice s.
    rusty s.
    s. smear
squama, pl. **squamae**
    frontal s.
    s. frontalis
    occipital s.
    s. occipitalis, occipital s.
    temporal s.
    s. temporalis
squamate
squamatization
squame
squamocellular
squamocolumnar
    s. junction
squamofrontal
squamomastoid
    s. suture
squamo-occipital
squamoparietal
    s. suture
squamopetrosal
squamosa, pl. **squamosae**
squamosal
squamosphenoid
squamotemporal
squamotympanic
    s. fissure

squamous
 s. alveolar cells
 s. border
 s. border of parietal bone
 s. border of sphenoid bone
 s. cell
 s. cell hyperplasia
 s. margin
 s. metaplasia
 s. metaplasia of amnion
 s. odontogenic tumor
 s. part of frontal bone
 s. part of occipital bone
 s. part of temporal bone
 s. pearl
 s. suture
squamozygomatic
square
 least s.'s
 s. matrix
 s. wave stimuli
squarrose, squarrous
squint
 convergent s.
 divergent s.
 external s.
 s. hook
 internal s.
squinting eye
squirrel plague conjunctivitis
S romanum
stab
 s. cell
 s. culture
 s. drain
 s. neutrophil
 s. wound
stabilate
stabilimeter
stability
 denture s.
 detrusor s.
 dimensional s.
stabilized baseplate
stabilizer
 endodontic s.
stabilizing
 s. circumferential clasp arm
 s. fulcrum line
stable
 s. equilibrium
 s. factor
 s. fracture
staccato speech
Staderini's nucleus
stadiometer
stadium, pl. **stadia**

staff
 attending s.
 s. cell
 consulting s.
 house s.
Stafne bone cyst
stage
 algid s.
 Arneth s.'s
 bell s.
 bud s.
 cap s.
 cold s.
 defervescent s.
 end s.
 eruptive s.
 exoerythrocytic s.
 genital s.
 imperfect s.
 incubative s.
 intuitive s.
 s. of invasion
 s.'s of labor
 latent s.
 perfect s.
 preconceptual s.
 prodromal s.
 resting s.
 Tanner s.
 trypanosome s.
 tumor s.
 vegetative s.
stagger
staghorn calculus
staging
 Jewett and Strong s.
 TNM s.
stagnant
 s. anoxia
 s. hypoxia
stagnation
 s. mastitis
Stahl's ear
stain
 Abbott's s. for spores
 aceto-orcein s.
 acid s.
 Ag-AS s.
 Albert's s.
 Altmann's anilin-acid fuchsin s.
 auramine O fluorescent s.
 basic s.
 basic fuchsin-methylene blue s.
 Bauer's chromic acid
  leucofuchsin s.
 Becker's s. for spirochetes
 Bennhold's Congo red s.
 Berg's s.

S

stain *(continued)*
Best's carmine s.
Bielschowsky's s.
Biondi-Heidenhain s.
Birch-Hirschfeld s.
Bodian's copper-PROTARGOL s.
Borrel's blue s.
Bowie's s.
Brown-Brenn s.
Cajal's astrocyte s.
carbol-thionin s.
C-banding s.
centromere banding s.
chromate s. for lead
chrome alum hematoxylin-phloxine s.
Ciaccio's s.
contrast s.
Da Fano's s.
Dane's s.
DAPI s.
diazo s. for argentaffin granules
Dieterle's s.
differential s.
double s.
Ehrlich's acid hematoxylin s.
Ehrlich's aniline crystal violet s.
Ehrlich's triacid s.
Ehrlich's triple s.
Einarson's gallocyanin-chrome alum s.
Eranko's fluorescence s.
Feulgen s.
Field's rapid s.
Fink-Heimer s.
Flemming's triple s.
fluorescence plus Giemsa s.
fluorescent s.
Fontana-Masson silver s.
Fontana's s.
Foot's reticulin impregnation s.
Fouchet's s.
Fraser-Lendrum s. for fibrin
Friedländer's s. for capsules
G-banding s.
Giemsa s.
Giemsa chromosome banding s.
Glenner-Lillie s. for pituitary
Golgi's s.
Gomori-Jones periodic acid-methenamine-silver s.
Gomori's aldehyde fuchsin s.
Gomori's chrome alum hematoxylin-phloxine s.
Gomori's methenamine-silver s.'s, GMS s.
Gomori's nonspecific acid phosphatase s.
Gomori's nonspecific alkaline phosphatase s.
Gomori's one-step trichrome s.
Gomori's silver impregnation s.
Goodpasture's s.
Gordon and Sweet s.
Gram's s.
green s.
Gridley's s.
Gridley's s. for fungi
Grocott-Gomori methenamine-silver s.
Hale's colloidal iron s.
Heidenhain's azan s.
Heidenhain's iron hematoxylin s.
hematoxylin and eosin s.
hematoxylin-malachite green-basic fuchsin s.
hematoxylin-phloxine B s.
Hirsch-Peiffer s.
Hiss' s.
Holmes' s.
Hortega's neuroglia s.
Hucker-Conn s.
immunofluorescent s.
India ink capsule s.
intravital s.
iodine s.
Jenner's s.
Kasten's fluorescent Feulgen s.
Kasten's fluorescent PAS s.
Kinyoun s.
Kleihauer's s.
Klinger-Ludwig acid-thionin s. for sex chromatin
Klüver-Barrera Luxol fast blue s.
Kossa s.
Kronecker's s.
Laquer's s. for alcoholic hyalin
lead hydroxide s.
Leishman's s.
Lendrum's phloxine-tartrazine s.
Lepehne-Pickworth s.
Levaditi s.
Lillie's allochrome connective tissue s.
Lillie's azure-eosin s.
Lillie's ferrous iron s.
Lillie's sulfuric acid Nile blue s.
Lison-Dunn s.
Loeffler's s.
Loeffler's caustic s.
Luna-Ishak s.
Macchiavello's s.
MacNeal's tetrachrome blood s.
malarial pigment s.
Maldonado-San Jose s.
Mallory's s. for actinomyces

Mallory's aniline blue s.
Mallory's collagen s.
Mallory's s. for hemofuchsin
Mallory's iodine s.
Mallory's phloxine s.
Mallory's phosphotungstic acid
  hematoxylin s.
Mallory's trichrome s.
Mallory's triple s.
Mann's methyl blue-eosin s.
Marchi's s.
Masson-Fontana ammoniacal
  silver s.
Masson's argentaffin s.
Masson's trichrome s.
Maximow's s. for bone marrow
Mayer's hemalum s.
Mayer's mucicarmine s.
Mayer's mucihematein s.
May-Grünwald s.
metachromatic s.
methyl green-pyronin s.
Mowry's colloidal iron s.
MSB trichrome s.
multiple s.
Nakanishi's s.
Nauta's s.
negative s.
Neisser's s.
neutral s.
Nicolle's s. for capsules
ninhydrin-Schiff s. for proteins
Nissl's s.
Noble's s.
nuclear s.
Orth's s.
Padykula-Herman s. for myosin
  ATPase
Paget-Eccleston s.
panoptic s.
Papanicolaou s.
Pappenheim's s.
paracarmine s.
PAS s.
periodic acid-Schiff s.
Perls' Prussian blue s.
peroxidase s.
phosphotungstic acid s.
picrocarmine s.
picro-Mallory trichrome s.
picronigrosin s.
plasma s., plasmatic s., plasmic s.
plastic section s.
port-wine s.
positive s.
Prussian blue s.
PTA s.
Puchtler-Sweat s.'s

Puchtler-Sweat s. for basement
  membranes
Puchtler-Sweat s. for hemoglobin
  and hemosiderin
Q-banding s.
quinacrine chromosome banding s.
Rambourg's chromic acid-
  phosphotungstic acid s.
Rambourg's periodic acid-chromic
  methenamine-silver s.
R-banding s.
Romanowsky's blood s.
Roux's s.
Schaeffer-Fulton s.
Schmorl's ferric-ferricyanide
  reduction s.
Schmorl's picrothionin s.
Schultz s.
selective s.
silver s.
silver-ammoniacal silver s.
silver protein s.
Stirling's modification of Gram's s.
supravital s.
Taenzer's s.
Takayama's s.
telomeric R-banding s.
thioflavine T s.
Tizzoni's s.
Toison's s.
trichrome s.
trypsin G-banding s.
Unna-Pappenheim s.
Unna's s.
Unna-Taenzer s.
uranyl acetate s.
urate crystals s.
van Ermengen's s.
van Gieson's s.
Verhoeff's elastic tissue s.
vital s.
von Kossa s.
Wachstein-Meissel s. for calcium-
  magnesium-ATPase
Warthin-Starry silver s.
Weigert-Gram s.
Weigert's s. for actinomyces
Weigert's s. for elastin
Weigert's s. for fibrin
Weigert's iron hematoxylin s.
Weigert's s. for myelin
Weigert's s. for neuroglia
Wilder's s. for reticulum
Williams' s.
Wright's s.
Ziehl-Neelsen s.
Ziehl's s.

S

staining
>progressive s.
>regressive s.

stains-all

staircase
>s. phenomenon

stalk
>allantoic s.
>body s.
>connecting s.
>s. of epiglottis
>infundibular s.
>optic s.
>pineal s.
>pituitary s.
>yolk s.

stalked hydatid

stammer

stammering
>s. of the bladder

Stamnosoma

standard
>s. bicarbonate
>s. deviation
>s. error of difference
>s. error of the mean
>s. limb lead
>s. score
>s. serologic tests for syphilis
>s. urea clearance

standardization
>s. of a test

standardized mortality ratio

standby pulse generator

standing
>s. plasma test
>s. test

standstill
>atrial s.
>auricular s.
>cardiac s.
>sinus s.
>ventricular s.

Stanford-Binet intelligence scale

Stanley
>S. cervical ligaments
>S. Way procedure

Stannius ligature

stapedectomy

stapedes (*pl. of* stapes)

stapedial
>s. artery
>s. branch of stylomastoid artery
>s. fold
>s. membrane

stapedii (*pl. of* stapedius)

stapediotenotomy

stapediovestibular

stapedius, pl. stapedii
>s. muscle

stapes, pl. stapes, stapedes

staphylectomy

staphyledema

staphyline

staphylion

staphylococcal
>s. enterotoxin
>s. pneumonia
>s. scalded skin syndrome

staphylococcemia

staphylococci (*pl. of* staphylococcus)

staphylococcia

staphylococcic

staphylococcolysin

staphylococcolysis

Staphylococcus
>*S. aureus*
>*S. epidermidis*
>*S. food poisoning*
>*S. haemolyticus*
>*S. hominis*
>*S. hyicus*
>*S. pyogenes albus*
>*S. pyogenes aureus*
>*S. saprophyticus*
>*S. simulans*

staphylococcus, pl. staphylococci

staphyloderma

staphylodermatitis

staphylodialysis

staphylohemia

staphylohemolysin

staphylolysin

staphyloma
>annular s.
>anterior s.
>ciliary s.
>corneal s.
>equatorial s.
>intercalary s.
>posterior s.
>Scarpa's s.
>scleral s.
>uveal s.

staphylomatous

staphylo-opsonic index

staphylopharyngorrhaphy

staphyloplasty

staphyloplegia

staphyloptosis

staphylorrhaphy

staphylotoxin

stapling
>gastric s.

star
- daughter s.
- lens s.'s
- mother s.
- polar s.
- venous s.
- Verheyen's s.'s
- Winslow's s.'s

starch-eating

starch equivalent

starch-iodine test

stare
- postbasic s.

Stargardt's disease

Starling's
- S. curve
- S. hypothesis
- S. law
- S. reflex

Starr-Edwards valve

starting friction

startle
- s. epilepsy
- s. reaction
- s. reflex

starvation
- s. acidosis
- s. diabetes

starve

stasimorphia

stasis, pl. **stases**
- s. cirrhosis
- s. dermatitis
- s. eczema
- intestinal s.
- papillary s.
- pressure s.
- s. ulcer
- venous s.

state
- absent s.
- anxiety tension s.
- apallic s.
- carrier s.
- central excitatory s.
- convulsive s.
- decerebrate s.
- decorticate s.
- dreamy s.
- eunuchoid s.
- s. hospital
- hypnoid s.
- hypnotic s.
- hypometabolic s.
- imperfect s.
- lacunar s.
- local excitatory s.
- multiple ego s.'s

- perfect s.
- refractory s.
- twilight s.

state-dependent learning

stathmokinesis

static
- s. arthropathy
- s. ataxia
- s. bone cyst
- s. compliance
- s. friction
- s. gangrene
- s. hysteresis
- s. infantilism
- s. perimetry
- s. reflexes
- s. refraction
- s. relations
- s. scoliosis
- s. sense
- s. system
- s. tremor

statim

station
- s. test

stationary
- s. anchorage
- s. cataract

statistical
- s. genetics
- s. model
- s. power
- s. significance

statistics
- descriptive s.
- inferential s.
- vital s.

statoacoustic
- s. nerve

statoconia, sing. **statoconium**

statoconial membrane

statokinetic
- s. reflex

statokinetics

statoliths

statometer

statosphere

statotonic reflexes

stature

status
- s. anginosus
- s. arthriticus
- s. asthmaticus
- s. choleraicus
- s. choreicus
- s. convulsivus
- s. cribrosus
- s. criticus

status *(continued)*
- s. dysmyelinisatus
- s. dysraphicus
- s. epilepticus
- s. hemicranicus
- s. hypnoticus
- s. lacunaris
- s. lymphaticus
- s. marmoratus
- s. nervosus
- s. praesens
- s. raptus
- s. spongiosus
- s. sternuens
- s. thymicolymphaticus
- s. thymicus
- s. typhosus
- s. vertiginosus

statuvolence

statuvolent

Staub-Traugott
- S.-T. effect
- S.-T. phenomenon

Stauffer's syndrome

staurion

steal
- coronary s.
- iliac s.
- s. phenomenon
- renal-splanchnic s.
- subclavian s.

steam-fitter's asthma

Stearns alcoholic amentia

stearrhea

steatocystoma
- s. multiplex

steatogenesis

steatonecrosis

steatopyga, steatopygia

steatopygous

steatorrhea
- biliary s.
- intestinal s.
- pancreatic s.

steatosis
- s. cardiaca
- s. cordis
- hepatic s.

steatozoon

Steele-Richardson-Olszewski
- S.-R.-O. disease
- S.-R.-O. syndrome

Steell's murmur

steeple skull

steering wheel injury

stege

stegnosis

Steinberg thumb sign

Steinert's disease

Stein-Leventhal syndrome

Steinmann pin

Stein's test

stella, pl. **stellae**
- s. lentis hyaloidea
- s. lentis iridica

stellate
- s. abscess
- s. block
- s. cataract
- s. cells of cerebral cortex
- s. cells of liver
- s. fracture
- s. ganglion
- s. hair
- s. ligament
- s. neuroretinitis
- s. reticulum
- s. skull fracture
- s. veins
- s. venules

stellectomy

stellula, pl. **stellulae**
- stellulae vasculosae
- stellulae verheyenii
- stellulae winslowii

Stellwag's sign

stem
- brain s.
- s. bronchus
- s. cell
- s. cell leukemia
- infundibular s.

Stender dish

Stenger test

stenion

stenobregmatic

stenocardia

stenocephalia

stenocephalous, stenocephalic

stenocephaly

stenochoria

stenocompressor

stenocrotaphy, stenocrotaphia

stenopeic, stenopaic
- s. disk
- s. iridectomy
- s. spectacles

stenosal
- s. murmur

Steno's duct

stenosed

stenosis, pl. **stenoses**
- aortic s.
- buttonhole s.
- calcific nodular aortic s.
- congenital pyloric s.

coronary ostial s.
Dittrich's s.
double aortic s.
fish-mouth mitral s.
hypertrophic pyloric s.
idiopathic hypertrophic subaortic s.
infundibular s.
laryngeal s.
mitral s.
muscular subaortic s.
pulmonary s.
pyloric s.
subaortic s.
subvalvar s.
subvalvular aortic s.
supravalvar s.
supravalvular s.
tricuspid s.
stenostenosis
stenostomia
stenothorax
stenotic
stenoxenous
stenoxous parasite
Stensen's
S. duct
S. experiment
S. foramen
S. plexus
S. veins
stent
Stent graft
Stenvers
S. projection
S. view
step
Krönig's s.'s
Rønne's nasal s.
stephanial
stephanion
Stephanofilaria
S. stilesi
Stephanofilaria stilesi
Stephanurus dentatus
steppage
s. gait
stercolith
stercoraceous
s. vomiting
stercoral
s. abscess
s. appendicitis
s. ulcer
stercoroma
stercorous
stercus
stereoagnosis
stereoanesthesia

stereoarthrolysis
stereocampimeter
stereocilium, pl. **stereocilia**
stereocinefluorography
stereocolpogram
stereocolposcope
stereoelectroencephalography
stereoencephalometry
stereoencephalotomy
stereognosis
stereognostic
stereogram
stereograph
stereography
stereology
stereo-orthopter
stereopathy
stereophantoscope
stereophorometer
stereophoroscope
stereophotomicrograph
stereopsis
stereoradiography
stereoroentgenography
stereoscope
stereoscopic
s. acuity
s. microscope
s. parallax
s. vision
stereoscopy
stereotactic, stereotaxic
s. cordotomy
s. instrument
s. surgery
stereotaxis
stereotaxy
stereotropic
stereotropism
negative s.
positive s.
stereotypy
oral s.
sterigma, pl. **sterigmata**
sterile
s. abscess
s. cyst
sterility
aspermatogenic s.
dysspermatogenic s.
female s.
male s.
normospermatogenic s.
sterilization
discontinuous s.
fractional s.
intermittent s.
sterilize

S

sterilizer
    glass bead s.
    hot salt s.
sterna (*pl. of* sternum)
sternad
sternal
    s. angle
    s. arteries
    s. articular surface of clavicle
    s. bar
    s. branches of internal thoracic
       artery
    s. cartilage
    s. end of clavicle
    s. extremity of clavicle
    s. joints
    s. line
    s. membrane
    s. muscle
    s. notch
    s. part of diaphragm
    s. plane
    s. puncture
sternalgia
sternalis
    s. muscle
Sternberg
    S. cells
    S. sign
Sternberg-Reed cells
sternebra, pl. **sternebrae**
sternen
sterni (*gen. of* sternum)
sternobrachial reflex
sternochondral separation
sternochondroscapularis
sternochondroscapular muscle
sternoclavicular
    s. angle
    s. articular disk
    s. disk
    s. joint
    s. ligament
    s. muscle
sternoclavicularis
sternocleidal
sternocleidomastoid
    s. branch of occipital artery
    s. branch of superior thyroid artery
    s. muscle
    s. region
    s. vein
sternocleidomastoideus
sternocostal
    s. articulations
    s. head of pectoralis major muscle
    s. joints
    s. part of pectoralis major muscle

    s. surface of heart
    s. triangle
sternocostalis muscle
sternodynia
sternofascialis
sternoglossal
sternohyoideus
sternohyoid muscle
sternoid
sternomanubrial junction
sternomastoid
    s. artery
    s. muscle
sternopagia
sternopericardial
    s. ligament
sternoschisis
sternothyroideus
sternothyroid muscle
sternotomy
    median s.
sternotracheal
sternotrypesis
sternovertebral
Stern's posture
sternum, gen. **sterni**, pl. **sterna**
sternutation
steroid
    s. acne
    s. diabetes
    s. fever
    s. metabolic clearance rate
    s. production rate
    s. secretory rate
    s. ulcer
    s. withdrawal syndrome
steroidogenic diabetes
stertor
    hen-cluck s.
stertorous
    s. breathing
    s. respiration
stethalgia
stetharteritis
stethocyrtograph
stethocyrtometer
stethogoniometer
stethograph
stethokyrtograph
stethomyitis
stethomyositis
stethoparalysis
stethoscope
    binaural s.
    Bowles type s.
    differential s.
stethoscopic
    s. phonocardiograph

stethoscopy
stethospasm
Stevens-Johnson syndrome
Stewart-Hamilton
    S.-H. method
    S.-H. principle
Stewart-Holmes sign
Stewart-Morel syndrome
Stewart's test
Stewart-Treves syndrome
sthenia
sthenic
sthenometer
sthenometry
stichochrome
    s. cell
Sticker's disease
Stickler's syndrome
Stieda's process
Stierlin's sign
sties (*pl. of* sty)
stiff
    s. heart syndrome
    s. neck
    s. toe
stiff-man syndrome
stigma, pl. stigmas, stigmata
    follicular s.
    malpighian stigmas
    s. ventriculi
stigmata
stigmatic
stigmatism
stigmatization
Stiles-Crawford effect
stilet, stilette
stillbirth
    s. rate
stillborn
    s. infant
Still-Chauffard syndrome
Stilling
    S. canal
    S. color tables
    S. column
    S. gelatinous substance
    S. nucleus
    S. raphe
still layer
Still's
    S. disease
    S. murmur
stimulation
    dorsal column s.
    Ganzfeld s.
    percutaneous s.
    photic s.

stimulator
    long-acting thyroid s.
stimulus, pl. stimuli
    adequate s.
    aversive s.
    conditioned s.
    s. control
    discriminant s.
    s. generalization
    heterologous s.
    heterotopic s.
    homologous s.
    inadequate s.
    liminal s.
    maximal s.
    s. sensitive myoclonus
    square wave stimuli
    subliminal s.
    s. substitution
    subthreshold s.
    supramaximal s.
    s. threshold
    threshold s.
    train-of-four s.
    unconditioned s.
    s. word
stingers
stippled
    s. epiphysis
    s. tongue
stippling
    geographic s. of nails
    Ziemann's s.
Stirling's modification of Gram's stain
stirrup
stitch
    s. abscess
ST junction
St. Louis encephalitis virus
Stobo antigen
stochastic
    s. independence
    s. process
stock
    s. culture
    s. strain
Stocker's line
Stockholm syndrome
stocking anesthesia
Stoerk's blennorrhea
Stoffel's operation
stoker's cramps
Stokes-Adams
    S.-A. disease
    S.-A. syndrome
Stokes amputation
stolon
stoma, pl. stomas, stomata

S

stoma *(continued)*
  Fuchs' stomas
  loop s.
stomach
  s. ache
  bilocular s.
  s. bubble
  cascade s.
  drain-trap s.
  hourglass s.
  leather-bottle s.
  miniature s.
  Pavlov s.
  s. pump
  s. reefing
  sclerotic s.
  thoracic s.
  s. tooth
  trifid s.
  s. tube
  wallet s.
  water-trap s.
stomachal
stomachalgia
stomachodynia
stomal
  s. ulcer
stomas (*pl. of* stoma)
stomata (*pl. of* stoma)
stomatal
stomatalgia
stomatic
stomatitis
  angular s.
  aphthous s.
  epidemic s.
  fusospirochetal s.
  gangrenous s.
  gonococcal s.
  lead s.
  s. medicamentosa
  mercurial s.
  nicotine s.
  primary herpetic s.
  recurrent aphthous s.
  recurrent herpetic s.
  recurrent ulcerative s.
  ulcerative s.
stomatocyte
stomatocytosis
stomatodeum
stomatodynia
stomatodysodia
stomatognathic
  s. system
stomatologic
stomatologist
stomatology

stomatomalacia
stomatomycosis
stomatonecrosis
stomatonoma
stomatopathy
stomatoplastic
stomatoplasty
stomatorrhagia
stomatoscope
stomatosis
stomion
stomocephalus
stomodeal
stomodeum
stone
  s. basket
  bladder s.'s
  s. heart
  pulp s.
  skin s.'s
  tear s.
  vein s.
stone-mason's disease
Stookey-Scarff operation
stool
  butter s.'s
  fatty s.
  rice-water s.
  spinach s.'s
  Trélat's s.'s
stops
storage
  s. disease
  s. oscilloscope
storiform
  s. neurofibroma
storm
  thyroid s.
Stout's wiring
strabismal
strabismic
  s. amblyopia
strabismologist
strabismometer
strabismus
  A-s.
  accommodative s.
  alternate day s.
  alternating s.
  A-pattern s.
  comitant s.
  concomitant s.
  convergent s.
  cyclic s.
  s. deorsum vergens
  divergent s.
  external s.
  incomitant s.

internal s.
kinetic s.
manifest s.
mechanical s.
monocular s.
paralytic s.
s. sursum vergens
vertical s.
X-s.
strabotome
strabotomy
straddling embolism
straight
s. back syndrome
s. gyrus
s. jacket
s. part of cricothyroid muscle
s. seminiferous tubule
s. sinus
s. tubule
s. venules of kidney
strain
auxotrophic s.'s
carrier s.
cell s.
congenic s.
s. fracture
s. gauge
HFR s., Hfr s.
hypothetical mean s.
isogenic s.
lysogenic s.
neotype s.
prototrophic s.'s
pseudolysogenic s.
recombinant s.
stock s.
type s.
wild-type s.
strains
strait
inferior s.
superior s.
straitjacket
strand
minus s.
plus s.
strangalesthesia
strangle
strangulated
s. hernia
strangulation
strangury
strap
s. cell
s. muscles
Strassburg's test
Strassman's phenomenon

strata (*pl. of* stratum)
strati (*gen. of* stratum)
stratification
stratified
s. ciliated columnar epithelium
s. epithelium
s. sample
s. squamous epithelium
s. thrombus
stratiform fibrocartilage
stratigraphy
stratum, gen. **strati**, pl. **strata**
s. aculeatum
s. album profundum
s. basale
s. basale epidermidis
s. cerebrale retinae
s. cinereum colliculi superioris
s. circulare membranae tympani
s. circulare tunicae
s. circulare tunicae muscularis coli
s. circulare tunicae muscularis
gastricae
s. circulare tunicae muscularis
intestini tenuis
s. circulare tunicae muscularis recti
s. circulare tunicae muscularis
ventriculi
s. compactum
s. corneum epidermidis
s. corneum unguis
s. cutaneum membranae tympani
s. cylindricum
s. disjunctum
s. fibrosum
s. functionale
s. ganglionare nervi optici
s. ganglionare retinae
s. gangliosum cerebelli
s. germinativum
s. germinativum unguis
s. granulosum cerebelli
s. granulosum epidermidis
s. granulosum folliculi ovarici
vesiculosi
s. granulosum ovarii
s. griseum colliculi superioris
s. griseum medium
s. griseum profundum
s. griseum superficiale
s. interolivare lemnisci
s. lemnisci
s. longitudinale tunicae muscularis
s. longitudinale tunicae muscularis
coli
s. longitudinale tunicae muscularis
gastricae

S

stratum *(continued)*
s. longitudinale tunicae muscularis intestini tenuis
s. longitudinale tunicae muscularis recti
s. longitudinale tunicae muscularis ventriculi
s. lucidum
malpighian s.
s. moleculare
s. moleculare cerebelli
s. moleculare retinae
s. neuroepitheliale retinae
s. neuronorum piriformium
s. nucleare externum et internum retinae
s. nucleare externum retinae
s. nucleare internum retinae
s. opticum
s. papillare corii
s. pigmenti bulbi
s. pigmenti corporis ciliaris
s. pigmenti iridis
s. pigmenti retinae
s. plexiforme externum et internum retinae
s. radiatum membranae tympani
s. reticulare corii
s. reticulare cutis
s. spinosum epidermidis
s. spongiosum
s. subcutaneum
s. synoviale
s. zonale
Straus' sign
straw-bed itch
strawberry
s. birthmark
s. gallbladder
s. hemangioma
s. mark
s. nevus
s. tongue
straw itch
streak
s. culture
germinal s.
s. gonad
gonadal s.
s. hyperostosis
Knapp's s.'s
meningitic s.
Moore's lightning s.'s
primitive s.
stream
hair s.'s
streaming
s. movement

streblodactyly
Streeter's
S. bands
S. developmental horizon(s)
stremma
strength
associative s.
biting s.
fatigue s.
ultimate s.
yield s.
strength-duration curve
strephosymbolia
strepitus
strepticemia
Streptobacillus
streptococcal
s. empyema
s. pneumonia
streptococcemia
streptococci
streptococci (*pl. of* streptococcus)
streptococcic
streptococcosis
Streptococcus
S. acidominimus
S. agalactiae
S. anginosus
S. bovis
S. constellatus
S. durans
S. equinus
S. lactis
S. M antigen
S. mitis
S. mutans
S. pneumoniae
S. pyogenes
S. salivarius
S. sanguis
S. viridans
S. zooepidemicus
streptococcus, pl. streptococci
α-streptococci
group A streptococci
group B streptococci
β-hemolytic streptococci
hemolytic streptococci
streptoderma
streptodermatitis
streptolysin
s. O
Streptomyces
S. albus
S. gibsonii
S. somaliensis
Streptomycetaceae
streptomycete

streptomycosis
streptosepticemia
streptothrichosis
streptotrichiasis
streptotrichosis
stress
    s. breaker
    s. echocardiography
    s. fracture
    s. immunity
    s. inoculation
    life s.
    s. reaction
    s. riser
    shear s.
    s. shielding
    tensile s.
    s. test
    s. ulcers
    s. urinary incontinence
    yield s.
stress-bearing area
stress-strain curve
stretch
    s. marks
    s. receptors
    s. reflex
stretcher
stria, gen. and pl. **striae**
    acoustic striae
    striae atrophicae
    auditory striae
    brown striae
    striae ciliares
    striae cutis distensae
    diagonalis s.
    s. fornicis
    Gennari's s.
    striae gravidarum
    Knapp's striae
    striae lancisi
    Langhans' s.
    lateral longitudinal s.
    s. longitudinalis lateralis
    s. longitudinalis medialis
    s. mallearis
    medial longitudinal s.
    striae medullares ventriculi quarti
    s. medullaris thalami
    medullary striae of fourth ventricle
    medullary s. of thalamus
    s. nasi transversa
    Nitabuch's s.
    striae olfactoriae
    olfactory striae
    striae parallelae
    striae retinae
    Retzius' striae

    Rohr's s.
    s. spinosa
    s. tecta
    tectal s.
    terminal s.
    s. terminalis
    s. vascularis of cochlea
    s. vascularis ductus cochlearis
    s. ventriculi tertii
    Wickham's striae
    striae of Zahn
striatal
striate
    s. area
    s. atrophy of skin
    s. body
    s. cortex
    s. keratopathy
    s. veins
striated
    s. border
    s. duct
    s. membrane
    s. muscle
    s. muscular sphincter
striation
    basal s.'s
    tabby cat s.
    tigroid s.
striatonigral
    s. fibers
striatum
stricture
    anastomotic s.
    annular s.
    bridle s.
    contractile s.
    functional s.
    Hunner's s.
    organic s.
    permanent s.
    recurrent s.
    spasmodic s.
    temporary s.
    urethral s.
stricturoplasty
stricturotome
stricturotomy
strident
stridor
    congenital s.
    s. dentium
    expiratory s.
    inspiratory s.
    laryngeal s.
    s. serraticus
stridulous

S

string
    auditory s.'s
    s. sign
    s. test
stringed instrument theory
strionigral fibers
strip
    abrasive s.
    amalgam s.
    celluloid s.
    lightning s.
stripe
    s. of Gennari
    Hensen's s.
    mallear s.
    Mees' s.'s
    pleural s.
    tracheal wall s.
    vascular s.
stripper
    s.'s asthma
    vein s.
strobila, pl. **strobilae**
strobilocercus
strobiloid
stroboscope
stroboscopic
    s. disk
    s. microscope
Stroganoff's method
stroke
    heart s.
    heat s.
    s. output
    spinal s.
    sun s.
    s. volume
    s. work index
stroking
stroma, pl. **stromata**
    s. glandulae thyroideae
    s. iridis
    s. of iris
    lymphatic s.
    nerve s.
    s. ovarii
    s. of ovary
    s. plexus
    Rollet's s.
    s. of thyroid gland
    s. of vitreous
    s. vitreum
stromal
    s. hyperthecosis
stromatolysis
stromatosis
stromic

stromuhr
    Ludwig's s.
    thermo-s.
Strong vocational interest test
strongyle
Strongylidae
Strongyloidea
Strongyloides
Strongylus
    S. asini
    S. edentatus
    S. equinus
    S. radiatus
    S. ventricosus
    S. vulgaris
strophocephaly
strophosomia
strophulus
    s. candidus
    s. intertinctus
    s. pruriginosus
Stroud's pectinated area
structural
    s. interface
    s. pleiotropy
structuralism
structure
    denture-supporting s.'s
    fine s.
    tuboreticular s.
structured noise
struma, pl. **strumae**
    s. aberrata
    s. colloides
    Hashimoto's s.
    ligneous s.
    s. lymphomatosa
    s. maligna
    s. medicamentosa
    s. ovarii
    Riedel's s.
strumectomy
    median s.
strumiform
strumitis
strumous
Strümpell-Marie disease
Strümpell's
    S. disease
    S. phenomenon
    S. reflex
Strümpell-Westphal disease
struvite calculus
Stryker
    S. frame
    S. saw
Stryker-Halbeisen syndrome
S-T segment

STS for syphilis
Stuart factor
Stuart-Prower factor
stuck finger
student nurse
Student's *t* **test**
study
analytic s.
blind s.
case control s.
cohort s.
cross-over s.
cross-sectional s.
diachronic s.
double blind s.
follow-up s.
Framingham Heart S.
longitudinal s.
multivariate s.'s
synchronic s.
stump
s. cancer
s. hallucination
s. neuralgia
stun
stunned myocardium
stupe
stupor
benign s.
catatonic s.
depressive s.
malignant s.
stuporous
s. catatonia
Sturge-Kalischer-Weber syndrome
Sturge-Weber
S.-W. disease
S.-W. syndrome
Sturmdorf's operation
Sturm's
S. conoid
S. interval
stutter
stuttering
urinary s.
s. urination
sty, stye, pl. **sties, styes**
meibomian s.
zeisian s.
style
stylet, stylette
endotracheal s.
styliform
styloauricularis
styloauricular muscle
styloglossus
s. muscle
stylohyal

stylohyoid
s. branch of facial nerve
s. ligament
s. muscle
styloid
s. cornu
s. process of fibula
s. process of radius
s. process of temporal bone
s. process of third metacarpal bone
s. process of ulna
s. prominence
styloiditis
stylolaryngeus
stylomandibular
s. ligament
stylomastoid
s. artery
s. foramen
s. vein
stylomaxillary
s. ligament
stylopharyngeal muscle
stylopharyngeus
s. muscle
stylopodium
styloradial reflex
stylostaphyline
stylosteophyte
Styloviridae
stylus tracing
stype
Stypven time test
subabdominal
subabdominoperitoneal
subacromial
s. bursa
s. bursitis
subacute
s. bacterial endocarditis
s. combined degeneration of the spinal cord
s. glomerulonephritis
s. granulomatous thyroiditis
s. hepatitis
s. inclusion body encephalitis
s. inflammation
s. lymphocyte thyroiditis
s. migratory panniculitis
s. necrotizing encephalomyelopathy
s. necrotizing myelitis
s. nephritis
s. rheumatism
s. sclerosing leukoencephalitis
s. sclerosing panencephalitis
s. spongiform encephalopathy
subadventitial fibrosis
subalimentation

S

subanal
subanconeus muscle
subaortic
    s. lymph nodes
    s. stenosis
subapical
    s. segment
subaponeurotic
subarachnoid
    s. anesthesia
    s. cavity
    s. hemorrhage
    s. space
subarachnoidal cisterns
subarcuate
    s. fossa
subareolar
    s. duct papillomatosis
subastragalar
    s. amputation
subaural
subauricular
subaxial
subaxillary
subbasal
subbrachycephalic
subcalcarine
subcallosal
    s. area
    s. fasciculus
    s. gyrus
subcapital fracture
subcapsular
    s. cataract
subcardinal
subcartilaginous
subcecal
    s. fossa
subcellular
subception
subceruleus nucleus
subchondral
subchorial
    s. lake
    s. space
subchorionic
subchoroidal
subclass
subclavian
    s. artery
    s. duct
    s. groove
    s. loop
    s. lymphatic trunk
    s. muscle
    s. nerve
    s. periarterial plexus
    s. plexus

    s. steal
    s. steal syndrome
    s. sulcus
    s. triangle
    s. vein
subclavicular
subclavius
    s. muscle
subclinical
    s. diabetes
    s. seizure
subcollateral
subcommissural organ
subconjunctival
subconjunctivitis
subconscious
    s. memory
    s. mind
subconsciousness
subcoracoid
    s. bursa
subcoracoid-pectoralis minor tendon
    syndrome
subcorneal
    s. pustular dermatitis
    s. pustular dermatosis
subcoronal hypospadias
subcortex
subcortical
    s. arteriosclerotic encephalopathy
subcostal
    s. artery
    s. groove
    s. line
    s. muscle
    s. nerve
    s. plane
subcostalgia
subcostosternal
subcranial
subcrepitant
    s. rale
subcrepitation
subcrestal pocket
subcruralis
subcrural muscle
subcrureus
subculture
subcurative
subcutaneous
    s. acromial bursa
    s. bursa of the laryngeal
      prominence
    s. bursa of lateral malleolus
    s. bursa of medial malleolus
    s. bursa of tibial tuberosity
    s. calcaneal bursa
    s. emphysema

s. fat necrosis of newborn
s. flap
s. implantation
s. infrapatellar bursa
s. mastectomy
s. myiasis
s. olecranon bursa
s. operation
s. part of external anal sphincter
s. phycomycosis
s. portion of external anal sphincter
s. ring
s. tenotomy
s. tissue
s. transfusion
s. veins of abdomen
s. wound
subcuticular
s. suture
subcutis
subdelirium
subdeltoid
s. bursa
s. bursitis
subdental
subdermic
subdiaphragmatic
s. abscess
s. pyopneumothorax
subdigastric node
subdorsal
subduce, subduct
subdural
s. cavity
s. cleavage
s. cleft
s. hematoma
s. hematorrhachis
s. hemorrhage
s. hygroma
s. space
subendocardial
s. layer
s. myocardial infarction
subendothelial
s. layer
subendothelium
subendymal
subependymal
s. giant cell astrocytoma
subependymoma
subepidermal, subepidermic
s. abscess
s. bulla
subepithelial
subepithelium
suberosis

subfalcial herniation
subfamily
subfascial
s. prepatellar bursa
subfertility
subfissure
subfolium
subfornical organ
subgaleal
s. emphysema
s. hemorrhage
subgemmal
subgenus
subgerminal cavity
subgingival
s. calculus
s. curettage
s. space
subglenoid
subglossal
subglottic
subgranular
subgrundation
subhepatic
s. abscess
s. recess
subhyaloid
subhyoid, subhyoidean
s. bursa
subicteric
subicular
subiculum, pl. **subicula**
s. promontorii
subiliac
subilium
subinfection
subinflammatory
subinguinal
s. fossa
s. triangle
subintegumental
subintimal
subintrant
subinvolution
subjacent
subject
subjective
s. assessment data
s. fremitus
s. insomnia
s. probability
s. psychology
s. sensation
s. sign
s. symptom
s. synonyms
s. vertigo
s. vision

S

subjugal
subkingdom
sublation
sublenticular
    s. limb of internal capsule
    s. part of internal capsule
sublethal
subleukemia
subleukemic
    s. leukemia
    s. myelosis
subliminal
    s. self
    s. stimulus
    s. thirst
sublimis
sublingual
    s. artery
    s. bursa
    s. caruncula
    s. crescent
    s. cyst
    s. fold
    s. fossa
    s. ganglion
    s. gland
    s. nerve
    s. pit
    s. vein
sublobular
sublumbar
subluminal
subluxation
sublymphemia
submammary
    s. mastitis
submandibular
    s. duct
    s. fossa
    s. ganglion
    s. gland
    s. lymph nodes
    s. triangle
submarginal
submaxilla
submaxillary
    s. duct
    s. fossa
    s. ganglion
    s. gland
    s. triangle
submedial, submedian
submembranous
submental
    s. artery
    s. lymph nodes
    s. triangle
    s. vein

    s. vertex projection
    s. vertex radiograph
submentovertex radiograph
submentovertical projection
submerged
    s. tonsil
submetacentric
    s. chromosome
submicronic
submicroscopic
submorphous
submucosa
submucosal
    s. implant
    s. plexus
submucous
subnasal
    s. point
subnasion
subneural
    s. apparatus
subnormal
subnormality
subnotochordal
subnucleus
suboccipital
    s. decompression
    s. muscles
    s. nerve
    s. neuralgia
    s. neuritis
    s. part of vertebral artery
    s. region
    s. triangle
    s. venous plexus
suboccipitobregmatic diameter
suboccluding ligature
subocclusal surface
suboptimal
suborbital
suborder
subpapillary
    s. layer
    s. network
subpapular
subparietal
    s. sulcus
subpatellar
subpectoral
subpellicular
    s. fibril
    s. microtubule
subpelviperitoneal
subpericardial
subperiodic periodicity
subperiosteal
    s. abscess
    s. amputation

s. fracture
s. implant
subperitoneal
s. appendicitis
s. fascia
subperitoneoabdominal
subperitoneopelvic
subpetrosal
subpharyngeal
subphrenic
s. abscess
s. pyopneumothorax
s. recesses
subphylum
subpial
subplacental
subplasmalemmal dense zone
subpleural
subplexal
subpopliteal recess
subpreputial
subpubic
s. angle
subpulmonary
subpulmonic effusion
subpyloric
s. lymph nodes
s. node
subpyramidal
subquadricipital muscle
subretinal
subsartorial
s. canal
s. fascia
subscapular
s. artery
s. branches of axillary artery
s. bursa
s. fossa
s. group of axillary lymph nodes
s. muscle
s. nerves
subscapularis
s. muscle
subscleral
subsclerotic
subsegmental atelectasis
subseptate uterus
subserous, subserosal
s. layer
s. plexus
subsibilant
subsidence
subsidiary atrial pacemaker
subsistence diet
subspinale
subspinous
substage

substance
s. abuse disorders
alpha s.
anterior perforated s.
autacoid s.
bacteriotropic s.
basophil s.
basophilic s.
blood group s.
central gray s.
central and lateral intermediate s.
chromidial s.
chromophil s.
compact s.
cortical s.
s. dependence
filar s.
gelatinous s.
glandular s. of prostate
gray s.
innominate s.
interspongioplastic s.
s. of lens of eye
medullary s.
müllerian inhibiting s.
muscular s. of prostate
neurosecretory s.
Nissl s.
posterior perforated s.
proper s.
reticular s.
Rolando's gelatinous s.,
  Rolando's s.
Schwann's white s.
sensitizing s.
slow-reacting s., slow-reacting s. of
  anaphylaxis
spongy s.
Stilling's gelatinous s.
threshold s.
tigroid s.
vasodepressor s.
white s.
zymoplastic s.
substance-induced organic mental
  disorders
substantia, pl. **substantiae**
s. adamantina
s. alba
s. basophilia
s. cinerea
s. compacta
s. compacta ossium
s. corticalis
s. eburnea
s. ferruginea
s. gelatinosa
s. gelatinosa centralis

S

substantia *(continued)*
s. glandularis prostatae
s. grisea
s. grisea centralis
s. innominata
s. intermedia centralis et lateralis
s. lentis
s. medullaris
s. muscularis prostatae
s. nigra
s. ossea dentis
s. perforata anterior
s. perforata posterior
s. propria of cornea
s. propria corneae
s. propria membranae tympani
s. propria sclerae
s. reticularis
s. reticulofilamentosa
s. spongiosa
s. trabecularis
s. vitrea
substernal
s. angle
s. goiter
substernomastoid
substitute
blood s.
volume s.
substitution
stimulus s.
symptom s.
s. therapy
s. transfusion
substitutive therapy
substratum
substructure
implant denture s.
subsultus
s. clonus
s. tendinum
subsuperior segment
subsurface cisterna
subtalar joint
subtarsal
subtegumental
subtemporal decompression
subtendinous
s. bursa of gastrocnemius muscle
s. bursa of the tibialis anterior muscle
s. iliac bursa
s. prepatellar bursa
subtentorial
subterminal
subtetanic

subthalamic
s. fasciculus
s. nucleus
subthalamus
subthreshold stimulus
subthyroideus
subtotal
s. hysterectomy
s. thyroidectomy
subtraction
subtrapezial
subtribe
subtrochanteric
subtrochlear
subtuberal
subtympanic
subumbilical
subungual, subunguial
s. abscess
s. exostosis
s. melanoma
suburethral
subvaginal
subvalvar, subvalvular
s. stenosis
subvertebral
subvirile
subvitrinal
subvocal speech
subvolution
subwaking
subzonal
subzygomatic
succedaneous
s. dentition
s. tooth
succenturiate placenta
successive contrast
succorrhea
succubus
succuss
succussion
hippocratic s.
s. sound
suck
sucking
s. cushion
s. louse
s. pad
s. wound
suckle
Sucquet-Hoyer
S.-H. anastomoses
S.-H. canals
Sucquet's
S. anastomoses
S. canals
sucrose hemolysis test

sucrosemia
sucrosuria
suction
    s. cup
    s. drainage
    s. ophthalmodynamometer
    s. plate
    posttussive s.
    Wangensteen s.
suctorial
    s. pad
sudamen, pl. **sudamina**
sudamina
sudaminal
Sudan
    S. black B
    S. brown
    S. III
    S. red III
    S. yellow
sudanophilia
sudanophilic
sudanophobic
    s. zone
sudation
sudden
    s. death
    s. infant death syndrome
Sudeck's
    S. atrophy
    S. critical point
    S. syndrome
sudomotor
    s. fibers
    s. nerves
sudor
    s. anglicus
    s. sanguineus
    s. urinosus
sudoral
sudoresis
sudoriferous
    s. duct
    s. glands
sudorific
sudorikeratosis
sudoriparous
    s. abscess
sudorometer
sudorrhea
sufficient cause
suffocate
suffocation
suffocative goiter
suffusion
sugar
    s. cataract
    s. tumor

sugar-coated spleen
sugar-icing liver
suggestibility
suggestible
suggestion
    posthypnotic s.
suggestive
    s. psychotherapy
    s. therapeutics
suggillation
    postmortem s.
Sugiura procedure
suicide
    s. gesture
suicidology
suid herpesvirus
suit
    anti-G s.
sulcal
    s. artery
sulcate
sulci (*gen. and pl. of* sulcus)
sulciform
sulcomarginal tract
sulcular
    s. epithelium
    s. fluid
sulculus, pl. **sulculi**
sulcus, gen. and pl. **sulci**
    alveolobuccal s.
    alveololabial s.
    alveololingual s.
    s. ampullaris
    ampullary s.
    s. angularis
    anterior intermediate s.
    anterior parolfactory s.
    anterolateral s.
    s. anthelicis transversus
    aortic s.
    s. aorticus
    s. arteriae occipitalis
    s. arteriae temporalis mediae
    s. arteriae vertebralis
    sulci arteriosi
    atrioventricular s.
    s. auriculae anterior
    s. auriculae posterior
    basilar s.
    s. basilaris pontis
    basilar pontine s.
    s. bicipitalis lateralis
    s. bicipitalis medialis
    calcaneal s.
    s. calcanei
    calcarine s.
    s. calcarinus
    callosal s.

S

sulcus *(continued)*
  callosomarginal s.
  s. callosomarginalis
  s. caroticus
  carotid s.
  s. carpi
  central s.
  s. centralis
  cerebellar sulci
  cerebral sulci
  sulci cerebri
  chiasmatic s.
  cingulate s.
  s. cinguli
  s. of cingulum
  circular s. of insula
  s. circularis insulae
  circular s. of Reil
  collateral s.
  s. collateralis
  s. coronarius
  coronary s.
  s. corporis callosi
  s. of corpus callosum
  s. costae
  s. costae arteriae subclaviae
  costophrenic s.
  s. cruris helicis
  sulci cutis
  s. ethmoidalis
  external spiral s.
  fimbriodentate s.
  s. fimbriodentatus
  s. frontalis inferior
  s. frontalis medius
  s. frontalis superior
  s. frontomarginalis
  gingival s.
  s. gingivalis
  gingivobuccal s.
  gingivolabial s.
  gingivolingual s.
  s. gluteus
  s. for greater palatine nerve
  habenular s.
  s. hamuli pterygoidei
  hippocampal s.
  s. hippocampi
  hypothalamic s.
  s. hypothalamicus
  inferior frontal s.
  inferior petrosal s.
  inferior temporal s.
  s. infraorbitalis
  infrapalpebral s.
  s. infrapalpebralis
  s. intermedius anterior
  s. intermedius posterior

internal spiral s.
interparietal s.
intertubercular s.
  s. intertubercularis
  s. interventricularis anterior
  s. interventricularis cordis
  s. interventricularis posterior
intragracile s.
  s. intragracilis
intraparietal s.
  s. intraparietalis
intraparietal s. of Turner
labial s.
labiodental s.
  s. lacrimalis
lateral cerebral s.
  s. lateralis anterior
  s. lateralis cerebri
  s. lateralis posterior
lateral occipital s.
  s. limitans
  s. limitans fossae rhomboideae
limiting s.
limiting s. of Reil
limiting s. of rhomboid fossa
lip s.
longitudinal s. of heart
malleolar s.
  s. malleolaris
  s. matricis unguis
medial s. of crus cerebri
  s. medialis cruris cerebri
median s. of fourth ventricle
median frontal s.
  s. medianus linguae
  s. medianus posterior medullae
    oblongatae
  s. medianus posterior medullae
    spinalis
  s. medianus ventriculi quarti
mentolabial s.
  s. mentolabialis
middle frontal s.
middle temporal s.
  s. for middle temporal artery
Monro's s.
  s. musculi subclavii
  s. mylohyoideus
  s. nasolabialis
  s. nervi oculomotorii
  s. nervi petrosi majoris
  s. nervi petrosi minoris
  s. nervi radialis
  s. nervi spinalis
  s. nervi ulnaris
nymphocaruncular s.
  s. nymphocaruncularis
nymphohymenal s.

s. obturatorius
s. of occipital artery
s. occipitalis lateralis
s. occipitalis superior
s. occipitalis transversus
occipitotemporal s.
s. occipitotemporalis
s. of the oculomotor nerve
s. olfactorius
s. olfactorius cavum nasi
olfactory s.
olfactory s. of nasal cavity
orbital sulci
sulci orbitales
s. palatinus, pl. sulci palatini
s. palatinus major
s. palatovaginalis
sulci paracolici
paraglenoid s.
s. paraglenoidalis
parieto-occipital s.
s. parieto-occipitalis
s. parolfactorius anterior
s. parolfactorius posterior
periconchal s.
s. popliteus
postcentral s.
s. postcentralis
posterior intermediate s.
posterior median s. of medulla
  oblongata
posterior median s. of spinal cord
posterior parolfactory s.
posterolateral s.
preauricular s.
precentral s.
s. precentralis
prechiasmatic s.
s. prechiasmatis
s. promontorii cavitatis tympanicae
s. of promontory of tympanic
  cavity
s. of pterygoid hamulus
s. pterygopalatinus
s. pulmonalis
pulmonary s.
rhinal s.
s. rhinalis
sagittal s.
s. of sclera
s. sclerae
scleral s.
sigmoid s.
s. sinus petrosi inferioris
s. sinus petrosi superioris
s. sinus sagittalis superioris
s. sinus sigmoidei
s. sinus transversi

s. spinosus
s. spiralis externus
s. spiralis internus
subclavian s.
s. subclavianus
s. subclavius
subparietal s.
s. subparietalis
superior frontal s.
superior longitudinal s.
superior occipital s.
superior petrosal s.
superior temporal s.
supra-acetabular s.
s. supra-acetabularis
talar s.
s. tali
sulci temporales transversi
s. temporalis inferior
s. temporalis medius
s. temporalis superior
s. tendinis musculi fibularis longi
s. tendinis musculi flexoris hallucis
  longi
s. tendinis musculi peronei longi
terminal s.
s. terminalis
tonsillolingual s.
transverse occipital s.
s. for transverse sinus
transverse temporal sulci
s. tubae auditivae
Turner's s.
s. tympanicus
s. of umbilical vein
s. for vena cava
s. venae cavae
s. venae cavae cranialis
s. venae subclaviae
s. venae umbilicalis
sulci venosi
s. ventralis
s. for vertebral artery
s. verticalis
vomeral s.
s. vomeralis
s. vomeris
s. vomerovaginalis
sulfatide lipidosis
sulfatidosis
sulfhemoglobinemia
sulfindigotic acid
sulforhodamine B
sulfosalicylic acid turbidity test
Sulzberger-Garbe
  S.-G. disease
  S.-G. syndrome

S

summation
   s. beat
   s. gallop
   s. of stimuli
summer
   s. asthma
   s. diarrhea
   s. itch
   s. prurigo
   s. rash
Sumner's sign
sump
   s. drain
   s. syndrome
sunburn
sundowning
sunflower cataract
sunstroke, sun stroke
superabduction
superacidity
superacromial
superactivity
superacute
superalimentation
superanal
superantigen
superciliary
   s. arch
   s. ridge
supercilium, pl. supercilia
superconducting magnet
superdicrotic
superdistention
superduct
superego
supereruption
superexcitation
superextension
superfetation
superficial
   s. angioma
   s. back muscles
   s. brachial artery
   s. branch
   s. branch of the lateral plantar nerve
   s. branch of the medial plantar artery
   s. branch of the radial nerve
   s. branch of the superior gluteal artery
   s. branch of the transverse cervical artery
   s. branch of the ulnar nerve
   s. burn
   s. cardiac plexus
   s. cerebral veins
   s. cervical artery

s. cervical nerve
s. circumflex iliac artery
s. circumflex iliac vein
s. cleavage
s. dorsal sacrococcygeal ligament
s. dorsal veins of clitoris
s. dorsal veins of penis
s. ectoderm
s. epigastric artery
s. epigastric vein
s. fascia
s. fascia of penis
s. fascia of perineum
s. fibular nerve
s. flexor muscle of fingers
s. gray layer of superior colliculus
s. head of flexor pollicis brevis muscle
s. inguinal lymph nodes
s. inguinal pouch
s. inguinal ring
s. lamina
s. layer
s. layer of deep cervical fascia
s. layer of the levator palpebrae superioris muscle
s. layer of temporalis fascia
s. linear keratitis
s. lingual muscle
s. lymphatic vessel
s. middle cerebral vein
s. origin
s. palmar (arterial) arch
s. palmar artery
s. palmar branch of radial artery
s. palmar venous arch
s. parotid lymph nodes
s. part of duodenum
s. part of external anal sphincter
s. part of masseter muscle
s. part of parotid gland
s. perineal pouch
s. perineal space
s. peroneal nerve
s. posterior sacrococcygeal ligament
s. punctate keratitis
s. pustular perifolliculitis
s. reflex
s. spreading melanoma
s. temporal artery
s. temporal branch of auriculotemporal nerve
s. temporal plexus
s. temporal veins
s. transverse metacarpal ligament
s. transverse metatarsal ligament
s. transverse muscle of perineum
s. transverse perineal muscle

s. vein
s. volar artery
superficialis
s. volae
superficies
superflexion
superfuse
superfusion
supergenual
superimposed
s. eclampsia
s. preeclampsia
superimpregnation
superinduce
superinfection
superinvolution
superior
s. aberrant ductule
s. alveolar nerves
s. anastomotic vein
s. angle of scapula
s. articular facet of atlas
s. articular pit of atlas
s. articular process of sacrum
s. articular surface of tibia
s. auricular muscle
s. azygoesophageal recess
s. basal vein
s. belly of omohyoid muscle
s. border
s. border of pancreas
s. border of petrous part of temporal bone
s. border of scapula
s. border of spleen
s. border of suprarenal gland
s. branch
s. branches
s. branch of the oculomotor nerve
s. branch of the pubic bone
s. branch of the right and left inferior pulmonary veins
s. branch of the superior gluteal artery
s. branch of the transverse cervical nerve
s. bursa of biceps femoris
s. carotid triangle
s. central tegmental nucleus
s. cerebellar artery
s. cerebellar artery syndrome
s. cerebellar peduncle
s. cerebral veins
s. cervical cardiac branches of vagus nerve
s. cervical cardiac nerve
s. cervical ganglion
s. choroid vein

s. cistern
s. cluneal nerves
s. colliculus
s. constrictor muscle of pharynx
s. costal facet
s. costal pit
s. costotransverse ligament
s. dental arch
s. dental branches of superior dental plexus
s. dental nerves
s. dental plexus
s. dental rami
s. duodenal fold
s. duodenal fossa
s. duodenal recess
s. epigastric artery
s. epigastric veins
s. esophageal sphincter
s. extensor retinaculum
s. extremity
s. facial index
s. fascia of pelvic diaphragm
s. fascia of urogenital diaphragm
s. flexure of duodenum
s. fovea
s. frontal convolution
s. frontal gyrus
s. frontal sulcus
s. ganglion of glossopharyngeal nerve
s. ganglion of vagus nerve
s. gastric lymph nodes
s. gemellus muscle
s. gingival branches of superior dental plexus
s. gluteal artery
s. gluteal nerve
s. gluteal veins
s. hemorrhagic polioencephalitis
s. hemorrhoidal artery
s. hemorrhoidal plexus
s. hemorrhoidal vein
s. horn of falciform margin of saphenous opening
s. horn of thyroid cartilage
s. hypogastric plexus
s. hypophysial artery
s. ileocecal recess
s. intercostal artery
s. intercostal vein
s. internal parietal artery
s. labial artery
s. labial branches of infraorbital nerve
s. labial vein
s. laryngeal artery
s. laryngeal cavity

S

superior (*continued*)
s. laryngeal nerve
s. laryngeal vein
s. laryngotomy
s. lateral brachial cutaneous nerve
s. lateral genicular artery
s. ligament of epididymis
s. ligament of incus
s. ligament of malleus
s. limb
s. limbic keratoconjunctivitis
s. lingular branch of lingular branch of superior lobar left pulmonary artery
s. lingular segment
s. lobe of lung
s. longitudinal fasciculus
s. longitudinal muscle of tongue
s. longitudinal sinus
s. longitudinal sulcus
s. macular arteriole
s. macular venule
s. maxillary nerve
s. medial genicular artery
s. mediastinum
s. medullary velum
s. mesenteric artery
s. mesenteric artery syndrome
s. mesenteric ganglion
s. mesenteric lymph nodes
s. mesenteric plexus
s. mesenteric vein
s. nasal arteriole of retina
s. nasal concha
s. nasal venule of retina
s. nuchal line
s. oblique muscle
s. oblique muscle of head
s. occipital gyrus
s. occipital sulcus
s. olivary nucleus
s. olive
s. omental recess
s. ophthalmic vein
s. orbital fissure
s. palpebral veins
s. pancreaticoduodenal artery
s. paraplegia
s. parietal gyrus
s. parietal lobule
s. part of diaphragmatic surface of liver
s. part of duodenum
s. part of lingular branch of left pulmonary vein
s. part of vestibular ganglion
s. part of vestibulocochlear nerve
s. pelvic aperture

s. petrosal sinus
s. petrosal sulcus
s. phrenic artery
s. phrenic lymph nodes
s. phrenic veins
s. pole
s. pole of kidney
s. pole of testis
s. polioencephalitis
s. posterior serratus muscle
s. pubic ligament
s. pubic ramus
s. pulmonary sulcus tumor
s. quadrigeminal brachium
s. radioulnar joint
s. recess of lesser peritoneal sac
s. recess of tympanic membrane
s. rectal artery
s. rectal lymph nodes
s. rectal plexus
s. rectal vein
s. rectus muscle
s. retinaculum of extensor muscles
s. root of ansa cervicalis
s. root of vestibulocochlear nerve
s. sagittal sinus
s. salivary nucleus
s. salivatory nucleus
s. segment
s. segmental artery of kidney
s. semilunar lobule
s. strait
s. suprarenal arteries
s. surface of cerebellar hemisphere
s. surface of talus
s. tarsal muscle
s. tarsus
s. temporal arteriole of retina
s. temporal convolution
s. temporal fissure
s. temporal gyrus
s. temporal line
s. temporal sulcus
s. temporal venule of retina
s. thalamostriate vein
s. thoracic aperture
s. thoracic artery
s. thyroid artery
s. thyroid notch
s. thyroid plexus
s. thyroid tubercle
s. thyroid vein
s. tibial articulation
s. tibiofibular joint
s. tracheobronchial lymph nodes
s. transverse scapular ligament
s. triangle sign
s. trunk of brachial plexus

s. turbinated bone
s. tympanic artery
s. ulnar collateral artery
s. veins of cerebellar hemisphere
s. vein of vermis
s. vena cava
s. vena cava syndrome
s. vesical artery
s. vestibular area
s. vestibular nucleus
s. wall of orbit

superiority complex
superlactation
superligamen
supermedial
supermotility
supernormal recovery phase
supernumerary
s. breast
s. kidney
s. mamma
s. organs
s. placenta

supernutrition
superolateral
s. cerebral surface
s. surface of cerebrum

superomedial margin
superovulation
superparasite
superparasitism
superpetrosal
superpigmentation
superscription
supersonic
s. rays
s. waves

superstructure
implant denture s.

supertension
supertraction conus
supinate
supination
s. of the foot
s. of the forearm
s. reflex

supinator
s. crest
s. jerk
s. longus reflex
s. muscle
s. reflex

supine
s. hypotensive syndrome
s. position

suppedanium, pl. **suppedania**
supplemental
s. air

s. groove
s. lobe
s. ridge

supplementary
s. menstruation
s. motor area epilepsy
s. motor cortex

support
advanced life s.
basic life s.

supporter
supporting
s. area
s. cell
s. reactions
s. reflexes

supportive psychotherapy
suppressed menstruation
suppression
s. amblyopia
intergenic s.
intragenic s.

suppressor cells
suppurate
suppuration
suppurative
s. appendicitis
s. arthritis
s. cerebritis
s. choroiditis
s. encephalitis
s. gingivitis
s. hepatitis
s. hyalitis
s. inflammation
s. mastitis
s. necrosis
s. nephritis
s. periodontitis
s. pleurisy
s. pneumonia
s. pulpitis
s. synovitis

supra-acetabular
s.-a. groove
s.-a. sulcus

supra-acromial
supra-anal
supra-arytenoid cartilage
supra-auricular
s.-a. point

supra-axillary
suprabuccal
suprabulge
supracallosal gyrus
supracardinal
supracerebellar
supracerebral

S

supracervical hysterectomy
suprachoroid
    s. lamina
    s. layer
suprachoroidea
supraciliary
supraclavicular
    s. lymph nodes
    s. muscle
    s. part of brachial plexus
    s. triangle
supraclavicularis
supraclinoid aneurysm
supracondylar
    s. fracture
    s. process
supracondyloid
supracostal
supracotyloid
supracrestal
    s. line
    s. plane
supracristal
    s. plane
supradiaphragmatic
supraduction
supraduodenal artery
supraepicondylar
    s. process
supragingival calculus
supraglenoid
    s. tubercle
supraglottic
suprahepatic
    s. spaces
suprahisian block
suprahyoid
    s. branch of lingual artery
    s. gland
    s. muscles
suprainguinal
suprainterparietal bone
supraintestinal
supraliminal
supralumbar
supramalleolar
supramammary
supramandibular
supramarginal
    s. convolution
    s. gyrus
supramastoid
    s. crest
    s. fossa
supramaxilla
supramaxillary
supramaximal stimulus

suprameatal
    s. pit
    s. spine
    s. triangle
supramental
supramentale
supranasal
    s. point
supraneural
supranormal
    s. conduction
    s. excitability
supranuclear
    s. lesion
    s. paralysis
supraocclusion
supraoptic
    s. commissures
    s. nucleus
    s. nucleus of hypothalamus
supraopticohypophysial tract
supraorbital
    s. arch
    s. artery
    s. foramen
    s. margin
    s. nerve
    s. neuralgia
    s. notch
    s. point
    s. reflex
    s. ridge
    s. vein
supraorbitomeatal
    s. plane
suprapatellar
    s. bursa
    s. reflex
suprapelvic
supraperiosteal implant
suprapineal recess
suprapleural membrane
suprapubic
    s. cystotomy
    s. lithotomy
suprapyloric
    s. lymph node
    s. node
suprarenal
    s. body
    s. capsule
    s. cortex
    s. gland
    s. impression
    s. medulla
    s. plexus
    s. veins

suprascapular
    s. artery
    s. ligament
    s. nerve
    s. notch
    s. vein
suprascleral
suprasellar
    s. cyst
supraspinal
supraspinalis
    s. muscle
supraspinatus
    s. muscle
    s. syndrome
supraspinous
    s. fossa
    s. ligament
    s. muscle
suprastapedial
suprasternal
    s. bone
    s. notch
    s. plane
    s. pulsation
    s. space
suprasylvian
suprasymphysary
supratemporal
supratentorial
suprathoracic
supratonsillar
    s. fossa
    s. recess
supratragic tubercle
supratrochlear
    s. artery
    s. nerve
    s. veins
supraturbinal
supratympanic
supraumbilical reflex
supravaginal
    s. portion of cervix
supravalvar
    s. aortic stenosis-infantile
      hypercalcemia syndrome
    s. aortic stenosis syndrome
    s. stenosis
supravalvular
    s. stenosis
supraventricular
    s. crest
    s. extrasystole
    s. tachycardia
supravergence
supraversion
supravesical fossa

supravital stain
supreme
    s. concha
    s. intercostal artery
    s. intercostal vein
    s. nasal concha
    s. turbinated bone
sura
sural
    s. artery
    s. nerve
    s. region
suralimentation
surdocardiac syndrome
surface
    acromial articular s. of clavicle
    s. anatomy
    anterior s.
    anterior s. of arm
    anterior articular s. of dens
    anterior s. of cornea
    anterior s. of elbow
    anterior s. of eyelids
    anterior s. of forearm
    anterior s. of iris
    anterior s. of kidney
    anterior s. of leg
    anterior s. of lens
    anterior s. of lower limb
    anterior s. of maxilla
    anterior s. of pancreas
    anterior s. of patella
    anterior s. of petrous part of
      temporal bone
    anterior s. of prostate
    anterior s. of radius
    anterior s. of suprarenal gland
    anterior talar articular s. of
      calcaneus
    anterior s. of thigh
    anterior s. of ulna
    anterolateral s. of shaft of humerus
    anteromedial s. of shaft of
      humerus
    articular s.
    articular s. of acromion
    articular s. of arytenoid cartilage
    articular s. of head of fibula
    articular s. of head of rib
    articular s. of patella
    articular s. of temporal bone
    articular s. of tubercle of rib
    arytenoidal articular s. of cricoid
    auricular s. of ilium
    auricular s. of sacrum
    axial s.
    balancing occlusal s.
    basal s.

S

surface *(continued)*
    buccal s.
    calcaneal articular s. of talus
    carpal articular s. of radius
    cerebral s.
    s. coil
    colic s. of spleen
    contact s. of tooth
    costal s.
    costal s. of lung
    costal s. of scapula
    cuboidal articular s. of calcaneus
    denture basal s.
    denture foundation s.
    denture impression s.
    denture occlusal s.
    denture polished s.
    diaphragmatic s.
    distal s. of tooth
    dorsal s.
    dorsal s. of digit
    dorsal s. of sacrum
    dorsal s. of scapula
    s. epithelium
    external s.
    external s. of frontal bone
    external s. of parietal bone
    facial s. of tooth
    fibular articular s. of tibia
    gastric s. of spleen
    glenoid s.
    gluteal s. of ilium
    grinding s.
    incisal s.
    inferior articular s. of tibia
    inferior s. of cerebellar hemisphere
    inferior cerebral s.
    inferior s. of pancreas
    inferior s. of petrous part of temporal bone
    inferior s. of tongue
    inferolateral s. of prostate
    infratemporal s. of maxilla
    interlobar s.'s of lung
    internal s.
    internal s. of frontal bone
    internal s. of parietal bone
    intestinal s. of uterus
    labial s.
    lateral s.
    lateral s. of arm
    lateral s. of fibula
    lateral s. of finger
    lateral s. of leg
    lateral s. of lower limb
    lateral malleolar s. of talus
    lateral s. of ovary
    lateral s. of testis
    lateral s. of tibia
    lateral s. of toe
    lateral s. of zygomatic bone
    lingual s. of tooth
    lunate s. of acetabulum
    malleolar articular s. of fibula
    malleolar articular s. of tibia
    masticating s.
    masticatory s.
    maxillary s. of greater wing of sphenoid bone
    maxillary s. of palatine bone
    medial s.
    medial s. of arytenoid cartilage
    medial cerebral s.
    medial s. of cerebral hemisphere
    medial s. of fibula
    medial s. of lung
    medial malleolar s. of talus
    medial s. of ovary
    medial s. of testis
    medial s. of tibia
    medial s. of toes
    medial s. of ulna
    mediastinal s. of lung
    mesial s. of tooth
    middle talar articular s. of calcaneus
    s. mucous cells of stomach
    nasal s. of maxilla
    nasal s. of palatine bone
    navicular articular s. of talus
    occlusal s.
    orbital s.
    palatine s. of horizontal plate of palatine bone
    palmar s. of fingers
    patellar s. of femur
    pelvic s. of sacrum
    plantar s. of toe
    popliteal s. of femur
    posterior s.
    posterior s. of arm
    posterior articular s. of dens
    posterior s. of arytenoid cartilage
    posterior s. of cornea
    posterior s. of elbow
    posterior s. of eyelids
    posterior s. of fibula
    posterior s. of forearm
    posterior s. of iris
    posterior s. of kidney
    posterior s. of leg
    posterior s. of lens
    posterior s. of lower limb
    posterior s. of pancreas
    posterior s. of petrous part of temporal bone

posterior s. of prostate
posterior s. of radius
posterior s. of shaft of humerus
posterior s. of suprarenal gland
posterior talar articular s. of
  calcaneus
posterior s. of thigh
posterior s. of tibia
posterior s. of ulna
pulmonary s. of heart
renal s. of spleen
renal s. of the suprarenal gland
renal s. of suprarenal gland
sacropelvic s. of ilium
sternal articular s. of clavicle
sternocostal s. of heart
subocclusal s.
superior articular s. of tibia
superior s. of cerebellar hemisphere
superior s. of talus
superolateral cerebral s.
superolateral s. of cerebrum
symphysial s. of pubis
talar articular s. of calcaneus
temporal s.
tentorial s.
s. thalamic veins
s. thermometer
thyroidal articular s. of cricoid
urethral s. of penis
ventral s. of digit
vesical s. of uterus
vestibular s. of tooth
visceral s. of liver
visceral s. of the spleen
working occlusal s.'s

surgeon
attending s.
dental s.
s. general
house s.
s. knot
oral s.

surgery
ambulatory s.
aseptic s.
closed s.
cosmetic s.
craniofacial s.
esthetic s.
featural s.
keratorefractive s.
laparoscopic s.
laparoscopically assisted s.
major s.
microscopically controlled s.
minimally invasive s.
minor s.

Mohs' s.
Mohs' micrographic s.
open heart s.
oral s.
orthognathic s.
orthopaedic s.
plastic s.
reconstructive s.
stereotactic s.
stereotaxic s.
thoracoscopic s.
transsexual s.
video-assisted thoracic s.

surgical
s. abdomen
s. anatomy
s. anesthesia
s. appliance
s. ciliated cyst
s. diathermy
s. emphysema
s. eruption
s. erysipelas
s. ligation
s. maggot
s. microscope
s. neck of humerus
s. orthodontics
s. pathology
s. prosthesis
s. splint
s. template

surrenal
surrogate
mother s.
s. mother
sursanure
sursumduction
sursumversion
surveillance
immune s.
immunological s.
post-marketing s.
survey
field s.
s. line
skeletal s.
surveying
surveyor
survival
s. analysis
s. time
susceptibility
s. testing
suspension
chromic phosphate P 32
  colloidal s.

S

suspension *(continued)*
    Coffey s.
    s. laryngoscopy
suspensory
    s. bandage
    s. ligament of axilla
    s. ligament of clitoris
    s. ligament of esophagus
    s. ligament of eyeball
    s. ligament of gonad
    s. ligament of lens
    s. ligament of ovary
    s. ligament of penis
    s. ligaments of breast
    s. ligaments of Cooper
    s. ligament of testis
    s. ligament of thyroid gland
    s. muscle of duodenum
sustentacular
    s. cell
    s. fibers of retina
sustentaculum, pl. **sustentacula**
    s. lienis
    s. tali
susurrus
    s. aurium
Sutton's
    S. disease
    S. nevus
    S. ulcer
sutura, pl. **suturae**
    s. coronalis
    suturae cranii
    s. ethmoidolacrimalis
    s. ethmoidomaxillaris
    s. frontalis
    s. frontoethmoidalis
    s. frontolacrimalis
    s. frontomaxillaris
    s. frontonasalis
    s. frontozygomatica
    s. incisiva
    s. infraorbitalis
    s. intermaxillaris
    s. internasalis
    s. interparietalis
    s. lacrimoconchalis
    s. lacrimomaxillaris
    s. lambdoidea
    s. metopica
    s. nasofrontalis
    s. nasomaxillaris
    s. notha
    s. occipitomastoidea
    s. palatina mediana
    s. palatina transversa
    s. palatoethmoidalis
    s. palatomaxillaris

    s. parietomastoidea
    s. plana
    s. sagittalis
    s. serrata
    s. sphenoethmoidalis
    s. sphenofrontalis
    s. sphenomaxillaris
    s. spheno-orbitalis
    s. sphenoparietalis
    s. sphenosquamosa
    s. sphenovomeriana
    s. sphenozygomatica
    s. squamosa
    s. squamosomastoidea
    s. temporozygomatica
    s. zygomaticofrontalis
    s. zygomaticomaxillaris
    s. zygomaticotemporalis
sutural
    s. bones
    s. cataract
    s. ligament
suture
    Albert's s.
    apposition s.
    approximation s.
    atraumatic s.
    blanket s.
    bridle s.
    Bunnell's s.
    buried s.
    button s.
    catgut s.
    coaptation s.
    cobbler's s.
    Connell's s.
    continuous s.
    control release s.
    coronal s.
    cranial s.'s
    Cushing's s.
    Czerny-Lembert s.
    Czerny's s.
    delayed s.
    dentate s.
    doubly armed s.
    Dupuytren's s.
    end-on mattress s.
    ethmoidolacrimal s.
    ethmoidomaxillary s.
    Faden s.
    false s.
    far-and-near s.
    figure-of-8 s.
    frontal s.
    frontoethmoidal s.
    frontolacrimal s.
    frontomaxillary s.

frontonasal s.
frontozygomatic s.
Frost s.
Gély's s.
glover's s.
Gould's s.
Gussenbauer's s.
Halsted's s.
harmonic s.
implanted s.
incisive s.
infraorbital s.
intermaxillary s.
internasal s.
interparietal s.
interrupted s.
Jobert de Lamballe's s.
s. joint
lacrimoconchal s.
lacrimomaxillary s.
lambdoid s.
Lembert s.
lens s.'s
s. ligature
mattress s.
median palatine s.
metopic s.
nasomaxillary s.
nerve s.
neurocentral s.
occipitomastoid s.
palatoethmoidal s.
palatomaxillary s.
Pancoast's s.
Paré's s.
parietomastoid s.
Parker-Kerr s.
petrosquamous s.
plane s.
pledgetted s.
premaxillary s.
purse-string s.
quilted s.
relaxation s.
retention s.
sagittal s.
secondary s.
serrate s.
shotted s.
sphenoethmoidal s.
sphenofrontal s.
sphenomaxillary s.
spheno-occipital s.
spheno-orbital s.
sphenoparietal s.
sphenosquamous s.
sphenovomerine s.
sphenozygomatic s.

spiral s.
squamomastoid s.
squamoparietal s.
squamous s.
subcuticular s.
temporozygomatic s.
tendon s.
tension s.
transfixion s.
transverse palatine s.
tympanomastoid s.
uninterrupted s.
wedge-and-groove s.
zygomaticomaxillary s.
zygomaticotemporal s.
suturectomy
Suzanne's gland
SV40-adenovirus hybrid
swab
swage
swallow
gastrografin s.
hypaque s.
somatic s.
s. syncope
visceral s.
swallowing
s. reflex
s. threshold
swamp
s. fever virus
s. itch
Swan-Ganz catheter
Swann antigens
swan-neck deformity
Sw^a antigen
swarming
sweat
colliquative s.
s. duct
s. gland carcinoma
s. glands
night s.'s
s. pore
red s.
s. test
sweating
s. test
Swediauer's disease
Swedish
S. gymnastics
S. movements
sweep
Sweet's disease
swelling
albuminous s.
arytenoid s.
brain s.

swelling (*continued*)
    Calabar s.
    cloudy s.
    fugitive s.
    genital s.'s
    hunger s.
    labial s.
    labioscrotal s.'s
    lateral lingual s.'s
    levator s.
    Neufeld capsular s.
    scrotal s.
    Spielmeyer's acute s.
Swift's disease
swimmer's
    s. ear
    s. itch
swimming
    s. pool conjunctivitis
    s. pool granuloma
swine
    s. encephalitis virus
    s. fever virus
    s. influenza viruses
swineherd's disease
swinepox virus
swing
    mood s.
swinging light test
Swiss
    S. cheese endometrium
    S. mouse leukemia virus
    S. type agammaglobulinemia
swollen
    s. belly disease
    s. belly syndrome
swordfish test
Swyer-James-MacLeod syndrome
Swyer-James syndrome
sycoma
sycosiform
sycosis
    s. frambesiformis
    lupoid s.
    s. nuchae necrotisans
Sydenham's
    S. chorea
    S. disease
Sydney
    S. crease
    S. line
syllabic speech
syllable-stumbling
Sylvest's disease
Sylvian
    S. cistern
sylvian
    s. angle

    s. aqueduct
    s. fissure
    s. line
    s. point
    s. valve
    s. ventricle
symballophone
symbion, symbiont
symbiosis
    dyadic s.
    triadic s.
symbiote
symbiotic
symblepharon
    anterior s.
    posterior s.
symblepharopterygium
symbolia
symbolism
symbolization
symbrachydactyly
Syme's
    S. amputation
    S. operation
Symington's anococcygeal body
symmelia
Symmers'
    S. clay pipestem fibrosis
    S. fibrosis
symmetric
    s. adenolipomatosis
    s. asphyxia
    s. distal neuropathy
symmetrical gangrene
symmetry
    inverse s.
sympathectomy
    chemical s.
    periarterial s.
    presacral s.
sympathetectomy
sympathetic
    s. branch to submandibular ganglion
    s. formative cell
    s. ganglia
    s. heterochromia
    s. hypertonia
    s. imbalance
    s. iridoplegia
    s. iritis
    s. nerve
    s. nervous system
    s. ophthalmia
    s. part
    s. plexuses
    s. reflex dystrophy
    s. root of ciliary ganglion

S

s. saliva
s. segment
s. symptom
s. trunk
s. uveitis
sympathetoblast
sympathetoblastoma
sympathic
sympathicectomy
sympathicoblast
sympathicoblastoma
sympathicogonioma
sympathiconeuritis
sympathicopathy
sympathicotonia
sympathicotonic
sympathicotripsy
sympathicotropic cells
sympathism
sympathist
sympathizer
sympathizing eye
sympathoadrenal
sympathoblast
sympathoblastoma
sympathochromaffin cell
sympathogonia
sympathogonioma
sympathy
symperitoneal
sympexis
symphalangism, symphalangy
symphyseotome (*var. of* symphysiotome)
symphyseotomy (*var. of* symphysiotomy)
symphyses (*gen. of* symphysis)
symphysial, symphyseal
s. surface of pubis
symphysic
s. teratosis
symphysion
symphysiotome, symphyseotome
symphysiotomy, symphyseotomy
symphysis, gen. **symphyses**
cardiac s.
intervertebral s.
s. intervertebralis
s. mandibulae
manubriosternal s.
s. manubriosternalis
mental s.
s. mentalis
s. menti
pubic s.
s. pubica
s. pubis
s. sacrococcygea
symplasmatic
symplast

sympodia
symptom
abstinence s.'s
accessory s.
accidental s.
assident s.
Baumès s.
Bezold's s.
Bolognini's s.
cardinal s.
s. complex
concomitant s.
constitutional s.
deficiency s.
Demarquay's s.
Epstein's s.
equivocal s.
first rank s.'s
Fischer's s.
s. formation
Frenkel's s.
Gordon's s.
Griesinger's s.
s. group
Haenel's s.
incarceration s.
induced s.
Kerandel's s.
Kussmaul's s.
local s.
localizing s.
Macewen's s.
objective s.
Oehler's s.
pathognomonic s.
Pratt's s.
presenting s.
rainbow s.
reflex s.
Romberg-Howship s.
Romberg's s.
schneiderian first rank s.'s
Schneider's first rank s.'s
s. score
Sklowsky s.
subjective s.
s. substitution
sympathetic s.
Trendelenburg's s.
Uhthoff s.
Wartenberg's s.
withdrawal s.'s
symptomatic
s. epilepsy
s. erythema
s. fever
s. headache
s. impotence

symptomatic *(continued)*
  s. indication
  s. myeloid metaplasia
  s. nanism
  s. neuralgia
  s. porphyria
  s. pruritus
  s. reaction
  s. tetany
  s. torticollis
  s. treatment
  s. ulcer
  s. varicocele
symptomatology
symptomatolytic
symptomolytic
symptosis
sympus
  s. apus
  s. dipus
  s. monopus
Syms tractor
synadelphus
synalgia
synalgic
synanastomosis
synanthem, synanthema
synaphoceptors
synapse, pl. **synapses**
  axoaxonic s.
  axodendritic s.
  axosomatic s.
  electrotonic s.
  pericorpuscular s.
synapsis
synaptic
  s. boutons
  s. cleft
  s. conduction
  s. endings
  s. phase
  s. resistance
  s. terminals
  s. trough
  s. vesicles
synaptinemal complex
synaptology
synaptosome
synarthrodia
synarthrodial
  s. joint
synarthrophysis
synarthrosis, pl. **synarthroses**
syncanthus
syncaryon
syncephalus
  s. asymmetros
syncephaly

syncheilia
syncheiria
synchilia
synchiria
synchondrodial joint
synchondroseotomy
synchondrosis, pl. **synchondroses**
  anterior intraoccipital s.
  s. arycorniculata
  arycorniculate s.
  cranial synchondroses
  synchondroses cranii
  s. epiphyseos
  s. intraoccipitalis anterior
  s. intraoccipitalis posterior
  s. manubriosternalis
  neurocentral s.
  s. petro-occipitalis
  posterior intraoccipital s.
  sphenoethmoidal s.
  s. sphenoethmoidalis
  spheno-occipital s.
  s. spheno-occipitalis
  s. sphenopetrosa
  sphenopetrosal s., sphenopetrous s.
  s. xiphosternalis
synchondrotomy
synchorial
synchronia
synchronic
  s. study
synchronism
synchronized intermittent mandatory ventilation
synchronous
  s. reflex
synchrony
  bilateral s.
synchysis
  s. scintillans
syncinesis
synclinal
synclitic
synclitism
synclonic spasm
synclonus
syncopal
syncope
  Adams-Stokes s.
  cardiac s.
  carotid sinus s.
  hysterical s.
  laryngeal s.
  local s.
  micturition s.
  postural s.
  swallow s.
  tussive s.

vasodepressor s.
vasovagal s.
syncopic
syncretio
syncyanin
syncytial
    s. bud
    s. knot
    s. sprout
    s. trophoblast
syncytium, pl. **syncytia**
syndactyl, syndactyle
syndactylia, syndactylism
syndactylous
syndactyly
syndesis
syndesmectomy
syndesmectopia
syndesmitis
    s. metatarsea
syndesmochorial
syndesmodial
    s. joint
syndesmography
syndesmologia
syndesmology
syndesmopexy
syndesmophyte
syndesmoplasty
syndesmorrhaphy
syndesmosis, pl. **syndesmoses**
    radioulnar s.
    s. radioulnaris
    tibiofibular s.
    s. tibiofibularis
    s. tympanostapedia
    tympanostapedial s.
syndesmotic
    s. joint
syndesmotomy
syndrome
    Aarskog-Scott s.
    abdominal muscle deficiency s.
    Achard s.
    Achard-Thiers s.
    Achenbach s.
    acquired immunodeficiency s.
      (AIDS)
    acrofacial s.
    acroparesthesia s.
    acute organic brain s.
    acute radiation s.
    Adams-Stokes s.
    adaptation s. of Selye
    addisonian s.
    adherence s.
    Adie s.
    adiposogenital s.

adrenal cortical s.
adrenal virilizing s.
adrenogenital s.
adult respiratory distress s.
afferent loop s.
aglossia-adactylia s.
Ahumada-Del Castillo s.
Aicardi's s.
Albright's s.
alcohol amnestic s.
Aldrich s.
Alezzandrini's s.
Alice in Wonderland s.
Allen-Masters s.
Alport's s.
Alström's s.
amenorrhea-galactorrhea s.
amnestic s.
amniotic fluid s.
Amsterdam s.
Angelman s.
Angelucci's s.
angio-osteohypertrophy s.
ankyloglossia superior s.
anorectal s.
anterior chamber cleavage s.
anterior tibial compartment s.
antibody deficiency s.
Anton's s.
anxiety s.
aortic arch s.
apallic s.
Apert's s.
s. of approximate relevant answers
Argonz-Del Castillo s.
Arndt-Gottron s.
Arnold-Chiari s.
arterial thoracic outlet s.
Ascher's s.
Asherman's s.
asplenia s.
ataxia telangiectasia s.
auriculotemporal nerve s.
autoerythrocyte sensitization s.
Avellis' s.
A-V strabismus s.
Ayerza's s.
Babinski's s.
baby bottle s.
Balint's s.
Bamberger-Marie s.
Bannwarth's s.
Banti's s.
Bardet-Biedl s.
bare lymphocyte s.
Barlow s.
Barrett's s.
Bart's s.

S

syndrome *(continued)*

Bartter's s.
basal cell nevus s.
Basan's s.
Bassen-Kornzweig s.
battered child s.
battered spouse s.
Bauer's s.
Bazex's s.
Beckwith-Wiedemann s.
Behçet's s.
Behr's s.
Benedikt's s.
Beradinelli's s.
Bernard-Horner s.
Bernard-Sergent s.
Bernard-Soulier s.
Bernhardt-Roth s.
Bernheim's s.
Besnier-Boeck-Schaumann s.
Beuren s.
Biemond s.
billowing mitral valve s.
Bjornstad's s.
Blatin's s.
blind loop s.
Bloch-Sulzberger s.
Bloom's s.
blue toe s.
Boerhaave's s.
Bonnier's s.
Böök s.
Börjeson-Forssman-Lehmann s.
bowel bypass s.
bradytachycardia s.
Briquet's s.
Brissaud-Marie s.
Brock's s.
Brown's s.
Brown-Séquard's s.
Brugsch's s.
Budd-Chiari s.
Budd's s.
Bürger-Grütz s.
burner s.
Burnett's s.
burning vulva s.
Buschke-Ollendorf s.
Caffey-Kempe s.
Caffey's s.
Caffey-Silverman s.
camptomelic s.
Capgras' s.
Caplan's s.
carcinoid s.
cardiofacial s.
Caroli's s.
carotid sinus s.

carpal tunnel s.
Carpenter's s.
cataract-oligophrenia s.
cat-cry s. (*var. of* cri-du-chat s.)
cat's cry s.
cat's-eye s.
cauda equina s.
cavernous sinus s.
Ceelen-Gellerstedt s.
celiac s.
cellular immunity deficiency s.
central cord s.
cerebellar s.
cerebellomedullary malformation s.
cerebellopontine angle s.
cerebrohepatorenal s.
cervical compression s.
cervical disc s.
cervical fusion s.
cervical rib s.
cervical rib and band s.
cervical tension s.
cervico-oculo-acoustic s.
Cestan-Chenais s.
chancriform s.
Chandler s.
Charcot's s.
Charcot-Weiss-Baker s.
Chauffard's s.
Cheney s.
cherry-red spot myoclonus s.
Chiari-Budd s.
Chiari-Frommel s.
Chiari II s.
Chiari's s.
chiasma s.
Chilaiditi's s.
CHILD s.
Chinese restaurant s.
Chotzen's s.
Christian's s.
Christ-Siemens-Touraine s.
chromosomal s.
chromosomal instability s.'s,
  chromosomal breakage s.'s
chronic hyperventilation s.
Churg-Strauss s.
Clarke-Hadfield s.
classic cervical rib s.
Claude's s.
click s.
climacteric s.
cloverleaf skull s.
Cobb s.
Cockayne's s.
Coffin-Lowry s.
Coffin-Siris s.
Cogan-Reese s.

Cogan's s.
Collet-Sicard s.
combined immunodeficiency s.
compartmental s.
compression s.
congenital rubella s.
Conn's s.
Cornelia de Lange s.
corpus luteum deficiency s.
Costen's s.
costochondral s.
costoclavicular s.
Cotard's s.
Crandall's s.
CREST s.
cri-du-chat s., cat-cry s., cri du
  chat s.
Crigler-Najjar s.
crocodile tears s.
Cronkhite-Canada s.
Crouzon's s.
crush s.
Cruveilhier-Baumgarten s. *cystic duct s.*
cryptophthalmus s.
Cushing's s.
Cushing's s. medicamentosus
cutaneomucouveal s.
DaCosta's s.
Dandy-Walker s.
dead fetus s.
Debré-Sémélaigne s.
de Clerambault s.
Degos' s.
Dejerine-Klumpke s.
Dejerine-Roussy s.
de Lange s.
Del Castillo s.
de Morsier's s.
dengue shock s.
depersonalization s.
depressive s.
dermatitis-arthritis-tenosynovitis s.
De Sanctis-Cacchione s.
De Toni-Fanconi s.
s. of deviously relevant answers
dialysis disequilibrium s.
dialysis encephalopathy s.
Diamond-Blackfan s.
diencephalic s. of infancy
DiGeorge s.
Di Guglielmo's s.
disconnection s.
disk s.
disputed neurogenic thoracic
  outlet s.
Donohue's s.
Doose s.
Dorfman-Chanarin s.

Down's s.
Dressler's s.
dry eye s.
Duane's s.
Dubin-Johnson s.
Dubreuil-Chambardel s.
Duchenne's s.
dumping s.
Dyggve-Melchior-Clausen s.
dyskinesia
dysmnesic s.
dysplastic nevus s.
Eagle s.
Eagle-Barrett s.
Eaton-Lambert s.
ectopic ACTH s.
Edwards' s.
effort s.
egg-white s.
Ehlers-Danlos s.
Eisenlohr's s.
Eisenmenger's s.
Ekbom s.
Ellis-van Creveld s.
E-M s.
EMG s.
encephalotrigeminal vascular s.
eosinophilia-myalgia s.
episodic dyscontrol s.
erythrodysesthesia s.
euthyroid sick s.
Evans' s.
exfoliation s.
extrapyramidal s.
Faber's s.
familial aortic ectasia s.
Fanconi's s.
Farber's s.
Favre-Racouchot s.
Felty's s.
female urethral s.
fetal aspiration s.
fetal face s.
fetal hydantoin s.
fetal trimethadione s.
fibrinogen-fibrin conversion s.
Fiessinger-Leroy-Reiter s.
Figueira's s.
first arch s.
Fisher's s.
Fitz-Hugh and Curtis s.
flashing pain s.
flecked retina s.
floppy valve s.
Flynn-Aird s.
Foix-Alajouanine s.
Foix-Cavany-Marie s.
folded-lung s.

S

syndrome *(continued)*
    Forbes-Albright s.
    Foster Kennedy's s.
    Foville's s.
    fragile X s.
    Fraley s.
    Franceschetti-Jadassohn s.
    Franceschetti's s.
    Fraser's s.
    Freeman-Sheldon s.
    Frenkel's anterior ocular
      traumatic s.
    Frey's s.
    Friderichsen-Waterhouse s.
    Fröhlich's s.
    Froin's s.
    Fuchs' s.
    functional prepubertal castration s.
    G s.
    Gaisböck's s.
    Ganser's s.
    Gardner-Diamond s.
    Gardner's s.
    gastrocardiac s.
    gastrojejunal loop obstruction s.
    gay bowel s.
    Gélineau's s.
    gender dysphoria s.
    general adaptation s.
    Gerstmann s.
    Gerstmann-Sträussler s.
    Gianotti-Crosti s.
    Gilbert's s.
    Gilles de la Tourette's s.
    glucagonoma s.
    Goldenhar's s.
    gold-myokymia s.
    Goltz s.
    Goodman's s.
    Goodpasture's s.
    Gopalan's s.
    Gorlin-Chaudhry-Moss s.
    Gorlin's s.
    Gorman's s.
    Gougerot-Carteaud s.
    Gowers' s.
    gracilis s.
    Gradenigo's s.
    Graham Little s.
    gray s., gray baby s.
    Greig's s.
    Grönblad-Strandberg s.
    Gubler's s.
    Guillain-Barré s.
    Gulf War s.
    Gunn's s.
    gustatory sweating s.
    Haber's s.

Hallermann-Streiff s.
Hallermann-Streiff-François s.
Hallervorden s.
Hallervorden-Spatz s.
Hallgren's s.
Hamman-Rich s.
Hamman's s.
hand-and-foot s.
Hanhart's s.
happy puppet s.
Harada's s.
Harris s.
Hartnup s.
Hayem-Widal s.
head-bobbing doll s.
Hegglin's s.
HELLP s.
Helweg-Larssen s.
hemangioma-thrombocytopenia s.
hemolytic uremic s.
Henoch-Schönlein s.
hepatorenal s., hepatonephoric s.
Herlitz s.
Hermansky-Pudlak s. type VI
Herrmann's s.
Hinman s.
Hirschowitz s.
holiday s.
holiday heart s.
Holmes-Adie s.
Holt-Oram s.
Horner's s.
Houssay s.
Hughes-Stovin s.
Hunter's s.
Hunt's s.
Hurler's s.
Hutchinson-Gilford s.
Hutchison s.
hyaline membrane s.
hydralazine s.
17-hydroxylase deficiency s.
hyperabduction s.
hyperactive child s.
hypereosinophilic s.
hyperimmunoglobulin E s.
hyperkinetic s.
hyperkinetic heart s.
hypersensitive xiphoid s.
hyperventilation s.
hyperviscosity s.
hypometabolic s.
hypoparathyroidism s.
hypophysial s.
hypophysio-sphenoidal s.
hypoplastic left heart s.
immotile cilia s.
immunodeficiency s.

s. of inappropriate secretion of antidiuretic hormone
indifference to pain s.
internal capsule s.
inversed jaw-winking s.
iridocorneal s.
iridocorneal endothelial s.
iris-nevus s.
Irvine-Gass s.
Isaac's s.
Ivemark's s.
Jadassohn-Lewandowski s.
Jahnke's s.
jaw-winking s.
Jeghers-Peutz s.
Jervell and Lange-Nielsen s.
Jeune's s.
Job s.
Joubert's s.
jugular foramen s.
Kallmann's s.
Kanner's s.
Kartagener's s.
Kasabach-Merritt s.
Katayama s.
Kawasaki's s.
Kearns-Sayre s.
Kennedy's s.
Kimmelstiel-Wilson s.
Kleine-Levin s.
Klippel-Feil s.
Klippel-Trenaunay-Weber s.
Klüver-Bucy s.
Kniest s.
Kocher-Debré-Sémélaigne s.
Koenig's s.
Koerber-Salus-Elschnig s.
Kohlmeier-Degos s.
Korsakoff's s.
Kostmann s.
Kuskokwim s.
Laband's s.
Labbé's neurocirculatory s.
LAMB s.
Lambert-Eaton s.
Lambert's s.
Landau-Kleffner s.
Landry s.
Landry-Guillain-Barré s.
Larsen's s.
Lasègue's s.
lateral medullary s.
Launois-Bensaude s.
Launois-Cléret s.
Laurence-Moon-Biedl s.
Lawrence-Seip s.
Lejeune s.
Lenègre's s.

Lennox s.
Lennox-Gastaut s.
LEOPARD s.
Leriche's s.
Leri-Weill s.
Lermoyez' s.
Lesch-Nyhan s.
Lev's s.
Libman-Sacks s.
Li-Fraumeni cancer s.
Lignac-Fanconi s.
liver kidney s.
locked-in s.
loculation s.
Löffler's s.
Lorain-Lévi s.
Louis-Bar s.
Lowe's s.
Lowe-Terrey-MacLachlan s.
Lown-Ganong-Levine s.
low salt s., low sodium s.
lupus-like s.
Lutembacher's s.
Lyell's s.
Macleod's s.
Mad Hatter s.
Maffucci's s.
Magendie-Hertwig s.
malabsorption s.
malignant carcinoid s.
malignant mole s.
Mallory-Weiss s.
mandibulofacial dysotosis s.
mandibulo-oculofacial s.
Marañón's s.
Marchiafava-Micheli s.
Marcus Gunn s.
Marfan's s.
Marie-Robinson s.
Marinesco-Garland s.
Marinesco-Sjögren s.
Maroteaux-Lamy s.
Marshall s.
Martorell's s.
MASS s.
massive bowel resection s.
maternal deprivation s.
Mauriac's s.
Mayer-Rokitansky-Küster-Hauser s.
May-White s.
McArdle's s.
McCune-Albright s.
Meadows' s.
Meckel s.
Meckel-Gruber s.
meconium blockage s.
megacystic s.
megacystitis-megaureter s.

S

syndrome (*continued*)

megacystitis-microcolon-intestinal
hypoperistalsis s.
Meigs' s.
Melkersson-Rosenthal s.
Melnick-Needles s.
Mendelson's s.
Ménétrier's s.
Ménière's s.
Menkes' s.
menopausal s.
metastatic carcinoid s.
Meyenburg-Altherr-Uehlinger s.
Meyer-Betz s.
middle lobe s.
Mikulicz' s.
milk-alkali s.
Milkman's s.
Millard-Gubler s.
minimal-change nephrotic s.
Mirizzi's s.
mitral valve prolapse s.
Möbius' s.
Mohr's s.
Monakow's s.
Morgagni-Adams-Stokes s.
Morgagni's s.
morning glory s.
Morquio's s.
Morton's s.
Mounier-Kuhn s.
Mucha-Habermann s.
Muckle-Wells s.
mucocutaneous lymph node s.
Muir-Torre s.
multiple endocrine deficiency s.
multiple glandular deficiency s.
multiple hamartoma s.
multiple lentigines s.
multiple mucosal neuroma s.
Munchausen s.
Munchausen s. by proxy
Münchhausen s.
myasthenic s.
myeloproliferative s.'s
myofacial pain-dysfunction s.
myofascial s.
Naegeli s.
Naffziger s.
nail-patella s.
NAME s.
Nelson s.
nephritic s.
nephrotic s.
Netherton's s.
neural crest s.
neurocutaneous s.
neuroleptic malignant s.

Nezelof s.
Nieden's s.
Noack's s.
nonsense s.
Noonan's s.
Nothnagel's s.
nystagmus blockage s.
OAV s.
ocular-mucous membrane s.
oculobuccogenital s.
oculocerebrorenal s.
oculocutaneous s.
oculomandibulofacial s.
oculopharyngeal s.
oculovertebral s.
oculovestibulo-auditory s.
OFD s.
Ogilvie's s.
Omenn's s.
Oppenheim's s.
orbital s.
organic brain s.
organic mental s.
organic mood s.
orofaciodigital s.
osteomyelofibrotic s.
Ostrum-Furst s.
Othello s.
otomandibular s.
otopalatodigital s.
ovarian vein s.
pacemaker s.
pachydermoperiostosis s.
Paget-von Schrötter s.
painful-bruising s.
paleostriatal s.
pallidal s.
Pancoast s.
papillary muscle s.
Papillon-Léage and Psaume s.
Papillon-Lefèvre s.
paraneoplastic s.
Parinaud's s.
Parinaud's oculoglandular s.
Parsonage-Turner s.
Patau's s.
Paterson-Brown-Kelly s.
Paterson-Kelly s.
pathologic startle s.'s
Pellizzi's s.
Pendred's s.
Pepper s.
pericolic membrane s.
Persian Gulf s.
persistent müllerian duct s.
pertussis s.
pertussis-like s.
petrosphenoidal s.

Peutz-Jeghers s.
Peutz's s.
Pfaundler-Hurler s.
Pfeiffer's s.
pharyngeal pouch s.
phospholipid s.
Picchini's s.
Pick's s.
pickwickian s.
Pierre Robin s.
Pins' s.
placental dysfunction s.
Plummer-Vinson s.
PNP s. (*var. of* psychogenic
  nocturnal polydipsia s.)
POEMS s.
Poland's s.
polycystic ovary s.
polyendocrine deficiency s.,
  polyglandular deficiency s.
polysplenia s.
popliteal entrapment s.
postadrenalectomy s.
postcardiotomy s.
postcholecystectomy s.
postcommissurotomy s.
postconcussion s.
posterior inferior cerebellar
  artery s.
postgastrectomy s.
postmaturity s.
postmyocardial infarction s.
postpartum pituitary necrosis s.
postpericardiotomy s.
postphlebitic s.
postrubella s.
postthrombotic s.
posttraumatic s.
posttraumatic neck s.
posttraumatic stress s.
Potter's s.
Prader-Willi s.
precordial catch s.
preexcitation s.
preinfarction s.
premature senility s.
premenstrual s.
premenstrual salivary s.
premenstrual tension s.
premotor s.
prune belly s.
psychogenic nocturnal polydipsia s.,
  PNP s.
pterygium s.
pulmonary dysmaturity s.
punchdrunk s.
Putnam-Dana s.
radial aplasia-thrombocytopenia s.

radicular s.
Raeder's paratrigeminal s.
Ramsay Hunt's s.
Raynaud's s.
Refetoff s.
Refsum's s.
Reifenstein's s.
Reiter's s.
REM s.
Rendu-Osler-Weber s.
Renpenning's s.
residual ovary s.
resistant ovary s.
respiratory distress s. of the
  newborn
restless legs s.
retraction s.
Rett's s.
Reye's s.
Rh null s.
Richards-Rundle s.
Richter's s.
Rieger's s.
right ovarian vein s.
Riley-Day s.
Roaf's s.
Roberts s.
Robinow's s.
Robin's s.
Rokitansky-Küster-Hauser s.
Romano-Ward s.
Romberg's s.
Rothmund's s.
Rothmund-Thomson s.
Rotor's s.
Roussy-Lévy s.
Rubinstein-Taybi s.
Rud's s.
runting s.
Russell's s.
Saethre-Chotzen s.
Sakati-Nyhan s.
salt depletion s.
salt-losing s.
Samter's s.
Sanchez Salorio s.
Sanfilippo's s.
Savage s.
scalded skin s.
scalenus anterior s.
scapulocostal s.
Schanz s.
Schaumann's s.
Scheie's s.
Schmid-Fraccaro s.
Schmidt's s.
Schönlein-Henoch s.
Schüller's s.

S

syndrome *(continued)*
    Schwartz s.
    Seckel s.
    Secrétan's s.
    Senear-Usher s.
    Sertoli-cell-only s.
    Sézary s.
    Sheehan's s.
    Shone's s.
    short-bowel s.
    shoulder-girdle s.
    shoulder-hand s.
    Shulman's s.
    Shwachman s.
    Shy-Drager s.
    sicca s.
    sick building s.
    sick euthyroid s.
    sick sinus s.
    Silver-Russell s.
    Silverskiöld's s.
    sinus venosus s.
    Sipple's s.
    Sjögren-Larsson s.
    Sjögren's s.
    sleep apnea s.
    sleep phase delay s.
    SLE-like s.
    slit ventricle s.
    Smith-Lemli-Opitz s.
    Smith-Riley s.
    Sneddon's s.
    Sohval-Soffer s.
    Sorsby's s.
    Sotos' s.
    space adaptation s.
    Spens' s.
    splenic flexure s.
    staphylococcal scalded skin s.
    Stauffer's s.
    Steele-Richardson-Olszewski s.
    Stein-Leventhal s.
    steroid withdrawal s.
    Stevens-Johnson s.
    Stewart-Morel s.
    Stewart-Treves s.
    Stickler's s.
    stiff heart s.
    stiff-man s.
    Still-Chauffard s.
    Stockholm s.
    Stokes-Adams s.
    straight back s.
    Stryker-Halbeisen s.
    Sturge-Kalischer-Weber s.
    Sturge-Weber s.
    subclavian steal s.

    subcoracoid-pectoralis minor tendon s.
    sudden infant death s.
    Sudeck's s.
    Sulzberger-Garbe s.
    sump s.
    superior cerebellar artery s.
    superior mesenteric artery s.
    superior vena cava s.
    supine hypotensive s.
    supraspinatus s.
    supravalvar aortic stenosis s.
    supravalvar aortic stenosis-infantile hypercalcemia s.
    surdocardiac s.
    swollen belly s.
    Swyer-James s.
    Swyer-James-MacLeod s.
    tachybradycardia s.
    tachycardia-bradycardia s.
    Takayasu's s.
    Tapia's s.
    TAR s. *(var. of* thrombocytopenia-absent radius s.)
    tarsal tunnel s.
    Taussig-Bing s.
    tegmental s.
    temporomandibular s.
    temporomandibular joint pain-dysfunction s.
    tendon sheath s.
    Terry's s.
    tethered cord s.
    thalamic s.
    Thiemann's s.
    third and fourth pharyngeal pouch s.
    thoracic outlet s.
    Thorn's s.
    thrombocytopenia-absent radius s., TAR s.
    thrombopathic s.
    thyrohypophysial s.
    Tietze's s.
    Tolosa-Hunt s.
    tooth-and-nail s.
    TORCH s.
    Tornwaldt's s.
    Torre's s.
    Torsten Sjögren's s.
    Tourette s.
    toxic shock s.
    transplant lung s.
    transurethral resection s.
    Treacher Collins' s.
    trichorhinophalangeal s.
    triple X s.
    trisomy 8 s.

trisomy 13 s.
trisomy 18 s.
trisomy 20 s.
trisomy 21 s.
trisomy C s.
trisomy D s.
trochanteric s.
tropical splenomegaly s.
Trousseau's s.
true neurogenic thoracic outlet s.
tumor lysis s.
TUR s.
Turcot s.
twiddler's s.
Uhthoff s.
Ullmann's s.
Ulysses s.
unroofed coronary sinus s.
urethral s.
Usher's s.
uveocutaneous s.
uveo-encephalitic s.
uveomeningitis s.
VACTERL s.
van Buchem's s.
van der Hoeve's s.
vanished testis s.
vanishing lung s.
vasculocardiac s. of
  hyperserotonemia
vasovagal s.
Verner-Morrison s.
Vernet's s.
vertical retraction s.
vibration s.
virus-associated hemophagocytic s.
vitreoretinal choroidopathy s.
vitreoretinal traction s.
Vogt s.
Vogt-Koyanagi s.
Vohwinkel s.
von Hippel-Lindau s.
vulnerable child s.
Waardenburg s.
Wagner's s.
Waldenström's s.
Wallenberg's s.
Ward-Romano s.
wasting s.
Waterhouse-Friderichsen s.
WDHA s.
Weber-Cockayne s.
Weber's s.
Weill-Marchesani s.
Wells' s.
Werner's s.
Wernicke-Korsakoff s.
Wernicke's s.

West's s.
Weyers-Thier s.
whistling face s.
white-out s.
Widal's s.
Wildervanck s.
Williams' s.
Wilson-Mikity s.
Wilson's s.
Wiskott-Aldrich s.
Wissler's s.
Wolff-Parkinson-White s.
Wright's s.
Wyburn-Mason s.
XO s.
XXY s.
XYY s.
yellow nail s.
Zellweger s.
Zieve's s.
Zollinger-Ellison s.
syndromic
synechia, pl. **synechiae**
  annular s.
  anterior s.
  s. pericardii
  peripheral anterior s.
  posterior s.
  total s.
synechiotomy
synechotome
synectenterotomy
synencephalocele
syneresis
synergic control
synergistic muscles
synesthesia
  s. algica
synesthesialgia
Syngamidae
Syngamus
syngamy
syngeneic
  s. graft
syngenesioplasty
syngenesiotransplantation
syngenesis
syngenetic
syngenic
syngnathia
syngraft
synidrosis
synizesis
synkaryon
synkinesis
synkinetic
synonychia

S

synonym
    objective s.'s
    senior s.
    subjective s.'s
synophrys
synophthalmia
synophthalmus
synoptophore
synorchidism, synorchism
synoscheos
synosteology
synosteosis
synostosis
    sagittal s.
    tribasilar s.
synostotic
synotia
synovectomy
synovia
synovial
    s. bursa
    s. cell
    s. chondromatosis
    s. crypt
    s. cyst
    s. fluid
    s. fold
    s. frena
    s. frenula
    s. fringe
    s. glands
    s. hernia
    s. joint
    s. ligament
    s. membrane
    s. mesenchyme
    s. osteochondromatosis
    s. sarcoma
    s. sheath
    s. sheaths of digits of foot
    s. sheaths of digits of hand
    s. tendon sheath
    s. trochlear bursa
    s. tufts
    s. villi
synovioma
    malignant s.
synoviparous
synovitis
    bursal s.
    chronic hemorrhagic villous s.
    dry s.
    filarial s.
    pigmented villonodular s.
    purulent s.
    serous s.
    s. sicca
    suppurative s.

    tendinous s.
    vaginal s.
synovium
synpolydactyly
syntactical aphasia
syntactics
syntality
syntectic
syntenic
synteny
syntexis
synthermal
synthesis, pl. **syntheses**
    s. of continuity
synthetic dyes
synthorax
syntonic
    s. personality
syntrophism
syntrophoblast
syntropic
syntropy
    inverse s.
Syphacia
syphilemia
syphilid
    acneform s.
    acuminate papular s.
    annular s.
    bullous s.
    corymbose s.
    ecthymatous s.
    erythematous s.
    flat papular s.
    follicular s.
    frambesiform s.
    gummatous s.
    impetiginous s.
    lenticular s.
    macular s.
    miliary papular s.
    nodular s.
    nummular s.
    palmar s.
    papular s.
    papulosquamous s.
    pemphigoid s.
    pigmentary s.
    plantar s.
    pustular s.
    rupial s.
    secondary s.
    tertiary s.
    varioliform s.
syphilimetry
syphilionthus
syphilis
    cardiovascular s.

congenital s.
s. d'emblée
early s.
early latent s.
endemic s.
s. hereditaria
s. hereditaria tarda
hereditary s.
late s.
late benign s.
late latent s.
latent s.
meningovascular s.
nonvenereal s.
primary s.
quaternary s.
secondary s.
tertiary s.

syphilitic
s. abscess
s. aneurysm
s. aortitis
s. cirrhosis
s. fever
s. leukoderma
s. meningoencephalitis
s. nephritis
s. osteochondritis
s. retinitis
s. roseola
s. teeth
s. ulcer

syphiloderm, syphiloderma
syphiloid
syphilologist
syphilology
syphiloma
s. of Fournier
syphilomatous
Syriac ulcer
Syrian ulcer
syrigmus
syringadenoma
syringadenosus
syringe
air s.
chip s.
control s.
Davidson s.
dental s.
fountain s.
hypodermic s.
Luer s.
Luer-Lok s.
Neisser's s.
probe s.
ring s.

Roughton-Scholander s.
rubber-bulb s.
syringeal
syringectomy
syringitis
syringoadenoma
syringobulbia
syringocarcinoma
syringocele
syringocystadenoma
s. papilliferum
syringocystoma
syringoencephalomyelia
syringoid
syringoma
chondroid s.
syringomeningocele
syringomyelia
syringomyelic
s. dissociation
s. hemorrhage
syringomyelocele
syringomyelus
syringopontia
syringotome
syringotomy
syssarcosic
syssarcosis
syssarcotic
systaltic
system
absorbent s.
alimentary s.
anterolateral s.
arch-loop-whorl s.
association s.
autonomic nervous s.
Bethesda s.
blood group s.'s
blood-vascular s.
bulbosacral s.
cardiovascular s.
central nervous s.
cerebrospinal s.
chromaffin s.
circulatory s.
conducting s. of heart
craniosacral s.
dermal s., dermoid s.
digestive s.
ecological s.
endocrine s.
esthesiodic s.
exterofective s.
extrapyramidal motor s.
feedback s.
gamma motor s.
genital s.

S

system (*continued*)
    genitourinary s.
    glandular s.
    haversian s.
    hematopoietic s.
    hepatic portal s.
    hexaxial reference s.
    His-Tawara s.
    hypophyseoportal s.
    hypophysial portal s.
    hypophysioportal s.
    hypothalamohypophysial portal s.
    hypoxia warning s.
    immune s.
    indicator s.
    information s.
    integumentary s.
    intermediary s.
    interofective s.
    involuntary nervous s.
    kallikrein s.
    kinetic s.
    limbic s.
    lymphatic s.
    s. of macrophages
    masticatory s.
    metameric nervous s.
    mononuclear phagocyte s.
    muscular s.
    nervous s.
    neuromuscular s.
    nonspecific s.
    occlusal s.
    oculomotor s.
    parasympathetic nervous s.
    pedal s.
    peripheral nervous s.
    Pinel's s.
    portal s.
    pressoreceptor s.
    projection s.
    properdin s.
    Purkinje s.
    renal portal s.
    renin-angiotensin-aldosterone s.
    reproductive s.
    respiratory s.
    reticular activating s.
    reticuloendothelial s.
    second signaling s.
    skeletal s.
    somesthetic s.
    static s.
    stomatognathic s.
    sympathetic nervous s.
    T s.
    thoracolumbar s.
    triaxial reference s.

    urinary s.
    urogenital s.
    uropoietic s.
    vascular s.
    vegetative nervous s.
    vertebral-basilar s.
    vertebral venous s.
    visceral nervous s.

systema
    s. alimentarium
    s. digestorium
    s. lymphaticum
    s. nervosum
    s. nervosum autonomicum
    s. nervosum centrale
    s. nervosum periphericum
    s. respiratorium
    s. skeletale
    s. urogenitale

systematic
    s. anatomy
    s. bacteriology
    s. desensitization

systematization

systematized
    s. delusion
    s. nevus

systemic
    s. anaphylaxis
    s. anatomy
    s. autoimmune diseases
    s. blastomycosis
    s. chondromalacia
    s. circulation
    s. death
    s. febrile diseases
    s. heart
    s. hyalinosis
    s. lupus erythematosus
    s. mastocytosis
    s. myelitis
    s. sclerosis
    s. vascular resistance
    s. venous hypertension

systemoid

systole
    aborted s.
    s. alternans
    atrial s.
    auricular s.
    electrical s.
    electromechanical s.
    extra-s.
    late s.
    premature s.
    ventricular s.

systolic
    s. bruit

s. click
s. ejection fraction
s. gallop
s. gallop rhythm
s. gradient
s. honk
s. murmur
s. pressure
s. shock
s. thrill

s. time intervals
s. whoop
systolic/diastolic ratio
systolometer
systremma
syzygial
syzygiology
syzygium
syzygy

S

T

T agglutinogen
T antigens
T cell
T cell antigen receptors
T cell-rich, B cell lymphoma
T cytotoxic cells
T fiber
T helper cells
T lymphocyte
T myelotomy
T system
T tube
T tubule
T wave

T1
T2
t

t distribution
t test

tabanid
Tabanidae
Tabanus
tabardillo
tabatière anatomique
tabby cat striation
tabes

t. diabetica
t. dorsalis
t. ergotica
t. infantum
t. mesenterica
peripheral t.
t. spasmodica
t. spinalis

tabescence
tabescent
tabetic

t. arthropathy
t. crisis
t. cuirass
t. dissociation
t. neurosyphilis

tabetiform
tabic
tabid
tablature
table

Aub-DuBois t.
contingency t.
examining t.
Gaffky t.
inner t. of skull
life t.
occlusal t.

operating t.
outer t. of skull
Reuss' color t.'s
Stilling color t.'s
tilt t.
vitreous t.

taboo, tabu
taboparesis
tabular
Tac antigen
Tacaribe

T. complex of viruses
T. virus

tache

t. blanche
t. bleuâtre
t. cérébrale
t. laiteuse
t. méningéale
t. noire
t. spinale

tachetic
tachistesthesia
tachistoscope
tachogram
tachograph
tachography
tachometer
tachyarrhythmia
tachyauxesis
tachybradycardia syndrome
tachycardia

atrial t.
atrial chaotic t.
atrioventricular junctional t.
auricular t.
A-V junctional t.
bidirectional ventricular t.
Coumel's t.
double t.
ectopic t.
t. en salves
essential t.
t. exophthalmica
fetal t.
junctional t.
nodal t.
orthostatic t.
paroxysmal t.
reflex t.
sinus t.
supraventricular t.
ventricular t.
t. window

tachycardia-bradycardia syndrome

T

tachycardiac
tachycardic
tachycrotic
tachylalia
tachylogia
tachypacing
tachyphagia
tachyphasia
tachyphemia
tachyphrasia
tachypnea
tachyrhythmia
tachysystole
tachyzoite
tactile
    t. agnosia
    t. anesthesia
    t. cell
    t. corpuscle
    t. disk
    t. elevations
    t. fremitus
    t. hallucination
    t. hyperesthesia
    t. image
    t. meniscus
    t. organ
    t. papilla
    t. sense
taction
tactometer
tactor
tactual
    T. Performance Test
tadpole-shaped pupil
Taenia
    T. africana
    T. armata
    T. crassicollis
    T. demerariensis
    T. dentata
    T. equina
    T. hominis
    T. hydatigena
    T. madagascariensis
    T. minima
    T. ovis
    T. philippina
    T. pisiformis
    T. quadrilobata
    T. saginata
    T. solium
    T. taeniaeformis
taenia
Taeniarhynchus
taeniid
Taeniidae
taenioid

Taeniorhynchus
Taenzer's stain
tag
    anal skin t.
    epiploic t.'s
    sentinel t.
    skin t.
tagliacotian operation
Tahyna virus
tail
    t. bone
    t. bud
    t. of caudate nucleus
    t. of dentate gyrus
    t. of epididymis
    t. fold
    t. of helix
    t. of pancreas
    t. sheath
    t. vertebrae
tailgut
tailor's
    t. cramp
    t. muscle
    t. spasm
Tait's law
Takahara's disease
Takayama's stain
Takayasu's
    T. arteritis
    T. disease
    T. syndrome
take
talalgia
talar
    t. articular surface of calcaneus
    t. sulcus
talc operation
talcosis
    pulmonary t.
tali (*gen. of* talus)
talion
    t. dread
talipedic
talipes
    t. arcuatus
    t. calcaneovalgus
    t. calcaneovarus
    t. calcaneus
    t. cavus
    t. equinovalgus
    t. equinovarus
    t. equinus
    t. plantaris
    t. planus
    t. spasmodicus
    t. transversoplanus

t. valgus
t. varus
talipomanus
Tallerman treatment
talocalcaneal, talocalcanean
t. joint
t. ligament
talocalcaneonavicular joint
talocrural
t. articulation
t. joint
talofibular
talonavicular
t. joint
t. ligament
talon cusp
taloscaphoid
talotibial
talus, gen. **tali**
tambour
t. sound
Tamm-Horsfall
T.-H. mucoprotein
T.-H. protein
tampon
Corner's t.
tamponade, tamponage
cardiac t.
chronic t.
heart t.
tamponing, tamponment
tangentiality
tangential wound
tangent screen
Tangier disease
tangle
neurofibrillary t.
tank
Hubbard t.
t. respirator
tanned red cells
Tanner
T. growth chart
T. stage
tanner's ulcer
tantalum bronchography
tantrum
tanycyte
tanyphonia
tap
heel t.
mitral t.
pericardial t.
spinal t.
tape
tapered bougie
tapeta (*pl. of* tapetum)
tapetochoroidal

tapetoretinal
t. degeneration
tapetoretinopathy
tapetum, pl. **tapeta**
t. alveoli
t. nigrum
t. oculi
tapeworm
taphophilia
taphophobia
Tapia's syndrome
tapinocephalic
tapinocephaly
tapir mouth
tapotement
tapping
tar
t. acne
t. keratosis
tarantism
tarantula
American t.
black t.
European t.
Peruvian t.
Tardieu's
T. ecchymoses
T. petechiae
T. spots
tardive
cyanose t.
t. cyanosis
t. dyskinesia
target
t. behavior
t. cell
t. cell anemia
t. gland
t. organ
t. patient
t. response
Tarin's
T. space
T. tenia
T. valve
Tarlov's cyst
Tarnier's forceps
tarry cyst
tarsadenitis
tarsal
t. arch
t. bones
t. canal
t. cartilage
t. cyst
t. fold
t. glands
t. joints

T

tarsal *(continued)*
    t. ligaments
    t. plates
    t. sinus
    t. tunnel syndrome
tarsale, pl. **tarsalia**
tarsalgia
tarsalis
tarsectomy
tarsectopia, tarsectopy
tarsen
tarsi (*gen. and pl. of* tarsus)
tarsitis
tarsochiloplasty
tarsoclasia, tarsoclasis
tarsoepiphyseal aclasis
tarsomalacia
tarsomegaly
tarsometatarsal
    t. joints
    t. ligaments
tarso-orbital
tarsophalangeal
    t. reflex
tarsophyma
tarsorrhaphy
tarsotarsal
tarsotibial
    t. amputation
tarsotomy
tarsus, gen. and pl. **tarsi**
    t. inferior
    inferior t.
    t. superior
    superior t.
TAR syndrome
tart cell
tartrazine
taste
    after-t.
    t. blindness
    t. bud
    t. bulb
    t. cells
    color t.
    t. corpuscle
    t. deficiency
    franklinic t.
    t. hairs
    t. pore
    t. ridge
    voltaic t.
TATA box
tattoo
    amalgam t.
taurodontism

Taussig-Bing
    T.-B. disease
    T.-B. syndrome
tautomenial
tautomeric fibers
Tawara's node
taxis
    bipolar t.
    negative t.
    positive t.
Taylor's
    T. apparatus
    T. back brace
    T. disease
    T. splint
Tay-Sachs disease
Tay's cherry-red spot
T-cell
    T.-c. growth factor
    T.-c. growth factor-1
    T.-c. growth factor-2
^{99m}Tc pyrophosphate
T-dependent antigen
TDTH cells
teachers' nodes
teaching hospital
Teale's amputation
tear
    artificial t.'s
    bucket-handle t.
    crocodile t.'s
    t. film
    Mallory-Weiss t.
    t. sac
    t. stone
tearing
tease
teat
technetium-99
technetium-99m
    ^{99m}Tc diphosphonate
    ^{99m}Tc-DPTA
    ^{99m}Tc sulfur colloid
technic
technical error
technician
technique
    airbrasive t.
    air-gap t.
    atrial-well t.
    Barcroft-Warburg t.
    Begg light wire differential
      force t.
    cellulose tape t.
    direct t.
    Ficoll-Hypaque t.
    flicker fusion frequency t.
    fluorescent antibody t.

flush t.
Hampton t.
Hartel t.
high-kV t.
immunoperoxidase t.
indirect t.
Jerne t.
Judkins t.
long cone t.
McGoon's t.
Merendino's t.
microetching t.
Mohs' fresh tissue chemosurgery t.
PAP t.
rebreathing t.
Rebuck skin window t.
sealed jar t.
Seldinger t.
washed field t.

technocausis
technologist
technology
assisted reproductive t.
tecta (*pl. of* tectum)
tectal
t. nucleus
t. stria
tectiform
Tectiviridae
tectobulbar tract
tectocephalic
tectocephaly
tectology
tectonic
t. keratoplasty
tectopontine tract
tectorial
t. membrane
t. membrane of cochlear duct
tectorium
tectospinal
t. decussation
t. tract
tectum, pl. **tecta**
t. mesencephali
teeth (*pl. of* tooth)
teething
T-E fistula
tegmen, gen. **tegminis**, pl. **tegmina**
t. cruris
t. mastoideum
t. tympani
t. ventriculi quarti
tegmenta (*pl. of* tegmentum)
tegmental
t. decussations
t. fields of Forel
t. nuclei

t. syndrome
t. wall of middle ear
tegmentotomy
tegmentum, pl. **tegmenta**
t. mesencephali
mesencephalic t.
midbrain t.
t. of pons
t. rhombencephali
rhombencephalic t.
t. of rhombencephalon
tegmina (*pl. of* tegmen)
tegminis (*gen. of* tegmen)
tegument
tegumental, tegumentary
teichopsia
tela, gen. and pl. **telae**
t. choroidea
t. choroidea inferior
t. choroidea superior
t. choroidea ventriculi quarti
t. choroidea ventriculi tertii
choroid t. of fourth ventricle
choroid t. of third ventricle
t. conjunctiva
t. elastica
t. subcutanea
t. submucosa
t. submucosa pharyngis
t. subserosa
t. vasculosa
Teladorsagia davtiani
telalgia
telangiectasia
ataxia t., ataxia-t.
cephalo-oculocutaneous t.
essential t.
hereditary hemorrhagic t.
t. lymphatica
t. macularis eruptiva perstans
primary t.
secondary t.
spider t.
t. verrucosa
telangiectasis, pl. **telangiectases**
telangiectatic
t. angioma
t. angiomatosis
t. cancer
t. fibroma
t. glioma
t. lipoma
t. osteogenic sarcoma
t. wart
telangiectodes
telangioma
telangion
telangiosis

T

telecanthus
telecardiogram
telecardiophone
telecobalt
telediagnosis
telediastolic
telehopsias
telelectrocardiogram
telemetry
    cardiac t.
telencephalic
    t. flexure
    t. vesicle
telencephalization
telencephalon
teleology
teleomitosis
teleomorph
teleonomic
teleonomy
teleopsia
teleorganic
telepathy
telephone theory
teleradiography
teleradiology
teleradium
    t. therapy
telereceptor
telergy
teleroentgenography
teleroentgentherapy
telescopic
    t. denture
    t. spectacles
telesis
telesystolic
teletactor
teletherapy
television microscope
TeLinde operation
tellurism
telocentric chromosome
telodendron
telogen
    t. effluvium
teloglia
telognosis
telokinesia
telolecithal
    t. ovum
telomere
telomeric R-banding stain
telophase
Telosporea
Telosporidia
telotism
temper

temperament
temperance
temperate
    t. bacteriophage
    t. virus
temperature
    basal body t.
    maximum t.
    minimum t.
    optimum t.
    room t.
    t. sense
    t. spot
temperature-compensated vaporizer
template
    surgical t.
temple
tempora (*pl. of* tempus)
temporal
    t. aponeurosis
    t. apophysis
    t. arteritis
    t. bone
    t. branch of facial nerve
    t. canal
    t. contiguity
    t. cortex
    t. dispersion
    t. fascia
    t. fossa
    t. horn
    t. line
    t. lobe
    t. lobe epilepsy
    t. muscle
    t. plane
    t. pole
    t. pole of cerebrum
    t. process
    t. region of head
    t. ridge
    t. squama
    t. surface
    t. veins
    t. venules of retina
temporalis
    t. muscle
temporary
    t. base
    t. callus
    t. cartilage
    t. denture
    t. parasite
    t. restoration
    t. stricture
    t. tooth
temporis (*gen. of* tempus)
temporoauricular

temporofrontal tract
temporohyoid
temporomalar
temporomandibular
    t. arthrosis
    t. articular disk
    t. articulation
    t. joint
    t. joint dysfunction
    t. joint pain-dysfunction syndrome
    t. ligament
    t. nerve
    t. syndrome
temporomaxillary
    t. vein
temporo-occipital
temporoparietal
    t. muscle
temporoparietalis muscle
temporopontine
    t. tract
temporosphenoid
temporozygomatic
    t. suture
temps utile
tempus, gen. temporis, pl. tempora
tenacious
tenacity
    cellular t.
tenaculum, pl. tenacula
    t. forceps
    tenacula tendinum
tenalgia
    t. crepitans
tender
    t. lines
    t. points
    t. zones
tenderness
    pencil t.
    rebound t.
tendines (pl. of tendo)
tendinis (gen. of tendo)
tendinitis
tendinoplasty
tendinosuture
tendinous
    t. arch
    t. arch of levator ani muscle
    t. arch of pelvic fascia
    t. arch of soleus muscle
    t. chiasm of the digital tendons
    t. cords
    t. inscription
    t. intersection
    t. opening
    t. spot

    t. synovitis
    t. xanthoma
tendo, gen. tendinis, pl. tendines
    t. Achillis
    t. Achillis reflex
    t. calcaneus
    t. conjunctivus
    t. cricoesophageus
    t. oculi
    t. palpebrarum
tendolysis
tendon
    Achilles t.
    t. advancement
    t. bundle
    calcanean t.
    t. cells
    central t. of diaphragm
    central t. of perineum
    conjoined t.
    conjoint t.
    coronary t.
    cricoesophageal t.
    Gerlach's annular t.
    t. graft
    hamstring t.
    heel t.
    t. recession
    t. reflex
    t. sheath of abductor pollicis
      longus and extensor pollicis
      brevis muscles
    t. sheath of extensor carpi radialis
      muscles
    t. sheath of extensor carpi ulnaris
      muscle
    t. sheath of extensor digiti minimi
      muscle
    t. sheath of extensor digitorum and
      extensor indicis muscles
    t. sheath of extensor digitorum
      longus muscle of foot
    t. sheath of extensor hallucis
      longus muscle
    t. sheath of extensor pollicis
      longus muscle
    t. sheath of flexor carpi radialis
      muscle
    t. sheath of flexor digitorum
      longus muscle of foot
    t. sheath of flexor hallucis longus
      muscle
    t. sheath of flexor pollicis longus
      muscle
    t. sheath of superior oblique
      muscle
    t. sheath syndrome
    t. sheath of tibialis anterior muscle

T

tendon (*continued*)
    t. sheath of tibialis posterior
      muscle
    t. suture
    Todaro's t.
    t. transplantation
    trefoil t.
    Zinn's t.
tendonitis
tendophony
tendoplasty
tendosynovitis
tendotomy
tendovaginal
tendovaginitis
    radial styloid t.
tenectomy
tenesmic
tenesmus
ten Horn's sign
tenia, pl. **teniae**
    teniae acusticae
    t. choroidea
    teniae coli
    colic teniae
    t. fimbriae
    t. fornicis
    t. of the fornix
    t. of fourth ventricle
    free t.
    t. hippocampi
    t. libera
    medullary teniae
    mesocolic t.
    t. mesocolica
    omental t.
    t. omentalis
    t. semicircularis
    Tarin's t.
    t. tecta
    t. telae
    t. terminalis
    t. thalami
    thalamic t.
    teniae of Valsalva
    t. ventriculi quarti
    t. ventriculi tertii
tenial
teniasis
    somatic t.
teniform
tenifugal
tenioid
teniola
    t. corporis callosi
tennis
    t. elbow

    t. leg
    t. thumb
tenodesis
tenodynia
tenofibril
tenolysis
tenomyoplasty
tenomyotomy
tenonectomy
tenonitis
Tenon's
    T. capsule
    T. space
tenontitis
tenontodynia
tenontography
tenontolemmitis
tenontology
tenontomyoplasty
tenontomyotomy
tenontoplastic
tenontoplasty
tenontothecitis
tenophony
tenophyte
tenoplastic
tenoplasty
tenoreceptor
tenorrhaphy
tenositis
tenostosis
tenosuspension
tenosuture
tenosynovectomy
tenosynovitis
    t. crepitans
    localized nodular t.
    villonodular pigmented t.
    villous t.
tenotomy
    curb t.
    graduated t.
    subcutaneous t.
tenovaginitis
tense
    t. part of the tympanic membrane
    t. pulse
tensile stress
tensiometer
tension
    arterial t.
    t. curve
    t. headache
    interfacial surface t.
    ocular t.
    t. pneumothorax
    premenstrual t.

t. suture
tissue t.
tensor, pl. **tensores**
t. fasciae latae muscle
t. muscle of fascia lata
t. muscle of soft palate
t. muscle of tympanic membrane
t. tarsi muscle
t. tympani muscle
t. veli palati muscle
tent
oxygen t.
sponge t.
tenth cranial nerve
tentorial
t. angle
t. nerve
t. notch
t. sinus
t. surface
tentorium, pl. **tentoria**
t. cerebelli
t. of hypophysis
tephromalacia
tephrylometer
teras, pl. **terata**
teratic
teratism
teratoblastoma
teratocarcinoma
teratogenesis
teratogenic, teratogenetic
teratoid
t. tumor
teratologic
teratology
teratoma
t. orbitae
sacrococcygeal t.
triphyllomatous t.
teratomatous
t. cyst
teratophobia
teratosis
atresic t.
ceasmic t.
ectogenic t.
ectopic t.
hypergenic t.
symphysic t.
teratospermia
terebrant, terebrating
terebration
teres, gen. **teretis**, pl. **teretes**
t. major muscle
t. minor muscle
tergal
tergum

term
t. infant
terminad
terminal
t. artery
axon t.'s
t. bar
t. boutons
t. bronchiole
t. cisternae
t. crest
t. deletion
t. disinfection
t. endocarditis
t. filum
t. ganglion
t. hair
t. hematuria
t. hinge position
t. ileitis
t. ileus
t. infection
t. jaw relation record
t. leukocytosis
t. line
t. nerve corpuscles
t. nerves
t. notch of auricle
t. nuclei
t. part
t. plate
t. pneumonia
t. sinus
t. stria
t. sulcus
synaptic t.'s
t. thread
t. vein
t. ventricle
t. web
terminatio, pl. **terminationes**
terminationes nervorum liberae
termination
termino-terminal anastomosis
terminus, pl. **termini**
termini generales
termone
terrace
Terrien's
T. marginal degeneration
T. valve
territorial matrix
Terry's
T. nails
T. syndrome
Terson's glands
tertian
double t.

T

tertian (*continued*)
  t. fever
  t. malaria
  t. parasite
tertiarism, tertiarismus
tertiary
  t. amputation
  t. cortex
  t. dentin
  t. egg membrane
  t. medical care
  t. syphilid
  t. syphilis
  t. villus
  t. vitreous
Teschen disease virus
Tesla current
tessellated
  t. fundus
Tessier classification
test
  ABLB t. (*var. of* alternate binaural
    loudness balance t.)
  acetone t.
  achievement t.
  acidified serum t.
  acid perfusion t.
  acid phosphatase t. for semen
  acid reflux t.
  ACTH stimulation t.
  Addis t.
  adhesion t.
  Adler's t.
  Adson's t.
  agglutination t.
  Albarran's t.
  alkali denaturation t.
  Allen-Doisy t.
  Allen's t.
  Almén's t. for blood
  Alpha t.
  alternate binaural loudness
    balance t., ABLB t.
  alternate cover t.
  alternating light t.
  Ames t.
  Amsler t.
  Anderson-Collip t.
  Anderson and Goldberger t.
  anoxemia t.
  antibiotic sensitivity t.
  antiglobulin t.
  antihuman globulin t.
  antithrombin t.
  Apt t.
  aptitude t.
  Army Alpha t.
  Army Beta t.'s

Army General Classification T.
Aschheim-Zondek t.
Ascoli's t.
ascorbate-cyanide t.
association t.
Astwood's t.
atropine t.
augmented histamine t.
aussage t.
autohemolysis t.
A.-Z. t.
Bachman t.
Bachman-Pettit t.
Bagolini t.
BALB t.
Bárány's caloric t.
BEI t.
belt t.
Bender gestalt t.
Bender Visual Motor Gestalt t.
Benedict's t. for glucose
bentiromide t.
bentonite flocculation t.
benzidine t.
Bernstein t.
Berson t.
Beta t.'s
Betke-Kleihauer t.
Bettendorff's t.
bile acid tolerance t.
bile esculin t.
bile solubility t.
binaural alternate loudness
  balance t.
Binet t.
Binz' t.
biuret t.
blind t.
block design t.
Bonney t.
breath analysis t.
breath-holding t.
bromphenol t.
bromsulphalein t.
BSP t.
butanol-extractable iodine t.
California psychological inventory t.
Calmette t.
caloric t.
CAMP t.
cancer antigen 125 t.
capillary fragility t.
capillary resistance t.
capon-comb-growth t.
carbohydrate utilization t.
carotid sinus t.
Carr-Price t.
Casoni intradermal t.

Casoni skin t.
CF t.
Chick-Martin t.
chi-square t.
clomiphene t.
coccidioidin t.
coin t.
cold bend t.
cold pressor t.
colloidal gold t.
colorimetric caries susceptibility t.
comb-growth t.
complement-fixation t.
contraction stress t.
Coombs' t.
Corner-Allen t.
cover t.
cover-uncover t.
CO_2-withdrawal seizure t.
Crampton t.
t.'s of criminal responsibility
t. cross
cutaneous t.
cutaneous tuberculin t.
cutireaction t.
cyanide-nitroprusside t.
cytotropic antibody t.
DA pregnancy t.
d-dimer t.
Dehio's t.
dehydrocholate t.
Denver Developmental Screening T.
dexamethasone suppression t.
Dick t.
differential renal function t.
differential ureteral catheterization t.
dinitrophenylhydrazine t.
direct Coombs' t.
direct fluorescent antibody t.
Doerfler-Stewart t.
double (gel) diffusion precipitin t.
  in one dimension
double (gel) diffusion precipitin t.
  in two dimensions
Dragendorff's t.
drawer t.
D-S t.
Ducrey t.
Dugas' t.
Duke bleeding time t.
dye exclusion t.
Ebbinghaus t.
Ellsworth-Howard t.
E-rosette t.
erythrocyte adherence t.
erythrocyte fragility t.
ether t.
exercise t.

FANA t. (*var. of* fluorescent
  antinuclear antibody t.)
Farnsworth-Munsell color t.
fern t.
ferric chloride t.
Fevold t.
Finckh t.
finger-nose t.
finger-to-finger t.
Fishberg concentration t.
Fisher's exact t.
fistula t.
FIT t.
Fleitmann's t.
flocculation t.
fluorescein instillation t.
fluorescein string t.
fluorescent antinuclear antibody t.,
  FANA t.
fluorescent treponemal antibody-
  absorption t.
foam stability t.
Folin-Looney t.
Folin's t.
Fosdick-Hansen-Epple t.
Foshay t.
fragility t.
Frei t.
Fridenberg's stigometric card t.
FTA-ABS t.
fusion-inferred threshold t.
Gaddum and Schild t.
galactose tolerance t.
gel diffusion precipitin t.'s
gel diffusion precipitin t.'s in one
  dimension
gel diffusion precipitin t.'s in two
  dimensions
Gellé t.
Geraghty's t.
Gerhardt's t. for urobilin in the
  urine
germ tube t.
glucose oxidase paper strip t.
glucose tolerance t.
Gmelin's t.
Gofman t.
Goldscheider's t.
gold sol t.
Goodenough draw-a-man t.
goodness of fit t.
Göthlin's t.
Graham-Cole t.
group t.
guaiac t.
Guthrie t.
Gutzeit's t.
Ham's t.

T

test *(continued)*

t. handle instrument
Hardy-Rand-Ritter t.
Harrington-Flocks t.
Harris t.
Harris and Ray t.
head-dropping t.
heat coagulation t.
heat instability t.
heel-tap t.
heel-to-knee-to-toe t.
heel-to-shin t.
Heinz body t.
hemadsorption virus t.
hemagglutination t.
hemoccult t.
Hering's t.
Hess' t.
Hines-Brown t.
Hinton t.
Histalog t.
histamine t.
histoplasmin-latex t.
Hollander t.
Holmgren's wool t.
homovanillic acid t.
Hooker-Forbes t.
Howard t.
Huhner t.
HVA t.
17-hydroxycorticosteroid t.
hyperventilation t.
hypoxemia t.
immune adhesion t.
immunologic pregnancy t.
indirect t.
indirect Coombs' t.
indirect fluorescent antibody t.
indirect hemagglutination t.
indole t.
t. injection
inkblot t.
insulin hypoglycemia t.
intelligence t.
iodine t.
Ishihara t.
isopropanol precipitation t.
Ito-Reenstierna t.
^{131}I uptake t.
Ivy bleeding time t.
Jaffe's t.
Janet's t.
Jolles' t.
Jones' t.
Katayama's t.
ketogenic corticoids t.
17-ketogenic steroid assay t.
Kirby-Bauer t.

Knoop hardness t.
Kober t.
Kolmer t.
Korotkoff's t.
Kurzrok-Ratner t.
Kveim t.
Kveim-Stilzbach t.
Lachman t.
Landsteiner-Donath t.
Lange's t.
latex agglutination t.
latex fixation t.
LE cell t.
Legal's t.
leishmanin t.
lepromin t.
t. letter
leukocyte adherence assay t.
leukocyte bactericidal assay t.
Liebermann-Burchard t.
limulus lysate t.
lipase t.
Lombard voice-reflex t.
Lücke's t.
lupus band t.
lupus erythematosus cell t.
Machado-Guerreiro t.
Maclagan's t.
Maclagan's thymol turbidity t.
macrophage migration inhibition t.
Mantel-Haenszel t.
Mantoux t.
Marshall t.
Marshall-Marchetti t.
Master t.
Master's two-step exercise t.
Mauthner's t.
maximal Histalog t.
Mazzotti t.
McMurray t.
McNemar's t.
McPhail t.
t. meal
Meinicke t.
Meltzer-Lyon t.
metabisulfite t.
3-methoxy-4-hydroxymandelic
  acid t.
metrotrophic t.
MHA-TP t.
microhemagglutination-Treponema
  pallidum t.
microprecipitation t.
migration inhibition t.
migration inhibitory factor t.
Millon Clinical Multiaxial
  Inventory t.

Minnesota multiphasic personality inventory t.
mixed agglutination t.
mixed lymphocyte culture t.
MLC t.
Moloney t.
Montenegro t.
Mörner's t.
Moschcowitz t.
Mosenthal t.
motility t.
Motulsky dye reduction t.
mucin clot t.
multiple puncture tuberculin t.
multiple sleep latency t.
mumps sensitivity t.
Nagel's t.
neutralization t.
niacin t.
Nickerson-Kveim t.
nitroblue tetrazolium t.
nitroprusside t.
nonstress t.
nystagmus t.
Obermayer's t.
t. object
17-OH-corticoids t.
oral lactose tolerance t.
Ouchterlony t.
oxidase t.
Pachon's t.
Palmer acid t. for peptic ulcer
palmin t., palmitin t.
pancreozymin-secretin t.
Pandy's t.
Pap t.
Papanicolaou smear t.
parallax t.
parametric t.
passive cutaneous anaphylaxis t.
patch t.
Patrick's t.
Paul-Bunnell t.
Paul's t.
PBI t.
pentagastrin t.
performance t.
Perls' t.
personality t.
Perthes' t.
phenolsulfonphthalein t.
phentolamine t.
photo-patch t.
photostress t.
phrenic pressure t.
phthalein t.
Pirquet's t.
pivot shift t.

P-K t.
plasmacrit t.
platelet aggregation t.
polyuria t.
Porges-Meier t.
Porter-Silber chromogens t.
P and P t.
precipitation t.
precipitin t.
prism cover t.
prism vergence t.
t. profile
projective t.
protection t.
protein-bound iodine t.
prothrombin t.
prothrombin and proconvertin t.
provocative t.
provocative Wassermann t.
psychological t.'s
psychomotor t.'s
pulp t.
Q tip t.
Queckenstedt-Stookey t.
quellung t.
Quick's t.
quinine carbacrylic resin t.
Quinlan's t.
radioactive iodide uptake t.
radioallergosorbent t.
radioimmunosorbent t.
RAI t.
rapid plasma reagin t.
Rapoport t.
Rayleigh t.
red t.
red cell adherence t.
Reinsch's t.
Reiter t.
resorcinol t.
Reuss' t.
Rh blocking t.
Rickles t.
Rimini's t.
ring t.
ring precipitin t.
Rinne's t.
Romberg t.
Römer's t.
Ropes t.
Rorschach t.
rose bengal radioactive (^{131}I) t.
Rosenbach-Gmelin t.
Rosenbach's t.
rosette t.
Rose-Waaler t.
Ross-Jones t.
Rothera's nitroprusside t.

T

test *(continued)*
Rowntree and Geraghty t.
RPR t.
rubella HI t.
Rubin t.
Rubner's t.
Rumpel-Leede t.
Sabin-Feldman dye t.
Sachs-Georgi t.
Saundby's t.
scarification t.
Schaffer's t.
Schellong t.
Schick t.
Schiller's t.
Schilling t.
Schirmer t.
Schönbein's t.
Schwabach t.
scratch t.
screening t.
Seashore t.
secretin t.
Selivanoff's t.
shadow t.
shake t.
sickle cell t.
single (gel) diffusion precipitin t. in one dimension
single (gel) diffusion precipitin t. in two dimensions
SISI t.
situational t.
skin t.
skin-puncture t.
small increment sensitivity index t.
sniff t.
Snyder's t.
solubility t.
spironolactone t.
split renal function t.
spot t. for infectious mononucleosis
standard serologic t.'s for syphilis, STS for syphilis
standing t.
standing plasma t.
starch-iodine t.
station t.
Stein's t.
Stenger t.
Stewart's t.
Strassburg's t.
stress t.
string t.
Strong vocational interest t.
STS for syphilis (*var. of* standard serologic t.'s for syphilis)
Student's *t* t.

Stypven time t.
sucrose hemolysis t.
sulfosalicylic acid turbidity t.
sweat t.
sweating t.
swinging light t.
swordfish t.
t. symbols
t t.
Tactual Performance T.
thematic apperception t.
thermostable opsonin t.
Thompson's t.
Thormählen's t.
Thorn t.
three-glass t.
thymol turbidity t.
thyroid-stimulating hormone stimulation t., TSH stimulating t.
thyroid suppression t.
thyrotropin-releasing hormone stimulation t., TRH stimulation t.
tilt t.
tine t.
titratable acidity t.
tolbutamide t.
tone decay t.
Töpfer's t.
total catecholamine t.
tourniquet t.
TPHA t.
TPI t.
Trendelenburg's t.
Treponema pallidum hemagglutination t.
Treponema pallidum immobilization t., TPH t.
TRH stimulation t. (*var. of* thyrotropin-releasing hormone stimulation t.)
triiodothyronine uptake t.
TSH stimulating t. (*var. of* thyroid-stimulating hormone stimulation t.)
t. tube
tuberculin t.
T_3 uptake t.
two-glass t.
two-step exercise t.
two-tail t.
t. type
Tzanck t.
urea clearance t.
urease t.
urecholine supersensitivity t.
urinary concentration t.
vaginal cornification t.
vaginal mucification t.

Valentine's t.
Valsalva t.
van Deen's t.
van den Bergh's t.
van der Velden's t.
vanillylmandelic acid t.
VDRL t.
vitality t.
vitamin C t.
VMA t.
Volhard's t.
Vollmer t.
Wada t.
Waldenström's t.
Wang's t.
washout t.
Wassermann t.
Watson-Schwartz t.
Weber's t. for hearing
Webster's t.
Weil-Felix t.
Werner's t.
Wheeler-Johnson t.
Wurster's t.
x^2 t.
Xiphophorus t.
xylose t.
Yvon's t.
Zondek-Aschheim t.
Zsigmondy's t.
Testacealobosia
testalgia
testectomy
testes (*pl. of* testis)
testicle
testicular
    t. appendage
    t. artery
    t. cord
    t. duct
    t. dysgenesis
    t. feminization
    t. implant
    t. plexus
    t. prosthesis
    t. tubular adenoma
    t. veins
testiculus
testing
    bench t.
    genetic t.
    histocompatibility t.
    reality t.
    susceptibility t.
testis, pl. **testes**
    t. cords
    cryptorchid t.
    t. ectopia

ectopic t.
movable t.
retractile t.
undescended t.
testitis
testoid hyperthecosis
test-retest reliability
test-tube baby
test type
    Jaeger's t. t.'s
    point system t. t.
    Snellen's t. t.'s
tetania
    t. gastrica
    t. gravidarum
    t. neonatorum
    t. parathyreopriva
tetanic
    t. contraction
    t. convulsion
tetaniform
tetanigenous
tetanilla
tetanism
tetanization
tetanize
tetanode
tetanoid
tetanolysin
tetanometer
tetanomotor
tetanospasmin
tetanotoxin
tetanus
    acoustic t.
    anodal closure t.
    anodal duration t.
    anodal opening t.
    t. anticus
    apyretic t.
    benign t.
    cathodal closure t.
    cathodal duration t.
    cathodal opening t.
    cephalic t.
    cerebral t.
    complete t.
    t. dorsalis
    generalized t.
    head t.
    hydrophobic t.
    imitative t.
    incomplete t.
    intermittent t.
    local t.
    neonatal t.
    t. neonatorum
    t. posticus

T

tetanus *(continued)*
    postpartum t.
    puerperal t.
    Ritter's opening t.
    rose cephalic t.
    Rose's cephalic t.
    t. toxin
    traumatic t.
    uterine t.
tetany
    t. of alkalosis
    t. cataract
    duration t.
    epidemic t.
    gastric t.
    hyperventilation t.
    hypoparathyroid t.
    infantile t.
    latent t.
    manifest t.
    neonatal t.
    parathyroid t.
    parathyroprival t.
    phosphate t.
    postoperative t.
    rheumatic t.
    symptomatic t.
Tete viruses
tethered cord syndrome
tetra-amelia
tetrabrachius
tetrachirus
tetracoccus, pl. **tetracocci**
tetracrotic
tetracuspid
tetrad
    Fallot's t.
    narcoleptic t.
tetradactyl
tetragon, tetragonum
    t. lumbale
tetragonus
Tetrahymena pyriformis
tetralogy
    Eisenmenger's t.
    t. of Fallot
tetramastia
tetramastigote
tetramastous
tetramelus
Tetrameres
tetramethyl acridine
tetraotus
tetraparesis
tetraperomelia
tetraphocomelia
tetraplegia
tetraplegic

tetraploid
tetrapus
tetrascelus
tetrasomic
tetraster
tetrastichiasis
Tetratrichomonas
    T. ovis
tetrazolium
    nitroblue t.
tetrazonium salts
tetrotus
tetter
    branny t.
    crusted t.
    dry t.
    honeycomb t.
    humid t.
    milk t.
    moist t.
    scaly t.
    wet t.
Teutleben's ligament
text blindness
textiform
textural
texture
textus
Tg cells
TGE virus
thalamectomy
thalamencephalic
thalamencephalon
thalami (*pl. of* thalamus)
thalamic
    t. fasciculus
    t. gustatory nucleus
    t. syndrome
    t. tenia
thalamocortical
    t. fibers
thalamolenticular
thalamostriate veins
thalamotomy
thalamus, pl. **thalami**
    dorsal t.
thalassemia, thalassanemia
    α t.
    A_2 t.
    β t.
    β-δ t.
    F t.
    t. intermedia
    α t. intermedia
    Lepore t.
    t. major
    t. minor
thalassophobia

TFCC
Triangular fibrocartilag complix

thalassoposia
thalassotherapy
thallic
thallium
    t.-201
Thallophyta
thallophyte
thallospore
thallus
Thal procedure
thanatobiologic
thanatognomonic
thanatography
thanatoid
thanatology
thanatomania
thanatophobia
thanatophoric
    t. dwarfism
thanatopsy
thanatos
Thane's method
thaumatropy
Thayer-Martin
    T.-M. agar
    T.-M. medium
theaism
theater
thebesian
    t. circulation
    t. foramina
    t. valve
    t. veins
theca, pl. thecae
    t. cells of stomach
    t. cell tumor
    t. cordis
    t. externa
    t. folliculi
    t. interna
    t. interna cone
    t. lutein cell
    t. tendinis
    t. vertebralis
thecal
    t. abscess
    t. whitlow
thecitis
thecodont
thecoma
thecomatosis
thecostegnosia, thecostegnosis
Theden's method
Theileria
    T. bovis
    T. orientalis
    T. parva bovis
    T. parva lawrencei

    T. parva parva
    T. sergenti
Theileriidae
Theiler's
    T. mouse encephalomyelitis virus
    T. original virus
    T. virus
Theile's
    T. canal
    T. glands
    T. muscle
theinism, theism
thelarche
Thelazia
    T. callipaeda
thele
theleplasty
thelium, pl. thelia
theloncus
thelorrhagia
thematic
    t. apperception test
    t. paralogia
    t. paraphasia
thenad
thenal
thenar
    t. eminence
    t. prominence
    t. space
thenen
Theobald Smith's phenomenon
theomania
theophobia
theorem
    Bayes t.
    central limit t.
theory
    Altmann's t.
    Arrhenius-Madsen t.
    balance t.
    Bordeau t., Bordeu t.
    Bowman's t.
    Burn and Rand t.
    Cannon-Bard t.
    Cannon's t.
    catastrophe t.
    cellular immune t.
    celomic metaplasia t. of
      endometriosis
    chaos t.
    cloacal t.
    clonal deletion t.
    clonal selection t.
    cognitive dissonance t.
    Cohnheim's t.
    de Bordeau t.
    decay t.

T

theory *(continued)*
Dieulafoy's t.
dipole t.
duplicity t. of vision
Ehrlich's side-chain t.
emergency t.
emigration t.
Flourens' t.
Frerichs' t.
Freud's t.
game t.
gastrea t.
gate-control t.
germ t.
germ layer t.
gestalt t.
Haeckel's gastrea t.
Helmholtz t. of accommodation
Helmholtz t. of color vision
Helmholtz t. of hearing
hematogenous t. of endometriosis
Hering's t. of color vision
implantation t. of the production
  of endometriosis
incasement t.
information t.
instructive t.
James-Lange t.
kern-plasma relation t.
Ladd-Franklin t.
learning t.
libido t.
lymphatic dissemination t. of
  endometriosis
mass action t.
t. of medicine
membrane expansion t.
Metchnikoff's t.
miasma t.
migration t.
Miller's chemicoparasitic t.
mnemic t.
molecular dissociation t.
monophyletic t.
myoelastic t.
myogenic t.
neurochronaxic t.
Ollier's t.
overproduction t.
place t.
polyphyletic t.
recapitulation t.
Reed-Frost t. of epidemics
reed instrument t.
reentry t.
resonance t. of hearing
Ribbert's t.
Semon-Hering t.

sensorimotor t.
somatic mutation t. of cancer
Spitzer's t.
stringed instrument t.
telephone t.
two-sympathin t.
Warburg's t.
Wollaston's t.
Young-Helmholtz t. of color vision
theotherapy
thèque
therapeusis
therapeutic
t. abortion
t. anesthesia
t. angiography
t. community
t. crisis
t. electrode
t. fever
t. group
t. iridectomy
t. malaria
t. nihilism
t. optimism
t. pessimism
t. pneumothorax
therapeutics
ray t.
suggestive t.
therapeutist
therapia
t. magna sterilisans
therapist
therapy
alkali t.
analytic t.
anticoagulant t.
antisense t.
autoserum t.
aversion t.
behavior t.
client-centered t.
cognitive t.
collapse t.
conditioning t.
conjoint t.
convulsive t.
cytoreductive t.
depot t.
diathermic t.
electroconvulsive t.
electroshock t.
electrotherapeutic sleep t.
extended family t.
family t.
fever t.
foreign protein t.

functional orthodontic t.
gene t.
geriatric t.
gestalt t.
heterovaccine t.
hormone replacement t.
hyperbaric oxygen t.
implosive t.
individual t.
insulin coma t.
interstitial t.
intralesional t.
maintenance drug t.
marital t.
marriage t.
microwave t.
milieu t.
myofunctional t.
nonspecific t.
occupational t.
orthodontic t.
orthomolecular t.
oxygen t.
parenteral t.
photoradiation t.
physical t.
plasma t.
play t.
proliferation t.
protein shock t.
psychedelic t.
psychoanalytic t.
quadrangular t.
radiation t.
radium beam t.
rational t.
reflex t.
replacement t.
root canal t.
rotation t.
salvage t.
sclerosing t.
serum t.
shock t.
social t.
social network t.
solar t.
specific t.
substitution t.
substitutive t.
teleradium t.
thyroid t.
total push t.
ultrasonic t.
viral t.
x-ray t.
therencephalous
theriomorphism

thermal
    t. anesthesia
    t. burn
    t. sense
    t. spectrum
thermalgesia
thermalgia
thermanalgesia
thermanesthesia
thermatology
thermesthesia
thermesthesiometer
thermic
    t. anesthesia
    t. fever
    t. sense
thermoalgesia
thermoanalgesia
thermoanesthesia
thermocauterectomy
thermocautery
thermocoagulation
thermoduric
thermoesthesia
thermoesthesiometer
thermoexcitory
thermogenesis
thermogenetic, thermogenic
thermogenics
thermogenous
thermogram
thermograph
thermography
    infrared t.
    liquid crystal t.
thermohyperalgesia
thermohyperesthesia
thermohypesthesia
thermohypoesthesia
thermoinhibitory
thermointegrator
thermokeratoplasty
thermolabile opsonin
thermolamp
thermoluminescence dosimetry
thermomassage
thermometer
    axilla t.
    axillary t.
    clinical t.
    surface t.
thermoneurosis
thermopenetration
thermophile, thermophil
thermophilic
thermophobia
thermophore
thermophylic

T

thermoplacentography
Thermoplasma
    T. acidophilum
thermoplasma, pl. **thermoplasmata**
thermoplastic
thermoplegia
thermoprecipitin reaction
thermoreceptor
thermoset
thermostable
    t. opsonin
    t. opsonin test
thermosteresis
thermostromuhr
thermosystaltic
thermosystaltism
thermotactic, thermotaxic
thermotaxis
    negative t.
    positive t.
thermotherapy
thermotonometer
thermotropism
theroid
thesaurismosis
thesaurismotic
thesaurosis
theta
    t. antigen
    t. rhythm
    t. wave
Thezac-Porsmeur method
Thiara
thiazide diabetes
thiazin
    t. dyes
thickness
    Breslow's t.
Thiemann's
    T. disease
    T. syndrome
thiemia
Thiersch
    T. canaliculi
    T. graft
    T. graft operation
    T. method
    T. operation
thigh
    t. bone
    driver's t.
    Heilbronner's t.
    t. joint
thigmesthesia
thigmotaxis
thigmotropism
thinking
    abstract t.

    archaic-paralogical t.
    concrete t.
    creative t.
    magical t.
    prelogical t.
thinking through
thin-layer immunoassay
thin section
thioesters
thioflavine
    t. S
    t. T stain
thioflavin T
thionine
third
    t. corpuscle
    t. cranial nerve
    t. cuneiform bone
    t. degree burn
    t. degree prolapse
    t. disease
    t. finger
    t. and fourth pharyngeal pouch
       syndrome
    t. heart sound
    t. molar
    t. occipital nerve
    t. ovary
    t. parallel pelvic plane
    t. peroneal muscle
    t. sound
    t. temporal convolution
    t. tonsil
    t. trochanter
    t. ventricle
    t. ventriculostomy
third s (*var. of* labor)
thirst
    false t.
    t. fever
    insensible t.
    morbid t.
    subliminal t.
    true t.
Thiry's fistula
Thiry-Vella fistula
Thoma's
    T. ampulla
    T. fixative
    T. laws
Thomas splint
Thompson's
    T. ligament
    T. test
Thomsen's disease
Thomson's sign
thoracal
thoracalgia

thoracentesis
thoraces (*pl. of* thorax)
thoracic
    t. aorta
    t. aortic plexus
    t. axis
    t. cage
    t. cardiac branches of vagus nerve
    t. cardiac nerves
    t. cavity
    t. compliance
    t. duct
    t. fistula
    t. ganglia
    t. girdle
    t. glands
    t. goiter
    t. index
    t. interspinales muscles
    t. interspinal muscle
    t. intertransversarii muscles
    t. intertransverse muscles
    t. kidney
    t. limb
    t. longissimus muscle
    t. nucleus
    t. outlet syndrome
    t. part of aorta
    t. part of esophagus
    t. part of spinal cord
    t. part of thoracic duct
    t. respiration
    t. rotator muscles
    t. spinal nerves
    t. spine
    t. splanchnic nerves
    t. stomach
    t. veins
    t. vertebrae
    t. wall
thoracicoabdominal
thoracicoacromial
thoracicohumeral
thoracic-pelvic-phalangeal dystrophy
thoracis (*gen. of* thorax)
thoracoabdominal
    t. nerves
thoracoacromial
    t. artery
    t. trunk
    t. vein
thoracoceloschisis
thoracocentesis
thoracocyllosis
thoracocyrtosis
thoracodelphus

thoracodorsal
    t. artery
    t. nerve
thoracodynia
thoracoepigastric vein
thoracogastroschisis
thoracograph
thoracolaparotomy
thoracolumbar
    t. aponeurosis
    t. fascia
    t. system
thoracolysis
thoracomelus
thoracometer
thoracomyodynia
thoracopagus
thoracoparacephalus
thoracopathy
thoracoplasty
    conventional t.
thoracopneumoplasty
thoracoschisis
thoracoscope
thoracoscopic surgery
thoracoscopy
thoracostenosis
thoracostomy
    t. tube
thoracotomy
thoradelphus
thorax, gen. **thoracis**, pl. **thoraces**
    barrel-shaped t.
    Peyrot's t.
thorium emanation
Thormählen's test
Thorn
    T. syndrome
    T. test
thorn
    t. apple crystals
    dendritic t.'s
thought
    t. broadcasting
    t. insertion
    t. process disorder
    t. withdrawal
thread
    Simonart's t.'s
    terminal t.
threadworm
thready pulse
threatened abortion
three-chambered heart
three-cornered bone
three-day
    t.-d. fever
    t.-d. measles

T

913

three-dimensional record
three-glass test
thresher's lung
threshold
    absolute t.
    achromatic t.
    auditory t.
    t. body
    brightness difference t.
    t. of consciousness
    convulsant t.
    differential t.
    t. differential
    displacement t.
    double-point t.
    erythema t.
    fibrillation t.
    galvanic t.
    t. of island of Reil
    light differential t.
    minimum light t.
    t. of nose
    pain t.
    t. percussion
    phenotypic t.
    relational t.
    renal t.
    t. shift
    t. stimulus
    stimulus t.
    t. substance
    swallowing t.
    t. trait
    visual t., t. of visual sensation
thrill
    diastolic t.
    hydatid t.
    presystolic t.
    systolic t.
thrix
    t. annulata
throat
    sore t.
throb
thrombasthenia
    hereditary hemorrhagic t.
thrombectomy
thrombi (*pl. of* thrombus)
thrombinogen
thrombin time
thromboangiitis
    t. obliterans
thromboarteritis
thromboasthenia
thromboblast
thromboclastic
thrombocyst, thrombocystis
thrombocytasthenia

thrombocyte
thrombocythemia
thrombocytic series
thrombocytopathy
thrombocytopenia
    autoimmune neonatal t.
    essential t.
    immune t.
    isoimmune neonatal t.
thrombocytopenia-absent radius
    syndrome
thrombocytopenic purpura
thrombocytopoiesis
thrombocytosis
thromboelastogram
thromboelastograph
thromboembolectomy
thromboembolism
thromboendarterectomy
thromboendocarditis
thrombogen
thrombogene
thrombogenic
thromboid
thrombokatilysin
thrombokinase
thrombolic
thrombolus
thrombolymphangitis
thrombolysis
thrombolytic
thrombon
thrombonecrosis
thrombopathic syndrome
thrombopathy
    constitutional t.
thrombopenia
thrombopenic purpura
thrombophilia
thrombophlebitis
    t. migrans
    t. saltans
thromboplastid
thromboplastin
thromboplastinogen
thromboplastinogenase
thromboplastinogenemia
thrombopoiesis
thrombosed
thrombosis, pl. **thromboses**
    atrophic t.
    cerebral t.
    compression t.
    coronary t.
    creeping t.
    dilation t.
    effort-induced t.
    marantic t., marasmic t.

mural t.
placental t.
plate t., platelet t.
posttraumatic arterial t.,
    posttraumatic venous t.
thrombostasis
thrombosthenin
thrombotic
t. gangrene
t. hydrocephalus
t. infarct
t. microangiopathy
t. phlegmasia
t. thrombocytopenic purpura
thrombozyme
thrombus, pl. **thrombi**
agglutinative t.
agonal t.
antemortem t.
ball t.
ball-valve t.
bile t.
fibrin t.
globular t.
hyaline t.
infective t.
laminated t.
marantic t., marasmic t.
mixed t.
mural t.
obstructive t.
pale t.
parietal t.
postmortem t.
propagated t.
red t.
secondary t.
stratified t.
valvular t.
white t.
through
t. drainage
t. transfer imaging
through-and-through
t.-a.-t. laceration
t.-a.-t. myocardial infarction
thrush fungus
thumb
bifid t.
t. forceps
gamekeeper's t.
hitchhiker t.'s
t. lancet
t. reflex
tennis t.
thumbprinting
Thygeson's disease
thylacitis

thymectomy
thymelcosis
thymic
t. abscesses
t. agenesis
t. alymphoplasia
t. arteries
t. branches of internal thoracic
    artery
t. corpuscle
t. hypoplasia
t. veins
thymicolymphatic
thymitis
thymocyte
thymogenic
thymokinetic
thymol
t. blue
t. turbidity test
thymoma
thymoprival, thymoprivic, thymoprivous
thymus
t. gland
t. treatment
thymus-dependent zone
thymus-independent antigen
thyroadenitis
thyroaplasia
thyroarytenoid
t. muscle
thyrocardiac
t. disease
thyrocele
thyrocervical
t. trunk
thyrocolloid
thyroepiglottic
t. ligament
t. muscle
thyroepiglottidean
t. ligament
t. muscle
thyrofissure
thyrogenic, thyrogenous
thyroglossal
t. diverticulum
t. duct
t. duct cyst
thyrohyal
thyrohyoid
t. membrane
t. muscle
thyrohypophysial syndrome
thyroid
accessory t.
t. axis
t. body

T

thyroid (*continued*)
  t. bruit
  t. cartilage
  t. colloid
  t. crisis
  t. diverticulum
  t. eminence
  t. foramen
  t. gland
  t. ima artery
  t. insufficiency
  t. lymph nodes
  t. storm
  t. suppression test
  t. therapy
  t. veins
thyroidal articular surface of cricoid
thyroidea
  t. accessoria, t. ima
thyroidectomy
  "chemical" t.
  near-total t.
  subtotal t.
thyroiditis
  autoimmune t.
  chronic atrophic t.
  chronic fibrous t.
  chronic lymphadenoid t.
  chronic lymphocytic t.
  de Quervain's t.
  focal lymphocytic t.
  giant cell t.
  giant follicular t.
  Hashimoto's t.
  ligneous t.
  lymphocytic t.
  parasitic t.
  Riedel's t.
  subacute granulomatous t.
  subacute lymphocyte t.
thyroidology
thyroidotomy
thyroid-stimulating
  t.-s. hormone stimulation test
  t.-s. immunoglobulins
thyrointoxication
thyrolaryngeal
thyrolingual
  t. cyst
  t. duct
thyrolytic
thyromegaly
thyropalatine
thyroparathyroidectomy
thyropathy
thyropharyngeal
  t. part of inferior pharyngeal
    constrictor muscle

thyroplasty
thyroprival
thyroprivia
thyroprivic, thyroprivous
thyroptosis
thyrotomy
thyrotoxic
  t. coma
  t. complement-fixation factor
  t. crisis
  t. encephalopathy
  t. heart disease
  t. myopathy
  t. serum
thyrotoxicosis
  apathetic t.
  t. medicamentosa
thyrotoxin
thyrotroph
thyrotropin-producing adenoma
**thyrotropin-releasing hormone
  stimulation test**
Thysanosoma actinoides
TI
tibia, gen. and pl. **tibiae**
  saber t.
  t. valga
  t. vara
tibiad
tibial
  t. border of foot
  t. collateral ligament
  t. communicating nerve
  t. crest
  t. intertendinous bursa
  t. nerve
  t. phenomenon
  t. tuberosity
tibiale posticum
tibialgia
tibialis
  t. anterior muscle
  t. posterior muscle
tibiocalcaneal
  t. ligament
  t. part of deltoid ligament
tibiocalcanean
tibiofascialis
tibiofemoral
  t. index
tibiofibular
  t. ligament
  t. syndesmosis
tibionavicular
  t. ligament
  t. part of deltoid ligament
tibioperoneal
tibioscaphoid

tibiotarsal
tic
    convulsive t.
    t. de pensée
    t. douloureux
    facial t.
    glossopharyngeal t.
    habit t.
    local t.
    mimic t.
    psychic t.
    rotatory t.
    spasmodic t.
tick
    t. typhus
tick-borne
    t.-b. encephalitis (Central European subtype)
    t.-b. encephalitis (Eastern subtype)
    t.-b. encephalitis virus
    t.-b. virus
tickling
tic-tac
    t.-t. rhythm
    t.-t. sounds
tidal
    t. air
    t. drainage
    t. volume
    t. wave
tide
    acid t.
    alkaline t.
    fat t.
Tiedemann's
    T. gland
    T. nerve
tie-over dressing
Tierfellnaevus
Tietze's syndrome
tiger heart
tight junction
tigretier
tigroid
    t. bodies
    t. fundus
    t. retina
    t. striation
    t. substance
tigrolysis
tilorone
tilt
    t. table
    t. test
tilting
    t. disc valve
    t. disc valve prosthesis
timbre

time
    activated clotting t.
    activated partial thromboplastin t.
    A-H conduction t.
    association t.
    biologic t.
    bleeding t.
    circulation t.
    clot retraction t.
    clotting t.
    coagulation t.
    t. compensation gain
    t. constant
    euglobulin clot lysis t.
    fading t.
    t. of flight
    forced expiratory t.
    H-R conduction t.
    H-V conduction t.
    inertia t.
    intra-atrial conduction t.
    left ventricular ejection t.
    t. marker
    P-A conduction t.
    partial thromboplastin t.
    P-H conduction t.
    prothrombin t.
    reaction t.
    recognition t.
    repetition t.
    rise t.
    Russell's viper venom clotting t.
    sensation t.
    t. sense
    sinoatrial conduction t.
    sinoatrial recovery t.
    survival t.
    thrombin t.
    tissue thromboplastin inhibition t.
    utilization t.
time-compensated gain
time-gain compensation
time-varied
    t. v. gain
    t.-v. gain control
timothy-hay bacillus
tin-113
tinctable
tinction
tinctorial
tine
    t. test
tinea
    t. amiantacea
    t. barbae
    t. capitis
    t. circinata
    t. corporis

T

tinea *(continued)*
- t. cruris
- t. favosa
- t. glabrosa
- t. imbricata
- t. inguinalis
- t. kerion
- t. manus
- t. nigra
- t. pedis
- t. profunda
- t. sycosis
- t. tonsurans
- t. tropicalis
- t. unguium
- t. versicolor

Tinel's sign
tinfoil
tingibility
tingible
tingle
tingling
- distal t. on percussion

tinnitus
- t. aurium
- t. cerebri
- clicking t.
- Leudet's t.

tint
tinted
- t. denture base
- t. vision

tip
- t. of auricle
- t. of elbow
- t. of nose
- t. of posterior horn
- root t.
- t. of tongue
- t. of tooth root
- Woolner's t.

tipping
tiring
Tissierella praeacuta
Tissot spirometer
tissue
- adenoid t.
- adipose t.
- areolar t.
- t. basophil
- bone t.
- cancellous t.
- cardiac muscle t.
- cartilaginous t.
- cavernous t.
- chondroid t.
- chromaffin t.
- connective t.

t. culture
t. culture infectious dose
dartoic t.
t. displaceability
t. displacement
epithelial t.
erectile t.
fatty t.
fibrohyaline t.
fibrous t.
t. fluid
Gamgee t.
gelatinous t.
gingival t.'s
granulation t.
gut-associated lymphoid t.
Haller's vascular t.
hard t.
hemopoietic t.
indifferent t.
interstitial t.
investing t.'s
islet t.
t. lymph
lymphatic t., lymphoid t.
mesenchymal t.
mesonephric t.
metanephrogenic t.
t. molding
mucous connective t.
muscular t.
myeloid t.
nasion soft t.
nephrogenic t.
nervous t.
nodal t.
osseous t.
osteogenic t.
osteoid t.
periapical t.
t. registration
t. respiration
reticular t., retiform t.
rubber t.
skeletal muscle t.
smooth muscle t.
subcutaneous t.
t. tension
t. thromboplastin inhibition time
t. valve
t. weighting factor
tissue-bearing area
tissue-specific antigen
tissue-trimming
tissular
titillation
titratable acidity test
titubation

Tizzoni's stain
Tj antigen
Tm cells
TM-mode
T-mycoplasma
TNM staging
toad skin
to-and-fro
    t.-a.-f. anesthesia
    t.-a.-f. murmur
    t.-a.-f. sound
toasted shins
tobacco heart
Tobia fever
Tobruk splint
tocodynagraph
tocodynamometer
tocograph
tocography
tocology
tocometer
tocophobia
Todaro's tendon
Todd
    T. paralysis
    T. postepileptic paralysis
    T. unit
Tod's muscle
toe
    t. clonus
    great t.
    hammer t.
    Hong Kong t.
    t. itch
    painful t.
    t. phenomenon
    stiff t.
    webbed t.'s
toe-drop
toenail
    ingrowing t.
Togaviridae
togavirus
toilet
    pulmonary t.
    t. training
Toison's stain
Tokelau ringworm
tolbutamide test
Toldt's
    T. fascia
    T. membrane
tolerance
    acoustic t.
    t. dose
    frustration t.
    high dose t.
    immunologic t.

    immunological t.
    immunologic high dose t.
    impaired glucose t.
    nonresponder t.
    pain t.
    split t.
    vibration t.
tolerogenic
Tolosa-Hunt syndrome
toluidine
    alkaline t. blue O
toluylene red
Toma's sign
tomentum, tomentum cerebri
Tomes'
    T. fibers
    T. granular layer
    T. processes
Tommaselli's disease
tomogram
tomograph
tomography
    computed t. (CT)
    computerized axial t.
    conventional t.
    dynamic computed t.
    helical computed t.
    high resolution computed t.
    hypocycloidal t.
    nuclear magnetic resonance t.
    positron emission t.
    single photon emission computed t.
    spiral computed t.
    trispiral t.
tomolevel
tomomania
tonaphasia
tone
    affective t., emotional t.
    t. color
    t. decay test
    feeling t.
    fundamental t.
    heart t.'s
    Traube's double t.
toner
tongue
    baked t.
    bald t.
    beet-t.
    bifid t.
    black t.
    t. bone
    t. of cerebellum
    cleft t.
    coated t.
    t. crib
    t. depressor

T

tongue (*continued*)
    dotted t.
    fissured t.
    t. flap
    furred t.
    geographic t.
    grooved t.
    hairy t.
    hobnail t.
    magenta t.
    mandibular t.
    t. phenomenon
    raspberry t.
    red strawberry t.
    scrotal t.
    smoker's t.
    stippled t.
    strawberry t.
tongue-swallowing
tongue thrust
tongue-tie
tonic
    t. contraction
    t. control
    t. convulsion
    t. epilepsy
    t. pupil
    t. reflex
    t. seizure
    t. spasm
tonic-clonic seizure
tonicoclonic
toning
tonitrophobia
tonoclonic
    t. spasm
tonofibril
tonofilament
tonograph
tonography
tonometer
    applanation t.
    Gärtner's t.
    Goldmann's applanation t.
    Mackay-Marg t.
    Mueller electronic t.
    pneumatic t.
    Schiötz t.
tonometry
tonophant
tonoplast
tonoscillograph
tonotopic
tonotropic
tonsil
    cerebellar t.
    eustachian t.
    faucial t.

    Gerlach's t.
    laryngeal t.'s
    lingual t.
    Luschka's t.
    palatine t.
    pharyngeal t.
    submerged t.
    third t.
    tubal t.
tonsilla, pl. **tonsillae**
    t. adenoidea
    t. cerebelli
    t. intestinalis
    t. lingualis
    t. palatina
    t. pharyngealis
    t. tubaria
tonsillar, tonsillary
    t. branch of the facial artery
    t. branch of glossopharyngeal nerve
    t. calculus
    t. crypt
    t. fossa
    t. fossulae
    t. herniation
    t. ring
tonsillectomy
tonsillith
tonsillitis
    lacunar t.
    Vincent's t.
tonsillolingual sulcus
tonsillolith
tonsillopathy
tonsillotome
tonsillotomy
tonus
    baseline t.
    myogenic t.
    neurogenic t.
tooth, pl. **teeth**
    t. abrasion
    acrylic resin t.
    anatomic teeth
    ankylosed t.
    anterior teeth
    t. arrangement
    auditory teeth
    t. avulsion
    baby t.
    back teeth
    bicuspid t.
    buck t.
    t. bud
    canine t.
    t. cement
    cheek t.
    Corti's auditory teeth

crossbite teeth
cuspid t., cuspidate t.
cuspless t.
cutting teeth
dead t.
deciduous t.
devitalized t.
extruded teeth
eye t.
fluoridated teeth
t. form
fused teeth
geminated teeth
t. germ
ghost t.
green t.
Horner's teeth
Huschke's auditory teeth
Hutchinson's teeth
impacted t.
incisor t.
t. ligation
metal insert teeth
migrating teeth
milk t.
molar t.
mottled t.
multicuspid t.
natal t.
neonatal t.
nonanatomic teeth
nonvital t.
normally posed t.
notched teeth
oral teeth
pegged t.
permanent t.
perpetually growing t.
persistently growing t.
t. plane
plastic teeth
t. polyp
posterior teeth
premolar t.
primary t.
protruding teeth
t. pulp
pulpless t.
t. sac
sclerotic teeth
screwdriver teeth
second t.
t. socket
spaced teeth
t. spasms
stomach t.
succedaneous t.
syphilitic teeth

temporary t.
t. transplantation
tricuspid t.
tube teeth
Turner's t.
unerupted t.
vital t.
wisdom t.
zero degree teeth
toothache
tooth-and-nail syndrome
tooth-borne
    t.-b. base
toothed vertebra
topagnosis
topalgia
toper's nose
topesthesia
Töpfer's test
tophaceous
    t. gout
tophus, pl. **tophi**
    gouty t.
topical
    t. anesthesia
Topinard's
    T. facial angle
    T. line
topistic
topoanesthesia
topognosis, topognosia
topogometer
topographic anatomy
topography
topoisomerase
Topolanski's sign
topology
toponarcosis
toponym
toponymy
topopathogenesis
topophobia
topophylaxis
toposcope
topothermesthesiometer
toppling gait
TORCH syndrome
torcular herophili
Torek operation
tori (*pl. of* torus)
toric
    t. lens
Torkildsen shunt
tornado epilepsy
Tornwaldt's
    T. abscess
    T. cyst

T

Tornwaldt's *(continued)*
    T. disease
    T. syndrome
Toronto formula for pulmonary artery banding
torose, torous
torpid
torpidity
torpor
    t. retinae
torque
Torre's syndrome
torsade de pointes
torsiometer
torsion
    t. of appendage
    t. disease of childhood
    t. dystonia
    extravaginal t.
    t. fracture
    intravaginal t.
    t. neurosis
    perinatal t.
    t. spasm
    t. of testis
    t. testis
    t. of a tooth
torsional deformity
torsionometer
torsive occlusion
torsiversion
torso
torsoclusion
Torsten Sjögren's syndrome
torticollar
torticollis
    congenital t.
    dermatogenic t.
    dystonic t.
    fixed t.
    hysterical t.
    intermittent t.
    labyrinthine t.
    ocular t.
    psychogenic t.
    rheumatic t.
    spasmodic t.
    t. spastica
    spurious t.
    symptomatic t.
tortipelvis
tortuous
toruli (*pl. of* torulus)
toruloma
Torulopsis

torulopsosis
torulus, pl. toruli
    toruli tactiles
torus, pl. tori
    t. fracture
    t. frontalis
    t. levatorius
    mandibular t., t. mandibularis
    t. manus
    t. occipitalis
    palatine t., t. palatinus
    t. tubarius
    t. uretericus
    t. uterinus
total *in toto*
    t. acidity
    t. aphasia
    t. ascertainment
    t. body hypothermia
    t. body water
    t. breech extraction
    t. cataract
    t. catecholamine test
    t. cleavage
    t. cystectomy
    t. elasticity of muscle
    t. end-diastolic diameter
    t. end-systolic diameter
    t. energy
    t. facial index
    t. hematuria
    t. hyperopia
    t. joint arthroplasty
    t. keratoplasty
    t. lung capacity
    t. mastectomy
    t. necrosis
    t. parenteral nutrition
    t. or partial anomalous pulmonary venous connections
    t. pelvic exenteration
    t. peripheral resistance
    t. placenta previa
    t. push therapy
    t. refractory period
    t. sclerectasia
    t. spinal anesthesia
    t. synechia
    t. transfusion
totem
totemism
totemistic
totipotency, totipotence
totipotent, totipotential
    t. cell
touch
    t. cell

t. corpuscle
royal t.
Tourette
T. disease
T. syndrome
Tournay
T. phenomenon
T. sign
tourniquet
Dupuytren's t.
Esmarch t.
Rummel t.
t. test
Tourtual's
T. membrane
T. sinus
Touton giant cell
Tovell tube
TO virus
tower skull
Towne
T. projection
T. projection radiograph
T. view
toxanemia
Toxascaris leonina
toxemia
toxemic
t. jaundice
t. retinopathy of pregnancy
toxic
t. amaurosis
t. amblyopia
t. anemia
t. cataract
t. delirium
t. dementia
t. epidermal necrolysis
t. goiter
t. hemoglobinuria
t. hydrocephalus
t. megacolon
t. myocarditis
t. nephrosis
t. neuritis
t. psychosis
t. retinopathy
t. shock
t. shock syndrome
t. unit
toxicemia
toxicity
oxygen t.
toxicoderma
toxicodermatitis
toxicodermatosis
toxicogenic conjunctivitis
toxicophobia

toxigenic
toxigenicity
toxin
intracellular t.
t. spectrum
tetanus t.
t. unit
toxinic
toxinogenic
toxinogenicity
toxiphobia
Toxocara
T. canis
T. mystax
toxon, toxone
toxoneme
toxophore
toxophorous
Toxoplasmatidae
toxoplasmosis
acquired t. in adults
congenital t.
Toynbee's
T. corpuscles
T. muscle
T. tube
TPHA test
TPH test
TPI test
trabecula, gen. and pl. **trabeculae**
anterior chamber t.
arachnoid t.
trabeculae carneae
trabeculae of corpora cavernosa
trabeculae corporis spongiosi penis
trabeculae corporum cavernosorum
trabeculae of corpus spongiosum
trabeculae cranii
trabeculae lienis
septomarginal t.
t. septomarginalis
trabeculae of spleen
trabeculae splenicae
t. testis
trabecular
t. bone
t. carcinoma
t. meshwork
t. network
t. reticulum
t. zone
trabeculate
trabeculated bladder
trabeculation
trabeculectomy
trabeculoplasty
laser t.
trabeculotomy

T

trace
    t. conditioned reflex
    t. conditioning
    memory t.
tracer
trachea, pl. tracheae
    saber-sheath t.
    scabbard t.
tracheal
    t. branches
    t. cartilages
    t. fenestration
    t. fistula
    t. glands
    t. intubation
    t. lymph nodes
    t. mucosa
    t. ring
    t. triangle
    t. tube
    t. tug
    t. ulceration
    t. veins
    t. wall stripe
trachealgia
trachealis
    t. muscle
tracheitis
trachelagra
trachelalis
trachelectomy
trachelematoma
trachelian
trachelism, trachelismus
trachelitis
trachelobregmatic diameter
trachelocele
tracheloclavicular muscle
trachelocyrtosis
trachelodynia
trachelokyphosis
trachelology
trachelomastoid
trachelomyitis
trachelo-occipitalis
trachelopanus
trachelopexia, trachelopexy
trachelophyma
tracheloplasty
trachelorrhaphy
trachelos
tracheloschisis
trachelotomy
tracheoaerocele
tracheobiliary
    t. fistula
tracheobroncheopathia osteoplastica

tracheobronchial
    t. diverticulum
    t. dyskinesia
    t. groove
tracheobronchitis
tracheobronchomegaly
tracheobronchoscopy
tracheocele
tracheoesophageal
    t. fistula
    t. speech
tracheolaryngeal
tracheomalacia
tracheomegaly
tracheopathia, tracheopathy
    t. osteoplastica
tracheopharyngeal
tracheophonesis
tracheophony
tracheoplasty
tracheorrhagia
tracheoschisis
tracheoscope
tracheoscopic
tracheoscopy
tracheostenosis
tracheostoma
tracheostomy
tracheotome
tracheotomy
    t. hook
    t. tube
trachitis
trachoma
    t. bodies
    follicular t.
    t. glands
    granular t.
    t. virus
trachomatous
    t. conjunctivitis
    t. keratitis
    t. pannus
trachychromatic
trachyonychia
trachyphonia
tracing
    arrow point t.
    cephalometric t.
    Gothic arch t.
    needle point t.
    stylus t.
tract
    alimentary t.
    anterior corticospinal t.
    anterior pyramidal t.
    anterior spinocerebellar t.
    anterior spinothalamic t.

Arnold's t.
association t.
auditory t.
Burdach's t.
central tegmental t.
cerebellorubral t.
cerebellothalamic t.
Collier's t.
comma t. of Schultze
corticobulbar t.
corticopontine t.
corticospinal t.
crossed pyramidal t.
cuneocerebellar t.
dead t.'s
deiterospinal t.
dentatothalamic t.
descending t. of trigeminal nerve
digestive t.
direct pyramidal t.
dorsolateral t.
fastigiobulbar t.
Flechsig's t.
frontopontine t.
frontotemporal t.
gastrointestinal t.
geniculocalcarine t.
genital t.
t. of Goll
Gowers' t.
habenulointerpeduncular t.
habenulopeduncular t.
Hoche's t.
hypothalamohypophysial t.
iliopubic t.
iliotibial t.
James t.'s
lateral corticospinal t.
lateral pyramidal t.
lateral spinothalamic t.
Lissauer's t.
Loewenthal's t.
mamillothalamic t.
Marchi's t.
mesencephalic t. of trigeminal nerve
Monakow's t.
t. of Münzer and Wiener
nerve t.
occipitocollicular t.
occipitopontine t.
occipitotectal t.
olfactory t.
olivocerebellar t.
olivocochlear t.
olivospinal t.
optic t.
parietopontine t.

posterior spinocerebellar t.
prepyramidal t.
pyramidal t.
respiratory t.
reticulospinal t.
rubrobulbar t.
rubroreticular t.
rubrospinal t.
t. of Schütz
sensory t.
septomarginal t.
solitary t.
sphincteroid t. of ileum
spinal t.
spinal t. of trigeminal nerve
spinocerebellar t.'s
spinocervicothalamic t.
spino-olivary t.
spinoreticular t.
spinotectal t.
spinothalamic t.
spiral foraminous t.
Spitzka's marginal t.
sulcomarginal t.
supraopticohypophysial t.
tectobulbar t.
tectopontine t.
tectospinal t.
temporofrontal t.
temporopontine t.
trigeminothalamic t.
tuberoinfundibular t.
Türck's t.
urinary t.
uveal t.
ventral spinocerebellar t.
ventral spinothalamic t.
vestibulospinal t.
Waldeyer's t.

tractellum, pl. **tractella**
traction

t. alopecia
t. atrophy
axis t.
Bryant's t.
Buck's t.
t. diverticulum
t. epiphysis
external t.
halo t.
intermaxillary t.
internal t.
isometric t.
isotonic t.
maxillomandibular t.
Russell t.
Sayre's suspension t.

Ilizarov traction device

traction *(continued)*
    skeletal t.
    skin t.
tractor
    Lowsley t.
    Syms t.
    Young prostatic t.
tractotomy
    anterolateral t.
    intramedullary t.
    pyramidal t.
    Schwartz t.
    Sjöqvist t.
    spinal t.
    spinothalamic t.
    trigeminal t.
    Walker t.
tractus, gen. and pl. **tractus**
    t. centralis tegmenti
    t. cerebellorubralis
    t. cerebellothalamicus
    t. corticobulbaris
    t. corticopontini
    t. corticospinalis
    t. corticospinalis anterior
    t. corticospinalis lateralis
    t. descendens nervi trigemini
    t. dorsolateralis
    t. fastigiobulbaris
    t. frontopontinus
    t. habenulopeduncularis
    t. iliotibialis
    t. mesencephalicus nervi trigemini
    t. occipitopontinus
    t. olfactorius
    t. olivocerebellaris
    t. opticus
    t. parietopontinus
    t. pyramidalis
    t. pyramidalis anterior
    t. pyramidalis lateralis
    t. reticulospinalis
    t. rubrospinalis
    t. solitarius
    t. spinalis nervi trigemini
    t. spinocerebellaris anterior
    t. spinocerebellaris posterior
    t. spinotectalis
    t. spinothalamicus
    t. spinothalamicus anterior
    t. spinothalamicus lateralis
    t. spiralis foraminosus
    t. supraopticohypophysialis
    t. tectobulbaris
    t. tectopontinus
    t. tectospinalis
    t. tegmentalis centralis

    t. temporopontinus
    t. tuberoinfundibularis
    t. vestibulospinalis
tragal
tragi (*pl. of* tragus)
tragicus
    t. muscle
tragion
tragomaschalia
tragophonia, tragophony
tragus, pl. **tragi**
    accessory t.
trained reflex
training
    t. analysis
    assertive t.
    aversive t.
    avoidance t.
    escape t.
    t. group
    toilet t.
train-of-four stimulus
trainwheel rhythm
trait
    Bombay t.
    categorical t.
    chromosomal t.
    codominant t.
    dominant t.
    dominant lethal t.
    galtonian t.
    intermediate t.
    liminal t.
    marker t.
    mendelian t.
    nonpenetrant t.
    penetrant t.
    qualitative t.
    recessive t.
    sickle cell t.
    threshold t.
trajector
tram lines
trance
    t. coma
    death t.
    induced t.
    somnambulistic t.
transaction
transactional
    t. analysis
    t. psychotherapy
transanimation
transaudient
transaxial plane
transcalent
transcapsidation

transcellular
　t. fluids
　t. water
transcendental
　t. anatomy
　t. meditation
transcervical fracture
transcondylar
　t. fracture
transcortical
　t. aphasia
　t. apraxia
transcranial radiograph
transcriptionist
　medical t.
transcutaneous
transcytosis
transdermic
transduce
transducer
　t. cell
　piezoelectric t.
　ultrasound t.
transductant
transduction
　abortive t.
　complete t.
　general t.
　high frequency t.
　low frequency t.
　specialized t.
　specific t.
transduodenal sphincterotomy
transection
transesophageal echocardiography
transethmoidal
transfection
transfer
　cavernous t. of portal vein
　t. coping
　embryo t.
　Fourier t.
　t. genes
　t. imaging
　linear energy t.
transferase
transference
　counter t.
　extrasensory thought t.
　t. love
　negative t.
　t. neurosis
　passive t.
　positive t.
transferred
　t. ophthalmia
　t. sensation
transfix

transfixion
　t. suture
transform
　Fourier t.
transformant
transformation
　cell t.
　t. constant
　Haldane t.
　logit t.
　lymphocyte t.
　nodular t. of the liver
　t. zone
transformed lymphocyte
transforming
　t. agent
　t. gene
　t. growth factor α
　t. growth factor β
transfuse
transfusion
　arterial t.
　direct t.
　drip t.
　exchange t.
　exsanguination t.
　fetomaternal t.
　t. hepatitis
　immediate t.
　indirect t.
　intrauterine t.
　mediate t.
　t. nephritis
　peritoneal t.
　placental t.
　reciprocal t.
　subcutaneous t.
　substitution t.
　total t.
　twin-twin t.
transgenic mice
transhiatal
　t. esophagectomy
transient
　t. acantholytic dermatosis
　t. agammaglobulinemia
　t. albuminuria
　t. equilibrium
　t. global amnesia
　t. hypogammaglobulinemia of
　　infancy
　t. ischemic attack
　t. myopia
　t. retinopathy
transiliac
transilient
transillumination
transinsular

T

transischiac
transisthmian
transition
    cervicothoracic t.
    t. electron
transitional
    t. cell
    t. cell carcinoma
    t. cell papilloma
    t. convolution
    t. denture
    t. epithelium
    t. gyrus
    t. leukocyte
    t. zone
transjugular intrahepatic portosystemic shunt
translatory movement
translocation
    balanced t.
    t. carrier
    t. chromosome
    reciprocal t.
    robertsonian t.
    unbalanced t.
translucent
translumbar aortography
transmembrane
    t. potential
transmigration
    ovular t., direct ovular t., external ovular t., indirect ovular t., internal ovular t.
transmissible
    t. dementia
    t. gastroenteritis virus of swine
    t. plasmid
    t. turkey enteritis virus
transmission
    duplex t.
    horizontal t.
    iatrogenic t.
    neurohumoral t.
    transovarial t.
    transstadial t.
    vertical t.
transmitted light
transmural
    t. myocardial infarction
    t. pressure
transmutation
transneuronal atrophy
transnexus channel
transocular
transonance
transonic

transorbital
    t. leukotomy
    t. lobotomy
transosseous venography
transovarial transmission
transparent
    t. dentin
    t. septum
    t. ulcer of the cornea
transparietal
transperitoneal
trans phase
transpirable
transpiration
    pulmonary t.
transpire
transplacental
transplant
    Gallie's t.
    hair t.
    t. lung syndrome
transplantar
transplantation
    t. antigen
    bone marrow t.
    cardiopulmonary t.
    t. of cornea
    corneal t.
    t. genetics
    heart t.
    heart-lung t.
    pancreaticoduodenal t.
    renal t.
    tendon t.
    tooth t.
transpleural
transporionic axis
transport
    axoplasmic t.
    t. host
    t. maximum
    t. medium
    vesicular t.
transpose
transposition
    t. of arterial stems
    corrected t. of the great vessels
    t. of the great vessels
    penoscrotal t.
transpulmonary pressure
transpyloric plane
transsection
transsegmental
transseptal
    t. fibers
    t. orchiopexy
transsexual
    t. surgery

transsexualism
transsphenoidal
transstadial transmission
transsynaptic
    t. chromatolysis
    t. degeneration
transtentorial
    t. herniation
transthalamic
transthermia
transthoracic
    t. echocardiography
    t. esophagectomy
    t. pacemaker
    t. pressure
transthoracotomy
transubstantiation
transureteroureteral anastomosis
transureteroureterostomy
transurethral
    t. resection
    t. resection syndrome
transvaginal
transversalis
    t. fascia
transversarial part of vertebral artery
transverse
    t. abdominal incision
    t. amputation
    t. anthelicine groove
    t. arch of foot
    t. artery of neck
    t. arytenoid muscle
    t. atlantal ligament
    t. auricular muscle
    t. branches
    t. carpal ligament
    t. cervical artery
    t. cervical nerve
    t. cervical veins
    t. colon
    t. costal facet
    t. crest
    t. crest of internal acoustic meatus
    t. crural ligament
    t. diameter
    t. disk
    t. ductules of epoöphoron
    t. facial artery
    t. facial fracture
    t. facial vein
    t. fasciculi
    t. fissure of cerebellum
    t. fissure of cerebrum
    t. fissure of the lung
    t. foramen
    t. fornix
    t. fracture

t. genicular ligament
t. head
t. hermaphroditism
t. horizontal axis
t. humeral ligament
t. lie
t. ligament of acetabulum
t. ligament of the atlas
t. ligament of elbow
t. ligament of knee
t. ligament of leg
t. ligament of pelvis
t. ligament of perineum
t. lines of sacrum
t. metacarpal ligament
t. metatarsal ligament
t. muscle of abdomen
t. muscle of auricle
t. muscle of chin
t. muscle of nape
t. muscle of thorax
t. muscle of tongue
t. myelitis
t. nasal groove
t. nerve of neck
t. occipital sulcus
t. oval pelvis
t. palatine fold
t. palatine ridge
t. palatine suture
t. pancreatic artery
t. part of left branch of portal vein
t. part of nasalis muscle
t. pericardial sinus
t. perineal ligament
t. plane
t. pontine fibers
t. presentation
t. process
t. rectal folds
t. relaxation
t. rhombencephalic flexure
t. ridge
t. scapular artery
t. section
t. septum
t. sinus
t. sinus of pericardium
t. tarsal articulation
t. tarsal joint
t. temporal convolutions
t. temporal gyri
t. temporal sulci
t. tibiofibular ligament
t. vein of face
t. vein of scapula
t. veins of neck

T

transverse *(continued)*
    t. velum
    t. vesical fold
transversectomy
transversion
transversocostal
transversospinalis muscle
transversospinal muscle
transversourethralis
transversovertical index
transversus
    t. abdominis muscle
    t. menti muscle
    t. nuchae muscle
    t. thoracis muscle
transvestism
transvestite
transvestitism
Trantas' dots
Tr^a antigen
trapezia (*pl. of* trapezium)
trapezial
trapeziform
trapeziometacarpal
trapezium, pl. **trapezia, trapeziums**
    t. bone
trapezius
    t. muscle
trapezoid
    t. body
    t. bone
    t. ligament
    t. line
    t. ridge
Trapp-Häser formula
Trapp's formula
Traube-Hering
    T.-H. curves
    T.-H. waves
Traube's
    T. bruit
    T. corpuscle
    T. double tone
    T. dyspnea
    T. plugs
    T. semilunar space
    T. sign
trauma, pl. **traumata, traumas**
    birth t.
    t. from occlusion
    occlusal t.
    psychic t.
traumasthenia
traumatic
    t. alopecia
    t. amenorrhea
    t. amnesia
    t. amputation

    t. anemia
    t. anesthesia
    t. aneurysm
    t. asphyxia
    t. bone cyst
    t. cataract
    t. cervical discopathy
    t. dermatitis
    t. encephalopathy
    t. fever
    t. herpes
    t. meningocele
    t. myiasis
    t. neurasthenia
    t. neuritis
    t. neuroma
    t. neurosis
    t. occlusion
    t. orchitis
    t. pneumonia
    t. progressive encephalopathy
    t. psychosis
    t. retinopathy
    t. tetanus
traumatism
traumatize
traumatogenic occlusion
traumatology
traumatonesis
traumatopathy
traumatopnea
traumatopyra
traumatosepsis
traumatotherapy
Trautmann's triangular space
traveler's diarrhea
traverse
tray
    acrylic resin t.
    annealing t.
    impression t.
Treacher Collins' syndrome
treat
treatment
    active t.
    Carrel's t.
    causal t.
    conservative t.
    Dakin-Carrel t.
    t. denture
    dietetic t.
    empiric t.
    endodontic t.
    Goeckerman t.
    heat t.
    insulin coma t.
    insulin shock t.
    isoserum t.

Kenny's t.
light t.
medical t.
Mitchell's t.
moral t.
Nauheim t.
palliative t.
preventive t.
prophylactic t.
root canal t.
Schott t.
shock t.
solar t.
symptomatic t.
Tallerman t.
thymus t.
Tweed edgewise t.
Weir Mitchell t.

trefoil
t. polypeptide
t. tendon

Treitz's
T. arch
T. fascia
T. fossa
T. hernia
T. ligament
T. muscle

Trélat's
T. sign
T. stools

trema
Trematoda
trematode, trematoid
trembling
t. palsy
tremelloid, tremellose
tremogram
tremograph
tremophobia
tremor
action t.
alcoholic withdrawal t.
alternating t.
alternative t.
arsenical t.
t. artuum
ataxic t.
benign essential t.
coarse t.
continuous t.
essential t.
familial t.
fine t.
flapping t.
head t.'s
heredofamilial t.
hysterical t.

intention t.
kinetic t.
mercurial t.
metallic t.
t. opiophagorum
passive t.
persistent t.
physiologic t.
pill-rolling t.
postural t.
t. potatorum
progressive cerebellar t.
psychogenic t.
resting t.
saturnine t.
senile t.
static t.
t. tendinum
volitional t.

tremorgram
tremulor
tremulous
t. iris
trench
t. fever
t. foot
t. hand
t. lung
t. mouth
t. nephritis
Trendelenburg
T. operation
T. position
T. radiograph
T. sign
T. symptom
T. test
trend of thought
trepan
trepanation
corneal t., t. of cornea
trephination
trephine
t. biopsy
trephocyte
trepidant
trepidatio cordis
trepidation
Treponema
T. carateum
T. cuniculi
T. denticola
T. genitalis
T. hyodysenteriae
T. mucosum
T. pallidum
T. pallidum hemagglutination test
T. pallidum immobilization reaction

T

Treponema (*continued*)
    T. pallidum immobilization test
    T. pertenue
treponema-immobilizing antibody
treponemal antibody
treponematosis
treponeme
treponemiasis
treppe
Tresilian's sign
tresis
Treves' fold
Trevor's disease
TRH stimulation test
triad
    acute compression t.
    Beck's t.
    Bezold's t.
    Charcot's t.
    Fallot's t.
    hepatic t.
    Hull's t.
    Hutchinson's t.
    Kartagener's t.
    portal t.
    Saint's t.
triadic symbiosis
trial
    t. base
    Bernoulli t.
    t. case
    clinical t.
    t. denture
    t. frame
    t. lenses
    randomized controlled t.
trial and error
tri-amelia
triangle
    anal t.
    anterior t. of neck
    Assézat's t.
    auricular t.
    t. of auscultation
    axillary t.
    Béclard's t.
    Bonwill t.
    Bryant's t.
    Burger's t.
    Burow's t.
    Calot's t.
    cardiohepatic t.
    carotid t.
    cephalic t.
    cervical t.
    Codman's t.
    color t.
    crural t.

deltoideopectoral t.
digastric t.
Einthoven's t.
Elaut's t.
t. of elbow
facial t.
Farabeuf's t.
femoral t.
t. of fillet
frontal t.
Garland's t.
Gombault's t.
Grocco's t.
Grynfeltt's t.
Hesselbach's t.
iliofemoral t.
inferior carotid t.
inferior occipital t.
infraclavicular t.
inguinal t.
interscalene t.
Killian's t.
Koch's t.
Labbé's t.
laimer t.
Langenbeck's t.
Lesser's t.
Lesshaft's t.
Lieutaud's t.
lumbar t.
lumbocostoabdominal t.
Macewen's t.
Malgaigne's t.
Marcille's t.
muscular t.
occipital t.
omoclavicular t.
omotracheal t.
palatal t.
paravertebral t.
Petit's lumbar t.
Philippe's t.
Pirogoff's t.
posterior t. of neck
pubourethral t.
Reil's t.
sacral t.
t. of safety
Scarpa's t.
sternocostal t.
subclavian t.
subinguinal t.
submandibular t.
submaxillary t.
submental t.
suboccipital t.
superior carotid t.
supraclavicular t.

suprameatal t.
tracheal t.
Tweed t.
umbilicomammillary t.
urogenital t.
t. of vertebral artery
vesical t.
Ward's t.
Weber's t.
Wilde's t.

triangular
t. bandage
t. bone
t. cartilage
t. crest
t. disk of wrist
t. fascia
t. fold
t. fossa
t. fovea of arytenoid cartilage
t. lamella
t. ligament
t. ligaments of liver
t. muscle
t. nucleus
t. part
t. pit of arytenoid cartilage
t. recess
t. ridge
t. uterus

triangularis
triangulum
Triatoma
Triatominae
triaxial reference system
tribade
tribadism, tribady
tribasilar
t. synostosis
tribe
tribology
tribrachia
tribrachius
TRIC agents
tricephalus
triceps
t. brachii muscle
t. bursa
t. coxae muscle
t. muscle of arm
t. muscle of calf
t. muscle of hip
t. reflex
t. surae muscle
t. surae reflex
trichalgia
trichangion
trichatrophia

trichauxis
trichiasis
trichilemmal cyst
trichilemmoma
Trichina
trichina, pl. **trichinae**
Trichinella
T. spiralis
Trichinellicae
Trichinelloidea
trichiniferous
trichinization
trichinoscope
trichinous
trichion
trichite
trichitis
Trichocephalus
trichoclasia, trichoclasis
trichocryptosis
trichocyst
Trichodectes
Trichoderma
trichodiscoma
trichodynia
trichodystrophy
trichoepithelioma
acquired t.
desmoplastic t.
hereditary multiple t.
trichoesthesia
trichofolliculoma
trichogenous
trichoglossia
trichohyalin
trichoid
tricholemmoma
tricholith
trichologia
trichology
trichoma
trichomatose
trichomatosis
trichomatous
trichomegaly
trichomonad
Trichomonadidae
Trichomonas
T. buccalis
T. foetus
T. gallinarum
T. hominis
T. ovis
T. suis
T. tenax
T. vaginalis
trichomoniasis
t. vaginitis

T

trichomycetosis
trichomycosis
    t. axillaris
    t. chromatica
    t. nodosa
    t. nodularis
    t. palmellina
    t. pustulosa
trichonocardiosis
    t. axillaris
trichonodosis
trichonosis
trichonosus
    t. versicolor
trichopathic
trichopathophobia
trichopathy
trichophagy
trichophobia
trichophytic
trichophytid
Trichophyton
    T. concentricum
    T. megninii
    T. rubrum
    T. schoenleinii
    T. tonsurans
    T. violaceum
trichophytosis
    t. barbae
    t. capitis
    t. corporis
    t. cruris
    t. unguium
Trichopleuris
trichopoliodystrophy
trichopoliosis
Trichoptera
trichoptilosis
trichorhinophalangeal syndrome
trichorrhexis
    t. invaginata
    t. nodosa
trichoschisis
trichoscopy
trichosis
    t. carunculae
    t. sensitiva
    t. setosa
trichosomatous
Trichosporon
trichosporonosis
trichosporosis
trichostasis spinulosa
trichostrongyle
Trichostrongylidae
Trichostrongylus
    T. axei

T. capricola
T. colubriformis
T. longispicularis
T. tenuis
T. vitrinus
Trichothecium
trichothiodystrophy
trichotillomania
trichotomy
trichotoxin
trichotrophy
trichroic
trichroism
trichromat
trichromatic
trichromatism
    anomalous t.
trichromatopsia
trichrome stain
trichromic
trichterbrust
Trichuris
    T. trichiura
tricipital
tricorn
tricornute
tricrotic
tricrotism
tricrotous
Tricula
tricuspid, tricuspidal, tricuspidate
    t. area
    t. atresia
    t. incompetence
    t. insufficiency
    t. murmur
    t. orifice
    t. stenosis
    t. tooth
    t. valve
tridactylous
trident
    t. hand
tridentate
tridermic
tridermoma
tridigitate
tridymite
tridymus
trielcon
trifacial
    t. nerve
    t. neuralgia
trifid
    t. stomach
trifocal
    t. lens
trifurcation

trigastric
trigeminal
t. cave
t. cavity
t. crest
t. decompression
t. ganglion
t. impression
t. lemniscus
t. nerve
t. neuralgia
t. pulse
t. rhizotomy
t. rhythm
t. tractotomy
trigeminofacial reflex
trigeminothalamic tract
trigeminus
trigeminy
trigger
t. area
ECG t.
EKG t.
t. finger
t. point
t. zone
triggered activity
trigona (*pl. of* trigonum)
trigonal
trigone
t. of auditory nerve
t. of bladder
cerebral t.
collateral t.
deltoideopectoral t.
fibrous t.'s of heart
t. of fillet
t. of habenula
habenular t.
hypoglossal t.
t. of hypoglossal nerve
inguinal t.
t. of lateral ventricle
left fibrous t.
lemniscal t.
Lieutaud's t.
Müller's t.
olfactory t.
right fibrous t.
vagal t.
t. of vagus nerve
ventricular t.
vertebrocostal t.
trigonid
trigonitis
trigonocephalic
trigonocephaly
trigonum, pl. **trigona**

t. acustici
t. caroticum
t. cerebrale
t. cervicale
t. cervicale anterius
t. cervicale posterius
t. collaterale
t. colli
t. deltoideopectorale
t. femorale
trigona fibrosa cordis
t. fibrosum dextrum
t. fibrosum sinistrum
t. habenulae
t. hypoglossi
t. inguinale
t. lemnisci
t. lumbale
t. lumbocostale
t. musculare
t. nervi hypoglossi
t. nervi vagi
t. olfactorium
t. omoclaviculare
t. omotracheale
t. palati
t. sternocostale
t. submandibulare
t. submentale
t. ventriculi
t. vesicae
trihybrid
triiniodymus
triiodothyronine uptake test
trilabe
trilaminar
t. blastoderm
trilateral
trilobate, trilobed
trilocular
trilogy
t. of Fallot
trimalleolar fracture
trimastigote
trimester
trimethylaminuria
trimorphic
trimorphism
trimorphous
triophthalmos
triorchism
triotus
triphalangia
triphammer pulse
triphenylmethane dyes
triphyllomatous teratoma
Tripier's amputation

T

triplant
    t. implant
triple
    t. arthrodesis
    t. quartan
    t. response
    t. rhythm
    t. symptom complex
    t. vision
    t. X syndrome
triplegia
triploblastic
triploid
triploidy
triplopia
tripod
    t. fracture
    Haller's t.
    vital t.
tripodia
triprosopus
triquetral bone
triquetrous
    t. cartilage
triquetrum
triradial, triradiate
triradius
triskaidekaphobia
trismic
trismoid
trismus
    t. capistratus
    t. dolorificus
    t. nascentium
    t. neonatorum
    t. sardonicus
trisomic
trisomy
    t. C syndrome
    t. D syndrome
    t. 8 syndrome
    t. 13 syndrome
    t. 18 syndrome
    t. 20 syndrome
    t. 21 syndrome
trispiral tomography
trisplanchnic
tristichia
trisulcate
tritanomaly
tritanopia
triticeal cartilage
triticeoglossus
triticeous
triticeum
triton tumor
Tritrichomonas
tritubercular

trivalve
trizonal
trocar
    Hasson t.
trochanter
    greater t.
    lesser t.
    t. major
    t. minor
    t. reflex
    small t.
    t. tertius
    third t.
trochanterian, trochanteric
trochanterplasty
trochantin
trochantinian
trochlea, pl. **trochleae**
    t. femoris
    t. fibularis calcanei
    t. humeri
    t. of humerus
    t. muscularis
    peroneal t. of calcaneus
    t. peronealis
    t. phalangis
    t. tali
    t. of the talus
trochlear
    t. fossa
    t. fovea
    t. nerve
    t. notch
    t. nucleus
    t. pit
    t. process
    t. spine
    t. synovial bursa
trochleariform
trochlearis
trochleiform
trochocardia
trochoid
    t. articulation
    t. joint
trochorizocardia
Troglotrema salmincola
Troisier's
    T. ganglion
    T. node
troland
Trolard's vein
Tröltsch's
    T. corpuscles
    T. fold
    T. pockets
    T. recesses

Trombicula
>> T. akamushi
>> T. deliensis

trombiculid
Trombiculidae
Trombidiidae
Trömner's reflex
tropeolins
trophectoderm
trophesic
trophesy
trophic
>> t. changes
>> t. gangrene
>> t. nucleus
>> t. ulcer

trophicity
trophism
trophoblast
>> plasmodial t.
>> syncytial t.

trophoblastic
>> t. lacuna
>> t. operculum

trophoblastoma
trophochromatin
trophochromidia
trophocyte
trophoderm
trophodermatoneurosis
trophoneurosis
>> facial t.
>> lingual t.
>> muscular t.
>> Romberg's t.

trophoneurotic
>> t. atrophy
>> t. leprosy

trophonucleus
trophoplast
trophospongia
trophotaxis
trophotropic
>> t. zone of Hess

trophotropism
trophozoite
tropia
tropical
>> t. abscess
>> t. acne
>> t. anemia
>> t. boil
>> t. bubo
>> t. diarrhea
>> t. diseases
>> t. eczema
>> t. eosinophilia
>> t. hyphemia

>> t. lichen
>> t. mask
>> t. measles
>> t. medicine
>> t. myositis
>> t. pyomyositis
>> t. sore
>> t. splenomegaly
>> t. splenomegaly syndrome
>> t. sprue
>> t. typhus
>> t. ulcer

tropism
>> negative t.
>> positive t.
>> viral t.

tropometer
trough
>> gingival t.
>> Langmuir t.
>> synaptic t.

Trousseau-Lallemand bodies
Trousseau's
>> T. point
>> T. sign
>> T. spot
>> T. syndrome

true
>> t. aneurysm
>> t. ankylosis
>> t. cementoma
>> t. conjugate
>> t. diverticulum
>> t. dwarfism
>> t. glottis
>> t. hermaphroditism
>> t. hypertrophy
>> t. knot
>> t. knot of umbilical cord
>> t. muscles of back
>> t. neurogenic thoracic outlet
>>   syndrome
>> t. pelvis
>> t. ribs
>> t. thirst
>> t. uterine inertia
>> t. vertebra
>> t. vocal cord

truncal
truncate
>> t. ascertainment

truncus, gen. and pl. **trunci**
>> t. arteriosus
>> t. arteriosus communis
>> t. brachiocephalicus
>> t. bronchiomediastinalis
>> t. celiacus
>> t. corporis callosi

truncus (*continued*)
    t. costocervicalis
    t. fascicularis atrioventricularis
    t. inferior plexus brachialis
    trunci intestinales
    t. jugularis
    t. linguofacialis
    trunci lumbales
    t. lumbosacralis
    t. medius plexus brachialis
    persistent t. arteriosus
    trunci plexus brachialis
    t. pulmonalis
    t. subclavius
    t. superior plexus brachialis
    t. sympathicus
    t. thyrocervicalis
    t. vagalis
Trunecek's sign
trunk
    accessory nerve t.
    t. of atrioventricular bundle
    t.'s of brachial plexus
    brachiocephalic t.
    bronchomediastinal t.
    celiac t.
    t. of corpus callosum
    costocervical t.
    inferior t. of brachial plexus
    intestinal t.'s
    jugular lymphatic t.
    linguofacial t.
    lumbar t.'s
    lumbosacral t.
    middle t. of brachial plexus
    nerve t.
    pulmonary t.
    subclavian lymphatic t.
    superior t. of brachial plexus
    sympathetic t.
    thoracoacromial t.
    thyrocervical t.
    vagal t.
trusion
Trusler's rule for pulmonary artery
  banding
truss
try-in
trypanid
Trypanoplasma
Trypanosoma
    T. avium
    T. cruzi
    T. dimorphon
    T. escomelis
    T. hominis
    T. ignotum
    T. lewisi

    T. melophagium
    T. rangeli
    T. theileri
    T. triatomae
    T. ugandense
trypanosomatid
Trypanosomatidae
trypanosome
    t. fever
    t. stage
trypanosomiasis
    acute t.
    African t.
    American t.
    chronic t.
    Cruz t.
    East African t.
    Gambian t.
    Rhodesian t.
    South American t.
    West African t.
trypanosomic
trypanosomid
trypomastigote
trypsin G-banding stain
tryptonemia
tryptophanuria
    t. with dwarfism
tsetse
TSH stimulating test
tsutsugamushi
    t. disease
    t. fever
tuba, gen. and pl. **tubae**
    t. acustica
    t. auditiva
    t. auditoria
    t. eustachiana, t. eustachii
    t. fallopiana, t. fallopii
    t. uterina
tubage
tubal
    t. abortion
    t. air cells
    t. branch
    t. branch of the tympanic plexus
    t. branch of the uterine artery
    t. cartilage
    t. colic
    t. dysmenorrhea
    t. extremity of ovary
    t. folds of uterine tubes
    t. infantilism
    t. ligation
    t. pregnancy
    t. prominence
    t. tonsil
tubatorsion

tubba, tubbae
tube

Abbott's t.
air t.
auditory t.
Babcock t.
Bouchut's t.
Bourdon t.
bronchial t.'s
Cantor t.
cardiac t.
Carlen's t.
t. cast
cathode ray t.
Celestin t.
Coolidge t.
Crookes-Hittorf t.
digestive t.
drainage t.
Durham's t.
empyema t.
endobronchial t.
endotracheal t.
eustachian t.
fallopian t.
feeding t.
Ferrein's t.
field emission t.
Geiger-Müller t.
germ t.
Haldane t.
intratracheal t.
Levin t.
Martin's t.
medullary t.
Miescher's t.'s
Miller-Abbott t.
molybdenum target t.
Moss t.
nasogastric t.
nasotracheal t.
nephrostomy t.
neural t.
O'Dwyer's t.
orotracheal t.
otopharyngeal t.
pharyngotympanic t.
photomultiplier t.
Pitot t.
pus t.
rectifier t.
Rehfuss stomach t.
Robertshaw t.
roll t.
rotating anode t.
Ruysch's t.
Ryle's t.
Sengstaken-Blakemore t.

PEG Tube
All CAPS

Southey's t.'s
stomach t.
T t.
t. teeth
test t.
thoracostomy t.
Tovell t.
Toynbee's t.
tracheal t.
tracheotomy t.
tympanostomy t.
uterine t.
vacuum t.
Venturi t.
Wangensteen t.
x-ray t.
tubectomy
tubed

t. flap
t. pedicle flap

tuber, pl. **tubera**

t. anterius
ashen t.
calcaneal t.
t. calcanei
t. calcis
t. cincrcum
t. cochleae
t. corporis callosi
t. dorsale
eustachian t.
frontal t.
t. frontale
gray t.
t. ischiadicum
t. of ischium
t. maxillae
omental t.
t. omentale
parietal t.
t. parietale
t. radii
t. valvulae
t. of vermis
t. vermis
t. zygomaticum

tuberal nuclei
tubercle

accessory t.
acoustic t.
adductor t.
amygdaloid t.
anatomical t.
anterior t. of atlas
anterior t. of cervical vertebrae
t. of anterior scalene muscle
anterior thalamic t.
anterior t. of thalamus

tubercle *(continued)*
articular t. of temporal bone
ashen t.
auricular t.
t. bacillus
calcaneal t.
Carabelli t.
carotid t.
caseous t.
Chassaignac's t.
conoid t.
corniculate t.
crown t.
t. of cuneate nucleus
cuneiform t.
darwinian t.
dental t.
dissection t.
dorsal t. of radius
epiglottic t.
fibrous t.
genial t.
genital t.
Gerdy's t.
Ghon's t.
gracile t.
t. of gracile nucleus
gray t.
greater t. of humerus
hard t.
hyaline t.
iliac t.
t. of iliac crest
inferior thyroid t.
infraglenoid t.
intercolumnar t.
intercondylar t.
intervenous t.
jugular t.
labial t.
lateral t. of posterior process of
 talus
lesser t. of humerus
Lisfranc's t.
Lister's t.
Lower's t.
mamillary t.
mamillary t. of hypothalamus
marginal t.
marginal t. of zygomatic bone
medial t. of posterior process of
 talus
mental t.
Montgomery's t.'s
Morgagni's t.
Müller's t.
nuchal t.
t. of nucleus gracilis

obturator t.
olfactory t.
orbital t. of zygomatic bone
phallic t.
pharyngeal t.
posterior t. of atlas
posterior t. of cervical vertebrae
postmortem t.
Princeteau's t.
prosector's t.
pterygoid t.
pubic t.
t. of rib
Rolando's t.
t. of saddle
Santorini's t.
scalene t.
scalene t. of Lisfranc
t. of scaphoid bone
sebaceous t.
sinus t.
soft t.
superior thyroid t.
supraglenoid t.
supratragic t.
t. of tooth
t. of trapezium
t. of upper lip
wedge-shaped t.
Whitnall's t.
Wrisberg's t.
tubercula *(pl. of* tuberculum)
tubercular, tuberculate, tuberculated
tuberculation
tuberculid
nodular t.
papular t.
papulonecrotic t.
rosacea-like t.
tuberculin test
tuberculin-type hypersensitivity
tuberculitis
tuberculization
tuberculocele
tuberculoderma
tuberculofibroid
tuberculoid
t. leprosy
t. rosacea
tuberculoma
tuberculo-opsonic index
tuberculoprotein
tuberculosis
acute t.
acute miliary t.
adult t.
aerogenic t.
anthracotic t.

arrested t.
attenuated t.
basal t.
cerebral t.
childhood t.
childhood type t.
cutaneous t.
t. cutis
t. cutis follicularis disseminata
t. cutis luposa
t. cutis orificialis
t. cutis verrucosa
dermal t.
disseminated t.
enteric t.
exudative t.
general t.
healed t.
inactive t.
t. lymphadenitis
miliary t.
open t.
t. papulonecrotica
postprimary t.
primary t.
pulmonary t.
reinfection t.
secondary t.
t. ulcerosa

tuberculous
t. abscess
t. bronchopneumonia
t. enteritis
t. lymphadenitis
t. meningitis
t. nephritis
t. pericarditis
t. peritonitis
t. rheumatism
t. spondylitis
t. wart

tuberculum, pl. **tubercula**
t. adductorium
t. anterius atlantis
t. anterius thalami
t. anterius vertebrarum cervicalium
t. arthriticum
t. articulare ossis temporalis
t. auriculae
t. calcanei
t. caroticum
t. cinereum
t. conoideum
t. corniculatum
t. coronae
t. costae
t. cuneatum
t. cuneiforme

t. dentis
tubercula dolorosa
t. dorsale
t. epiglotticum
t. gracile
t. hypoglossi
t. iliacum
t. impar
t. infraglenoidale
t. intercondylare
t. intervenosum
t. jugulare
t. labii superioris
t. laterale processus posterioris tali
t. majus humeri
t. mallei
t. marginale ossis zygomatici
t. mediale processus posterioris tali
t. mentale
t. minus humeri
t. musculi scaleni anterioris
t. nuclei cuneati
t. nuclei gracilis
t. obturatorium
t. olfactorium
t. ossis scaphoidei
t. ossis trapezii
t. pharyngeum
t. posterius atlantis
t. posterius vertebrarum cervicalium
t. pubicum
t. sebaceum
t. sellae
t. septi narium
t. superius
t. supraglenoidale
t. supratragicum
t. syphiliticum
t. thyroideum inferius
t. thyroideum superius

tuberiferous
tuberoinfundibular tract
tuberose
tuberositas
t. coracoidea
t. costalis
t. deltoidea
t. glutea
t. iliaca
t. masseterica
t. musculi serrati anterioris
t. ossis cuboidei
t. ossis metatarsalis primi
t. ossis metatarsalis quinti
t. ossis navicularis
t. phalangis distalis
t. pterygoidea
t. radii

T

tuberositas *(continued)*
  t. sacralis
  t. tibiae
  t. ulnae
  t. unguicularis
tuberosity
  bicipital t.
  calcaneal t.
  coracoid t.
  costal t.
  t. of cuboid bone
  deltoid t.
  t. of distal phalanx
  t. of fifth metatarsal
  t. of first metatarsal
  gluteal t.
  greater t. of humerus
  iliac t.
  infraglenoid t.
  ischial t.
  lateral femoral t.
  lesser t. of humerus
  masseteric t.
  maxillary t.
  medial femoral t.
  t. of navicular bone
  pterygoid t.
  radial t.
  t. of radius
  t. reduction
  sacral t.
  scaphoid t.
  t. for serratus anterior muscle
  tibial t.
  t. of ulna
  ungual t.
tuberous
  t. sclerosis
tubi (*pl. of* tubus)
Tübinger perimeter
tuboabdominal
  t. pregnancy
tuboligamentous
tubo-ovarian
  t.-o. abscess
  t.-o. pregnancy
  t.-o. varicocele
tubo-ovariectomy
tubo-ovaritis
tuboperitoneal
tuboplasty
tuboreticular structure
tubotorsion
tubotympanic, tubotympanal
  t. canal
  t. recess
tubouterine
  t. pregnancy

tubovaginal
tubular
  t. adenoma
  t. aneurysm
  t. carcinoma
  t. cyst
  t. excretory mass
  t. forceps
  t. gland
  t. maximum
  t. respiration
  t. vision
tubule
  Albarran y Dominguez' t.'s
  collecting t.
  connecting t.
  convoluted t. of kidney
  convoluted seminiferous t.
  dental t.'s
  dentinal t.'s
  discharging t.
  Henle's t.'s
  Kobelt's t.'s
  malpighian t.'s
  mesonephric t.
  metanephric t.
  paragenital t.'s
  pronephric t.
  segmental t.
  seminiferous t.
  Skene's t.'s
  spiral t.
  straight t.
  straight seminiferous t.
  T t.
  uriniferous t.
  wolffian t.'s
tubuli (*pl. of* tubulus)
tubuliform
tubulization
tubuloacinar gland
tubuloalveolar gland
tubulocyst
tubulodermoid
tubulointerstitial nephritis
tubuloneogenesis
tubuloracemose
tubulorrhexis
tubulose, tubulous
tubulus, pl. **tubuli**
  tubuli biliferi
  t. contortus
  tubuli dentales
  tubuli epoöphori
  tubuli galactophori
  tubuli lactiferi
  tubuli paroöphori
  t. rectus

t. renalis contortus
t. renalis rectus
t. seminifer contortus
t. seminifer rectus
t. transversus

tubus, pl. **tubi**
t. digestorius
t. medullaris
t. vertebralis

Tucker-McLean forceps
tuffstone body
tuft
enamel t.
malpighian t.
synovial t.'s

tufted
t. cell
t. phalanx

tuftsin
tug, tugging
tracheal t.

tularemia
glandular t.
pulmonary t.
pulmonic t.

tularemic
t. chancre
t. conjunctivitis
t. pneumonia

tulle gras
Tullio's phenomenon
Tulpius' valve
Tulp's valve
tumefaction
tumefy
tumentia
tumescence
tumescent
tumid
tumor
acinar cell t.
acute splenic t.
adenoid t.
adenomatoid t.
adenomatoid odontogenic t.
adipose t.
ameloblastic adenomatoid t.
amyloid t.
t. angiogenic factor
angiomatoid t.
t. antigens
aortic body t.
Bednar t.
benign t.
blood t.
borderline t.
Brenner t.
Brooke's t.

brown t.
t. burden
Buschke-Löwenstein t.
calcifying epithelial odontogenic t.
carcinoid t.
carotid body t.
cellular t.
cerebellopontine angle t.
chemoreceptor t.
chromaffin t.
Codman's t.
collision t.
connective t.
dermal duct t.
dermoid t.
desmoid t.
dysembryoplastic neuroepithelial t.
eighth nerve t.
t. embolism
embryonal t., embryonic t.
embryonal t. of ciliary body
endocervical sinus t.
endodermal sinus t.
endometrioid t.
Erdheim t.
Ewing's t.
fecal t.
fibroid t.
giant cell t. of bone
giant cell t. of tendon sheath
glomus t.
glomus jugulare t.
Godwin t.
granular cell t.
granulosa cell t.   cyst
Grawitz' t.
Gubler's t.
haarscheibe t.
heterologous t.
hilar cell t. of ovary
histoid t.
homologous t.
Hürthle cell t.
hylic t.
innocent t.
interstitial cell t. of testis
Koenen's t.
Krukenberg's t.
Landschutz t.
Lindau's t.
low malignant potential t.
t. lysis syndrome
malignant t.
malignant mixed müllerian t.
t. marker
melanotic neuroectodermal t. of
infancy
Merkel cell t.

943

tumor (*continued*)
  mesonephroid t.
  mixed t.
  mixed mesodermal t.
  mixed t. of salivary gland
  mixed t. of skin
  mucoepidermoid t.
  t. necrosis factor-beta
  Nelson t.
  oil t.
  oncocytic hepatocellular t.
  organoid t.
  Pancoast t.
  papillary t.
  paraffin t.
  phantom t.
  phyllodes t.
  pilar t. of scalp
  Pindborg t.
  Pinkus t.
  placental site trophoblastic t.
  pontine angle t.
  potato t. of neck
  Pott's puffy t.
  pregnancy t.
  primitive neuroectodermal t.
  ranine t.
  Rathke's pouch t.
  Recklinghausen's t.
  retinal anlage t.
  Rous t.
  sand t.
  Sertoli cell t.
  solitary fibrous t.
  squamous odontogenic t.
  t. stage
  sugar t.
  superior pulmonary sulcus t.
  teratoid t.
  theca cell t.
  triton t.
  turban t.
  villous t.
  t. virus
  Warthin's t.
  Wilms' t.
  wing-beating t.
  yolk sac t.
  Zollinger-Ellison t.
tumoral calcinosis
tumor-associated antigen
tumorigenesis
  foreign body t.
tumorigenic
tumor-infiltrating lymphocytes
tumorlets
tumorous
tumor-specific transplantation antigens

tumultus cordis
Tunga penetrans
tungiasis
Tungidae
tungstate
  calcium t.
tungsten
  t. arc lamp
  t. carbide
tunic
  Bichat's t.
  Brücke's t.
  fibrous t. of corpus spongiosum
  fibrous t. of eye
  mucosal t.'s, mucous t.'s
  muscular t.'s
  muscular t. of gallbladder
  nervous t. of eyeball
  serous t.
  vascular t. of eye
tunica, pl. **tunicae**
  t. adventitia
  t. albuginea
  t. albuginea of corpora cavernosi
  t. albuginea corporis spongiosi
  t. albuginea corporum cavernosorum
  t. albuginea of corpus spongiosum
  t. albuginea oculi
  t. albuginea testis
  t. albuginea of testis
  t. carnea
  t. conjunctiva
  t. conjunctiva bulbi
  t. conjunctiva palpebrarum
  t. dartos
  t. elastica
  t. externa
  t. externa oculi
  t. externa thecae folliculi
  t. extima
  t. fibrosa
  t. fibrosa bulbi
  t. fibrosa hepatis
  t. fibrosa lienis
  t. fibrosa renis
  t. fibrosa splenis
  tunicae funiculi spermatici
  Haller's t. vasculosa
  t. interna bulbi
  t. interna thecae folliculi
  t. intima
  t. media
  t. mucosa
  t. mucosa bronchiorum
  t. mucosa cavitatis tympani
  t. mucosa coli
  t. mucosa ductus deferentis
  t. mucosa esophagi

t. mucosa gastrica [ventriculi]
t. mucosa intestini tenuis
t. mucosa laryngis
t. mucosa linguae
t. mucosa nasi
t. mucosa oris
t. mucosa pharyngis
t. mucosa tracheae
t. mucosa tubae auditivae
t. mucosa tubae uterinae
t. mucosa ureteris
t. mucosa urethrae femininae
t. mucosa uteri
t. mucosa vaginae
t. mucosa vesicae biliaris
t. mucosa vesicae felleae
t. mucosa vesicae urinariae
t. mucosa vesiculae seminalis
t. muscularis
t. muscularis bronchiorum
t. muscularis coli
t. muscularis ductus deferentis
t. muscularis esophagi
t. muscularis gastrica
t. muscularis intestini tenuis
t. muscularis pharyngis
t. muscularis recti
t. muscularis tracheae
t. muscularis tubae uterinae
t. muscularis ureteris
t. muscularis urethrae femininae
t. muscularis uteri
t. muscularis vaginae
t. muscularis ventriculi
t. muscularis vesicae biliaris
t. muscularis vesicae felleae
t. muscularis vesicae urinariae
t. nervea
t. propria
t. propria corii
t. propria lienis
t. reflexa
t. sclerotica
t. serosa
t. serosa coli
t. serosa gastrica
t. serosa hepatis
t. serosa intestini tenuis
t. serosa peritonei
t. serosa tubae uterinae
t. serosa uteri
t. serosa ventriculi
t. serosa vesicae biliaris
t. serosa vesicae felleae
t. serosa vesicae urinariae
t. submucosa
t. vaginalis communis
t. vaginalis testis

t. vasculosa
t. vasculosa bulbi
t. vasculosa lentis
t. vasculosa oculi
t. vasculosa testis
t. vitrea
tuning fork
tunnel
    aortico-left ventricular t.
    carpal t.
    t. cells
    Corti's t.
    t. vision
Tuohy needle
T_3 uptake test
turban tumor
Turbatrix
turbinal
    t. varix
turbinate
turbinated
    t. body
    t. bones
    t. crest
turbinectomy
turbinotome
turbinotomy
Türck's
    T. bundle
    T. column
    T. degeneration
    T. tract
Turcot syndrome
turgescence
turgescent
turgid
turgometer
turgor
    t. vitalis
turista
Türk
    T. cell
    T. leukocyte
turkey
    t. gobbler neck
    t. red
Turkish saddle
Turlock virus
turn
Turner's
    T. sulcus
    T. tooth
turnover flap
turpentine enema
turricephaly
TUR syndrome
turunda, pl. **turundae**
tussal

T

tussicular
tussiculation
tussigenic
tussis
tussive
    t. fremitus
    t. syncope
tutamen, pl. **tutamina**
    tutamina cerebri
    tutamina oculi
Tuttle's proctoscope
Tweed
    T. edgewise treatment
    T. triangle
tweezers
twelfth cranial nerve
twelfth-year molar
twenty-nail dystrophy
twiddler's syndrome
twig
twilight
    t. sleep
    t. state
    t. vision
twin
    allantoidoangiopagous t.'s
    t. cone
    conjoined t.'s
    conjoined asymmetrical t.'s
    conjoined equal t.'s
    conjoined symmetrical t.'s
    conjoined unequal t.'s
    t. crystal
    dichorial t.'s
    diovular t.'s
    dizygotic t.'s
    enzygotic t.'s
    fraternal t.'s
    heterologous t.'s
    identical t.'s
    incomplete conjoined t.'s
    t. method
    monoamniotic t.'s
    monochorial t.'s
    monovular t.'s
    monozygotic t.'s
    omphaloangiopagous t.'s
    parasitic t.
    t. placenta
    placental parasitic t.
    polyzygotic t.'s
    t. pregnancy
    Siamese t.'s
    uniovular t.'s
twinge
twinning
twin-twin transfusion
twisted hairs

twitch
two-bellied muscle
two-dimensional
    t.-d. echocardiography
    t.-d. immunoelectrophoresis
two-glass test
Twort-d'Herelle phenomenon
Twort phenomenon
two-step exercise test
two-sympathin theory
two-tail test
two-way catheter
tyle
tylectomy
tylion, pl. **tylia**
tyloma
    t. conjunctivae
tylosis, pl. **tyloses**
    t. ciliaris
    t. linguae
    t. palmaris et plantaris
tylotic
tympana (*pl. of* tympanum)
tympanal
tympanectomy
tympania
tympanic
    t. air cells
    t. antrum
    t. attic
    t. body
    t. bone
    t. canal
    t. canaliculus
    t. cavity
    t. cells
    t. enlargement
    t. ganglion
    t. gland
    t. groove
    t. incisure
    t. intumescence
    t. labium of limbus of spiral lamina
    t. lip of limbus of spiral lamina
    t. membrane
    t. nerve
    t. notch
    t. opening of auditory tube
    t. opening of canaliculi for chorda tympani
    t. opening of eustachian tube
    t. part of temporal bone
    t. plate of temporal bone
    t. plexus
    t. promontory
    t. ring
    t. scute

t. sinus
t. veins
t. wall of cochlear duct
tympanichord
tympanichordal
tympanicity
tympanism
tympanites
uterine t.
tympanitic
t. resonance
tympanitis
tympanocentesis
tympanoeustachian
tympanohyal
t. bone
tympanomalleal
tympanomandibular
tympanomastoid
t. fissure
t. suture
tympanomastoiditis
tympanomeatomastoidectomy
tympanophonia, tympanophony
tympanoplasty
tympanosquamosal
tympanosquamous fissure
tympanostapedial
t. junction
t. syndesmosis
tympanostomy
t. tube
tympanotemporal
tympanotomy
tympanous
tympanum, pl. **tympana, tympanums**
tympany
Skoda's t.
tyndallization
Tyndall phenomenon
type
t. A behavior
t. A personality
basic personality t.
t. B behavior
blood t.
t. B personality
buffalo t.
t. culture
t. 1 dextrocardia
t. 2 dextrocardia
t. 3 dextrocardia
t. 4 dextrocardia
T. 1 G_{MI} gangliosidosis
t. 1 glycogenosis
t. 2 glycogenosis
t. 3 glycogenosis
t. 4 glycogenosis

t. 5 glycogenosis
t. 6 glycogenosis
t. 7 glycogenosis
t. I
t. I acrocephalosyndactyly
t. I cells
t. I diabetes
t. I diabetes mellitus
t. I dip
t. I error
t. II
t. II acrocephalosyndactyly
t. II cells
t. II diabetes
t. II dip
t. II error
t. II familial hyperlipoproteinemia
t. III
t. III acrocephalosyndactyly
t. III familial hyperlipoproteinemia
t. III hypersensitivity reaction
t. III mucopolysaccharidosis
t. II mucopolysaccharidosis
t. IS mucopolysaccharidosis
t. IVA, B mucopolysaccharidosis
t. IV acrocephalosyndactyly
t. IV familial hyperlipoproteinemia
nomenclatural t.
t. species
t. strain
test t.
t. V acrocephalosyndactyly
t. V familial hyperlipoproteinemia
t. VIII mucopolysaccharidosis
t. VII mucopolysaccharidosis
t. VI mucopolysaccharidosis
t. V mucopolysaccharidosis
wild t.
typhinia
typhlectasis
typhlectomy
typhlenteritis
typhlitis
typhlodicliditis
typhloempyema
typhloenteritis
typhlolithiasis
typhlology
typhlomegaly
typhlon
typhlopexy, typhlopexia
typhlorrhaphy
typhlosis
typhlostomy
typhlotomy
typhoid
abdominal t.
ambulatory t.

T

typhoid *(continued)*
    apyretic t.
    t. bacillus
    t. bacteriophage
    bilious t. of Griesinger
    t. cholera
    t. fever
    latent t.
    t. pleurisy
    t. pneumonia
    provocation t.
    t. septicemia
    walking t.
typhoidal
typholysin
typhomania
typhosepsis
typhous
typhus
    Australian tick t.
    endemic t.
    epidemic t.
    European t.
    exanthematous t.
    flea-borne t.
    Indian tick t.
    louse-borne t.
    Manchurian t.
    Mexican t.
    mite t.
    mite-born t.
    t. mitior
    murine t.
    North Queensland tick t.
    prison fever t.
    Queensland tick t.

    recrudescent t.
    São Paulo t.
    scrub t.
    shop t.
    Siberian tick t.
    tick t.
    tropical t.
    urban t.
typical achromatopsia
typing
    bacteriophage t.
    DNA t.
    HLA t.
typist's cramp
tyrannism
tyremesis
Tyroglyphus longior
tyroid
tyroketonuria
tyroma
Tyrophagus putrescentiae
tyrosinase
    t. negative type
    t. positive type
tyrosinemia
tyrosinosis
tyrosinuria
tyrosis
tyrosyluria
Tyrrell's fascia
Tyson's glands
Tyzzeria
Tzanck
    T. cells
    T. test

U

U wave

Uhl anomaly

Uhthoff

U. symptom

U. syndrome

Uhthoff's sign

ulcer

acute decubitus u.

Aden u.

amputating u.

anastomotic u.

atonic u.

Buruli u.

chiclero u.

chrome u.

chronic u.

cockscomb u.

cold u.

constitutional u.

corrosive u.

creeping u.

Curling's u.

decubitus u.

dendritic corneal u.

dental u.

diphtheritic u.

distention u.

elusive u.

fascicular u.

Fenwick-Hunner u.

Gaboon u.

gastric u.

gravitational u.

groin u.

gummatous u.

hard u.

healed u.

herpetic u.

Hunner's u.

hypopyon u.

indolent u.

inflamed u.

Kurunegala u.'s

Lipschütz' u.

lupoid u.

Mann-Williamson u.

marginal ring u. of cornea

Marjolin's u.

Meleney's u.

Mooren's u.

Oriental u.

penetrating u.

peptic u.

perambulating u.

perforated u.

perforating u. of foot

phagedenic u.

phlegmonous u.

pudendal u.

recurrent aphthous u.'s

ring u. of cornea

rodent u.

Saemisch's u.

serpent u. of cornea

serpiginous u.

serpiginous corneal u.

simple u.

sloughing u.

soft u.

stasis u.

stercoral u.

steroid u.

stomal u.

stress u.'s

Sutton's u.

symptomatic u.

syphilitic u.

Syriac u., Syrian u.

tanner's u.

transparent u. of the cornea

trophic u.

tropical u.

undermining u.

varicose u.

venereal u.

Zambesi u.

ulcera (*pl. of* ulcus)

ulcerate

ulcerated

ulcerating granuloma of pudenda

ulceration

tracheal u.

ulcerative

u. colitis

u. pharyngitis

u. stomatitis

ulcerogenic

ulceroglandular

ulceromembranous

u. gingivitis

u. pharyngitis

ulcerous

ulcus, pl. **ulcera**

u. ambulans

u. hypostaticum

u. terebrans

u. venereum

u. vulvae acutum

ulectomy

U

ulegyria
ulerythema
    u. ophryogenes
    u. sycosiforme
uletomy
ulex europaeus
Ullmann's
    U. line
    U. syndrome
ulna, gen. and pl. **ulnae**
ulnad
ulnar
    u. artery
    u. branch of medial antebrachial
      cutaneous nerve
    u. bursa
    u. clubhand
    u. collateral ligament
    u. collateral ligament of elbow
    u. collateral ligament of wrist
    u. communicating branch of
      superficial radial nerve
    u. eminence of wrist
    u. extensor muscle of wrist
    u. flexor muscle of wrist
    u. head
    u. margin of forearm
    u. nerve
    u. notch
    u. reflex
    u. veins
ulnaris
ulnen
ulnocarpal
ulnoradial
ulodermatitis
uloid
ulotomy
ulotrichous
ultimate strength
ultimobranchial
    u. body
    u. pouch
ultimum moriens
ultrabrachycephalic
ultracytostome
ultradian
    u. rhythm
ultradolichocephalic
ultrafiltration
    u. coefficient
    u. hemodialyzer
ultraligation
ultramicroscope
ultramicroscopic
ultramicrotome
ultramicrotomy
ultrashortwave diathermy

ultrasonic
    u. cardiography
    u. cephalometry
    u. cleaning
    u. egg recovery
    u. lithotresis
    u. microscope
    u. rays
    u. scaler
    u. therapy
    u. waves
ultrasonics
ultrasonogram
ultrasonograph
ultrasonographer
ultrasonography
    Doppler u.
    duplex u.
    endovaginal u.
    gray-scale u.
    real-time u.
ultrasonosurgery
ultrasound
    u. cardiography
    diagnostic u.
    obstetric u.
    u. transducer
ultrastructural anatomy
ultrastructure
ultratherm
ultrathin section
ultraviolet
    u. A
    u. B
    u. C
    extravital u.
    intravital u.
    u. keratoconjunctivitis
    u. lamp
    u. microscope
    u. rays
    u. spectrum
    vital u.
ultravirus
ultromotivity
ultropaque method
ululation
Ulysses syndrome
umbilical
    u. artery
    u. cord
    u. cyst
    u. duct
    u. fissure
    u. fistula
    u. fossa
    u. fungus
    u. hernia

u. notch
u. part of left branch of portal vein
u. prevesical fascia
u. region
u. ring
u. souffle
u. vein
u. vesicle
umbilicate, umbilicated
umbilication
umbilici (*pl. of* umbilicus)
umbilicomammillary triangle
umbilicovesical fascia
umbilicus, pl. **umbilici**
umbo, gen. **umbonis,** pl. **umbones**
u. membranae tympani
u. of tympanic membrane
Umbre virus
unarmed rostellum
unavoidable hemorrhage
unbalanced translocation
uncal
u. herniation
unci (*pl. of* uncus)
unciform
u. bone
u. fasciculus
u. pancreas
unciforme
uncinariasis
uncinate
u. attack
u. bundle of Russell
u. epilepsy
u. fasciculus
u. fasciculus of Russell
u. fit
u. gyrus
u. pancreas
u. process of ethmoid bone
u. process of pancreas
uncinatum
uncipressure
uncompensated
u. acidosis
u. alkalosis
uncomplemented
unconditioned
u. reflex
u. response
u. stimulus
unconjugated bilirubin
unconscious
collective u.
u. homosexuality
unconsciousness
unco-ossified

uncovertebral
u. joints
uncrossed diplopia
unction
uncus, pl. **unci**
u. band of Giacomini
u. gyri parahippocampalis
underachievement
underachiever
underbite
undercut
u. gauge
underdrive pacing
undermining ulcer
undernutrition
undersensing
undershoot
understain
underventilation
Underwood's disease
undescended testis
undetermined nitrogen
undifferentiated
u. cell
u. cell adenoma
u. type fevers
undine
undinism
undiversion
undoing
undulate
undulating
u. fever
u. membrane
u. pulse
undulatory membrane
undulipodium, pl. **undulipodia**
unequal
u. cleavage
u. crossing-over
u. pulse
u. retinal image
unerupted tooth
unesterified free fatty acid
uneven crossing-over
unformed visual hallucination
ungual
u. phalanx
u. tuberosity
unguinal
unguis, pl. **ungues**
u. aduncus
u. avis
Haller's u.
u. incarnatus
uniarticular
uniaxial
u. joint

U

Uniblue A
unicameral, unicamerate
  u. bone cyst
  u. cyst
unicanalicular sphincter
unicellular
  u. gland
  u. sclerosis
unicentral
unicorn
  u. uterus
unicornous
unicuspid, unicuspidate
unidirectional
  u. block
  u. flux
unifamilial
uniflagellate
uniforate
uniform
unigerminal
uniglandular
unilaminar, unilaminate
unilateral
  u. anesthesia
  u. hemianopia
  u. hermaphroditism
  u. hyperlucent lung
  u. lobar emphysema
unilobar
unilocal
unilocular
  u. cyst
  u. fat
  u. hydatid cyst
  u. joint
uninhibited neurogenic bladder
uninterrupted suture
uninuclear, uninucleate
uniocular
  u. hemianopia
union
  autogenous u.
  faulty u.
  fibrous u.
  primary u.
  secondary u.
  vicious u.
unioval, uniovular
unipennate
  u. muscle
unipolar
  u. cell
  u. electrocardiogram
  u. leads
  u. neuron
uniseptate

unit
  alpha u.'s
  Bethesda u.
  u. character
  u. of convergence
  coronary care u.
  critical care u.
  CT u.
  u. fibrils
  Fishman-Lerner u.
  Holzknecht u.
  Hounsfield u.
  intensive care u.
  Karmen u.
  Kienböck's u.
  lung u.
  u. membrane
  motor u.
  u. of ocular convergence
  ostiomeatal u.
  physiologic u.
  u. of radioactivity
  roentgen u.
  Schwann cell u.
  Somogyi u.
  Todd u.
  toxic u.
  toxin u.
  volume u.
United States Public Health Service
uniting
  u. canal
  u. cartilage
  u. duct
univalent antibody
univentricular
  u. connections
  u. heart
universal
  u. appliance
  u. donor
  u. infantilism
unmedullated
unmodified zinc oxide-eugenol cement
unmyelinated
  u. fibers
  u. nerve
Unna-Pappenheim stain
Unna's
  U. disease
  U. mark
  U. stain
Unna-Taenzer stain
unpaired
  u. allosome
  u. chromosome
unphysiologic
unresolved pneumonia

unroofed coronary sinus syndrome
unsanitary
unsex
unsharp masking
unstable
    u. angina
    u. bladder
    u. equilibrium
    u. fracture
    u. hemoglobin hemolytic anemia
unstrained jaw relation
unstriated
    u. muscle
unstriped muscle
unsystematized delusion
ununited fracture
Unverricht's disease
unwinding proteins
upbeat nystagmus
upper
    u. abdominal periosteal reflex
    u. airway
    u. extremity
    u. extremity of fibula
    u. eyelid
    u. GI series
    u. jaw
    u. jaw bone
    u. lateral cutaneous nerve of arm
    u. lid
    u. limb
    u. lip
    u. lobe of lung
    u. motor neuron
    u. motor neuron lesion
    u. nodal extrasystole
    u. nodal rhythm
    u. subscapular nerve
    u. thoracic splanchnic nerves
    u. uterine segment
upsiloid
urachal
    u. cyst
    u. fistula
    u. fold
    u. ligament
urachus
uranin
uraniscochasm
uranisconitis
uraniscoplasty
uraniscorrhaphy
uraniscus
uranium nephritis
uranoplasty
uranorrhaphy
uranoschisis
uranostaphyloplasty

uranostaphylorrhaphy
uranostaphyloschisis
uranoveloschisis
uranyl acetate stain
uraroma
urarthritis
urate crystals stain
uratemia
uratoma
uratosis
uraturia
Urbach-Wiethe disease
urban
    u. cutaneous leishmaniasis
    u. typhus
Urban's operation
urceiform
urceolate
ur-defenses
urea
    u. clearance
    u. clearance test
    u. frost
    u. nitrogen
Ureaplasma
    U. urealyticum
ureapoiesis
urease test
urecchysis
urecholine supersensitivity test
uredema
uredo
urelcosis
uremia
    hypercalcemic u.
uremic
    u. breath
    u. colitis
    u. coma
    u. frost
    u. lung
    u. pericarditis
    u. pneumonia
    u. pneumonitis
    u. polyneuropathy
uremigenic
uresiesthesia
uresis
ureter
    curlicue u.
    ectopic u.
    postcaval u.
    retrocaval u.
    retroiliac u.
ureteral
    u. branches
    u. colic

U

ureteral *(continued)*
  u. meatus
  u. opening
ureteralgia
uretercystoscope
ureterectasia
ureterectomy
ureteric
  u. branches
  u. branches of the ovarian artery
  u. branches of the patent part of
    umbilical artery
  u. branches of the renal artery
  u. branches of the testicular artery
  u. bud
  u. dysmenorrhea
  u. fold
  u. orifice
  u. pelvis
  u. plexus
ureteritis
ureterocalicostomy
ureterocele
ureterocelorraphy
ureterocolic
ureterocolostomy
ureterocutaneous fistula
ureterocystoscope
ureterocystostomy
ureteroenteric
ureteroenterostomy
ureterography
ureterohydronephrosis
uretero-ileal anastomosis
ureteroileoneocystostomy
ureteroileostomy
ureterolithiasis
ureterolithotomy
ureterolysis
ureteroneocystostomy
ureteronephrectomy
ureteropathy
ureteropelvic
  u. junction
  u. junction obstruction
  u. obstruction
ureteroplasty
ureteroproctostomy
ureteropyelitis
ureteropyelography
ureteropyeloplasty
ureteropyelostomy
ureteropyosis
ureterorectostomy
ureterorenal reflux
ureterorrhagia
ureterorrhaphy
ureteroscope

ureterosigmoid
  u. anastomosis
ureterosigmoidostomy
ureterostenosis
ureterostomy
  cutaneous u.
  cutaneous loop u.
ureterotomy
ureterotrigonoenterostomy
ureterotubal anastomosis
ureteroureteral
  u. anastomosis
ureteroureterostomy
ureterovaginal fistula
ureterovesical
  u. obstruction
ureterovesicostomy
urethra
  anterior u.
  female u.
  u. feminina
  male u.
  u. masculina
  membranous u.
  u. muliebris
  penile u.
  posterior u.
  prostatic u.
  spongy u.
  u. virilis
urethral
  u. artery
  u. calculus
  u. carina of vagina
  u. caruncle
  u. crest
  u. crest of female
  u. crest of male
  u. dilation
  u. diverticulum
  u. fever
  u. glands
  u. groove
  u. hematuria
  u. lacuna
  u. openings
  u. papilla
  u. plate
  u. pressure profile
  u. stricture
  u. surface of penis
  u. syndrome
  u. valves
urethralgia
urethrectomy
urethremorrhagia
urethrism, urethrismus

urethritis
  anterior u.
  follicular u.
  gonorrheal u.
  granular u.
  nongonococcal u.
  nonspecific u.
  u. petrificans
  posterior u.
  simple u.
  specific u.
  u. venerea
urethrobulbar
urethrocele
urethrocystometrography
urethrocystometry
urethrocystopexy
urethrodynia
urethrography
urethrometer
urethropenile
urethropcrineal
urethroperineoscrotal
urethropexy
urethroplasty
  cecil u.
urethroprostatic
urethrorectal
urethrorrhagia
urethrorrhaphy
urethrorrhea
urethroscope
urethroscopic
urethroscopy
urethrospasm
urethrostaxis
urethrostenosis
urethrostomy
  perineal u.
urethrotome
urethrotomy
  external u.
  internal u.
  perineal u.
urethrovaginal
  u. fistula
urethrovesical
urethrovesicopexy
urge incontinence
urgency
  u. incontinence
  motor u.
  sensory u.
urhidrosis
uric acid infarct
uricolytic index
uricosuria
uricosuric

uridrosis
  u. crystallina
uriesthesia
urinal
urinalysis
urinary
  u. apparatus
  u. bladder
  u. calculus
  u. casts
  u. concentration test
  u. cyst
  u. exertional incontinence
  u. fever
  u. fistula
  u. nitrogen
  u. organs
  u. reflex
  u. sand
  u. schistosomiasis
  u. smear
  u. stuttering
  u. system
  u. tract
  u. tract infection
urinate
urination
  stuttering u.
urine
  ammoniacal u.
  black u.
  chylous u.
  cloudy u.
  crude u.
  febrile u.
  feverish u.
  gouty u.
  honey u.
  maple syrup u.
  milky u.
  nebulous u.
  residual u.
urinemia
uriniferous
  u. tubule
urinific
uriniparous
urinogenital
urinogenous
urinoma
urinometer
urinometry
urinoscopy
urinosexual
urinous
uriposia
uritis
uroammoniac

U

urobilinemia
urobilinuria
urocele
urocheras
urochesia
urocrisia
urocrisis
urocyanin
urocyanogen
urocyanosis
urocyst
urocystic
urocystis
urodynamics
urodynia
uroflowmeter
urofuscohematin
urogenital
   u. apparatus
   u. canal
   u. cleft
   u. diaphragm
   u. fistula
   u. membrane
   u. mesentery
   u. region
   u. ridge
   u. septum
   u. sinus
   u. system
   u. triangle
urogenous
uroglaucin
urogram
urography
   antegrade u.
   cystoscopic u.
   intravenous u., excretory u.
   retrograde u.
urogravimeter
urolagnia
urolith
urolithiasis
urolithic
urolithology
urologic, urological
urologist
urology
urometer
uroncus
uronephrosis
uronoscopy
uropathy
   obstructive u.
urophanic
urophein
uropoiesis

uropoietic
   u. system
uropsammus
uroradiology
urorectal
   u. fold
   u. membrane
   u. septum
urorubin
urorubrohematin
uroschesis
uroscopic
uroscopy
urosemiology
urosepsin
urosepsis
urothelium
urothorax
urticant
urticaria
   u. acuta
   acute u.
   u. bullosa
   cholinergic u.
   chronic u.
   u. chronica
   cold u.
   u. conferta
   congelation u.
   u. endemica, u. epidemica
   u. factitia
   factitious u.
   febrile u.
   u. febrilis
   giant u.
   heat u.
   u. hemorrhagica
   u. maculosa
   u. medicamentosa
   papular u.
   u. papulosa
   u. perstans
   u. pigmentosa
   pressure u.
   solar u.
   u. subcutanea
   u. tuberosa
   u. vesiculosa
   vibratory u.
urticarial, urticarious
   u. fever
   u. vasculitis
urticate
urtication
u-score method
Usher's syndrome

Ustilago
> *U. maydis*
> *U. zeae*

usual interstitial pneumonia of Liebow
usurpation
uta
uterectomy
uteri (*pl. of* uterus)
uterine
> u. appendages
> u. artery
> u. calculus
> u. cavity
> u. colic
> u. contraction
> u. dysmenorrhea
> u. extremity of ovary
> u. glands
> u. horn
> u. inertia
> u. insufficiency
> u. milk
> u. opening of uterine tubes
> u. ostium of uterine tubes
> u. part of uterine tube
> u. pregnancy
> u. relaxing factor
> u. sinus
> u. sinusoid
> u. souffle
> u. tetanus
> u. tube
> u. tympanites
> u. veins
> u. venous plexus

uterismus
uteritis
in utero
uteroabdominal
> u. pregnancy

uterocervical
uterocystostomy
uteroepichorial membrane
uterofixation
uterolith
uterometer
utero-ovarian
> u.-o. varicocele

uteroparietal
uteropelvic
uteroperitoneal fistula
uteropexy
uteroplacental
> u. apoplexy
> u. sinuses

uteroplasty
uterosacral
> u. ligament

uterosalpingography
uteroscope
uteroscopy
uterotomy
uterotubal
uterotubography
uterovaginal
> u. canal
> u. plexus

uteroventral
uterovesical
> u. fold
> u. ligament
> u. pouch

uterus, pl. **uteri**
> u. acollis
> anomalous u.
> arcuate u.
> u. arcuatus
> bicornate u.
> u. bicornate bicollis
> u. bicornate unicollis
> u. bicornis
> bifid u.
> u. bifidus
> biforate u.
> u. biforis
> u. bilocularis
> bipartite u.
> u. bipartitus
> capped u.
> cordiform u.
> u. cordiformis
> Couvelaire u.
> u. didelphys
> double-mouthed u.
> duplex u.
> u. duplex
> gravid u.
> heart-shaped u.
> incudiform u.
> u. incudiformis
> masculine u.
> u. masculinus
> one-horned u.
> u. parvicollis
> septate u.
> u. septus
> subseptate u.
> u. subseptus
> triangular u.
> u. triangularis
> unicorn u.
> u. unicornis

utility
utilization time
utricle
> prostatic u.

U

utricular
    u. cyst
    u. nerve
    u. reflexes
    u. spot
utriculi (*pl. of* utriculus)
utriculitis
utriculoampullar nerve
utriculosaccular
    u. duct
utriculus, pl. **utriculi**
    u. prostaticus
utriform
uvaeformis
uvea
uveal
    u. part of trabecular reticulum
    u. staphyloma
    u. tract
uveitic
uveitides
uveitis, pl. **uveitides**
    anterior u.
    Förster's u.
    Fuchs' u.
    heterochromic u.
    intermediate u.
    lens-induced u.
    phacoanaphylactic u.
    phacogenic u.
    posterior u.
    sympathetic u.
uveocutaneous syndrome
uveo-encephalitic syndrome

uveoencephalitis
uveomeningitis syndrome
uveoparotid fever
uveoscleritis
uviform
uviofast
uviol
    u. lamp
uviometer
uvioresistant
uviosensitive
uvula, pl. **uvuli**
    bifid u.
    u. of bladder
    u. cerebelli
    Lieutaud's u.
    u. palatina
    palatine u.
    u. vermis
    u. vesicae
uvulae muscle
uvulaptosis
uvular
uvularis
uvulatome
uvulectomy
uvuli (*pl. of* uvula)
uvulitis
uvulopalatopharyngoplasty
uvulopalatoplasty
uvuloptosis
uvulotome
uvulotomy
Uzbekistan hemorrhagic fever

V

V antigen
V lead
V wave

v̄
vaccinal
vaccinate
vaccination
vaccinator
vaccine

attenuated v.
v. bodies
Haemophilus influenzae type B v.
human diploid cell v.
v. lymph
poliomyelitis v.'s
split-virus v.
v. virus

vaccinia

v. gangrenosa
generalized v.
v. lymph
progressive v.
v. vaccinia
v. virus

vaccinist
vaccinization
vaccinogen
vaccinogenous
vaccinoid

v. reaction

vaccinostyle
V-A conduction
VACTERL syndrome
vacuolar

v. degeneration
v. nephrosis

vacuolate, vacuolated
vacuolating virus
vacuolation
vacuole

autophagic v.
contractile v.
parasitophorous v.

vacuolization
vacuome
vacutome
vacuum

v. aspirator
v. casting
v. disk phenomenon
v. extractor
v. flask
v. headache

v. investing
v. tube

vadum
vagabond's disease
vagal

v. attack
v. bradycardia
v. part
v. part of accessory nerve
v. trigone
v. trunk

vagectomy
vagi (*gen. and pl. of* vagus)
vagina, gen. and pl. **vaginae**

bipartite v.
v. bulbi
v. carotica
v. cellulosa
v. communis musculorum flexorum
v. externa nervi optici
vaginae fibrosae digitorum manus
vaginae fibrosae digitorum pedis
v. fibrosa tendinis
v. interna nervi optici
v. intertubercularis
v. masculina
v. mucosa tendinis
v. musculi recti abdominis
vaginae nervi optici
v. oculi
v. processus styloidei
septate v.
vaginae synoviales digitorum manus
vaginae synoviales digitorum pedis
v. synovialis tendinis
v. synovialis trochleae
v. tendinis musculi extensoris carpi ulnaris
v. tendinis musculi extensoris digiti minimi
v. tendinis musculi extensoris hallucis longi
v. tendinis musculi extensoris pollicis longi
v. tendinis musculi flexoris carpi radialis
v. tendinis musculi flexoris hallucis longi
v. tendinis musculi flexoris pollicis longi
v. tendinis musculi obliqui superioris
v. tendinis musculi peronei longi plantaris

V

vagina *(continued)*
    v. tendinis musculi tibialis
      anterioris
    v. tendinis musculi tibialis
      posterioris
    v. tendinum musculi extensoris
      digitorum pedis longi
    v. tendinum musculi flexoris
      digitorum pedis longi
    v. tendinum musculorum abductoris
      longi et extensoris brevis pollicis
    v. tendinum musculorum extensoris
      digitorum et extensoris indicis
    v. tendinum musculorum
      extensorum carpi radialium
    v. tendinum musculorum fibularium
      communis
    v. tendinum musculorum
      peroneorum communis
    vaginae vasorum
vaginal
    v. artery
    v. atresia
    v. celiotomy
    v. columns
    v. cornification test
    v. dysmenorrhea
    v. fornix
    v. gland
    v. hysterectomy
    v. hysterotomy
    v. introitus
    v. laceration
    v. lithotomy
    v. mucification test
    v. mucosa
    v. myomectomy
    v. nerves
    v. opening
    v. orifice
    v. pool
    v. portion of cervix
    v. process
    v. process of peritoneum
    v. process of sphenoid bone
    v. process of testis
    v. synovial membrane
    v. synovitis
    v. venous plexus
vaginapexy
vaginate
vaginectomy
vaginism
vaginismus
    posterior v.
vaginitis, pl. **vaginitides**
    v. adhesiva
    adhesive v.

    amebic v.
    atrophic v.
    v. cystica
    desquamative inflammatory v.
    v. emphysematosa
    Gardnerella v.
    nonspecific v.
    pinworm v.
    senile v.
    v. senilis
vaginoabdominal
vaginocele
vaginodynia
vaginofixation
vaginohysterectomy
vaginolabial
vaginomycosis
vaginopathy
vaginoperineal
vaginoperineoplasty
vaginoperineorrhaphy
vaginoperineotomy
vaginoperitoneal
vaginopexy
vaginoplasty
vaginoscopy
vaginosis
    bacterial v.
vaginotomy
vaginovesical
vaginovulvar
Vaginulus plebeius
vagitus uterinus
vagoaccessorius
vagoglossopharyngeal
vagolysis
vagomimetic
vagotomy
vagotonia
vagotonic
vagotropic
vagovagal
    v. reflex
vagrant's disease
vagus, gen. and pl. **vagi**
    v. area
    vagi eminentia
    v. nerve
    v. pulse
Valentine's
    V. position
    V. test
Valentin's
    V. corpuscles
    V. ganglion
    V. nerve
valetudinarianism
valgoid

valgus
valid
validation
    consensual v.
validity
    concurrent v.
    construct v.
    content v.
    criterion-related v.
    face v.
    predictive v.
valla (*pl. of* vallum)
vallate
    v. papilla
vallecula, pl. **valleculae**
    v. cerebelli
    epiglottic v.
    v. epiglottica
    v. sylvii
    v. unguis
vallecular dysphagia
Valleix's points
valley
    v. fever
vallis
vallum, pl. **valla**
    v. unguis
Valsalva
    V. antrum
    V. ligaments
    V. maneuver
    V. muscle
    V. sinus
    V. test
value
    homing v.
    maturation v.
    normal v.'s
    phenotypic v.
    predictive v.
    reference v.'s
valva, pl. **valvae**
    v. aortae
    v. atrioventricularis dextra
    v. atrioventricularis sinistra
    v. ileocecalis
    v. mitralis
    v. tricuspidalis
    v. trunci pulmonalis
valval, valvar
valvate
valve
    Amussat's v.
    anal v.'s
    anterior urethral v.
    aortic v.
    atrioventricular v.'s
    ball v.

Bauhin's v.
Béraud's v.
Bianchi's v.
bicuspid v.
bi-leaflet v.
Bjork-Shiley v.
Bochdalek's v.
Braune's v.
Carpentier-Edwards v.
caval v.
congenital v.
coronary v.
v. of coronary sinus
eustachian v.
v. of foramen ovale
Gerlach's v.
Guérin's v.
Hasner's v.
Heister's v.
Heyer-Pudenz v.
Hoboken's v.'s
Houston's v.'s
Huschke's v.
ileocecal v.
ileocolic v.
v. of inferior vena cava
Kerckring's v.'s
Kohlrausch's v.'s
Krause's v.
left atrioventricular v.
Mercier's v.
mitral v.
Morgagni's v.'s
nasal v.
v. of navicular fossa
nonrebreathing v.
O'Beirne's v.
v. of oval foramen
parachute mitral v.
porcine v.
posterior urethral v.'s
prosthetic v.'s
pulmonary v.
v. of pulmonary trunk
pulmonic v.
pyloric v.
rectal v.'s
reducing v.
right atrioventricular v.
Rosenmüller's v.
semilunar v.
spiral v. of cystic duct
Starr-Edwards v.
sylvian v.
Tarin's v.
Terrien's v.
thebesian v.
tilting disc v.

V

valve (*continued*)
   tissue v.
   tricuspid v.
   Tulp's v., Tulpius' v.
   urethral v.'s
   v. of Varolius
   venous v.
   v. of vermiform appendix
   vesicoureteral v.
   v. of Vieussens
   Vieussens' v.
valveless
valviform
valvoplasty
valvotomy
   v. knife
   mitral v.
   rectal v.
valvula, pl. **valvulae**
   Amussat's v.
   valvulae anales
   v. bicuspidalis
   valvulae conniventes
   v. foraminis ovalis
   v. fossae navicularis
   Gerlach's v.
   v. lymphatica
   v. processus vermiformis
   v. pylori
   valvulae pylori
   v. semilunaris
   v. semilunaris anterior valvae trunci pulmonalis
   v. semilunaris dextra valvae aortae
   v. semilunaris dextra valvae trunci pulmonalis
   v. semilunaris posterior valvae aortae
   v. semilunaris sinistra valvae aortae
   v. semilunaris sinistra valvae trunci pulmonalis
   v. semilunaris tarini
   v. sinus coronarii
   v. spiralis
   v. tricuspidalis
   v. venae cavae inferioris
   v. venosa
   v. vestibuli
valvular
   v. endocarditis
   v. incompetence
   v. insufficiency
   v. pneumothorax
   v. prolapse
   v. regurgitation
   v. sclerosis
   v. thrombus

valvule
   Foltz' v.
   lymphatic v.
valvulitis
   rheumatic v.
valvuloplasty
valvulotome
valvulotomy
van
   v. Bogaert encephalitis
   v. Buchem's syndrome
   v. Buren's disease
   v. Buren sound
   v. Deen's test
   v. den Bergh's test
   v. der Hoeve's syndrome
   v. der Kolk's law
   v. der Velden's test
   v. Ermengen's stain
   v. Gieson's stain
   v. Helmont's mirror
   v. Horne's canal
   V. Slyke apparatus
   V. Slyke's formula
vanillism
vanillylmandelic acid test
vanished testis syndrome
vanishing
   v. lung
   v. lung syndrome
vapor
   anesthetic v.
   v. density
vaporizer
   flow-over v.
   temperature-compensated v.
vaporthorax
vapotherapy
Vaquez' disease
variability
   baseline v. of fetal heart rate
variable
   continuous v.
   continuous random v.
   v. coupling
   v. deceleration
   dependent v.
   discrete v.
   discrete random v.
   independent v.
   intermediate v.
   intervening v.
   mixed discrete-continuous random v.
   moderator v.
   random v.
variable-interval reinforcement schedule

variance
- ball v. *DANDy-WALKER*
- v. ratio

variant
- v. angina pectoris
- v. hemoglobin
- inherited albumin v.'s
- L-phase v.'s

variate

variation
- beat-to-beat v. of fetal heart rate
- continuous v.

varication

variceal

varicella
- v. encephalitis
- v. gangrenosa

varicellation

varicella-zoster virus

varicelliform

varicelloid
- v. smallpox

varices (*pl. of* varix)

variciform

varicoblepharon

varicocele
- ovarian v.
- symptomatic v.
- tubo-ovarian v.
- utero-ovarian v.

varicocelectomy

varicography

varicoid

varicomphalus

varicophlebitis

varicose
- v. aneurysm
- v. eczema
- v. ulcer
- v. veins

varicosis, pl. varicoses

varicosity

varicotomy

varicula

varicule

variegate porphyria

variola
- v. benigna
- v. hemorrhagica
- v. major
- v. maligna
- v. miliaris
- v. minor
- v. pemphigosa
- v. sine eruptione
- v. vera
- v. verrucosa
- v. virus

variolar

variolate

variolation

variolic

varioliform
- v. syphilid

variolization

varioloid

variolous

varix, pl. varices
- v. anastomoticus
- aneurysmal v.
- cirsoid v.
- conjunctival v.
- esophageal varices
- gelatinous v.
- lymph v.
- turbinal v.

varnish (dental)

Varolius' sphincter

varus

vas, gen. vasis, gen. and pl. vasorum, pl. vasa
- v. aberrans hepatis, pl. vasa aberrantia hepatis
- v. aberrans of Roth
- vasa aberrantes
- v. afferens, pl. vasa afferentia
- v. anastomoticum
- vasa auris internae
- vasa brevia
- v. capillare
- vasa chylifera
- v. collaterale
- v. deferens, pl. vasa deferentia
- v. efferens, pl. vasa efferentia
- Ferrein's vasa aberrantia
- Haller's v. aberrans
- vasa lymphatica
- v. lymphaticum
- v. lymphaticum afferens
- v. lymphaticum efferens
- v. lymphaticum profundum
- v. lymphaticum superficiale
- vasa nervorum
- vasa previa
- v. prominens ductus cochlearis
- vasa recta
- vasa sanguinea retinae
- v. spirale
- vasa vasorum
- vasa vorticosa

vasal

vascula (*pl. of* vasculum)

vascular
- v. bud
- v. cataract
- v. circle

V

vascular *(continued)*
v. circle of optic nerve
v. cones
v. dementia
v. dentin
v. fold of the cecum
v. gland
v. headache
v. keratitis
v. lacuna
v. lamina of choroid
v. layer
v. layer of choroid coat of eye
v. leiomyoma
v. meninx
v. murmur
v. nerve
v. papillae
v. pedicle
v. plexus
v. polyp
v. ring
v. sclerosis
v. sheaths
v. spider
v. spur
v. stripe
v. system
v. tunic of eye
v. zone
vascularity
vascularization
vascularized
v. graft
vasculature
vasculitis
cutaneous v.
hypersensitivity v.
hypocomplementemic v.
leukocytoclastic v.
livedo v.
nodular v.
urticarial v.
vasculocardiac
v. syndrome of hyperserotonemia
vasculogenesis
vasculogenic impotence
vasculomotor
vasculomyelinopathy
vasculopathy
vasculum, pl. **vascula**
vasectomy
vasifaction
vasifactive
vasiform
vasis (*gen. of* vas)
vasitis
v. nodosa

[handwritten annotation: A — 2 words per txt]

vasoconstriction
active v.
passive v.
vasodentin
vasodepression
vasodepressor
v. substance
v. syncope
vasodilatation
vasodilation
active v.
passive v.
vasoepididymostomy
vasofactive
vasoformation
vasoformative
v. cell
vasoganglion
vasogenic shock
vasography
vasohypertonic
vasohypotonic
vasoinhibitory
vasolabile
vasoligation
vasomotion
vasomotor
v. angina
v. ataxia
v. center
v. epilepsy
v. fibers
v. imbalance
v. nerve
v. neurosis
v. paralysis
v. rhinitis
v. spasm
vasoneuropathy
vasoneurosis
vaso-orchidostomy
vasoparalysis
vasoparesis
vasopressin-resistant diabetes
vasopressor reflex
vasopuncture
vasoreflex
vasorelaxation
vasorum (*gen. and pl. of* vas)
vasosection
vasosensory
vasospasm
vasospastic
vasostomy
vasotomy
vasotonia
vasotrophic

vasovagal
v. attack
v. epilepsy
v. syncope
v. syndrome
vasovasostomy
vasovesiculectomy
vastoadductor fascia
vastus
v. intermedius muscle
v. lateralis muscle
v. medialis muscle
VATER complex
Vater-Pacini corpuscles
Vater's
V. ampulla
V. corpuscles
V. fold
vault
cranial v.
V-bends
VCE smear
VDRL test
vection
vectis
vector
biological v.
v. cardiography
instantaneous v.
v. loop
manifest v.
mean v.
mean manifest v.
mechanical v.
recombinant v.
spatial v.
vectorcardiogram
vectorcardiography
spatial v.
vectorial
vectors
VEE virus
vegetality
vegetal pole
vegetarian
vegetarianism
vegetation
bacterial v.'s
verrucous v.'s
vegetative
v. bacteriophage
v. endocarditis
v. life
v. nervous system
v. pole
v. reproduction
v. stage

veil
aqueduct v.
v. cell
Jackson's v.
Sattler's v.
veiled
v. cells
v. puff
veiling glare
Veillonella
V. alcalescens subsp. *alcalescens*
V. alcalescens subsp. *criceti*
V. alcalescens subsp. *dispar*
V. alcalescens subsp. *ratti*
V. alcalesens
V. atypica
V. parvula
V. parvula subsp. *atypica*
V. parvula subsp. *parvula*
V. parvula subsp. *rodentium*
V. rodentium
Veillonellaceae
vein
accessory cephalic v.
accessory hemiazygos v.
accessory saphenous v.
accessory vertebral v.
accompanying v.
accompanying v. of hypoglossal
nerve
anastomotic v.'s
angular v.
anonymous v.'s
anterior auricular v.
anterior cardiac v.'s
anterior cardinal v.'s
anterior cardinal v.'s (*var. of*
cardinal v.'s)
anterior cerebral v.
anterior facial v.
anterior intercostal v.'s
anterior jugular v.
anterior labial v.'s
anterior pontomesencephalic v.
anterior scrotal v.'s
anterior v. of septum pellucidum
anterior tibial v.'s
anterior vertebral v.
appendicular v.
aqueous v.
arciform v.'s of kidney
arcuate v.'s of kidney
arterial v.
ascending lumbar v.
auricular v.'s
axillary v.
azygos v.
basal v.'s

V

vein *(continued)*

basal v. of Rosenthal
basilic v.
basivertebral v.
Baumgarten's v.'s
Boyd communicating
  perforation v.'s
brachial v.'s
brachiocephalic v.'s
Breschet's v.
bronchial v.'s
Browning's v.
v. of bulb of penis
Burow's v.
capillary v.
cardiac v.'s
cardinal v.'s, anterior cardinal v.'s,
  common cardinal v.'s, posterior
  cardinal v.'s
v.'s of caudate nucleus
cavernous v.'s of penis
central v.'s of liver
central v. of retina
central v. of suprarenal gland
cephalic v.
cerebellar v.'s
v.'s of cerebellum
cerebral v.'s
cervical v.
choroid v.
choroid v.'s of eye
ciliary v.'s
circumflex v.'s
v. of cochlear aqueduct
v. of cochlear canaliculus
Cockett communicating
  perforating v.'s
colic v.'s
common basal v.
common cardinal v.'s (*var. of*
  cardinal v.'s)
common cardinal v.'s
common facial v.
common iliac v.
companion v.
companion v.'s
condylar emissary v.
conjunctival v.'s
coronary v.
v. of corpus striatum
costoaxillary v.
cutaneous v.
Cuvier's v.'s
cystic v.
deep cerebral v.'s
deep cervical v.
deep circumflex iliac v.
deep v.'s of clitoris

deep dorsal v. of clitoris
deep dorsal v. of penis
deep epigastric v.
deep facial v.
deep femoral v.
deep lingual v.
deep middle cerebral v.
deep v. of penis
deep temporal v.'s
digital v.'s
diploic v.
dorsal callosal v.
dorsal v.'s of clitoris
dorsal v. of corpus callosum
dorsal digital v.'s of foot
dorsal digital v.'s of toes
dorsal lingual v.
dorsal metacarpal v.'s
dorsal metatarsal v.'s
dorsal v.'s of penis
dorsal scapular v.
dorsispinal v.'s
emissary v.
epigastric v.'s
episcleral v.'s
esophageal v.'s
ethmoidal v.'s
external iliac v.
external jugular v.
external nasal v.'s
external pudendal v.'s
v.'s of eyelids
facial v.
femoral v.
fibular v.'s
frontal v.'s
v.'s of Galen
gastric v.'s
gastroepiploic v.'s
gluteal v.'s
great cardiac v.
great cerebral v.
great cerebral v. of Galen
great v. of Galen
great saphenous v.
hemiazygos v.
hemorrhoidal v.'s
hepatic v.'s
hepatic portal v.
highest intercostal v.
hypogastric v.
ileal v.'s
ileocolic v.
iliac v.'s
iliolumbar v.
inferior anastomotic v.
inferior basal v.
inferior cardiac v.

inferior v.'s of cerebellar
  hemisphere
inferior cerebral v.'s
inferior choroid v.
inferior epigastric v.
v.'s of inferior eyelid
inferior gluteal v.'s
inferior hemorrhoidal v.'s
inferior labial v.
inferior laryngeal v.
inferior mesenteric v.
inferior ophthalmic v.
inferior palpebral v.'s
inferior phrenic v.
inferior rectal v.'s
inferior thalamostriate v.'s
inferior thyroid v.
inferior ventricular v.
inferior v. of vermis
infrasegmental v.'s
innominate v.'s
innominate cardiac v.'s
insular v.'s
intercapitular v.'s
intercostal v.'s
interlobar v.'s of kidney
interlobular v.'s of kidney
interlobular v.'s of liver
intermediate antebrachial v.
intermediate basilic v.
intermediate cephalic v.
intermediate cubital v.
intermediate v. of forearm
internal auditory v.'s
internal cerebral v.'s
internal iliac v.
internal jugular v.
internal pudendal v.
internal thoracic v.
intersegmental v.'s
intervertebral v.
intrasegmental v.'s
jejunal and ileal v.'s
jugular v.'s
key v.
v.'s of kidney
v.'s of knee
Krukenberg's v.'s
Labbé's v.
labial v.'s
labyrinthine v.'s
lacrimal v.
large v.
large saphenous v.
laryngeal v.'s
Latarget's v.
lateral atrial v.
lateral circumflex femoral v.'s

lateral direct v.'s
lateral v. of lateral ventricle
v. of lateral recess of fourth
  ventricle
lateral sacral v.'s
lateral thoracic v.
left colic v.
left coronary v.
left gastric v.
left gastroepiploic v.
left gastroomental v.
left hepatic v.'s
left inferior pulmonary v.
left ovarian v.
left superior intercostal v.
left superior pulmonary v.
left suprarenal v.
left testicular v.
left umbilical v.
levoatrio-cardinal v.
lingual v.
long saphenous v.
long thoracic v.
lumbar v.'s
Marshall's oblique v.
masseteric v.'s
mastoid emissary v.
maxillary v.
Mayo's v.
medial atrial v.
medial circumflex femoral v.'s
medial v. of lateral ventricle
median antebrachial v.
median basilic v.
median cephalic v.
median cubital v.
median v. of forearm
median v. of neck
median sacral v.
mediastinal v.'s
medium v.
v.'s of medulla oblongata
meningeal v.'s
mesencephalic v.'s
mesenteric v.'s
metacarpal v.'s
middle cardiac v.
middle colic v.
middle hemorrhoidal v.'s
middle hepatic v.'s
middle meningeal v.'s
middle rectal v.'s
middle temporal v.
middle thyroid v.
musculophrenic v.'s
nasofrontal v.
oblique v. of left atrium
obturator v.

V

967

vein *(continued)*

occipital v.
occipital cerebral v.'s
occipital emissary v.
v. of olfactory gyrus
ophthalmic v.'s
ovarian v.'s
palatine v.
palmar digital v.'s
palmar metacarpal v.'s
palpebral v.'s
pancreatic v.'s
pancreaticoduodenal v.'s
paraumbilical v.'s
parietal v.'s
parietal emissary v.
parotid v.'s
pectoral v.'s
peduncular v.'s
perforating v.'s
pericardiacophrenic v.'s
pericardial v.'s
peroneal v.'s
petrosal v.
pharyngeal v.'s
phrenic v.'s
plantar digital v.'s
plantar metatarsal v.'s
v.'s of pons
pontine v.'s
popliteal v.
portal v.
posterior anterior jugular v.
posterior auricular v.
posterior cardinal v.'s *(var. of* cardinal v.'s)
posterior cardinal v.'s
posterior facial v.
v. of posterior horn
posterior intercostal v.'s
posterior labial v.'s
posterior v. of left ventricle
posterior marginal v.
posterior parotid v.'s
posterior pericallosal v.
posterior scrotal v.'s
posterior v. of septum pellucidum
posterior tibial v.'s
precentral cerebellar v.
prefrontal v.'s
prepyloric v.
v. of pterygoid canal
pudendal v.'s
pulmonary v.'s
pyloric v.
radial v.'s
renal v.'s
retromandibular v.

[handwritten: Soleal vein]

Retzius' v.'s
right colic v.
right gastric v.
right gastroepiploic v.
right gastroomental v.
right hepatic v.'s
right inferior pulmonary v.
right ovarian v.
right superior intercostal v.
right superior pulmonary v.
right suprarenal v.
right testicular v.
Rosenthal's v.
Ruysch's v.'s
sacral v.'s
Santorini's v.
saphenous v.'s
Sappey's v.'s
scleral v.'s
scrotal v.'s
v. of septum pellucidum
short gastric v.'s
short saphenous v.
sigmoid v.'s
small v.
small cardiac v.
smallest cardiac v.'s
small saphenous v.
spermatic v.
spinal v.'s
spiral v. of modiolus
splenic v.
stellate v.'s
Stensen's v.'s
sternocleidomastoid v.
v. stone
striate v.'s
v. stripper
stylomastoid v.
subclavian v.
subcutaneous v.'s of abdomen
sublingual v.
submental v.
superficial v.
superficial cerebral v.'s
superficial circumflex iliac v.
superficial dorsal v.'s of clitoris
superficial dorsal v.'s of penis
superficial epigastric v.
superficial middle cerebral v.
superficial temporal v.'s
superior anastomotic v.
superior basal v.
superior v.'s of cerebellar hemisphere
superior cerebral v.'s
superior choroid v.
superior epigastric v.'s

v.'s of superior eyelid
superior gluteal v.'s
superior hemorrhoidal v.
superior intercostal v.
superior labial v.
superior laryngeal v.
superior mesenteric v.
superior ophthalmic v.
superior palpebral v.'s
superior phrenic v.'s
superior rectal v.
superior thalamostriate v.
superior thyroid v.
superior v. of vermis
supraorbital v.
suprarenal v.'s
suprascapular v.
supratrochlear v.'s
supreme intercostal v.
surface thalamic v.'s
temporal v.'s
v.'s of temporomandibular joint
temporomaxillary v.
terminal v.
testicular v.'s
thalamostriate v.'s
thebesian v.'s
thoracic v.'s
thoracoacromial v.
thoracoepigastric v.
thymic v.'s
thyroid v.'s
tracheal v.'s
transverse cervical v.'s
transverse v. of face
transverse facial v.
transverse v.'s of neck
transverse v. of scapula
Trolard's v.
tympanic v.'s
ulnar v.'s
umbilical v.
v. of uncus
uterine v.'s
varicose v.'s
vertebral v.
v.'s of vertebral column
Vesalius' v.
vesical v.'s
vestibular v.'s
v. of vestibular aqueduct
v. of vestibular bulb
vidian v.
Vieussens' v.'s
vitelline v.
vortex v.'s
vorticose v.'s

veined

veinlet
Vejovis
vela (*pl. of* velum)
velamen, pl. **velamina**
    v. vulvae
velamentous
    v. insertion
velamentum, pl. **velamenta**
velamina (*pl. of* velamen)
Vel antigen
velar
veldt sore
veliform
Vella's fistula
vellicate
vellication
vellus
    v. hair
    v. olivae inferioris
velocity
    nerve conduction v.
velonoskiascopy
velopharyngeal
    v. closure
    v. insufficiency
    v. seal
    v. sphincter
velosynthesis
Velpeau's
    V. bandage
    V. canal
    V. fossa
    V. hernia
velum, pl. **vela**
    anterior medullary v.
    inferior medullary v.
    v. interpositum
    v. medullare inferius
    v. medullare superius
    v. palatinum
    v. pendulum palati
    posterior medullary v.
    v. semilunare
    superior medullary v.
    v. tarini
    v. terminale
    transverse v.
    v. transversum
    v. triangulare
velvet ant
vena, gen. and pl. **venae**
    v. advehens, pl. venae advehentes
    v. afferentes hepatis
    v. anastomotica inferior
    v. anastomotica superior
    v. angularis
    v. appendicularis
    v. aqueductus cochleae

V

vena *(continued)*

v. aqueductus vestibuli
venae arcuatae renis
v. arteriosa
venae articulares
  temporomandibulares
v. atrii lateralis
v. atrii medialis
v. auricularis anterior
v. auricularis posterior
v. axillaris
v. azygos
v. azygos major
v. azygos minor inferior
v. azygos minor superior
v. basalis
v. basalis communis
v. basalis inferior
v. basalis superior
v. basilica
v. basivertebralis
Billroth's venae cavernosae
venae brachiales
venae brachiocephalicae
venae bronchiales
v. bulbi penis
v. bulbi vestibuli
v. canaliculi cochleae
v. canalis pterygoidei
v. cardiaca magna
v. cava filter
v. cava inferior
v. caval foramen
v. cava superior
venae cavernosae penis
venae centrales hepatis
v. centralis glandulae suprarenalis
v. centralis retinae
v. cephalica
v. cephalica accessoria
venae cerebelli
venae cerebelli inferiores
venae cerebelli superiores
v. cerebri anterior
venae cerebri inferiores
venae cerebri internae
v. cerebri magna
v. cerebri media profunda
v. cerebri media superficialis
venae cerebri profundae
venae cerebri superficiales
venae cerebri superiores
v. cervicalis profunda
venae choroideae oculi
v. choroidea inferior
v. choroidea superior
venae ciliares
venae circumflexae femoris laterales
venae circumflexae femoris
  mediales
v. circumflexa iliaca profunda
v. circumflexa iliaca superficialis
v. colica dextra
v. colica media
v. colica sinistra
venae columnae vertebralis
v. comitans
v. comitans nervi hypoglossi
venae comitantes
venae conjunctivales
venae cordis anteriores
v. cordis magna
v. cordis media
venae cordis minimae
v. cordis parva
v. cornus posterioris
v. coronaria ventriculi
v. corporis callosi dorsalis
v. cutanea
v. cystica
venae digitales dorsales pedis
venae digitales palmares
venae digitales plantares
v. diploica
venae directae laterales
venae dorsales clitoridis
  superficiales
venae dorsales linguae
venae dorsales penis superficiales
v. dorsalis clitoridis profunda
v. dorsalis penis profunda
v. emissaria, pl. venae emissariae
v. emissaria condylaris
v. emissaria mastoidea
v. emissaria occipitalis
v. emissaria parietalis
venae epigastricae superiores
v. epigastrica inferior
v. epigastrica superficialis
venae episclerales
venae esophageae
venae ethmoidales
v. facialis
v. facialis anterior
v. facialis communis
v. facialis posterior
v. faciei profunda
v. femoralis
venae fibulares
venae frontales
v. gastrica dextra
venae gastricae breves
v. gastrica sinistra
v. gastro-omentalis dextra
v. gastro-omentalis sinistra
venae genus

venae gluteae inferiores
venae gluteae superiores
v. gyri olfactorii
v. hemiazygos
v. hemiazygos accessoria
venae hemispherii cerebelli inferiores
venae hemispherii cerebelli superiores
venae hemorrhoidales inferiores
venae hemorrhoidales mediae
v. hemorrhoidalis superior
venae hepaticae
venae hepaticae dextrae
venae hepaticae mediae
venae hepaticae sinistrae
v. hypogastrica
v. ileocolica
v. iliaca communis
v. iliaca externa
v. iliaca interna
v. iliolumbalis
inferior v. cava
v. innominata
venae insulares
venae intercapitales
venae intercostales anteriores
venae intercostales posteriores
v. intercostalis superior dextra
v. intercostalis superior sinistra
v. intercostalis suprema
venae interlobares renis
venae interlobulares hepatis
venae interlobulares renis
v. intermedia antebrachii
v. intermedia basilica
v. intermedia cephalica
v. intermedia cubiti
v. intervertebralis
venae jejunales et ilei
v. jugularis anterior
v. jugularis externa
v. jugularis interna
venae labiales anteriores
venae labiales posteriores
v. labialis inferior
v. labialis superior
venae labyrinthi
v. lacrimalis
v. laryngea inferior
v. laryngea superior
v. lienalis
v. lingualis
venae lumbales
v. lumbalis ascendens
v. mammaria interna
v. maxillaris, pl. venae maxillares
v. mediana antebrachii

v. mediana basilica
v. mediana cephalica
v. mediana cubiti
venae mediastinales
venae medullae oblongatae
venae meningeae
venae meningeae mediae
venae mesencephalicae
v. mesenterica inferior
v. mesenterica superior
venae metacarpeae dorsales
venae metacarpeae palmares
venae metatarseae dorsales
venae metatarseae plantares
venae musculophrenicae
venae nasales externae
v. nasofrontalis
venae nuclei caudati
v. obliqua atrii sinistri
v. obturatoria, pl. venae obturatoriae
venae occipitales
v. occipitalis
v. ophthalmica inferior
v. ophthalmica superior
v. ovarica dextra
v. ovarica sinistra
v. palatina
venae palpebrales
venae palpebrales inferiores
venae palpebrales superiores
venae pancreaticae
venae pancreaticoduodenales
venae paraumbilicales
venae parietales
venae parotidea
venae pectorales
venae pedunculares
venae perforantes
venae pericardiacae
venae pericardiacophrenicae
venae peroneae
v. petrosa
venae pharyngeae
venae phrenicae superiores
v. phrenica inferior, pl. venae phrenicae inferiores
venae pontis
v. pontomesencephalica anterior
v. poplitea
v. portae hepatis
v. portalis
v. posterior ventriculi sinistri
v. preauricularis
v. precentralis cerebelli
venae prefrontales
v. prepylorica
venae profundae clitoridis
v. profunda femoris

vena *(continued)*
v. profunda linguae
v. profunda penis
venae pudendae externae
v. pudenda interna
venae pulmonales
v. pulmonalis inferior dextra
v. pulmonalis inferior sinistra
v. pulmonalis superior dextra
v. pulmonalis superior sinistra
venae radiales
v. recessus lateralis ventriculi quarti
venae rectae
venae rectales inferiores
venae rectales mediae
v. rectalis superior
venae renales
venae renis
v. retromandibularis
v. revehens, pl. venae revehentes
venae sacrales laterales
v. sacralis mediana
v. saphena accessoria
v. saphena magna
v. saphena parva
v. scapularis dorsalis
venae sclerales
venae scrotales anteriores
venae scrotales posteriores
v. septi pellucidi anterior
v. septi pellucidi posterior
venae sigmoideae
venae spinales
v. spiralis modioli
venae cavernosae of spleen
v. splenica
venae stellatae
v. sternocleidomastoidea
venae striatae
v. stylomastoidea
v. subclavia
venae subcutaneae abdominis
v. sublingualis
v. submentalis
superior v. cava
v. supraorbitalis
v. suprarenalis dextra
v. suprarenalis sinistra
v. suprascapularis
venae supratrochleares
venae temporales profundae
venae temporales superficiales
v. temporalis media
v. terminalis
v. testicularis dextra
v. testicularis sinistra
venae thalamostriatae inferiores

v. thalamostriata superior
v. thoracica interna, pl. venae thoracicae internae
v. thoracica lateralis
v. thoracoacromialis
v. thoracoepigastrica, pl. venae thoracoepigastricae
venae thymicae
v. thyroidea ima
v. thyroidea inferior
v. thyroidea media
v. thyroidea superior
venae tibiales anteriores
venae tibiales posteriores
venae tracheales
venae transversae colli
v. transversa faciei
v. transversa scapulae
venae tympanicae
venae ulnares
v. umbilicalis sinistra
v. unci
venae uterinae
v. ventricularis inferior
v. ventriculi lateralis lateralis
v. ventriculi lateralis medialis
v. vermis inferior
v. vermis superior
v. vertebralis
v. vertebralis accessoria
v. vertebralis anterior
venae vesicales
venae vestibulares
v. vitellina
venae vorticosae
venacavography
Ven antigen
venation
venectasia
venectomy
veneer
venereal
v. bubo
v. disease
v. lymphogranuloma
v. sore
v. ulcer
v. wart
venereology
venereophobia
venesection
Venezuelan equine encephalomyelitis virus
venipuncture
Venn diagram
venocaval filter
venoclysis
venofibrosis

venogram
venography
> splenic portal v.
> transosseous v.
> vertebral v.

venom
> v. hemolysis
> kokoi v.

venomotor
veno-occlusive disease of the liver
venoperitoneostomy
venopressor
venorespiratory reflex
venosclerosis
venose
venosinal
venosity
venostasis
venostat
venostomy
venotomy
venous
> v. angioma
> v. angle
> v. artery
> v. blood
> v. capillary
> v. circle of mammary gland
> v. congestion
> v. embolism
> v. foramen
> v. gangrene
> v. grooves
> v. heart
> v. hum
> v. hyperemia
> v. insufficiency
> v. lakes
> v. ligament
> v. murmur
> v. occlusion plethysmography
> v. plexus
> v. plexus of bladder
> v. plexus of foramen ovale
> v. plexus of hypoglossal canal
> v. pulse
> v. return
> v. segments of the kidney
> v. segments of liver
> v. sinuses
> v. sinus of sclera
> v. star
> v. stasis
> v. valve

venous-stasis retinopathy
venovenostomy
vent

venter
> v. anterior musculi digastrici
> v. frontalis musculi occipitofrontalis
> v. inferior musculi omohyoidei
> v. occipitalis musculi occipitofrontalis
> v. posterior musculi digastrici
> v. propendens
> v. superior musculi omohyoidei

ventilate
ventilation
> alveolar v.
> artificial v.
> assist-control v.
> assisted v.
> continuous positive pressure v.
> controlled v.
> controlled mechanical v.
> intermittent mandatory v.
> intermittent positive pressure v.
> manual v.
> maximum voluntary v.
> mechanical v.
> v. meter
> pulmonary v.
> spontaneous intermittent mandatory v.
> synchronized intermittent mandatory v.
> wasted v.

ventilation/perfusion mismatch
ventilation/perfusion ratio
ventilation-perfusion scan
ventilatory compliance
ventplant
ventrad
ventral
> v. anterior nucleus of thalamus
> v. aortas
> v. border
> v. branch
> v. decubitus
> v. glands
> v. hernia
> v. horn
> v. intermediate nucleus of thalamus
> v. lateral nucleus of thalamus
> v. mesocardium
> v. mesogastrium
> v. nucleus of thalamus
> v. nucleus of trapezoid body
> v. pancreas
> v. part of pons
> v. plate
> v. plate of neural tube
> v. posterior intermediate nucleus of thalamus

V

ventral *(continued)*
    v. posterior lateral nucleus of thalamus
    v. posterior nucleus of thalamus
    v. posterolateral nucleus of thalamus
    v. posteromedial nucleus of thalamus
    v. primary rami of cervical spinal nerves
    v. primary rami of lumbar spinal nerves
    v. primary rami of sacral spinal nerves
    v. primary ramus of spinal nerve
    v. root
    v. sacrococcygeal ligament
    v. sacrococcygeal muscle
    v. sacrococcygeus muscle
    v. sacroiliac ligaments
    v. spinocerebellar tract
    v. spinothalamic tract
    v. splanchnic arteries
    v. surface of digit
    v. tegmental decussation
    v. thalamic peduncle
    v. tier thalamic nuclei
    v. white column
ventralis
ventricle
    Arantius' v.
    cerebral v.'s
    v. of cerebral hemisphere
    v. of diencephalon
    double outlet right v.
    Duncan's v.
    fifth v.
    fourth v.
    v.'s of heart
    laryngeal v.
    lateral v.
    left v.
    Morgagni's v.
    v. of rhombencephalon
    right v.
    single v.
    sixth v.
    sylvian v.
    v. of Sylvius
    terminal v.
    third v.
    Verga's v.
    Vieussens' v.
    Wenzel's v.
ventricose
ventricular
    v. aberration
    v. afterload

    v. aneurysm
    v. arteries
    v. assist device
    v. band of larynx
    v. bigeminy
    v. bradycardia
    v. capture
    v. complex
    v. conduction
    v. diastole
    v. diverticulum
    v. escape
    v. extrasystole
    v. fibrillation
    v. filling pressure
    v. fluid
    v. flutter
    v. fold
    v. fusion beat
    v. gradient
    v. inhibited pulse generator
    v. layer
    v. ligament
    v. loop
    v. plateau
    v. pre-excitation
    v. preload
    v. rhythm
    v. septal defect
    v. septum
    v. standstill
    v. synchronous pulse generator
    v. systole
    v. tachycardia
    v. triggered pulse generator
    v. trigone
ventricularis
ventricularization
ventricular ponderance
ventriculi (*pl. of* ventriculus)
ventriculitis
ventriculoatrial
    v. conduction
ventriculocisternostomy
ventriculography
    radionuclide v.
ventriculomastoidostomy
ventriculonector
ventriculophasic
ventriculoplasty
ventriculopuncture
ventriculoradial dysplasia
ventriculoscopy
ventriculostomy
    third v.
ventriculosubarachnoid
ventriculotomy
ventriculus, pl. ventriculi

v. cordis
v. dexter
v. laryngis
v. lateralis
v. quartus
v. quintus
v. sinister
v. terminalis
v. tertius
ventriduct
ventriduction
ventrobasal nucleus
ventrocystorrhaphy
ventrodorsad
ventroinguinal
ventrolateral
ventromedial nucleus of hypothalamus
ventromedian
ventroptosis, ventroptosia
ventroscopy
ventrotomy
Venturi
V. effect
V. meter
V. tube
venula, pl. venulae
v. macularis inferior
v. macularis superior
v. medialis retinae
v. nasalis retinae inferior
v. nasalis retinae superior
venulae rectae renis
venulae stellatae
v. temporalis retinae inferior
v. temporalis retinae superior
venular
venule
high endothelial postcapillary v.'s
inferior macular v.
inferior nasal v. of retina
inferior temporal v. of retina
medial v. of retina
nasal v.'s of retina
pericytic v.'s
postcapillary v.'s
stellate v.'s
straight v.'s of kidney
superior macular v.
superior nasal v. of retina
superior temporal v. of retina
temporal v.'s of retina
venulous
verbal
v. agraphia
v. apraxia
verbigeration
verbomania
verdoperoxidase

Veress needle
Verga's ventricle
verge
anal v.
vergence
v. of lens
vergeture
Verheyen's stars
Verhoeff's elastic tissue stain
vermes (*pl. of* vermis)
vermian fossa
vermicular
v. colic
v. movement
v. pulse
vermiculation
vermicule
vermiculose, vermiculous
vermiculus
vermiform
v. appendage
v. appendix
v. process
vermilion
v. border
v. transitional zone
v. zone
vermilionectomy
vermin
verminal
vermination
verminous
v. abscess
v. appendicitis
v. ileus
vermis, pl. vermes
v. folium
vermix
vernal
v. catarrh
v. conjunctivitis
v. encephalitis
v. keratoconjunctivitis
Verner-Morrison syndrome
Vernet's syndrome
Verneuil's neuroma
Vernier acuity
vernix
v. caseosa
Verocay bodies
verruca, pl. verrucae
v. acuminata
v. digitata
v. filiformis
v. glabra
v. mollusciformis
v. necrogenica
v. peruana, v. peruviana

V

verruca *(continued)*
    v. plana
    v. plana juvenilis
    v. plana senilis
    v. plantaris
    seborrheic v.
    v. senilis
    v. simplex
    v. vulgaris
verruciform
verrucose
verrucosis
    lymphostatic v.
verrucous
    v. carcinoma
    v. endocarditis
    v. hemangioma
    v. hyperplasia
    v. nevus
    v. scrofuloderma
    v. vegetations
    v. xanthoma
verruga
    v. peruana
versicolor
version
    bimanual v.
    bipolar v.
    Braxton Hicks v.
    cephalic v.
    combined v.
    external cephalic v.
    internal cephalic v.
    pelvic v.
    podalic v.
    postural v.
    Potter's v.
    spontaneous v.
    Wright's v.
versive seizure
vertebra, gen. and pl. **vertebrae**
    basilar v.
    block vertebrae
    butterfly v.
    cervical vertebrae
    vertebrae cervicales
    vertebrae coccygeae
    coccygeal vertebrae
    codfish vertebrae
    cranial v.
    v. dentata
    dorsal vertebrae
    false vertebrae
    hourglass vertebrae
    H-shape vertebrae
    ivory v.
    vertebrae lumbales
    lumbar vertebrae

    v. magna
    odontoid v.
    picture frame v.
    v. plana
    v. prominens
    rugger jersey v.
    sacral vertebrae
    vertebrae sacrales
    vertebrae spuriae
    tail vertebrae
    thoracic vertebrae
    vertebrae thoracicae
    toothed v.
    true v.
    v. vera
vertebral
    v. arch
    v. artery
    v. border of scapula
    v. canal
    v. column
    v. epidural space
    v. foramen
    v. formula
    v. fusion
    v. ganglion
    v. groove
    v. nerve
    v. notch
    v. part of the costal surface of the lungs
    v. part of diaphragm
    v. plexus
    v. polyarthritis
    v. pulp
    v. region
    v. ribs
    v. vein
    v. venography
    v. venous plexus
    v. venous system
vertebral-basilar system
vertebrarium
vertebrated
    v. catheter
    v. probe
vertebrectomy
vertebroarterial
    v. foramen
vertebrochondral
    v. ribs
vertebrocostal
    v. trigone
vertebrofemoral
vertebroiliac
vertebropelvic ligaments
vertebrosacral

vertebrosternal
    v. ribs
vertex, pl. **vertices**
    v. cordis
    v. of cornea
    v. corneae
    v. presentation
vertical
    v. axis
    v. banded gastroplasty
    v. dimension
    v. elastic
    v. growth phase
    v. heart
    v. hymen
    v. illumination
    v. index
    v. muscle of tongue
    v. nystagmus
    v. opening
    v. osteotomy
    v. overlap
    v. parallax
    v. plate
    v. retraction syndrome
    v. strabismus
    v. transmission
    v. vertigo
verticalis
vertices (*pl. of* vertex)
verticil
verticillate
Verticillium
verticomental
verticosubmental view
vertiginous
vertigo
    v. ab aure laeso
    auditory v.
    aural v.
    benign paroxysmal postural v.
    benign positional v.
    Charcot's v.
    chronic v.
    endemic paralytic v.
    epidemic v.
    gastric v.
    height v.
    horizontal v.
    hysterical v.
    labyrinthine v.
    laryngeal v.
    lateral v.
    mechanical v.
    nocturnal v.
    objective v.
    ocular v.
    organic v.

    paralyzing v.
    physiologic v.
    positional v. of Bárány
    postural v.
    sham-movement v.
    subjective v.
    vertical v.
vertometer
verumontanitis
verumontanum
vesalianum
Vesalius'
    V. bone
    V. foramen
    V. vein
vesica, gen. and pl. **vesicae**
    v. biliaris
    v. fellea
    v. prostatica
    v. urinaria
vesical
    v. calculus
    v. diverticulum
    v. fistula
    v. gland
    v. hematuria
    v. lithotomy
    v. plexus
    v. reflex
    v. surface of uterus
    v. triangle
    v. veins
vesicalis anus
vesicate
vesication
vesicle
    acoustic v.
    acrosomal v.
    air v.'s
    allantoic v.
    amniocardiac v.
    auditory v.
    Baer's v.
    blastodermic v.
    cerebral v.
    cervical v.
    encephalic v.
    forebrain v.
    germinal v.
    v. hernia
    hindbrain v.
    lens v.
    lenticular v.
    malpighian v.'s
    midbrain v.
    ocular v.
    ophthalmic v.
    optic v.

V

vesicle *(continued)*
   otic v.
   pinocytotic v.
   primary brain v.
   seminal v.
   synaptic v.'s
   telencephalic v.
   umbilical v.
vesicoabdominal
vesicobullous
vesicocele
vesicocervical
vesicoclysis
vesicocolic fistula
vesicocutaneous fistula
vesicointestinal
   v. fistula
vesicolithiasis
vesicoprostatic
vesicopubic
vesicopustular
vesicopustule
vesicorectal
vesicorectostomy
vesicosigmoid
vesicosigmoidostomy
vesicospinal
vesicostomy
vesicotomy
vesicoumbilical
   v. ligament
vesicoureteral
   v. reflux
   v. valve
vesicourethral
   v. canal
vesicouterine
   v. fistula
   v. ligament
   v. pouch
vesicouterovaginal
vesicovaginal
   v. fistula
vesicovaginorectal
   v. fistula
vesicovisceral
vesicula, gen. and pl. vesiculae
   v. fellis
   v. ophthalmica
   v. seminalis
   v. umbilicalis
vesicular
   v. appendage
   v. appendices of uterine tube
   v. exanthema of swine virus
   v. keratitis
   v. keratopathy
   v. mole

v. murmur
v. ovarian follicle
v. rale
v. resonance
v. respiration
v. rickettsiosis
v. stomatitis virus
v. transport
v. venous plexus
vesiculate
vesiculated
vesiculation
vesiculectomy
vesiculiform
vesiculitis
vesiculobronchial
vesiculocavernous
   v. respiration
vesiculography
vesiculopapular
vesiculoprostatitis
vesiculopustular
vesiculose
vesiculotomy
vesiculotubular
vesiculotympanic
vesiculotympanitic resonance
vesiculous
Vesiculovirus
Vesling's line
vessel
   absorbent v.'s
   afferent v.
   anastomosing v.
   blood v.
   capillary v.
   chyle v.
   collateral v.
   deep lymphatic v.
   efferent v.
   v.'s of internal ear
   lacteal v.
   lymph v.'s
   lymphatic v.'s
   nutrient v.
   superficial lymphatic v.
   v.'s of vessels
   vitelline v.'s
vestibula (*pl. of* vestibulum)
vestibular
   v. anus
   v. apparatus
   v. area
   v. blind sac
   v. branches of labyrinthine artery
   v. canal
   v. cecum of the cochlear duct
   v. crest

v. fissure of cochlea
v. fold
v. fossa
v. ganglion
v. glands
v. hair cells
v. labium of limbus of spiral lamina
v. labyrinth
v. ligament
v. lip of limbus of spiral lamina
v. membrane
v. nerve
v. neuronitis
v. nucleus
v. nystagmus
v. ocular reflex
v. organ
v. part of vestibulocochlear nerve
v. root
v. root of vestibulocochlear nerve
v. screen
v. surface of tooth
v. veins
v. wall of cochlear duct
v. window
vestibularis
vestibulate
vestibule
aortic v.
buccal v.
esophagogastric v.
gastroesophageal v.
labial v.
v. of larynx
v. of mouth
v. of nose
v. of omental bursa
oral v.
Sibson's aortic v.
v. of vagina
vestibulitis
vestibulocerebellar ataxia
vestibulocerebellum
vestibulocochlear
v. nerve
v. nuclei
v. organ
vestibulo-equilibratory control
vestibulopathy
idiopathic bilateral v.
vestibuloplasty
vestibulospinal
v. reflex
v. tract
vestibulotomy
vestibulourethral
vestibulum, pl. **vestibula**

v. aortae
v. bursae omentalis
v. laryngis
v. nasi
v. oris
v. pudendi
v. vaginae
vestige
v. of processus vaginalis
v. of vaginal process
vestigial
v. fold
v. muscle
v. organ
vestigium, pl. **vestigia**
v. processus vaginalis
vesuvin
Veterans Administration hospital
Vi
V. antibody
V. antigen
via, pl. **viae**
viability
viable
viae (*pl. of* via)
vibrating line
vibration
v. syndrome
v. tolerance
vibrative
vibrator
vibratory
v. massage
v. sensibility
v. urticaria
Vibrio
V. alginolyticus
V. cholerae
V. fetus
V. fluvialis
V. furnissii
V. hollisae
V. metschnikovii
V. mimicus
V. parahaemolyticus
V. sputorum
V. vulnificus
vibrio
El Tor v.
Nasik v.
vibrion septique
vibrissa, gen. and pl. **vibrissae**
vibrissal
vibrocardiogram
vibromasseur
vibrotherapeutics

V

vicarious
    v. hypertrophy
    v. menstruation
Vicat needle
vicious
    v. cicatrix
    v. circle
    v. union
Vicq
    V. d'Azyr's bundle
    V. d'Azyr's centrum semiovale
    V. d'Azyr's foramen
Victoria
    V. blue
    V. orange
Vidal's disease
video-assisted thoracic surgery
video fluoroscopy
videokeratoscope
vidian
    v. artery
    v. canal
    v. nerve
    v. vein
Vierra's sign
Vieussens'
    V. annulus
    V. ansa
    V. centrum
    V. foramina
    V. ganglia
    V. isthmus
    V. limbus
    V. loop
    V. ring
    V. valve
    V. veins
    V. ventricle
view
    axial v.
    base v.
    v. box _Grashey_
    Caldwell v.
    half axial v.
    long axis v.
    Stenvers v.
    Towne v.
    verticosubmental v.
    Waters' v.
vigil
    coma v.
vigilambulism
vigilance
villi (_pl. of_ villus)
villitis
villoma
villonodular pigmented tenosynovitis
villose

villositis
villosity
villous
    v. adenoma
    v. atrophy
    v. carcinoma
    v. papilloma
    v. placenta
    v. tenosynovitis
    v. tumor
villus, pl. villi
    anchoring v.
    arachnoid villi
    chorionic villi
    floating v.
    free v.
    intestinal villi
    villi intestinales
    villi pericardiaci
    pericardial villi
    peritoneal villi
    villi peritoneales
    pleural villi
    villi pleurales
    primary v.
    secondary v.
    synovial villi
    villi synoviales
    tertiary v.
villusectomy
Vincent's
    V. angina
    V. bacillus
    V. disease
    V. infection
    V. spirillum
    V. tonsillitis
    V. white mycetoma
vinculum, pl. vincula
    v. breve
    v. linguae
    vincula lingulae cerebelli
    long v.
    v. longum
    v. preputii
    short v.
    vincula tendinum
    vincula of tendons
Vineberg procedure
violaceous
violet
    Hoffman's v.
violinist's cramp
vipoma
Vipond's sign
viraginity
viral
    v. cystitis

v. dysentery
v. encephalomyelitis
v. envelope
v. gastroenteritis
v. hemagglutination
v. hemorrhagic fever
v. hemorrhagic fever virus
v. hepatitis
v. hepatitis type A
v. hepatitis type B
v. hepatitis type C
v. hepatitis type D
v. hepatitis type E
v. neutralization
v. pericarditis
v. probe
v. therapy
v. tropism
v. wart

Virchow-Hassall bodies
Virchow-Holder angle
Virchow-Robin space
Virchow's
V. angle
V. cells
V. corpuscles
V. crystals
V. disease
V. law
V. node
V. psammoma

viremia
vires (*pl. of* vis)
virga
virgin
v. generation
v. silk
virginal
v. membrane
virginity
virgophrenia
viricidal
viricide
viridans hemolysis
virile
v. member
virilescence
virilia
virilism
adrenal v.
virility
virilization
virilizing
viripotent
viroid
virologist
virology
viropexis

virtual
v. focus
v. image
virucidal
virucide
virucopria
virulence
virulent
v. bacteriophage
v. bubo
viruliferous
viruria
virus, pl. **viruses**
2060 v.
Abelson murine leukemia v.
adeno-associated v.
adenoidal-pharyngeal-conjunctival v.
adenosatellite v.
African horse sickness v.
v. A hepatitis
AIDS-related v.
Akabane v.
Aleutian mink disease v.
amphotropic v.
animal viruses
A-P-C v.
Argentine hemorrhagic fever v.
attenuated v.
Aujeszky's disease v.
Australian X disease v.
avian encephalomyelitis v.
avian erythroblastosis v.
avian influenza v.
avian leukosis-sarcoma v.
avian lymphomatosis v.
avian myeloblastosis v.
avian neurolymphomatosis v.
avian pneumoencephalitis v.
avian sarcoma v.
avian viral arthritis v.
B v.
B19 v.
bacterial v.
v. B hepatitis
Bittner v.
BK v.
v. blockade
bluetongue v.
Bolivian hemorrhagic fever v.
Borna disease v.
Bornholm disease v.
bovine leukemia v.
bovine leukosis v.
bovine papular stomatitis v.
bovine virus diarrhea v.
Bunyamwera v.
Bwamba v,
California v.

V

virus (*continued*)
canine distemper v.
Capim viruses
Caraparu v.
cattle plague v.
Catu v.
CELO v.
Central European tick-borne
  encephalitis v.
C group viruses
Chagres v.
v. C hepatitis
chicken embryo lethal orphan v.
chickenpox v.
chikungunya v.
Coe v.
cold v.
Colorado tick fever v.
Columbia S. K. v.
common cold v.
contagious ecthyma (pustular
  dermatitis) v. of sheep
contagious pustular stomatitis v.
cowpox v.
Coxsackie v.
Crimean-Congo hemorrhagic
  fever v.
croup-associated v.
cytopathogenic v.
defective v.
delta v.
dengue v.
distemper v.
DNA v.
dog distemper v.
duck hepatitis v.
duck influenza v.
duck plague v.
eastern equine encephalomyelitis v.
EB v.
Ebola v.
ECHO v.
ECMO v.
ecotropic v.
ECSO v.
ectromelia v.
EEE v.
EMC v.
emerging viruses
encephalitis v.
v. encephalomyelitis
encephalomyocarditis v.
enteric viruses
enteric cytopathogenic bovine
  orphan v.
enteric cytopathogenic human
  orphan v.

enteric cytopathogenic monkey
  orphan v.
enteric cytopathogenic swine
  orphan v.
enteric orphan viruses
enzootic encephalomyelitis v.
ephemeral fever v.
epidemic gastroenteritis v.
epidemic keratoconjunctivitis v.
epidemic myalgia v.
epidemic parotitis v.
epidemic pleurodynia v.
Epstein-Barr v.
equine abortion v.
equine arteritis v.
equine influenza viruses
equine rhinopneumonitis v.
FA v.
feline panleukopenia v.
feline rhinotracheitis v.
fibromatosis v. of rabbits
fibrous bacterial viruses
filamentous bacterial viruses
filtrable v.
fixed v.
Flury strain rabies v.
FMD v.
foamy viruses
foot-and-mouth disease v.
fowl erythroblastosis v.
fowl lymphomatosis v.
fowl myeloblastosis v.
fowl neurolymphomatosis v.
fowl plague v.
fowlpox v.
fox encephalitis v.
Friend v.
Friend leukemia v.
GAL v.
gallus adeno-like v.
gastroenteritis v. type A
gastroenteritis v. type B
German measles v.
Germiston v.
goatpox v.
Graffi's v.
green monkey v.
Gross' v.
Gross' leukemia v.
Guama v.
Guaroa v.
HA1 v.
HA2 v.
hand-foot-and-mouth disease v.
Hantaan v.
hard pad v.
helper v.
hemadsorption v. type 1

hemadsorption v. type 2
v. hepatitis
hepatitis A v.
hepatitis B v.
hepatitis C v.
hepatitis delta v.
hepatitis E v.
herpes v.
herpes simplex v.
herpes zoster v.
hog cholera v.
horsepox v.
human immunodeficiency v.
human papilloma v.
human T-cell
  lymphoma/leukemia v.
human T-cell lymphotropic v.
human T lymphotrophic v.
IBR v.
v. III of rabbits
Ilhéus v.
inclusion conjunctivitis viruses
infantile gastroenteritis v.
infectious arteritis v. of horses
infectious bronchitis v.
infectious ectromelia v.
infectious hepatitis v.
infectious papilloma v.
infectious porcine
  encephalomyelitis v.
influenza viruses
insect viruses
iridescent v.
Jamestown Canyon v.
Japanese B encephalitis v.
JC v.
JH v.
Junin v.
K v.
Kelev strain rabies v.
v. keratoconjunctivitis
Kilham rat v.
Kisenyi sheep disease v.
Koongol viruses
Korean hemorrhagic fever v.
Kyasanur Forest disease v.
La Crosse v.
lactate dehydrogenase v.
Lassa v.
latent rat v.
LCM v.
louping-ill v.
Lucké's v.
Lunyo v.
lymphadenopathy-associated v.
lymphocytic choriomeningitis v.
lymphogranuloma venereum v.
Machupo v.

maedi v.
malignant catarrhal fever v.
Maloney leukemia v.
mammary cancer v. of mice
mammary tumor v. of mice
Marburg v.
Marek's disease v.
marmoset v.
masked v.
Mason-Pfizer v.
Mayaro v.
measles v.
medi v.
Mengo v.
milker's nodule v.
mink enteritis v.
MM v.
Mokola v.
molluscum contagiosum v.
Moloney's v.
monkey B v.
mouse encephalomyelitis v.
mouse hepatitis v.
mouse leukemia viruses
mouse mammary tumor v.
mouse parotid tumor v.
mouse poliomyelitis v.
mousepox v.
mouse thymic v.
mucosal disease v.
mumps v.
murine sarcoma v.
Murray Valley encephalitis v.
Murutucu v.
MVE v.
myxomatosis v.
naked v.
ND v.
Neethling v.
negative strand v.
Negishi v.
neonatal calf diarrhea v.
neurotropic v.
Newcastle disease v.
non-A, non-B hepatitis v.
nonoccluded v.
Norwalk v.
occluded v.
Omsk hemorrhagic fever v.
oncogenic v.
o'nyong-nyong v.
orf v.
Oriboca v.
ornithosis v.
orphan viruses
Pacheco's parrot disease v.
panleukopenia v. of cats
pantropic v.

V

virus (*continued*)
papilloma v.
pappataci fever viruses
papular stomatitis v. of cattle
parainfluenza viruses
paravaccinia v.
parrot v.
Patois v.
pharyngoconjunctival fever v.
phlebotomus fever viruses
plant viruses
pneumonia v. of mice
poliomyelitis v.
polyoma v.
porcine hemagglutinating
  encephalomyelitis v.
Powassan v.
progressive pneumonia v.
pseudocowpox v.
pseudolymphocytic
  choriomeningitis v.
pseudorabies v.
psittacosis v.
PVM v.
quail bronchitis v.
Quaranfil v.
rabbit fibroma v.
rabbit myxoma v.
rabbitpox v.
rabies v., Flury strain
rabies v., Kelev strain
Rauscher leukemia v.
Rauscher's v.
REO v.
respiratory enteric orphan v.
respiratory syncytial v.
Rida v.
Rift Valley fever v.
rinderpest v.
RNA v.
RNA tumor viruses
Ross River v.
Rous-associated v.
Rous sarcoma v.
Rs v.
Rubarth's disease v.
rubella v.
rubeola v.
Russian autumn encephalitis v.
Russian spring-summer
  encephalitis v.
Salisbury common cold viruses
salivary v.
salivary gland v.
sandfly fever viruses
San Miguel sea lion v.
Sendai v.
serum hepatitis v.

v. shedding
sheep-pox v.
shipping fever v.
Shope fibroma v.
Shope papilloma v.
Simbu v.
simian v.
simian v. 40
simian vacuolating v. No. 40
Sindbis v.
slow v.
smallpox v.
snowshoe hare v.
soremouth v.
Spondweni v.
St. Louis encephalitis v.
swamp fever v.
swine encephalitis v.
swine fever v.
swine influenza viruses
swinepox v.
Swiss mouse leukemia v.
Tacaribe v.
Tahyna v.
temperate v.
Teschen disease v.
Tete viruses
TGE v.
Theiler's v.
Theiler's mouse
  encephalomyelitis v.
Theiler's original v.
tick-borne v.
tick-borne encephalitis v.
TO v.
trachoma v.
transmissible gastroenteritis v. of
  swine
transmissible turkey enteritis v.
tumor v.
Turlock v.
Umbre v.
vaccine v.
vaccinia v.
vacuolating v.
varicella-zoster v.
variola v.
VEE v.
Venezuelan equine
  encephalomyelitis v.
vesicular exanthema of swine v.
vesicular stomatitis v.
viral hemorrhagic fever v.
visceral disease v.
visna v.
VS v.
WEE v.
Wesselsbron disease v.

western equine encephalomyelitis v.
West Nile v.
West Nile encephalitis v.
v. X disease
xenotropic v.
Yaba v.
Yaba monkey v.
yellow fever v.
Zika v.

virus-associated hemophagocytic syndrome
virusoid
virus-transformed cell
vis, pl. **vires**
v. conservatrix
v. a fronte
v. a tergo
v. vitae, v. vitalis
viscance
viscera (*pl. of* viscus)
viscerad
visceral
v. anesthesia
v. arches
v. brain
v. cavity
v. cleft
v. cranium
v. crises
v. disease virus
v. disorder
v. epilepsy
v. inversion
v. larva migrans
v. layer
v. layer of serous pericardium
v. layer of tunica vaginalis of testis
v. leishmaniasis
v. lymph nodes
v. mesoderm
v. motor neuron
v. motor neurons
v. muscle
v. nerve
v. nervous system
v. nodes
v. pelvic fascia
v. pericardium
v. peritoneum
v. plate
v. pleura
v. pleurisy
v. sense
v. skeleton
v. surface of liver
v. surface of the spleen

v. swallow
v. traction reflex
visceralgia
viscerimotor
viscerocranium
cartilaginous v.
membranous v.
viscerogenic
v. reflex
viscerograph
visceroinhibitory
visceromegaly
visceromotor
v. reflex
visceroparietal
visceroperitoneal
visceropleural
visceroptosis, visceroptosia
viscerosensory
v. reflex
visceroskeletal
visceroskeleton
viscerosomatic
viscerotome
viscerotomy
viscerotonia
viscerotrophic
v. reflex
viscerotropic
viscidosis
viscosity
absolute v.
anomalous v.
apparent v.
dynamic v.
kinematic v.
newtonian v.
relative v.
viscus, pl. **viscera**
visibility acuity
visile
vision
achromatic v.
binocular v.
blue v.
central v.
chromatic v.
colored v.
cone v.
direct v.
double v.
facial v.
green v.
halo v.
haploscopic v.
indirect v.
multiple v.
night v.

vision (*continued*)
    oscillating v.
    peripheral v.
    photopic v.
    red v.
    rod v.
    scotopic v.
    stereoscopic v.
    subjective v.
    tinted v.
    triple v.
    tubular v.
    tunnel v.
    twilight v.
    yellow v.
visiting nurse
visna virus
visual
    v. acuity
    v. agnosia
    v. alexia
    v. angle
    v. aphasia
    v. area
    v. axis
    v. blackout
    v. cortex
    v. efficiency
    v. evoked potential
    v. extinction
    v. field
    functional v. loss
    v. image
    v. inattention
    v. orbicularis reflex
    v. organ
    v. pathway
    v. projection
    v. receptor cells
    v. threshold
visualize
visual-spatial agnosia
visuoauditory
visuognosis
visuomotor
visuopsychic
visuosensory
visuospatial
visuscope
vita glass
vital
    v. capacity
    v. center
    v. force
    v. index
    v. knot
    v. node
    v. pulp

    v. red
    v. signs
    v. stain
    v. statistics
    v. tooth
    y. tripod
    v. ultraviolet
vitalism
vitalistic
vitality
    v. test
vitalize
vitalometer
vitals
vitamin
    v. B_{12} neuropathy
    v. C test
    v. D-binding protein
    v. D-resistant rickets
vitellarium
vitelliform
    v. degeneration
vitelline
    v. artery
    v. cord
    v. duct
    v. fistula
    v. membrane
    v. pole
    v. reservoir
    v. sac
    v. vein
    v. vessels
vitelliruptive degeneration
vitellogenesis
vitellogenin
vitellointestinal
    v. cyst
    v. duct
vitellus
vitiation
vitiliginous
vitiligo, pl. **vitiligines**
    v. capitis
    Cazenave's v.
    Celsus' v.
    v. iridis
vitiligoidea
vitrectomy
    anterior v.
    posterior v.
vitreitis
vitreodentin
vitreoretinal
    v. choroidopathy syndrome
    v. traction syndrome
vitreoretinopathy
    exudative v.

vitreo-tapetoretinal dystrophy
vitreous
    v. body
    v. camera
    v. cell
    v. chamber of eye
    v. detachment
    v. hernia
    v. humor
    v. lamella
    v. membrane
    persistent anterior hyperplastic primary v.
    persistent posterior hyperplastic primary v.
    primary v.
    secondary v.
    v. table
    tertiary v.
vitreum
vitrification
in vitro **fertilization**
vivax
    v. fever
    v. malaria
vividialysis
vividiffusion
vivification
viviperception
in vivo **fertilization**
Vladimiroff-Mikulicz amputation
VMA test
vocal
    v. amusia
    v. cord
    v. cord nodules
    v. fold
    v. fremitus
    v. ligament
    v. muscle
    v. process
    v. process of arytenoid cartilage
    v. resonance
    v. shelf
vocalis muscle
Vogel's law
Voges-Proskauer reaction
Vogt
    V. angle
    V. cephalodactyly
    V. syndrome
Vogt-Koyanagi syndrome
Vogt-Spielmeyer disease
Vohwinkel syndrome
voice
    amphoric v.
    bronchial v.
    cavernous v.

    epigastric v.
    eunuchoid v.
    myxedema v.
void
    flow v.
    v. metal composite
    signal v.
voiding
    v. cystogram
    v. flow rate
Voigt's lines
vola
volar
    v. carpal ligament
    v. interosseous artery
    v. interosseous nerve
volaris
volatile anesthetic
vole bacillus
Volhard's test
volition
volitional
    v. tremor
Volkmann's
    V. canals
    V. cheilitis
    V. contracture
    V. spoon
volley
Vollmer test
Volpe-Manhold Index
volsella
voltage-gated channel
voltaic taste
Voltolini's disease
volume
    v. averaging
    closing v.
    distribution v.
    v. element
    end-diastolic v.
    end-systolic v.
    expiratory reserve v.
    extracellular fluid v.
    forced expiratory v.
    v. index
    inspiratory reserve v.
    mean corpuscular v.
    minute v.
    packed cell v.
    residual v.
    respiratory minute v.
    resting tidal v.
    stroke v.
    v. substitute
    tidal v.
    v. unit
volume-controlled respirator

V

volume-displacement plethysmograph
volumetric flask
voluntary
    v. dehydration
    v. guarding
    v. hospital
    v. muscle
    v. mutism
    v. nystagmus
voluptuous
volute
volutin
    v. granules
Volvox
volvulosis
volvulus
    cecal v.
    gastric v.
    sigmoid v.
vomer, gen. **vomeris**
    v. cartilagineus
vomeral
    v. groove
    v. sulcus
vomerine
    v. canal
    v. cartilage
vomeris (*gen. of* vomer)
vomerobasilar
    v. canal
vomeronasal
    v. cartilage
    v. organ
vomerorostral canal
vomerovaginal
    v. canal
    v. groove
vomica
vomicose
vomicus
vomit
    Barcoo v.
    bilious v.
    black v.
    coffee-ground v.
vomiting
    cerebral v.
    dry v.
    epidemic v.
    fecal v.
    morning v.
    pernicious v.
    v. of pregnancy
    projectile v.
    psychogenic v.
    v. reflex
    retention v.
    stercoraceous v.

vomition
vomiturition
vomitus
    v. cruentes
    v. marinus
    v. niger
von
    v. Economo's disease
    v. Gierke's disease
    v. Graefe's sign
    v. Hippel-Lindau syndrome
    v. Kossa stain
    v. Langenbeck's bipedicle
      mucoperiosteal flap
    v. Meyenburg's disease
    v. Recklinghausen disease
    v. Spee's curve
    v. Willebrand factor
    v. Willebrand's disease
Voorhoeve's disease
vortex, pl. **vortices**
    v. coccygeus
    v. cordis
    Fleischer's v.
    v. of heart
    v. lentis
    vortices pilorum
    v. veins
Vorticella
vorticose
    v. veins
Vossius' lenticular ring
vox
    v. choleraica
voxel
voyeur
voyeurism
VS virus
vulgaris
vulnerable
    v. child syndrome
    v. period
    v. period of heart
    v. phase
Vulpian's atrophy
vulsella, vulsellum
    v. forceps
vulva, pl. **vulvae**
vulvar, vulval
    v. dystrophy
    v. slit
vulvectomy
vulvismus
vulvitis
    chronic atrophic v.
    chronic hypertrophic v.
    follicular v.
    leukoplakic v.

vulvocrural
vulvodynia
vulvouterine
vulvovaginal
- v. anus
- v. cystectomy
- v. gland

vulvovaginitis
Vw antigen
V-Y
- V.-Y. flap
- V.-Y. procedure

V-Y plasty

V

W

W chromosome
W procedure
W rays
Waardenburg syndrome
Wachendorf's membrane
Wachstein-Meissel stain for calcium-magnesium-ATPase
Wada test
wadding
waddingtonian homeostasis
waddle
waddling gait
Wagner's
W. disease
W. syndrome
Wagstaffe's fracture
waist
w. of the heart
waiter's cramp
Walcher position
Waldenström's
W. macroglobulinemia
W. purpura
W. syndrome
W. test
Waldeyer's
W. fossae
W. glands
W. sheath
W. space
W. throat ring
W. tract
W. zonal layer
walk
Walker
W. chart
W. tractotomy
walking
chromosome w.
w. typhoid
walk-through angina
wall
anterior w. of middle ear
anterior w. of stomach
anterior w. of tympanic cavity
anterior w. of vagina
axial w.'s of the pulp chambers
carotid w. of middle ear
cavity w.
cell w.
chest w.
enamel w.
external w. of cochlear duct
inferior w. of orbit
inferior w. of tympanic cavity
jugular w. of middle ear
labyrinthine w. of middle ear
lateral w. of middle ear
lateral w. of orbit
lateral w. of tympanic cavity
mastoid w. of middle ear
medial w. of middle ear
medial w. of orbit
medial w. of tympanic cavity
membranous w. of middle ear
membranous w. of trachea
w. of nail
parietal w.
posterior w. of middle ear
posterior w. of stomach
posterior w. of tympanic cavity
posterior w. of vagina
pulpal w.
splanchnic w.
superior w. of orbit
tegmental w. of middle ear
thoracic w.
tympanic w. of cochlear duct
vestibular w. of cochlear duct
Wallenberg's syndrome
wallerian
w. degeneration
w. law
wallet stomach
wall-eye
Walthard's cell rest
Walther's
W. canals
W. dilator
W. ducts
W. ganglion
W. plexus
waltzed flap
wandering
w. abscess
w. cell
w. erysipelas
w. goiter
w. kidney
w. liver
w. organ
w. pacemaker
w. pneumonia
Wangensteen
W. drainage
W. suction
W. tube
Wangiella
Wang's test

W

warble botfly
Warburg's
    W. apparatus
    W. theory
ward
Ward-Romano syndrome
Wardrop's
    W. disease
    W. method
Ward's triangle
warehouseman's itch
warm
    w. agglutinins
    w. autoantibody
warm-cold hemolysin
war neurosis
Warren shunt
wart
    anatomical w.
    asbestos w.
    common w.
    digitate w.
    fig w.
    filiform w.
    flat w.
    fugitive w.
    genital w.
    Henle's w.'s
    infectious w.'s
    moist w.
    mosaic w.
    necrogenic w.
    Peruvian w.
    pitch w.
    plane w.
    plantar w.
    pointed w.
    postmortem w.
    prosector's w.
    seborrheic w.
    senile w.
    soft w.
    soot w.
    telangiectatic w.
    tuberculous w.
    venereal w.
    viral w.
Wartenberg's symptom
Warthin-Finkeldey cells
Warthin-Starry silver stain
Warthin's tumor
wartpox
warty
    w. dyskeratoma
    w. horn
washed field technique
washerman's mark
washerwoman's itch

washout
    w. cannula
    w. test
Wasmann's glands
wasserhelle cell
Wassermann
    W. antibody
    W. reaction
    W. test
Wassermann-fast
wasted ventilation
wasting
    w. disease
    w. palsy
    w. paralysis
    salt w.
    w. syndrome
watchmaker's cramp
water
    w. aspirator
    w. bed
    w. canker
    w. depletion
    w. diuresis
    w. dressing
    gentian aniline w.
    w. immersion
    w. intoxication
    w. itch
    w. sore
    total body w.
    transcellular w.
    w. wheel murmur
water-clear cell of parathyroid
waterfall
water-hammer pulse
Waterhouse-Friderichsen syndrome
watering-can
    w.-c. perineum
    w.-c. scrotum
waterpox
Waters'
    W. operation
    W. projection
    W. view
    W. view radiograph
waters
    bag of w.
    false w.
watershed
    w. infarction
Waterston
    W. operation
    W. shunt
water-trap stomach
waterwheel sound
water-whistle sound
watery eye

Watson-Schwartz test
wave
- A w.
- acid w.
- alkaline w.
- alpha w.
- arterial w.
- B w.
- beta w.
- brain w.
- C w., c w.
- cannon w.
- D w.
- delta w.
- dicrotic w.
- electrocardiographic w.
- excitation w.
- F w.'s, ff w.'s
- fibrillary w.'s
- fibrillatory w.'s
- flat top w.'s
- fluid w.
- flutter-fibrillation w.'s
- w. form
- w. number
- overflow w.
- P w.
- percussion w.
- postextrasystolic T w.
- pulse w.
- Q w.
- R w.
- random w.'s
- recoil w.
- retrograde P w.
- S w.
- sonic w.'s
- supersonic w.'s
- T w.
- theta w.
- tidal w.
- Traube-Hering w.'s
- U w.
- ultrasonic w.'s
- V w.
- x w.
- y w.

(handwritten: pArvus tardus wAve foRms)

wavelength
waveshape
wax
- baseplate w.
- boxing w.
- casting w.
- ear w.
- w. expansion
- w. form
- grave w.
- inlay w.
- w. model denture
- w. pattern

waxing, waxing-up
wax-tipped bougie
waxy
- w. cast
- w. degeneration
- w. fingers
- w. kidney
- w. liver
- w. spleen

WDHA syndrome
wear
- occlusal w.

weaver's cough
web
- esophageal w.
- w. eye
- w. of fingers/toes
- terminal w.

Webb antigen
webbed
- w. fingers
- w. neck
- w. penis
- w. toes

webbing
Weber-Christian disease
Weber-Cockayne syndrome
Weber-Fechner law
Weber's
- W. experiment
- W. glands
- W. law
- W. organ
- W. paradox
- W. point
- W. sign
- W. syndrome
- W. test for hearing
- W. triangle

Webster's
- W. operation
- W. test

Wechsler-Bellevue scale
Wechsler intelligence scales
weddellite calculus
Wedensky
- W. effect
- W. facilitation
- W. inhibition

wedge
- w. biopsy
- w. bone
- dental w.
- w. pressure
- w. resection
- w. spirometer

W

wedge-and-groove
    w.-a.-g. joint
    w.-a.-g. suture
wedge-shaped
    w.-s. fasciculus
    w.-s. tubercle
weekend hospital
Weeks' bacillus
weeping eczema
WEE virus
Wegener's granulomatosis
Wegner's
    W. disease
    W. line
Weibel-Palade bodies
Weichselbaum's coccus
Weidel's reaction
Weigert-Gram stain
Weigert's
    W. iodine solution
    W. iron hematoxylin stain
    W. law
    W. stain for actinomyces
    W. stain for elastin
    W. stain for fibrin
    W. stain for myelin
    W. stain for neuroglia
weight
    birth w.
    w. sense
weightlessness
Weil-Felix
    W.-F. reaction
    W.-F. test
Weill-Marchesani syndrome
Weil's
    W. basal layer
    W. basal zone
    W. disease
Weinberg's reaction
Weingrow's reflex
Weir
    W. Mitchell's disease
    W. Mitchell treatment
    W. operation
Weisbach's angle
weismannism
Weiss' sign
Weitbrecht's
    W. cartilage
    W. cord
    W. fibers
    W. foramen
    W. ligament
Welch's bacillus
Welcker's angle

welder's
    w. conjunctivitis
    w. lung
well counter
well-differentiated lymphocytic lymphoma
Wells' syndrome
welt
wen
Wenckebach
    W. block
    W. period
    W. phenomenon
Wenzel's ventricle
Wepfer's glands
Werdnig-Hoffmann
    W.-H. disease
    W.-H. muscular atrophy
Werlhof's disease
Wernekinck's
    W. commissure
    W. decussation
Werner's
    W. syndrome
    W. test
Wernicke-Korsakoff
    W.-K. encephalopathy
    W.-K. syndrome
Wernicke's
    W. aphasia
    W. area
    W. center
    W. disease
    W. encephalopathy
    W. field
    W. radiation
    W. reaction
    W. region
    W. sign
    W. syndrome
    W. zone
Wertheim's operation
Werther's disease
Wesselsbron disease virus
West
    W. African fever
    W. African sleeping sickness
    W. African trypanosomiasis
    W. Indian smallpox
    W. Nile encephalitis virus
    W. Nile fever
    W. Nile virus
    W. syndrome
Westberg's space
Westergren method
Westermark's sign
Western
    W. blot, W. blotting

W. blot analysis
Western W., Western W.
western equine encephalomyelitis virus
Westphal-Erb sign
Westphal-Piltz phenomenon
Westphal's
    W. disease
    W. phenomenon
    W. pseudosclerosis
    W. pupillary reflex
    W. sign
Westphal-Strümpell pseudosclerosis
wet
    w. beriberi
    w. compress
    w. cup
    w. cutaneous leishmaniasis
    w. dream
    w. gangrene
    w. lung
    w. nurse
    w. pack
    w. pleurisy
    w. shock
    w. tetter
Wetzel grid
Wever-Bray phenomenon
Weyers-Thier syndrome
whale fingers
Wharton's
    W. duct
    W. jelly
wheal
wheal-and-erythema reaction
wheal-and-flare reaction
wheat germ
Wheatstone's bridge
wheel
    Burlew w.
Wheeler-Johnson test
Wheeler method
Wheelhouse's operation
wheeze
    asthmatoid w.
"w" hernia
whetstone crystals
whewellite calculus
whip bougie
whiplash
    w. injury
Whipple's
    W. disease
    W. operation
whipworm
whisper
whispered
    w. bronchophony
    w. pectoriloquy

whispering pectoriloquy
whistle
    Galton's w.
whistle-tip catheter
whistling
    w. deformity
    w. face syndrome
    w. rale
white
    w. bile
    w. blood cell
    w. blood cell cast
    w. cell cast
    w. commissure
    w. corpuscle
    w. of eye
    w. fat
    w. fiber
    w. fingers
    w. forelock
    w. gangrene
    w. graft
    w. infarct
    w. leg
    w. line
    w. line of anal canal
    w. line of Toldt
    w. lung
    w. matter
    w. muscle
    w. piedra
    w. pulp
    w. pupillary reflex
    w. rami communicantes
    w. sponge nevus
    w. spot
    w. spot disease
    w. substance
    w. thrombus
    w. yolk
whitegraft reaction
whitehead
Whitehead deformity
Whitehead's operation
white-out syndrome
whitepox
whites
whiting
whitlow
    herpetic w.
    melanotic w.
    thecal w.
Whitman's frame
Whitmore's bacillus
Whitnall's tubercle
whole-body
    w.-b. counter
    w.-b. titration curve

W

whoop
    systolic w.
whooping cough
whorl
    coccygeal w.
    digital w.
    hair w.'s
whorled
    w. enamel
WI-38 cells
Wickham's striae
Widal's
    W. reaction
    W. syndrome
wide
    w. field ocular
    w. plane
    w. spectrum
wide-latitude film
widow's peak
width
    orbital w.
    window w.
Wigand maneuver
Wildermuth's ear
Wilder's
    W. diet
    W. law of initial value
    W. sign
    W. stain for reticulum
Wildervanck syndrome
Wilde's
    W. cords
    W. triangle
wildfire
    w. rash
wild type
wild-type strain
Wilhelmy balance
Wilkie's
    W. artery
    W. disease
Willett's forceps
Williams'
    W. stain
    W. syndrome
Willis'
    W. centrum nervosum
    W. cords
    W. pancreas
    W. paracusis
    W. pouch
Williston's law
Wilms' tumor
Wilson
    W. block
    W. disease
    W. lichen

    W. method
    W. muscle
    W. syndrome
Wilson-Mikity syndrome
windage
windburn
Windigo psychosis
window
    aortic w.
    aorticopulmonary w.
    aortic-pulmonic w.
    aortopulmonary w.
    cochlear w.
    w. level
    lung w.
    mediastinal w.
    oval w.
    round w.
    soft tissue w.
    tachycardia w.
    vestibular w.
    w. width
windpipe
wing
    angel's w.
    ashen w.
    w. cell
    w. of crista galli
    gray w.
    greater w. of sphenoid bone
    w. of ilium
    Ingrassia's w.
    lesser w. of sphenoid bone
    w. of nose
    w. plate
    w. of sacrum
    w. of vomer
wing-beating tumor
winged
    w. catheter
    w. scapula
Winiwarter-Buerger disease
wink
    w. reflex
winking spasm
Winkler's disease
Winslow's
    W. foramen
    W. ligament
    W. pancreas
    W. stars
winter
    w. eczema
    w. itch
Winterbottom's sign
Winternitz' sound
Wintersteiner rosettes

wire
    arch w.
    w. arch
    guide w.
    Kirschner's w.
    ligature w.
    separating w.
    w. splint
    wrought w.
wire-loop lesion
wiring
    circumferential w.
    continuous loop w.
    craniofacial suspension w.
    Gilmer w.
    Ivy loop w.
    perialveolar w.
    pyriform aperture w.
    Stout's w.
Wirsung's
    W. canal
    W. duct
wiry
    w. pulse
wisdom tooth
Wiskott-Aldrich syndrome
Wissler's syndrome
witch's milk
withdrawal
    w. reflex
    w. symptoms
    though w.
witkop
Wittigo psychosis
witzelsucht
Wohlfart-Kugelberg-Welander disease
Wolfe
    W. graft
    W. method
Wolfe-Krause graft
Wolff-Chaikoff
    W.-C. block
    W.-C. effect
wolffian
    w. body
    w. cyst
    w. duct
    w. duct carcinoma
    w. rest
    w. ridge
    w. tubules
Wolff-Parkinson-White syndrome
Wolff's law
Wölfler's gland
Wolf-Orton bodies
Wolfring's glands
Wolinella

Wollaston's
    W. doublet
    W. theory
Wolman's
    W. disease
    W. xanthomatosis
womb
    falling of the w.
wood
    orange w.
woodcutter's encephalitis
wooden resonance
wooden-shoe heart
Wood's
    W. glass
    W. lamp
    W. light
woolly hair
woolly-hair nevus
Woolner's tip
woolsorter's, wool-sorter's
    w. disease
    w. pneumonia
word
    w. blindness
    w. deafness
    w. salad
    stimulus w.
Woringer-Kolopp disease
working
    w. bite
    w. contacts
    w. occlusal surfaces
    w. occlusion
    w. out
    w. side
    w. side condyle
    w. through
workstation
World Health Organization
worm
    w. abscess
    caddis w.
    fleece w.
    Manson's eye w.
    meal w.
wormian bones
Worth's amblyoscope
wound
    abraded w.
    avulsed w.
    w. botulism
    w. clip
    crease w.
    w. dehiscence
    w. fever
    glancing w.
    gunshot w.

W

wound *(continued)*
    gutter w.
    incised w.
    w. myiasis
    nonpenetrating w.
    open w.
    penetrating w.
    perforating w.
    puncture w.
    septic w.
    seton w.
    stab w.
    subcutaneous w.
    sucking w.
    tangential w.
woven bone
W-plasty
Wr^a antigen
wrap
    cardiac muscle w.
wreath
    ciliary w.
Wright
    W. antigens
    W. respirometer
    W. stain
    W. syndrome
    W. version

wrinkle
wrinkler muscle of eyebrow
Wrisberg's
    W. cartilage
    W. ganglia
    W. ligament
    W. nerve
    W. tubercle
wrist
    w. clonus
    w. clonus reflex
    w.-drop
    w. joint
    w. sign
wrist-drop
writer's cramp
writing
    w. hand
    skin w.
wrought wire
wryneck, wry neck
Wuchereria
    W. bancrofti
    W. malayi
wuchereriasis
Wurster's test
Wyburn-Mason syndrome

[handwritten annotation: SLAC - ALL cAPS]

X

   X body
   X chromosome
   X zone

x

   x wave

xanchromatic

xanthelasma

   generalized x.
   x. palpebrarum

xanthemia

xanthene dyes

xanthinuria

xanthism

xanthiuria

xanthoastrocytoma

   pleomorphic x.

xanthochroia

xanthochromatic

xanthochromia

xanthochromic

xanthochroous

xanthoderma

xanthodont

xanthogranuloma

   juvenile x.
   necrobiotic x.

xanthogranulomatous

   x. cholecystitis
   x. pyelonephritis

xanthoma

   x. diabeticorum
   x. disseminatum
   eruptive x.
   fibrous x.
   x. multiplex
   x. palpebrarum
   x. planum
   tendinous x.
   x. tuberosum
   x. tuberosum simplex
   verrucous x.

xanthomatosis

   biliary x.
   x. bulbi
   chronic idiopathic x.
   familial hypercholesteremic x.
   normal cholesteremic x.
   Wolman's x.

xanthomatous

Xanthomonas

   X. *maltophilia*

xanthopathy

xanthopsia

xanthopsydracia

xanthosis

xanthous

xanthurenic acid

xanthuria

xenodiagnosis

xenogeneic

xenogenic

xenogenous

xenograft

xenon-133

xenon-arc photocoagulator

xenoparasite

xenophobia

xenophonia

xenophthalmia

Xenopsylla

xenotropic virus

xeransis

xerantic

xerasia

xerochilia

xeroderma

   x. pigmentosum

xerogram

xerography

xeroma

xeromammography

xeromenia

xeromycteria

xeronosus

xerophagia, xerophagy

xerophthalmia

xerophthalmus

xeroradiograph

xeroradiography

xerosis

   x. parenchymatosus

xerostomia

xerotes

xerotic

   x. degeneration
   x. keratitis

xerotripsis

Xg

   Xg antigen
   Xg blood group

X-inactivation

xiphisternal

   x. crunching sound
   x. joint

xiphisternum

xiphocostal

xiphodynia

X

xiphoid
- x. cartilage
- x. process

xiphoidalgia

xiphoiditis

xiphopagus

Xiphophorus test

X-linked
- X-l. gene
- X-l. hypogammaglobulinemia
- X-l. infantile hypogammaglobulinemia
- X-l. inheritance
- X-l. locus

XO
- XO female
- XO gonadal dysgenesis
- XO syndrome

x-omat

x-radiation

x-ray
- x-r. dosimetry
- x-r. generator
- x-r. microscope
- x-r. therapy
- x-r. tube

x^2 **test**

XX
- XX gonadal dysgenesis
- XX male

XXX female

XXY
- XXY male
- XXY syndrome

XY gonadal dysgenesis

xylene
- x. cyanol FF

xylidine

xylose test

L-xylulosuria

xyrospasm

xysma

XYY
- XYY male
- XYY syndrome

y
- y body
- y cartilage
- y chromosome
- y wave

Yaba
- Y. monkey virus
- Y. virus

Yangtze
- Y. edema
- Y. Valley fever

yaw
- mother y.

yawn

yawning

yaws
- bosch y.
- bush y.
- crab y.
- foot y.
- forest y.
- guinea corn y.
- ringworm y.

years of potential life lost

yeast
- y. extract agar
- y. fungus

yellow
- y. atrophy of the liver
- y. body
- y. bone marrow
- butter y.
- y. cartilage
- chrome y.
- y. corallin
- corralin y.
- y. disease
- y. fever
- y. fever virus
- y. fibers
- y. hepatization
- hydrazine y.
- y. ligament
- y. nail
- y. nail syndrome

- y. skin
- y. spot
- y. vision
- y. yolk

Yersinia
- *Y. enterocolitica*
- *Y. frederiksenii*
- *Y. intermedia*
- *Y. kristensenii*
- *Y. pestis*

yersiniosis

yield
- y. strength
- y. stress

Y-linkage

Y-linked
- Y.-l. gene
- Y.-l. inheritance
- Y.-l. locus

yoke
- alveolar y.
- y. bone

yolk
- y. cells
- y. cleavage
- y. membrane
- y. sac
- y. sac carcinoma
- y. sac tumor
- y. stalk
- white y.
- yellow y.

Yorke's autolytic reaction

Young
- Y. modulus
- Y. prostatic tractor
- Y. rule

Young-Helmholtz theory of color vision

ypsiliform

Y-shaped
- Y.-s. cartilage
- Y.-s. ligament

Yt^a antigen

Yvon's test

Z

Z band
Z chromosome
Z disk
Z filament
Z line
Z procedure
Zaglas' ligament
Zahn's infarct
Zambesi ulcer
Zappert counting chamber
zebra body
Zeeman effect
Zeis' glands
zeisian sty
Zeitgeist
Zellweger syndrome
zelophobia
zelotypia
Zenker's

Z. degeneration
Z. diverticulum
Z. fixative
Z. necrosis
Z. paralysis
zero

z. degree teeth
z. end-expiratory pressure
z. gravity
Patient Z.
zeta

z. potential
z. sedimentation ratio
zetacrit
Ziehen-Oppenheim disease
Ziehl-Neelsen stain
Ziehl's stain
Ziemann's

Z. dots
Z. stippling
Zieve's syndrome
Zika

Z. fever
Z. virus
Zimany's bilobed flap
Zimmerlin's atrophy
Zimmermann's

Z. corpuscle
Z. elementary particle
Z. granule
zinc

z. colic
z. fume fever
z. phosphate cement

z. sulfate flotation centrifugation
method
Zinn's

Z. artery
Z. corona
Z. ligament
Z. membrane
Z. ring
Z. tendon
Z. vascular circle
Z. zonule
zirconium granuloma
zoacanthosis
zoanthropic
zoanthropy
zoetic
zoic
zoite
Zollinger-Ellison

Z.-E. syndrome
Z.-E. tumor
Zöllner's lines
zona, pl. zonae

z. arcuata
z. ciliaris
z. corona
z. dermatica
z. epithelioserosa
z. facialis
z. fasciculata
z. glomerulosa
z. hemorrhoidalis
z. ignea
z. incerta
z. medullovasculosa
z. ophthalmica
z. orbicularis
z. pectinata
z. pellucida
z. perforata
z. pupillaris
z. radiata
z. reticularis
z. serpiginosa
z. striata
z. tecta
z. vasculosa
zonal

z. necrosis
zonary

z. placenta
zonate
Zondek-Aschheim test
zone

abdominal z.'s

Z

zone (*continued*)
  androgenic z.
  arcuate z.
  Barnes' z.
  cervical z.
  cervical z. of tooth
  ciliary z.
  comfort z.
  z.'s of discontinuity
  dolorogenic z.
  entry z.
  ependymal z.
  epileptogenic z.
  equivalence z.
  erogenous z.'s, erotogenic z.'s
  fetal z.
  gingival z.
  Golgi z.
  grenz z.
  Head's z.'s
  hemorrhoidal z.
  interpalpebral z.
  intertubular z.
  language z.
  latent z.
  Lissauer's marginal z.
  Looser's z.'s
  mantle z.
  Marchant's z.
  marginal z.
  motor z.
  neutral z.
  nucleolar z.
  Obersteiner-Redlich z.
  orbicular z.
  pectinate z.
  pellucid z.
  peritubular z.
  polar z.
  protective z.
  pupillary z.
  reflexogenic z.
  secondary X z.
  segmental z.
  Spitzka's marginal z.
  subplasmalemmal dense z.
  sudanophobic z.
  tender z.'s
  thymus-dependent z.
  trabecular z.
  transformation z.
  transitional z.
  trigger z.
  trophotropic z. of Hess
  vascular z.
  vermilion z., vermilion
    transitional z.
  Weil's basal z.
  Wernicke's z.
  z. 1, 2, 3, 4 of West
  X z.

zonesthesia
zonifugal
zoning
zonipetal
zonography
zonoskeleton
zonula, pl. **zonulae**
  z. adherens
  z. ciliaris
  z. occludens
zonular
  z. band
  z. cataract
  z. fibers
  z. layer
  z. scotoma
  z. spaces
zonule
  ciliary z.
  Zinn's z.
zonulitis
zonulolysis, zonulysis
zooblast
zooerastia
zoofulvin
zooglea
zoograft
zoografting
zoolagnia
zoom
zoomania
Zoomastigina
Zoomastigophorasida
Zoomastigophorea
zoomylus
zoonotic cutaneous leishmaniasis
Zoon's erythroplasia
zoophilia
zoophilism
  erotic z.
zoophobia
zooplastic graft
zooplasty
zoosadism
zoospermia
zoster
  z. encephalomyelitis
  geniculate z.
zosteriform
zosteroid
Z-plasty
Zsigmondy's test
Z-tract injection
Zubrod scale
zuckergussleber

Zuckerkandl's
- Z. bodies
- Z. convolution
- Z. fascia

zwieback

zygal
- z. fissure

zygapophysial, zygapophyseal

zygapophysis, pl. **zygapophyses**

zygion

zygoma

zygomatic
- z. arch
- z. bone
- z. border of greater wing of sphenoid bone
- z. branch of facial nerve
- z. diameter
- z. fossa
- z. margin of greater wing of sphenoid bone
- z. nerve
- z. process of frontal bone
- z. process of maxilla
- z. process of temporal bone
- z. region

zygomaticoauricular
- z. index

zygomaticoauricularis

zygomaticofacial
- z. branch of zygomatic nerve
- z. foramen

zygomaticofrontal

zygomaticomaxillary
- z. suture

zygomatico-orbital
- z.-o. artery
- z.-o. foramen

zygomaticosphenoid

zygomaticotemporal
- z. branch of zygomatic nerve
- z. foramen
- z. suture

zygomaticus
- z. major muscle
- z. minor muscle

zygomaxillare

zygomaxillary
- z. point

Zygomycetes

zygomycosis

zygon

zygonema

zygopodium

zygosis

zygosity

zygosperm

zygospore

zygote

zygotene

zygotic

zygotoblast

zygotomere

zymogenic cell

zymoplastic substance

zymotic papilloma

Z

Appendix 1

Hyphenation: The Mark of Quality

Today, work printed from computer-generated files is often unhyphenated—especially if lines can be automatically justified. Nevertheless, hyphenation is necessary and useful in many cases.

End-of-line hyphenation tends to serve as a measurement of the care with which a given document—page, letter, book, journal, or other written record—has been produced. It also serves as a measure of overall quality.

Some medical words are so long that they must be broken to avoid a very obvious space at the right of the page. Sometimes, setting up narrow columns, tables, or graphs requires breaking words. Finally, formal publication in a journal or book often requires decisions about end-of-line breaks.

Determining End-of-Line Breaks

When guidance on hyphenation is available, choices still need to be made among the possible end-of-line breaks available for a particular word. Determining which to choose is usually a simple process that involves accepted pronunciation and readability.

How Pronunciation Affects Hyphenation

Pronunciation is generally, but not always, the most widely accepted factor used in setting end-of-line hyphenation in the United States. Yet pronunciations vary, so even when dictionaries show more than one pronunciation for a word, they will still show a single version of the end-of-line break for the word.

Hyphenate for Readability

Think from the reader's point of view. Keep the broken word as intelligible as possible. Be sure that the chosen break will not mislead the reader by suggesting another word.

Five Major Rules of Hyphenation

Rule 1: **A word pronounced as a single sound may not be broken.**

	NOT PERMITTED
cast	ca- st
cause	cau- se

Rule 2: **Do not leave a single letter at the end of a line or at the beginning of a line.**

	NOT PERMITTED
a#car*di*ac	a- cardiac
car*di*o*pho*bi#a	cardiophobi- a

Rule 3: **Use at least two letters for an end-of-line break.**

Note: Three or four letters increase readability and are strongly recommended

	MINIMUM	BETTER
car*bol*ic	carbol- ic	car- bolic

Rule 4: **When a spelling hyphen is part of the word being broken, use the spelling hyphen as the end-of-line break, if at all possible**

Note: Very long compound medical words may force a break at a place other than at the spelling hyphen. When this is necessary, be sure to consider readability first.

	BEST	OR(see Rule 5)
car*bo*hy*drate-in*duced	carbohydrate- induced	carbo- hydrate-induced
cli*ent-cen*tered	client- centered	
McCune-Albright	McCune- Albright	

Rule 5: **For words composed of one or more combining forms, but do not include spelling hyphens, hyphenate at the end of a combining form.**

Note: Very long compound medical words may force a break at a place other than at the spelling hyphen. When this is necessary, be sure to consider readability first.

	BEST	OR
car*di*o*ky*mo*gram	cardio- kymogram	cardiokymo- gram

Note: To see the proper hyphenation of terms in this word book, refer to your *Stedman's Medical Dictionary, 26th edition.*

Appendix 3
Medical Prefixes, Suffixes, and Combining Forms

a- not, without, less

ab- from, away from, off

abs- from, away from, off

ad- increase, adherence, motion toward; very

-ad toward, in the direction of; -ward

alge- pain

algesi- pain

algio- pain

algo- pain

ambi- around, on (both) sides, on all sides, both

amyl- starch, polysaccharide nature or origin

amylo- starch, polysaccharide nature or origin

an- not, without, -less

ana- up, toward, apart

ante- before

anti- 1 against, opposing; 2 curative; 3 an antibody

apo- separated from, derived from

arteri- artery

arterio- artery

arthr- a joint, an articulation

arthro- a joint, an articulation

-ase an enzyme

-ate a salt or ester of an "[ib]-ic" acid

aut- self, same

auto- self, same

bacteri- bacteria

bacterio- bacteria

bi- twice, double

bio- life

blasto- budding by cells or tissue

bronch- bronchus

bronchi- bronchus

broncho- bronchus

carcin- cancer

carcino- cancer

cardi- 1 the heart; 2 esophageal opening of stomach

cardio- 1 the heart; 2 esophageal opening of stomach

cata- down

cephal- the head

cephalo- the head

chem- chemistry

chemo- chemistry

chlor- 1 green; 2 chlorine

chloro- 1 green; 2 chlorine

chol- bile

chondrio- 1 cartilage; 2 granular; 3 gritty

chondro- 1 cartilage; 2 granular; 3 gritty

chrom- color

chromat- color

chromo- color

-cidal killing, destroying

-cide killing, destroying

cis- on this side, on the near side

co- with, together, in association, very, complete

col- with, together, in association, very, complete

com- with, together, in association, very, complete

con- with, together, in association, very, complete

cor- with, together, in association, very, complete

crani- cranium

cranio- cranium

cry- cold

cryo- cold

cycl- 1 a circle, a cycle; 2 the ciliary body

cyst- the bladder; the cystic duct; a cyst

cysti- the bladder; the cystic duct; a cyst

cysto- the bladder; the cystic duct; a cyst

cyt- cell

-cyte cell

cyto- cell

dactyl- the fingers, the toes

dactylo- the fingers, the toes

de- away from, cessation

derm- skin

derma- skin
dermat- skin
dermato- skin
dermo- skin
dextr- toward or on the right side
dextro- right, toward or on the right side
di- separation, taking apart, reversal, not, un-
dif- separation, taking apart, reversal, not, un-
dir- separation, taking apart, reversal, not, un-
dis- separation, taking apart, reversal, not, un-
duodeno- the duodenum
-dynia pain
dynamo- force, energy
dys- bad, difficult
ect- outer, on the outside
ecto- outer, on the outside
encephal- the brain
encephalo- the brain
end- within, inner
endo- within, inner
enter- the intestines
entero- the intestines
epi- upon, following, subsequent to
ergo- work
erythr- red, redness
erythro- red, redness
esthesio- sensation, perception
eu- good, well
ex- out of, from, away from
exo- exterior, external, outward
extra- without, outside of
ferri- the presence in a compound of a ferric ion
ferro- metallic iron, the divalent ion Fe^2
fibr- fiber
fibro- fiber
-form in the form or shape of
galact- milk
galacto- milk
-gen 1 producing, coming to be; **2** precursor of
gen- 1 producing, coming to be; **2** precursor of

gloss- the tongue
glosso- the tongue
gluco- glucose
glyco- sugars
gnath- the jaw
gnatho- the jaw
-gram a recording
granul- granular, granule
granulo- granular, granule
-graph a recording instrument
gyn- woman
gyne- woman
gyneco- woman
gyno- woman
hem- blood
hema- blood
hemat- blood
hemato- blood
hemi- one-half
hemo- blood
hepat- the liver
hepatico- the liver
hepato- the liver
hidr- sweat
hidro- sweat
hist- tissue
histio- tissue
histo- tissue
hydr- water; hydrogen
hydro- water; hydrogen
hyper- excessive, above normal
hypo- beneath; diminution, deficiency; the lowest
hyster- 1 uterus; hysteria; **2** late, following
hystero- 1 uterus; hysteria; **2** late, following
-ia a condition
-iasis a condition, a state
-ic pertaining to
-ics organized knowledge, practice, treatment
ileo- the ileum
infra- below
inter- between, among
intra- within
irid- the iris

irido- the iris
ischi- the ischium
ischio- the ischium
-ism 1 condition, disease; 2 a practice, doctrine
-ismus spasm; contraction
iso- 1 equal, like; 2 "isomer of"; 3 sameness
-ite the nature of, resembling
-ites -y, -like
-itides plural of -itis
-itis inflammation
karyo- nucleus
kerat- the cornea
kerato- the cornea
kin- movement
kine- movement
kinesi- motion
kinesio- motion
kineso- motion
kino- movement
lact- milk
lacti- milk
lacto- milk
laryng- the larynx
laryngo- the larynx
latero- lateral, to one side, a side
-lepsis a seizure
-lepsy seizure
lepto- light, slender, thin, frail
leuk- white
leuko- white
linguo- the tongue
lip- fat, lipid
lipo- fat, lipid
lith- a stone, calculus, calcification
litho- a stone, calculus, calcification
-log speech, words
log- speech, words
-login 1 study of; 2 collecting
logo- speech, words
-logy 1 study of; 2 collecting
lymph- lymph
lympho- lymph
lys- lysis, dissolution
lyso- lysis, dissolution
macr- large; long

macro- large; long
mast- breast
masto- breast
meg- 1 large, oversize; 2 one million
mega- 1 large, oversize; 2 one million
megal- large
megalo- large
-megaly large
melan- black
melano- black
mening- meninges
meningo- meninges
mes- 1 middle, mean, intermediacy; 2 mesentery
meso- 1 middle, mean, intermediacy; 2 mesentery
meta- 1 after, behind; 2 joint action, sharing
micr- 1 smallness; 2 one-millionth; 3 microscopic
micro- 1 smallness; 2 one-millionth; 3 microscopic
mon- single
mono- single
morph- form, shape, structure
morpho- form, shape, structure
myx- mucus
myxo- mucus
necr- death, necrosis
necro- death, necrosis
nephr- the kidney
nephro- the kidney
neur- a nerve, the nervous system
neuri- a nerve, the nervous system
neuro- a nerve, the nervous system
oculo- eye, ocular
odont- tooth
odonto- tooth
odyn- pain
odyno- pain
-oid resemblance to
olig- few, little
oligo- few, little
-oma tumor, neoplasm
-omata plural of -oma
oncho- onco-
onco- tumor, bulk, volume

-one a ketone (–CO–) group
onych- fingernail, toenail
onycho- fingernail, toenail
oo- egg, ovary
oophor- ovary
oophoro- ovary
ophthalm- the eye
ophthalmo- the eye
orchi- testis
orchido- testis
orchio- testis
-oses plural of -osis
-osis process, condition, state
ossi- bone
osseo- bony
ost- bone
oste- bone
osteo- bone
ovari- ovary
ovario- ovary
ovi- egg
ovo- egg
oxa- the presence or addition of oxygen
  atom(s)
oxo- addition of oxygen
oxy- sharp; acid; acute; shrill; quick;
  oxygen
pachy- thick
pan- all, entire
pant- all, entire
panto- all, entire
para- 1 abnormal; 2 involvement of two
  like parts
path- disease
patho- disease
-pathy disease
ped- 1 child; 2 foot
pedi- 1 child; 2 foot
pedo- 1 child; 2 foot
-penia deficiency
per- through, thoroughly, intensely
peri- around, about
-pexy fixation, usually surgical
phaco- 1 lens-shaped; 2 relation to a lens
-phage eating, devouring
-phagia eating, devouring
phago- eating, devouring

-phagy eating, devouring
pharmaco- drugs, medicine
pharyng- the pharynx
pharyngo- the pharynx
phleb- vein
phlebo- vein
phon- sound, speech
phono- sound, speech
phor- carrying, bearing; a carrier, a
  bearer; phoria
phoro- carrying, bearing; a carrier, a
  bearer; phoria
phos- light
phot- light
photo- light
phren- 1 diaphragm; 2 the mind; 3 phrenic
phreni- 1 diaphragm; 2 the mind;
  3 phrenic
-phrenia of mind
phrenico- 1 diaphragm; 2 the mind;
  3 phrenic
phreno- 1 diaphragm; 2 the mind;
  3 phrenic
physi- 1 physical; 2 natural; 3 the science
  of physics
physio- 1 physical; 2 natural; 3 the
  science of physics
physo- 1 tendency to swell or inflate;
  2 air, gas
phyt- plants
phyto- plants
-plasia formation
plasma- plasma
plasmat- plasma
plasmato- plasma
plasmo- plasma
-plegia paralysis
pleur- rib, side, pleura
pleura- rib, side, pleura
pleuro- rib, side, pleura
pluri- several, more
-pnea breath, respiration
pneo- breath, respiration
pneum- 1 air, gas; 2 the lungs;
  3 breathing
pneuma- 1 air, gas; 2 the lungs;
  3 breathing

pneumat- 1 air, gas; 2 the lungs; 3 breathing

pneumato- 1 air, gas; 2 the lungs; 3 breathing

pod- foot, foot-shaped

-pod foot, foot-shaped

podo- foot, foot-shaped

-poiesis production

poly- 1 multiplicity; 2 "polymer of"

post- after, behind, posterior

pre- anterior, before

pro- 1 before, forward; 2 precursor of

proct- the anus, the rectum

procto- the anus, the rectum

psych- the mind

psyche- the mind

psycho- the mind

pyel- (renal) pelvis

pyelo- (renal) pelvis

pyo- suppuration, an accumulation of pus, pus

pyreto- fever

pyro- fire, heat, fever

rachi- the spine

rachio- the spine

radio- 1 radiation, chiefly x-ray; 2 radius

re- again, backward

rect- the rectum

recto- the rectum

retro- backward, behind

rhin- the nose

rhino- the nose

-rrhagia discharge

-rrhaphy surgical suturing

-rrhea a flowing, a flux

salping- a tube

salpingo- a tube

sarco- muscular substance, flesh-like

schisto- split, cleft

schiz- split, cleft, division

schizo- split, cleft, division

scler- hardness (induration), sclerosis, the sclera

sclero- hardness (induration), sclerosis, the sclera

-scope an instrument for viewing

-scopy the use of an instrument for viewing

semi- one-half; partly

sial- saliva, the salivary glands

sialo- saliva, the salivary glands

sigmoid- sigmoid, the sigmoid colon

sigmoido- sigmoid, the sigmoid colon

sito- food, grain

somat- the body, bodily

somato- the body, bodily

somatico- the body, bodily

spasmo- spasm

spermato- semen, spermatozoa

spermo- semen, spermatozoa

sperma- semen, spermatozoa

splanchn- the viscera

splanchni- the viscera

splanchno- the viscera

splen- the spleen

spleno- the spleen

staphyl- a grape, a bunch of grapes; staphylococci

staphylo- a grape, a bunch of grapes; staphylococci

-stat an agent to prevent changing or moving

steno- narrowness, constriction

stheno- strength, force, power

stom- mouth

stoma- mouth

stomat- mouth

stomato- mouth

sub- beneath, less than normal, inferior

super- in excess, above, superior, in the upper part

sy- together

syl- together

sym- together

syn- together

sys- together

thel- the nipples

thelo- the nipples

therm- heat

thermo- heat

thorac- the chest, the thorax

thoracico- the chest, the thorax

thoraco- the chest, the thorax

thromb- blood clot
thrombo- blood clot
thyr- the thyroid gland
thyro- the thyroid gland
toco- childbirth
-tome 1 a cutting instrument; 2 a
    segment, section
-tomy a cutting operation
tono- tone, tension, pressure
top- place, topical
topo- place, topical
tox- a toxin, a poison
toxi- a toxin, a poison
toxico- a toxin, a poison
toxo- a toxin, a poison
trache- the trachea
tracheo- the trachea
trans- across, through, beyond
trich- the hair, a hairlike structure
trichi- the hair, a hairlike structure

-trichia the hair, a hairlike structure
tricho- the hair, a hairlike structure
-trophic food, nutrition
tropho- food, nutrition
-trophy food, nutrition
-tropic turning toward, affinity
uri- uric acid
uric- uric acid
urico- uric acid
vas- a duct, a blood vessel
vasculo- a blood vessel
vaso- a duct, a blood vessel
vesic- a vesica, a vesicle
vesico- a vesica, a vesicle
xanth- yellow, yellowish
xantho- yellow, yellowish
zo- an animal, animal life
zoo- an animal, animal life
zym- fermentation, enzymes
zymo- fermentation, enzymes